Evidence-based Dermatology

SECOND EDITION

We, the editors, dedicate this book to our patients who have helped us to understand the meaning of skin disease and to better understand which research questions really matter to them. We owe much to our patients for their contribution to clinical research both as participants of studies and as active collaborators, helping to design better and more relevant research to tackle the enormous gaps in knowledge on the treatment of skin disease.

Evidence-based Dermatology: Companion Website

Additional resources to accompany this book are available at:

www.evidbasedderm.com

Included on the site:

- **Additional chapters:**

  Molluscum contagiosum
  Jochen Schmitt and Thomas Diepgen

  Pityriasis Versicolor
  Michael Bigby and Carlo Casulo

- **Extra tables of trial results**

- **Glossary of terms**

Updates and futher new chapters will also be posted on the site.

Evidence-based Dermatology

SECOND EDITION

EDITED BY

Hywel Williams

Centre of Evidence-Based Dermatology
Nottingham University Hospital NHS Trust
Queen's Medical Centre
Nottingham, UK

ASSOCIATE EDITORS

Michael Bigby

Department of Dermatology
Harvard Medical School and Beth Israel Deaconess Medical Center
Boston, MA, USA

Thomas Diepgen

Department of Social Medicine, Occupational and Environmental Dermatology
University of Heidelberg
Heidelberg, Germany

Andrew Herxheimer

Emeritus Fellow, UK Cochrane Centre

Luigi Naldi

Centro Studi GISED
Department of Dermatology
Ospedali Riuniti
Bergamo, Italy

Berthold Rzany

Division of Evidence Based Medicine (dEBM)
Klinik für Dermatologie
Charité- Universitätsmedizin Berlin
Campus Charité Mitte
Berlin, Germany

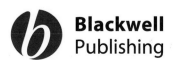 **Blackwell** Publishing

BMJ|Books

© BMJ Publishing Group 2003
© 2008 by Blackwell Publishing

BMJ Books is an imprint of the BMJ Publishing Group Limited, used under licence
Blackwell Publishing, Inc., 350 Main Street, Malden, Massachusetts 02148-5020, USA
Blackwell Publishing Ltd, 9600 Garsington Road, Oxford OX4 2DQ, UK
Blackwell Publishing Asia Pty Ltd, 550 Swanston Street, Carlton, Victoria 3053, Australia

First published 2003
Second edition 2008

1   2008

Library of Congress Cataloging-in-Publication Data
   Evidence-based dermatology / edited by Hywel C. Williams ; associate editors,
Michael Bigby . . . [et al.]. – 2nd ed.
      p. ; cm.
   Includes bibliographical references and index.
   ISBN 978-1-4051-4518-3
   1. Evidence-based dermatology.   I. Williams, Hywel C.
   [DNLM: 1. Skin Diseases.   2. Evidence-Based Medicine.   WR 140 E93 2008]

   RL71.E95 2008
   616.5–dc22

                                                    2007050632

ISBN: 978-1-4051-7070-3
A catalogue record for this title is available from the British Library

Set in 9.25/12pt Palatino by Graphicraft Limited, Hong Kong
Printed and bound in Singapore by Utopia Press Pte Ltd

Commissioning Editor: Mary Banks
Development Editor: Victoria Pittman
Production Controller: Debbie Wyer

For further information on Blackwell Publishing, visit our website:
http://www.blackwellpublishing.com

Contents

Contents

Part IV: The future of evidence-based dermatology
Luigi Naldi, Editor

*Additional chapters and resources are published on the book's web site
(www.evidbasedderm.com)*

Contributors

Joerg Albrecht, MD
Resident Internal Medicine
Department of Internal Medicine
John H Stroger Jr Hospital of Cook County
Chicago, ILL, USA

Fiona Bath-Hextall, BSc (Hon), PhD
Associate Professor
Centre for Evidence-based Dermatology
University of Nottingham
Nottingham, UK

Kapila Batta, FRCP, MRCGP
Consultant Dermatologist
Department of Dermatology
Watford General Hospital
Watford, Hertfordshire, UK

Michael Bigby, MD
Associate Professor of Dermatology
Department of Dermatology
Harvard Medical School and Beth Israel
    Deaconess Medical Center
Boston, MA, USA

Ulrike Blume-Peytavi, MD
Universiäts Professor
Clinical Research Center for Hair and Skin
    Physiology
Klinik für Dermatologie
Charité-Universitätsmedizin Berlin
Berlin, Germany

Jenna E. Bowen, MSc, HBSc
Research Scientist
Mediprobe Research Inc.,
London, Ontario, Canada

Ian F. Burgess, BSc, MSc, MPhil, FRES, FRSH, FADO
Director,
Medical Entomology Centre,
Insect Research & Development Limited,
Shepreth, Royston, UK

Jeffrey P. Callen, MD
Professor of Medicine (Dermatology) and
    Chief, Division of Dermatology,
University of Louisville School of Medicine
Louisville, Kentucky, USA

Norma Cameli, MD
Dermatologist
Department of Aesthetic Dermatology
San Gallicano Dermatological Institute
Rome, Italy

Paolo Carli, MD
Late of Department of Dermatology,
University of Florence
Firenze, Italy

Ciara S. Casey, BSc (Hon), PhD
Laboratory Manager/Lecturer
Department of Biological Science,
    University of Lincoln
Lincoln, UK

Carlo Casulo, BA
Harvard Medical School
Boston, MA, USA

Robert J.G. Chalmers, MB, FRCP
Consultant Dermatologist
Dermatology Centre
University of Manchester School of
    Medicine
Manchester, UK

Carolyn Charman, MRCP, MD
Special Lecturer, Centre of Evidence Based
    Dermatology
University of Nottingham
Queen's Medical Centre
Nottingham, UK

Suephy C. Chen, MD, MS
Assistant Professor of Dermatology and
    Director of the Dermatology Clinical
    and Outcomes Research Unit
Emory University
Staff Physician,
Department of Health Services Research and
    Development
Division of Dermatology
Atlanta VA Medical Center
Atlanta, Georgia, USA

Olivier Chosidow, MD, PhD
Professor Therapeutics and Dermatology
Department of Dermatology
Hospital Tenon, Paris, France

Pieter-Jan Coenraads, MD, PhD, MPH
Professor of Occupational and
    Environmental Dermatology
Department of Dermatology
University Medical Centre,
Groningen, The Netherlands

Avanta P. Collier, MD
Dermatology Research Fellow,
University of Colorado
Denver School of Medicine
Denver, CO, USA

Elizabeth A Cooper, BESc, HBSc
Senior Clinical Research Manager
Senior Research Scientist
Mediprobe Research Inc.,
London, Ontario, Canada

Rosamaria Corona, DSc, MD
Attending Dermatologist
Division of Immunodermatology
Istituto Dermopatico dell'Immacolata
Via dei Monti di Creta 104, Rome, Italy

Neil H. Cox, BSc (Hons), MB, ChB, FRCP (Lond & Edin)
Consultant Dermatologist
Cumberland Infirmary
Carlisle, UK

Fay Crawford, DPodM, MSc, PhD
DH/CSO Post-Doctoral Fellow
Division of Community Health Sciences:
General Practice Section
The University of Edinburgh
Edinburgh, UK

Bernard Cribier, MD, PhD
Head of Department
Department of Dermatology
Hôpitaux Universitaires de Strasbourg
Strasbourg, France

Thomas Crosby, MB, BS, MRCP, FRCR
Consultant Clinical Oncologist
Velindre Cancer Centre
Cardiff, UK

Luis Gabriel Cuervo-Amore, MD, MSc
Pan American Health Organization
(PAHO/WHO)
Washington, DC, USA

Robert S. Dawe, MBChB, MD, FRCP
Consultant Dermatologist & Honorary
Senior Lecturer
Ninewells Hospital & Medical School
Dundee, UK

Finola Delamere, BSc (Hons), PhD
Trials Search Coordinator
Cochrane Skin Group
Centre of Evidence-Based Dermatology
King's Meadow Campus
University of Nottingham
Nottingham, UK

Robert P. Dellavalle, MD, PhD, MSPH
Associate Professor Dermatology and
Preventative Medicine and Biometrics
University of Colorado
Denver School of Medicine and Department
of Veterans Affairs Medical Center
Denver, CO, USA

Mayda Delma Villalta Alvarez
Pediatrician
Private Practice
San Salvador, El Salvador

Laura K. DeLong, MD, MPH
Outcomes Research Fellow
Dermatology Clinical and Outcomes
Research Unit
Emory Department of Dermatology
Atlanta, Georgia, USA

Jean-Paul Deslypere,
Business Development Manager Asia-Pacific
Clinical Research
SGS Testing & Control Services
Singapore

Thomas Diepgen, MD
Professor Dermatology
Department of Social Medicine
Occupational and Environmental
Dermatology
University of Heidelberg
Germany

Joseph C. English III, MD
Associate Professor of Dermatology
Residency Program Director
Department of Dermatology
University of Pittsburgh
Pennsylvania, USA

James Ferguson, MR, FRCP
Professor of Dermatology
Photobiology Unit
Ninewells Hospital and Medical School
Dundee, UK

David F. Fiorentino, MD, PhD
Assistant Professor
Departments of Dermatology and Medicine
(Rheumatology)
Stanford University School of Medicine
Stanford, California, USA

Scott R. Freeman, MD
Dermatology Research Fellow
University of Colorado
Denver School of Medicine
Denver, CO, USA

Natalie Garcia-Bartels, MD
Oberärztin
Clinical Research Center for Hair and Skin
Physiology
Klinik für Dermatologie Chariét -
Universitätsmedizin
Berlin, Berlin, Germany

Pierre-Dominique Ghislain, MD
Cliniques Universitaires St-Luc
Service de Dermatologie
Brussels, Belgium

Sam Gibbs, MD
Consultant Dermatologist
Department of Dermatology
Ipswich Hospital NHS Trust
Ipswich, UK

Urbà Gonzalez, MD, PhD
Dermatologist, Senior Consultant
Department of Dermatology,
Clinica Plató
Barcelona, Spain

Malcolm W. Greaves, MD, PhD, FRCP, FAMS
Emeritus Professor of Dermatology
Guy's, Kings and St Thomas' Schools of
Medicine and Dentistry London
and Clinical Professor
Faculty of Medicine
National University of Singapore
Singapore

Christopher E.M. Griffiths, MD, FRCP, FRCPath
Professor of Dermatology
Dermatology Center
University of Manchester
Manchester, UK

Aditya K. Gupta, MD, PhD, FRCP
Professor of Dermatology
Division of Dermatology
Department of Medicine
Sunnybrook Health Sciences Center
University of Toronto, Toronto, Canada
and Mediproble Research Inc.,
London, Canada

Conrad Hauser, MD
Associate Professor
Head, Allergy Unit,
Division of Immunology and Allergy
Consultant, Department of Dermatology
Hôpitaux Universitaires et Faculté de
Médecine de Genève
Geneva, Switzerland

Roderick J. Hay, MD
Dean, Faculty of Medicine and Health
Sciences
School of Medicine and Dentistry
Queens University
Belfast UK

Andrew Herxheimer, MB, FRCP
Emeritus Fellow
UK Cochrane Centre

Contributors

Leonid Izlkson, MD
Resident in Dermatology
Department of Dermatology
University of Pittsburgh
Pittsburgh, USA

Susan Jessop, MB, ChB, FFDermCSA
Senior Consultant Dermatologist
Groote Schuur Hospital
Observatory
South Africa

Jonathan Kantor, MD, MSCE
North Florida Dermatology Associates
Jacksonville, FL, USA

Gudula Kirtschig, MD
Consultant Dermatologist
Department of Dermatology
VU Medisch Centrum
Amsterdam, The Netherlands

Nonhlanhla P. Khumalo, MBChB, FCDerm, PhD
Dermatologist
Division of Dermatology
Groote Schuur Hospital and the University of Cape Town
South Africa

Sandra R. Knowles, Bsc Phm
Drug Safety Pharmacist and Lecturer
Sunnybrook Health Sciences Center and University of Toronto
Toronto, Ontario, Canada

Sander Koning, MD, PhD
General Practitioner
Department of General Practice
Erasmus MC-University Medical Center
Rotterdam, The Netherlands

Shamez Ladhani, MRCPCH (UK)
National Grid Trainee
Paediatric Infectious Diseases Unit
St Georges Hospital
London, UK

Sinéad Langan, MD, FRP, DCH
Research Fellow
Centre of Evidence-Based Dermatology
Queen's Medical Centre
Nottingham, UK

Sean W. Lanigan, MB, FRP, DCH
Consultant Dermatologist
The Birmingham Regional Skin Laser Centre
Birmingham Skin Centre
City Hospital, Birmingham, UK

Belen Lardizabal-Dofitas, MD, MSc
Consultant Dermatologist
Section of Dermatology
Department of Medicine
St Luke's Medical Center
Quezon City and Clinical Assistant Professor
University of the Philippines College of Medicine & Philippine General Hospital
Metro Manila, Philippines

Laurence Le Cleach, MD
Practicien Hospitalier
Service de Dermatologie
Corbeil Essonnes, France

Tina Leonard, BSc, PhD
Managing Editor and Review Group Coordinator
Cochrane Skin Group
Centre of Evidence-Based Dermatology
King's Meadow Campus
University of Nottingham
Nottingham, UK

Nanette J. Liegeois, MD, PhD
Assistant Professor Dermatology
Johns Hopkins University
Baltimore MD, USA

Dennis Linder, MD, MSc
Lecturer in Psychodermatology
Department of Dermatology
University Hospital of Padua
Padua, Italy

Vera Mahler, MD
Department of Dermatology
University Hospital Erlangen
Friedrich-Alexander-University
Erlangen-Nuremberg, Germany

Juan Jorge Manriquez, MD
Department of Dermatology
Pontificia Universidad Catolica de Chile, Chile

David J. Margolis, MD, PhD
Associate Professor Dermatology
Associate Professor of Epidemiology
Senior Scholar in the Center for Epidemiology and Biostatistics
University of Pennsylvania
Philadelphia, USA

Linda K. Martin, MBBS
Dermatology Fellow
Department of Dermatology
St George Hospital
Sydney, Australia

Russell N. Moule, MRCP, FRCR
Mount Vernon Cancer Centre
Northwood, Middlesex, UK

Dedee F. Murrell, MA, BMBCh, MD, FAAD
Chair, Department of Dermatology
St George Hospital, Associate Professor
University of New South Wales Medical School
Sydney, Australia

Luigi Naldi, MD
Director, Centro Studi GISED
Department of Dermatology
Ospedali Riuniti
Bergamo, Italy

Suzanne Olbricht, MD
Chair, Department of Dermatology
Lahey Clinic
Burlington MA Associate Professor Dermatology
Harvard Medical School USA

William Perkins, MB, BS, FRCP
Consultant Dermatologist
Department of Dermatology
Nottingham University Hospitals
Nottingham, UK

Mauro Picardo, MD
Director, Unit of Cutaneous Fisopathology
San Gallicano Dermatological Institute
Rome, Italy

Peterson Pierre, MD
Private Practice
Agoura Hilla
California, USA

Magdalena Radulescu, MD
Dermatologist
Allergologist Department of Clinical Social Medicine
Occupational and Environmental Dermatology
University Hospital Heidelberg
Heidelberg, Germany

Jane Ravenscroft, MRCP, MRCGP, MB, ChB
Consultant Dermatologist
Queen's Medical Centre
Nottingham, UK

Alfredo Rebora, MD
Professor Emeritus
Department of Endrocrinological and
    Metabolic Sciences
University of Genoa, Italy

Mónica Rengifo-Pardo, MD
Specialist in Dermatology
Member of the Cochrane Skin Group
Kensington, Maryland, USA

Dafydd Roberts, MB, BS, MBBS, FRCP
Consultant Dermatologist and Clinical
    Director
National Clinical Lead for Skin Cancer
Singleton Hospital, Swansea, UK

Jean-Claude Roujeau, MD, PhD
Henri Mondor Hospital
University Paris XII
Créteil, France

Berthold Rzany, MD, ScM
Division of Evidence Based Medicine (dEBM)
Klinik für Dermatologie
Charité-Universitätsmedizin Berlin, Berlin,
    Germany

Asad Salim, MRCP
Dermatology Department
Mid Staffordshire Hospitals,
Staffordshire, UK

Camilla Salvini, MD
Medical Doctor, specialized in dermatology
Department of Dermatology,
University of Florence, Firenze, Italy

Miny Samuel
Senior Evidence-based Medicine Analyst
Co-Director of Singapore Branch of the
    Australasian Cochrane Centre
Clinical Trials & Epidemiology Research
    Unit
Singapore

Torsten Schäfer, MPH, MD
Professor in Clinical Epidemology
Institute of Social Medicine
Medical University
Lübeck, Germany

Jochen Schmitt, MD, MPH
Dermatologist
Department of Dermatology
Medical Faculty Carl Gustav Carus
Technical University Dresden, Dresden,
    Germany

Peter Schnider, MD
Universitäts Professor
Klinik für Neurologie
Hocheggerstrasse 88
Grimmenstein Hochegg, Austria

Su-Jean Seo, MD, PhD
Fellow in Dermatopathology
Harvard Medical School
Boston, MA, USA

Neil H. Shear, MD, FRCPC
Professor and Chief of Dermatology
Sunnybrook Health Sciences Center and
    University of Toronto Medical School
Torono, Ontario, Canada

Rod Sinclair, MBBS, MD, FACD
Professor and Director of Dermamtology
St Vincent's Hospital
Melbourne, Victoria, Australia

Seaver L. Soon, MD
Department of Dermatology
Emory University
Atlanta, USA

Brian R. Sperber, MD, PhD
Private Practice
Colorado Springs
Colorado, CO, USA

Margaret F. Spittle, FRCP, FRCR
Consultant Clinical Oncologist
University College London Hospital
London, UK

Thomas Sycha, MD
Universitäts Professor
Universitats Klinik für Neurologie
Medizinische Universität Wien
Währinger Gürlel 18–20
Wien, Austria

Yee Jen Tai, MBBS
Dermatology Registrar
Department of Dermatology
St Vincent's Hospital
Melbourne, Victoria, Australia

Philip Taramarcaz, MD
Consultant, Allergy Unit,
Division of Immunology and Allergy
Hôpitaux Universitaires de Genève
Geneva, Switzerland

Kim Thomas, BSc (Hons), PhD
Associate Professor
Centre of Evidence-based Dermatology

University of Nottingham
Nottingham, UK

A. Marco van Coevorden, MD
Dermatologist
Department of Dermatology
Gelre Hospital
Apeldoorn
The Netherlands

Johannes C. van der Wouden, PhD
Senior Lecturer
Department of General Practice
Erasmus MC—University Medical Center
    Rotterdam
Rotterdam, The Netherlands

Lisette W.A. van Suijlekom-Smit, MD, PhD
Senior Pediatrician
Department of Pediatrics
Erasmus MC—University Medical
    Center/Sophia Children's Hospital
Rotterdam, The Netherlands

Vanessa Venning, BM, BCh, DM, FRCP
Consultant Dermatologist
Department of Dermatology
The Churchill
Oxford Radcliffe Hospitals NHS Trust and
    University of Oxford
Oxford, UK

Sam Vincent, MSc
Head of Information
InferMed Ltd
London, UK

Elke Weisshaar, MD
Consultant, Dermatologist, Department of
    Social Medicine Occupational and
    Environmental
Dermatology, University Hospital of
    Heidelberg, Germany

Victoria P. Werth, MD
Professor of Dermatology and Medicine
University of Pennsylvania School of Medicine
Philadelphia, PA, USA

Ros Weston, PhD, MA
Focus Freelance Writing & Research
Salisbury, Wiltshire, UK

David Whitelaw, MB, ChB, PhD, FCP (SA)
Senior Consultant Rheumatologist
Department of Medicine

Contributors

Tygerberg Hospital
Parow Valley, South Africa

Sean Whittaker, MB, MD, FRCP
Clinical Director for Dermatology
Allergy and Sexual Health
St Johns Institute of Dermatology
Guy's and St Thomas Hospital, Head Skin
   Cancer Unit, Division of Genetics and
   Molecular
Medicine, King's College London, UK

Maxine Whitton, BA (hons), MSc
Consumer Contributor
Cochrane Skin Group
London, UK

Hywel C. Williams, MSC, PhD, FRCP
Professor Dermato-Epidemiology and
   Co-ordinating Editor of the Cochrane
   Skin Group
Centre of Evidence-Based Dermatology
University Hospital
Queen's Medical Centre,
Nottingham, UK

Fenella Wojnarowska, DM, FRCP
Professor of Dermatology, Department of
   Dermatology
The Churchill
Oxford Radcliffe Hospitals NHS Trust and
   University of Oxford
Oxford, UK

Hans Wolff, MD
Universitäts Professor
Klinik und Poliklinik für Dermatologie und
   Allergologie
Universität Müchen, Germany

Weiya Zhang, PhD
Associate Professor
Academic Rheumatology Medical & Surgical
   Sciences University of Nottingham City
Hospital, Nottingham, UK

Hendrik Zielke, MD
Resident
Klinik für Anásthesiokigue und operative
   Intensivmedizin
Charité-Universitätsmedizin Berlin, Berlin,
   Germany

Foreword

Twenty years ago, when drafting an introductory chapter for a book on the effects of care during pregnancy and childbirth,[1] I decided to use contrasting quotations from a distinguished statistician and a distinguished dermatologist. In 1952, Austin Bradford Hill had written:

"In my indictment of the statistician, I would argue that he may tend to be a trifle too scornful of the clinical judgement, the clinical impression. Such judgements are, I believe, in essence, statistical. The clinician is attempting to make a comparison between the situation that faces him at the moment and a mentally recorded but otherwise untabulated past experience."[2]

Twenty years later, Sam Shuster coined the memorable phrase:

"Lies, damned lies and clinical impressions"[3]

My draft went on to discuss the fundamental importance and great dangers of clinical impressions: in obstetric practice they have led both to important therapeutic discoveries and to iatrogenic disasters. I doubt that people treating skin disease have the capacity to do unintended harm on the scale achieved by obstetricians and neonatologists, but I also doubt there is any justification for complacency in matters of dermatological therapy.

The huge variability that exists in the management of common chronic skin diseases is clear evidence of collective uncertainty about the effects of alternative management strategies, even if a majority of individual clinicians are certain that they are doing the right thing. For example, I gather that fumaric acid esters have been used widely to treat psoriasis for nearly 40 years in Germany and the Netherlands, but that, although their use is supported by good evidence,[4] they have hardly been used at all anywhere else. Some patients with warts are being put to the inconvenience (and expense) of attending hospital for cryotherapy; yet there is no strong evidence to suggest that they would be worse off treating their warts at home with salicylic acid paints.[5] Topical corticosteroid preparations like bethamethasone valerate are traditionally used twice daily, yet there is no good evidence to show that twice daily is more effective than once daily applications. Furthermore, once daily applications are easier for people with eczema, they may result in less side effects and they are also less costly.[6] As professionals concerned to do more good than harm to their patients, all who treat skin disease have a duty to reduce uncertainty about the relative merits of alternative treatments by paying attention to the results of well-designed research.

To do right by their patients, people treating skin disease need to know what they know and what they don't know. This book tries to help them. Unlike traditional textbooks, it contains a toolbox section that describes the methods that have been used to review the evidence upon which conclusions about the effects of treatments have been based, and gives references to more detailed reports of the systematic reviews on which much of the text has drawn.

There is no consensus about the materials and methods that should be used to assemble evidence to support treatment recommendations published in textbooks and review articles, nor even about the principles of systematic reviews. One senior dermatologist, for example, has written:

"The idea of a systematic review is a nonsense, and the sooner those advocates of it are tried at the International Court of Human Rights at the Hague (or worse still, sent for counselling), the better."[7]

Unfortunately, those who express reservations about applying systematic approaches to the synthesis of research evidence tend not to outline the alternative strategies that they implicitly deem preferable. This is a serious matter because it has been shown that reviews using explicit methods reach conclusions that differ from traditional reviews, with implications that can be matters of life or death.[8] In dermatology, too, the conclusions of reviews in which efforts have been made to reduce biases and the effects of chance can differ from those reached in traditional reviews,[9] and Cochrane reviews have been shown to be higher quality than other systematic reviews.[10] In the light of this evidence, I believe that continued acquiescence in reviews that have not attempted to minimise biases and, where possible and appropriate, the effects of chance, is not only scientifically unacceptable but also ethically highly questionable.[11]

The contributors to this book have tried to control biases and—where they judged it appropriate—they have also reduced the play of chance by using statistical synthesis to analyse the results of similar but separate studies. As ways of improving the materials and methods used in such research synthesis are developed further, researchers will apply them, taking advantage of the potential offered by electronic media to publish full and transparent accounts of their work, and to respond to new data and suggestions for improving their analyses.

This second edition of *Evidence-Based Dermatology* has extended coverage of topics from the first edition to include several additional and important skin disorders, such as cellulitis, port wine stains, and herpes simplex. And in the penultimate chapter, the editors have drawn attention to randomised controlled trials of treatments for less common skin diseases. In laying bare just how much cannot be known on the basis of reliable evidence, the contributors to this book have also posed a very great challenge to everyone involved in treating skin disease. Can it be that a modest reduction in 'doctor-assessed itch' is really the only demonstrable beneficial effect of the widespread use of evening primrose oil for people with eczema?[12] The book exposes the dearth of reliable studies addressing questions and outcomes that matter to patients, and it reveals the extent to which perverse incentives distort the dermatological research agenda. Those suffering from skin disease have every right to expect more from clinicians, researchers, and those who fund research. This book should help to provoke them to do better.

References

1 Chalmers I. Evaluating the effects of care during pregnancy and childbirth. In: Chalmers I, Enkin M, Keirse MJNC, eds. *Effective care in pregnancy and childbirth*. Oxford: Oxford University Press, 1989: 3–38.
2 Bradford Hill A. The clinical trial. New England Journal of Medicine 1952;**247**:113–119.
3 Shuster S. Primary cutaneous virilism or idiopathic hirsuties? BMJ 1972;**2**:285–286.
4 Griffiths CEM, Clark CM, Chalmers RJG, Li Wan Po A, Williams HC. A systematic review of treatments for severe psoriasis. Health Technology Assessment 2000;**4**:40.
5 Gibbs S, Harvey I. Topical treatments for cutaneous warts. Cochrane Database of Systematic Reviews 2006, Issue 3. Art. No.: CD001781. DOI: 10.1002/14651858.CD001781.pub2.
6 Williams HC. Established corticosteroid creams should be applied only once daily in patients with atopic eczema. BMJ 2007;**334**: 1272.
7 Rees JL. Two cultures? Journal of the American Academy of Dermatology 2002;**46**:313–314.
8 Antman EM, Lau J, Kupelnick B, Mosteller F, Chalmers TC. A comparison of results of meta-analyses of randomized control trials and recommendations of clinical experts. JAMA 1992;**268**: 240–48.
9 Ladhani S, Williams HC. The management of established postherpetic neuralgia: a comparison of the quality and content of traditional vs. systematic reviews. British Journal of Dermatology 1998;**139**:66–72.
10 Collier A, Heilig L, Schilling L, Williams H, Dellavalle RP. Cochrane Skin Group systematic reviews are more methodologically rigorous than other systematic reviews in dermatology. British Journal of Dermatology 2006;**155**:1230–5.
11 Chalmers I, Hedges LV, Cooper H. A brief history of research synthesis. Evaluation and the Health Professions 2002;**25**:12–37.
12 Hoare C, Li Wan Po A, Williams H. Systematic review of treatments for atopic eczema. Health Technology Assessment 2000;**4**: 37.

Iain Chalmers, Coordinator, James Lind Initiative

Preface

Evidence-based dermatology is no longer a dirty word in dermatology. Nowadays, all dermatologists are practicing evidence-based dermatology to some degree. Rather than just mutter the word "evidence" every now and again at meetings, the real challenge is to improve the skills of integrating the best external evidence to clinical care of individual patients. This book may help you.

For those of you new to *Evidence-Based Dermatology*, you will find it a *different* sort of book to the usual textbook. Different in that we have introduced the whole rationale for evidence-based dermatology in a section at the start of the book. Different in that we then provide you, the reader, with a detailed "toolbox" to help you understand some of the basic concepts of *practicing* evidence-based dermatology. But the biggest difference is in the way we have encouraged our chapter contributors to follow a common structure when summarizing the evidence base for different skin diseases—the "meat" of the book. That structure begins with a clinical scenario, followed by clinical questions that lead to an evidence summary, based on the best possible evidence such as systematic reviews and randomized controlled trials. The summary includes a description of the efficacy and drawbacks of individual treatment approaches followed by a viewpoint on the clinical implications of that evidence. It is a lot more work writing in such a structured way than letting experts write what they like, but the success of the first edition of this book suggests that you, the reader, appreciate such an approach. We have taken care, where possible, to separate the evidence found in studies from our opinions about that evidence, and we have tried to help the reader by summarizing the key points at the end of each chapter. The book also differs from others in that it is accompanied by a website (http://www. evidbasedderm.com) which will include additional chapters and updates and will grow between this and the next edition.

For those of you familiar with the first edition of *Evidence-Based Dermatology*, welcome back. In addition to providing evidence updates to all of the chapters from the first edition, several new chapters in this edition deal with important diseases such as cellulitis, port wine malformations and herpes simplex, plus new methodological chapters on issues such as how to critically appraise case series—something that we see a lot of in dermatology. Finally, we have tried to scoop up near the end of the book a number of less common skin conditions where at least some trial evidence exists. Our ambition is to eventually find a home for every randomized controlled trial that has been conducted in dermatology in this book and its accompanying website as it progresses through subsequent editions.

This second edition of *Evidence-Based Dermatology* has been a labor of love for me, my associate editors and chapter contributors and I wish to thank them all for their efforts. We have strived to keep the book grounded in reality by making it as patient-based as possible by discussing the evidence around commonly encountered real patient scenarios. That is because at the end of the day, it is patients who are at the heart of evidence-based dermatology. Please keep and use this book in your clinic, and not in the library.

Hywel Williams

The concept of evidence-based dermatology

Andrew Herxheimer, Editor

1 The field and its boundaries

Luigi Naldi

Evidence-based medicine (EBM) represents the best way of linking and integrating clinical research with clinical practice. The results of clinical research should inform clinical practice. Ideally, whenever there is no satisfactory answer for a clinical question, it should be addressed by clinical research. Since clinical questions are innumerable and resources are limited, the process needs some control, and priorities should be set using explicit and verifiable criteria. The public and purchasers have to be involved at this stage, and health needs and expectations in any given clinical area should be analyzed and taken into account. In many instances, confirmatory studies are needed, and systematic reviews can be used to summarize study results or to explore results in specific subgroups with a view to further research. The results of clinical research should be applied back to the individual patients in the light of their personal values and preferences. Communicational skills and patient understanding are key issues in this respect. In the real world, forces other than those involved in such an ideal process often distort research priorities and questions. For example, strong industrial and economic interests may partly explain the lack of data on rare disorders, or on common disorders if they occur mainly in less developed countries. This book may help identify the more urgent questions that lack satisfactory answers by summarizing for physicians (and patients) the best evidence available for the management of a large number of skin disorders. It may thus provide a starting-point for rethinking the clinical research priorities in patient-oriented dermatology.

What is special about dermatology

The skin is not a simple, inert covering of the body, but a sensitive dynamic boundary, and it is an important organ of social and sexual contact. Body image, which is deeply rooted in the culture of any given social group, is profoundly affected by the appearance of the skin and its associated structures. The role that skin appearance plays in any given society is best understood from an anthropological perspective and using a narrative qualitative approach. This area is rather neglected in dermatological curricula.

Extensive disorders affecting the skin may disrupt its homeostatic functions, ultimately resulting in "skin failure," requiring intensive care. This is rare, but may happen—for example, with extensive bullous disorders or exfoliative dermatitis. The commonest health consequence of skin disorders is connected with the discomfort of symptoms, such as itching and burning or pain, which frequently accompany skin lesions and interfere with everyday life and sleep, and with the loss of confidence and disruption of social relations that visible lesions may cause. Feelings of stigmatization and major changes in lifestyle caused by a chronic skin disorder such as psoriasis have been repeatedly documented in population surveys.[1]

A vast array of clinical entities

Unlike most other organs, which are usually associated with around 50–100 diseases, the skin has a complement of 1000–2000 conditions, and over 3000 dermatological categories can be found in the International Classification for Disease version 9 (ICD-9). Part of the reason for this is that the skin is a large and visible organ. In addition to disorders primarily affecting the skin, most of the major systemic diseases (e.g., of vascular and connective tissue) have cutaneous manifestations. Currently, the widespread use of symptom-based or purely descriptive terms such as parapsoriasis or pityriasis rosea reflects our limited understanding of the causes and pathogenetic mechanisms of a large number of skin disorders. We still lack consensus on a detailed lexicon of dermatological terms to be used in research and everyday clinical practice.

An effort to improve consensus has recently been taken with three very significant initiatives:
• The *Dermatologischer Diagnosenkatalog* (DDK), published in the German-speaking countries by the *Deutsche*

Dermatologische Gesellschaft and published in English by the International League of Dermatological Societies (ILDS).

- The British Association of Dermatologists' Diagnostic Index (BAD Index), first published in 1994 and updated annually since then.
- The Dermatology Lexicon Project, developed with a grant from the U.S. National Institutes of Health, first published in 2005 and now supported by the American Academy of Dermatology.

It is expected that in the not too distant future, a single instrument meeting dermatologists' requirements will become available.[2]

Extremely common disorders

Skin diseases are very common in the general population. Prevalence surveys have shown that skin disorders may affect 20–30% of the general population at any one time. The most common diseases are also the most trivial ones. They include such conditions as mild eczematous lesions, mild to moderate acne, benign tumors, and angiomatous lesions. More severe skin disorders, which can cause physical disability or even death, are rare or very rare. They include, among others, bullous diseases such as pemphigus, severe pustular and erythrodermic psoriasis, and such malignant tumors as malignant melanoma and lymphoma. The disease frequency may vary according to age, sex, and geographic area. In many cases, skin diseases are trivial health problems in comparison with more serious medical conditions. However, as already noted, because skin manifestations are visible, they may distress people more than more serious medical problems do. The issue is complicated, because many skin disorders are not a "yes-or-no" phenomenon, but occur with a spectrum of severity. The public's perception of what constitutes a "disease" requiring medical advice may vary according to cultural issues, the social context, resources, and time. Minor changes in health policy may have a large health and financial impact simply because a large number of people may be affected. For example, most of the campaigns conducted to raise public awareness of skin cancer have led to a big increase in the number of people having benign skin conditions such as benign melanocytic nevi evaluated and excised.

Large variations in terms of health-care organization

Countries differ greatly in the way in which their health services deal with skin disorders. These variations are roughly indicated by the density of dermatologists—ranging, in Europe, from about one in 20 000 in Italy and France to one in 150 000 in the United Kingdom.

In general, only a minority of people with skin diseases seek medical help, while many opt for self-medication. Pharmacists have a key role in advising the public on the use of over-the-counter products. Primary-care physicians seem to treat the majority of people among those seeking medical advice. Primary care of dermatological problems is not precisely defined and overlaps with specialist activity. Everywhere, the dermatologist's workload is concentrated in the outpatient department. Despite the vast number of skin diseases, just a few categories account for about 70% of all dermatological consultations.

Generally speaking, dermatology requires a low-technology clinical practice. Clinical expertise depends mainly on the ability to recognize a skin disorder quickly and reliably, and this in turn depends largely on awareness of a given clinical pattern, based on previous experience and on the practised eye of a visually literate physician.[3] The process of developing "visual skill" and a "clinical eye" is poorly understood, and these skills are not formally taught.

Topical treatment is often possible

A peculiar aspect of dermatology is the possible option for topical treatment. This treatment modality is ideally suited to localized lesions, the main advantage being the restriction of the effect to the site of application and the limitation of systemic side effects. A topical agent is usually described as consisting of a vehicle and an active substance, with the vehicles being classified as powder, grease, liquid, or combinations such as pastes and creams.

Much traditional topical therapy in dermatology has been developed empirically with so-called magistral formulations. Most of these products appear to rely on physical rather than chemical properties for their effects, and it may be an arbitrary decision to consider one specific ingredient as being the "active" one. Physical effects of topical agents may include detersion, hydration, and removal of keratotic scales. The border between pharmacological and cosmetic effects may be blurred, and the term "cosmeceuticals" is sometimes used.[4] In addition to drug treatment, various non-drug treatment modalities exist, including phototherapy or photochemotherapy and minor surgical procedures such as electrodesiccation and cryotherapy. Wide variations in the treatment modalities used for the same condition mainly reflect local traditions and preferences.[5,6]

Limitations of clinical research

As in other disciplines, the last few decades have seen an impressive increase in clinical research in dermatology. However, the upsurge of clinical research has not been paralleled by methodological refinements and, for example, the quality of randomized control trials (RCTs) in dermatology appears to fall well below the usually accepted standards.[7] Innovative thinking is needed in dermatology to make clinical research address the important issues and not simply ape the scientific design.

Disease rarity

In at least a thousand rare or very rare skin conditions, no single randomized trial has been conducted. These conditions are also those that carry a higher burden of physical disability and mortality. Many of them have an annual incidence rate of below one case per 100 000 and frequently below one case per million. International collaboration and institutional support is clearly needed, but so far such efforts are very few.

Patients' preferences

One alleged difficulty with mounting randomized clinical trials in dermatology is the visibility of skin lesions and the consideration that much more than in other areas, patients self-monitor their disease and may have preconceptions and preferences about specific treatment modalities.[8] The decision to treat is usually dictated by subjective issues and personal feelings. Physicians and the public need to be educated about the value of randomized trials to assess interventions in dermatology. Motivations and expectations are likely to influence clinical outcomes of all treatments, but they may have a more crucial role in situations in which "soft end points" matter, as in dermatology. Commonly, more than 20% of patients with psoriasis entering randomized clinical trials improve on placebo independently of the initial disease extension. Motivations are equally important in pragmatic trials that evaluate different management packages, such as the comparison of a self-administered topical product for psoriasis with hospital-based forms of treatment such as phototherapy. Traditionally, motivation is seen as a characteristic of the patient that is assumed not to change with the nature of the intervention. However, it has been argued that it is more realistic to view motivation in terms of the "fit" between the nature of the treatment and the patient's wishes and perceptions—especially with complex interventions that require the patient's active participation. The public is inundated with uncontrolled and sometimes misleading or unrealistic messages on how to improve the body's appearance. It is important to ensure that patient information and motivations are properly considered in the design and analysis of clinical trials on skin disorders.

The use of placebo in randomized controlled trials

Too many placebo-controlled RCTs are conducted in dermatology even when alternative therapies exist. As a consequence, a large number of similar molecules used for the same clinical indications can be found in some areas—e.g., topical steroids. Many regulatory agencies still consider placebo controls as the "gold standard." Criteria are needed for the use of placebos in dermatology. They should be developed with the active and informed participation of the public, and ethics committees and regulatory agencies should consider them. "Pragmatic" randomized trials conducted in conditions close to clinical practice and contrasting alternative therapeutic regimens are urgently needed in order to guide clinical decisions.

Long-term outcome of chronic disorders

Several major skin disorders are chronic conditions for which a cure does not at present exist. Whenever a definite cure is not reasonably attainable, it is common to distinguish between short, intermediate (usually measurable within months), and long-term outcomes. Long-term results are not simply predictable from short-term outcomes. Many skin disorders wax and wane over time, and it is not easy to define what represents a clinically significant long-term change in the disease status. This is even more difficult than defining the outcome for other clinical conditions, such as cancer or ischemic heart disease, in which death or major hard clinical end points (e.g., myocardial infarction) are of particular interest. In the long term, the way the disease is controlled and the treatment side effects are vitally important, and simply and cheaply measured outcomes applicable in all patients seem to be preferable. These may include the number of patients in remission, the number of hospital admissions or outpatient consultations, and major disease flare-ups. Drop-outs merit special attention, since they may strongly reflect dissatisfaction with treatment.

Self-control design

Study designs that are often used at a preliminary stage in drug development are *within-patient control studies*—i.e., crossover and self-controlled studies or simultaneous within-patient control studies. In dermatology they are also used, albeit improperly, at a more advanced stage. In a survey of more than 350 published RCTs of psoriasis (unpublished data), a self-controlled design accounted for one-third of all the studies examined and was relied on at some stage in drug development. The main advantage of a within-patient study over a parallel concurrent study is a statistical one. A within-patient study obtains the same statistical power with far fewer patients, and at the same time reduces variability between the populations confronted. Within-patient studies may be useful when studying conditions that are uncommon or show a high degree of patient-to-patient variability. On the other hand, within-patient studies impose restrictions and artificial conditions, which may undermine the validity and generalizability of results and may also raise some ethical concerns. The wash-out period of a crossover trial, as well as the treatment schemes of a self-controlled design, which entails applying different treatments to various parts of the body, do not seem to be fully justifiable from an ethical point of view. Clearly, the impractical treatment modalities in self-controlled studies or the wash-out period in crossover studies may be difficult for the patient to accept. Drop-outs may have more pronounced effects in a within-patient study than in other study designs, because each patient contributes a large proportion of the total information. The situation is compounded in self-controlled studies, where a patient may drop out from the study having noticed a difference in treatment effect between the parts into which she or he has been "split up." In this case, given that drop-outs are related to a difference in treatment effect between interventions, the effect of the intervention is liable to be underestimated.

The increasing role of industry-sponsored trials

The influence of the pharmaceutical industry on medical research has increased enormously in recent decades. Dermatology does not appear be an exception. As indicated by the European Dermatoepidemiology Network (EDEN) psoriasis project, only a quarter of all randomized clinical trials published on psoriasis from 1977 to 2000 were conducted independently of direct pharmaceutical company sponsorship, and the proportion of sponsored trials has been increasing dramatically since then.[9] Systematic reviews indicate that published studies funded by pharmaceutical companies are several times more likely to have results favoring the company than studies funded from other sources.[10] As indicated by the recent development of "biological agents" in psoriasis, placebo-controlled randomized trials and the use of surrogate outcome measures over a short period of time, rather than clinically relevant outcomes over a significant time span, are means of increasing the chances of obtaining favorable results.[11] Selective presentation of scientific data, statements by opinion leaders in sponsored symposia, and involvement of patient organizations in sponsored campaigns are among the promotional strategies adopted to expand the market once limited clinical evidence has been collected on a new agent. Heavy marketing competition has been paralleled by a cycle of increasing dependency between physicians, academic opinion leaders, patients' organizations, researchers, and industrial interests.[12] In Italy, the recognition of the problems involved with new drug registration and lack of data on effectiveness and safety in situations in which alternative conventional treatments already exist have prompted the launch of post-marketing surveillance programs linking prescription to the provision of patient data at first drug prescription and regularly thereafter during a predefined follow-up period. One example of such a program on psoriasis is the Psocare program (www.psocare.it).

The limitations of systematic reviews

The large number of clinical studies in dermatology and the lack of consensus on the management of many skin disorders suggest systematic reviews as a way of improving the evidence and guiding clinical decisions. However, systematic reviews alone cannot be expected to overcome the methodological limitations in dermatological research described above. On the contrary, it seems that systematic reviews, if not properly guided by important clinical questions, may amplify the unimportant issues and may result in a rather misleading scale of evidence to guide clinical decisions. Since most RCTs are performed by pharmaceutical companies, data-driven systematic reviews might well reflect the priorities of pharmaceutical companies and not necessarily those of the public and clinicians. Without a change in regulatory procedures, pharmaceutical companies will continue to pay little attention to comparative RCTs and will continue to assess drugs for lucrative indications, neglecting rare but clinically important disorders.

Systematic reviews alone cannot fill the gap, and we urgently need primary research and high-quality and relevant clinical trials.

Evidence-based medicine: where do we go from here?

An EBM approach should permeate medical education and inform academic medicine. It is only if such a change is promoted that EBM can become central to clinical practice and not trivialized to become "cookbook" medicine. If EBM is successfully integrated into everyday practice, it may become easier to conduct primary clinical research based on clinical needs rather than on commercial interests.

In primary research, more imaginative and effective research instruments are needed, and research strategies should be developed that take account of the peculiarities of dermatology as compared with other disciplines. Qualitative research should not be neglected. It is the key to understanding intercultural variations in body image and of the ways in which health needs for skin diseases are expressed and perceived in different situations.

Acknowledgment

This chapter is based on Luigi Naldi and Cosetta Minelli, "Dermatology," in Machin D, Day S, Green S, eds., *Textbook of Clinical Trials*, 2nd ed., Chichester: Wiley, 2006: 263–85.

References

1 McKenna KE, Stern RS. The outcomes movement and new measures of the severity of psoriasis. *J Am Acad Dermatol* 1996;**34**:534–8.

2 Papier A, Chalmers RJG, Byrnes JA, Goldsmith LA. Framework for improved communication: the Dermatology Lexicon Project. *J Am Acad Dermatol* 2004;**50**:630–4.

3 Webster GF. Is dermatology slipping into its anec-dotage? *Arch Dermatol* 1995;**131**:149–50.

4 Vermeer BJ, Gilchrest BA. Cosmeceuticals: a proposal for rational definition, evaluation, and regulation. *Arch Dermatol* 1996;**132**:337–40.

5 Peckham PE, Weinstein GD, McCullough JL. The treatment of severe psoriasis: a national survey. *Arch Dermatol* 1987;**123**:1303–7.

6 Farr PM, Diffey BL. PUVA treatment of psoriasis in the United Kingdom. *Br J Dermatol* 1991;**124**:365–7.

7 Williams HC, Seed P. Inadequate size of "negative" clinical trials in dermatology. *Br J Dermatol* 1993;**128**:317–26.

8 Van de Kerkhof PCM, De Hoop D, De Korte J, Cobelens SA, Kuipers MV. Patient compliance and disease management in the treatment of psoriasis in the Netherlands. *Dermatology* 2000;**200**:292–8.

9 Naldi L, Svensson A, Diepgen T, *et al.* Randomized clinical trials for psoriasis 1977–2000: the EDEN survey. *J Invest Dermatol* 2003;**120**:738–41.

10 Lexchin J, Bero LA, Djulbegovic B, Clark O. Pharmaceutical industry sponsorship and research outcome and quality. *BMJ* 2003;**326**:1167–70.

11 Naldi L. A new era in the management of psoriasis? Promises and facts. *Dermatology* 2005;**210**:179–81.

12 Williams HC, Naldi L, Paul C, Vahlquist A, Schroter S, Jobling R. Conflicts of interest in dermatology. *Acta Derm Venereol* 2006;**86**:485–97.

2 The rationale for evidence-based dermatology

Hywel Williams, Michael Bigby

What is evidence-based dermatology?

Definitions

Sackett, a clinical epidemiologist and one of the founders of modern evidence-based medicine (EBM), defined the latter as "the conscientious, explicit and judicious use of current best evidence about the care of individual patients."[1] Sackett's definition reflects a number of key concepts:

• "Conscientious" implies an *active* process that requires learning, doing, and reflection.

• "Explicit" implies that we can describe and replicate the *process* that we use to practice EBM.

• "Judicious" denotes the need for clinical judgment in applying evidence.

• "Current" implies being *up to date.*

• "Best" implies that we should seek the most *reliable* evidence source to inform practice.

As Chapter 14 elaborates, perhaps the most important and frequently forgotten phrase in this definition is "the care of individual patients." The place for EBM is not in trying to score intellectual points in the literature or in humiliating colleagues at journal clubs; it is at the bedside or in the outpatient consulting room. As Chapter 68 emphasizes, EBM is a way of thinking and working, with improved health of our patients as its central aim.

Nowadays, the term "evidence-based practice" is often used instead of EBM. The term "evidence-based practice" reflects *doing* rather than *talking* about EBM, and may be defined as integrating one's clinical expertise with the best external evidence from systematic research.[2] Evidence-based dermatology simply implies the application of EBM principles to people with skin problems.[3]

What evidence-based dermatology is not

Despite the above clear definitions, the purpose of evidence-based dermatology (EBD) is often misunderstood in the

---

BOX 2.1 What evidence-based dermatology is not

• Something that ignores patients' values.
• A promotion of a cookbook approach to medicine.
• An ivory-tower concept that can only be understood and practised by an exclusive club of aficionados.
• A tool designed solely to cut costs.
• A reason for therapeutic nihilism in the absence of randomized controlled trials.
• The same as guidelines.
• A way of denigrating the value of clinical expertise.
• A restriction on clinical freedom, if this is defined as doing the best for one's patients.

---

literature.[4] Some of these misinterpretations are shown in Box 2.1. First, EBD does not tell dermatologists what to do.[1] Even the best external evidence has limitations in informing the care of individual patients. To use R.E. Clerk's metaphor, external evidence is just one leg of a three-legged stool—the other two being the clinician's expertise and the patient's values and preferences. Such clinical expertise and discussion of patient factors will always be at the heart of applying evidence during a dermatology consultation. EBM is not a cookbook of recipes to be followed slavishly, but an approach to medicine that is patient-driven from its outset. Patients are the best sources for generating the important clinical questions, answers to which then need to be applied back to such patients.[5]

Just as ordinary patients are at the heart of framing evidence-based questions, so too are ordinary clinical dermatologists at the heart of the practice of EBD. EBM is not something that only an exclusive club of academics with statistical expertise can understand and practise, but rather it is something that all dermatologists can practise with appropriate training. Being able to critically appraise a published clinical trial or systematic review about a new dermatological treatment is a core competency that is as basic to being a dermatologist as the ability to examine and diagnose.

Contrary to popular belief, the prime purpose of EBM is not to cut costs. Like any information source, selective use of evidence can be twisted to support different economic arguments. Thus, the relative lack of randomized clinical trial (RCT) evidence for the efficacy of methotrexate in psoriasis should not imply that methotrexate should not be used or purchased for patients with severe disease when there is so much other evidence and long-term clinical experience to support its use. But this is not to say that a clinical trial comparing methotrexate against other systemic agents such as acitretin or fumarates would not be desirable at some stage.[6]

EBM should not be viewed as a restriction on clinical freedom, if clinical freedom is defined as the opportunity to do the best for your patients, as opposed to making the same mistakes with increasing confidence. Searching for relevant information for your patients frequently opens up *more* rather than fewer treatment options.[7] Shared decision-making through a physician–patient partnership is free to choose or discard the various options in whatever way gives the most desirable outcome.

Guidelines are not the same as EBM, although the two are frequently confused.[8] Guidelines may or may not be evidence-based, but guidelines are just that—guidelines. Many dermatology guidelines now incorporate a grading system that describes the quality of evidence used to make recommendations and their strength.[9]

Problems with other sources of evidence

Working things out on the basis of mechanism and logic
Many physicians base clinical decisions on an understanding of the etiology and pathophysiology of disease and logic.[10,11] This paradigm is problematic, because the accepted hypothesis for the etiology and pathogenesis of disease changes over time, and so the logically deduced treatments change too. For example, in the past 20 years, hypotheses about the etiology of psoriasis have shifted from a disorder of keratinocyte proliferation and homeostasis, to abnormal signaling of cyclic adenosine monophosphate, to aberrant arachidonic acid metabolism, to aberrant vitamin D metabolism, to the current favorite: a T-cell–mediated autoimmune disease. Each of these hypotheses led to logically deduced treatments. The efficacy of many of these treatments has been substantiated by rigorous RCTs, whereas other treatments are used even in the absence of systematically collected observations. We thus have many options for treating patients with severe psoriasis (for example, ultraviolet B, Goeckerman treatment, psoralen–ultraviolet A, methotrexate, ciclosporin, and anti-interleukin-2 receptor antibodies) and mild to moderate psoriasis (for example,

dithranol, topical corticosteroids, calcipotriol, and tazarotene). However, we do not know which is best, in what order they should be used, or in what combinations.

Treatments based on logical deduction from pathophysiology can have unexpected consequences. For example, the observation that antiarrhythmic drugs could prevent abnormal ventricular depolarization after myocardial infarction logically led to their use to prevent sudden death after myocardial infarction. However, RCTs showed increased mortality in patients treated with antiarrhythmic drugs in comparison with placebo.[12,13] So although patients' electrocardiograms looked a lot happier and smoother, more people died whilst on treatment. This example highlights the dangers of using surrogate outcome measures, such as electrocardiograms, for more meaningful outcomes such as disability or death, simply because the surrogate measurements are easily made. The challenge with surrogate outcome measures is to ensure that they measure important things rather than trying to make measurable things important. Another classic example of the dangers in basing our treatments on empirical observations of "scientific" mechanisms is the clinical trial of thalidomide for toxic epidermal necrolysis (TEN).[14] On the basis of observations that TEN is associated with high levels of tumor necrosis factor-α (TNF-α), a trial of thalidomide (a drug that inhibits the actions of TNF-α) was commenced. The trial was stopped early because 10 out of 12 patients in the thalidomide group died, in comparison with three of 10 on placebo treatment. It was also found that those in the thalidomide group had an unexpected increase in TNF-α levels during treatment.

Some "designer" drugs, such as topical tazarotene, were promoted on the basis of their molecular mechanisms of action and may have appeared attractive at launch, but have been less exciting when tested in practice.[5] It might also be argued that the frequent narration of the superantigen story as a mechanism for antistaphylococcal treatments for atopic eczema is a smokescreen that obscures the real lack or uncertainty of evidence of clear benefit for such agents.[5]

Given these lessons, many dermatologists have become less interested in *how* treatments work and are now daring to ask questions such as: "*Does* it work?" and—more important than a demonstration of statistically significant efficacy in comparison with placebo—"How *well* does it work in comparison with existing, more established treatments?"

Personal experience

Although personal experience is an invaluable part of becoming a competent physician, the pitfalls of relying too heavily on personal experience have been widely documented.[15–17] These include:
• Overemphasis on vivid, anecdotal occurrences and underemphasis on statistically significant strong evidence.

- Bias in recognizing, remembering, and recalling evidence that supports preexisting knowledge structures (for example, ideas about disease etiology and pathogenesis) and parallel failure to recognize, remember, and recall evidence that is more valid but does not fit preexisting knowledge or beliefs.
- Failure to characterize population data accurately because of ignorance of statistical principles—including sample size, sample selection bias, and regression to the mean.
- Inability to detect and distinguish statistical association and causality.
- Persistence of beliefs despite overwhelming contrary evidence.[17]

Nisbett and Ross[18] provide examples of these pitfalls from controlled clinical research, and simple clinical examples abound. Physicians may remember patients assuming that those who did not return for follow-up improved, and conveniently forget the patients who did not improve. A patient treated with a given medication may develop a severe life-threatening reaction. On the basis of this single undesirable experience, the physician may avoid using that medication for many future patients, even though on average it may be more efficacious and less toxic than the alternative treatments that the physician chooses. Few physicians keep adequate, easily retrievable records to codify the results of treatments with a particular agent or of a particular disease, and even fewer actually carry out analyses. Few physicians make provisions for tracking those patients who are lost to follow-up. Thus, statements made about a physician's "clinical experience" may be biased. Finally, for many conditions, a single physician sees far too few patients to draw reasonably firm conclusions about the response to treatments. For example, suppose a physician who treated 20 patients with lichen planus with tretinoin found that 12 (60%) had an excellent response. The confidence interval for this response rate (i.e., the true response rate for this treatment in the larger population from which this physician's sample was obtained) ranges from 36% to 81%. Thus, the true response rate might well be substantially less (or more) than the physician concludes from personal experience.[10,19] Personal experience alone is also unlikely to pick up smaller treatment differences between active treatments. A new treatment must be substantially better than an existing treatment for a physician to notice. If, in the above example of lichen planus, standard treatment with topical corticosteroids resulted in a response rate of 55%, then the physician would need to treat 20 patients on average (number needed to treat = the reciprocal of 60% minus 50%) to notice one additional success from tretinoin.

Expert opinion

Expert opinion can be valuable, particularly for rare conditions in which the expert has the most experience or when other forms of evidence are not available. However, several studies have demonstrated that expert opinion often lags significantly behind conclusive evidence.[15] Experts suffer from relying on bench research, pathophysiology, and treatments based on logical deduction from pathophysiology, and from the same pitfalls noted for relying on personal experience.[19]

Textbooks can be valuable, particularly for rare conditions and for conditions for which the evidence does not change rapidly over time. However, textbooks have several well-documented shortcomings. They tend to reflect the biases and shortcomings of the experts who write them. By virtue of the way in which they are written, produced, and distributed, most are at least 2 years out of date at the time of publication. Also, many textbook chapters are narrative reviews that do not consider the quality of the evidence reported.[15,19,20]

Uncontrolled data

Empirical, uncontrolled and unsystematically collected data form the basis of much of dermatology practice. This situation is justified by its advocates by two erroneous assumptions. The first is that it is acceptable to use such data because better evidence is not available—an assumption that is often not true. There is a surprisingly large body of high-quality evidence that is useful for the care of patients with skin disease, as exemplified by the growing body of evidence-based treatments discussed in this book. The second erroneous assumption is that the majority of dermatologists already base their practice on the best evidence that is already available. The base of knowledge for the practice of medicine is expanding exponentially. It is estimated that to keep up with the best evidence available, a general physician would have to examine 19 articles a day, 365 days a year.[2] Therefore, keeping up to date by reading the primary literature is now an impossible task for most practising physicians.[21] The burden for dermatologists is no less daunting.[5] The challenge is to know how to find information efficiently, appraise it critically, and use it well. Knowing the best sources and methods for searching the literature allows a dermatologist to find the most current and most useful information in the most efficient manner, when it is needed. The techniques and skills needed to find, critically appraise, and use the best evidence available for the care of individual patients have been developed over two centuries. These techniques and skills are currently best known as EBM.[10]

The process of evidence-based dermatology

Having discussed the definition and rationale of EBD, how does one actually do it? This process is best considered in five steps (Box 2.2), although in real life they tend to merge

BOX 2.2 The five steps of practising evidence-based dermatology

1. Asking an answerable structured question generated from a patient encounter.
2. Searching for valid external evidence.
3. Critically appraising that evidence for relevance and validity.
4. Applying the results of that appraisal of evidence back to the patient.
5. Recording the information for the future.

and become iterative.[5] These steps are elaborated in subsequent chapters.

Step 1: asking an answerable structured question

Developing a structured question that can be answered requires practice. An example of a useless question would be, "Are diets any good in eczema?" A better question, generated from a real clinical encounter, would be, "In children with established moderate to severe atopic dermatitis, how effective is a dairy-free diet in comparison with standard treatment in inducing and maintaining a remission?" Such a question includes four key elements:
- The patient population to which one wishes to generalize.
- The intervention.
- Its comparator.
- The outcomes that might make you change your practice.[22]
Unless one uses such a structure, it would be easy to waste time discussing and searching for data on the role of diets in preventing atopic disease, the effects of dietary supplements such as fish oil, studies that evaluate only short-term clinical signs, and those that deal with a "ragbag" of different types of eczema in adults and children. Rzany and Bigby discuss further examples of framing answerable questions in more detail in Chapter 5.

Step 2: searching for the best external information

Publication of biomedical information has now expanded so much that it is hard to contemplate searching for relevant information without some form of electronic bibliographic search, followed by reading the original key papers. Most of us (including the authors) are not experts at performing complex electronic searches, and need to learn such skills. These skills are dealt with in more detail by Bigby and Corona in Chapter 6. As pointed out earlier, traditional expert reviews are risky, because often they have not been done systematically, and the links between the author's conclusions and

the data are often unclear.[23] If one is searching for trials, then the Medline and Embase databases are also hazardous sources unless one is proficient, because simply searching by the "clinical trials" type can miss up to half of the relevant trials due to coding problems.[24] The world's most comprehensive database of trials is now the Cochrane Central Register of Controlled Clinical Trials (www.thecochranelibrary.com), containing almost half a million trials in 2007. Thankfully, it is also the easiest to search.

Step 3: sifting information for relevance and quality

The usefulness of an article is a product of its clinical relevance, multiplied by its validity, divided by its accessibility.[25] Information sources need to be near the clinical area if they are to be used for patients. Becoming distracted by irrelevant but interesting citations is also a real hazard when reading search results. Two filters need to be applied if one is to keep practising EBD—the first is to discard irrelevant information, and the second is to spend more time looking at a few high-quality papers. It is timely at this point to mention the concept of the hierarchy of evidence,[26] which is discussed in more detail in Chapter 7. This means that if a randomized controlled trial is found that deals with the question of interest (for example, dietary exclusion in childhood atopic dermatitis), or better still a systematic review dealing with the same topic, one should critically appraise these sources rather than dilute what little time one has by reading lots of case series and case reports.

Step 4: applying the evidence back to the patient

This is usually the most important step, although the least well developed in EBD. Key points to note here are:
- To consider how similar the patients in the studies are to the patient facing you now.
- Whether the outcome measures used in those studies are clinically meaningful for both you as a practicing doctor and the patient.
- How large the treatment benefits were.
- What the drawbacks of the intervention were.
- How the evidence fits in with your patient's past experience and current preferences.
This difficult area is discussed in more detail in Chapter 14.

Step 5: recording the information for the future

Having done so much work pursuing the above "evidence-based prescription" from question to patient, it might be useful to others and yourself to make a record of that information for future use as a critically appraised topic (CAT), although these have a limited lifespan if not updated.[2] Such CATs could become the norm in dermatology journal clubs all over the world, replacing unstructured chats about articles selected for unclear reasons.

The key point to remember about the process of EBD is that it *starts and ends with patients*. A problem highlighted during an encounter with a patient is the best generator of an EBM problem.[27] Even if one then searches and critically appraises the best data in the world, the utility of this exercise would be zero if it were not then applied back to that patient or other similar patients. Developing the skills to undertake evidence-based prescription requires practice.

Dermatologists will participate in the practice of EBD to different degrees depending on their enthusiasm, skills, time pressures and interest.[26] Some will be "doers," implying that they undertake at least steps 1–4 highlighted in Box 2.2. Others will be more inclined to adopt a "using mode," relying on searching for evidence-based summaries such as systematic reviews that others have constructed, thereby skipping step 3, at least to some degree. Finally, some will incorporate evidence into their practice in a "replicating mode," following decisions of respected leaders (i.e., skipping steps 2 and 3). These categories bear some similarity to those of deduction, induction, and seduction that Sackett used to describe the methods that physicians employ to make decisions about therapy.[15] Such categories are not mutually exclusive, since even the most enthusiastic EBM practitioners in "doing" mode will flit to "user" and "replicating" mode according to whether they are dealing with a common or rare clinical problem.

Conclusions

Few dermatologists would argue that their overarching professional role is to provide their patients with the best health care. To do so, a dermatologist must be able to assess the patient's physical condition, know the best and most current information about diagnosis, prevention, therapy, prognosis, and potential harm, and then apply that knowledge of universals to the individual patients.[28] Medicine is advancing very rapidly, creating major changes in the way we treat our patients. We must keep up with such changes. We need to be up to date with such new external evidence. We frequently fail to do this if we rely on passive means or an occasional flick through the main journals, and our knowledge gradually deteriorates with time. Attempts to overcome this deficiency by attending clinical education programs fail to improve our performance, whereas the practice of EBM has been shown to keep its practitioners up to date. EBM is a way of thinking that is intended to help accomplish these objectives. If we stick to thinking about patients' welfare when contemplating EBM, we are less likely to get things wrong.[5,10]

References

1 Sackett DL, Rosenberg WM, Gray JA, Haynes RB, Richardson WS. Evidence based medicine: what it is and what it isn't. *BMJ* 1996;**312**:71–2.

2 Sackett DL, Richardson WS, Rosenberg Q, Haynes RB. *Evidence-based Medicine. How to Practise and Teach EBM*. London: Churchill Livingstone, 1997.

3 Bigby M. Snake oil for the 21st century. *Arch Dermatol* 1998; **134**:1512–4.

4 Rees J. Evidence-based medicine: the epistemology that isn't. *J Am Acad Dermatol* 2000;**43**:727–9.

5 Williams HC. Evidence-based dermatology: a bridge too far? *Clin Exp Dermatol* 2001;**26**:714–24.

6 Griffiths CEM, Clark CM, Chalmers RJG, Li Wan Po A, Williams HC. A systematic review of treatments for severe psoriasis. *Health Technol Assess* 2000;**4**:1–125.

7 Hoare C, Li Wan Po A, Williams H. Systematic review of treatments for atopic eczema. *Health Technol Assess* 2000;**4**(37):1–191.

8 Seidman D. Compliance with guidelines is not the same as evidence-based medicine. *J Pediatr* 2001;**138**:299–300.

9 Hanifin JM, Cooper KD, Ho VC, *et al*. Guidelines of care for atopic dermatitis, developed in accordance with the American Academy of Dermatology (AAD)/American Academy of Dermatology Association "Administrative Regulations for Evidence-Based Clinical Practice Guidelines." *J Am Acad Dermatol* 2004;**50**:391–404.

10 Bigby M. Paradigm lost. *Arch Dermatol* 2000;**136**:26–7.

11 Klovning A. Seminar 3: an introduction to evidence-based practice (http://www.shef.ac.uk/uni/projects/wrp/sem3.html.)

12 Echt DS, Liebson PR, Mitchell LB, *et al*. Mortality and morbidity in patients receiving encainide, flecainide, or placebo: the Cardiac Arrhythmia Suppression Trial. *N Engl J Med* 1991;**324**:781–8.

13 The Cardia Arrhythmia Suppression Trial II Investigators. Effects of the antiarrhythmic agent moricizine on survival after myocardial infarction. *N Engl J Med* 1992;**327**:227–33.

14 Wolkenstein P, Latarjet J, Roujeau JC, *et al*. Randomised comparison of thalidomide versus placebo in toxic epidermal necrolysis. *Lancet* 1998;**352**:1586–9.

15 Sackett DL, Haynes RB, Guyatt GH, Tugwell P. *Clinical Epidemiology: A Basic Science for Clinical Medicine*. Boston: Little, Brown, 1991: 441.

16 Bigby M, Gadenne AS. Understanding and evaluating clinical trials. *J Am Acad Dermatol* 1996;**34**:555–90.

17 Hines DC, Goldheizer JW. Clinical investigation: a guide to its evaluation. *Am J Obstet Gynecol* 1969;**105**:450–87.

18 Nisbett R, Ross L. *Human Inference: Strategies and Shortcomings of Social Judgment*. Englewood Cliffs, NJ: Prentice-Hall, 1980: 330.

19 Bigby M, Szklo M. Evidence-based dermatology. In: Freedberg I, Eisen AZ, Katz SI, *et al.*, eds. *Dermatology in General Medicine*. New York: McGraw Hill, 2003: 2301–2311.

20 Greenhalgh T. *How to Read a Paper. The Basics of Evidence Based Medicine*. London: BMJ Books, 1997: 196.

21 Guyatt GH, Sackett DL, Cook DJ. Users' guides to the medical literature, II. How to use an article about therapy or prevention, B. What were the results and will they help me in caring for my patients? *JAMA* 1994;**271**:59–63.

22 Straus SE, Sackett DL. Bringing evidence to the clinic. *Arch Dermatol* 1998;**134**:1519–20.

23 Ladhani S, Williams HC. The management of established post-herpetic neuralgia: a comparison of the quality and content of traditional *v.* systematic reviews. *Br J Dermatol* 1998;**139**:66–72.

24 Delamere FM, Williams HC. How can hand searching the dermatological literature help people with skin problems? *Arch Dermatol* 2001;**137**:332–5.

25 Shaughnessy AF, Slawson DC, Bennett JH. Becoming an informa-tion master: a guidebook to the medical information jungle. *J Fam Pract* 1994;**39**:489–99.

26 Bigby M. Evidence-based medicine in dermatology. *Dermatol Clin* 2000;**18**:261–76.

27 Shaughnessy AF, Slawson DC, Becker L. Clinical jazz: harmoniz-ing clinical experience and evidence-based medicine. *J Fam Pract* 1998;**47**:425–8.

28 Cook HJ. What stays constant at the heart of medicine. *Br Med J* 2006;**333**:1281–2.

3

The role of the consumer and the public in evidence-based dermatology

Maxine Whitton, Andrew Herxheimer

Bridging the communication gap

Dermatologists, like other doctors, now recognize the therapeutic value of an alliance with their patients (the "therapeutic alliance"), and the need to explain their advice and, as far as possible, to share management decisions with the patient. Different people may have very different values and preferences, and it is often wrong to assume agreement without explanation and discussion. Medical terms are often unfamiliar to patients. For example, to hear a rash or spot called an "eruption" or a "lesion" can be disconcerting. Using language the patient can understand, clinicians need to be able to explain the condition, its implications and treatment, as well as possible side effects, and the consequences of not using the medication. If this can be achieved, then patients are more likely to accept the requirements of the treatment and a true care partnership with the professional can be established. This could save time and lead to quicker recovery and greater mutual trust. Unfortunately, most consultations offer too little time to do this adequately, especially since some of the concepts that underlie diagnosis and treatment are unfamiliar to most patients and many lack the necessary background knowledge. It is important to bridge this communication gap from both ends, by helping dermatologists and those working with them to become more fluent and understanding of the patient's perspective, and by developing training and education for their current and future patients—or "consumers."

The many roles of patients, the public, and consumers in health care

It is difficult to find a term that encompasses the idea of a member of the public who uses or receives health care or is a carer or parent of a patient. Different terms have different connotations for people from different countries and backgrounds, so no one term will be acceptable to everyone. We have used the term "consumer" throughout this chapter, as it is widely used in the Cochrane Collaboration, while fully recognizing that it is not ideal.

Patients, consumers, and the public have many roles:
- To play an active part in self-care as far as one's capacity allows;
- To work together with professionals in one's own care and in the care of others in the family, the workplace, and the locality;
- To communicate to health professionals and the healthy community the points of view, needs, and wishes of people affected by a disease;
- To take part with professionals in the development and governance of health institutions (for example, hospitals and nursing homes) and organizations, such as providers of primary care;
- To contribute to research policy and practice by helping decide research priorities and funding, and helping to improve the design of research;
- To help recruit participants for worthwhile research;
- To help disseminate important research findings;
- To contribute one's own experiences of illness to inform and educate other patients and professionals.

The skin shows: it matters psychologically and socially

All the above roles are relevant to dermatology, but not special to it. What distinguishes skin disease from other kinds of illnesses is its greater visibility. This means that its social effects are often far greater than for other illnesses of comparable seriousness, and that the patient's self-image is often harmed. Healthy people, including many health professionals, do not sufficiently understand these aspects, and do not cope adequately with them. Consumers and patients can help them understand and learn what matters to people with various skin conditions. In the case of vitiligo, for example, doctors sometimes base treatment decisions on how they perceive the degree of distress. Many think that white patients suffer less than those with darker skins, but studies as well as anecdotal experience have shown that this may not be true.[1] Nor is the extent of the disease always the most important factor in the patient's suffering. Self-esteem, self-image, the site of the lesions, the degree to which the patient feels disabled by the disease, and the support networks available to the patient all need to be considered. A study of psoriasis has found that the patient's opinion of disease severity can differ from the physician's and that the degree of distress depends on how much the disease affects everyday life.[2] These findings underline that the assessment of psoriasis (whether by doctor or patient) influences the choice of treatment. Patients may well prefer treatments that will mitigate the disfiguring social effects of the disease to those that reduce the size of the lesions.

The importance of the psychosocial impact of skin disease has always been recognized, but not adequately addressed. It could be argued that some patient-support groups perform this role. However, although they can provide opportunities for members to share experiences and give practical advice, most are not equipped to offer either medical advice or in-depth psychological help. More could be done to ensure that dermatology patients are given the opportunity for referral to professional psychological help as an integral part of disease management.[3] It should also be part of treatment guidelines. This approach is crucial for vitiligo, a disease that has no significant physical symptoms but can be psychologically devastating. In spite of this, a recent Cochrane review of interventions for vitiligo[4] found only one study of psychological therapies.[5]

Changing Faces, a UK charity that supports people with disfigurement from birth, accident, or disease such as skin disease, directly helps individuals and families through information, workshops, counseling, and disfigurement life skills. It has published a booklet to help patients with a skin disorder cope with their disease: "When a medical skin condition affects the way you look." The charity is also contributing to research into disfigurement. In 1998, Changing Faces and the University of the West of England set up the world's first and only Center for Appearance Research (CAR) to enhance understanding of the psychosocial, educational, and cultural aspects of disfigurement and concerns related to appearance.

A program for psoriasis patients in Manchester, England, represents an important development that could be a model for other skin diseases. As well as medical treatment, they are offered a program of cognitive behavioral therapy that includes education about the disease, its treatments, and the implications. The results are encouraging.[6]

A recent study from Germany has shown how a tailored program of educational and psychological support for young people with eczema and their parents can result in sustained improvement in eczema severity and quality of life.[7]

The skin has a dual function as both a large and important organ and the superficial covering of the body, which can lead to its association with cosmetics and cosmetic surgery. Some skin conditions, such as acne and vitiligo, are apt to be trivialized as cosmetic problems, particularly by some general practitioners. The boundaries between treatment, prevention, and aggravation of skin problems are often blurred.

Education and information for self-care

Before patients with skin disease can hope to manage their own treatment, they have to learn about the condition and about the principles that underlie its treatment and how to apply them in everyday life. When this is achieved, the patient has much greater control and is more confident and self-reliant, especially with a chronic skin disease—although of course some advice and help from professionals will still be needed at times.

Many self-help groups or patient-support groups (PSGs) are founded by people who have been given no information about their condition, or whose questions have not been answered adequately. They may have difficulty asking the questions that most concern them, or may be too embarrassed, or feel that the subject is too trivial and wastes the doctor's time. Often a PSG can resolve the practical everyday problems that clinicians are not aware of or avoid dealing with through either embarrassment or a lack of understanding.

PSGs have a clear role in providing just such information, through fact sheets, leaflets, newsletters, in confidence on the telephone, CDs, videos, or increasingly through their web sites, so reaching wider international audiences. Most of this information is of course not yet rigorously evidence-based, but as consumers acquire the skills of critical appraisal and an understanding of levels of evidence—for example, by working within the Cochrane Consumer Network—information should become better and more reliable.

The UK Vitiligo Society is unique in publishing a book on all aspects of vitiligo, its management and current research.[8] Most self-help organizations have developed a raft of fact sheets, written in good lay language but with professional input where necessary to ensure accuracy. These help not only patients, but also professionals. Leaflets and fact sheets can be tailored to different groups, such as children, parents, teachers, health and other professionals, as well as to the general public.

Information from PSGs can cover a wide range of topics, including diet, clothing, complementary therapies, and useful tips on various aspects of managing the disease. Some of this information may not be easily found elsewhere—for example:

- The UK Raynaud's and Scleroderma Association gives information on heating aids and on how to keep warm, including the use of electrically heated gloves and socks provided by the UK National Health Service. Few patients know about this.
- The UK Psoriasis Association includes personal tips from members in its journal, as well as publishing various leaflets and fact sheets—including, for example, information about treatments abroad for psoriasis.
- The UK National Eczema Society publishes booklets on psoralen and ultraviolet A (PUVA) treatment, itching and scratching, and wet wraps, as well as the psychological aspects of eczema and fact sheets on diet, topical steroids, sun protection, and the use of Chinese herbs for eczema.

PSGs state explicitly that they do not recommend alternative treatments, but they give sound advice on what to look out for to minimize trouble—for example, checking that alternative practitioners have appropriate qualifications.

Self-help groups can also make valuable contributions by helping to collect patients' own personal experiences of illness—which often raise issues that medical accounts do not consider. These narratives can be systematically analyzed and made accessible to patients, professionals, and students so that everyone can be much better informed. The Database of Individual Patients' Experiences of illness (DIPEx) is an ambitious project that is establishing such collections for a wide range of diseases.[9] So far, it does not include experiences of skin disease; that is planned for the future.

The importance of all this work to the patient cannot be overstated. An understanding of the disease enhances the patient's ability to cope. An informed patient can begin to take responsibility for his/her disease and learn to manage it more confidently. It is not uncommon for some patients to be better informed than their family doctor about their disease and its treatment, especially for less common genetic disorders. This can lead to problems in the doctor–patient relationship if it is not handled properly, but it can also contribute to much better collaboration between the patient and the doctor.

Consumers and research

Consumer involvement in clinical research is still rare in dermatology. On the one hand, many investigators and clinicians are not convinced of the value of public involvement in research, and on the other, dermatology patients don't realize that they can play a vital role in the research process. Nonetheless, examples of successful patient participation do exist in other disease areas—for example, the Quality Research in Dementia program. Two studies conducted in the Netherlands show that patients can prioritize research needs and pose questions not considered by

researchers. One of the studies used focus groups and questionnaires with patients suffering from asthma and chronic obstructive pulmonary disease to assess their ability to prioritize research.[10] The other study searched the literature for examples of patient involvement and also interviewed scientists, patients, representatives from patient organizations and clinicians.[11] The findings suggest that patients' experiential knowledge can contribute to the relevance and validity of research.

Most PSGs among other things aim to support and encourage research. Many strive towards finding a "cure" for their particular condition, however unrealistic this may seem to health professionals. In general, however, PSGs tend to give financial support to projects that researchers (mainly university-based academics) have already chosen. Such research is often of high quality, but the resulting "basic science" discoveries rarely find their way back to the patient. Patient organizations vary in the priority they give to research over support and education.

Dermatology PSGs do fund research, but the sums are modest compared with other disease areas. Among the UK skin groups, the biggest funder of research is the Psoriasis Association. Like many other PSGs, the association has a Medical and Research Committee to vet projects for research funding. Its lay members help ensure that the patient's perspective is included in their discussions. Projects are always referred to the National Council for a final decision and at this stage are sometimes passed back to the Medical and Research Committee for review, often for a more patient-based approach.

Pharmaceutical companies fund the highest proportion of dermatological research projects, and they have been reluctant to involve consumers in such research in any meaningful way until recently. Companies can establish strong relationships with groups and sometimes work with them to devise quality-of-life questionnaires. Although these studies are mainly for marketing purposes, the results may also influence the choice of research topics and the design of clinical studies. For the most part, pharmaceutical companies tend to approach PSGs mainly for help with recruiting patients for trials, and most PSGs have contributed in this way. Because companies often regard some of the data contained in their protocol as being commercially sensitive, PSGs rarely get much information to give to potential participants. Often participants are not thanked for their involvement and are not told about the outcome of the trial. Skin diseases are by and large chronic illnesses with much higher morbidity than mortality. Patients who have been managing their disease and living with it for many years have in some ways become experts. PSGs, because of the cumulative and combined experience of their members, have good insights into what research is needed. More recently, concerns have been raised about companies that have developed new drugs for specific skin conditions (e.g., biologics for psoriasis) who then donate large funds to PSGs in order to create increased awareness of the disease. Whilst this might seem like a wonderful gift to PSGs at the start, given that most PSGs want to increase awareness of the disease, they have to take great care to avoid inadvertently becoming yet another marketing arm for a pharmaceutical company.

Some organizations, such as the Raynaud's and Scleroderma Association, are beginning to suggest areas of research based on their members' experience. For example, the association decided to offer funding for a project on calcinosis—a big problem for many people with the disease. This is not a particularly attractive topic and can be difficult to tackle. After several months waiting for a worthwhile proposal, a project was started in 2002. The association is also keen to fund a study of the causes of childhood scleroderma.

The UK National Eczema Society supported and funded the double-blinded controlled study at Liverpool University of the effect of house-dust mites in adults and children with eczema.[12] Other organizations, such as the National Eczema Association for Science and Education based in the USA, have set up and supported international research meetings.

Two specific dermatology research initiatives involve patients: the UK Dermatology Clinical Trials Network (UK DCTN) and the European Vitiligo Task Force (EVTF). The UK DCTN was established in 2002 to conduct high-quality multicenter clinical trials of skin diseases addressing questions that matter to clinicians and patients. It involves a collaborative network of dermatologists, dermatology nurses, health services researchers, and patients in the UK and Ireland. It invites suggestions for trials from anyone, including patients, and is committed to involving patients in research wherever possible—from the design of the trial right through to the dissemination of the results.

The EVTF was formed in 2003 by a group of scientists and dermatologists to develop global standards for vitiligo research. Uniquely, the group invited representatives from patient groups to its first symposium in Reston, Virginia, in 2005, held as a satellite meeting of the International Pigment Cell Conference. Unanswered questions gathered from people with vitiligo were discussed and patient delegates could speak of their experience of the disease. This symposium afforded a rare and valuable opportunity for dialogue between scientists, patients, and clinicians.

PSGs can play an important role in educating patients about ways in which they can become involved in clinical research. The National Eczema Society recognized this and encouraged its members and other dermatology patient groups to volunteer to join the Cochrane Skin Group (see Chapter 4) as consumer representatives. Under the auspices of an umbrella organization of UK skin support groups called the Skin Care Campaign (formerly a project of the National Eczema Society), a meeting was held to inform consumers about the Cochrane Collaboration and how they as consumers could contribute to its work. Some consumers subsequently contributed by hand-searching journals, commenting on protocols and reviews, translating reviews, and co-authoring a review (on vitiligo). This meeting led to a focus group to help identify suitable questions for eczema research. The mutual benefits for consumers and doctors working together in the Cochrane Skin Group have been documented elsewhere.[13]

More general organizations committed to encouraging more consumer involvement in research should also be mentioned. The organization known as Involve (formerly Consumers in NHS Research) was set up in 1996 to advise the UK National Health Service (NHS) on how best to involve consumers in research and development (R&D). Members are drawn from the voluntary sector, research organizations, health information providers, and health and social services management. The group aims "to ensure that consumer involvement in R&D in the NHS improves the way that research is prioritized, commissioned, undertaken and disseminated." This includes persuading researchers of the importance and value of consumer involvement by indicating ways in which consumers can be part of the research process, and offering information, advice, and support to consumers, researchers, and NHS employees through the support unit. The James Lind Alliance (JLA) was established to build a coalition of patient organizations and clinicians working together to identify and prioritize important treatment uncertainties. The resulting JLA Working Partnership is a unique first step in encouraging well-designed research projects on answerable questions to address the mismatch between research and the clinical needs of both patients and doctors. The Database of Uncertainties about the Effects of Treatments (DUETs) is a resource of the JLA that publishes questions by patients and clinicians which existing systematic reviews do not answer.

The Cochrane Consumer Network is a part of the Cochrane Collaboration. Its members include individual consumers as well as community organizations around the world. The network gives much-needed support and training to consumers, encouraging them to take part in the work of the collaboration by helping identify questions for review from the viewpoint of the person with the health problem, searching for the trials, commenting on drafts of reviews and protocols, and helping to disseminate the reviews. It works to keep consumers informed, develops training materials, helps demystify scientific jargon to make reviews more accessible to the general public, and publishes a digest of new additions to the Cochrane Library, including full consumer summaries of reviews. Its web site provides a means of commenting on issues and reviews and has links with other sources of evidence-based health care on the Internet.

Consumer involvement in the process of evidence-based dermatology

Given the important and diverse roles that a consumer may play in the therapeutic alliance with his/her physician, how do these roles become translated into the practice of evidence-based dermatology? This can be best answered by considering the four steps of evidence-based practice: 1, asking an answerable question; 2, searching for relevant information; 3, appraising the validity of that information; and then 4, applying it back to the patient.

1. *Asking an answerable question.* By definition, the question generated within an "evidence-based prescription" is derived from a patient encounter. For example, a woman aged 32 with facial acne may want to know whether it is safe to take a combined antiandrogen/estrogen pill, as opposed to continuing to use an oral antibiotic. Further discussion may reveal that she worries mainly about deep vein thrombosis, which a family member suffered. The structured evidence-based question arising from this discussion would then be, "What is the increased risk for a woman in her thirties to suffer a deep vein thrombosis when taking the combined antiandrogen/estrogen pill for her acne when compared with taking an oral antibiotic?" This will of course depend on other factors such as whether she smokes, her weight, exercise profile, etc., but it nevertheless illustrates how an evidence-based question needs to be tailored in a structured way around a particular individual.

2. *Searching for relevant information.* This may at first seem to be the domain of the clinician, yet the advent of the Internet and many high-quality skin information web sites has transformed this. Many patients now come to their first dermatology consultation armed with pages printed out from the Internet. They sometimes correctly self-diagnose conditions such as "cold urticaria" when even their family doctor was unsure. Whilst it is true that much of the information on the Internet is of dubious value as a result of various vested interests and the lack of explicit criteria used to develop it, the Internet can be a useful source of information for many rare and common skin diseases. Some web sites, such as DermNetNZ and e-medicine, produce excellent and comprehensive information about skin disorders, including rare ones. Other sites, such as the UK National Health Service skin disorders specialist library, serve as a public "one-stop shop" for quality-appraised web resources on skin disorders that is freely available for health professionals and patients. In this sense, consumers can play a useful role by helping their dermatologists search for information that may be relevant to the question.

3. *Appraising the quality of the data.* Again, although it might seem that only the clinician can appraise the validity of the data by checking for things such as adequacy of conceal-

ment of the randomization schedule, and issues of blinding and intention-to-treat analysis, such an assessment is of little value if the clinician examines reported outcomes in a trial that means little to the patient. Consumers are ideally placed to help inform their physicians about which aspect of the disease is important to them. For example, in patients with atopic eczema, is it short-term control of itching, duration or frequency of remissions, healing painful cracks in the fingers, coping skills, or ability to take part in sport and social activities?

4. *Applying the information back to the patient.* An "evidence-based prescription" is useless if that information is not then presented back to the patient who generated it. Patients are the only people who can ultimately decide if the treatment options they are offered fit in with their belief systems and expectation for improvement, willingness to be inconvenienced by side effects and frequent consultations, and so on.

Thus, the consumer clearly has a central role in driving and informing the entire process of evidence-based dermatology, in that the important questions begin and end with the patient. The dermatologist is seen as the patient's advocate, guiding and interpreting the evidence and applying it to the patient's unique circumstances through a caring and trusting partnership.

Conclusions

Given that many skin diseases are chronic, many patients and their carers want to know as much as possible about the causes and prognosis of their skin disease, and of the costs and benefits of the many treatments available to them. In many circumstances, doctors have trivialized the psychological effects of skin disease, and until now consumers have been minimally involved in skin research.

Yet there is a huge opportunity for clinicians to work more closely and in partnership with consumers, particularly in the field of skin disease. Consumers are often in the best position to guide clinicians and researchers on what matters most to them in terms of therapeutic benefit, and they can provide psychological support and useful written information to fellow patients in ways that doctors cannot. The "expert patient" with a chronic skin condition might also be well placed to deliver health-care support to organizations such as hospitals, and they may be helpful in teaching medical students about their skin disorder. Consumers are also well placed to help prioritize relevant research in dermatology by framing the research questions that are most important to them, by helping researchers choose meaningful outcome measures, and by recruiting patients through their networks. Consumer groups are also ideally placed to disseminate research findings, and many are increasingly funding their own research.

Further information

Details of the PSGs and other organizations mentioned in this chapter are listed below. Dermatology web resources that have been appraised for quality can all be found in one place in the UK national skin disorders specialist library (www.library.nhs.uk/skin).

Health on the Net and other organizations have developed ethical principles to aid consumers and evaluate the quality of health-related information. For a more comprehensive list of UK-based PSGs, contact the Skin Care Campaign. There may be similar organizations in other countries, but the authors do not have reliable information on PSGs in other parts of the world. The web site of the International Alliance of Patients' Organizations (IAPO) lists many (www.patientsorganizations.org).

- *Changing Faces*: The Squire Centre, 33–37 University Street, London WC1E 6JN, UK (www.changingfaces.org.uk).
- *Cochrane Consumer Network* (www.cochrane.org/consumers/homepage.htm, e-mail: ccnet-contact@cochrane.de).
- *Database of Uncertainties about the Effects of Treatments* (DUETs) (www.duets.nhs.uk).
- DeimNetNZ www.dermnetnz.org
- *eMedicine* (http://www.emedicine.com/derm).
- *Involve* (Consumers in NHS Research Support Unit): Wessex House, Upper Market St., Eastleigh, Hampshire SO50 9FD UK. Tel: +44-(0)2380-651088 (www.invo.org.uk).
- *National Eczema Association for Science and Education* (USA): 1220 SW Morrison, Suite 433, Portland, OR 97205, USA. Tel.: +503-228-4430 or +800-818-7546; fax: +503-224-3363 (www.eczema-assn.org).
- *National Eczema Society (UK)*: Hill House, Highgate Hill, London N19 5NA, UK. Tel.: 44-(0)20-7281 3553; fax: 44-(0)-20-7281 6395 (www.eczema.org).
- *New Zealand Dermatological Society* (www.dermnetnz.org).
- *Psoriasis Association*: Milton House, 7 Milton Street, Northampton NN2 7JG, UK. Tel.: +44-(0)1604-711129; fax: +44-(0)-1604-792894 (www.psoriasis-association.org.uk).
- *Raynaud's and Scleroderma Association*: 112 Crewe Road, Alsager, Cheshire ST7 2JA, UK. Tel.: +44-(0)1270-872776; fax: +44-(0)-1270-883556 (www.raynauds.demon.co.uk).
- *Skin Care Campaign*: address as National Eczema Society, UK (www.skincarecampaign.org).
- *The UK Dermatology Clinical Trials Network* (UK DCTN) (www.ukdctn.org.uk).
- *Vitiligo Society*: 125 Kennington Road, London SE11 6SF, UK. Tel.: 0800-018-2631; fax: +44-(0)20-7840 0866 (www.vitiligosociety.org.uk).

References

1 Porter JR, Beuf AH. Racial variation in reaction to physical stigma: a study of degree of disturbance by vitiligo among black and white patients. *J Health Soc Behav* 1991;**32**:192–204.

2 Root S, Kent G, Al'Abadie MSK. The relationship between disease severity, disability and psychological distress in patients undergoing PUVA treatment for psoriasis. *Dermatology* 1994;**189**:234–7.

3 Gupta MA, Gupta AK. Psychiatric and psychological co-morbidity in patients with dermatological disorders: epidemiology and management. *Am J Clin Dermatol* 2003;**4**: 833–42.

4 Whitton ME, Ashcroft DM, Barrett CW, Gonzalez U. Interventions for vitiligo. *Cochrane Database Syst Rev* 2006;(1):CD003263.

5 Papadopoulos L, Walker CJ, Anthis L. Living with vitiligo: a controlled investigation into the effects of group cognitive-behavioural and humanistic therapies. *Dermatol Psychosom* 2004;**5**:172–4.

6 Fortune DG, Richards HL, Kirby B, Bowcock S, Main CJ, Griffiths CEM. A cognitive-behavioural symptom management programme as an adjunct in psoriasis therapy. *Br J Dermatol* 2002;**146**:458–65.

7 Staab D, Diepgen TL, Fartasch M, *et al.* Age related, structured educational programmes for the management of atopic dermatitis in children and adolescents: multicentre, randomized controlled trial. *BMJ* 2006;**332**:933–8.

8 Lesage M. *Vitiligo: Understanding the Loss of Skin Colour.* London: The Vitiligo Society, 2002.

9 Herxheimer A, Ziebland S. The DIPEx project: collecting personal experiences of illness and health care. In: Hurwitz B, Greenhalgh T, Skultans V, eds. *Narrative Research in Health and Illness.* Malden, MA: Blackwell and BMJ Books, 2004:115–131.

10 Tan BB, Weald D, Strickland I, Friedmann PS. Double-blind controlled trial of effect of housedust-mite allergen avoidance on atopic dermatitis. *Lancet* 1996;**347**:15–8.

11 Caron-Flinterman JF, Broerse JEW, Bunders JFG. Patients' priorities concerning health research: the case of asthma and COPD research in the Netherlands. *Health Expect* 2005;**8**:253–63.

12 Caron-Flinterman JF, Broerse JEW, Teerling J, Bunders JFG. The experiential knowledge of patients: a new resource for biomedical research? *Soc Sci Med* 2005;**60**:2575–84.

13 Collier A, Johnson K, Heilig L, Leonard T, Williams H, Dellavalle RP. A win–win proposition: fostering US health care consumer involvement in the Cochrane Collaboration Skin Group. *J Am Acad Dermatol* 2005;**53**:920–1.

4   The Cochrane Skin Group

Tina Leonard, Finola Delamere, Dedee Murrell

Background

The Cochrane Skin Group (CSG) is one of 50 collaborative review groups that together make up the Cochrane Collaboration. This international organization has developed in response to a challenge issued by Archie Cochrane, a British epidemiologist, who in 1972 pointed out the deficiencies of reviews of the medical literature and the lack of access to up-to-date information about health care.[1] Later, he wrote: "It is surely a great criticism of our profession that we have not organized a critical summary, by specialty or sub-specialty, adapted periodically, of all relevant randomized controlled trials."[2]

Archie Cochrane recognized that there was a great collective ignorance about the effects of health care. The amount of information available to both professionals and the public was overwhelming, much of it was not evidence-based, and some was contradictory. A systematic approach to organizing and evaluating the information available from clinical trials was sorely needed. In 1987, Cochrane admiringly described a systematic review of randomized controlled trials (RCTs) of care during pregnancy and childbirth as "a real milestone in the history of randomized trials and in the evaluation of care," and suggested that other specialties should copy the methods used.[3] This suggestion was taken up by the UK's Research and Development Programme, which had been set up to support the National Health Service (NHS). Funds were provided to establish a "Cochrane center" that would collaborate with researchers both in the UK and elsewhere to facilitate the production of systematic reviews of RCTs across all areas of health care.[4,5] The first Cochrane center opened in Oxford in October 1992, and 6 months later the New York Academy of Sciences organized a meeting to discuss the possibility of an international collaboration.[6] In October 1993, 77 people from 11 countries then met to set up the Cochrane Collaboration. This meeting was the first in what became a series of annual Cochrane Colloquia.

The Cochrane Collaboration is guided by ten principles:
- Collaboration
- Building on the enthusiasm of individuals
- Avoiding duplication
- Minimizing bias
- Keeping up to date
- Ensuring relevance
- Ensuring access
- Continually improving the quality of its work
- Continuity
- Enabling wide participation

Structure of the Cochrane Collaboration

The structure of the Cochrane Collaboration is summarized in Figure 4.1.

Collaborative review groups. The Collaboration has grown rapidly, and the 50 review groups between them cover all the important areas of health care. Their main outputs are:
- Systematic reviews, published electronically in the Cochrane Library and updated regularly.
- A specialized register of clinical trials in each group's subject area.

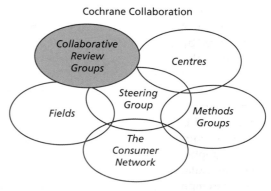

Figure 4.1 The structure of the Cochrane Collaboration.

Cochrane methods groups. Authors are supported by the work of various groups specializing in methodology—for example, in the fields of statistics, economics, non-randomized studies, and patient-reported outcomes.

Cochrane fields/networks. These are groupings that represent a population, group, or type of care that overlaps multiple review group areas—for example, primary health care, child health, complementary medicine, vaccines, and cancer.

The Consumer Network. Participation by consumers (the users or recipients of health care) is essential to the Collaboration, and the Consumer Network's core function is to provide consumer input into Cochrane systematic reviews by:
- Providing links for consumers to Cochrane groups
- Developing training materials and workshops to facilitate effective consumer participation
- Maintaining a web site
- Publishing regular newsletters
- Providing an avenue for consumer representation

Steering Group. This is the policy-making body of the Cochrane Collaboration.

The Cochrane Library. This is the main output of the Collaboration. It is the single best source of reliable evidence about the effects of health-care interventions. It is updated quarterly and is available on the Internet (www.thecochranelibrary.org). Residents in a number of countries have free use of the Cochrane Library through a national provision, which gives them access to the full-text versions of nearly 3298 completed Cochrane systematic reviews (as of issue 4, 2007). Several programs also provide free access in Latin America and low-income countries (details available at http://www3.interscience.wiley.com/cqi-bin/mrwhome/106568753/AccessCochraneLibrary.html). The Cochrane Library is also available on CD-ROM.

The Cochrane Library includes several databases:
- The Cochrane Database of Systematic Reviews (CDSR) contains protocols and reviews prepared and maintained by collaborative review groups. It includes a feedback system to enable users to improve the quality of Cochrane reviews.
- The Database of Abstracts of Reviews of Effectiveness (DARE), produced by the NHS Centre for Reviews and Dissemination in England, contains critical assessments and structured abstracts of other high-quality systematic reviews.
- The Cochrane Central Register of Controlled Trials (C) contains bibliographic information on over 522 340 controlled trials (as of issue 4, 2007), including reports from conference proceedings and many other sources not listed in other bibliographic databases.
- The Cochrane Database of Methodology Reviews (CDMR) summarizes the empirical basis for decisions about methods for systematic reviews and evaluations of health care.

- The NHS Economic Evaluation Database is a register of published economic evaluations of healthcare interventions.
- The Cochrane Methodology Register is a bibliography of publications which report on methods used in the conduct of controlled trials.
- The Health Technology Assessment Database contains information on healthcare technology assessments.
- The About the Cochrane Collaboration database contains information on the groups that make up The Cochrane Collaboration.

The Cochrane Library also includes a handbook on how to perform a systematic review and a glossary of terms.

The Cochrane Skin Group

The CSG aims to provide the best evidence about the effects (beneficial and harmful) of interventions for skin diseases, so that professionals and consumers can make well-informed decisions about treatment.

History and structure

The CSG was established in 1997.[7] The founder of the group and its coordinating editor, Prof. Hywel Williams, works at the University of Nottingham, UK, which is also the editorial base. The other team members are Dr. Tina Leonard (managing editor and group coordinator), Dr. Finola Delamere (trials search coordinator), Helen Nankervis (editorial assistant) and Diane Horstey (administrative assistant).

The editors include Dr. Michael Bigby (USA), Dr. Robert Dellavalle (USA), Dr. Sarah Garner (UK), Dr. Sam Gibbs (UK), Dr. Sue Jessop (South Africa), Dr. Jo Leonardi-Bee (UK), Philippa Middleton (Australia), Prof. Dédée Murrell (Australia), and Prof. Luigi Naldi (Italy). The group's feedback editor is Dr. Urbà González (Spain). A particular strength of the CSG has been the involvement of consumers, who help in many diverse ways. The Group now supports about 470 authors worldwide and receives funding from the NHS Research and Development Program in the UK.

Scope

Over 1000 skin conditions are listed on the CSG's web site at www.csg.cochrane.org. The CSG's scope also includes cosmetic skin care products and the effectiveness of different models for delivering health care for skin diseases. It excludes sexually transmitted diseases, now a separate medical specialty; some overlap exists with other review groups, such as the musculoskeletal group, the neuromuscular disease group, and the wounds group.

Topics for review are chosen by potential authors with encouragement and support from the editorial base, and the editors also identify priority areas. All authors are volunteers, but public authorities in some countries give grants for specific topics. The CSG accepts no funding from pharmaceutical companies.

Systematic reviews benefit dermatology in three ways:
• By providing a much more comprehensive literature search than a standard review. For example, when issues of *Clinical and Experimental Dermatology* from 1976 to 1997 were hand-searched, 96 clinical trials were identified; Medline listed only 47.[8]
• By helping people with skin diseases to make informed decisions. For example, the review on "local treatments for cutaneous warts" found that simple topical treatments containing salicylic acid appear to be both effective and safe. There was no clear evidence that any other treatments have higher cure rates and/or fewer adverse effects.[9]
• By providing evidence on which to base clinical decisions. A recent review examined all 26 systematic reviews relevant to dermatology in the CDSR and found sufficient evidence for recommending treatments in at least half of them.[10] Even when evidence is lacking, Cochrane reviews identify gaps in knowledge and frame the future research agenda. For example, the review on "Drugs for discoid lupus erythematosus" highlighted the need for RCTs comparing potent topical steroids and chloroquine/hydroxy-chloroquine.[11]

Editorial process

Each review is prepared in a defined manner to ensure consistency and high quality, using the Collaboration's own free software. First, the authors submit a protocol that includes a background section, search strategy, and the methods for study selection, data extraction, and analysis. When the protocol is complete, it is peer-reviewed by an editor, an external content expert, the statistical and methods editors, and a consumer. Necessary revisions must be made and accepted by the editors before the protocol is published in the Cochrane Library.

A review takes on average 2 years to complete. The required papers and other information have to be gathered, and two independent coauthors decide which papers meet the inclusion criteria. The scientific quality of these papers is assessed, the data are extracted and analyzed, with a meta-analysis if appropriate, and conclusions are drawn. The completed review is then submitted and is again peer-reviewed and revised as necessary. Authors are expected to update their reviews at least every 2 years.

The role of consumers

The CSG has always involved people with skin diseases, their families and carers (consumers).[12] Skin disease greatly affects people's quality of life, but much of the trial work in

skin disease has addressed questions that are important to pharmaceutical companies. Consumers help us to redress that imbalance. In late 2007, the CSG had 123 teams of authors working on topics, both common and rare, such as acne, alopecia, bullous pemphigoid, eczema, excessive sweating, psoriasis and skin cancer. About 100 active consumers are involved at many levels. Initially, they came mainly through the National Eczema Society and the Vitiligo Society, but since we now always include a relevant consumer in the peer-review process, and often as a coauthor, many others have joined the CSG. A review on vitiligo led by a consumer author has recently been published.

Our experience of consumer involvement is both positive and challenging. Consumers have little or no access to the support systems and infrastructure that professionals take for granted (e.g., information technology, administration, photocopying, etc.). They have to meet many expenses themselves, from travel to telephone bills, and often funding is a major problem. However, their enthusiasm is boundless and infectious. Our consumers are highly motivated, and several of them have won stipends to attend Cochrane colloquia. Many also attend local meetings of the Collaboration and the annual meeting of the CSG. In particular, consumers help us to ensure that our reviews are relevant to people with skin diseases and written in language accessible to intelligent lay people.

Two comments from Skin Group consumers

"The strong consumer involvement in the Skin Group is well known within the Cochrane Collaboration. Many groups don't have a consumer on each review team as we do. As a consumer, the inspiring aspects of working with the CSG are:
• Working with clinicians and researchers who are dedicated to finding the evidence to help people with skin conditions.
• Seeing quality-of-life issues being taken seriously.
• Having my views and suggestions accepted.
• Being able to meet consumers and researchers from around the world at national and international meetings.
I have been involved in training other consumers and have given talks about our work to patients, medical students, and postgraduates. But outside the Collaboration, the idea that consumers can contribute significantly to systematic reviews is still seen as unusual. Why? We're the ones with the condition! We know what matters to us about it and what questions we want answered. There is still a long way to go . . ."

"Being the lead author of a Cochrane systematic review of interventions for vitiligo has been one of the most amazing experiences of my life, driving me to the depths of despair and frustration, but also bringing a great sense of achievement. It has also brought invitations to speak about the review at meetings and to join the British Association of Dermatologists Guidelines Committee for vitiligo, which accepted a poster presentation of the review for its annual meeting. I have had vitiligo for more than 50 years, and I decided to write the review from a growing awareness of the need to highlight the lack of good, effective treatment for vitiligo. Having retired early from my job as an academic librarian at a university, I had no easy access to basic resources. I lacked experience of scientific writing, and the lack of support during parts of the process also caused problems. On the plus side, I now realize the importance of good, unbiased evidence and the value of a supportive collaboration with coauthors. Writing the review has given me confidence. It has certainly been worth it."

Trials register

The CSG maintains the Skin Group Specialized Register, a comprehensive international register of reports of controlled trials in dermatology. It contains reports of both RCTs and controlled clinical trials (CCTs) and is a valuable resource for those preparing systematic reviews on dermatology topics.

The Specialized Register is submitted to the Cochrane Library every quarter for incorporation into the Cochrane Central Register of Controlled Trials (Central), which is the world's single most important source of reports of RCTs.

The search for trials

Each report is included in the Register only after its trial status has been checked in the full publication. Several criteria must be met:
• A trial must be planned in advance and be a comparison of two or more interventions (where one may be a placebo).
• A trial must involve a single original population of human beings, or groups of human beings, or parts of their body.
If the allocation of the interventions to the single population is randomized and explicitly stated to be so, this is classified as an RCT. However, many reports are of trials using quasi-randomization, or trials in which double-blinding was used but randomization was not mentioned. These reports are classified as CCTs. The quality of the random allocation varies greatly even among RCTs, so inevitably many CCTs turn out to be unreliable sources of evidence.

Each review group develops its own search strategies related to its medical scope to find reports of trials relevant to its discipline. These may be electronic searches of databases, web-based searches, hand-searching, searches of conference proceedings, searches of the "gray literature," searches for ongoing trials, etc. In addition to the contributions from the review groups, the Collaboration has developed sensitive search strategies for finding reports of clinical trials in all medical disciplines. These are used to search Medline and Embase in order to filter out the clinical trials from all the many other types of studies present in these databases. The results of these searches and those applied to other databases are downloaded into Central.

Hand-searching

The Cochrane Collaboration aims to identify reports of trials back to 1948. If an article was not written with a clear indication in the title or abstract that it describes a clinical trial, or if the journal has not been entered into an electronic database, then electronic searching will miss reports of these trials.[13]

The Collaboration is engaged in a one-off systematic trawl of the medical literature worldwide for reports of trials not found by electronic searches. This exercise is known as hand-searching, as it refers to the task of physically turning each page of a journal looking for indications that the article is about a trial, which may sometimes only be found in the methods sections of papers or in the correspondence pages.

To prevent duplication of the considerable effort involved in hand-searching, the Collaboration holds a master list of the journals that are being searched. The need for hand-searching, particularly of English-language journals, is diminishing as the searching of older journals is completed.

Many of the over 200 international dermatology publications (see www.csg.cochrane.org/Handsearch/dermjnls01.htm for a list of those identified so far) are not on electronic databases. Currently, 35 dermatology journals have been hand-searched by the Skin Group for all or part of their years of publication. The Skin Group also hand-searches the meeting abstracts from dermatology conferences. The hand-searching progress of the Cochrane Skin Group can be viewed on the Internet by going to: The Cochrane Library > About > Skin Group > Specialized Register.

Ongoing trials

The hand-searching exercise only finds trials that have already been completed. To make it easier to find out what research is already being done, the International Committee of Medical Journal editors (ICMJE) issued a statement[14] that all ongoing trials would have to register a minimum data set, in a public trials registry, to be considered for publication. The World Health Organization (WHO) supports this initiative. The CSG invites dermatology trialists to lodge the (minimal) details of their clinical trial, with their proposed outcome measures, on its Ongoing Skin Trials Register (www.nottingham.ac.uk/ongoingskintrials). This then provides a source of trial information for a review author.

Other web-based clinical trial registries that contain ongoing dermatology trials are:

- The *meta*Register of Current Controlled Trials, an international searchable database (http://www.controlled-trials.com/mrct/).
- ClinicalTrials.gov, a service of the U.S. National Institutes of Health (www.clinicaltrials.gov).
- The Australian Clinical trials Registry (www.actr.org.au/).
- The World Health Organisation Search Portal (www.who.int/trialsearch/).

The future

The need for hand-searching will diminish over the years as searching of older journals is completed. Also, journal editors are adopting the CONSORT guidelines (*Con*solidated *S*tandards *of R*eporting *T*rials),[15] which will improve the standard of reporting of trials in publications and make it much easier to find trials electronically with simple search terms.

Other sources also need to be examined for valuable information about trials that have been performed. This gray literature includes Ph.D. and M.D. theses, pharmaceutical company records, conference proceedings, etc. It is known that trials with statistically significant results tend to be published before those with less clear results,[16] so that authors of reviews need to examine unpublished data that may contain valuable negative information about an intervention.

The Specialized Skin Register is now a database of trial reports. But many trials, especially multicenter studies, result in several publications from the same trial. We aim to gather together these reports to make the Register study-based rather than report-based.

The Cochrane Collaboration is international, but it is still dominated by English-language publications, which may introduce their own bias.[17] As more studies in other languages are found and are incorporated into systematic reviews, all will gain a broader and more balanced view about the value of interventions.

Lessons learnt

As the group has grown and more reviews are being written, we have had to reduce the amount of one-to-one support that we can offer authors, so we can no longer support a team consisting entirely of inexperienced authors. We ask about a potential review team's experience and expertise, and encourage each team to include a statistician or methodologist, and a consumer.

We are keen to help authors in developing countries and offer to find a native English speaker to join their team if this is likely to help. We facilitate the inclusion of isolated authors in teams and do our best to ensure that inexperienced authors work with more experienced ones. Often the Skin Group way of working is a novel experience for authors from other countries, especially the experience of working with a consumer coauthor. We have found that authors from developing countries are very excited by the opportunity to collaborate with people from across the globe and that the experience is described as being "useful for preparing other reviews and treatment guidelines, and the network we develop fosters our professional growth."

We have been able to improve the quality of the submitted protocols by providing a model protocol, which is updated as we learn from problems encountered in earlier reviews. For example, we now insist on much clearer definition of the outcomes, as this simplifies both data extraction and analysis. We always try to find ways to improve rather than reject reviews, and the editorial base can provide a mentor if asked.

We provide support at various stages of writing the review. We have a guide for lead authors writing a protocol, another guide for the review stage, and a third guide for coauthors. The guides include information on the editorial process and methodologies. Authors are also encouraged to attend training courses run by their local Cochrane center.

Although we tend to favor combining all interventions for a particular skin condition together into one review, some complex reviews are easier for readers if split into smaller reviews. Recently, we have suggested that our consumer peer referees work in pairs or small groups. This has much improved consumer comments.

The core functions of the editorial base are funded by the UK National Health Service Research and Development Programme. Additional funding for administrative support would improve the speed and capacity of our group in managing our essential processes. To this end, we are working with a group of American colleagues led by Dr. Bob Dellavalle to try and develop a satellite in the United States for the Skin Group in the United States. This satellite would encourage and supporting more high-quality reviews from North American authors.

Contacting the CSG

If you would like to help the CSG in any way, more information about the CSG and the Cochrane Collaboration, including contact details, can be found on our web site.

Useful web sites

- Cochrane Skin Group: http://www.csg.cochrane.org
- Ongoing Skin Trials Register: www.nottingham.ac.uk/ongoingskintrials

- Cochrane centers: http://www.cochrane.org/contact/entities.htm
- Cochrane Library: http://www.thecochranelibrary.org
- Author's handbook: http://www.cochrane.org/resources/handbook/
- Cochrane Consumer Network: http://www.cochrane.org/consumers/homepage.htm

References

1 Cochrane AL. *Effectiveness and Efficiency: Random Reflections on Health Services*. London: Nuffield Provincial Hospitals Trust, 1972. (Reprinted in 1989 in association with the BMJ.)

2 Cochrane AL. 1931–1971: a critical review, with particular reference to the medical profession. In: *Medicines for the Year 2000*. London: Office of Health Economics, 1979: 1–11.

3 Cochrane AL. Foreword. In: Chalmers I, Enkin M, Keirse MJNC, eds. *Effective Care in Pregnancy and Childbirth*. Oxford: Oxford University Press, 1989.

4 Chalmers I, Dickersin K, Chalmers TC. Getting to grips with Archie Cochrane's agenda. *BMJ* 1992;**305**:786–8.

5 Editorial. Cochrane's legacy. *Lancet* 1992;**340**:1131–2.

6 Chalmers I. The Cochrane collaboration: preparing, maintaining, and disseminating systematic reviews of the effects of health care. *Ann N Y Acad Sci* 1993;**703**:156–63.

7 Collier A, Johnson KR, Delamere F, *et al.* The Cochrane Skin Group: promoting the best evidence. *J Cutan Med Surg* 2005;**9**:324–31.

8 Delamere FM, Williams HC. How can hand searching the dermatological literature help people with skin problems? *Arch Dermatol* 2001;**137**:332–5.

9 Gibbs S, Harvey I, Sterling JC, Stark R. Local treatments for cutaneous warts. *Cochrane Database Syst Rev* 2003;(3):CD001781. [Update in: *Cochrane Database Syst Rev* 2006;**3**:CD001781.]

10 Parker ER, Schilling LM, Diba V, Williams HC, Dellavalle RP. What is the point of databases of reviews for dermatology if all they compile is "insufficient evidence"? *J Am Acad Dermatol* 2004;**50**:635–9.

11 Jessop S, Whitelaw D, Jordaan F. Drugs for discoid lupus erythematosus. *Cochrane Database Syst Rev* 2001;(1):CD002954.

12 Collier A, Johnson K, Heilig L, Leonard T, Williams H, Dellavalle RP. A win–win proposition: fostering US health care consumer involvement in the Cochrane Collaboration Skin Group. *J Am Acad Dermatol* 2005;**53**: 920–1.

13 Adetugbo K, Williams H. How well are randomized controlled trials reported in the dermatology literature? *Arch Dermatol* 2000;**136**:381–5.

14 De Angelis C, Drazen JM, Frizelle FA, *et al.* Clinical trial registration: a statement from the International Committee of Medical Journal Editors. *Ann Intern Med* 2004;**141**:477–8.

15 Moher D, Schulz KF, Altman DG, *et al.* The CONSORT statement: revised recommendations for improving the quality of reports of parallel-group randomized trials. *Ann Intern Med* 2001;**134**: 657–62.

16 Clarke M, Hopewell S. Time lag bias in publishing results of clinical trials: a systematic review. [Paper presented at the 3rd Symposium on Systematic Reviews: Beyond the Basics, Oxford: Centre for Statistics in Medicine, 2000.]

17 Sterne JAC, Bartlett C, Juni P, Egger M. Do we need comprehensive literature searches? A study of publication and language bias in meta-analyses of controlled trials. [Paper presented at the 3rd Symposium on Systematic Reviews: Beyond the Basics, Oxford: Centre for Statistics in Medicine, 2000.]

The critical appraisal toolbox

Michael Bigby, Editor

5 Formulating well-built clinical questions

Berthold Rzany, Michael Bigby

Practicing evidence-based medicine (EBM) centers on trying to find answers to clinically relevant questions that arise in caring for individual patients. Asking well-built clinical questions may be the most important step in practicing EBM.

Structuring well-built clinical questions

A well-built clinical question has four elements: a patient or problem; an intervention; a comparison intervention (if necessary); and an outcome.[1–3] Well-built clinical questions about individual patients can be grouped into several categories: etiology, diagnosis, therapy, prevention, prognosis, and harm.

The first component of a well-built clinical question is an accurate description of the patient or problem. The next two components are accurate descriptions of the intervention or interventions. Interventions can be etiologic factors, diagnostic tests, treatments, prognostic factors, or harmful exposures. Several interventions (e.g., many treatments for psoriasis) might be appropriate for inclusion in the question. When the focus is on treatment, the comparative intervention may be an established treatment, another treatment, or a placebo. The final component of the well-built clinical question is a clinically relevant outcome measure that is important to the patient and treating dermatologist. One easy way of remembering these key components is the acronym PICO: *p*atient, *i*ntervention, *c*omparator, and *o*utcome.

For example, a 71-year-old man presents with a painful cluster of vesicles on an erythematous base on his cheek. You suspect he has herpes zoster, although herpes simplex is in your differential diagnosis. Examples of well-built clinical questions about diagnosis, therapy, and prognosis would be:

1 In an elderly man presenting with a vesicular eruption, is a viral culture or direct fluorescence antibody (DFA) slide test more useful in establishing a diagnosis of herpes zoster?

2 In an elderly man with acutely painful herpes zoster, would treatment with antivirals, or antivirals and corticosteroids, lead to more rapid resolution of pain and more rapid return to a normal quality of life?

3 If an elderly man who presents with acutely painful herpes zoster is treated with antivirals and corticosteroids or is left untreated, how likely is he to develop postherpetic neuralgia? Examples of poorly structured questions about this same patient would be:

4 How do you make a diagnosis of herpes zoster?

5 What is the best treatment for herpes zoster?

6 What is the prognosis of herpes zoster?

In most clinical situations, several well-built clinical questions are possible using the PICO structure (Table 5.1). It is up to the physician and the patient to determine what are the most important questions.

The advantages of well-built clinical questions

A well-formed clinical question has two strong advantages. A major benefit of careful and thoughtful question-forming is that it makes the search for evidence—and the critical appraisal of the evidence found—easier. The well-formed question makes it relatively straightforward to elicit and combine the appropriate terms needed to represent your need for information in the query language of whichever database search service you choose (e.g., Medline, Embase, or the Cochrane Library). Having to formulate well-built clinical questions will also train you to clearly define your patient, be specific about the interventions used, and choose carefully described and precise desired outcomes.

Questions like questions 4, 5, and 6 above will certainly lead to answers. However, obtaining the answer would require a considerable amount of time searching and validating a vast amount of literature. Structuring the question as in questions 1, 2, and 3 above would lead to more specific answers in considerably less time.

Table 5.1 The four elements of a well-built clinical question using the PICO (patient, intervention, comparator, and outcome) structure

Element	Patient or problem	Intervention	Comparison intervention (if necessary)	Clinically relevant outcome(s)
Description	Description of the patient based on demographic factors, past history, and clinical presentation	Interventions can be etiologic factors, diagnostic tests, treatments, prognostic factors, or harmful exposures	Interventions can be etiologic factors, diagnostic tests, treatments, prognostic factors, or harmful exposures	Clinically relevant outcome measure that is important to the patient
Example 1 (diagnostic procedure)	In an elderly man presenting with a vesicular eruption,	. . . is viral culture . . .	. . . or a direct fluorescence antibody (DFA) slide test . . .	. . . more useful in establishing a diagnosis of herpes zoster?
Example 2 (therapeutic intervention)	In an elderly man with acutely painful herpes zoster,	. . . would treatment with antivirals . . .	. . . or antivirals and corticosteroids . . .	. . . lead to more rapid resolution of pain and more rapid return to a normal quality of life?
Example 3 (prognosis)	If an elderly man with acutely painful herpes zoster . . .	. . . is treated with antivirals and corticosteroids . . .	. . . or is left untreated,	. . . how likely is he to develop post-herpetic neuralgia?

For example, consider the difference between searching Medline for questions 2 and 5 above. Searching Medline to answer question 5 using the search string "herpes zoster and treatment" yields 5467 references, many of which are narrative review articles, bench research, and case reports. Even limiting the search to randomized controlled clinical trials yields 246 references, many of which have poor-quality evidence. In contrast, searching Medline to answer question 2 using the search string "herpes zoster and (corticosteroid* or pred*) and (acyclovir or valacyclovir or famciclovir)" yields 52 references. Limiting the search to randomized controlled clinical trials yields one reference, which is a randomized controlled trial of the treatment of acute herpes zoster with acyclovir alone for 7 or 21 days and acyclovir plus prednisolone for 7 or 21 days.[4]

What factors are important in generating well-built questions in a dermatology consultation? The patient's characteristics—such as age, sex, past therapy, general health, or allergies—are important. A well-built and relevant question can only be generated if there has been an accurate initial evaluation of the patient, which includes a detailed history and examination to establish an accurate diagnosis. Understanding which factors are important to the patient (e.g., efficacy of treatment, difficulty of treatment regimen, potential side effects, or affordability) is also crucial. Specifying an outcome that is meaningful to the patient is also important. For example, consider a 28-year-old man with psoriasis who is desperate for a remission of the visible plaques on his body, as he was planning to go for a once-in-a-lifetime holiday to the coast, where he wanted to expose his skin at the beach. Finding trials that only mention a 50% reduction in Psoriasis Area and Severity Index (PASI) scores as their sole outcome measure would be of little value. What would be of most interest to this man are those trials that specify the percentage of patients achieving complete or nearly complete clearing after a course of therapy.

Asking a clinically relevant well-built question is not as easy as it might appear. It takes practice and is a learnable skill. Ultimately it saves time, and it is more likely to provide useful answers in caring for individual patients. Formulating well-built clinical questions is essential for the next steps in practicing evidence-based dermatology.

References

1 Sackett DL, Richardson WS, Rosenberg Q, Haynes RB. *Evidence-Based Medicine: How to Practice and Teach EBM.* London: Churchill Livingstone, 1997.

2 Bigby M. Evidence-based medicine in dermatology. *Dermatol Clin* 2000;**18**:261–76.

3 Richardson WS, Wilson MC, Nishikawa J, Hayward RS. The well-built clinical question: a key to evidence-based decisions. *ACP J Club* 1995;**123**:A12–3.

4 Wood MJ, Johnson RW, McKendrick MW, Taylor J, Mandal BK, Crooks J. A randomized trial of acyclovir for 7 days or 21 days with and without prednisolone for treatment of acute herpes zoster. *N Engl J Med* 1994;**330**:896–900.

6 Finding the best evidence

Michael Bigby, Rosamaria Corona

The ability to find the best evidence to answer clinical questions is crucial for practicing evidence-based medicine. Finding evidence requires access to electronic searching, searching skills, and available resources. Methods for finding systematic reviews and evidence about etiology (harm), diagnosis, therapy, prognosis, and clinical prediction guides have been well developed.[1,2]

Evidence about therapy is the easiest to find. The best sources for finding the best evidence about treatment include:

- The Cochrane Library
- Searching the Medline and Embase databases
- Primary journals
- Secondary journals
- Evidence-based dermatology and evidence-based medicine books (e.g., Clinical Evidence)
- The National Guideline Clearinghouse (http://www.jcaai.org)
- The National Institute for Health and Clinical Excellence (NICE) (www.nice.org.uk)

The Cochrane Library

The Cochrane Library contains the Cochrane Database of Systematic Reviews of the Treatment of Diseases, the Database of Abstracts of Reviews of Effectiveness (DARE), the Cochrane Central Register of Controlled Trials (Central), and the Health Technology Assessment (HTA) database. Volunteers, according to strict guidelines developed by the Cochrane Collaboration, write the systematic reviews in the Cochrane Library. The last issue of the Cochrane Library (2007, issue 1, accessed January 25th, 2007) contained 4655 completed systematic reviews. The number of reviews of dermatological topics is steadily increasing.

Central is a database of over 489 000 controlled clinical trials. It is compiled by searching the Medline and Embase databases and hand-searching many journals. Hand-searching journals to identify controlled clinical trials and randomized controlled clinical trials was undertaken because members of the Cochrane Collaboration noticed that many trials were incorrectly classified in the Medline database. As an example, Dr. Finola Delamere of the Cochrane Skin Group hand-searched *Archives of Dermatology* from 1990 through 1998 and identified 99 controlled clinical trials. Nineteen of the trials were not classified as controlled clinical trials in Medline, and 11 trials that were not controlled clinical trials were misclassified as controlled clinical trials in Medline.[3]

DARE is a database of abstracts of systematic reviews published in the medical literature. It contained abstracts and bibliographic details on 5931 published systematic reviews. DARE is the only database to contain abstracts of systematic reviews that have been quality-assessed. Each abstract includes a summary of the review, together with a critical commentary about the overall quality.

HTA consists of completed and ongoing health technology assessments (studies of the medical, social, ethical, and economic implications of health-care interventions) from around the world. The aim of the database is to improve the quality and cost-effectiveness of health care.

The Cochrane Library is the best source for evidence about treatment. It can be easily searched using simple Boolean combinations of search terms and by more sophisticated search strategies. The Cochrane Database of Systematic Reviews, DARE, Central, and HTA can be searched simultaneously. The Cochrane Library is available on a personal or institutional subscription basis on CD, and on the Internet from Wiley InterScience (http://www3.interscience.wiley.com/cgi-bin/mrwhome/106568753/home). Subscriptions to the Cochrane library are updated quarterly. The Cochrane Library is offered free of charge in many countries by national provision and by many medical schools in the United States. It should be available at any medical library.

Medline and Embase databases and how to perform efficient searches

The second-best method for finding evidence about treatment, and the best source for finding most other types of best evidence in dermatology, is by searching the Medline database by computer.[2,4] Medline is the bibliographic database of the National Library of Medicine (NLM), covering the fields of medicine, nursing, dentistry, veterinary medicine, the health-care system, and the preclinical sciences. The Medline file contains bibliographic citations and author abstracts from approximately 5000 current biomedical journals published in the United States and 80 other countries. The file contains approximately 15 million records, dating back to the mid-1950s.[5]

Medline searches have inherent limitations that make their reliability less than ideal.[2] For example, Spuls *et al.* conducted a systematic review of systemic treatments for psoriasis.[6] The treatments analyzed included ultraviolet B, psoralen ultraviolet A (PUVA), methotrexate, cyclosporin A, and retinoids. The authors used an exhaustive strategy to find relevant references, including Medline searches, contacting pharmaceutical companies, polling leading authorities, reviewing abstract books of symposia and congresses, and reviewing textbooks, reviews, editorials, guideline articles, and the reference lists of all papers identified. Of 665 studies found, 356 (54%) were identified by Medline search (range 30–70% for different treatment modalities). Of 23 authorities contacted, the 17 who responded provided no references beyond those identified by Medline searching.

The key to Medline searching is to find relevant articles and to exclude irrelevant citations. Several useful techniques can greatly aid in the ability to accomplish this goal. Searches are generally done on the basis of Boolean combinations of search terms. For example, a search for best evidence about drug treatment of onychomycosis might read: "[onychomycosis and (terbinafine or itraconazole or fluconazole) not case reports]." (The convention used throughout for search entries is that Boolean operations within parentheses are executed first.) This search would identify articles on onychomycosis using any of the listed drugs and excluding case reports.[1,2]

It is important to understand the difference between text word and Medical Subject Headings (MeSH) searching and to be able to do both. Many of the programs used to search the Medline database automatically do text word and MeSH searches. MeSH terms include all of the terms in *Medical Subject Headings,* a controlled vocabulary of keywords used to index Medline. Each Medline citation is given a group of MeSH terms that relate to the subject of the paper from which it is drawn. Frequently, MeSH terms will have an additional subheading, which further defines how the MeSH term relates to the article with which it is associated. This subheading is appended to the MeSH term —e.g., "onychomycosis diagnosis."

Indexing articles is not an exact science. The MeSH headings assigned by the NLM may not coincide with the intent of the author or the majority of searchers, for several reasons. Authors may not clearly express their intent, indexers are usually not experts in the field of the article they are indexing, and the mistakes associated with doing repetitive tasks occur.[2] Relevant articles may be missed when they are not assigned the appropriate MeSH heading. Irrelevant articles may be included in a MeSH search if they are assigned to the wrong MeSH heading. For example, the Cochrane Collaboration identified major problems in the Medline indexing of randomized controlled trials.[2]

Text word searches allow one to search articles for words within the title and abstract that are important to and coincide with the intent of the author. However, text word searches are subject to several problems. Authors may not describe their methods or objectives well, or may make errors in spelling and errors of omission or commission.[2] The problem of misspelling can be illustrated by doing a text word search for "pruritis" (pruritus spelled incorrectly). This search will yield over 40 references in which the word has been misspelled. Many of these references may not be detected in a search for pruritus (spelled correctly).[2]

Boolean topic searches will often contain too many references or too few. They may contain many irrelevant citations and miss many relevant citations. Several techniques will help make searches more sensitive (i.e., pick up relevant citations) and more specific (i.e., exclude irrelevant citations).[2] To increase the sensitivity of searches, searching both text word and MeSH headings, exploding MeSH headings, and using truncation may be helpful. MeSH term searches can be "exploded" to include all terms that are logical subsets of the term entered.[2] For example, exploding the MeSH term "onychomycosis" will retrieve all of the articles that use that MeSH term, whether they have subheadings or not. Many of the programs used to search the Medline database automatically explode searches of MeSH terms or MeSH major topics.

Truncation refers to searching using the root of a word to allow variants of the word to be detected. For example, a search of "onychomycosis" and "controlled clinical trial" will detect fewer studies than a search for "onychomycosis and control*" (where "control*" contains a wild card that will allow detection of all words that begin with the root "control"). Truncation can be performed on text word and MeSH heading searches.

To increase the specificity of searches, selecting specific subheadings of MeSH terms and limiting the search may be helpful. MeSH heading terms can be limited to specific subheadings, to help narrow search results to relevant articles. For example, "onychomycosis" has subheadings that restrict retrieved articles to ones dealing with diagnosis or drug treatment.[2] Searches can be limited in many ways, including publication type, language, human subjects, and date of publication. Restricting the publication type to randomized controlled trials or case–control studies is useful for limiting retrieved articles to those of the highest quality.

Performing a sensitive or specific search from scratch is often a time-consuming task. Arriving at an efficient search strategy to suit one's particular needs is sometimes a work of art. Once accomplished, it is important to be able to edit, save, and retrieve the search strategy. The saved strategy can then be used in future searches of different subjects without having to rethink or retype the whole search procedure. The methods for performing these techniques (text word and MeSH searching, exploding, truncation, using subheadings, limiting and saving) vary depending on the platform used. Mastering them will greatly improve searching efficiency.

Specific search strategies known as "filters" have been developed to help find relevant references and exclude irrelevant references for best evidence about etiology, diagnosis, therapy, prognosis, and clinical prediction guides, and for finding systematic reviews (http://www.ncbi.nlm. nih.gov/entrez/query/static/clinicaltable.html).[7,8] Each type of search can be made narrow (specific) or broad (sensitive). These filters have been incorporated into the PubMed Clinical Queries search engine at the National Library of Medicine and are available at http://www.ncbi.nlm.nih. gov/entrez/query/static/clinical.shtml.[5] PubMed Clinical Queries is the preferred method for searching the Medline database for the best, clinically relevant evidence. It can be freely used by anyone with Internet access.

Embase is Excerpta Medica's database covering drugs, pharmacology, and biomedical specialties.[9] Embase has better coverage of European and non–English-language sources and may be more up to date.[9] The overlap in journals covered by Medline and Embase is about 34% (range 10–75%, depending on the subject).[2] Embase contains over 11 million records from 1974 to the present. Embase is available online (http://www.embase.com/). Personal and institutional subscriptions are available. Embase.com performs simultaneous searches of Embase and Medline databases and eliminates duplicate records. The filters that are incorporated into the PubMed Clinical Queries search engine can be used to perform clinically relevant searches of Embase, with some modification.[2,7,8]

Secondary publications and other resources

Structured abstracts of articles are published in secondary journals (e.g., the section on evidence-based dermatology published quarterly in *Archives of Dermatology*). The articles are strictly selected on the basis of methodological quality and are accompanied by commentary putting the information

into clinical perspective. Clinical Evidence is a compendium of evidence on the effects of common clinical interventions, updated every 6 months. Twenty-three skin-related diseases were included in the latest issue (Issue 15, June 2006). It is available through the American College of physicians and the British Medical Association (http://clinicalevidence. org/ceweb/index.jsp).

Full-text versions of many primary journals are now available on the Internet. Available vendors include Ovid Online (http://www.ovid.com/site/index.jsp), ScienceDirect (http://www.sciencedirect.com/), and STN (http://www. cas.org/stn.html), among others.

The National Guideline Clearinghouse maintains a database of guidelines for the treatment of diseases, written by panels of experts following strict guidelines of evidence. The database is accessible through the Internet (http:// www.guideline.gov/index.asp). The current coverage of dermatological topics is limited.

The National Institute for Clinical Excellence (NICE) produces guidance on public health, health technologies, and clinical practice based on the best available evidence. It is accessible online at www.nice.org.uk, and includes guidance for treating atopic eczema, a final appraisal determination on the use of calcineurin inhibitor for atopic dermatitis, the use of biologics for psoriasis, and a full set of guidelines for skin cancer, including melanoma.

References

1 Bigby M, Szklo M. Evidence-based dermatology. In: Freedberg IM, Eisen AZ, Wolff K, Austen KF, Goldsmith LA, Katz SI, eds. *Fitzpatrick's Dermatology in General Medicine*, 6th ed. New York: McGraw-Hill, 2003: 2301–11.

2 Bigby M. Evidence-based medicine in a nutshell: a guide to finding and using the best evidence in caring for patients. *Arch Dermatol* 1998;**134**:1609–18.

3 Delamere FM, Williams HC. How can hand searching the dermatological literature benefit people with skin problems? *Arch Dermatol* 2001;**137**:332–5.

4 Oxman AD, Sackett DL, Guyatt GH. Users' guides to the medical literature. I. How to get started. The Evidence-Based Medicine Working Group. *JAMA* 1993;**270**:2093–5.

5 http://www.ncbi.nlm.nih.gov/entrez/query/static/overview. html. Last update December 6, 2006 (accessed January 25, 2007).

6 Spuls PI, Witkamp L, Bossuyt PM, Bos JD. A systematic review of five systemic treatments for severe psoriasis. *Br J Dermatol* 1997;**137**:943–9.

7 Haynes RB, Wilczynski N, McKibbon KA, Walker CJ, Sinclair JC. Developing optimal search strategies for detecting clinically sound studies in MEDLINE. *J Am Med Inform Assoc* 1994;**1**:447–58.

8 Haynes B. PubMed clinical queries using research methodology filters. http://www.nlm.nih.gov/pubs/techbull/jf04/cq_info.html. Last update January 2005 (accessed January 25, 2007).

9 Greenhalgh T. *How to Read a Paper: the Basics of Evidence Based Medicine*. London: BMJ, 1997.

7 The hierarchy of evidence

Michael Bigby

Once appropriate questions have been formulated, what are the sources for the best evidence to answer these questions? Potential sources include personal experience, colleagues or experts, textbooks, and articles published in journals. An important principle of evidence-based medicine (EBM) is that the quality (strength) of evidence is based on the concept of a *hierarchy of evidence*. The hierarchy of evidence consists of the results of one or more well-designed studies, the results of large case series, expert opinion, case reports, and personal experience, in descending order.[1,2] Systematic reviews are scientific summaries of the quality, direction, magnitude, and precision of the evidence, but they should not be considered as evidence *per se* in the hierarchy of evidence (Figure 7.1). The ordering of the hierarchy of evidence has been widely discussed, actively debated and sometimes hotly contested.[3–7]

Well-conducted systematic reviews of well-performed clinical studies (especially if the studies have results of similar magnitude and direction, and if there is statistical homogeneity) are most likely to have results that are true and useful. A systematic review is an overview that answers a specific clinical question, contains a thorough, unbiased search of the relevant literature, explicit criteria for assessing studies, and a structured presentation of the results. A systematic review that uses quantitative methods to summarize results is a meta-analysis.[3,8] Meta-analysis is credited with allowing recognition of important treatment effects by combining the results of small trials that individually lacked the power to demonstrate differences among treatments. For example, the benefits of intravenous streptokinase in acute myocardial infarction were recognized by the results of a cumulative meta-analysis of smaller trials

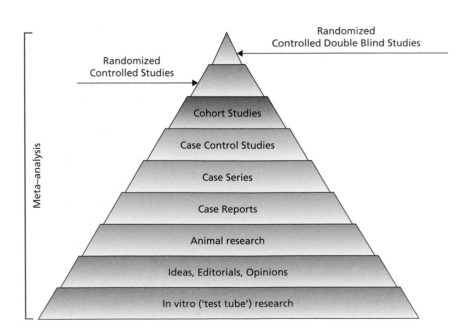

Figure 7.1 The evidence pyramid (reproduced with permission from SUNY Downstate Medical Center, Medical Research Library of Brooklyn Guide to Research Methods. The Evidence Pyramid. SUNY Health Sciences, Evidence Based Medicine Course http://servers. medlib.hscbklyn.edu/ebm/2100.htm

at least a decade before it was recommended by experts and before it was demonstrated to be efficacious in large clinical trials.[3,4] Meta-analysis has been criticized for the discrepancies between the results of meta-analysis and from the results of large clinical trials.[3,5–7] For example, the results of a meta-analysis of 14 small studies of calcium to treat preeclampsia showed that treatment was beneficial, whereas a large trial failed to show a treatment effect.[3] The frequency of discrepancies ranges from 10% to 23%.[3] Discrepancies can often be explained by differences in treatment protocols, heterogeneity of study populations, or changes that occur over time.[3] Not all systematic reviews and meta-analyses are equal. Systematic reviews conducted within the Cochrane Collaboration are rated among the best, but even then, up to a third may contain significant problems.[9,10] Methods for assessing the quality of each type of analysis are available.[2,11]

The type of clinical study that constitutes best evidence is determined by the category of the question being asked (Table 7.1).[12] Questions about diagnosis are best addressed

Table 7.1 Oxford Centre for Evidence-based Medicine levels of evidence (May 2001)

Level	Therapy/prevention, etiology/harm	Prognosis	Diagnosis
1a	SR (with homogeneity*) of RCTs	SR (with homogeneity*) of inception cohort studies; CDR† validated in different populations	SR (with homogeneity*) of level 1 diagnostic studies; CDR† with 1b studies from different clinical centers
1b	Individual RCT (with narrow confidence interval‡)	Individual inception cohort study with ≥ 80% follow-up; CDR† validated in a single population	Validating** cohort study with good††† reference standards; or CDR† tested within one clinical center
1c	All or none§	All or none case series	Absolute SpPins and SnNouts††
2a	SR (with homogeneity*) of cohort studies	SR (with homogeneity*) of either retrospective cohort studies or untreated control groups in RCTs	SR (with homogeneity*) of level > 2 diagnostic studies
2b	Individual cohort study (including low-quality RCT; e.g., < 80% follow-up)	Retrospective cohort study or follow-up of untreated control patients in an RCT; derivation of CDR† or validated on split sample§§§ only	Exploratory** cohort study with good††† reference standards; CDR† after derivation, or validated only on split sample§§§ or databases
2c	"Outcomes" research; ecological studies	"Outcomes" research	
3a	SR (with homogeneity*) of case–control studies		SR (with homogeneity*) of level 3b and better studies
3b	Individual case–control study		Nonconsecutive study; or without consistently applied reference standards
4	Case series (and poor-quality cohort and case–control studies§§)	Case series (and poor-quality prognostic cohort studies***)	Case–control study, poor or nonindependent reference standard
5	Expert opinion without explicit critical appraisal, or based on physiology, bench research, or "first principles"	Expert opinion without explicit critical appraisal, or based on physiology, bench research, or "first principles"	Expert opinion without explicit critical appraisal, or based on physiology, bench research, or "first principles"

Produced by Bob Phillips, Chris Ball, Dave Sackett, Doug Badenoch, Sharon Straus, Brian Haynes, Martin Dawes since November 1998.

Users can add a minus-sign ("−") to denote the level of that fails to provide a conclusive answer because of *either* a single result with a wide confidence interval (such that, for example, an ARR in an RCT is not statistically significant but whose confidence intervals fail to exclude clinically important benefit or harm); *or* a systematic review with troublesome (and statistically significant) heterogeneity. Such evidence is inconclusive, and therefore can only generate grade D recommendations.

* By homogeneity, we mean a systematic review that is free of worrisome variations (heterogeneity) in the directions and degrees of results between individual studies. Not all systematic reviews with statistically significant heterogeneity need be worrisome, and not all worrisome heterogeneity need be statistically significant. As noted above, studies displaying worrisome heterogeneity should be tagged with a "−" at the end of their designated level.

† Clinical decision rule: these are algorithms or scoring systems that lead to a prognostic estimation or a diagnostic category.

‡ See note for advice on how to understand, rate, and use trials or other studies with wide confidence intervals.

§ Met when *all* patients died before the treatment became available, but some now survive on it; or when some patients died before the treatment became available, but *none* now die on it.

§§ By a poor-quality *cohort* study, we mean one that failed to clearly define comparison groups and/or failed to measure exposures and outcomes in the same (preferably blinded), objective way in both exposed and nonexposed individuals, and/or failed to identify or appropriately control known confounders and/or failed to carry out a sufficiently long and complete follow-up of patients. By a poor-quality *case–control* study, we mean one that failed to clearly define comparison groups and/or failed to measure exposures and outcomes in the same (preferably blinded), objective way in both cases and controls and/or failed to identify or appropriately control known confounders.

§§§ Split-sample validation is achieved by collecting all the information in a single tranche, then artificially dividing this into "derivation" and "validation" samples.

†† An "absolute SpPin" is a diagnostic finding whose specificity is so high that a *positive* result rules *in* the diagnosis. An "absolute SnNout" is a diagnostic finding whose sensitivity is so high that a *negative* result rules *out* the diagnosis.

‡‡ Good, better, bad, and worse refer to the comparisons between treatments in terms of their clinical risks and benefits.

††† *Good* reference standards are independent of the test, and applied blindly or objectively to applied to all patients. *Poor* reference standards are haphazardly applied, but still independent of the test. Use of a nonindependent reference standard (where the "test" is included in the "reference," or where the "testing" affects the "reference") implies a level 4 study.

†††† Better-value treatments are clearly as good but cheaper, or better at the same or reduced cost. Worse-value treatments are as good and more expensive, or worse and equally or more expensive.

** Validating studies test the quality of a specific diagnostic test, based on prior evidence. An exploratory study collects information and trawls the data (e.g., using a regression analysis) to find which factors are "significant."

*** By a poor-quality prognostic cohort study, we mean one in which sampling was biased in favor of patients who already had the target outcome, or the measurement of outcomes was accomplished in < 80% of the study patients, or outcomes were determined in an unblinded, nonobjective way, or there was no correction for confounding factors.

**** Good follow-up in a differential diagnosis study is > 80%, with adequate time for alternative diagnoses to emerge (e.g., 1–6 months acute, 1–5 years chronic).

Grades of recommendation:
A Consistent level 1 studies.
B Consistent level 2 or 3 studies, or extrapolations from level 1 studies.
C Level 4 studies, or extrapolations from level 2 or 3 studies.
D Level 5 evidence, or troublingly inconsistent or inconclusive studies of any level.
"Extrapolations" are where data is used in a situation that has potentially clinically important differences from the original study situation.

by comparisons with a reference standard evaluated in an appropriate spectrum of patients in whom the test is likely to be used.[2,11,13,14] Questions about therapy and prevention are best addressed by randomized controlled trials.[2,11,15,16] Cohort studies or case control studies best address questions about prognosis, harm, and disease etiology.[2,11,17,18] Methods for assessing the quality of each type of evidence are available.[2,9]

The randomized controlled clinical trial became the gold standard for determining treatment efficacy in 1948, with the publication of the trial that demonstrated that streptomycin was effective in the treatment of tuberculosis.[19] Over 489 000 randomized controlled trials (RCTs) have been recorded in the Cochrane Controlled Trials Registry, and thousands more exist in an unpublished form.[20] Large, inclusive trials that have concealed randomization, are fully blinded, have clinically relevant outcomes, intention-to-treat analysis, and equal treatment of randomized groups are likely to provide the best possible evidence about effectiveness.[21–23] Studies have demonstrated that failure to use randomization or adequate concealment of allocation resulted in larger estimates of treatment effects, predominantly caused by a poorer prognosis in nonrandomly

selected control groups in comparison with randomly selected control groups.[23]

Expert opinion can be valuable, particularly for rare conditions in which the expert has the most experience or when other forms of evidence are not available. However, several studies have demonstrated that expert opinion often lags significantly behind conclusive evidence.[1] Experts should be aware of the quality of evidence that exists.

Whereas personal experience is an invaluable part of becoming a competent physician, the pitfalls of relying too heavily on personal experience have been widely documented.[1,24,25] Nisbett and Ross extensively reviewed people's ability to draw inferences from personal experience and documented several pitfalls.[26] They include:
• Overemphasis of vivid anecdotal occurrences and underemphasis of significant statistically strong evidence.
• Bias in recognizing and accepting evidence that supports one's own beliefs, and parallel failure to recognize or accept evidence that contradicts one's own beliefs.
• Persistence of beliefs in spite of overwhelming evidence presented against them.

Whereas textbooks appear to be a valuable source of evidence, they have several well-documented shortcomings.

First, by virtue of the way in which they are written, produced, and distributed, most are about 2 years out of date at the time of publication. Most textbook chapters are narrative reviews that do not consider the quality of the evidence reported.[1,2] They tend to reflect the biases and shortcomings of the experts who write them.

More detailed studies of the relationship of study type and the direction and magnitude of purported benefit are needed in dermatology in order to guide dermatologists on the relative merits of different study designs. In the meantime, the hierarchy of evidence should not be conceptualized as a linear phenomenon (i.e., as a scale going from "good" to "bad"). The quality and relevance of evidence should be considered. Thus, a well-conducted large cohort study may be more reliable than a small RCT that has violated most aspects of good RCT design and reporting. Similarly, a small RCT of moderate quality dealing with the exact problem that the patient is complaining about (e.g., lipodermatosclerosis) is likely to be more useful than a large RCT dealing with a different problem (e.g., venous stasis ulcer).

References

1 Sackett DL, Haynes RB, Guyatt GH, Tugwell P. *Clinical Epidemiology: A Basic Science for Clinical Medicine.* Boston: Little, Brown, 1991: 441.

2 Greenhalgh T. *How to Read a Paper: the Basics of Evidence Based Medicine.* London: BMJ Publishing Group, 1997: 196.

3 Lau J, Ionnidis JPA, Schmid CH. Summing up evidence: one answer is not always enough. *Lancet* 1998;**351**:123–7.

4 Lau J, Antman EM, Jimenez-Silva J, Kupelnick B, Mosteller F, Chalmers TC. Cumulative meta-analysis of therapeutic trials for myocardial infarction. *N Engl J Med* 1992;**327**:248–54.

5 Villar J, Carroli G, Belizan JM. Predictive ability of meta-analyses of randomised controlled trials. *Lancet* 1995;**345**:772–6.

6 Cappelleri JC, Ioannidis JP, Schmid CH, *et al.* Large trials vs. meta-analysis of smaller trials: how do their results compare? *JAMA* 1996;**276**:1332–8.

7 LeLorier J, Gregoire G, Benhaddad A, Lapierre J, Derderian F. Discrepancies between meta-analyses and subsequent large randomized, controlled trials. *N Engl J Med* 1997;**337**:536–42.

8 Chalmers I, Altman D, eds. *Systematic Reviews.* London: BMJ Publishing, 1995.

9 Jadad AR, Moher M, Browman GP, Booker L, Sigouin C, Fuentes M. Systematic reviews and meta-analyses on treatment of asthma: critical evaluation. *BMJ* 2000;**320**:537–40.

10 Olsen O, Middleton P, Ezzo J, *et al.* Quality of Cochrane reviews: assessment of sample from 1998. *BMJ* 2001;**323**:829–32.

11 Sackett D, Richardson W, Rosenberg W, Haynes R. *Evidence-Based Medicine: How to Practice and Teach EBM.* Edinburgh: Churchill Livingstone, 1996: 250.

12 Phillips B, Ball C, Sackett D, *et al.* Levels of evidence and grades of recommendations. Available at: http://www.cebm.net/levels_of_evidence.asp. Last update May 2001 (accessed 31 March 2007).

13 Jaeschke R, Guyatt G and Sackett DL. Users' guides to the medical literature, III. How to use an article about a diagnostic test, A. Are the results of the study valid? *JAMA* 1994;**271**:389–91.

14 Jaeschke R, Guyatt GH, Sackett DL. Users' guides to the medical literature, III. How to use an article about a diagnostic test, B. What are the results and will they help me in caring for my patients? *JAMA* 1994;**271**:703–7.

15 Guyatt GH, Sackett DL, Cook DJ. Users' guides to the medical literature, II. How to use an article about therapy or prevention, A. Are the results of the study valid? *JAMA* 1993;**270**:2598–601.

16 Guyatt GH, Sackett DL, Cook DJ. Users' guides to the medical literature, II. How to use an article about therapy or prevention, B. What were the results and will they help me in caring for my patients? JAMA 1994;**271**:59–63.

17 Levine M, Walter S, Lee H, Haines T, Holbrook A, Moyer V. Users' guides to the medical literature, IV. How to use an article about harm. JAMA 1994;**271**:1615–9.

18 Laupacis A, Wells G, Richardson WS, Tugwell P. Users' guides to the medical literature, V. How to use an article about prognosis. JAMA 1994;**272**:234–8.

19 Anonymous. Medical Research Council Streptomycin in Tuberculosis Trials Committee. Streptomycin treatment of pulmonary tuberculosis. *BMJ* 1948;**ii**:769–82.

20 Higgins JPT, Green S, eds. Cochrane Handbook for Systematic Reviews of Interventions 4.2.6 [updated September 2006]. http://www.cochrane.org/resources/handbook/hbook.htm (accessed 29 March 2007).

21 Barton S. Which clinical studies provide the best evidence: the best RCT still trumps the best observational study. *BMJ* 2000;**321**:255–6.

22 Pocock SJ, Elbourne DR. Randomized trials or observational tribulations? *N Engl J Med* 2000;**342**:1907–9.

23 Kunz R, Oxman AD. The unpredictability paradox: review of empirical comparisons of randomised and non-randomised clinical trials. *BMJ* 1998;**317**:1185–90.

24 Bigby M, Gadenne AS. Understanding and evaluating clinical trials. *J Am Acad Dermatol* 1996;**34**:555–90.

25 Hines DC, Goldheizer JW. Clinical investigation: a guide to its evaluation. *Am J Obstet Gynecol* 1969;**105**:450–87.

26 Nisbett R, Ross L. *Human Inference: Strategies and Shortcomings of Social Judgment.* Englewood Cliffs, NJ: Prentice-Hall, 1980: 330.

8 Appraising systematic reviews and meta-analyses

Michael Bigby, Hywel Williams

Introduction

A systematic review is an overview that answers a specific clinical question, contains a thorough, unbiased search of the relevant literature, explicit criteria for assessing studies, and structured presentation of the results. Put simply, a systematic review is a review that is done systematically. Many systematic reviews incorporate a meta-analysis—i.e., a quantitative pooling of several similar studies to produce one overall summary of treatment effect.[1,2] Meta-analysis provides an objective and quantitative summary of evidence that is amenable to statistical analysis.[1] Meta-analysis allows recognition of important treatment effects by combining the results of small trials that individually might have lacked the power to consistently demonstrate differences among treatments. Meta-analysis has been criticized for discrepancies between the results of meta-analyses and the results of large clinical trials.[3–6] The frequency of discrepancies ranges from 10% to 23%.[3] Discrepancies can often be explained by differences in treatment protocols, differences in study populations, or changes that occur over time.[3] In conducting a meta-analysis, the authors should recognize the importance of having clear objectives, explicit criteria for study selection, an assessment of the quality of included studies, and prior consideration of which studies to combine. These items are the essential features of a systematic review. Meta-analysis is not appropriate if the included studies are very different. Meta-analyses that are not conducted within the context of a systematic review should be viewed with great caution.[7]

A systematic review can be viewed as a scientific and systematic examination of the available evidence. A good systematic review will have explicitly stated objectives (the focused clinical question, materials (the relevant medical literature), and methods (the way in which studies are assessed and summarized). The steps taken during a systematic review are shown in Table 8.1. Just like good randomized controlled trials, protocols describing the plans

Table 8.1 The six steps involved in undertaking a systematic review

1 Asking a clear, focused question
2 An explicit and thorough search of the literature*
3 Data extraction
4 Critical appraisal of the quality of the primary studies
5 Quantitative pooling of the data, if appropriate
6 Interpretation of the data, including implications for clinical practice and further research

* Should ideally include searching several electronic bibliographic databases, no language restrictions, scrutiny of citation lists in retrieved articles, hand-searching for conference reports, prospective trial registers, contacting key researchers, authors, and drug companies.

of a systematic review should be published in the public domain before the review is undertaken, in order to avoid data-driven reviews. Such is the practice of the Cochrane Collaboration, where protocols and completed reviews can be compared (www.thecochranelibrary.com).

Not all systematic reviews and meta-analyses are equal. A systematic review should be conducted in a manner that will include all of the relevant trials (including unpublished trials), minimize the introduction of bias, and synthesize the results to be as truthful as possible and as useful to clinicians as possible. The criteria for critically appraising systematic reviews and meta-analyses are shown in Table 8.2. In general, these criteria are similar to the criteria used to appraise the individual studies that make up the systematic review. Detailed explanations of each criterion are available.[1,8] The quality of reporting of systematic reviews is highly variable. One cross-sectional study of 300 systematic reviews published in Medline by Moher *et al.* showed that over 90% were reported in specialty journals.[9] Funding sources were not reported in 40% of reviews, and only two-thirds reported the years that trials were searched for. Around a third of reviews failed to provide a quality

Table 8.2 Critical appraisal of a systematic review

Are the results of this systematic review valid?
- Did the review address a focused clinical question?*
- Were the criteria used to select articles for inclusion appropriate?*
- Is it unlikely that important, relevant studies were missed?†
- Was the validity of the included studies appraised?†
- Were assessments of studies reproducible?†
- Were the results similar from study to study?†

Are the valid results of this systematic review important?
- What are the overall results of the review in terms of magnitude of benefit or harm?
- How precise were the results?

Can you apply this valid, important evidence in caring for your patient?
- Can the results be applied to my patient's care?
- Were all clinically important outcomes considered?
- Are the benefits worth the harms and costs?

From: Sackett D, Richardson W, Rosenberg W, Haynes R, *Evidence-Based Medicine: How to Practice and Teach EBM* (Edinburgh: Churchill Livingstone, 1996).
* Primary guides.
† Secondary guides.

assessment of the included studies, and only half of the reviews included the term "systematic review" or "meta-analysis" in the title. Guidelines for better reporting of systematic reviews were established in 1999 by the Quality of Reporting of Meta-Analyses (QUORUM) initiative, and many journals now insist on reporting systematic reviews in accordance with the QUORUM checklist.[10]

Asking a clear question

The validity criteria are designed to ensure that the systematic review is conducted in a manner that will minimize the introduction of bias. Like the well-built clinical question for individual studies, a focused clinical question for a systematic review should contain four elements:
- A patient, group of patients, or problem
- An intervention
- Comparison interventions
- Specific outcomes[11]

The patient populations should be similar to the majority of patients seen in the population to which one wishes to apply the results of the systematic review. The interventions studied should be those commonly available in practice. Outcomes reported should be those that are most relevant to physicians and patients. Main outcomes should be previously specified in a published protocol, in order to avoid problems with *post hoc* data dredging.

Sources of evidence within a systematic review

The overwhelming majority of systematic reviews involve therapy. Randomized, controlled clinical trials should therefore be used for systematic reviews of therapy if they are available, because they are generally less susceptible to selection and information bias in comparison with other study designs. The quality of included trials is assessed using the criteria that are used to evaluate individual randomized controlled clinical trials. The quality criteria commonly used include concealed, random allocation; groups similar in terms of known prognostic factors; equal treatment of groups; and accounting for all patients entered into the trial when analyzing the results (intention-to-treat design).

Randomized controlled trials are rarely a reliable source for identifying adverse reactions, unless they are very common. Evidence sources such as case–control studies, case reports, and post-marketing surveillance studies should therefore be examined. Systematic reviews of treatment efficacy should always include a thorough assessment of common and serious adverse events as well as efficacy, in order to come to an informed and balanced decision about the utility of a treatment. A thorough assessment of adverse events should include data from randomized controlled trials, case–control and post-marketing surveillance studies, and some of the other sources shown in Table 8.3.

The hazards of "quick" searches

A sound systematic review can be performed only if most or all of the available data are examined. Simply performing a quick Medline search using "clinical trial" as the publication type is rarely adequate, because complex and sensitive search strategies are needed in order to identify all potential trials, and because some clinical trials will be missed if they are published in a journal not listed by Medline.[12] Potential sources for finding studies about treatment include: the Cochrane Controlled Trials Registry (CCTR), which is part of the Cochrane Library, Medline, Embase, bibliographies of studies, review articles and textbooks, symposia proceedings, pharmaceutical companies, and contacting experts in the field.

The CCTR is a database of over 495 000 controlled clinical trials (April 2007) and is now the largest and most complete database of clinical trials worldwide. The Cochrane Controlled Trials Registry has been compiled through several complex searches of the Medline and Embase databases, and by hand-searching many journals—a process that is quality controlled and monitored by the Cochrane Collaboration in Oxford, England. Hand-searching journals

Table 8.3 Other sources for data on adverse reactions to drugs

Resource	Source	Comments
Meyler's *Side Effects of Drugs*	http://www.elsevier.com	Data 1–2 years old
Side Effects of Drugs annuals	http://www.elsevier.com	Data 1–2 years old
Reactions Weekly and Reactions Database	ADIS Press: http://www.ovid.com	Requires registration and fee
Current Problems in Pharmacovigilance	http://www.mhra.gov.uk/home/idcplg?IdcService=SS_GET_PAGE&nodeId=368	Drug safety bulletin of the MHRA and the Commission on Human Medicines (CHM). Issues freely searchable
Australian Adverse Drug Reactions Bulletin	http://www.tga.gov.au/adr/aadrb.htm	Back issues and free e-mail subscription available
European Public Assessment Reports	http://www.emea.europa.eu/index/indexh1.htm	Free, searchable database of reports
MedWatch	http://www.fda.gov/medwatch/	Searchable database of spontaneous reports of adverse reactions to drugs, maintained by the US Food and Drug Administration

to identify controlled clinical trials and randomized, controlled clinical trials was undertaken because members of the Cochrane Collaboration noticed that many trials were incorrectly classified in the Medline database. As an example, Adetugbo *et al.* hand-searched the journal *Clinical and Experimental Dermatology* for randomized controlled trials from its inception in 1976 through 1997 and identified 73 controlled clinical trials, yet only 31 of these could be identified from a Medline search using "clinical trial" as the publication type.[13]

Medline is the National Library of Medicine (NLM) bibliographic database covering the fields of medicine, nursing, dentistry, veterinary medicine, the health-care system, and the preclinical sciences. The Medline file contains bibliographic citations and author abstracts from approximately 5000 current biomedical journals published in the United States and 80 other countries. The file contains approximately 15 million records, dating back to the mid-1950s.[14]

Embase is Excerpta Medica's database covering drugs, pharmacology, and biomedical specialties.[1] Embase has better coverage of European and non–English-language sources and may be more up to date.[1] The overlap in journals covered by Medline and Embase is about 34% (range 10–75%, depending on the subject).[15,16] Embase contains over 11 million records from 1974 to the present. Embase is available online (http://www.embase.com). Personal and institutional subscriptions are available. Embase.com performs simultaneous searches of the Embase and Medline databases and eliminates duplicate records.

Publication bias

Publication bias—i.e., the tendency that studies that are easy to locate are more likely to show "positive" effects—is an important concern for systematic reviews, and a useful review of this subject can be found elsewhere.[17] It results from allowing factors other than the quality of the study to influence its acceptability for publication. Several studies have shown that factors such as the sample size, the direction and statistical significance of findings, or the investigators' perception of whether the findings are "interesting," are related to the likelihood of publication.[18,19]

Language bias may also be a problem—i.e., the tendency for studies that are "positive" to be published in an English-language journal and also more quickly than inconclusive or negative studies.[20] A thorough systematic review should therefore include a search for high-quality unpublished trials and should not restrict itself to journals published in English.

Studies with small samples are less likely to be published, especially if they have negative results.[18,19] By emphasizing only those studies that are positive, this type of publication bias jeopardizes one of the main goals of meta-analysis (i.e., an increase in power when pooling the results of small studies). The creation of study registers (e.g., http://clinicaltrials.gov) and advance publication of research designs have been proposed as ways to prevent publication bias (see http://prsinfo.clinicaltrials.gov/icmje.html).[20–22]

Publication bias can be detected by using a simple graphic test (funnel plot), by calculating the "fail-safe N, Begg's rank correlation method, Egger regression method and others."[23,24] These techniques are of limited value when less than 10 randomized controlled trials are included. Testing for publication bias is almost never possible in systematic reviews of skin diseases, due to the limited number and sizes of trials.

For many diseases, the studies published are dominated by drug company–sponsored trials of new, expensive treatments. Such studies are almost always "positive."[25,26] This bias in publication can result in data-driven systematic reviews that draw more attention to those medicines. In contrast, question-driven systematic reviews answer the clinical questions of most concern to practitioners. In many cases, studies that are of most relevance to doctors and patients have not been done in the field of dermatology, due to inadequate sources of independent funding. Systematic reviews that have been sponsored directly or indirectly by industry are also prone to bias through over-inclusion of unpublished "positive" studies that are kept "on file" by that company.[27] Until it becomes mandatory to register all clinical trials conducted on human beings in a central registry and to make all of the results available in the public domain, distortions may occur due to selective withholding or release of data. Thankfully, some dermatology journals now require all their published trials to have been registered beforehand.

Generally, reviews that have been conducted by volunteers in the Cochrane Collaboration are of better quality than non-Cochrane reviews.[27,28] However, potentially serious errors have been noted in up to a third of such reviews.[29]

Data abstraction

In general, the studies included in systematic reviews are reviewed by at least two reviewers for eligibility, according to pre-specified inclusion and exclusion criteria. Data such as the numbers of people entered into studies, numbers lost to follow-up, effect sizes and quality criteria are recorded on pre-designed data abstraction forms by at least two reviewers. Differences among reviewers are usually settled by consensus or by a third arbitrator. A systematic review in which there are large areas of disagreement among reviewers should lead the reader to question the validity of the review.

Pooling results

Results in the individual clinical trials that make up a systematic review may be similar in magnitude and direction (e.g., they may all indicate that treatment A is superior to treatment B by a similar magnitude). Assuming that publication bias can be excluded, systematic reviews with studies that have results that are similar in magnitude and direction provide results that are most likely to be true and useful. It may be impossible to draw firm conclusions from systematic reviews in which studies have results of widely different magnitude and direction.

The magnitude of the difference between the treatment groups in achieving meaningful outcomes is the most useful summary result of a systematic review. The most easily understood measures of the magnitude of the treatment effect are the difference in response rate and the its reciprocal, the number needed to treat (NNT).[1,8] The NNT represents the number of patients one would need to treat in order to achieve one additional cure. Whereas the interpretation of NNT might be straightforward within one trial, interpretation of NNT requires some caution within a systematic review, as this statistic is highly sensitive to baseline event rates. For example, if a treatment A is 30% more effective than treatment B for clearing psoriasis, and 50% of people on treatment B are cleared with therapy, then 65% will clear with treatment A. These results correspond to a rate difference of 15% (65–50) and an NNT of seven (1/0.15). This difference sounds quite worthwhile clinically. But if the baseline clearance rate for treatment B in another trial or setting is only 30%, the rate difference will be only 9% and the NNT now becomes 11, and if the baseline clearance rate is 10%, then the NNT for treatment A will be 33, which is perhaps less worthwhile. In other words, it rarely makes sense to provide one NNT summary measure within a systematic review, because "control" or baseline event rates usually differ considerably between studies, due to differences in study populations, interventions, and trial conditions.[30] Instead, a range of NNTs for a range of plausible control event rates that occur in different clinical settings should be given, along with their 95% confidence intervals. Further examples of NNTs in dermatology are to be found elsewhere.[31]

The precision of the estimate of the differences among treatments should be estimated. The confidence interval provides a useful measure of the precision of the treatment effect.[1,8,32,33] The calculation and interpretation of confidence intervals has been extensively described.[34] In simple terms, the reported result (known as the "point estimate") provides the best estimate of the treatment effect. The population or "true" response to treatment will most likely lie near the middle of the confidence interval and will rarely be found at or near the ends of the interval. The population or true response to treatment has only a one in 20 chance of being outside of the 95% confidence interval.

Certain conditions must be met when meta-analysis is performed to synthesize results from different trials. The trials should have conceptual homogeneity. They must involve similar patient populations, have used similar treatments, and have measured results in a similar fashion at a similar point in time. There are two main statistical methods by which results are combined: using random-effects models and fixed-effects models. Random-effects models assume that the different studies' results may come from different populations with varying responses to treatment. Fixed-effects models assume that each trial represents a random sample of a single population with a single response to treatment. In general, random-effects models are more conservative (i.e., random-effects models are less likely to show statistically significant results than fixed-effects models). When the combined studies have statistical homogeneity (i.e., when the studies are reasonably similar in direction, magnitude, and variability), random-effects and fixed-effects models give similar results.

The key principle when considering combining results from several studies together is that conceptual homogeneity precedes statistical homogeneity. In other words, results of several different studies should not be combined if it does not make sense to combine them—e.g., if the patient groups or interventions studied are not sufficiently similar to each other. Although what constitutes "sufficiently similar" is a matter of judgment, the important thing is to be explicit about one's decision to combine or not combine different studies. Tests for statistical heterogeneity are typically of very low power, so that statistical homogeneity does not mean clinical homogeneity. When there is evidence of heterogeneity, reasons for heterogeneity between studies—such as different disease subgroups, intervention dosage, or study quality—should be sought.[35]

Sometimes, the robustness of an overall meta-analysis is tested further by means of a sensitivity analysis. In a sensitivity analysis, the data are re-analyzed, excluding those studies that are of low quality or because of certain patient factors such as disease subtype, to see whether their exclusion makes a substantial difference in the direction or magnitude of the main original results. In some systematic reviews in which a large number of trials have been performed, it is possible to evaluate whether certain subgroups (e.g., children versus adults) are more likely to benefit than others. Subgroup analysis is rarely possible in dermatology, because few trials are available. Subgroup analyses should always be pre-specified in a systematic review protocol in order to avoid spurious *post hoc* claims.

The conclusions in the discussion section of a systematic review should closely reflect the data that have been presented within that review. The authors should make it clear which of the treatment recommendations are based on the review data and which reflect their own judgments. In addition to making clinical recommendations of therapies when evidence exists, many reviews in dermatology find little evidence to address the questions posed. This lack of conclusive evidence does not mean that the review is a waste of time, especially if the question addressed appears to be an important one.[36] For example, the systematic review of antistreptococcal therapy for guttate psoriasis provided the authors with an opportunity to call for primary research in this area, and to make recommendations on study design and outcomes that might help future researchers.[37]

Applying evidence summarized in a systematic review to specific patients requires the same processes that are used to apply the results of individual controlled clinical trials to patients (see Chapter 14).

References

1 Greenhalgh T. *How to Read a Paper: the Basics of Evidence Based Medicine*. London: BMJ Publishing Group, 1997: 196.

2 Chalmers I, Altman D, eds. *Systematic Reviews*. London: BMJ Publishing, 1995.

3 Lau J, Ionnidis JPA, Schmid CH. Summing up evidence: one answer is not always enough. *Lancet* 1998;**351**:123–7.

4 Villar J, Carroli G, Belizan JM. Predictive ability of meta-analyses of randomised controlled trials. *Lancet* 1995;**345**:772–6.

5 Cappelleri JC, Ioannidis JP, Schmid CH, *et al*. Large trials vs. meta-analysis of smaller trials: how do their results compare? *JAMA* 1996;**276**:1332–8.

6 LeLorier J, Gregoire G, Benhaddad A, *et al*. Discrepancies between meta-analyses and subsequent large randomized, controlled trials. *N Engl J Med* 1997;**337**:536–42.

7 Egger M, Smith GD, Sterne JA. Uses and abuses of meta-analysis. *Clin Med* 2001;**1**:478–84.

8 Sackett D, Richardson W, Rosenberg W, Haynes R. *Evidence-Based Medicine: How to Practice and Teach EBM*. Edinburgh: Churchill Livingstone, 1996: 250.

9 Moher D, Tetzlaff J, Tricco AC, Sampson M, Altman DG. Epidemiology and reporting characteristics of systematic reviews. *PLoS Med* 2007;**4**:e78.

10 Moher D, Cook DJ, Eastwood S, Olkin I, Rennie D, Stroup DF. Improving the quality of reports of meta-analyses of randomised controlled trials: the QUOROM statement. Quality of Reporting of Meta-analyses. *Lancet* 1999;**354**:1896–900.

11 Richardson W, Wilson M, Nishikawa J, Hayward R. The well-built clinical question: a key to evidence-based decisions [editorial]. *ACP J Club* 1995;**123**:A12–3.

12 Delamere FM, Williams HC. How can hand searching the dermatological literature benefit people with skin problems? *Arch Dermatol* 2001;**137**:332–5.

13 Adetugbo K, Williams H. How well are randomized controlled trials reported in the dermatology literature? *Arch Dermatol* 2000; **136**:381–5.

14 PubMed Overview. http://www.ncbi.nlm.nih.gov/entrez/query/static/overview.html (last updated 6 December 2006, last accessed 29 March 2007).

15 Smith B, Darzins P, Quinn M, Heller R. Modern methods of searching the medical literature. *Med J Aust* 1992;**157**:603–11.

16 Higgins JPT, Green S, eds. Cochrane Handbook for Systematic Reviews of Interventions, 4.2.6 [updated September 2006]. http://www.cochrane.org/resources/handbook/hbook.htm (accessed 29 March 2007).

17 Sterne JA, Egger M, Smith GD. Systematic reviews in health care: Investigating and dealing with publication and other biases in meta-analysis. *BMJ* 2001;**323**:101–5.

18 Dickersin K, Min YI, Meinert CL. Factors influencing publication of research results. Follow-up of applications submitted to two institutional review boards. *JAMA* 1992;**267**:374–8.

19 Easterbrook PJ, Berlin JA, Gopalan R, Matthews DR. Publication bias in clinical research. *Lancet* 1991;**337**:867–72.

20 Bassler D, Antes G, Egger M. Non-English reports of medical research. *JAMA* 2000;**284**:2996–7.

21 Dickersin K. Report from the panel on the Case for Registers of Clinical Trials at the Eighth Annual Meeting of the Society for Clinical Trials. *Control Clin Trials* 1988;**9**:76–81.

22 Piantadosi S, Byar DP. A proposal for registering clinical trials. *Control Clin Trials* 1988;**9**:82–4.

23 Macaskill P, Walter SD, Irwig L. A comparison of methods to detect publication bias in meta-analysis. *Stat Med* 2001;**20**:641–54.

24 Sutton AJ, Duval SJ, Tweedie RL, Abrams KR, Jones DR. Empirical assessment of effect of publication bias on meta-analyses. *BMJ* 2000;**320**:1574–7.

25 Smith R. Conflicts of interest: how money clouds objectivity. In: Smith R, ed. *The Trouble with Medical Journals*. London: Royal Society of Medicine, 2006: 125–38.

26 Perlis CS, Harwood M, Perlis RH. Extent and impact of industry sponsorship conflicts of interest in dermatology research. *J Am Acad Dermatol* 2005;**52**:967–71.

27 Melander H, Ahlqvist-Rastad J, Meijer G, Beermann B. Evidence b(i)ased medicine—selective reporting from studies sponsored by pharmaceutical industry: review of studies in new drug applications. *BMJ* 2003;**326**:1171–3.

28 Jadad AR, Cook DJ, Jones A, *et al.* Methodology and reports of systematic reviews and meta-analyses: a comparison of Cochrane reviews with articles published in paper-based journals. *JAMA* 1998;**280**:278–80.

29 Olsen O, Middleton P, Ezzo J, *et al.* Quality of Cochrane reviews: assessment of sample from 1998. *BMJ* 2001;**323**:829–32.

30 Ebrahim S, Smith GD. The "number need to treat": does it help clinical decision making? *J Hum Hypertens* 1999;**13**:721–4.

31 Manriquez JJ, Villouta MF, Williams HC. Evidence-based dermatology: number needed to treat and its relation to other risk measures. *J Am Acad Dermatol* 2007;**56**:664–71.

32 Gardner MJ, Altman DG. Estimating with confidence. In: Gardner MJ, Altman DG, eds. *Statistics with Confidence*. London: British Medical Journal, 1989: 3–5.

33 Gardner MJ, Altman DG. Estimation rather than hypothesis testing: confidence intervals rather than P values. In: Gardner MJ, Altman DG, eds. *Statistics with Confidence*. London: British Medical Journal, 1989: 6–19.

34 Gardner MJ, Altman DG, eds. *Statistics with Confidence*. London: British Medical Journal, 1989: 140.

35 Fletcher J. What is heterogeneity and is it important? *BMJ*. 2007;**334**:94–6.

36 Parker ER, Schilling LM, Diba V, Williams HC, Dellavalle RP. What is the point of databases of reviews for dermatology if all they compile is "insufficient evidence"? *J Am Acad Dermatol* 2004;**50**:635–9.

37 Owen CM, Chalmers RJ, O'Sullivan T, Griffiths CE. Antistreptococcal interventions for guttate and chronic plaque psoriasis. *Cochrane Database Syst Rev* 2000;(**2**):CD001976.

How to critically appraise a randomized controlled trial

Hywel Williams

The place of randomized controlled trials

The rationale for the randomized controlled trial is covered extensively in The James Lind Library (www.JamesLindLibrary.org), a nonprofit organization and free online resource that charts out the development of fair tests in history. Although numerous examples of attempts at fair tests can be found, such as the controlled trial by James Lind in 1762 on the value of lemons in preventing scurvy for British sailors, many recognize the first well- documented randomized controlled trial (RCT) as that performed by the Medical Research Council on the use of streptomycin for the treatment of pulmonary tuberculosis in 1948.[1] Many variants of clinical trials have developed since then, yet the basic principle of using concealed randomization as the fairest method of allocating study participants to an experimental versus control treatment has remained essentially the same. The RCT remains the most robust study to minimize the effects of bias when trying to assess the degree of effectiveness of a clinical intervention. Yet, as with any study design, there are good and bad RCTs, and this chapter aims to guide the reader on how to tell them apart. As discussed by Naldi in Chapter 10, RCTs are not the best source of study design to assess the potential harms of new treatments, especially for less common adverse effects.[2]

It should be mentioned at the outset of this chapter that, as highlighted in Chapter 7, the RCT should ideally be interpreted within the context of a high-quality systematic review of *all* relevant RCTs. The results of single RCTs, even when published in highly prestigious journals, can be hazardous when read in isolation. Thus, Ioannidis showed that of 49 original clinical research studies (almost all were RCTs) published in three major journals and cited over 1000 times, the effectiveness claims of around a third appeared to be exaggerated or contradicted by subsequent research.[3] Such studies underline the notion that one RCT is seldom enough. The practicing dermatologist should aim to refer to high-quality systematic reviews as their first port of call when available.

Definitions of quality, validity, and bias

Quality, when referring to randomized controlled trials (RCTs), is a multidimensional concept that includes appropriateness of design, conduct, analysis, reporting, and its perceived clinical relevance.[4-7] Validity refers to the extent to which the study results relate to the "truth." Validity may be internal (i.e., are the results of *this* trial true?) or external (to what extent do the results of this trial apply to *my* patients?). Factors affecting external validity are discussed further in Chapter 15. It is no good starting to examine factors affecting external validity unless the reader is assured of the internal validity of an RCT—in other words, internal validity is a prerequisite for external validity.

Most readers will be familiar with the need to estimate the role of chance when interpreting results from RCTs. Once the basic lessons in interpreting P values and confidence intervals have been achieved, the role of chance as an alternative explanation of study results is usually an easy exercise, especially since such information is usually accessible in almost all published RCTs. In addition to assessing the role of chance, a crucial component in appraising the internal validity of a trial is assessment of its potential for bias. Bias denotes a systematic error resulting in an incorrect estimation of the true effect. Unlike the role of chance, which is usually explicit and well highlighted within RCT reports, the role of bias needs to be specifically explored. With respect to clinical trials, bias may be best understood in terms of:
• Selection bias—resulting in an imbalance in treatment groups.
• Performance bias—treating one group of people differently from the other.
• Detection bias—biased assessment of outcome resulting from lack of blinding.

• Attrition bias—biased handling of deviations from the study protocol and those lost to follow-up.

How to tell a good dermatological RCT from a bad one

Quality criteria derived from research

Three main factors related to study reporting have been associated with altering the estimation of the risk estimate, usually by inflating the claimed benefit.[6] These are shown in Box 9.1, and are still considered today as the three most important indicators of RCT quality.

Generation and concealment of treatment allocation

Generation and concealment of treatment allocation are two interrelated steps in the crucial process of randomization. The first refers to the method used to generate the

---

BOX 9.1 Factors to consider when assessing the validity of clinical trials in dermatology

The "big three" that should always be assessed
• Is the method of generating the randomization sequence and subsequent concealment of allocation of participants clearly described and appropriate?
• Were participants and study assessors blind to the intervention?
• Were all those who originally entered the study accounted for in the results and analysis (i.e. was an intention-to-treat analysis performed)?

Other factors worth looking for
• Did the study investigators use an adequate disease definition?
• Were the treatment groups similar with respect to predictors of treatment response at baseline?
• Were the main outcome measures declared a priori, or did the investigators "data dredge" amongst many outcomes for a statistically significant result?
• Were the outcome measures clinically meaningful to you and your patient?
• Did the investigators do an appropriate statistical test?
• Did the investigators test the right thing (i.e., between-group differences rather than just differences from baseline)?
• Have the authors misinterpreted no evidence of an effect as being evidence of no effect?
• Were the groups treated equally except for the interventions studied?
• Who sponsored the study? Could sponsorship have affected the results or the way they were reported?
• Is the trial clearly and completely reported by CONSORT standards?

BOX 9.2 Adequacy of generation and concealment of randomization sequence

Generation of the randomization code
• Adequate: random numbers generated by computer program, table of random numbers, flipping a coin.
• Inadequate: quasi-randomization methods (for example, date of birth, alternate records, date of attendance at clinic).

Concealing the sequence from recruiters
• Adequate: if investigators and patients cannot foresee the assignment to intervention groups (i.e., numbered and coded identical sealed boxes prepared by central pharmacy, sealed opaque envelopes).
• Inadequate: allocation schedule open for recruiting physician to view beforehand, unsealed envelopes.

---

randomization sequence. The second refers to the subsequent steps taken by the trialists to conceal the allocation of participants to the intervention groups from those recruiting trial participants. Both aspects are designed to minimize selection bias, so that participants in a trial are allocated to one treatment or another on the basis of chance only.

Suggestions for adequate and inadequate definitions of the generation of randomization and subsequent concealment are shown in Box 9.2. Additional guidance is available in the Cochrane Handbook.[8] Studies that do not describe how the randomization sequence was generated should be viewed with some suspicion, given that humans frequently subvert the intended aims of randomization.[9]

Concealing the allocation of interventions from those recruiting participants is a crucial step in the progress of an RCT. The randomization list should be kept away from enrollment sites (for example, by a central clinical trials office or pharmacy). Internet randomization by a third party, whereby details of a new potentially eligible trial participant are entered irrevocably onto a trial database before an allocation code is offered, is another very secure way of concealing allocation. Less ideally, sealed opaque envelopes are used—a method that is still susceptible to tampering by opening the envelopes or holding them up against a bright light.[9] Failure to conceal such allocation means that those recruiting patients can foresee which treatment a patient is about to have. Such lack of concealment can result in selective enrolment of patients on the basis of prognostic factors,[10] and loss of the "even playing field" that randomization was designed to achieve.

Motives for interfering with the randomization schedule include a desire on the part of investigators to ensure that their new treatment is successful by deliberately allocating patients in a better prognostic group to the new treatment. Another reason may be that a doctor wants to ensure that particular patients for whom they have sympathy are not allocated to a control or placebo group if their belief in the experimental treatment is high. Such selective recruitment is a form of selection bias, resulting in an unfair comparison of the interventions under evaluation. Trials in which concealment of allocation was judged to have been inadequate were found to have inflated the estimates of benefit by about 30% in comparison with studies reporting adequate concealment.[6] Although concealment of allocation may help with subsequent blinding of assessors and patients when recording outcomes, it refers to a process that occurs *before* participants enter the trial, and its prime purpose is to ensure that the groups to be compared are as similar as possible to each other. Whereas blinding of participants and assessors is sometimes not possible—for example, in some surgical procedures in which a sham operation might be considered unethical—concealment of allocation is always possible.

Blinding (masking) the intervention

Blinding or masking is the extent to which trial participants and others involved in the study assessments are kept unaware of treatment allocation. Blinding can refer to at least four groups of people: those recruiting patients, the study participants themselves, those assessing the outcomes in study participants, and those analyzing the results.[11] The term "double blind" traditionally refers to a study in which both the participants and the investigators are "blind" to the study intervention allocation, but the term is ambiguous unless qualified by a statement as to who exactly was blinded.

Blinding is less of an issue with objective outcomes such as death, but it is especially important with subjective outcomes such as the opinion of participants or assessment of disease activity, as happens in many dermatology trials. Blinding may be achieved by a range of techniques, such as ensuring that placebo tablets look, feel, smell, and taste the same as the active tablets,[12] or, in the case of ointments, by using the same vehicle or base in which the active ingredient is formulated.[13] Even skin outcomes that may at first seem very difficult to blind—such as parents' views on the effects of laser treatment versus observation only for their child's hemangioma—can be blinded by taking digital photographs and then asking a panel of independent parents to judge the therapeutic response whilst concealing the identity of the intervention groups.[14] Judging whether a study has been truly blinded can be tricky and relies on a clear description in the methods section of the steps taken to ensure blinding, such as the use of placebos. Just because a study is described as being "double-blinded" does not necessarily mean that blinding was achieved. For example, placebo-controlled RCTs of oral retinoids (which have predictable adverse effects of mucosal dryness in nearly all those given the active drug) are impossible to blind effectively, despite studies regularly referring to them as

"double-blinded."[15] The same applies to controlled trials of topical capsaicin, which creates a burning sensation when applied to the skin.[16] Some trials test the effectiveness of their blinding methods by asking study participants at the end of the study to guess which treatment they had been allocated to.[13]

It is important to emphasize the difference between allocation concealment and blinding, although they may superficially appear to be the same. Failure to conceal the randomization sequence may result in unequal groups and is a form of selection bias, whereas failure to mask the intervention once a fair randomization has taken place represents a form of detection or information bias. Both can result in an incorrect estimate of the effects of a treatment. Studies that are not double-blinded typically overestimate treatment effects by about 14% in comparison with studies that are double-blinded.[6]

Accounting for all those randomized

The whole point of randomization is to create two or more groups that are as similar to each other as possible, the only exception being the intervention under study. In this way, the additional effects of the intervention can be assessed.[17] A potentially serious violation of this principle is the failure to take into account all those who were randomized when conducting the final main analysis—for example, participants who deviate from the study protocol, those who do not adhere to the interventions, and those who subsequently drop out for other reasons. People who drop out of trials differ from those who remain in them in several ways.[18] People may drop out because they die, encounter adverse events, get worse (or no better), or simply because the proposed regimen is too complicated for a busy person to follow. They may even drop out because the treatment works so well. Ignoring participants who have dropped out in the analysis is not acceptable, as their very reason for dropping out is likely to be related in some direct or indirect way to the study interventions. Excluding participants who drop out after randomization potentially biases the results. One way to reduce bias is to perform an intention-to-treat (ITT) analysis, in which all those initially randomized in the final analysis are included.[18,19]

Unless one has detailed information on why participants dropped out of a study, it cannot be assumed that an analysis of those remaining in the study to the end is representative of those randomized to the groups at the beginning. Failure to perform an ITT analysis may inflate or deflate estimates of treatment effect.[7] Performing an ITT analysis is often regarded as a major criterion by which the quality of an RCT is assessed.

It may be entirely appropriate to conduct an analysis of all those who remained at the end of a study (a "per-protocol" analysis) alongside the ITT analysis.[19] Discrepancies between the results of ITT and per-protocol analyses may indicate the potential benefit of the intervention in ideal compliance conditions and the need to explore ways of reformulating the intervention so that fewer participants drop out of the trial. Discrepancies may also indicate serious flaws in the study design. A good discussion of when and where it might be appropriate to exclude trial participants from the main analysis may be found elsewhere.[20]

Quality scales

It has been shown that faulty reporting generally reflects faulty trial methods, although sometimes space in journals has been suggested as a reason for not including vital information such as sample size calculation that could be found in original study protocols.[6,9,21] A number of scales have been developed for assessing study trial quality over the past 15 years. These vary in the dimensions covered and in their complexity.[5] Generally, the recent trend has been to use the few quality criteria given in Box 9.1, plus a few more that the appraiser considers important in relation to the condition being studied.[6] It is now considered unwise to use summary quality scores in an attempt to "adjust" the potentially biased treatment estimate, because the effects of such adjustment vary with the scale used and the way in which the components of each scale are weighted.[22] Instead, greater emphasis is placed on using the components of the scale as a checklist and considering how each may affect the results.[6]

Additional empirical criteria

Disease definition

Whilst it may seem simple to apply the three criteria of randomization generation/concealment, blinding, and ITT to judge the quality of RCTs, it is still uncertain how far these three factors can reliably discriminate between "good" and "bad" RCTs in dermatology. Other factors that are disease-specific and rely on content knowledge/expertise are likely to be equally important in determining the quality of some dermatology trials. The influence of such disease-specific factors in dermatology is an area that requires further systematic research.

A clear description of the disease being studied may be important. For example, when referring to a child with atopic dermatitis, I would not trust a study that claimed a beneficial effect for a new treatment if the study included both children and adults with diverse eczematous dermatoses,[23] as people with such conditions might respond differently.[24] And if the study did refer to atopic dermatitis, I would like to see a clear description of how the disease was defined.

Similarity of groups for baseline differences

In addition to helping to balance known predictors of treatment response, such as baseline disease severity (which

could serve as confounders when evaluating treatment efficacy between groups), it has also been suggested that randomization will balance against unknown confounders.[6] This statement is superficially appealing, but is difficult to verify if these confounders are indeed unknown. Yet simple randomization, even when perfectly implemented on small sample sizes, may still result in imbalances in possible cofactors that can affect the treatment response. In other words, randomization is not a guarantee against imbalance, although more sophisticated methods of randomization, such as blocking and stratification, can help minimize such imbalances.[11]

It is quite common for the first table in the results section of an RCT report to show a long list of demographic characteristics of the participants in the different treatment groups, along with a statement to the effect that "the two groups did not differ statistically at baseline." Such a statement is problematic for two reasons:
• It is inappropriate to perform such multiple statistical tests without prior hypotheses—indeed, many of the variables recorded may be totally irrelevant to predicting treatment response.
• There may still be no arbitrary 5% statistically significant differences even for gross imbalances in treatment groups, simply because the groups are so small.
Before reading such tables, the most important thing to do is to ask oneself, "What are the most important factors that may predict the treatment response?" and then to see whether they have been recorded. If there are major imbalances, such as in the baseline severity score, then these can and should be allowed for in a number of ways during analysis—for example, with a multivariate analysis adjusting for baseline severity as a covariate.[11]

Data dredging

Many trials report as many as 10 different outcome measures recorded at several different time points. Even by chance, at least one in 20 of such outcomes will be "significant" at the 5% level. It is therefore important in studies that use multiple outcomes to ensure that the trialists are not data dredging—that is, performing repeated statistical tests for a range of outcome measures and then emphasizing only the one that is "significant" at the "magic" 5% level. Such a practice is akin to throwing a dart and drawing a dartboard around it. Instead, trialists should declare up front what they would regard as a single "success criterion" for a particular trial. This way, it is more credible if that main success criterion is indeed fulfilled—as opposed to some secondary or tertiary outcome measure that turns out to be "significant" at one particular assessment time point. Sometimes, trialists will try to save face by emphasizing a range of less clinically significant biological markers of success when in fact the main clinical comparisons look disappointing. The problem of data dredging could be eliminated by trialists selecting and declaring their main outcome measure initially, and by registering their clinical trial protocols in the public domain on prospective trial registries—now a requirement by the major general and specialist journals.[25-27]

Related to data dredging, although perhaps worse, is the phenomenon of selective reporting of outcome measures—i.e., not mentioning at all some outcomes that were part of the original study protocol. The issue of outcome reporting bias has been well documented by Chan and Altman in 519 trials with 553 publications relating to 10 557 outcomes identified in trial protocols.[28] Chan, a dermatologist, found that on average, 20% of the outcomes measured in parallel group studies were incompletely reported, and that such incompletely reported outcomes had higher odds of being nonsignificant in comparison with fully reported outcomes (odds ratio 2.0; 95% confidence interval, 1.6 to 2.7). Chan and Altman suggested that the medical literature therefore represents a selective and biased subset of study outcomes —further underlining the need for trial protocols to be made publicly available on trial registers.[28]

"Sensible" outcome measures

In evaluating a clinical trial, look for clinical outcome measures that are clear-cut and clinically meaningful to you and your patients.[29] For example, in a study of a systemic treatment for warts, complete disappearance of warts is a meaningful outcome, whereas a decrease in the volume of warts is not.[30] The development of scales and indices for cutaneous diseases and testing their validity, reproducibility, and responsiveness has been inadequate.[29,31] A lack of clearly defined and clinically useful outcome variables remains a major problem in interpreting clinical trials in dermatology. Usually, dermatology clinical trials need at least three outcomes: a patient-centered outcome that seeks the views of trial participants on the "success" or otherwise of the study treatments; an objective and validated outcome measure that has not been tampered with; and a validated quality-of-life scale.

Until better scales are developed, trials with the simplest and most objective outcome variables are probably the most useful. Categorical outcomes are usually widely understood by clinicians and patients alike. Thus, trials in which a comparison is made between death and survival, patients with recurrence of disease and those without recurrence, or patients who are cured and those who are not cured, are studies whose outcome variables are easily understood and verified. For trials in which the outcomes are less clear-cut and more subjective, a simple ordinal scale is probably the best choice. The best ordinal scales involve a minimum of human judgment, have a precision that is much smaller than the differences being sought, and are sufficiently standardized to enable others to use them and produce similar results.[29,31]

Doing the wrong tests

It is quite common for continuous data such as acne spot counts to have a skewed frequency distribution. It may then be inappropriate to use parametric tests such as the Student t-test without first transforming the data. Alternatively, nonparametric tests that do not rely on the assumption of a normal distribution can be used. A quick way to check whether a continuous variable is normally distributed is to determine whether the mean minus two standard deviations is less than zero. If it is, the data are likely to be skewed.

Testing the wrong thing

Performing a statistical test on something other than the main outcome of interest is a subtle but not uncommon error in dermatology trials.[32,33] When comparing a continuous outcome measure such as a decrease in acne spots between treatment A and treatment B, the correct summary statistic to challenge the null hypothesis of no difference between the treatments is to examine the *difference between the two treatments* in terms of the change in the spot count from baseline. Sometimes the investigators simply perform a statistical test on whether the acne lesion count falls from baseline in the two groups independently. If the fall in spot count reaches the 5% level in one group but not in the other, then the authors may conclude that "therefore treatment A is more effective than treatment B". Perhaps the P value for change in spot count from baseline is 0.04 in one group (i.e., significant) and 0.06 in the other (i.e., conventionally nonsignificant). This practice is clearly inappropriate, since the difference between the two treatments has not been tested.

Interpreting trials with negative results

Misinterpreting trials with negative results is a common error in dermatology clinical trials.[34] Failure to find a statistically significant difference between treatments should not be interpreted as showing that "treatment is ineffective." Put another way, no evidence of effect is not the same as evidence of no effect.[35] In many dermatology trials, the sample sizes are too small to detect clinically important differences. Providing 95% confidence intervals around the main response estimates allows readers to see what kind of effects might have been missed. For example, in an RCT of famotidine versus diphenhydramine for acute urticaria, itch as measured by a 100-mm visual analogue scale decreased by 36 mm in the famotidine group and by 54 mm in the diphenhydramine group, a difference of 18 mm (54 − 36) in favor of diphenhydramine. Although the statistical test for this difference of 18 mm between the two treatment groups was not significant at the 5% level, there was a trend towards a greater reduction in itch in the diphenhydramine group. The 95% confidence interval around the 18-mm difference between the groups was from −3 to 38. In other words, the results were compatible with a difference of as little as 3 mm in favor of famotidine and as much as 38 mm in favor of diphenhydramine.[36]

The trial environment

Once randomized, it is important that the two intervention groups are followed up in similar ways. Previous studies have shown the nonspecific benefits of being included in a clinical trial, even in placebo groups.[37] Part of the benefit might be the result of better ancillary care and motivation prompted by frequent follow-ups and being "fussed over" by study assessors.[11] It is important therefore to scrutinize whether the treatment groups have been treated equally in terms of the frequency and duration of follow-up and whether they have been afforded identical privileges except for the treatment under investigation. Sometimes, especially in surgical trials, the effects of the expertise of the surgeon undertaking the procedure can result in an unfair estimation of treatment effect—a phenomenon that can be overcome by ensuring that participants are randomized to clinicians who are expert on delivering the intervention.[38]

Sponsorship issues

It is natural to assume that a clinical trial of a dermatological drug that has taken years of development investment by a pharmaceutical will strive to demonstrate that the drug is successful. Indeed, millions of dollars of profit may rely on convincing opinion leaders in dermatology of a new drug's worth. Yet the influence of sponsorship on efficacy claims has not been adequately explored in dermatology RCTs. Drug companies and trialists have many opportunities to influence journal readers when the results of their trial are published (Box 9.3).

Conflicts of interest are not unique to the pharmaceutical industry, although some of the best examples of distorting the scientific record have emerged from company-sponsored studies.[39] Those conducting trials for government agencies might hope to show that a new drug is less cost-effective than standard therapy. Some independent clinicians with preformed conclusions about an existing treatment may be equally susceptible to being influenced by their own prejudices when testing and writing up the results for that treatment. In assessing a study, readers should always consider who sponsored the study and ask themselves whether such sponsorship could have influenced the results or the way that they are presented. Empirical research from general medicine trials suggests that inclusion of a clear statement of pharmaceutical sponsorship does influence a clinician's interpretation of results. Absence of declared sponsorship may not mean absence of sponsorship.[40]

Other factors

This short chapter can only touch on some of the bigger issues in interpreting clinical trials. For most of the chapter, I have referred to single pharmacological interventions.

BOX 9.3 Ways to enhance the impact of positive studies or reduce the impact of negative studies

- Withhold "negative" trials from being published at all by keeping them as "data on file."
- Delay release of such "negative" studies into the public domain.
- Stopping a trial early at a "random high."
- Publish negative studies in an obscure or non-English-language journal.
- Deliberately select outcome measures that show the treatment in a better light—e.g. Psoriasis Area and Severity Index (PASI) 50 instead of PASI 75.
- "Torture" the data by performing multiple statistical tests on subgroups.
- Use many statistical techniques until you find one that shows the results in the best light.
- Divert attention from the main "negative" findings by emphasizing biomedical markers and "mechanism of action."
- Incorrectly interpret inconclusive studies as equivalence studies—for example, by suggesting that two drugs are the same when the confidence intervals surrounding their differences are large.
- Use a comparator that other studies have not used in order to avoid a head-to-head comparison with a current established treatment.
- Use the comparator drug at the wrong dose or frequency to show the active drug in a better light.
- Avoid mentioning significant adverse events in the abstract and discussion sections.
- Flood the literature with lots of placebo-controlled studies that make the new drug look impressive. Few doctors use placebos in clinical practice, and most would like to know how a new drug compares with the best existing active therapy.
- Use optimistic language and writing styles when discussing essentially negative studies—for example, repetition of positive results such as "nonsignificant trend in favor of," or use percentage relative treatment benefits when the absolute degree of improvement is small.
- Publish positive study results in duplicate or triplicate—overtly or even covertly.

Other more complex interventions, such as educational classes for eczema families, consist of several defined components such as the educational package itself, who delivers it, how it is delivered and reinforced, etc., and may require additional special interpretation.[41] Guidance on the evaluation of RCTs of complex interventions are discussed elsewhere.[42] The reader is referred to other resources to learn more about variations in study design, such as pragmatic versus explanatory trials,[43,44] and crossover studies or internally controlled right/left limb studies, which are frequently used in dermatology.[45] Issues on the unit of randomization are relevant to some areas of dermatology, where the failure to consider the whole person as opposed to number of warts can have a distorting effect on trial conclusions.[46]

Attempts to overcome limitations in the conduct, reporting, and publication of clinical trials

At this point, the reader might despair at the many hazards in interpreting clinical trial reports and in the way that they have been published over the years. But nearly all of the issues described can and have been overcome by strict reporting guidelines and the compulsory registration of clinical trials. The need for better standards of reporting of trials have led to the Consolidated Standards of Reported Trials (CONSORT) statement.[47] CONSORT contains a structured checklist for reporting the details of clinical trials, including methods of randomization and concealment, blinding, ITT analysis, and a flow diagram to illustrate the progress of trial participants. Several dermatology journals now require that submitted clinical trial reports meet CONSORT standards in order to be published.[48,49]

Whereas CONSORT may help with better reporting of trials that find their way into the pubic domain, it does not overcome the pervasive effect of publication bias.[50] The creation of prospective clinical trial registers accessible in the public domain is becoming a powerful tool to ensure that *all* trials are eventually published in some form, or at least that their presence can be determined by those doing systematic reviews of all available evidence.[25–28] Trial registers with fully accessible study protocols minimize publication bias, data dredging, and outcome reporting bias. Publishing trial protocols in the public domain may also minimize the increasing problem of covert ghost authorship writing, which may occur in up to 75% of industry-sponsored trials.[51] Thankfully, several leading dermatology journals now require RCTs to have been registered in accordance with the International Committee of Medical Journal Editors statement.[25–27]

References

1 Medical Research Council. Streptomycin treatment of pulmonary tuberculosis. *Br Med J* 1948;**ii**:769–82.
2 Vandenbroucke JP. Benefits and harms of drug treatments. *BMJ* 2004;**329**:2–3.
3 Ioannidis JP. Contradicted and initially stronger effects in highly cited clinical research. *JAMA* 2005;**294**:218–28.
4 Jadad AR, Cook DJ, Jones A, *et al.* Methodology and reports of systematic reviews and meta-analyses: a comparison of Cochrane reviews with articles published in paper-based journals. *JAMA* 1998;**280**:278–80.
5 Moher D, Jadad AR, Nichol G, Penman M, Tugwell P, Walsh S. Assessing the quality of randomized controlled trials: an annotated bibliography of scales and checklists. *Control Clin Trials* 1995; **16**:62–73.
6 Juni P, Altman DG, Egger M. Systematic reviews in health care: Assessing the quality of controlled clinical trials. *BMJ* 2001;**323**: 42–6.
7 Juni P, Altman DG, Egger M. Assessing the quality of controlled clinical trials. *Br Med J* 2001;**323**:42–6.
8 Higgins JPT, Green S, editors. *Cochrane Handbook for Systematic Reviews of Interventions* 4.2.6 [updated September 2006]. In: *The Cochrane Library*, Issue 4. Chichester, UK: Wiley, 2006.
9 Schulz KF. Subverting randomization in controlled trials. *JAMA* 1995;**274**:1456–8.
10 Schulz KF. Randomised trials, human nature, and reporting guidelines. *Lancet* 1996;**348**:596–8.
11 Pocock SJ. *Clinical Trials: a Practical Approach.* New York: Wiley, 1983.
12 Karlowski TR, Chalmers TC, Frenkel LD, Kapikian AZ, Lewis TL, Lynch JM. Ascorbic acid for the common cold: a prophylactic and therapeutic trial. *JAMA* 1975;**231**:1038–42.
13 Thomas KS, Armstrong S, Avery A, Li Wan Po A, O'Neill C, Williams HC. Randomised controlled trial of short bursts of a potent topical corticosteroid versus more prolonged use of a mild preparation, for children with mild or moderate atopic eczema. *BMJ* 2002;**324**:768–71.
14 Batta K, Goodyear HM, Moss C, Williams HC, Hiller L, Waters R. Randomised controlled study of early pulsed dye laser treatment of uncomplicated childhood haemangiomas: results of a 1-year analysis. *Lancet* 2002;**360**:521–7.
15 Naldi L, Svensson A, Diepgen T, *et al.* Randomized clinical trials for psoriasis 1977–2000: the EDEN survey. *J Invest Dermatol* 2003;**120**:738–41.
16 Tarng DC, Cho YL, Liu HN, Huang TP. Hemodialysis-related pruritus: a double-blind, placebo-controlled, crossover study of capsaicin 0.025% cream. *Nephron* 1996;**72**:617–22.
17 Altman DG, Bland JM. Statistics notes. Treatment allocation in controlled trials: why randomise? *BMJ* 1999;**318**:1209.
18 Hollis S, Campbell F. What is meant by intention to treat analysis? Survey of published randomised controlled trials. *BMJ* 1999;**319**: 670–4.
19 Williams HC. Are we going OTT about ITT? *Br J Dermatol* 2001;**144**:1101–2.
20 Fergusson D, Aaron SD, Guyatt G, Hebert P. Post-randomisation exclusions: the intention to treat principle and excluding patients from analysis. *BMJ* 2002;**325**:652–4.
21 Soares HP, Daniels S, Kumar A, *et al.* Bad reporting does not mean bad methods for randomised trials: observational study of randomised controlled trials performed by the Radiation Therapy Oncology Group. *BMJ* 2004;**328**:22–4.
22 Juni P, Witschi A, Bloch R, Egger M. The hazards of scoring the quality of clinical trials for meta-analysis. *JAMA* 1999;**282**:1054–60.
23 English JS, Bunker CB, Ruthven K, Dowd PM, Greaves MW. A double-blind comparison of the efficacy of betamethasone dipropionate cream twice daily versus once daily in the treatment of steroid responsive dermatoses. *Clin Exp Dermatol* 1989;**14**:32–4.
24 Hoare C, Li Wan Po A, Williams H. Systematic review of treatments for atopic eczema. *Health Technol Assess* 2000;**4**:1–191.
25 Williams HC, Goldsmith L. The JID opens its doors to high quality randomised controlled clinical trials. *J Invest Dermatol* 2006;**126**:1683–4.
26 Ormerod AD, Williams HC. Compulsory registration of trials. *Br J Dermatol* 2005;**152**:859–60.

27 Rennie D. Trial registration: a great idea switches from ignored to irresistible. *JAMA* 2004;**292**:1359–62.

28 Chan AW, Altman DG. Identifying outcome reporting bias in randomised trials on PubMed: review of publications and survey of authors. *BMJ* 2005;**330**:753–6.

29 Bigby M, Gadenne AS. Understanding and evaluating clinical trials. *J Am Acad Dermatol* 1996;**34**:555–90.

30 Gibbs S. Breakthrough in the treatment of warts? *Arch Dermatol* 2006;**142**:767–8.

31 Allen AM. Clinical trials in dermatology, part 3: measuring responses to treatment. *Int J Dermatol* 1980;**19**:1–6.

32 Williams HC. Hywel Williams' top 10 deadly sins of clinical trial reporting. *Ned Tijdschr Derm Venereol* 1999;**9**:372–3.

33 Harper J. Double-blind comparison of an antiseptic oil-based bath additive (Oilatum Plus) with regular Oilatum (Oilatum Emollient) for the treatment of atopic eczema. In: Lever R, Levy J, eds. *The Bacteriology of Eczema.* London: Royal Society of Medicine Press, 1995: 42–7.

34 Williams HC, Seed P. Inadequate size of "negative" clinical trials in dermatology. *Br J Dermatol* 1993;**128**:317–26.

35 Altman DG, Bland JM. Absence of evidence is not evidence of absence. *BMJ* 1995;**311**:485.

36 Watson NT, Weiss EL, Harter PM. Famotidine in the treatment of acute urticaria. *Clin Exp Dermatol* 2000;**25**:186–9.

37 Braunholtz DA, Edwards SJ, Lilford RJ. Are randomized clinical trials good for us (in the short term)? Evidence for a "trial effect." *J Clin Epidemiol* 2001;**54**:217–24.

38 Devereaux PJ, Bhandari M, Clarke M, *et al.* Need for expertise based randomised controlled trials. *BMJ* 2005;**330**:88.

39 House of Commons Health Committee. The influence of the pharmaceutical industry. http://www.parliament.the-stationery-office.co.uk/pa/cm200405/cmselect/cmhealth/42/42.pdf (accessed 16 February 2007).

40 Davidoff F, DeAngelis CD, Drazen JM, *et al.* Sponsorship, authorship, and accountability. *Lancet* 2001;**358**:854–6.

41 Williams HC. Educational programmes for young people with eczema: one size does not fit all. *BMJ* 2006;**332**:923–4.

42 Hawe P, Shiell A, Riley T. Complex interventions: how "out of control" can a randomised controlled trial be? *BMJ* 2004;**328**:1561–3.

43 Ozolins M, Eady EA, Avery AJ, *et al.* Comparison of five antimicrobial regimens for treatment of mild to moderate inflammatory facial acne vulgaris in the community: randomised controlled trial. *Lancet* 2004;**364**:2188–95.

44 Helms PJ. "Real world" pragmatic clinical trials: what are they and what do they tell us? *Pediatr Allergy Immunol* 2002;**13**:4–9.

45 Naldi L, Minelli C. Dermatology. In: Machin D, Day S, Green S, eds. *Textbook of Clinical Trials* Chichester, UK: Wiley, 2004: 211–32.

46 Gibbs S, Harvey I. Topical treatments for cutaneous warts. *Cochrane Database Syst Rev* 2006;**3**:CD001781.

47 Moher D, Schulz KF, Altman DG, Lepage L. The CONSORT statement: revised recommendations for improving the quality of reports of parallel-group randomised trials. *Lancet* 2001;**357**:1191–4.

48 Cox NH, Williams HC. Can you COPE with CONSORT? *Br J Dermatol* 2000;**142**:1–3.

49 Weinstock MA. The JAAD adopts the CONSORT statement. *J Am Acad Dermatol* 1999;**41**:1045–7.

50 Stern JM, Simes RJ. Publication bias: evidence of delayed publication in a cohort study of clinical research projects. *BMJ* 1997;**315**:640–5.

51 Gotzsche PC, Hrobjartsson A, Johansen HK, Haahr MT, Altman DG, Chan AW. Ghost authorship in industry-initiated randomised trials. *PLoS Med* 2007;**4**:e19 [Epub ahead of print].

10 How to assess the evidence concerning the safety of medical interventions

Luigi Naldi

Introduction

As for any other human activities, medical interventions may carry a risk of unintended adverse events. Whenever a physician prescribes a drug, there is a potential for an adverse reaction connected with drug use. Despite limited accurate data, a widely cited meta-analysis of 39 prospective studies in hospitals in the USA from 1966 to 1996 found that the incidence of severe adverse drug reactions —i.e., life-threatening reactions and reactions prolonging hospitalization—among in-patients was 6.7%, with 0.32% of them having a fatal reaction.[1] Despite these impressive figures, the rate of severe adverse reactions for any given drug is usually very low. In addition, the system works in such a way that even a small increase in the incidence of a clinically severe reaction may prompt the withdrawal from the market of the implicated drug.

It is commonly stated that clinical decisions should balance the benefit with the risk of the available options. A difficulty stems from the fact that data on the benefits and risks of medical interventions are usually derived from different study designs and information sources. A large part of our discussion will be focused on the safety of drug use. While systems to survey the safety of medications are well established, that is not the case for other medical interventions—e.g., surgical procedures or invasive diagnostic tests. It is well accepted that no *in vitro* or animal models may accurately predict adverse events associated with drug use before the same drug is employed in humans. Advances in the understanding of adverse reaction causation—e.g., pharmacogenomics—may in the future enable us to predict the risk in individual patients in a more reliable way.[2-4]

Data sources

The limitation of randomized clinical trials

The great strength of randomized clinical trials is their ability to provide an unbiased estimate of treatment effect by controlling not only for the determinants of outcome we know about, but also for those we do not know about. If randomized clinical trials demonstrate an important relationship between an agent and an adverse event, then we can be confident of the results. However, randomized clinical trials are usually designed to document frequent events—i.e., those associated with the intended effect of a treatment. With the usual sample size, which rarely exceeds a few thousand people, randomized clinical trials are not suited to accurately document the safety of medical intervention for uncommon events.[5,6] Besides the statistical power issue, additional limitations include the usual short duration of most clinical trials and the careful selection of the eligible population (restriction in patient selection according to age and co-morbidity). All in all, when an intervention has been proved to be effective in a randomized clinical trial, the safety issue still remains to be resolved. Pharmaceutical companies may strive to work out the adverse effect profile of a drug before licensing, but because only a limited number of selected individuals can be exposed to the drug before it is released, only common adverse events can be accurately documented and the complete range of adverse events remains to be elucidated in the post-marketing phase. This is particularly true for delayed reactions and rare but severe acute events.

The value of suspicion: case reports and case series

As opposed to randomized clinical trials, individual cases or case series do not provide any comparison with a control group and are unable to produce reliable risk estimates. In spite of their limitations, astute clinical observations are still fundamental to describe new disease entities and to raise new hypotheses concerning disease causation, including the effects of medical interventions. Case reports still represent a first-line modality for detecting new adverse reactions after a drug has been marketed.[7] Spontaneous surveillance

Table 10.1 Criteria for signal assessment in spontaneous surveillance systems

1 Number of case reports
2 Presence of a characteristic feature or pattern and absence or rarity of converse findings
3 Site, timing, dose–response relationship, reversibility
4 Rechallenge
5 Biological plausibility
6 Laboratory findings (e.g., drug-dependent antibodies)
7 Previous experience with related drugs

Table 10.2 Examples of pharmacoepidemiologic methods

- Intensive hospital monitoring
- Prescription event monitoring (PEM)
- Cohort studies
- Case–control studies and case–control surveillance
- Case–crossover design
- Record linkage

systems, such as the International Drug Monitoring Program of the World Health Organization (WHO), capitalize on the collection and periodical analysis of spontaneous reports of suspected adverse drug reactions.[8] All physicians are expected to take an active part in promoting the safety of medical interventions and to contribute by reporting any suspected adverse events they observe in association with drug use.[9] Such a collection of reported adverse events may be explored to raise signals (Table 10.1) to be validated by more formal study designs—i.e., studies providing estimates of incidence rates and quantifying risks.[10,11] Spontaneous reporting should be seen as an early warning system for possible unknown adverse events and may be prone to all sorts of bias.[12] Case reports may be more effective in revealing unusual or rare acute adverse events. In general, they do not reliably detect adverse drug reactions that occur widely separated in time from the original use of the drug, or that represent an increased risk of an adverse event that occurs commonly in populations not exposed to the drug.

Epidemiological studies: the most comprehensive source of data

Quantitative estimates of risks associated with drug use may be obtained from analytic epidemiology studies—i.e., cohort and case–control studies[13]—and from a number of modifications of these traditional study designs pertaining to the broad area of pharmacoepidemiology (Table 10.2). These observational (nonrandomized) studies provide less stringent results than randomized clinical trials, being prone to unmeasured confounders and biases. On the other hand, these study designs may represent in the "real world" the only practical option for obtaining risk estimates once a new drug has entered the market. Cohort studies are studies in which groups are defined according to their exposure status (e.g., users of a drug and nonusers) and are followed up, with subsequent events being recorded and compared.[14,15] In contrast, case–control studies are studies in which groups are defined according to their experience

of an outcome of interest (e.g., patients with cases of toxic epidermal necrolysis and their neighboring controls), and prior exposures are ascertained retrospectively and compared.[16] A crucial point for the validity of a case–control study is the choice of appropriate controls. In principle, controls should be an unbiased sample of those individuals composing the so-called "study base." Controls for cases arising in the ambulatory population with resultant hospitalization (community cases) may be represented by patients admitted to the same hospitals with cases of an acute condition or for an elective procedure not suspected of being related to drugs.[17]

Generally speaking, cohort studies are better suited to the study of rare exposures and common events, while case–control studies are suited to the assessment of rare outcomes and relatively common exposures. In addition, while cohort studies allow the assessment of several outcomes for one specific exposure, case–control studies make it possible to assess the role of a range of different exposures on the development of a single specific outcome. Cohort studies are not feasible when dealing with rare events, because millions of drug users have to be observed for years. In these conditions, case–control studies with a very large population base are the most feasible methods. For example, it is intuitive that only a case–control study would be feasible for assessing the pharmacological risk for a disease such as toxic epidermal necrolysis, with an expected rate in the general population of one case per million people per year.[18,19]

It is important that outcome and exposure should be measured in the same way in the groups being compared in observational studies. On the other hand, even if investigators document the comparability of potential confounding variables in the groups being analyzed (exposed and nonexposed cohorts, or cases and controls) or use statistical techniques to adjust for such variables, there may be an important imbalance that the investigators do not know about or simply have not measured that may be responsible for any observed difference. The presence of unaccounted-for imbalances is the main limitation of observational studies in comparison with randomized clinical trials. It is usually considered that such analytical studies should be developed with the aim of testing a specific predefined hypothesis. In the last few decades, modifications of traditional cohort and case–control studies have been developed to explore new associations and to raise signals. Record linkage is based on the linkage of data on exposure and outcome from large electronic databases, while case–control surveillance is the ongoing collection of cases of prespecified rare and severe acute events and of suitable controls, to look for new associations of the events with drug exposure.[20]

The association of an exposure with a given event is usually expressed in terms of a relative risk or odds ratio (an estimate of the relative risk obtained from case–control studies) (Table 10.3). The relative risk is a measure of the size of an association in relative terms. It refers to the ratio of the incidence of the outcome among exposed individuals to that among those not exposed. Values greater than one represent an increase in risk associated with the exposure, while values less than one represent a reduction in risk. A relative risk of two, for example, tells us that the event under study occurs two times more often in exposed people than in those not exposed. For rare events, even a large relative risk may translate to the occurrence of a few additional drug reactions. The total incidence of an outcome among exposed individuals is a combination of the baseline incidence plus the excess of incidence due to the exposure. The excess risk (or risk difference, or absolute risk reduction) is calculated as the difference between the incidence among exposed individuals and the incidence among individuals not exposed. It measures the occurrence of an outcome among exposed individuals that can be attributed to the exposure. As such, it is a better measure of the impact of different outcomes than the relative risk, and a more informative measure from the point of view of an individual physician and of public health. Measures of excess risk are directly calculated in cohort studies and—provided that data on the incidence of the outcome are available in

the underlying unexposed population—they can also be derived from case–control studies.

Back to the individual patient

What is the risk of extraspinal hyperostosis in a psoriasis patient treated for several months with acitretin? Does psoralen–ultraviolet A therapy increase the risk of nonmelanoma skin cancer in a patient being treated for mycosis fungoides? What is the chance of severe depression in an adolescent on 13-*cis*-retinoic acid for acne? To address these questions, physicians must effectively search for evidence and be able to assess the validity of the available data, to consider the strength of any documented association, and the relevance when the issue is to apply the evidence back to an individual patient.[21]

We have already considered that many different sources of information should be looked for and that the search should not be limited to randomized clinical trials.[22] When data from randomized clinical trials are scrutinized, the statistical power to rule in or rule out any important adverse event should be taken into account. When dealing with observational studies, it should be carefully considered whether they provide reliable quantitative risk estimates or simply generate signals needing further validation. The optimal study design should be one assuring unbiased comparison between exposed and unexposed groups. Comparison groups should be similar with respect to important determinants of outcome. Outcome and exposure should be measured in the same way in the groups being compared, and the exposure should clearly precede the adverse outcome. In addition, follow-up should be sufficiently long and complete and the study should have sufficient statistical power to document the association of interest.

When risk estimates from several studies are available, it should be determined whether they are roughly in the same direction or if there are discrepancies among the studies. If there are discrepancies, the reasons for the discrepancies should be considered. Systematic reviews may help in summarizing the study results.[23] Unfortunately, the value of meta-analyses of observational studies is not as stringent as that of randomized clinical trials.[24] Once an association has been established, the magnitude of the risk should be taken into account and expressed in understandable terms if it is to be of practical use to clinicians. We have already considered that, from the perspective of a physician deciding about the risk of prescribing a particular drug, the excess risk (or risk difference) is a more informative measure than the relative risk. In the context of randomized clinical trials, Sackett *et al.* proposed a method for converting risk differences into a more intuitive quantity. This quantity was named the number needed to treat (NNT = 1/excess risk).[25] This is the number of people who have to be treated in order

Table 10.3 Measures of association

Patients	Adverse event (cases)	No adverse event (controls)
Exposed	a	b
Not exposed	c	d

Relative risk = [a/(a + b)]/[c/(c + d)]
Odds ratio = (a/c)/(b/d)
Excess risk* = [a/(a + b)] − [c/(c + d)]
Number needed to treat (NNT) = 1/excess risk
NNT from case–control studies = 1/[(odds ratio −1) (unexposed event rate)]
* The excess risk may be also referred to as the "risk difference" or the "absolute risk reduction."

for one clinical event to be prevented by the treatment at issue (e.g., the number of people to be treated to avoid one patient experiencing a relapse of psoriasis). The "number needed to harm" (NNH) or "number of patients needing to be treated for one additional patient to be harmed" (NNTH)[26] is the number of people exposed to a given treatment such that, on average and over a given follow-up period, one additional person experiences an adverse effect of interest because of the treatment. In randomized clinical trials and cohort studies, NNH is directly calculated as the reciprocal of the excess risk. Recently, a formula has been proposed using odds ratios from case–control studies and data on the event rate in the unexposed population (Table 10.3).[27] According to the formula, given an odds ratio of 3 and an unexposed event rate of one per 1 000 000 people, the NNTH can be calculated as 500 000 (i.e., 500 000 people have to be treated for one additional adverse effect to be experienced with the treatment).

After estimates have been derived for the potential harm of an intervention, they should be weighted against the expected benefits of the same intervention. The adverse consequences of not withholding the intervention should be carefully considered. A final decision should try to integrate probability issues with the patient's values and preferences about therapy. Integration requires patient education about the benefits and risks of alternatives tailored to the particular patient's risk profile.

To conclude, not only should physicians be able to retrieve and critically assess the evidence concerning the safety of any given intervention, but also they should take an active part in promoting safety by contributing to surveillance programs once an intervention is proposed to the medical community.

References

1 Lazarou J, Pomeranz B, Corey D, et al. Incidence of adverse drug reactions in hospitalized patients: a meta-analysis of prospective studies. JAMA 1998;279:1200–5.
2 Phillips KA, Veenstra DL, Oren E, Lee JK, Sadee W. Potential role of pharmacogenomics in reducing adverse drug reactions. A systematic review. JAMA 2001;286:2270–9.
3 Knowles SR, Uetrecht J, Shear NH. Idiosyncratic drug reactions: the reactive metabolite syndromes. Lancet 2000;356:1587–91.
4 Meyer UA. Pharmacogenetics and adverse drug reactions. Lancet 2000;356:1667–71.
5 Eypasch E, Lefering R, Kum CK, Troidl H. Probability of adverse events that have not yet occurred: a statistical reminder. BMJ 1995;311:619–20.
6 Hanley JA, Lippman-Hand A. If nothing goes wrong, is everything all right? Interpreting zero numerators. JAMA 1983;249:1743–5.
7 Brewer T, Colditz GA. Postmarketing surveillance and adverse drug reactions: current perspectives and future trends. JAMA 1999;281:824–9.
8 Venning GR. Identification of adverse reactions to new drugs. II. How were 18 important adverse reactions discovered and with what delays? BMJ 1983;286:289–92, 365–8.
9 Gruchalla RS. Clinical assessment of drug-induced disease. Lancet 2000;356:1505–11.
10 Edwards R, Lindquist M, Wiholm BE, et al. Quality criteria for early signals of possible adverse drug reactions. Lancet 1990;336:156–8.
11 Meyboom RHB, Egherts ACG, Edwards JR, et al. Principles of signal detection in pharmacovigilance. Drug Saf 1997;16:355–65.
12 Belton KJ, Lewis SC, Payne S, Rawlins MD, Wood SM. Attitudinal survey of adverse reaction reporting by medical practitioners in the United Kingdom. Br J Pharmacol 1995;39:223–6.
13 Kaufman DW, Shapiro S. Epidemiological assessment of drug-induced disease. Lancet 2000;356:1339–43.
14 Van der Linden PD, van der Lei J, Vlug AE, Stricker BH. Skin reactions to antibacterial agents in general practice. J Clin Epidemiol 1998;51:703–8.
15 Fellay J, Boubaker K, Ledergerber B, et al. Prevalence of adverse events associated with potent antiretroviral treatment: Swiss HIV Cohort Study. Lancet 2001;358:1322–7.
16 Roujeau JC, Kelly JP, Naldi L, et al. Medication use and the risk of Stevens–Johnson syndrome or toxic epidermal necrolysis. N Engl J Med 1995;333:1600–7.
17 Kelly JP, Auqier A, Rzany B, et al. An international collaborative case–control study of severe cutaneous adverse reactions (SCAR). Design and methods. J Clin Epidemiol 1995;48:1099–108.
18 Roujeau JC, Guillaume JC, Fabre JP, Penso D, Flechet ML, Girre JP. Toxic epidermal necrolysis (Lyell's syndrome): incidence and drug etiology in France 1981–1985. Arch Dermatol 1990;126:37–42.
19 Schöpf E, Stühmer A, Rzany B, Victor N, Zentgraf R, Kapp JF. Toxic epidermal necrolysis and Stevens–Johnson syndrome: an epidemiologic study from West Germany. Arch Dermatol 1991;127:839–42.
20 Kaufman DW, Rosenberg L, Mitchell AA. Signal generation and clarification: use of case–control data. Pharmacoepidemiol Drug Saf 2001;10:197–203.
21 Levine M, Walter S, Lee H, et al. Users' guides to the medical literature, IV. How to use an article about harm. JAMA 1994;271:1615–9.
22 Maistrello M, Morgutti M, Rossignoli A, Posca M. A selective guide to pharmacovigilance resources on the internet. Pharmacoepidemiol Drug Saf 1998;7:183–8.
23 Bigby M. Rates of cutaneous reactions to drugs. Arch Dermatol 2001;137:765–70.
24 Temple R. Meta-analysis and epidemiologic studies in drug development and postmarketing surveillance. JAMA 1999;281:841–4.
25 Laupacis A, Sackett DL, Roberts RS. An assessment of clinically useful measures of the consequences of treatment. N Engl J Med 1998;318:1728–33.
26 Altman DG. Confidence intervals for the number needed to treat. BMJ 1998;317:1309–12.
27 Bjerre LM, LeLorier J. Expressing the magnitude of adverse effects in case–control studies: "the number of patients needed to treat for one additional patient to be harmed." BMJ 2000;320:503–6.

11 What makes a good case series?

Joerg Albrecht, Michael Bigby

Case reports and case series are often the first available evidence for the effectiveness of a treatment, or for rare adverse effects of interventions. They may remain the only evidence for the effectiveness of treatment if controlled clinical trials are not available.[1] In dermatology, the most common reasons for controlled clinical trials not being available are necessity, feasibility, and scale.

• *Necessity.* The first and most obvious reason for a lack of clinical trials is that treatments are so clearly effective that controlled clinical trials seem unnecessary (e.g., the use of insulin for type 1 diabetes).[2] Such "all-or-none" treatments are acknowledged to have achieved the highest level of clinical evidence, even without randomized clinical trials. All-or-none conditions are met when all or most patients died before the treatment became available, but some or many survived on treatment; or when some patients died before the treatment became available, but none or few died when receiving it.[3] This "all-or-none" effect is exceedingly rare in dermatology, but the use of systemic corticosteroids in pemphigus vulgaris may fall into the category.

• *Feasibility.* Studies that challenge the clinical perceptions of participants can be very difficult or impossible to conduct, because participation and recruitment of patients cannot be achieved. If therapies are strongly believed to work, there is most likely little interest in funding or conducting trials of their effectiveness. This state of affairs is unfortunate, because the history of medicine is full of reports of established practices that were found to be ineffective or even harmful when subjected to clinical trials.

• *Scale.* In dermatology, there are treatments for more than 2000 syndromes or diseases. Many of these diseases are so uncommon that trials would have to be conducted on a multicenter basis and would be very expensive. It is often impossible to find funding for such studies of rare skin disorders, which may need to be conducted in several countries, and pharmaceutical companies have almost no financial incentive to develop new drugs for rare diseases. Many treatments in dermatology are not very good and have low response rates, and this inflates the study sizes needed to

demonstrate clinically meaningful and statistical differences. It therefore seems likely that many skin diseases and their treatments will never be subjected to clinical trials, purely for reasons of scale. In dermatology, the majority of diseases are unlikely to be the object of primary licensing trials. Thus, for a long (or even indefinite) period, the only evidence for newly licensed drugs available may come in the form of case series or case reports.

For these reasons, as the present book illustrates, case series continue to provide important clinical evidence in dermatology, since they are often the only source of available evidence.

Methodology of case series

Some characteristics of good case series are traditional methodological features associated with clinical trials (Table 11.1). In general, as for clinical trials, it is essential for the report to allow full understanding of what happened to the patients. The ideal case series for the reader is one that constitutes an uncontrolled clinical trial and is ideally preplanned, with blinded outcome observations. These trials are rare, however, because the majority of case reports in dermatology are published in the form of consecutive cases of patients in whom the standard treatment has failed. Usually, the treatment is compassionate, and it is therefore not usually administered according to a standard protocol.

The purpose of this chapter is to delineate the characteristics of high-quality case series, always keeping in mind that phase 3 randomized controlled clinical trials may never come. The literature on how to improve case reporting and case series is limited, but includes papers by Moses[2] and Abel,[4] and most comprehensively Jenicek's book *Clinical Case Reporting in Evidence-Based Medicine*.[5] The recommendations offered in this chapter rely heavily on this literature, which in essence uses the experience gained from cohort studies to improve case reports.

Table 11.1 Methodology of case series

Diagnosis	Are the diagnostic criteria clearly identified and met by the patients included in the series?
Inclusion and exclusion criteria	Are inclusion and exclusion criteria clearly stated?
Informed consent	Has the patient consent been documented? For prospective studies: is institutional review board approval documented?
Consecutive cases	Are all consecutive patients treated by one physician or at one institution included?
Natural course of the disease	Is there any reference to the natural course of the disease, or, if applicable, the course on standard treatment?
Dosages	Are the dosage, duration, and titration of the treatment described adequately?
Outcome measures	Are the outcomes of the therapy well defined and clinically relevant?
Patient perception	Is there any documentation of the patient's perception of the outcome of treatment?
Safety	Do the authors explain the toxicology and safety issues associated with the treatment? Do they abstain from unfounded claims about safety?

Diagnosis

The authors of any case report or case series must explicitly state the diagnostic criteria used to establish the diagnosis of each patient reported, so that others wishing to replicate the study may do so with similar patients. The diagnostic criteria may include histological confirmation, which should also be described in detail. Appropriate testing to exclude other entities in the differential diagnosis should be performed and reported.

Inclusion and exclusion criteria

At the core of any description of case series is the delineation of exclusion and inclusion criteria. These criteria are often important to understand the authors' clinical reasoning. They help readers to apply the findings of the series to their patients and to define the external validity and generalizability of the findings, as they delineate the population to whom the observations are applicable. Inclusion and exclusion criteria are often used to increase the power of clinical trials by restricting studies to populations of patients who are most likely to respond on the basis of their age, the stage of the disease, or lack of concomitant diseases. While these selection criteria are likely to improve the outcome of any treatment, they introduce selection bias and seriously reduce the external validity of the study.

Detailing exclusion criteria can help to ensure clinical safety, in that they describe who should not receive the treatment in question. For example, patients with renal failure, children, or pregnant women may need to be excluded. The treatments that need to have failed before the experimental

treatment is tried should be specified. Explicit inclusion and exclusion criteria are helpful and illustrative even in case reports, where they help the reader identify which patients the authors think are not suitable for the therapy, due to theoretical considerations or knowledge of the treatment's side-effect profile.

Informed consent

Case reports and series are often the result of compassionate use rather than preplanned clinical trials. For the latter, informed consent and approval by an institutional review board (IRB) is required. IRB approval is not mandatory for compassionate use, but informed consent needs to be sought from the patient for any novel treatment. IRB approval indicates that the series has been collected prospectively, which is likely to signal higher quality by potentially reducing selection bias, which is likely in retrospective trials. It should be documented that informed consent was obtained. As in any treatment, the authors should note that they have explained the risks and benefits, and particularly the experimental nature of the treatment, to the patients and that they have consented.

Consecutive cases

The greatest threat to the credibility of case series is uncontrolled selection bias. All consenting, eligible patients at an institution or in the care of one physician should therefore be included in the series. Feinstein showed rather elegantly that even this approach has inherent limitations, since the patient introduces bias by choosing the investigator, rather than vice versa.[6] In spite of this potential pitfall, reporting "selected cases" introduces significant bias and severely limits the validity of such case series. If eligible patients refused to participate in the study or for other reasons did not receive the treatment, it should be noted, and the reader should learn about the outcome for these patients. If patients were lost to follow-up, it should be documented. The patients who cannot be followed may differ significantly from those who come back. The former may be better, worse, or unchanged in comparison with the patients reported. If a number of patients are not accounted for, the series becomes a series of "selected cases."[2]

Natural course of the disease

The implicit comparison for case series is either the natural course of the disease or the course when receiving an established treatment. Quite often, the authors go to great lengths to describe a litany of failed treatments in order to describe the treatment-resistant nature of their patients' condition, which they then go on to cure. However, many—if not most—dermatological diseases have a waxing and waning natural course. A knowledge of what may happen to the patient without the intervention is essential for the reader. For example, many interventions have been shown to halt the progression of toxic epidermal necrolysis. This disease-arresting effect was observed usually after several "ineffective" treatment attempts had been tried in the patient. However, in untreated patients, the average duration of progression is less than 4 days, which makes the interpretation of treatment that is initiated at or after this point impossible.[7]

Dosages

Information on dosages is an essential part of any treatment regimen. This applies not only to systemic and topical treatment, but also to laser or other surgery as well. The dosage, duration, and titration of the treatment should be described adequately. For systemic treatments, the amount (total or per kilogram), the number of times per day, and the duration are important. For topical treatments, the preparation, concentration, vehicle, number of times per day, and duration are important. For laser treatment, "dosage" refers not only to the adjustments and types of laser, but also to the number of sessions that are needed to achieve a certain result. The authors should ideally treat all patients with the same treatment regimen, which may well include a protocol or policy for dose escalation or reduction—for example, steroid tapering. The reader needs to understand what dosages patients received and whether there were any differences among patients, such as why some received more or less treatment than others.

Outcome measures

The outcomes of the therapy should be well defined and clinically relevant. Very often, authors claim clear-cut disappearance of the skin lesions, and this outcome is a well-defined end point. However, not all (and in most cases, very few) patients in case series are cured, and the demonstration of clinical improvement is much more challenging. Ideally, the patients are assessed with established outcome measures, such as the Psoriasis Area and Severity Index (PASI), the Scoring Index of Atopic Dermatitis (SCORAD), or the Cutaneous Lupus Erythematosus Disease Area and Severity Index (CLASI). These instruments all have inherent and well-recognized limitations, and are not part of normal clinical practice. While desirable, the baseline assessment may be missing for patients treated compassionately. Treating physicians may fear that documenting these baseline characteristics would constitute clinical research, when initially the focus of the treatment is only on patient care. In addition, many dermatologic diseases cannot be measured with available scales or instruments, and the definition and description of the outcome is challenging.

It is not uncommon for authors to make statements about the therapeutic effect based on percentage improvement. This approach has its pitfalls, particularly if the disease, like most, has more than one dimension (e.g., a combination of pruritus, erythema, and scaling). More often than not, the authors do not describe what constitutes a 50% improvement, and often the content of this improvement remains unclear. The assessment of the involved area of the skin surface is notoriously difficult and inexact. Although reference to the surface area involved gives an impression of precision, the accuracy and the intraobserver and interobserver reliability of these measurements is very low.[8]

Patient perception

The patients' perception of the outcome of treatment should be documented. The patients' perception of treatment is especially important, given the difficulties in measuring and reporting outcomes noted above. Many dermatological treatments are tedious and expensive, and it is therefore of great importance for clinicians to report whether patients were content with their treatment and if they were not, what they did not like. If patients discontinue treatment, the reasons should be documented if they are known to the investigators.

Safety

Safety data derived from small case series are rarely helpful and may be misleading. The data may be misleading if the author implies that the observation that no adverse events were observed in a series is relevant. As a general rule, the estimate of frequency of events derived from case series is imprecise. This imprecision can be estimated even for series without adverse reactions. The upper 95% confidence interval of the frequency of adverse reactions can be determined by referring to available tables, or a reasonable approximation of the rate can be calculated by dividing 3 by the number of patients studied.[9] The results illustrate that the small numbers found in case series do not document safety very well. For example, if no adverse events occur in a case series of 10 patients (3/10 = 0.30), an underlying adverse event rate of 30% cannot be excluded. No events in 100 (3/100 = 0.03) can still mean a 3% rate of adverse events. Thus, case series add little to knowledge about safety, because they are unlikely to detect rare events and frequently miss common ones.

Usually, large cohort studies, case–control studies, or post-surveillance studies are needed to describe the risks associated with any treatment with authority.[10] Thus, to claim safety on the basis of an absence of adverse effects in series with a small sample size is inappropriate. However, the reader should be informed about adverse events or the absence of them. We think that for case series, it is appropriate to give further guidance on expected side effects on the basis of what is known from the literature and previous experience with the treatment.

Conclusions

Simply because of their quantity, case series are important sources of information about dermatological therapies; this is rather unfortunate, but it is unlikely to change in the near future. Due to the lack of control groups, case series can demonstrate the efficacy of treatment only in rare circumstances (e.g., when the effect is dramatic and no other effective therapy is available). Given their low level of evidence and the many reasons for being skeptical about their findings (Table 11.2), it is mandatory that case series should be very well reported. If they are well designed, executed, and reported, case series can provide important clinical evidence that allows us to learn about alternative treatments

Table 11.2 Reasons to be sceptical about case reports and case series

Lack of test to placebo or vehicle control or standard treatment	Better than placebo or vehicle, or just the result of the natural history in a fluctuating condition? Would this treatment perform better than the standard treatment? Case reports and series cannot be used to compare treatments to either placebo, vehicle, or standard
Recruitment bias	Were the patients chosen only on the basis of their likelihood to respond to the treatment?
Information bias	Were the observers not blinded, and thus potentially more likely to report favorable outcomes? Third-party assessment may partially overcome this bias
Survival bias	Were some patients not reported who were originally enrolled? Patients in whom treatment failed may never have come back, or may have died
Publication bias	The tendency to publish only positive results. Are there negative case series for the treatment in question?
Confounding	Could there be a systematic influence, beyond the treatment, that might have influenced the outcome? Confounding is hard to assess and cannot be adjusted for in the absence of a control group
Chance	Could the results have occurred by chance? Hypothesis testing is not possible for case series, and thus it is not possible to assess whether the result might reflect chance. While the population response rate or the overall natural course of the disease, is helpful, it may not reflect the particular selected cases. Ideally, the reporter would not publish two or three dramatic cures, but use these successes as a starting-point for further observations, which would not include these first ones
Regression to the mean	Were the patients recruited during a particularly bad phase of a fluctuating disease that would in most cases improve over time? Such effects are well documented in placebo-controlled studies
Lack of formalized quality control	Is there any external formalized quality control to exclude fraud or data manipulation? Is there any conflict of interest?
Retrospective collection	Was the study only a retrospective collection of cases? Did the authors make sure that all patients in the institution who met the inclusion criteria were included?

before controlled trials, and perhaps in the absence of them. A poorly reported case series is likely to be unconvincing at best and misleading at worst, and thus it is important to stress that controlled high-quality clinical trials should be conducted if feasible.

Acknowledgment

We are grateful to Prof. Hywel Williams for valuable suggestions and editorial comments.

References

1 Black N. Why we need observational studies to evaluate the effectiveness of health care. *BMJ* 1996;**312**:1215–8.

2 Moses LE. The series of consecutive cases as a device for assessing outcomes of intervention. *N Engl J Med* 1984;**311**:705–10.

3 Oxford Centre for Evidence-based Medicine. Levels of evidence (2001). http://www.cebm net/levels_of_evidence.asp (accessed September 3, 2006).

4 Abel U. Erkenntnisgewinn mittels nichtrandomisierter Therapiestudien gaining understanding through nonrandomised therapeutic studies. *Ellipse* 1999;**15**:48–58.

5 Jenicek M. *Clinical Case Reporting in Evidence-Based Medicine,* 2nd ed. London: Arnold, 2001.

6 Feinstein AR. Clinical biostatistics. II. Statistics versus science in design of experiments. *Clin Pharmacol Ther* 1970;**11**:282–92.

7 Roujeau JC, Stern RS. Severe adverse cutaneous reactions to drugs. *N Engl J Med* 1994;**331**:1272–85.

8 Charman CR, Venn AJ, Williams HC. Measurement of body surface area involvement in atopic eczema: an impossible task? *Br J Dermatol* 1999;**140**:109–11.

9 Eypasch E, Lefering R, Kum CK, Troidl H. Probability of adverse events that have not yet occurred: a statistical reminder. *BMJ* 1995;**311**:619–20.

10 Albrecht J, Bigby M. The meaning of "safe and effective." *J Am Acad Dermatol* 2003;**48**:144–7.

12 What makes a good prevalence survey?

Magdalena Radulescu, Thomas Diepgen, Hywel Williams

In addition to providing an estimate of the burden of skin disease in a given community, prevalence surveys make it possible to estimate the potential demand for medical facilities and the economic impact of a disorder. Comparison of data from prevalence surveys conducted in different populations with varying dietary and lifestyle habits may allow tentative inferences to be drawn about the association between a certain disease and its possible triggering factors.[1]

Prevalence surveys, like other study designs, are prone to bias. It is important to draw inferences only from high-quality surveys. But how do you tell a good prevalence survey from a bad one? This chapter discusses criteria that can be used to assess the quality and relevance of publications that report on the prevalence of a disease. The proposed criteria have been derived from a systematic search of the general medical literature (Box 12.1), supplemented by our own experience in assessing the quality of prevalence surveys of psoriasis in Europe (Table 12.1).[2–23]

Quality criteria

The most comprehensive guideline for evaluating the quality of prevalence surveys was that published in 1998 by Loney et al.[24] They proposed eight main quality criteria. On the basis of this publication, we developed seven quality criteria, some of which are identical to those suggested by Loney et al. (Box 12.1).

We discuss each criterion in more detail below with reference to prevalence surveys of psoriasis, in order to illustrate the way in which these principles can be applied to a common skin disease.

Specification of the target population

Published prevalence surveys should give a definition of the target population, which is the population to whom the researchers wish to generalize their results. Information about the geographical area covered, as well as age and

> **BOX 12.1** Criteria to consider when assessing the quality of prevalence surveys in dermatology
>
> **Seven criteria that should always be assessed (adapted from Loney et al.[24]):**
> - Was the target population specified?
> - Which sampling method was employed? Is the survey based on a random sample or a whole population?
> - Was the sample size adequate?
> - Was the response rate adequate?
> - Was information given on nonresponders?
> - Was a valid and repeatable disease definition given?
> - Have reasonable efforts been made to reduce observer bias?
>
> **Other factors worth looking for:**
> - Were inclusion criteria specified?
> - Was information on persons actually studied reported in detail?
> - Were known and validated instruments used for measurement of the health outcome?
> - Were the terms "incidence" and "prevalence" correctly applied?
> - Were confidence intervals or standard errors presented for the estimates of prevalence?

gender, should be included. Whether certain population subgroups are excluded (e.g., certain ethnic groups) should be mentioned.

Employment of adequate sampling methods

In most cases, it is impossible to survey the whole population of interest. It is therefore necessary to draw a sample that is representative of the population of interest. The best sampling technique is random sampling, in which a group of people are selected at random for study from a larger group (population). Each person is chosen entirely by chance, thereby reducing the likelihood of a selection bias favoring one group of people over another.

Table 12.1 Critical appraisal of studies of the prevalence of psoriasis in Europe, 1975–February 2006

First author, year (ref.) Setting	Sample size (n)	Sample design	Measures	Prevalence rates	Present quality criteria	Limitations
Barisic-Drusko (1989)[2] Yugoslavia (Croatia)	8416	Urban and rural communities, factory employees	Clinical examination	Point prevalence: 1.6%	Target population specified Random sample Sample size adequate	No information on response rate and non-responders No valid disease definition No information with reference to reduction of observer bias
Braathen (1993)[3] Norway	13 438	Random sample of the Norwegian population	Questionnaire	Point prevalence: 1.4%	Target population specified Random sample Sample size and response rate adequate Observer bias reduced	No information on nonresponders No valid disease definition
Brandrup (1981)[4] Denmark	4977	Random sample of the Danish population	Interviews	Lifetime prevalence: 2.8%	Target population specified Random sample Sample size and response rate adequate Observer bias reduced	No information on nonresponders No valid disease definition
Broadley (2000)[5] UK (Cambridge)	753	First-degree relatives of patients with multiple sclerosis	Questionnaire, confirmation from general practitioner	Lifetime prevalence: 2.8%	Target population specified Response rate adequate Information on nonresponders Observer bias reduced	Convenience sample Sample size too small No valid disease definition Not a population-based survey
Cellini (1994)[6] Italy (Recanati)	426	Agricultural workers authorized to use pesticides	Clinical examination	Point prevalence: 1.2%	Target population specified Response rate adequate Observer bias reduced	Convenience sample Sample size too small No valid disease definition Not a population-based survey
Cribier (1998)[7] France (Strasbourg)	100	Hepatitis C–infected patients	Clinical examination by dermatologists	Point prevalence: 4.0%	Target population specified Response rate adequate Observer bias reduced	Convenience sample Sample size too small No valid disease definition Not a population-based survey
Ferrandiz (2001)[8] Spain	12 938	Stratified random sample of the Spanish population; persons responding to phone calls	Phone interview	Lifetime prevalence: 1.4%	Target population specified Random sample Sample size and response rate adequate Observer bias reduced	No information on nonresponders No valid disease definition
Formicone (2005)[9] Italy (L'Aquila)	109	Kidney transplant recipients between June 2000 and August 2004	Clinical examination by a dermatologist	4-year prevalence: 4.6%	Target population specified Response rate adequate	Convenience sample Sample size too small No valid disease definition No information about reduction of observer bias Not a population-based survey

Table 12.1 *Cont'd*

First author, year (ref.) Setting	Sample size (n)	Sample design	Measures	Prevalence rates	Present quality criteria	Limitations
Jensen (1995)[10] Norway (Oslo)	140	Heart transplant recipients still alive 1 year after surgery	Clinical examination by a dermatologist	Point prevalence: 7.0%	Target population specified Response rate adequate Information on nonresponders Observer bias reduced	Convenience sample Sample size too small No valid disease definition Not a population-based survey
Larsson (1980)[11] Sweden (AC County)	9615	Adolescents aged 12–16, attending grades 7–9 of compulsory schooling in AC County	Clinical dermatological examination	Point prevalence: 0.3%	Target population specified Whole population Sample size and response rate adequate Information on nonresponders Observer bias reduced	No valid disease definition
Lee (1990)[12] UK (Blackpool)	136	Patients with Crohn's disease attending a colitis clinic	Clinical examination, confirmation by a dermatologist in case of doubt	Point prevalence: 9.6%	Target population specified Response rate adequate	Convenience sample Sample size too small No valid disease definition No information about reduction of observer bias Not a population-based survey
Naldi (2004)[13] Italy	3660	Italian population aged 45 or older	Face-to-face interview by specifically trained interviewers	Lifetime prevalence: 3.1%	Target population specified Random sample (proportional stratified sample) Sample size adequate Observer bias reduced	No valid disease definition No information on response rate and nonresponders
Olsen (2005)[14] Norway	12 701	Norwegian twins born between 1967 and 1979	Questionnaire	Lifetime prevalence: 4.2%	Target population specified Whole population Sample size adequate Observer bias reduced	Response rate too low No information on nonresponders No valid disease definition
Paoletti (2002)[15] Italy (Rome)	96	Patients with chronic HCV infection	Clinical dermatological examination	3-year prevalence: 1%	Target population specified Response rate adequate	Convenience sample Sample size too small No valid disease definition No information about reduction of observer bias Not a population-based survey
Popescu (1999)[16] Romania (Bucharest)	1265	Schoolchildren in Bucharest, grades 1–4	Clinical dermatological examination; questionnaire for additional data	Point prevalence: 0.3%	Target population specified Random sample Sample size and response rate adequate Information on nonresponders Observer bias reduced	No valid disease definition

Table 12.1 *Cont'd*

First author, year (ref.) Setting	Sample size (n)	Sample design	Measures	Prevalence rates	Present quality criteria	Limitations
Rea (1976)[17] UK (Lambeth)	1200	Stratified random sample of population of Lambeth, aged 15–74	1, screening with a questionnaire; 2, clinical examination by dermatologists, other doctors, or trained nurses of 75% of individuals responding positive and 20% of individuals responding negative to questionnaire	Point prevalence: 1.6%	Target population specified Random sample Sample size and response rate adequate Information on nonresponders	No valid disease definition No information with reference to reduction of observer bias
Romano (1998)[18] Italy (Messina)	457	Patients with diabetes mellitus attending an outpatient clinic	Clinical dermatological examination	Point prevalence: 5.3%	Target population specified Response rate adequate Observer bias reduced	Convenience sample Sample size too small No valid disease definition Not a population-based survey
Schäfer (2001)[19] Germany (Augsburg)	2539	Stratified random sample of all registered residents of Augsburg aged 25–74	Clinical dermatological examination	Point prevalence: 3.8%	Target population specified Random sample Sample size adequate	Response rate too low No information on nonresponders No valid disease definition No information with reference to reduction of observer bias
Siragusa (1999)[20] Italy (Troina)	1500	All individuals admitted to the Dept. of Geriatrics at the Oasi Institute	Clinical dermatological examination	Point prevalence: 1.9%	Target population specified Sample size and response rate adequate	Convenience sample No valid disease definition No information with reference to reduction of observer bias
Susitaival (1995)[21] Finland (Pielavesi)	1052	All registered farmers aged 18–64 in two municipalities	Validated questionnaire	Point prevalence: 1.8%	Target population specified Sample size and response rate adequate	Cluster sample No information on nonresponders No valid disease definition No information with reference to reduction of observer bias
Van Romunde (1984)[22] Netherlands (Zoetermeer)	4691	Inhabitants of two residential areas in Zoetermeer	Questionnaire, clinical dermatological examination	Point prevalence: 1.1%	Target population specified Whole population Sample size adequate Observer bias reduced	Response rate too low No information on nonresponders No valid disease definition
Weismann (1980)[23] Denmark (Copenhagen)	584	Individuals living at a municipal old people's home in Copenhagen	Clinical examination	Point prevalence: 2.9%	Target population specified Response rate adequate	Convenience sample Sample size too small No valid disease definition No information with reference to reduction of observer bias

Based on a Medline search using the terms "psoriasis" and "prevalence." European studies published in English, German, French, and Italian were included. Studies of hospital patients and disease registers were excluded.

Cluster sampling—i.e., sampling clusters of people, such as a random sample of villages within a region—is acceptable provided that the methods are clearly described and that the precision of the final prevalence estimate incorporates the clustering effect. Convenience samples—e.g., a street survey or interviewing lots of people at a public gathering—do not provide a representative sample of the base population.

Adequate sample size

The larger the sample, the narrower will be the confidence interval around the prevalence estimate, making the results more precise.[1] As no observed sample value exactly equals the population value, the confidence interval is a necessary parameter that describes the range of plausible values for the population parameter.[24] Often, a "95% confidence interval" is quoted. The figure of 95% reflects the strength of belief that the computed interval actually contains the unknown parameter value.[25]

The sample size required to estimate the prevalence of a disease with a certain degree of precision can be calculated. For example, following a review of surveys concerning the prevalence of psoriasis, we calculated that if the prevalence of psoriasis is assumed to be 2%, a sample size of 753 would be needed in order to obtain an error rate of ±1% at the 95% confidence level. So with this sample size, and a real psoriasis prevalence of 2%, the prevalence value resulting from a survey could vary between 1% and 3%.

The accepted error rate could vary depending on the assumed absolute prevalence of a disease. If a disease has a prevalence of around 10%, an error rate of 2% could be acceptable, resulting in a prevalence estimate with 95% confidence intervals varying between 8% and 12%. As the prevalence of psoriasis is not assumed to be that high, though, an error rate higher than 1% could result in imprecise outcomes.

In order to guarantee the defined confidence level and error rate, and therefore ensure a specified degree of precision, it is necessary to define the actual final sample size by subtracting the nonresponders from the initially determined sample size. For example, in our review of European prevalence surveys for psoriasis (Table 12.1), we considered the sample size adequate if the total number accounted for at least 753 participants after subtracting the nonresponders.

Adequate response rate

If only a proportion of the invited people participate in a survey, selection bias may occur, thus affecting the validity of the findings.[26] Individuals affected by a certain disease could either respond more often than healthy people, or rather tend towards nonparticipation. For population surveys, a response rate of 66–75% has been recommended as generalizable in the literature.[27] In our rating of prevalence surveys for psoriasis, we considered a response rate of 70% or higher as adequate.

Information on nonresponders

It is necessary to obtain information about nonresponders in order to make sure that they do not systematically differ from survey responders in terms of factors such as sociodemographic characteristics or the presence of disease. Researchers should try to follow up individuals who do not consent to participate in a survey and ascertain their reasons for nonresponse. In our review of prevalence surveys for psoriasis, any attempt by the researchers to obtain and present information about the reasons for nonparticipation and the characteristics of the group of nonresponders was regarded as a quality asset.

Valid and repeatable disease definition

An important quality criterion for prevalence surveys is the presence of a standardized definition of the disease under investigation. A good disease definition is valid and repeatable. The term "validity" refers to the sensitivity (discerning as many cases of disease as possible) and specificity (excluding as many noncases as possible) of the definition.[28] A disease definition's validity has to be tested on an independent sample before it can be used on the study population.

Ideally, a repeatable disease definition leads to similar results between several observers or within replicate measurements taken by the same observer. Testing of this criterion is also necessary before adopting a disease definition.

In the field of dermatology, valid and repeatable disease definitions are rarely to be found in prevalence surveys. As our rating of prevalence surveys for psoriasis shows (Table 12.1), not one of the 22 surveys assessed contained a valid disease definition—reflecting a research need to develop valid and reliable diagnostic criteria for psoriasis in population surveys.

Reduction of observer bias

Observer bias may occur when a prevalence survey is based on clinical examination or on interviews. If there are several observers, their assessment concerning the presence or absence of a disease or of its severity could vary considerably. Even if only one examiner is responsible for the whole survey, observer bias may occur—e.g., if the examiner has a lower threshold for diagnosing borderline cases of psoriasis in comparison with others, or if he or she has a personal interest in a certain outcome (e.g., a company with a new psoriasis product that wishes to show that psoriasis is a big problem).

Thus, an attempt to minimize observer bias is mandatory for every prevalence survey. This task may be accomplished by adequate training of the examiners and by teaching them to rate the presence or absence of a disorder in the same standardized way. A comparison of the results of all observers may also show whether there is any interobserver variability. If there is only one observer, it should be made clear before the onset of the survey that he or she has no personal interest in a particular outcome. Other methods of reducing observer bias include the use of photographs, which can then be assessed by an independent panel.

Additional criteria

In addition to the above-mentioned quality criteria, several other factors should be taken into account when a prevalence survey is planned.

Specification of inclusion criteria for the study population

To allow for comparability between different prevalence surveys, it is important to specify inclusion criteria. These should comprise information about the age range and, if appropriate, gender and ethnic group of the individuals to be studied.

Information on studied individuals

In addition to specifying inclusion criteria to denote who is eligible for study, a good prevalence survey should give basic demographic information about the individuals actually studied. Given that nonresponse is common, data on the population that is actually studied might differ from the specified inclusion criteria. For example, if a survey of psoriasis sets out to include all adults between 20 and 80 years of age, but individuals older than 75 years do not participate, the age range of the actually studied persons runs from 20 to 75 years. Valuable information about the studied individuals comprises at least the age range, ethnic group, and sex distribution.

Measurement with valid instruments

A good prevalence survey describes the examination methods which led to its results. Furthermore, the instruments employed should be valid, displaying a high sensitivity and specificity. If an agreed standard measurement of a disease exists, with tested validity and reliability, it should either be employed, or any other instruments used should have been tested previously in relation to the standard instrument.

In prevalence surveys, one method of measurement is clinical examination of the study population, especially when dealing with surveys of visible dermatological diseases. If this examination is performed by one or more trained specialists, a valid measurement is often assumed, since specialists are often used as a reference standard where no objective tests are available as in psoriasis. Other common methods are questionnaires and interviews. Ideally, employed questionnaires should have been tested for validity before being used on the study population.

Correct application of epidemiological terms

It cannot be assumed that published prevalence surveys always apply the correct epidemiological terms for their findings. Sometimes, the terms "prevalence" and "incidence" are misused, the one being applied when in fact the other has been determined. A careful evaluation of the results with regard to their correct epidemiological relevance is therefore necessary.

In our review of prevalence surveys, one out of 22 surveys applied the term "incidence" (number of new cases per unit time) to its findings, when in fact the prevalence (number of cases existing at one point in time) had been determined.

Confidence intervals or standard errors

The results for the prevalence of a disease derived from a prevalence survey provide only an estimate of the true prevalence in the larger population. Confidence intervals provide a range that contains the true population prevalence estimate with a certain degree of assurance, thus indicating the level of confidence one can have in the estimates. The degree of assurance commonly used is 95%.

Confidence intervals are influenced by the sample size. The larger the sample, the narrower the confidence interval and the more precise the estimate.[25] By calculating and mentioning confidence intervals for their prevalence estimates, quality prevalence surveys indicate their precision.

The standard error as a measure of the amount of sampling variability is also influenced by the sampling size.[25] The standard error reflects how much the estimate for prevalence fluctuates from sample to sample. A small standard error shows that different samples do not highly affect the estimate for prevalence derived from the survey.

Thus, both confidence intervals and standard error are important for describing the reliability of the outcome of prevalence surveys. One of them should be computed and always reported in the results of a prevalence survey.

Conclusion

Cross-sectional prevalence surveys are useful for estimating disease burden and costs, and they are sometimes very straightforward to undertake. As in any other study, it is possible to do a good or bad quality prevalence survey, and the factors outlined in Box 12.1 should be heeded when designing and setting up a prevalence survey. A good study design and execution does not always mean that those reporting the results have included the important features. Better reporting of the quality factors outlined in this chapter is therefore crucial in order to allow readers to decide whether the results of a prevalence survey are valid and relevant to their population.

References

1 Strachan DP. The nature of epidemiological studies. In: Williams HC, Strachan DP, eds. *The Challenge of Dermato-Epidemiology*, Boca Raton: CRC Press, 1997: 3–12.

2 Barisic-Drusko V, Paljan D, Kansky A, Vujasinovic S. Prevalence of psoriasis in Croatia. *Acta Derm Venereol Suppl (Stockh)* 1989; **146**:178–9.

3 Braathen LR, Botten G, Bjerkedal T. Prevalence of psoriasis in Norway. *Acta Derm Venereol Suppl (Stockh)* 1989;**142**:5–8.

4 Brandrup F, Green A. The prevalence of psoriasis in Denmark. *Acta Derm Venereol* 1981;**61**:344–6.

5 Broadley SA, Deans J, Sawcer SJ, Clayton D, Compston DA. Autoimmune disease in first-degree relatives of patients with multiple sclerosis. A UK survey. *Brain* 2000;**123**:1102–11.

6 Cellini A, Offidani A. An epidemiological study on cutaneous diseases of agricultural workers authorized to use pesticides. *Dermatology* 1994;**189**:129–32.

7 Cribier B, Samain F, Vetter D, Heid E, Grosshans E. Systematic cutaneous examination in hepatitis C virus infected patients. *Acta Derm Venereol* 1998;**78**:355–7.

8 Ferrandiz C, Bordas X, Garcia-Patos V, Puig S, Pujol R, Smandia A. Prevalence of psoriasis in Spain (Epiderma Project: phase I). *J Eur Acad Dermatol Venereol* 2001;**15**:20–3.

9 Formicone F, Fargnoli MC, Pisani F, Rascente M, Famulari A, Peris K. Cutaneous manifestations in Italian kidney transplant recipients. *Transplant Proc* 2005;**37**:2527–8.

10 Jensen P, Clausen OP, Geiran O, *et al.* Cutaneous complications in heart transplant recipients in Norway 1983–1993. *Acta Derm Venereol* 1995;**75**:400–3.

11 Larsson PA, Liden P. Prevalence of skin diseases among adolescents 12–16 years of age. *Acta Derm Venereol* 1980;**60**:415–23.

12 Lee FI, Bellary SV, Francis C. Increased occurrence of psoriasis in patients with Crohn's disease and their relatives. *Am J Gastroenterol* 1990;**85**:962–3.

13 Naldi L, Colombo P, Benedetti Placchesi E, Piccitto R, Chatenoud L, La Vecchia C. Study design and preliminary results from the pilot phase of the PraKtis Study: self-reported diagnoses of selected skin diseases in a representative sample of the Italian population. *Dermatology* 2004;**208**:38–42.

14 Olsen AO, Grjibovski A, Magnus P, Tambs K, Harris JR. Psoriasis in Norway as observed in a population-based Norwegian twin panel. *Br J Dermatol* 2005;**153**:346–51.

15 Paoletti V, Mammarella A, Basili S, *et al.* Prevalence and clinical features of skin diseases in chronic HCV infection. *Panminerva Med* 2002;**44**:349–52.

16 Popescu R, Popescu CR, Williams HC, Forsea D. The prevalence of skin conditions in Romanian schoolchildren. *Br J Dermatol* 1999;**140**:891–6.

17 Rea JN, Newhouse ML, Halil T. Skin disease in Lambeth. A community study of prevalence and use of medical care. *Br J Prev Soc Med* 1976;**30**:107–14.

18 Romano G, Moretti G, Di Benedetto A, *et al.* Skin lesions in diabetes mellitus: prevalence and clinical correlations. *Diabetes Res Clin Pract* 1998;**39**:101–6.

19 Schäfer T, Bohler E, Ruhdorfer S, *et al.* Epidemiology of contact allergy in adults. *Allergy* 2001;**56**:1192–6.

20 Siragusa M, Schepis C, Palazzo R, *et al.* Skin pathology findings in a cohort of 1500 adult and elderly subjects. *Int J Dermatol* 1999; **38**:361–6.

21 Susitaival P, Husman L, Hollmen A, Horsmanheimo M. Dermatoses determined in a population of farmers in a questionnaire-based clinical study including methodology validation. *Scand J Work Environ Health* 1995;**21**:30–5.

22 Van Romunde LK, Valkenburg HA, Swart-Bruinsma W, Cats A, Hermans J. Psoriasis and arthritis. I. A population study. *Rheumatol Int* 1984;**4**:55–60.

23 Weismann K, Krakauer R, Wanscher B. Prevalence of skin diseases in old age. *Acta Derm Venereol* 1980;**60**:352–3.

24 Loney PL, Chambers LW, Bennett KJ, Roberts JG, Stratford PW. Critical appraisal of the health research literature: prevalence or incidence of a health problem. *Chron Dis Can* 1998;**19**:170–6.

25 Jolley DJ. Chance. In: Williams HC, Strachan DP, eds. *The Challenge of Dermato-Epidemiology*, Boca Raton: CRC Press, 1997: 61–74.

26 Bobak M. Bias—the silent menace. In: Williams HC, Strachan DP, eds. *The Challenge of Dermato-Epidemiology*, Boca Raton: CRC Press, 1997: 87–98.

27 Marshall V. Factors affecting response and completion rates in some Canadian studies. *Can J Aging* 1987;**6**:217–27.

28 Williams HC. Defining cases. In: Williams HC, Strachan DP, eds. *The Challenge of Dermato-Epidemiology*, Boca Raton: CRC Press, 1997: 13–24.

13 Critical appraisal of pharmacoeconomic studies

Laura K. DeLong, Suephy C. Chen

Dermatologists are increasingly interested in pharmacoeconomic studies, with the realization that funds for health care are limited. This chapter outlines the four fundamental types of pharmacoeconomic study (Table 13.1), gives dermatological examples, and concludes with a discussion of the necessary items for such studies. Readers can then critically appraise these studies.

Cost analysis

Cost analyses are the most fundamental pharmacoeconomic study; they deal solely in costs of therapeutic interventions. Researchers can derive costs from either microcosting or macrocosting. Microcosting involves enumerating each component of a therapeutic strategy and then determining the cost of each component. Bialy et al. compared the cost of Mohs micrographic surgery and traditional surgical excision

(TSE) performed by otolaryngologists for the treatment of facial and auricular nonmelanoma skin cancer.[1] They itemized costs of the surgery, pathologic analysis, reconstruction, facility fees, and follow-up visits. They concluded that Mohs is cost-comparable to two sequential TSEs with permanent section in the office and much less costly than facility-based TSE with frozen section in this patient population.

Ramrakha-Jones et al. sought to identify which current treatment for Bowen's disease incurred the lowest costs to the National Health Service in the UK.[2] Assuming equal efficacy across all treatments, they calculated direct medical costs of procedures and equipment and concluded that a single lesion of Bowen's disease is most cheaply treated by curettage (£200) or excision biopsy (£200) under local anesthetic, and most expensively treated by photodynamic therapy (£456.72).

Macrocosting determines the overall cost to care for a particular disease, usually with a population-based approach.

Table 13.1 Summary of the advantages and disadvantages of different types of pharmacoeconomic analysis

Type of pharmacoeconomic analysis	Advantages	Disadvantages
Cost analysis	Sources of rigorous cost accounting Basis of other pharmacoeconomic studies	Does not account for outcomes and side effects Does not measure the value of the therapy
Cost-effectiveness analysis	Accounts for outcomes and side effects Measures value of the therapy	Outcomes are not standardized across disease processes Results are not weighted according to importance
Cost-utility analysis*	Accounts for outcomes and measures value of therapy Results are standardized	Need to invoke some external criterion of value to interpret results
Cost–benefit analysis	Accounts for outcomes and measures value of therapy Does not need external criterion of value to interpret results	Assigning monetary value to health may be offensive May be difficult to measure benefits in monetary terms for expensive and complex therapies

* Often called "cost-effectiveness analysis."

Kirsner *et al.* evaluated the cost of hospitalization for dermatology-specific and diagnosis-related groups (DRGs) using the Medicare Provider Analysis and Review 1990–1996 database, which contains information for all Medicare beneficiaries using hospital in-patient services.[3] The authors used codes for various dermatologic conditions and found that in 1996, Medicare reimbursement was $52 million for dermatology-specific DRGs and $840 million for dermatology-related DRGs, a combined total of $892 million.

Cost analyses are useful as a source of rigorous cost accounting and as the basis for other pharmacoeconomic studies. However, they do not account for outcomes and potential side effects. Without accounting for the outcomes, the value of the therapeutic intervention cannot be easily measured. A costly medication that does not work well and does not provide quality outcomes has very little value. On the other hand, a costly medication that routinely improves lives may have very high value.

Cost-effectiveness analysis

Cost-effectiveness analyses (CEAs) are a form of pharmacoeconomic analysis that incorporates both costs and outcome. The results of CEAs are presented as a cost-effectiveness ratio (CE ratio), with costs in the numerator and health outcomes in the denominator. The ratio is a measure of value; the smaller the ratio, the fewer the resources required for a given unit of health outcome. Costs are determined in the same manner as for cost analyses, as discussed above. The health outcomes are generally measured by some biological unit, such as intraocular pressure for glaucoma interventions, or by life-years saved for cancer chemotherapy.

CEAs compare at least two therapies; usually, a new therapy is compared with a currently available therapy. A CEA that compares two therapies is called an incremental CEA; the additional costs that one therapy would entail are compared with the additional benefits that it provides. This is in contrast to an average CEA, in which the therapy in question is not compared with anything. However, this approach does not provide useful information to the policy-maker or the clinician unless the currently available therapy is to do nothing.

Bergstrom *et al.* published a CEA comparing the foam and cream/solution combination forms of topical clobetasol propionate for the treatment of psoriasis.[4] They used the Psoriasis Area and Severity Index (PASI) score to measure their outcome. They did not find a statistically significant difference in cost per change of one PASI unit using foam vs. cream/solution ($21.60 vs. $16.42 per PASI unit, respectively).

CEAs provide information about the value of the therapeutic intervention in question by accounting for the outcomes of the therapy. However, the outcome measure is not standardized and therefore cannot be used to make comparisons with other disease processes. For example, a reasonable outcome measure for a new therapy for seborrheic dermatitis might be dollars per clear scalp. However, this measure cannot be used to compare with the cost-effectiveness ratio of new therapies for disparate diseases such as onychomycosis, venous ulcers, or acne. Even if "clear skin" is used as the outcome measure, it cannot be used to make comparisons with nondermatological problems. Another problem with CEA is that the outcomes are not weighted according to their importance. For instance, let us assume that new therapies for scalp psoriasis, onychomycosis, and venous ulcers were cost-effective compared with their respective current therapies. Policy-makers may not be able to incorporate all the therapies into their formulary because of budgetary constraints. They would need to decide which is the most important outcome: clear scalp, smooth nails, or healed ulcer. A better situation would be to have the outcomes standardized and weighted according to value, so that policy-makers could compare CEA results across disease processes.

Cost-utility analysis

Cost-utility analyses (CUAs) provide outcomes that are standardized and weighted. CUAs give rise to a ratio similar to that of a CEA, except that the outcomes are measured in quality-adjusted life-years (QALYs). It should be noted that many health-care researchers use the two terms CUA and CEA synonymously.[5] QALYs reflect both the additional quantity of life that a therapy provides and also the quality of that additional amount of life. The latter measurement is particularly important in dermatology, where therapeutic interventions rarely save lives but often improve the quality of life. In the QALY approach, quality of life is measured by a set of weights called utilities, one for each possible health state, that reflect the relative desirability of the health state. The reader is encouraged to consult other references for detailed explanations of utilities.[5,6] By incorporating quality of life and by standardizing the outcome measure with QALYs, a dermatology CUA such as acne therapy can be compared with a mortality-impacting CUA such as breast cancer therapy. There are few published dermatological CUAs, but a recent paper providing dermatologic utilities will provide a strong foundation for future CUAs.[7]

Freedberg *et al.* published a CUA comparing a one-time screening strategy for melanoma with a no-screening strategy.[8] They primarily used life-years saved as their outcome measure, but they also used an estimate of utilities to estimate a QALY outcome. They found the cost-effectiveness ratio for the screening program to be $29 170 per life-year saved and $30 360 per QALY. While the strategy of screening once in a lifetime may not mimic reality, the analysis was a good beginning for investigating the cost-effectiveness of melanoma screening. Before interpreting the QALY result ($30 360 per QALY), readers should realize that the criterion for cost-effectiveness, known as the cost-effectiveness threshold, is arbitrary and open to debate. A cost-effective therapy is one that delivers more QALYs per dollar (or costs fewer dollars per QALY) in comparison with some benchmark. Researchers consider therapies less than $50 000 per QALY to be relatively cost-effective, whereas those greater than $175 000 per QALY are not.[9–11]

Cost–benefit analysis

Cost–benefit analysis (CBAs) differs from CEA and CUA in that the results are reported as differences between the costs and health benefits of the therapeutic program. The health benefits are represented in monetary terms, usually by asking patients how much they would be willing to pay for the therapy. The interpretation of a CBA is also different from that of a CEA or CUA. The CEA/CUA results give the value of a particular therapy relative to a standard therapy. However, in order to decide whether the new therapy is worth adopting at the expense of forgoing a different therapy, readers must invoke some external criterion of value, such as the cost-effectiveness threshold. The CBA, in contrast, allows the investigator to determine whether the therapy is worth the costs without an external criterion, since all benefits in CBAs are valued in monetary terms.

We compared Goeckerman therapy with methotrexate for psoriasis using CBA in addition to the CUA described above.[12] We queried a sample of "society" for the amount that they would be willing to pay for each therapy if their insurance company did not provide for it. We found that there was no net benefit of Goeckerman over methotrexate. When we compared each therapy with a "do nothing" approach for different severity levels of psoriasis, only methotrexate produced net benefits for severe psoriasis.

Detractors of CBA cite a wariness about assigning monetary value to health, because of moral and ethical issues.[6] However, proponents of the method point out that decision-makers who use the CEA/CUA implicitly place a monetary value on the health outcome, since they choose some threshold below which they consider that the outcome is worth the cost.[5] Another disadvantage to the CBA method lies in the validity of the "willingness to pay" estimate of the value of the health benefits. Fortunately, many dermatological interventions are neither overly expensive nor complex, and thus it is reasonable to expect patients to be able to conceptualize how much they would be willing to pay for a dermatological therapy.

Guidelines for critical appraisal of pharmacoeconomic studies (Box 13.1)

Framework

To evaluate any pharmacoeconomic analysis, readers must bear in mind several points about the framework of the study. Firstly, the study needs to be clear about the perspective of the analysis. Three main perspectives of a pharmacoeconomic analysis include the individual patient, the third-party payer, and society. The perspective dictates the cost used in the analysis (see below). The Panel on Cost-Effectiveness in Health and Medicine has recommended including an analysis from the societal perspective.[13] Secondly, the target population to which the intervention is directed should be explicitly stated. Finally, all pharmacoeconomic studies should be incremental analyses, comparing at least two therapies unless no standard of care exists. Pure cost analyses can be an exception to this guideline, since they can be used purely to account for cost.

Data and methods

Pharmacoeconomic studies should detail the pathway of the health intervention being analyzed, preferably with diagrams. In this way, readers can determine whether the

---

BOX 13.1 Checklist for readers of pharmacoeconomic analyses (adapted from Siegel *et al.*[13])

Framework
- Perspective of analysis
- Target population for intervention
- Description of comparator programs

Data and methods
- Diagram of pathway of health intervention
- Type of outcome used
- Methods for obtaining cost, effectiveness and quality of life
- Costs are market rates and not charges
- Critique of data quality
- Assumptions for input data are tested with sensitivity analysis
- Inflation and discount rates noted

Results
- Societal perspective (reference case)
- Sensitivity analysis

Discussion
- Summary of reference case
- Implications of sensitivity analysis
- Limitations
- Relevance to health-policy decisions

proposed flow of health care is comparable to their own. If not, then the analysis may not be relevant. The study should be explicit in the type of outcomes used in the analysis, whether it is QALYs, life-years saved, or a disease-specific outcome. The methods for obtaining cost, effectiveness, and quality-of-life measures should also be clear. If primary data are not available, the assumptions for using secondary data must be clearly stated and a sensitivity analysis performed to ensure that the results are robust to these assumptions. A critique of the quality of the input data should also be explicit.

Several points about cost should be mentioned. The perspective of the study influences the costs used in the analysis. If an analysis is performed from the perspective of the individual patient, then only the costs relevant to the patient should be considered. These costs would include the co-payment involved in the physician visit and the drug, and the time off from work that is needed to see the doctor. Assuming that the drug is covered by insurance, the actual cost of the drug would not be factored, since it is irrelevant from the perspective of the patient. On the other hand, third-party payers would be concerned about the cost of the drug as well as the cost of the physician, but not the co-payment or the time off from work. The analysis performed from the societal perspective would factor in costs that affect all members of society: the cost of the drug, the physician, and the time off from work, as well as any impact on family members.

It is also useful to consider the categories of cost when evaluating a pharmacoeconomic analysis. Direct health-care costs are the cost of the resources that directly provide the therapy. These include physicians, medications, laboratory monitoring, and radiography, for example. Indirect costs are those resources that are related to time and productivity. Indirect costs include the cost of the consumption of the time that the patient took from work, volunteer time, and family leisure time. It can also include costs associated with the loss of or impaired ability to work secondary to illness. Opmeer *et al.* performed a detailed cost analysis of treatment of patients with moderate to severe psoriasis from a societal perspective.[14] They outlined not only direct costs, but also indirect costs including productivity loss due to absence from work and time spent by patients or relatives in personal care.

The theoretically correct method of estimating cost is by determining the opportunity cost. Opportunity costs consist of the value of forgone benefits; some other program must have been forsaken in order to pay for a particular therapeutic regimen. For instance, in a developing country, it might be necessary to sacrifice an education program in order to implement a vaccination program. However, sometimes one cannot assume perfect competition between two programs, so that health-care prices may not approximate true opportunity costs. Instead, health economists

use existing market prices to estimate costs. Readers should be wary of analyses that use charges to estimate costs, since charges rarely approximate the market prices of services. In general, analyses performed from the societal perspective approximate the cost of physician and hospital services by using the Medicare reimbursement rate and estimate the cost of medication using the average wholesale price.

If the study analyzes the therapy over a long time course, then there needs to be an explanation of methods to account for inflation. Also, because people generally prefer to have money and benefits now rather than in the future, future costs and benefits in the analysis must be discounted. Experts recommend using a 3% discount rate.[13]

Results and discussion

Results should, at the minimum, be reported from the societal perspective. Results of sensitivity analysis should also be discussed. When assumptions have been made for the input data, those variables should be varied within reasonable clinical parameters. If the results change with variations in those variables, then readers should be wary of the robustness of the results. Finally, the relevance and limitations of the results to health policy issues need to be discussed.

References

1 Bialy TL, Whalen J, Veledar E, *et al.* Mohs micrographic surgery vs. traditional surgical excision: a cost comparison analysis. *Arch Dermatol* 2004;**140**:736–42.

2 Ramrakha-Jones VS, Herd RM. Treating Bowen's disease: a cost-minimization study. *Br J Dermatol* 2003;**148**:1167–72.

3 Kirsner R, Yang D, Kerdel F. Dermatologic disease accounts for a large number of hospital admissions annually. *J Am Acad Dermatol* 1999;**41**:970–3.

4 Bergstrom KG, Arambula K, Kimball AB. Medication formulation affects quality of life: a randomized single-blind study of clobetasol propionate foam 0.05% compared with a combined program of clobetasol cream 0.05% and solution 0.05% for the treatment of psoriasis. *Cutis* 2003;**72**:407–11.

5 Drummond M, O'Brien B, Stoddart G, Torrance G. *Methods for the Economic Evaluation of Health Care Programmes,* 2nd ed. Toronto: Oxford Medical Publishers, 1998.

6 Gold M, Siegel J, Russell L, Weinstein M, editors. *Cost-Effectiveness in Health and Medicine.* New York: Oxford University Press, 1996.

7 Chen SC, Bayoumi AM, Soon SL, *et al.* A catalog of dermatology utilities: a measure of the burden of skin diseases. *J Investig Dermatol Symp Proc* 2004;**9**:160–8.

8 Freedberg K, Geller G, Miller D, Lew R, Koh H. Screening for malignant melanoma: a cost-effectiveness analysis. *J Am Acad Dermatol* 1999;**41**:738–45.

9 Owens D. Interpretation of cost-effectiveness analyses. *J Gen Intern Med* 1998;**13**:716–7.

10 Hlatky MA, Owens DK. Cost-effectiveness of tests to assess the risk of sudden death after acute myocardial infarction. *J Am Coll Cardiol* 1998;**31**:1490–2.

11 Goldman L, Garber A, Grover S, Hlatky M. Cost-effectiveness of assessment and management of risk factors. *J Am Coll Cardiol* 1996;**27**:1020–30.

12 Chen S, Shaheen A, Garber A. Cost-effectiveness and cost-benefit analysis of using methotrexate vs. Goeckerman therapy for psoriasis: a pilot study. *Arch Dermatol* 1998;**134**:1602–8.

13 Siegel J, Weinstein M, Russell L, Gold M. Recommendations for reporting cost-effectiveness analyses. *JAMA* 1996;**276**:1339–41.

14 Opmeer BC, Heydendael VM, De Borgie CA, *et al.* Costs of treatment in patients with moderate to severe plaque psoriasis: economic analysis in a randomized controlled comparison of methotrexate and cyclosporine. *Arch Dermatol* 2004;**140**:685–90.

14 Applying the evidence back to the patient

Hywel Williams

Applying the external evidence back to the patient sitting in front of you is perhaps one of the most difficult and least discussed steps of evidence-based medicine.[1,2] Having unearthed some relevant, high-quality, and valid information from clinical trials in relation to a clinical question generated by a patient encounter, five questions now need to be asked in order to guide the application of such information to that patient.[3] They are listed in Box 14.1 and discussed in turn below (Figure 14.1).

How similar are the study participants to my patient?

Trial participants are sometimes atypical

Participants in clinical trials may be different from the patient who originally prompted you to ask an evidence-based question—in obvious biological ways such as age, sex, and clinical disease type.[4] In most circumstances, these differences do not prevent you from making some useful generalizations from the literature. For example, I would be quite happy to generalize from a randomized controlled trial (RCT) of topical corticosteroids for atopic eczema in the absence of strict diagnostic criteria, provided that the description of that disease made sense to me—for example, with phrases such as "itchy red flexural eczema."

Occasionally, the description of the clinical trial participants may render it difficult to extrapolate study results to the patient in front of you. For example, it may be unrealistic to generalize the results of an RCT dealing with high-dose ultraviolet A (UVA) in the treatment of young women with an acute flare of atopic eczema to a man with chronic lichenified atopic eczema. In such circumstances, perhaps more weight should be given to one trial of chronic eczema in adult men than to several trials conducted in younger women.

Perhaps one of the most frequent problems encountered is that of having to generalize trials of adult therapy to

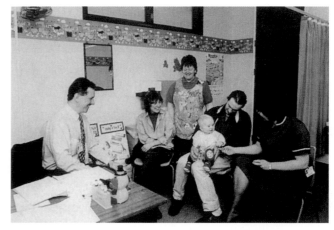

Figure 14.1 Clinical trial evidence is all very well, but what if the patient in front of you says, "I don't want that treatment"—what then?

children, in whom RCTs are rarely performed. Yet children can suffer almost all of the "adult" skin diseases, and practitioners frequently have no choice but to use adult-based data as a guide.

Another difficulty is that treatments that appear promising when tested in enthusiastic and healthy clinical trial volunteers often turn out to be less effective when applied to a wider group of patients with other comorbidities and levels of compliance. Such a divergence between study participants and real patients has been termed the difference between efficacy and effectiveness.[5] A regimen that involves applying creams three times a day may be attainable under the special conditions of a clinical trial, with continuous encouragement from the study assessors (and sometimes financial inducements). However, when it is tried in everyday life, it may simply be too much trouble. These effects can often be explored by looking at the dropout rate for different interventions and reasons for such dropouts. Finding such effects should not deter the reader from using the evidence, but rather make him or her more aware of the factors that need to be taken into account when describing

BOX 14.1 Questions that need to be considered when generalizing from studies to a patient

Are the patients in these trials sufficiently similar to mine?
- Do they differ in certain biological characteristics, such as age and sex?
- Do they differ in terms of disease subtypes—for example, pustular versus plaque psoriasis?
- Are there social factors that may diminish compliance?
- Does the patient suffer from other comorbidities, such as renal disease?
- Does the patient have a similar baseline risk of benefit or adverse events as the trial participants?

Do the outcomes make clinical sense to me?
- If a composite scale of signs and symptoms has been used, do you know what it means?
- Has the scale been deliberately selected or modified to enhance the apparent treatment effect?
- Are the main outcomes measured at an appropriate time point—e.g., months for a chronic skin disease, or days for an infectious one?
- Has the patient's perception of the intervention been considered?

Is the magnitude of benefit likely to be worthwhile for my patient?
- In addition to seeing whether a treatment produces statistically significant gain over its comparator, is the magnitude of that gain clinically worthwhile?
- Does the patient consider the magnitude of gain adequate to justify the risk and expense?
- Have you translated the magnitude of benefit into the number needed to treat for that patient's baseline risk—do you still think it is worthwhile?

What are the adverse effects?
- Why did patients drop out of the studies?
- Have you considered rare side effects that might not show up in the trials?
- How will you communicate this risk of adverse events to your patient?
- How will you involve your patient in weighing up the pros and cons of the treatment choices?

Does the treatment fit in with my patient's values and beliefs?
- What is the patient's prior belief about the proposed intervention?
- Does the patient prefer a topical or systemic medication?
- Would the patient prefer no pharmacological treatment at all?
- What treatments has the patient had before?

the potential efficacy of a treatment for the patient. One type of trial design—namely, the pragmatic clinical trial—overcomes the "ideal patient" effect by recruiting as wide a mix of patients as possible and by capturing the effects of poor compliance in the final analysis.[6]

Groups are different from individuals

Even if the person in front of you is a woman with acute atopic eczema, the results of the trial may not translate into real clinical benefit to her, for several reasons. Firstly, because the treatment effects reported in clinical trials—whether the outcome is a mean change in severity score or the proportion of people cleared—refer to *groups* of people. In a group of patients with a summary treatment effect such as a mean change in the Scoring Index of Atopic Dermatitis (SCORAD) of 5 points, there will be some individuals with score improvements of 10 or 15 points, some with changes of 3 or 4, some with no change, and possibly some whose disease has worsened. For example, closer inspection of the trial data on sildenafil (Viagra) for the treatment of erectile dysfunction[7] suggested that some men had all the fun! It follows that the patient sitting in front of you might benefit a lot or very little from the proposed treatment, and one has little way of knowing, apart from trying the treatment and seeing what happens. Similarly, telling your patient that "on average 60% of patients clear with this treatment" may not be very helpful if the patient then asks, "Am I in that 60%, doctor?"

One way forward is to see whether treatment response varies according to different study subgroups. However, it is unusual for dermatology RCTs to be large enough to include such subgroup analysis, and care has to be taken to be aware of "data dredging" in studies with many subgroup analyses. Conducting a series of "n of 1" trials on that patient may appear to be one way forward,[8] but such an approach is only suitable for stable chronic diseases and for treatments that do not affect the response to subsequent treatments. Pharmacogenetic testing offers one way of predicting whether an individual will respond to a drug. For example, measurement of thiopurine methyltransferase levels predicts who will develop serious bone-marrow suppression from oral azathioprine.[9]

Triumph of the aggregate

It is easy to misinterpret the application of aggregate data to individuals by equating group probabilities to individuals.[10] Thus, if a trial of excisional surgery for melanoma showed that 95% of participants (similar to your patient) were clear of the disease after 5 years, one cannot then tell the patient "You have a 95% chance of being clear at 5 years with this treatment," since this 95% refers to the group and not the individual. The patient in front of you will either clear or not clear—the patient's fate or response is already determined at that moment by that patient's microdisease and other cofactors such as immunological status, much of which may be under genetic influence. However, it is correct to tell that patient that "95% of people similar to you are clear at 5 years".

This inability to directly apply aggregate data directly to individuals is not unique to RCTs—it applies to most basic science.[11] Our everyday "clinical experience" with a particular drug is, after all, a form of aggregation of data based on recollection of treatment responses amongst *groups* of previous patients. The same difficulties in predicting whether the next patient will respond to that drug, and by how much, exist more in anecdote-based clinical practice than in an evidence-based practice approach.

Conclusions

Thus, it is important to consider a number of factors when thinking about study participants and the patient in front of you.[4] There may be pathophysiological differences that could lead to a diminished treatment response. For example, people with atopic eczema may not respond well to reduction of house dust mites if they were not allergic to house dust mite in the first place. There may be important social and economic differences that may diminish treatment compliance and hence response. For example, a single parent with four children and a full-time job may not have the time to diligently apply short-contact dithranol to his or her widespread plaque psoriasis every day. Comorbidities such as renal disease might also affect the treatment response, either directly by affecting drug metabolism and clearance or indirectly through drug interaction and compliance. Many doctors practice this process "automatically," without labeling it as "evidence-based medicine". Sometimes, the patient's baseline risk of adverse events also profoundly affects the effectiveness of the treatment being contemplated. These factors do not mean that it is impossible to apply the results of RCTs to your patient; they are simply prompts to think about when generalizing from a published study.

Do the outcomes make sense to me?

Even though you might have specified which outcomes would change your practice in your structured evidence-based question—for example, "the proportion of patients cleared at 6 months"—very often the studies will contain a number of other short-term outcomes.[12] You then have to decide whether these outcomes provide useful clinical information. In most circumstances, there will be at least some information that makes some clinical sense to you.

Take care in interpreting composite scales

Particular care should be taken in interpreting quantitative scales. Scales that combine several objective clinical signs and symptoms into an overall score are commonly used in dermatology RCTs. Despite their appearance of objectivity, most of them have rarely been tested for validity.[13] More importantly, such composite scales are often difficult to translate into clinical practice. What, for instance, does a difference of eight units ($P < 0.05$) as the mean change in the Psoriasis Area and Severity Index (PASI) score from baseline between two treatments mean to you? Such scales are not linear (i.e., a patient with a PASI score of 30 is not "twice as bad" as a patient with a score of 15). A lot of psoriasis over the covered areas of the body does not mean more distress than a little bit of psoriasis on the backs of the hands and face.

Sensitive scales amplify effects

Scales that are very sensitive to change amplify statistically significant changes that may be clinically unimportant. Take, for example, the trial of 2% minoxidil against placebo for androgenetic alopecia in women.[14] This study found a statistically significant increase in non-vellus target area hairs in the minoxidil-treated group in comparison with the vehicle-treated group after 32 weeks ($P = 0.006$), although the "subjects discerned no difference." The study, which was otherwise well conducted, should have concluded "something seems to be happening, but it is not clinically useful." However, the authors' conclusion was that "Two percent minoxidil appears to be effective in the treatment of female androgenetic alopecia." Effective for whom?

Too many scales and too many short-term studies

Given the profusion of scales used in dermatology (there are at least 13 named and at least 30 unnamed scales in atopic eczema alone),[15] it is quite easy to introduce bias by choosing a scale containing features that will enhance one's own product in comparison with competing products. Introduction of a new scale is another potential source of bias, since they can increase the likelihood of showing a treatment benefit.[16] Lack of suitable long-term outcomes is another problem frequently encountered in dermatology clinical trials. For example, atopic eczema is a long-term condition for most sufferers, yet of the 272 RCTs conducted to date, most have been less than 6 weeks in duration.[12] Other factors, such as the frequency and duration of the remission, are key components in assessing the value of therapy. It is therefore important when reading a trial report to think of the time frame for outcomes as well as the type of outcome.

So what would I go for?

Although composite scales may be useful in the early development of a drug, in that they may show that something is happening, the key question within the framework of pursuing an evidence-based prescription is whether something *useful* is happening. Given the limitations of quantitative composite scales in dermatology, what should one look for in terms of outcomes that can best inform practice? My starting position would be to see what the patients who participated in the trials thought of their treatment, using simple measures such as the proportion of participants with a "good or excellent" response, or other categorical measures such as percentage cleared. Did the patients' quality of life improve? Although such measures are subjective, is not such subjective distress the precise treatment goal for many chronic skin diseases with significant psychological effects? Objective measures are of course also needed, alongside measures that help generalize the meaning of such subjective responses across cultures, since it is possible that some cultural groups may complain less about symptoms. Objective measures are also more useful in some diseases (for example, to assess the response to treatments for basal cell carcinoma). Again, the objective outcomes need to be simple enough for most physicians and their patients to understand (for example, the proportion of recurrences within 5 years, rather than hazard ratios for first recurrence).

Magnitude of treatment effects

How big?

Even if a trial yields a result that is clinically meaningful, it is important to ask, "Is the *size* of that benefit likely to be helpful for *my patient*?" Even when the study benefits are of large magnitude, they may still not be enough. Consider a patient with a facial port-wine stain who is treated with pulsed tunable dye laser, and who achieves a 70% reduction in the total surface area involved. We might be impressed by such a magnitude of gain, but if the patient is still unhappy because he or she feels that the stigma associated with the residual lesion is just as disabling, or that the odd pattern of circular pale holes left by the laser within the lesion draws even more attention to it, then this is a treatment failure.

Thus, it is crucial to consider not only whether a treatment is effective in a published report, but also *how* effective it is. It follows that an important part of the discussion with the patient is to agree on what is possible or not possible in terms of realistic treatment objectives.

Number needed to treat

Because many interventions in medicine are of only modest effect, their apparent benefit may not be that noticeable after one has tried the intervention on a few patients. One way to understand the magnitude of benefit in relation to baseline risk is to use the concept of "number needed to treat" (NNT).[17] NNT refers to the number of patients that you would need to treat in order to see one additional success in the new treatment in comparison with another treatment. NNT is calculated simply as the reciprocal of the difference in success rates between the treatments being compared. Thus, a new treatment that results in clearing of psoriasis in 40% of patients, compared with 30% for the conventional treatment, translates into a risk difference of 10% (40 − 30) and an NNT of 10 (1/0.10). In other words, one needs to treat 10 patients to clear one additional patient.

Patients' and physicians' views regarding the threshold for what might constitute a useful NNT may differ significantly. Thus, in a study of perspectives of physicians and patients on anticoagulation for atrial fibrillation, patients placed significantly more value on the avoidance of bleeding than did doctors.[18] Again, the message here is not to think of NNT as belonging exclusively to doctors—patients also need to be incorporated into the decision-making process in determining what is useful and important.

It is also important that the dermatologist and patient decide for themselves what might constitute a useful NNT, rather than accepting the conventions that have been derived from acute medicine. For example, it may be perfectly justifiable to treat 200 patients with low-dose aspirin in order to prevent one stroke. I would certainly not be willing to work with such an NNT for a new antibiotic if the gain was just one extra short-term remission of acne. In a pressurized health service, I might even question the value of a new treatment for plaque psoriasis with an NNT of 20. Perhaps the opportunity costs associated with seeing the extra 20 patients needed in order to achieve one extra response from the new treatment could be better spent discussing other treatment options with them, or assessing other new patients. Despite these caveats, the NNT is a more useful tool than relative risk or odds ratios for translating the evidence back to the patient.

Adverse events

Trials are not a useful source of rare but serious side effects

As highlighted in Chapter 10, adverse events are often overshadowed by an emphasis on the positive treatment benefits in clinical trials. Details of reasons for withdrawals are frequently missing from trial reports altogether, and failure to perform an intention-to-treat analysis may compound this omission, as dropouts may be related to lack of efficacy or to adverse events that are not obviously related to the trial medication.[19] Rare side effects are unlikely to show up in small clinical trials and often emerge as subsequent case reports or during post-marketing surveillance. Simply stating that no serious liver problems occurred in 100 patients taking traditional Chinese herbs for atopic eczema is still compatible with an upper 95% confidence limit of 3% if a larger population were tested.[20]

Particular efforts should therefore be made to scrutinize trials for a list of the frequency and severity of adverse events, as discussed in Chapter 10. As the events surrounding the thalidomide tragedy remind us, caution should be exercised when using new treatments that have not been tested on thousands of patients. Additional literature sources and post-marketing surveillance studies need to be scrutinized before one can reassure patients on side-effect issues with a reasonable degree of certainty.

Limitations of aggregate data

Just as for assessing treatment benefits, aggregate data on side effects can be misleading. Thus, when comparing two types of corticosteroid, one may find that the mean decrease in skin thickness is similar in the two groups. However, if further scrutiny of the individual data shows that two children in one group developed skin thinning with noticeable visible striae, then that observation might influence your decision not to use such a treatment, despite the relative reassurance provided by the group means.

Communicating risks

How to communicate risk presents its own problems, with different conclusions being reached by doctors and their patients, depending on how the information is presented in terms of relative or absolute risk.[21] Paling and others suggest that supplementing verbal data with numerical data is key.[22,23] Absolute numbers, rather than relative or percentage changes, should be used, and the same denominator should be used to compare with other risks in order to provide context. Risk should be communicated in straightforward numbers that are easily understood, such as one in 1000, and the figures should relate to a specific time period—e.g., per year or lifetime. Visual aids, such as those depicting what can happen amongst a group of a thousand people undergoing an intervention, can be especially helpful.[22]

Even when the risks are understood, weighing up the pros and cons of an intervention is a highly variable affair. It depends not only on the type of information presented to the patient, but also on the manner in which the information is presented. Thus, a doctor who believes that a patient with psoriasis needs ciclosporin A may play down the possibility of permanent kidney damage by his or her body language and by saying that he or she has treated hundreds of patients without any problem. However, for another patient who has requested the same treatment, but for whom the doctor considers ciclosporin A inappropriate, he or she may use the very same potential adverse event as a "threat" to dissuade the patient.

Decision-analysis approaches to weighing up risks and benefits

Combining the values of treatment benefits versus risks for individual patients has been tackled using approaches such as decision analysis—a process in which the sequential choices faced by patents are made explicit.[24] Patients are then invited to place their own values on the various potential gains and losses. These methods have been used extensively in areas such as amniocentesis for detecting fetal abnormalities, but less so in dermatology.[25] Simplifications of a decision-analysis approach, such as the likelihood of being helped or harmed, have been advocated by others.[26]

What are the patient's values?

Values and belief models

Even if the external evidence suggests a good treatment for your patient, he or she might have a number of reasons for choosing or not choosing that treatment. For example, a teenager who consults you with acne, whose friend developed hepatitis whilst taking oxytetracycline, might initially refuse that treatment option. If that drug is really the best choice, the dermatologist can explain how rare such an event is and reach a joint decision with the patient. Another patient with acne might come demanding treatment with isotretinoin simply because his or her friend at school had similar treatment with excellent long-term results and tolerable side effects. Although such a declaration might influence the consultation, it does not automatically mean that the dermatologist will concede to such a request if he or she feels that the treatment is not in the patient's best interest (for example, very mild disease or a history of several unplanned pregnancies). Application of the best external evidence requires a dialogue with the patient in order to explore their values and expectations.

Patients sometimes prefer to use something that they perceive to be more "natural"—for example, evening primrose oil rather than synthetic topical corticosteroids for atopic eczema. Sometimes patients prefer to forgo pharmacological treatment and instead undertake various measures to manipulate their environment. Others just prefer to take a few pills and forget about it. Some like creams, others like ointments. Some people do not wish to be involved in lengthy discussions of treatment options if indeed they believe that their doctor is the best person to help them choose a treatment option. For example, a person with a basal cell carcinoma may be happy to be recommended surgical excision rather than debate the 10 or so treatment options available to treat such lesions.

These issues of personal perception, belief models, locus of control, and personal experience should be part of a consultation with the patient. Although patients' treatment choices may at times appear to be at odds with the external trial reports, patients are human beings who have their own sets of preferences and values, and these preferences need to be respected and understood.[27]

And if the treatment still does not work?

After agreeing on a treatment, a patient may return saying that the treatment does not work. After obvious issues have been explored, such as compliance and whether adverse events can be avoided (e.g., the presumed "allergic reaction" from topical benzoyl peroxide may be a predictable irritant reaction that could be circumvented by less frequent or vigorous application), other treatment options are often discussed. If several treatments fail in a particular patient, the patient may belong to a subset with refractory disease, making it even more difficult to generalize from clinical trials of people with more responsive forms of the disease. Dermatologists frequently face the problem of trying several drugs in succession. External trial evidence could be improved by better descriptions of study participants in terms of previous treatments, and by means of sequential RCTs that try different treatment approaches following failure of a treatment.

Conclusions

Applying evidence back to the patient is often the most difficult and neglected step in the practice of evidence-based dermatology. The question of how best to relate universals to the particular has always been the real doctor's dilemma. Clinical judgment is at the heart of this process.[28] This step requires consideration of several factors, including an appraisal of the magnitude and meaning of the treatment benefit and adverse events in relation to the patient's values and preferences. Presenting the evidence back to the patient is a complex process requiring good communication skills and an appreciation of the limitations of the generalizability of trial data in terms of trial participants, relevance, and size of benefits.

Having illustrated the chapter with examples of some of the difficulties in applying evidence to individual patients, I would like to close with an example of how easy and fruitful practicing evidence-based dermatology can be. I was recently called to see a young woman with cutaneous larva migrans that was causing intense itching on her feet. My first-line treatment would have been oral albendazole, probably because I had been involved in writing up a case series several years earlier.[29] I was just about to recommend it when I reminded myself to practice what I preached by conducting a search of Medline using the term "cutaneous larva migrans" as a sensitive text word search. To my sur-

prise, I quickly found a small but good RCT published in the *American Journal of Tropical Medicine and Hygiene* (not a journal I read every week) suggesting that a single 12-mg dose of ivermectin was more effective than albendazole.[30] And so ivermectin is what I recommended. The itching stopped within 24 hours and the visible eruption was cleared within a few days.

References

1 Mant D. Can randomised trials inform clinical decisions about individual patients? *Lancet* 1999;**353**:743–6.

2 Eypasch E. The individual patient and evidence-based medicine —a conflict? *Langenbecks Arch Surg* 1999;**384**:417–22.

3 Williams H. Dowling Oration 2001. Evidence-based dermatology —a bridge too far? *Clin Exp Dermatol* 2001;**26**:714–24.

4 Dans AL, Dans LF, Guyatt GH, Richardson S. Users' guides to the medical literature: XIV. How to decide on the applicability of clinical trial results to your patient. Evidence-Based Medicine Working Group. *JAMA* 1998;**279**:545–9.

5 Li Wan Po A. *Dictionary of Evidence-based Medicine*. Abingdon, UK: Radcliffe Medical Press, 1998: 52.

6 Roberts RJ, Casey D, Morgan DA, Petrovic M. Comparison of wet combing with malathion for treatment of head lice in the UK: a pragmatic randomised controlled trial. *Lancet* 2000;**356**:540–4.

7 Virag R. Indications and early results of sildenafil (Viagra) in erectile dysfunction. *Urology* 1999;**54**:1073–7.

8 Nikles CJ, Glasziou PP, Del Mar CB, Duggan CM, Mitchell G. N of 1 trials. Practical tools for medication management. *Aust Fam Physician* 2000;**29**:1108–12.

9 Lennard L. Therapeutic drug monitoring of cytotoxic drugs. *Br J Clin Pharmacol* 2001;**52**(Suppl 1):75S–87S.

10 Bakan D. The general and the aggregate: a methodological distinction. *Percept Mot Skills* 1955;**5**:211–2.

11 Straus SE, McAlister FA. Evidence-based medicine: a commentary on common criticisms. *Can Med Assoc J* 2000;**163**:837–41.

12 Hoare C, Li Wan Po A, Williams H. Systematic review of treatments for atopic eczema. *Health Technol Assess* 2000;**4**(37):1–191.

13 Charman C, Williams H. Outcome measures of disease severity in atopic eczema. *Arch Dermatol* 2000;**136**: 763–9.

14 Olsen EA. Topical minoxidil in the treatment of androgenetic alopecia in women. *Cutis* 1991;**48**:243–8.

15 Charman C, Williams HC. The problem of un-named scales for measuring atopic eczema. *J Invest Dermatol* [in press].

16 Marshall M, Lockwood A, Bradley C, Adams C, Joy C, Fenton M. Unpublished rating scales: a major source of bias in randomised controlled trials of treatments for schizophrenia. *Br J Psychiatry* 2000;**176**:249–52.

17 Cook RJ, Sackett DL. The number needed to treat: a clinically useful measure of treatment effect. *BMJ* 1995;**310**:452–4.

18 Devereaux PJ, Anderson DJ, Gardner MJ, *et al.* Differences between perspectives of physicians and patients on anticoagulation in patients with atrial fibrillation: an observational study. *BMJ* 2001;**323**:1218–22.

19 Hollis S, Campbell F. What is meant by intention to treat analysis? Survey of published randomised controlled trials. *BMJ* 1999;**319**: 670–4.

20 Eypasch E, Lefering R, Kum CK, Troidl H. Probability of adverse events that have not yet occurred: a statistical reminder. *BMJ* 1995;**311**:619–20.

21 Levine M, Whelan T. Decision-making process-communicating risk/benefits: is there an ideal technique? *J Natl Cancer Inst Monogr* 2001;**30**:143–5.

22 Paling J. Strategies to help patients understand risks. *BMJ* 2003;**327**:745–8.

23 [No authors listed.] On risk. *Bandolier* February 2006;144-3 (available at: http://www.jr2.ox.ac.uk/bandolier/band144/b144-3.html; accessed 12 March 2007).

24 Thornton JG, Lilford RJ, Johnson N. Decision analysis in medicine. *BMJ* 1992;**304**:1099–103.

25 Ashcroft DM, Li Wan Po A, Williams HC, Griffiths CE. Cost-effectiveness analysis of topical calcipotriol versus short-contact dithranol in the treatment of mild to moderate plaque psoriasis. *Pharmacoeconomics* 2000;**18**:469–76.

26 McAlister FA, Straus SE, Guyatt GH, Haynes RB. Users' guides to the medical literature: XX. Integrating research evidence with the care of the individual patient. Evidence-Based Medicine Working Group. *JAMA* 2000;**283**:2829–36.

27 Gibbs S. Losing touch with the healing art: dermatology and the decline of pastoral doctoring. *J Am Acad Dermatol* 2000;**43**:875–8.

28 Cook HJ. What stays constant at the heart of medicine. *BMJ*. 2006;**333**:1281–2.

29 Williams HC, Monk B. Creeping eruption stopped in its tracks by albendazole. *Clin Exp Derm* 1989;**14**:355–6.

30 Caumes E, Carriere J, Datry A, Gaxotte P, Danis M, Gentilini M. A randomized trial of ivermectin versus albendazole for the treatment of cutaneous larva migrans. *Am J Trop Med Hygiene* 1993;**49**:641–4.

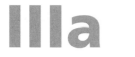

IIIa Common inflammatory skin diseases

Luigi Naldi, Editor

Additional chapters are published on the book's web site (http://www.evidbasedderm.com).

15   Acne vulgaris

Avanta P. Collier, Scott R. Freeman, Robert P. Dellavalle

Web tables referred to in this chapter are published on the book's web site (http://www.evidbasedderm.com).

Background

Definition

Acne vulgaris is a pervasive disease of the pilosebaceous follicles of the skin, which are located on the face, back, and chest. The disease has a range of clinical expression and can be classified according to the predominant lesion type:

• Noninflammatory or comedonal acne is primarily composed of open comedones (blackheads) and closed comedones (whiteheads), with little or no inflammatory involvement.

• Inflammatory acne is characterized by inflamed lesions (pustules, papules, and nodules) and can be further subdivided into papulopustular, nodular, and conglobate, depending on the predominant lesion type.

• Conglobate or nodulocystic acne is characterized by inflammatory lesions that have progressed to form abscesses or granulomas.[1] Acne fulminans is a severe form of conglobate acne.

Incidence/prevalence

Estimates of the overall prevalence vary considerably and depend on the study populations and epidemiological methodology used. The disease is defined by a continuum of severity, along which members of the adolescent population are placed; it is estimated that up to 30% of teenagers have acne of sufficient severity to warrant medical treatment.[1] An increasing number of women in their twenties develop late-onset acne, and surveys of adults over the age of 25 years have reported prevalences of 22% in males and 40% in females.[2,3]

Etiology/risk factors

Acne results from pathological changes in the pilosebaceous duct (PSD). Thickening of the follicular stratum corneum (hypercornification) leads to blockage and accumulation of sebum, which is produced in large quantities in response to the androgen surges that accompany puberty. The resident skin commensal bacterium, *Propionibacterium acnes*, proliferates in the lipid-rich sebaceous follicles, causing accumulation of bacterial metabolites, sebum, and dead cellular material. Follicular occlusion blocks discharge, and an inflammatory response ensues. The extent and duration of the inflammation, and hence the severity of the acne, may be determined by individual variation in the immune response to *P. acnes*. The onset of acne is associated with adrenarche, although androgen markers and mild comedonal acne have been detected in children under 10 years of age,[4,5] particularly in girls who have an earlier onset of puberty.[6] Although the overall incidence is roughly equal in both sexes, with the peak rates occurring at 17 years of age,[7] boys tend to have more severe disease.[8] There is no evidence that ethnic or racial differences influence the development of acne, although blacks have a higher incidence of disease.[9] Whilst genetic factors are also thought to influence susceptibility to acne,[10,11] the mode of inheritance has not been determined.

Prognosis

Most cases of adolescent acne clear spontaneously over time. There are, however, two common forms of postadolescent acne: persistent acne commences in adolescence, but does not resolve and is generally resistant to antibiotic therapy, and late-onset acne is generally less severe, evolves more commonly in women after 25 years of age, and has been linked to abnormalities in plasma androgens.[11,12]

The total burden of acne extends beyond financial costs; the impact on the individual can be devastating, as the disease occurs at an age when its effects are acutely felt. The cosmetic changes associated with acne have been linked to anxiety, depression, social isolation, and interpersonal difficulties.[13]

Aims of treatment

Treatment aims to alleviate symptoms and accelerate healing of lesions in the short term, and in the longer term to limit disease activity, scarring, and the impact of the disease on quality of life.

Treatment options are commonly classified according to route of delivery and mode of action. The comparative data on various therapies are limited and individual trials have obtained contradictory results, largely because of inadequate trial design and unfair comparisons in terms of dosage. Isotretinoin is the only acne treatment that can induce persistent remissions. All other acne treatments are palliative, and whilst improvement of symptoms and control of disease progression is possible, prolonged therapy is needed.

Relevant outcomes

Disease severity is assessed by a visual assessment of the number of lesions and extent of disease. Although numerous visual assessment methods of varying complexity exist, at the basic level they can be subdivided into grades or counts. In both cases, there are three levels at which assessment can be made:

1 An overall or "global" evaluation.
2 Subdivision according to the predominant morphological component (i.e., inflammatory or noninflammatory).
3 Separate evaluations of individual lesion type—for example, comedones, papules, and pustules.

The results are generally expressed as an absolute or percentage change from the onset of therapy and are commonly transformed to give the numbers of individuals attaining a given level of improvement—for example, 50%.

Other important outcomes include changes in quality of life, scarring, patient satisfaction, tolerability and adverse events, speed of action, and treatment-free interval.

Search methods

In the previous edition of this book, this chapter used a systematic review prepared for the Agency for Healthcare Research and Quality (AHRQ)[14] as the primary source of evidence, supplemented by evidence located by searches in the following databases: Cochrane Library (issue 1, 2002), Cochrane Skin Group Specialist Trial Register, Medline (1966 to February 2002), and Embase (1980 to February 2002). The updated chapter includes searches of each of these databases from 2002 to February 2006 for systematic reviews and randomized controlled trials.

Questions

Is there any evidence to support the routine use of skin cleansers and/or abrasives in the management of mild to moderate acne?

The impact of detergent bases on the control of sebum has not been ascertained, although it has been hypothesized that removal of sebum may enhance the activity of topically applied antibacterials. There is also controversy as to whether exfoliation using abrasives clears blocked PSDs and speeds up lesion healing, or whether associated irritancy and drying may aggravate inflamed skin. Antibacterial agents reduce surface bacteria, but there is little evidence to suggest that they penetrate the PSD.

Efficacy

The AHRQ review included four relevant RCTs,[15–17] and additional searches provided four individual trials and a review that included two RCTs.[18–22] Five of the studies were double-blinded (Table 15.1); only two studies enrolled more than 100 patients.

The largest RCT showed that an acidic soap-free syndet was less irritant than soap and reduced both inflamed lesions (ILs) and noninflamed lesions (NILs) in 120 patients with mild acne who were not taking any other anti-acne

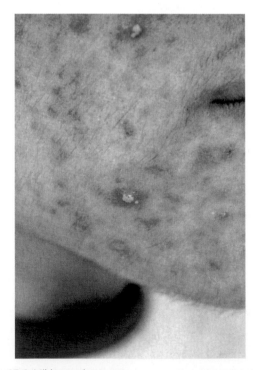

Figure 15.1 Mild to moderate acne.

Table 15.1 Randomized controlled trials of skin cleansers and abrasives

First author, ref.	Comparators	Patients (n)	Severity	Duration (weeks)	Blinding	Results	Comments
Bettley (1976)[15]	1. Hexachlorophene 2. Triclosan	34	1/2/3	6/6	0	No significant differences; drug improved: 21/28 vs. 22/28; local reaction: 11 vs. 9	6 LTF; not ITT; crossover study; no wash-out period
Fulghum (1982)[18]	1. Sulfur/salicylic acid cleanser with polyethylene granules 2. Sulfur/salicylic acid cleanser	53	1/2	8	0	Both reduced ILs and NILs; no significant differences; equal sensitivity	7 LTF; not ITT; split half-face study; no concomitant therapy
Kanof (1971, part 2)[19]	1. Antibacterial soap 2. Soap	51	3	>12	A, P	Flare 13/30 vs. 22/31	Tetracycline responders; no details on concomitant therapy
Kanof (1971, Part 1)[19]	1. Antibacterial soap 2. Soap	86	3	4	A, P	Response 30/44 v 31/42	All tetracycline 250 mg 2 or 3 times daily; no details on concomitant therapy; not ITT
Korting (1995)[16]	1. Acidic syndet bar 2. Soap	120	1	12	0	1 reduced ILs and NILs; 2 increased ILs and NILs; no intergroup comparison	2-week wash-out; 6 LTF; ITT analysis; soap 5 dropouts exacerbation; no concomitant therapy
Milikan (1976, A)[17]	1. Povidone–iodine cleanser 2. Vehicle	30	1	12–16	A, P	Improved 9/10 vs. 3/7; intolerance 1 = 2	13 LTF; not ITT
Milikan (1976, B)[17]	1. Povidone-iodine cleanser 2. Vehicle	30	2	12–16	A, P	10/13 vs. 12/14 improved; 0 intolerance	3 LTF; all tetracycline 250 mg 1 or 2 times daily
Stoughton (1987, A)[20]	1. Chlorhexidine gluconate cleanser 4% 2. Benzoyl peroxide 5%	50	2	12	A	No significant differences in ILs or NILs	3 LTF; not ITT; no concomitant therapy; twice-daily application
Stoughton (1987, B)[20]	1. Chlorhexidine gluconate cleanser 1.4% 2. Vehicle	110	2	12	A	1 > 2 ILs and NILs; dry skin: 3 vs. 1	17 LTF; not ITT; no concomitant therapy; twice-daily application
Millikan (1981)[240]	1. Buf-Puf 2. No abrasion	50	2	12	A	No intergroup comparisons; suggestion that abrasion better, but no data	2 LTF; not ITT; all patients received 5% benzoyl peroxide; split-face study
Subramanyan (2004)[21]	1. Benzamycin with or with out Differen + soap 2. Benzamycin with or without Differen + syndet bar	50	2	4	AP	Patients in soap group had increased rates of peeling, dryness Reduced scores for syndet group in itching, acne, and oiliness	
Subramanyan (2003)[23]	1. Current medications + mild cleansing lotion (Dove) 2. Current medications	25	1	4	AP	Significant reductions in NILs, ILs, erythema, dryness	

Table 15.1 *Cont'd*

First author, ref.	Comparators	Patients (n)	Severity	Duration (weeks)	Blinding	Results	Comments
Boutli (2003)[22]	1. Chloroxylenol 0.5% + salicylic acid 2% cream 2. BP 5% gel	37	1/2	12	AP	At week 12, both groups significant in ILs and NILs (60% and 54% for BP group and 56% and 56% for chloroxylenol + salicylic acid group)	Chloroxylenol + salicylic acid slightly stronger keratolytic activity. No difference in reduction of papules. Erythema and photosensitivity significantly lower in chloroxylenol + salicylic acid group

Severity: 1, mild; 2, moderate; 3, severe; blinding: 0, open; A, assessor; P, patient. BP, benzoyl peroxide; LTF, lost to follow-up; ITT, intention-to-treat; ILs, inflamed lesions; NILs, noninflamed lesions.

medication.[16] There were no significant differences between the groups, although the individuals using soap experienced a mean increase in both NILs and ILs over 12 weeks and 23 of 57 experienced irritation, compared with one of 57 in the soap-free group. Similar results were also obtained in more recent studies.[21] A double-blind RCT included 50 patients with moderate acne currently using topical Benzamycin (benzoyl peroxide) or Benzamycin plus adapalene.[23] After 4 weeks of additional treatment with soap or a mild syndet bar, patients using soap had more peeling, dryness, and irritation, whereas those using syndet soap had no significant changes in skin irritation. The mild cleanser was more effective in reducing the severity scores of negative characteristics such as acne, itching, and oiliness. Another RCT included 25 acne patients using prescription medications (topical antibiotics, tretinoin, or benzoyl peroxide) who were instructed to use a mild cleansing lotion while also continuing current therapy.[24] After 4 weeks of cleansing lotion use, patients had significant decreases in the number of inflammatory and noninflammatory lesions. These results demonstrate the compatibility between mild cleansing lotions and these various treatment options.

Cleansers containing the antibacterial hexachlorophene produced improvement in equivalent numbers of patients to triclosan in a 12-week crossover trial with 34 patients,[15] although no wash-out period was permitted. Eleven patients experienced local reactions to triclosan and nine to hexachlorophene; hexachlorophene is now not recommended. Chlorhexidine was shown to produce equivalent significant reductions in NILs and ILs in 50 patients with moderate acne in comparison with 5% benzoyl peroxide at 12 weeks. It also produced significantly greater reductions in ILs and NILs than in those treated with the vehicle alone in 110 individuals, again at 12 weeks.[20] Chloroxylenol 0.5% in combination with 2% salicylic acid was as effective as 5%

benzoyl peroxide in reducing NILs and ILs in 37 patients with mild to moderate acne when applied to the face twice a day.[22] Patients in the combination group experienced significantly less erythema and photosensitivity than those using benzoyl peroxide.

In individuals treated with tetracycline, 500 mg twice daily, additional use of antibacterial soap in a 4-week period offered no benefit over the use of normal soap. However, it was shown to significantly reduce the incidence of acne flare in responders to 4-week tetracycline therapy in a 90-day follow-up (13/30 flared vs. 22/31).[19]

After 12–14 weeks in a double-blind RCT, povidone–iodine skin cleanser led to improvement in nine of 10 patients with mild acne, compared with three of seven in the vehicle group. The results are invalidated, however, by the high losses to follow-up.[17] The results in a second group of patients with more severe acne who also received tetracycline, 250 mg once or twice daily, were equivocal (10/13 compared with 12/14).[17] Only one case of mild itching was experienced.

The addition of abrasives to a combination of sulfur and salicylic acid in a split-half-face study in 44 patients did not show any difference in either efficacy or tolerability after 8 weeks. The potential for the effects of the active ingredients to mask all other effects must be considered.[18] One split-face study evaluated the use of additional abrasion to 5% benzoyl peroxide therapy, but there were no intergroup comparisons to validate the authors' claim that the side of the face treated with abrasion showed better results.[25]

Adverse effects

Soaps are of alkaline pH and are known irritants, causing itching, dryness, and redness; acidic soap-free cleansers may therefore be preferable. Aggressive use of abrasives may irritate skin, and for that reason common sense suggests that they should not be used in conjunction with topical agents such as benzoyl peroxide, which sensitize the skin, unless tolerance has initially been demonstrated. Dermatological reactions are idiosyncratic and cannot be predicted, and the patient should be advised to discontinue use immediately if irritation develops. Like any topical agent, it is possible that antibacterial cleansers and abrasives are less suitable in individuals with sensitive skin. The literature does not support a link between the use of topical antimicrobials and the emergence of antiseptic or antibiotic resistance.[26]

Comment

The number of propionibacteria on the skin surface is increased by soap and decreased by synthetic detergents.[27] This may be due to the changes in skin pH, which is increased by soap.[27] There is no evidence either for or against the use of abrasive agents, either alone or in combination with topical treatments. There is evidence to suggest that antibacterial skin cleansers may be effective in the management of mild acne,[17] and may produce similar outcomes to benzoyl peroxide in moderate acne.[20] However, the long-term benefits of "step-up" management strategies versus aggressive therapy from onset have not been examined. There is no evidence that antibacterial cleansers offer additional benefits when used in conjunction with oral antibiotics in individuals with more severe acne, but they may help maintain improvement following the termination of antibiotic therapy.[19] The impact of increased contact time during washing has not been examined.

Implications for clinical practice

In individuals with mild acne whose disease is not adversely affecting their quality of life, antibacterial washes should be considered in the choice of first-line management strategies in step-up approaches. They should also be considered in the maintenance of patients who have ceased therapy following response. They should not be prescribed routinely in patients who are receiving more aggressive therapy, as there is no evidence of any additional benefit. Alkaline syndet bars may be preferable to soap in skin care routines.

What is the role of topical nonantibiotic agents in the treatment of mild primarily noninflammatory acne?

Mild acne consisting of open and closed comedones with a few inflammatory lesions is commonly treated with topical agents. A number of options have been effective in placebo-controlled RCTs, and all can be used either alone or in combination. Options include the topical retinoids (isotretinoin, tretinoin, adapalene, and tazarotene), benzoyl peroxide, salicylic acid, and azelaic acid.

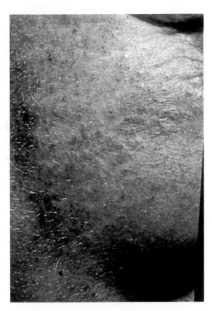

Figure 15.2 Noninflammatory lesions (reproduced by kind permission of Dr Carolyn Charman).

Topical retinoids

Topical retinoids reduce abnormal growth and development of keratinocytes within the PSD. This inhibits microcomedo formation and therefore subsequently reduces the number of comedones and inflamed lesions.

Efficacy

Evidence for the efficacy of topical retinoids was available from two systematic reviews,[14,28] which examined 20 RCTs and split-face studies.[29–47] Fourteen further studies were located through searching[48,49] (web table 15.1). Focusing only on comparisons that had at least two RCTs of acceptable quality showing moderate to strong statistical evidence, the authors of the AHRQ review concluded that 0.1% adapalene and 0.025% tretinoin were equally efficacious and that motretinide and tretinoin were equally effective. The second review[28] evaluated five RCTs of 0.1% adapalene gel versus 0.025% tretinoin.[33–35,38,50] All RCTs were investigator-blind, and a total of 900 individuals with mild to moderate acne were enrolled. Using data collected from intention-to-treat (ITT) analyses, equivalent efficacy against total lesion counts was demonstrated, with adapalene showing greater activity at 1 week.

Of the RCTs that presented data,[33,34,37,38,50–54] mean percentage reductions in NILs ranged from 36% to 88% in the 0.1% adapalene group, from 33% to 83% in the 0.025% tretinoin group, and 50% to 86.9% in the 0.05% tretinoin and isotretinoin groups at 12 weeks. Percentage reductions in ILs were 35–69% and 38–71%, respectively. Higher-strength adapalene (0.5%) was investigated in one 25-patient split-face study and was shown to have greater activity than

0.1% adapalene against both ILs and NILs, but was associated with more erythema.[49] Two strengths of adapalene (0.1% and 0.03%) were evaluated in five studies enrolling a total of 1053 patients with mild to severe acne.[32,33,53,54,55] The higher strength produced greater reductions in IL and NIL counts, but was associated with more irritation in some studies, whereas others showed similar rates of erythema.

Topical tazarotene is more effective than other topical retinoids, including adapalene and tretinoin, in the treatment of mild to moderate acne. An RCT compared daily-use tazarotene 0.1% gel with daily 0.1% tretinoin in 169 patients. Tazarotene was more cost-effective and was associated with greater reduction of NILs.[56] Both regimens were well tolerated. A meta-analysis of data from six multicenter, double-blind RCTs included data on 688 patients who used tazarotene 0.1% gel or cream once daily for 12 weeks. Tazarotene was effective and well tolerated, regardless of the patients' acne severity, skin type, sex, or ethnicity.[57] One RCT comparing 0.1% tazarotene to 0.1% adapalene showed mean NIL reductions of 68% in the tazarotene group and 36% in the adapalene group at 12 weeks.[58] The percentage reductions in ILs were 62% and 50%, respectively. Another study compared tazarotene monotherapy with three tazarotene combination therapies and clindamycin monotherapy in 440 patients with mild to moderate acne. Tazarotene alone was as effective in reducing NILs as tazarotene in combination with the erythromycin–benzoyl peroxide combination and clindamycin.[59] All tazarotene-containing regimens were more effective than clindamycin alone. For ILs, tazarotene plus erythromycin–benzoyl peroxide combination therapy was significantly more effective than all other treatments. Twice-daily use of tazarotene appeared more effective than once-daily use or vehicle alone in patients with mild to moderate acne,[60] with similar pharmacokinetics in patients with acne or photodamaged skin.[61]

Few comparative data for retinoids against other agents were found. In 77 patients with mild to moderate acne, 0.05% isotretinoin applied twice daily was slightly less effective than 5% benzoyl peroxide against ILs and NILs and was slower to resolve ILs.[46] The results for tretinoin against benzoyl peroxide[62–64] were equivocal, and there were no differences in the rate of adverse events. Another study compared topical adapalene with 4% benzoyl peroxide in 178 patients with mild to moderate acne.[65] Adapalene was more effective against both NILs and ILs at 11 weeks, with no significant adverse events noted in either treatment group.

Adverse effects

Topical retinoids induce local reactions and should be discontinued if the reaction is severe. All studies presenting data suggested that 0.1% adapalene causes less local irritation than 0.025% tretinoin[49] and that the rate of local reactions with both agents increases with concentration.[32,33,49,55,66]

Retinoids increase the sensitivity of skin to ultraviolet light and should therefore be applied at night and washed off in the morning. Rarely, eye irritation, edema, and blistering of the skin occur, and hypopigmentation may result from tretinoin use.

Comment

There remains uncertainty as to whether retinoids applied topically cause birth defects, and whilst minimal absorption has been demonstrated following topical application,[67] it is recommended that they should not be used during pregnancy or by women of childbearing age who are not taking adequate contraceptive precautions.

Implications for practice

The comedolytic action of topical retinoids suggests that they should be used in the treatment of mild acne. However, as this activity halts subsequent lesion formation, they are also suitable for moderate to severe acne and can be used in conjunction with topical and oral antibiotics. Benzoyl peroxide inactivates tretinoin, so the two agents should not be applied simultaneously; if used in combination, one should be applied in the morning and one at night. All topical retinoids cause local sensitivity reactions, which are less common with adapalene. To limit local sensitivity, topical retinoid therapy should start at a lower strength, be applied every third night, and increase gradually.

Benzoyl peroxide

The lipid solubility of benzoyl peroxide allows it to penetrate the PSD. It has comedolytic, anti-inflammatory and bactericidal activity and is therefore suitable for management of individuals with mild inflammatory or mixed acne. It can be bought over the counter from pharmacies and is available in a number of formulations, in strengths of 2.5–10.0%.

Efficacy

The AHRQ systematic review[14] examined seven placebo-controlled RCTs in patients with mild to severe acne[46,68–73] (web table 15.2). Changes in both NILs and ILs were consistently significantly superior in the active group. Two RCTs reported mean reductions in lesion counts with 5% benzoyl peroxide: 52% and 60% for ILs and 30% and 52% for NILs.[46,70] The reductions in the vehicle comparator arms were less than 10% in each case. Four RCTs compared different dosages of benzoyl peroxide,[62,68,74] and no evidence was found to support a dose–response effect (Table 15.2).

Three RCTs compared topical tretinoin with 5% benzoyl peroxide.[63,64,75] Tretinoin was more effective against NILs up to 12 weeks, but benzoyl peroxide had a greater impact on ILs. Compared with topical 0.05% isotretinoin, 5% benzoyl peroxide had a greater effect on ILs at 8 weeks but not 12 weeks, and a similar effect on NILs at all time points

Table 15.2 Benzoyl peroxide (BP) dose response randomized controlled trials

First author, ref.	Comparators	Patients (n)	Severity	Duration (weeks)	Blinding	Outcomes	Comments
Mills (1986, 2)[68]	1. BP 2.5% 2. BP 5%	53	1/2	8	P, A	Equivalent efficacy and burning, peeling and erythema; ILs: 56% vs. 58% reduction	2 LTF; not clear if randomized
Mills (1986, 3)[68]	1. BP 10% 2. BP 2.5%	50	1/2	8	P, A	Equivalent efficacy but 10% more burning, erythema and peeling. ILs: 45% vs. 47% reduction	No LTF; not clear if randomized
Yong (1979)[74]	1. BP 2.5% 2. BP 5%	200	1/2/3	4–18	0	> 50% reduction in lesion counts 64/96 vs. 74/98 (no SSD); erythema 45 vs. 50; desquamation 22 vs. 28; itching/burning 16 vs. 10; no SSD overall	Variable duration of treatment
Handojo (1979)[62]	1. Tretinoin 0.05% 2. BP 5% 3. BP 10% 4. Tretinoin 0.05%/BP 5% 5. Tretinoin 0.05%/BP 10%	250	1/2/3	10	0	Overall change greater in 5% combination group; rate of local intolerance 20% in both groups, but greater in 10% group; > 50% reduction in NILs: 34/47 vs. 37/45 vs. 33/47 vs. 45/50 vs. 44/50; > 50% reduction in ILs: 27/36 vs. 34/42 vs. 28/41 vs. 34/44 vs. 39/49; no SSD between BP concentrations	11 LTF; not ITT; 47 patients reactions
Marsden (1985)[212]	1. BP 5% 2. BP 5%/0.5 g OT 3. BP 5%/1 g OT 4. BP 5%/1.5 g OT	82	1/2/3	16	A	Patient adequate response: 2/23 vs. 6/24 vs. 8/19 vs. 12/17; 10 BP patients local intolerance; ILs: 56 vs. 70 vs. 75% vs. 78% reduction	Assume randomized but not stated; previous failure to treatment; 10 LTF; not ITT
Fyrand (1986)[241]	1. BP 5% (alcohol) 2. BP 5% (water)	48	–	8	P, A	No difference in clinical effect, but less irritation with water-based preparation	Abstract only

Severity: 1, mild; 2, moderate; 3, severe; blinding: 0, open; A, assessor; P, patient. BP, benzoyl peroxide; LTF, lost to follow-up; ITT, intention-to-treat; ILs, inflamed lesions; NILs, noninflamed lesions; SSD, statistically significant difference.

in 77 patients with mild to moderate acne;[46] 5% benzoyl peroxide has similar efficacy to 20% azelaic acid in mild acne.[76] A fourth trial compared 0.1% tretinoin alone with 0.1% tretinoin in combination with 6% benzoyl peroxide treatment in 56 patients and showed significant reductions in total lesions counts for the combination group after 12 weeks of treatment.[77]

Adverse effects

Benzoyl peroxide is commonly associated with local irritation that presents as erythema, peeling, dryness, burning, stinging, itching, and soreness. Use of an emollient or water-based gel may reduce these reactions. Allergic contact dermatitis, characterized by erythema, small papules, and pruritus, may occur rarely. RCT evidence shows that the side-effect profile of a 2.5% preparation is similar to that of 5%[68,74] and less than 10% preparations.[68] Combinations of benzoyl peroxide with antibiotics are unstable because of degradation of the antibiotic by benzoyl peroxide. Benzoyl peroxide will bleach hair and fabrics, and patients should therefore be counseled accordingly. It is safe for use during pregnancy. There were concerns that benzoyl

Table 15.3 Randomized controlled trials of salicylic acid

First author, ref.	Comparators	Patients (n)	Severity	Duration (weeks)	Blinding	NIL	IL	Outcomes	Comments
Shalita (1981)[83]	1. Salicylic acid 2% cleanser 2. BP 10% wash	30	2 + 2	1/2	0 20	34		No side effects reported	Crossover; no wash-out period; no LTF; results not valid as phase 1 only 2 weeks and no wash-out period; BP group higher NIL count at baseline; short contact
Eady (1996)[66]	1. Salicylic acid 2% 2. Vehicle	114	12	1/2	2	46* 26	28* 9	1 > 2 all lesions; irritant dermatitis both groups but greater incidence in 1; % decrease total lesions: 40 vs. 16*	15 LTF; not ITT; both in alcoholic lotion
Roth (1964)[84]	1. Salicylic acid 1.5% 2. Placebo	30	10	1/2	0			Salicylic acid reported as greater reduction, but no intergroup comparison; burning in 10/15 in salicylic acid group	

Severity: 1, mild; 2, moderate; 3, severe; blinding: 0, open; A, assessor; P, patient; BP, benzoyl peroxide; LTF, lost to follow-up; ITT, intention-to-treat; ILs, inflamed lesions; NILs, noninflamed lesions; *, statistically significantly superior ($P < 0.05$).

peroxide might promote skin cancer,[78,79] but these have been refuted.[80]

Comment

A major concern with the continued use of antibiotics, topical and oral, is the promotion of *P. acnes* resistance. Benzoyl peroxide has a broad-spectrum bactericidal action, which does not select for resistance during long-term use. It is therefore recommended that it is used intermittently during courses of antibiotics, to eliminate any resistant propionibacteria.[81,82]

Implications for practice

Benzoyl peroxide is an effective treatment for mild to moderate acne vulgaris, as a result of its activity against both ILs and NILs. Some individuals find benzoyl peroxide highly irritating on initial application. Tolerance is generally developed with prolonged exposure, and individuals should be counseled accordingly. Low-strength benzoyl peroxide is recommended, as higher strengths are more irritant and there is no evidence to suggest that 10% in general is more effective than 5%. It is common practice for patients to apply benzoyl peroxide to individual lesions alone; clinicians should advise patients to apply it in a thin layer to all areas to prevent the formation of new lesions.

Salicylic acid

Salicylic acid is an exfoliant and chemical irritant.

Efficacy

The AHRQ review[14] located three RCTs (Table 15.3).[82–84] Two percent salicylic acid was more effective in reducing all lesion types than the alcoholic lotion vehicle at 12 weeks in 114 paired individuals with mild to moderate acne.[82] The second study enrolled 30 individuals and had major losses to follow-up;[84] 1.5% salicylic acid was more beneficial than placebo. One further crossover RCT in 30 individuals with mild acne compared a 2% cleanser with a 10% benzoyl peroxide facial wash; neither product was therefore in prolonged contact with the skin.[83] The results of the study cannot be considered as valid evidence, however, because the trial was only 4 weeks in total and there was no wash-out period between the 2-week treatment periods.

Adverse effects

Salicylic acid is known to cause skin irritation that presents as erythema, dryness, and peeling; this was evident in the RCT evidence located.

Implications for practice

There is no evidence to support the routine use of salicylic acid in preference to other topical therapies.

Azelaic acid

Azelaic acid has been shown to normalize the increased keratinocyte production and keratinization associated with acne and to inhibit *P. acnes*.[85] A direct anti-inflammatory effect has also been demonstrated.[86]

Efficacy

The AHRQ review[14] located eight RCTs of azelaic acid in mild to moderate acne (web table 15.3). The comparators used were placebo,[87] vehicle,[88] benzoyl peroxide,[75] tretinoin,[88] oral tetracycline,[89,90] and in combination with glycolic acid versus tretinoin.[91] One further RCT published in German evaluated its efficacy against 2% erythromycin.[92,93]

In papulopustular acne, 20% azelaic acid has similar efficacy at 5 or 6 months to 0.05% tretinoin,[88] 5% benzoyl peroxide,[76] 2% topical erythromycin,[93] and oral tetracycline 1 g/day,[89,90] with consistent percentage reductions in median ILs of 80–84%. Across the studies, good to excellent improvement occurred in 71–82% of individuals. In comedonal acne, 20% azelaic acid had similar activity to 0.05% topical isotretinoin, with 79% and 82% reductions in comedonal counts, respectively, and good or excellent improvement in 59% and 63% of the 289 patients at 6 months.[88]

Adverse effects

In common with other topical agents, azelaic acid induces cutaneous reactions, which occur in approximately one-third of individuals.[93] The incidence is highest in the first 4 weeks of therapy and, in the RCTs examined, only 5–10% of reactions were categorized as "marked." In the clinical studies, which also included post-marketing evaluations, 0–5% of individuals experienced scaling, 5–23% burning, and 13–29% itching. Azelaic acid is not known to cause photosensitivity, and sublethal doses do not promote *P. acnes* resistance.[94] Azelaic acid is better tolerated than benzoyl peroxide[76] and tretinoin,[88,91] and it does not bleach clothing or hair. It is used in hyperpigmentary skin disorders, but has not been shown to have depigmentatory effects in acne patients,[94] suggesting that it preferentially targets abnormal melanocytes.

Comments

There are no known incompatibilities between azelaic acid and other topical anti-acne agents.

Implications for practice

Azelaic acid is an effective therapy for mild to moderate papulopustular acne and as effective as 0.05% isotretinoin in comedonal acne. The onset of action is slower than that seen with benzoyl peroxide. Patients should be counseled to expect a delayed response. Anecdotal reports have suggested that azelaic acid may reduce the incidence of postinflammatory hyperpigmentation, which is possibly attributable to its activity on abnormal melanocytes.[95]

Darker-skinned patients should be monitored for signs of hypopigmentation.

Summary

All of the agents reviewed are effective in the treatment of mild and moderate acne vulgaris. There are very few data to support the use of one agent over another, and there has only been one RCT on the use of the agents in combination, which showed that benzoyl peroxide and tretinoin in combination are superior to either agent alone.[62] Adapalene is better tolerated than tretinoin, and the RCT evidence reviewed suggests that azelaic acid may be better tolerated overall than other agents, but there will be considerable variation between individual patients. A number of RCTs compare these agents against and in combination with topical antibiotics; these are considered in the next section.

What is the role of antibiotics in the management of acne vulgaris?

The role of antibiotics in the management of acne is still debated, and although much evidence has been collected on the efficacy of individual agents, there are very few good-quality comparative data. Oral antibiotics were used initially in the 1950s because it was assumed that acne occurred as a result of bacterial infection. Whilst activity against *P. acnes* has been clearly demonstrated, there is evidence of an anti-inflammatory effect,[96] which is still being investigated.

Three systematic reviews provided evidence on the role of antibiotics.[14,97,98] The conclusions of the AHRQ review are based only on comparisons, where there are at least two trials of acceptable quality showing moderate to strong statistical evidence for a clinically meaningful end point and effect. Of the oral antibiotics, the only clear evidence was located for tetracycline. Topical clindamycin and erythromycin were superior to vehicle in the treatment of mild to moderate acne, and topical tetracycline was ineffective. The Cochrane review[97] of minocycline examined 27 RCTs and concluded that while minocycline is likely to produce similar outcomes to other first-generation and second-generation tetracyclines, it should not be used as a firstline agent, because of uncertainty over its safety and higher cost in comparison with older tetracyclines. There was no evidence to suggest that it is superior to other tetracyclines, and its efficacy relative to other acne therapies could not be reliably determined because of inadequacies in the studies examined. The third systematic review[98] evaluated all randomized and nonrandomized clinical trials (n = 45) investigating topical therapy with erythromycin or clindamycin alone for inflammatory acne. A significant decrease in the treatment effect of topical erythromycin occurred over time, suggesting the development of antibiotic resistance.

Oral antibiotics

The AHRQ report reviewed 11 placebo-controlled trials of oral antibiotics,[99–109] and five others were located by searches[110–114] (web table 15.4). All but five RCTs investigated tetracycline; one evaluated minocycline, two doxycycline,[115] one roxithromycin,[112] and one lymecycline.[113] All were double-blinded, and most included patients with moderate to severe acne. Only five provided data at 12 weeks or more,[102,105,106,113,114] and only four included more than 50 patients in each arm.[106,108,110,113] Tetracycline at total daily doses of 500 mg and 1 g was consistently superior to placebo in terms of overall grade and reduction in ILs. Lymecycline 150 mg b.i.d. and lymecycline 300 mg q.o.d. were equally efficacious in the treatment of moderate to severe acne, and both were superior to placebo at all points during a 12-week study[113] A small RCT (n = 46) reported a significant decrease in median acne scores in comparison with placebo in patients taking roxithromycin 150 mg b.i.d. during the 10-week study. Data on NILs were from two doxycycline RCTs.[114,115] One reported comparable efficacy[115] at 4 weeks, but this is expected, given the delayed onset of activity associated with oral antibiotics. A second RCT designed to evaluate subantimicrobial dosing of doxycycline (20 mg b.i.d.) showed statistically significant decreases in combined IL and NIL counts, comedones, and total lesion counts at 6 months.[114]

Nine head-to-head RCTs of the currently used oral antibiotics were included in the AHRQ review;[116–124] the Cochrane review located a further nine,[125–133] and further search located two additional studies[134,135] (web table 15.5). The majority of the trials had problems with design and execution. No oral antibiotic was demonstrated to be superior to any other, although equivalence cannot be conclusively stated, as none of the studies was adequately powered to demonstrate it. Percentage reductions in ILs were consistently greater than 50% at 12 weeks. Percentage reductions in NILs were more variable, with only three RCTs reporting more than 50% reductions at 12 weeks.[130,133,135] The results consistently showed an improvement in 70–90% of individuals at 12 weeks.

Topical antibiotics

The AHRQ review located 31 RCTs comparing a topical antibiotic with its vehicle, and a further eight RCTs were located by independent searches (web table 15.6). Nine of the RCTs also included other comparators. The antibiotics investigated were clindamycin (13 RCTs),[73,107,108,136–145] erythromycin (14 RCTs),[146–154] erythromycin/zinc (three RCTs),[109,155,156] 2% fusidic acid (two RCTs),[157,158] meclocycline,[159] metronidazole,[160] triclosan,[161] and tetracycline (three RCTs).[104–106] Among the studies for which details were available, all but two used twice-daily application.[73,145] Many of the studies were underpowered to conclusively state that there were no significant differences between the compar-

ators. A systematic review[98] designed to assess the efficacy of the topical antibiotics erythromycin and clindamycin over time included 45 studies; 22 double-blind intention-to-treat studies, 10 placebo-controlled trials, 12 single-blind trials and one open, randomized trial. The duration of treatment in the trials included varied between 8 and 12 weeks for erythromycin and between 8 and 16 weeks for clindamycin, with 12 weeks being most common for both medications. Erythromycin concentrations varied in studies from 1.5% to 4% (most common concentrations were 1.5% and 2%), while clindamycin concentrations remained stable during the analysis period at between 1% and 1.2%. Comparisons of studies longitudinally only included trials using the same antibiotic dosage.

The AHRQ review concluded that although clindamycin tended to produce greater reductions in ILs than its vehicle, the results were rarely statistically significant; global measures more consistently indicated superiority to placebo. The evidence available does not support the effectiveness of clindamycin against NILs. Erythromycin similarly had a greater impact on ILs. A 12-week study of clindamycin 1% foam vs. clindamycin 1% gel applied once daily also included vehicle comparators.[145] This study reported a statistically significant advantage in total lesions, ILs, and NILs with foam over gel and superior efficacy in comparison with the vehicle. A 24-week study of 2% erythromycin gel versus vehicle, designed primarily to detect bacterial resistance to treatment over time,[154] found no difference in acne outcomes at any point during the study. Highly resistant erythromycin-specific susceptibility profiles were found among patients randomly assigned to the erythromycin treatment arm. Fusidic acid was more active than vehicle against ILs at 6 weeks in one study, but not at 12 weeks in a second study, which also did not show any difference in its activity against NILs. The two meclocycline studies also showed decreases in ILs, with no data for NILs. The 0.75% metronidazole RCT showed that it was no more active than placebo in mild to moderate acne, producing statistically significant reductions in neither ILs or NILs. The three tetracycline RCTs demonstrated that 0.5% tetracycline was approximately 50% more active than vehicle in terms of change in acne grade from baseline, although no intergroup statistical analyses were performed. Only one trial provided data on differential lesion counts; the results suggested again that tetracycline was active against ILs but not NILs. In the larger RCTs, a 55–60% mean reduction in ILs was consistently seen at 12 weeks.[14]

The AHRQ review located 14 head-to-head trials of topical antibiotics, and further search yielded four additional RCTs (web table 15.7). There were no differences in efficacy between clindamycin hydrochloride and phosphate,[139,140,144] or between different formulations[143,162,163] in the six RCTs examined in the AHRQ. Clindamycin 1% foam was superior to clindamycin 1% gel for total lesions and IL and NIL outcomes at 12 weeks.[145] Two additional RCTs reported no difference between clindamycin formulations.[164,165] Four large RCTs[156,166-168] and one smaller study[169] compared clindamycin and erythromycin; all enrolled subjects had mild to severe acne. Several of the trials reported differences between the topical antibiotics for certain outcomes at certain time points, but there were no consistent differences overall. In comparison with tetracycline of unspecified concentration, the two located studies[170,171] reported insignificant or inconsistent differences in lesion counts. However, both trials demonstrated a significant difference in favor of clindamycin in the overall measures of acne severity or improvement. No difference between clindamycin and nicotinamide was shown in the RCT located, but it was underpowered to conclusively state equivalence.[172] An additional 12-week RCT[173] compared a 2% topical azithromycin preparation to 2% topical erythromycin. Comparable decreases in inflammatory lesions counts were seen in both groups, though the study included only 19 patients in the acne treatment arm and no placebo group.

One systematic review[98] longitudinally evaluated RCTs comparing treatment efficacies of erythromycin vs. clindamycin. This study concluded that while topical erythromycin remains a viable option in the treatment of acne, a significant decrease in the effect of topical erythromycin over time (1974–2002) has occurred. The efficacy of topical clindamycin remained stable during the study period (1976–2003).

Oral versus topical antibiotics

The two systematic reviews located also provided comparative data on the use of oral versus topical antibiotics.[14,97] A number of other nonsystematic reviews and individual RCTs were also located, giving a total of 21 studies,[150,174-187] six of which also included a placebo control arm[104-109] (web table 15.8). Twelve used double-dummy designs to maintain blinding. Oral antibiotics have a delayed onset of activity; studies of shorter duration may therefore be biased in favor of the topical agent.

The evidence from three RCTs suggests that minocycline, 50 mg twice daily, produces results against both NILs and ILs that are comparable with 1% clindamycin applied twice daily.[180-182] All but one trial[187] enrolled fewer than 100 patients, and they were therefore underpowered to conclusively state equivalence.

Six RCTs compared oral tetracycline 250 mg twice daily with 1% clindamycin twice daily.[107,108,150,174-176] Only one RCT was longer than 8 weeks in duration,[176] and only one study was adequately powered (305 patients), but it was of inadequate duration.[108] This study found that at 8 weeks, there was no significant difference in the percentage reductions obtained with either tetracycline 250 mg twice daily or 1% clindamycin applied twice daily in pustules (68% versus 76%) and papules (63% versus 68%) in patients with moderate to severe acne. However, the physician rated the clindamycin therapy as good to excellent in a greater number of cases—86 of 105 in comparison with 66 of 103 ($P < 0.05$). Four of the other studies failed to detect any significant differences between the therapies, with the fifth finding that clindamycin caused significantly greater percentage reductions in ILs (57% versus 72%; $P < 0.001$) at 8 weeks in patients with mild acne.[107] The 12-week study found no difference.[176]

Tetracycline, 250 mg twice daily, produced similar changes in lesion counts at 12 weeks to topically applied 1.5% erythromycin in a single RCT of 54 patients with moderate to severe acne.[179] Although erythromycin produced greater percentage changes numerically, these were not significant. None of the four RCTs located found any differences in overall grade between oral tetracycline, 250 mg twice daily, and topically applied 1.5% meclocycline twice daily; both were superior to placebo in the three studies that also used a placebo control.[178] None of the studies used ITT analysis. At 8–12 weeks, oral tetracycline 250 mg twice daily was found to produce similar reductions in overall grade to topical 0.5% tetracycline, with one trial finding no effect on comedones.[104-106]

Combination therapy

A number of RCTs have investigated oral and topical antibiotics either against or in combination with other agents (web table 15.9), the rationale for this being that treatments that attack more than one factor implicated in the pathogenesis of acne will be more effective. The different mechanisms of action are summarized in Table 15.4.[188]

Efficacy

Two RCTs were located that compared an oral antibiotic with benzyl peroxide.[185,187] Although one study was underpowered to conclusively state equivalence, similar efficacy was found between 5% benzyl peroxide and oral oxytetracycline, 250 mg twice daily, at 6 weeks.[186] The oral agent was more effective against acne of the trunk. A large (n = 649) randomized 18-week study compared five antibacterial regimens: oxytetracycline plus topical placebo; oral Monocline (doxycycline) plus topical placebo; topical benzyl peroxide plus oral placebo; topical erythromycin and benzyl peroxide combination plus oral placebo; and topical erythromycin and benzyl peroxide separately plus oral placebo.[187] Topical benzyl peroxide and benzyl peroxide–erythromycin combinations showed similar efficacy to oral oxytetracycline and minocycline. The AHRQ review located eight RCTs that compared topical antibiotics with 5% benzoyl peroxide, and searches found one additional trial.[73,153,185,189-193] In the three RCTs located, 5% benzoyl peroxide was found more active against NILs in moderate acne than 1% clindamycin[73,189,190] over 10–12 weeks. Two

Table 15.4 Targets of acne therapies (adapted from Gollnick[188])

	Sebum excretion	Keratinization	Follicular *Propionibacterium acnes*	Inflammation
Benzoyl peroxide	–	(+)	+++	(+)
Tretinoin	–	++	(+)	–
Clindamycin	–	–	++	–
Antiandrogens	++	–	–	–
Azelaic acid	–	++	++	+
Tetracyclines	–	–	++	+
Erythromycin	–	–	++	–
Isotretinoin	+++	++	(+)	++

studies also found that it was more active against ILs,[189,190] although the third found no difference.[73] Benzoyl peroxide was also more active against both NILs and ILs than 1% meclocycline.[192] Compared with erythromycin, benzoyl peroxide was more active against NILs and similarly active against ILs.[153,191] All RCTs providing data showed that benzoyl peroxide caused more local irritation.

Three RCTs compared 20% azelaic acid with oral tetracycline (variable dose)[89,90] in patients with mild to severe acne. No significant differences were reported in any lesion counts, except in the smallest trial, which was very small and suffered from high drop-out rates in the azelaic acid group. A 20-week RCT of 20% azelaic acid in comparison with 2% topical erythromycin was located through additional searches.[92] No differences between the comparators were found.

Use of combination therapies

Ten RCTs were located that examined combinations of 0.025% tretinoin and 1% clindamycin against either tretinoin,[194] clindamycin,[194,195] or both[196–198] (web table 15.10). One additional RCT compared 2% erythromycin/0.05% tretinoin against both agents individually.[199] Numerically, the combination produced greater mean percentage reductions in NILs than either agent alone, but the only statistically significant results were against clindamycin in two studies.[194,195] Against ILs, the combination showed greater activity numerically than either agent, but it reached significance only against tretinoin.[194] One study reported similar efficacy and improved tolerability of clindamycin–benzoyl peroxide in comparison with clindamycin–benzoyl peroxide applied in the morning plus tretinoin and clindamycin applied in the evening.[198]

Four trials compared 0.1% adapalene plus antibiotic combinations to antibiotic alone.[200–203] In the first trial of 242 patients with moderate to severe acne, adapalene plus 300 mg of lymecycline showed a greater reduction in NILs

and ILs at 12 weeks than lymecycline plus vehicle. Side-effect profiles were similar for both treatment groups.[200] The second trial included 467 patients with severe acne who were randomly assigned to either the adapalene plus doxycycline group or doxycycline treatment alone for 12 weeks. Percentage reductions in NILs were 60 and 41% respectively.[201] There was also a greater reduction in the combination group for ILs (65% vs. 59%). Both treatments were well tolerated. The third and fourth trials compared the efficacy of clindamycin alone and in combination with adapalene in a total of 549 patients with mild to moderate acne.[202,203] Both trials showed significant reductions in NILs and ILs in the combination group by week 12. The fourth trial also demonstrated a significant reduction in all lesion counts during the maintenance phase in patients receiving adapalene (42%) in comparison with an increase for all lesion counts in the control group (92.1%). A fifth trial that compared a retinoid in combination with an antibiotic with 5% benzoyl peroxide in combination with 3% erythromycin in 188 patients with mild to moderate acne showed comparable efficacy after 12 weeks.[204]

A trial that compared a hydrogen peroxide cream and 0.1% adapalene gel combination with a benzoyl peroxide cream and adapalene gel combination showed equivalent reductions in NILs.[205] Significant reductions in ILs and better tolerability were noted for the hydrogen peroxide plus adapalene group at week 8 in patients with mild to moderate acne. The use of adapalene and benzoyl peroxide alone and in combination reduced NILs and ILs at 24 weeks, with no significant differences in erythema, dryness, or burning.

Combinations of antibiotics and benzoyl peroxide were examined in 11 RCTs (web table 15.11); the antibiotics were clindamycin,[73,189,206] erythromycin,[153,207–210] meclocycline,[192] and metronidazole.[193] In the six studies that used an antibiotic alone as a comparator, the combination was more active against both ILs and NILs.[73,153,189,206,207] Six studies used benzoyl peroxide alone as a comparator.[73,153,189,192,193,210]

The data were equivocal, with some studies showing a greater effect for the combination and others showing no difference. Combinations of 5% benzoyl peroxide with 3% erythromycin have greater activity against *P. acnes* than 3% erythromycin and result in significantly greater clinical improvement.[82] One study[211] included 327 patients with moderate to severe acne who were randomly assigned to four treatment groups (single-use combination of erythromycin–benzoyl peroxide package, vehicle control package, original reconstituted erythromycin–benzoyl peroxide combination packaged in a jar, and matching vehicle control in a jar) and showed that the new formulation was comparable to the original jar formulation in reducing acne lesions, in the physicians' global acne severity scores, and in the end-of-treatment patient evaluation of global improvement. The results of this 8-week trial demonstrate that this new single-use erythromycin–benzoyl peroxide formulation has promise for improving the convenience of using the combination product. Refrigeration is no longer required and patients can mix the two gels included in the single-use package, thus eliminating the need for the pharmacist to compound the two medications. Another study compared 5% benzoyl peroxide plus 2% metronidazole against an oral antibiotic (oxytetracycline), but because it was of only 6 weeks' duration, it unfairly biased the results against the oral antibiotic.[193] A 16-week study was the only one that compared concomitant use of 5% benzoyl peroxide with an oral antibiotic (oxytetracycline 0.5 g, 1 g, and 1.5 g), but it did not clearly state whether patients were randomly allocated to treatment.[212] The response was considered adequate in two of 23 patients with 5% benzoyl peroxide alone and in six of 24, eight of 19, and 12 of 17 patients using 5% benzoyl peroxide plus oxytetracycline 0.5 g, 1 g, and 1.5 g, respectively.

Harms

All antibiotics are associated with individual side effects that are well documented and must be considered. The potential systemic side effects are theoretically reduced by topical application, as usually less than 10% absorption occurs.[213] However, prolonged and extensive application to the skin, which is a good medium for gene exchange amongst bacteria,[214] may facilitate the spread of resistance.[215] This has implications for clinical practice, as *P. acnes* resistance is associated with a poor therapeutic response to antibiotics and the efficacy of some antibiotics is decreasing over time. Of greater importance, however, is the spread of resistance to other microorganisms, and there have been calls for policies to restrict the prescribing of antibiotics in acne.[81,216] One systematic review examined *P. acnes* resistance to systemic antibiotics.[217] The 12 articles examined demonstrated an overall increase in *P. acnes* resistance, from 20% in 1978 to 62% in 1996. Resistance was most commonly reported to erythromycin, clindamycin, tetracycline,

doxycycline, and trimethoprim; resistance to minocycline was rare. The authors concluded that long-term rotational antibiotics are inappropriate and that treatment should be adjusted when therapeutic failure becomes evident. Antibiotic–benzoyl peroxide combination therapies can be useful, as these regimens were not affected by *P. acnes* antibiotic resistance.[187]

Comment

A proportion of individuals fail to respond to antibiotics; epidemiological studies have estimated that the figure is between 10%[218] and 17%[219] of individuals. Theories that have been proposed include individual differences in the absorption, distribution, and elimination of the antibiotic, as well as poor compliance, the follicular microenvironment, and *P. acnes* resistance.[218] The underlying severity of the disease may also determine the response to antibiotics, as severe acne and acne of the trunk have been shown to respond less well than moderate acne,[220,221] possibly as a result of the higher sebum excretion rate[222] diluting follicular drug concentrations.[218] Clinically, another important impact of alteration in cutaneous microflora is the possibility of Gram-negative folliculitis developing, which presents with profuse superficial pustules around the nose and deep cystic lesions on the face and neck, usually colonized by *Proteus, Enterobacter.* or *Klebsiella* species.[223]

Implications for practice

There is no conclusive evidence of the superiority of one antibiotic over another, nor of any advantages for either oral or topical application. The choice of agent should therefore be based on the patient's preference, with consideration of the individual side effects of the antibiotics and the cost. The formulation of the topical antibiotic may also be important—for example, alcohol bases are likely to be more drying and therefore more suitable for oilier skins. Patients with more extensive disease, particularly those with acne of the trunk, may prefer oral treatment rather than having to apply topical agents to extensive areas. It is vital that patients should be properly counseled on how to use their medication, as inappropriate use has been shown to reduce effectiveness.[212]

Second-generation tetracyclines—such as minocycline, doxycycline, and lymecycline—have been described as being more active, because their greater lipophilicity results in greater sebum penetration and PSD concentration. This review has not found any evidence to support this, and their superiority has not been demonstrated. These agents are easier for patients to take, however, as they can be taken once daily and the absorption may be less affected by food.[224–226] However, tetracycline need not be taken four times a day: its half-life of approximately 9 hours in plasma is likely increased in the skin. Furthermore, subantimicrobial doses of doxycycline may be as effective as standard dosages. Maintaining serum antibiotic concentrations at steady state does not appear necessary for clinical efficacy or moderating anti-inflammatory effects.

It is recognized that antibiotics have less activity than other agents against NILs, which makes them less suitable for use in patients with primarily noninflammatory acne. The evidence for the comparative efficacy of antibiotics and benzoyl peroxide against ILs is equivocal, and further research is required to establish their relative place in acne therapy. The studies reviewed found that combinations of antibiotics with benzoyl peroxide were more effective than antibiotics alone, which can probably be attributed in part to the lack of activity of antibiotics against NILs. However, the irritancy of benzoyl peroxide may make it unacceptable to some patients. There is no compelling evidence for the combined use of antibiotics and retinoids. There is no benefit in concomitant use of oral and topical antibiotics, and this practice may select for resistant strains. Intermittent use of benzoyl peroxide is recommended during extended antibiotic therapy, to eliminate any resistant strains.[227]

What dose of oral antibiotics should be prescribed?

Historically, antibiotics have been used for the treatment of acne vulgaris at doses that are lower than those used for other infections. Although the exact origin and rationale of this convention is not known, the most likely explanation is that doses were reduced initially in response to concerns over maintaining patients on high-dose antibiotics for long periods of time. When it was subsequently observed that lesions did not recur when the dose was reduced and that patients relapsed as soon as therapy was discontinued, dose reduction would have become standard practice.[228] Low doses of antibiotics were therefore used in early trials.[102,111,229,230] Guidelines recommended that full antibiotic doses should be used initially for 3–4 weeks and then reduced gradually until the patient can be maintained on the lowest possible dose.[231,232] Despite the fact that there are no adequate dose–response studies to support it, this use of low-dose antibiotics has remained standard practice for many years.

Only three RCTs were located that investigated the use of different doses of antibiotics. One study failed to find any clinical difference after 8 weeks of therapy between patients maintained on an initial starting dose of minocycline 100 mg daily and those in whom the initial dosage was reduced to 50 mg daily after 4 weeks.[233] Minocycline may not be typical of all antibiotics, however, because there is considerable variation between individuals in the serum levels attained after oral administration.[234] Eight weeks may also be an inadequate period to examine comparative efficacy. In the second study, roxithromycin 300 mg was more effective

than 150 mg over 8 weeks in 30 patients with severe acne.[235] A third study evaluated subantimicrobial doses of doxycycline (20 mg b.i.d.) in comparison with placebo for 6 months and found statistically significant decreases in combined IL and NIL counts, total lesion counts, and comedones in patients randomly assigned to doxycycline.[114] Other evidence located included a series of nonrandomized studies in 420 individuals with moderate to severe acne. In a nonrandomized controlled study of 152 patients matched for age, sex, site of involvement, and severity, those maintained on erythromycin, 1 g daily, and 5% benzoyl peroxide showed a significantly greater response in comparison with those receiving 0.5 g and 5% benzoyl peroxide. The improvements in acne grade at 6 months were 35% and 79% in men and 59% and 79% in women. The relapse rates within 1 year were also significantly lower in the high-dose group: 31% versus 60% in women and 82% versus 39% in men. A similar group of 296 patients did not show higher rates of gastrointestinal side effects at the higher dose.[220] Individuals with severe acne, acne of the trunk, and high sebum excretion rates responded less well to combined treatment with 5% benzoyl peroxide and erythromycin 250 mg twice daily over 6 months.[220]

There are also reports in the literature that higher daily doses of tetracycline[236] and oxytetracycline[212] are more effective in patients with severe acne or acne that is recalcitrant to standard therapy. The results of these studies are questionable, however, as both have serious methodological flaws and used concomitant topical therapy. A cohort of 80 patients with nodulocystic and conglobate acne who had not responded to standard antibiotic doses showed improvement with 1.5–3.0 g tetracycline.[237] A second similar cohort of 31 patients with severe acne or acne resistant to standard-dose antibiotics received up to 3.5 g with concomitant topicals, and 27 of the patients showed great improvement. Fifteen individuals suffered adverse events and two had to discontinue therapy because of raised serum creatinine phosphokinase, emphasizing the need for ongoing renal and hepatic monitoring. The onset of improvement ranged from 1 to 6 months. Flare occurred in nine patients on reduced dose, despite the use of topicals.[236]

A prospective case series of 68 patients with moderate to "cystic" acne, in whom the dose was titrated according to the response, found that in a period of up to 2.5 years, 51 of the 58 patients who improved required only 250 mg tetracycline daily.[230] Increased severity of acne was an indicator for higher dose and nonresponse. In 10 cases, tetracycline had no effect, regardless of dose.

For how long should antibiotic therapy be continued?

This question was not addressed in either of the systematic reviews, and no specific RCT evidence was located. The literature contains a number of recommendations, few of which are backed by hard evidence. The consensus of opinion is that although the effects of antibiotics on inflammatory lesions are visible after a few days, a minimum of 3 weeks is required before any improvement can be categorically stated,[106,232] and therapy should therefore be continued for a minimum of 3 months, and 6 months for maximum benefit.[1] As antibiotics do not expel existing comedones, the effect on these lesions only becomes evident after a few months of continual use; it takes approximately 8 weeks for a microcomedo to develop into a visible lesion. Relapse occurs in nearly half of the patients up to 8 weeks after stopping therapy,[238] necessitating additional courses.[219] In patients who relapse immediately, the antibiotic used should be rotated every 6 months.[239] Two RCTs that included intermediate assessments showed that improvement continued beyond 4–6 weeks to 3 months.[102,120]

An observational cohort study of 543 patients with moderate acne who were treated with erythromycin, 1 g/day, combined with 5% benzoyl peroxide suggested that the median percentage improvement at 6 months was 78% (interquartile range 67–90%); 408 of 492 individuals showed an over 50% reduction in acne grade; 247 of 279 who continued with benzoyl peroxide alone maintained improvement; 174 individuals who continued with combination for a further 6 months showed no additional benefit, but this group also included a subgroup of responders, nonresponders, and those switched to alternative antibiotics. Therapy was continued in 31 patients who had not shown 50% improvement within the 6-month period; the percentage improvement was greater in the 29 individuals treated with minocycline.

Key points

- Antibacterial washes should be considered in the first-line management of mild acne and in the maintenance of individuals who have improved following other therapy. They should not be used routinely in conjunction with other therapies. There is no evidence to support the use of abrasives, which may further irritate already sensitized skin. Alkaline syndet bars are less irritant than soap for cleansing.

- Topical retinoids can be used in both noninflammatory and inflammatory acne and in conjunction with oral and topical antibiotics. The evidence suggests that adapalene is less irritant than other retinoids.

- Azelaic acid is effective in mild to moderate acne and may be less irritant than topical retinoids, but has a slower onset of response.

- Benzoyl peroxide is an effective treatment in mild to moderate acne, but causes an initial sensitization that may persist in some individuals. Higher-strength benzoyl peroxide is in general no more effective than at lower strength, but is associated with more irritation.

- Antibiotics are more effective against inflamed lesions than noninflamed lesions. There is no evidence to support a difference in efficacy between any of the agents, either oral or topical, although topical therapies are more cost-effective.

- There is no good-quality evidence to support recommendations about either the dose or duration of antibiotic therapy; further research is needed.

- Benzoyl peroxide appears to have similar activity to antibiotics against inflamed lesions and greater activity against noninflamed lesions, but causes local irritation. The evidence suggests that combined use of antibiotics with retinoids is more active than either agent alone, and whilst benzoyl peroxide combinations are more effective than antibiotics alone, the data against benzoyl peroxide alone are equivocal.

- Given concerns about the development of resistance, further research is urgently required to assess the efficacy of antibiotics relative to other agents and to provide data for an appropriate assessment of the risks and benefits associated with their continued use. Benzoyl peroxide should be used intermittently during extended antibiotic therapy to eliminate any resistant strains.

References

1 Cunliffe WJ. *Acne*. London: Dunitz, 1989.

2 Newton JN, Edwards C. Epidemiology and treatment of acne in primary care. *J Eur Acad Dermatol Venereol* 1997;**9**(Suppl 1):S81.

3 Poli F, Dreno B, Verschoore M. An epidemiological study of acne in female adults: results of a survey conducted in France. *J Eur Acad Dermatol Venereol* 2001;**15**:541–5.

4 Lucky AW, Biro FM, Huster GA, Leach AD, Morrison JA, Ratterman J. Acne vulgaris in premenarchal girls: an early sign of puberty associated with rising levels of dehydroepiandrosterone. *Arch Dermatol* 1994;**130**:308–14.

5 Lucky AW, Biro FM, Simbarti LA, Morrison JA, Sorg NW. Predictors of severity of acne vulgaris in young adolescent girls: results of a five-year longitudinal study. *J Pediatr* 1997;**130**:30–9.

6 Stewart ME, Downing DT, Cook JS, Hansen JR, Strauss JS. Sebaceous gland activity and serum dehydroepiandrosterone sulfate levels in boys and girls. *Arch Dermatol* 1992;**128**:1345–8.

7 Burton JL, Cunliffe WJ, Stafford I, Shuster S. The prevalence of acne vulgaris in adolescence. *Br J Dermatol* 1971;**85**:119–26.

8 Cunliffe WJ, Gould DJ. Prevalence of facial acne vulgaris in late adolescence and in adults. *BMJ* 1979;**i**:1109–10.

9 Siemens HW. [The treatment and control of patients with acne; in German]. *Münch Med Wochenschr* 1965;**107**:1652–5.

10 Walton S, Wyatt R, Cunliffe WJ. Genetic control of sebum excretion and acne: a twin study. *Br J Dermatol* 1988;**18**:393–6.

11 Goulden V, McGeown CH, Cunliffe WJ. The familial risk of adult acne: a comparison between first-degree relatives of affected and unaffected individuals. *Br J Dermatol* 1999;**141**:297–300.

12 Goulden V, Clark SM, Cunliffe WJ. Post-adolescent acne: a review of clinical features. *Br J Dermatol* 1997;**136**:66–70.

13 Layton, AM. A review on the treatment of acne vulgaris. *Int J Clin Pract* 2006;**60**:64–72.

14 Lehmann HP, Andrews JS, Robinson KA, *et al. Management of Acne*. Rockville, MD: Agency for Healthcare Research and

Quality, 2001. (Evidence Report/Technology Assessment, 17; AHRQ publication no. 01–E019).

15 Bettley FR, Dale TL. The local treatment of acne. *Br J Clin Pract* 1976;**30**:67–9.

16 Korting HC, Ponce-Poschl E, Klovekorn W, Schmotzer G, Arens-Corell M, Braun-Falco O. The influence of the regular use of a soap or an acidic syndet bar on pre-acne. *Infection* 1995;**23**:89–93.

17 Milikan LE. A double-blind study of Betadine skin cleanser in acne vulgaris. *Cutis* 1976;**17**:394–8.

18 Fulghum DD, Catalano PM, Childers RC, Cullen SI, Engel MF. Abrasive cleansing in the management of acne vulgaris. *Arch Dermatol* 1982;**118**:658–9.

19 Kanof NB. Acne control with an antibacterial soap bar: a double-blind study. *Cutis* 1971;**7**:57–61.

20 Stoughton RB, Leyden JJ. Efficacy of 4 percent chlorhexidine gluconate skin cleanser in the treatment of acne vulgaris. *Cutis* 1987;**39**:551–3.

21 Subramanyan K. Role of mild cleansing in the management of patient skin. *Dermatol Ther* 2004;**17**:26–34.

22 Boutli F, Zioga M, Koussidou T, Ioannides D, Mourellou O. Comparison of chloroxylenol 0.5% plus salicylic acid 2% cream and benzoyl peroxide 5% gel in the treatment of acne vulgaris: a randomized double-blind study. *Drugs Exp Clin Res* 2003;**29**:101–5.

23 Subramanyan K, Johnson AW. Role of mild cleansing in the management of sensitive skin. [Poster presented at the American Academy of Dermatology 61st Annual Meeting, San Francisco, March 21–26, 2003.]

24 Data on file, Unilever HPC NA, September 2003.

25 Millikan LE, Ameln R. Use of Buf-Puf and benzoyl peroxide in the treatment of acne. *Cutis* 1981;**28**:201–5.

26 Vaughan Jones SA, Hern S, Black MM. Neutrophil folliculitis and serum androgen levels. *Clin Exp Dermatol* 1999;**24**:392–5.

27 Korting HC, Kober M, Mueller M, Braun-Falco O. Influence of repeated washings with soap and synthetic detergents on pH and resident flora of the skin of forehead and forearm. *Acta Derm Venereol* 1987;**67**:41–7.

28 Cunliffe WJ, Poncet M, Loesche C, Verschoore M. A comparison of the efficacy and tolerability of adapalene 0.1% gel versus tretinoin 0.025% gel in patients with acne vulgaris: a meta-analysis of five randomized trials. *Br J Dermatol* 1998;**139**(Suppl 52):48–56.

29 Caron D, Sorba V, Kerrouche N, Clucas A. Split-face comparison of adapalene 0.1% gel and tretinoin 0.025% gel in acne patients. *J Am Acad Dermatol* 1997;**36**(6 Pt 2):S110–2.

30 Dunlap FE, Mills OH, Tuley MR, Baker MD, Plott RT. Adapalene 0.1% gel for the treatment of acne vulgaris: its superiority compared to tretinoin 0.025% cream in skin tolerance and patient preference. *Br J Dermatol* 1998;**139**(Suppl 52):17–22.

31 Galvin SA, Gilbert R, Baker M, Guibal F, Tuley MR. Comparative tolerance of adapalene 0.1% gel and six different tretinoin formulations. *Br J Dermatol* 1998;**139**(Suppl 52):34–40.

32 Verschoore M, Langner A, Wolska H, Jablonska S, Czernielewski J, Schaefer H. Efficacy and safety of CD 271 alcoholic gels in the topical treatment of acne vulgaris. *Br J Dermatol* 1991;**124**:368–71.

33 Alirezai M, Meynadier J, Jablonska S, Czernielewski J, Verschoore M. [Comparative study of the efficacy and tolerability of 0.1 and 0.03 p.100 adapalene gel and 0·025 p.100 tretinoin gel in the treatment of acne; in French.] *Ann Dermatol Venereol* 1996;**123**:165–70.

34 Grosshans E, Marks R, Mascaro JM, *et al.* Evaluation of clinical efficacy and safety of adapalene 0.1% gel versus tretinoin 0.025% gel in the treatment of acne vulgaris, with particular reference to the onset of action and impact on quality of life. *Br J Dermatol* 1998;**139**(Suppl 52):26–33.

35 Berger RS, Griffin E, Jones L, *et al.* Clinical safety and efficacy evaluation of 0.1% CD271 gel versus 0.025% Retin A gel and CD271 gel vehicle. 2002. [Unpublished data, CIRD Galderma.]

36 Clucas A, Verschoore M, Sorba V, Poncet M, Baker M, Czernielewski J. Adapalene 0.1% gel is better tolerated than tretinoin 0.025% gel in acne patients. *J Am Acad Dermatol* 1997;**36**(6 Pt 2):S116–18.

37 Ellis CN, Millikan LE, Smith EB, *et al.* Comparison of adapalene 0.1% solution and tretinoin 0.025% gel in the topical treatment of acne vulgaris. *Br J Dermatol* 1998;**139**(Suppl 35):41–7.

38 Shalita A, Weiss JS, Chalker DK, *et al.* A comparison of the efficacy and safety of adapalene gel 0.1% and tretinoin gel 0.025% in the treatment of acne vulgaris: a multicenter trial. *J Am Acad Dermatol* 1996;**34**:482–5.

39 Christiansen JV, Gadborg E, Ludvigsen K, *et al.* Topical vitamin A acid (Airol) and systemic oxytetracycline in the treatment of acne vulgaris: a controlled clinical trial. *Dermatologica* 1974;**149**:121–8.

40 Krishnan G. Comparison of two concentrations of tretinoin solution in the topical treatment of acne vulgaris. *Practitioner* 1976;**216**:106–9.

41 Schafer-Korting M, Korting HC, Ponce-Poschl E. Liposomal tretinoin for uncomplicated acne vulgaris. *Clin Invest* 1994;**72**:1086–91.

42 Dominguez J, Hojyo MT, Celayo JL, Dominguez-Soto L, Teixeira F. Topical isotretinoin vs. topical retinoic acid in the treatment of acne vulgaris. *Int J Dermatol* 1998;**37**:54–5.

43 Elbaum DJ. Comparison of the stability of topical isotretinoin and topical tretinoin and their efficacy in acne. *J Am Acad Dermatol* 1988;**19**:486–91.

44 Christiansen J, Holm P, Reymann F. Treatment of acne vulgaris with the retinoic acid derivative Ro 11–1430: a controlled clinical trial against retinoic acid. *Dermatologica* 1976;**153**:172–6.

45 Christiansen J, Holm P, Reymann F. The retinoic acid derivative Ro 11–1430 in Acne vulgaris: a controlled multicenter trial against retinoic acid. *Dermatologica* 1977;**154**:219–27.

46 Hughes BR, Norris JF, Cunliffe WJ. A double-blind evaluation of topical isotretinoin 0·05%, benzoyl peroxide gel 5% and placebo in patients with acne. *Clin Exp Dermatol* 1992;**17**:165–8.

47 Nordin K, Fredriksson T, Rylander C. Ro 11–1430, a new retinoic acid derivative for the topical treatment of acne. *Dermatologica* 1981;**162**:104–11.

48 Shalita AR, Chalker DK, Griffith RF, *et al.* Tazarotene gel is safe and effective in the treatment of acne vulgaris: a multicenter, double-blind, vehicle-controlled study. *Cutis* 1999;**63**:349–54.

49 Pierard-Franchimont C, Henry F, Fraiture AL, Fumal I, Pierard GE. Split-face clinical and bio-instrumental comparison of 0.1% adapalene and 0·05% tretinoin in facial acne. *Dermatology* 1999;**198**:218–22.

50 Cunliffe WJ, Caputo R, Dreno B, *et al.* Efficacy and safety comparison of adapalene (CD271) gel and tretinoin gel in the topical

treatment of acne vulgaris: a European multicentre trial. *J Dermatolog Treat* 1997;**8**:173–8.

51 Thiboutot D, Pariser DM, Egan N, et al. Adapalene gel 0.3% for the treatment of acne vulgaris: a multicenter, randomized, double-blind, controlled, phase III trial. *J Am Acad Dermatol* 2006;**54**:242–50.

52 Ioannides D, Rigopoulos D, Katsambas A. Topical adapalene gel 0.1% vs. isotretinoin gel 0.05% in the treatment of acne vulgaris: a randomized open-label clinical trial. *Br J Dermatol* 2002;**147**:523–7.

53 Cunliffe WJ, Danby FW, Dunlap F, Gold MH, Gratton D, Greenspan A. Randomised, controlled trial of the efficacy and safety of adapalene gel 0.1% and tretinoin cream 0.05% in patients with acne vulgaris. *Eur J Dermatol* 2002;**12**:350–4.

54 Pariser DM, Thiboutot DM, Clark SD, et al. The efficacy and safety of adapalene gel 0.3% in the treatment of acne vulgaris: a randomized, multicenter, investigator-blinded, controlled comparison study versus adapalene gel 0.1% and vehicle. *Cutis* 2005;**76**:145–51.

55 Dunlap FE, Baker MD, Plott RT, Verschoore M. Adapalene 0.1% gel has low skin irritation potential even when applied immediately after washing. *Br J Dermatol* 1998;**139**(Suppl 35):23–5.

56 Leyden JJ, Tanghetti EA, Miller B, Ung M, Berson D, Lee J. Once-daily tazarotene 0.1% gel versus once-daily tretinoin 0.1% microsponge gel for the treatment of facial acne vulgaris: a double-blind randomized trial. *Cutis* 2002;**69**(2 Suppl):12–9.

57 Leyden JJ. Meta-analysis of topical tazarotene in the treatment of mild to moderate acne. *Cutis* 2004;**74**(Suppl 4):9–15.

58 Shalita A, Miller B, Menter A, Abramovits W, Loven K, Kakita L. Tazarotene cream versus adapalene cream in the treatment of facial acne vulgaris: a multicenter, double-blind, randomized, parallel-group study. *J Drugs Dermatol* 2005;**4**(2):153–8.

59 Draelos ZD, Tanghetti EA, Tazarotene Combination Leads to Efficacious Acne Results (CLEAR) Trial Study Group. Optimizing the use of tazarotene for the treatment of facial acne vulgaris through combination therapy. *Cutis* 2002;**69**(2 Suppl):20–9.

60 Bershad S, Kranjac Singer G, Parente JE, Tan MH, Sherer DW, Persaud AN, Lebwohl M. Successful treatment of acne vulgaris using a new method: results of a randomized vehicle-controlled trial of short-contact therapy with 0.1% tazarotene gel. *Arch Dermatol* 2002;**138**:481–9.

61 Yu Z, Sefton J, Lew-Kaya DA, Walker PS, Yu D, Tang-Liu DDS. Pharmacokinetics of tazarotene cream 0.1% after a single dose and after repeat topical applications at clinical or exaggerated application rates in patients with acne vulgaris or photodamaged skin. *Clin Pharmacokinet* 2003;**42**:921–9.

62 Handojo I. The combined use of topical benzoyl peroxide and tretinoin in the treatment of acne vulgaris. *Int J Dermatol* 1979;**18**:489–96.

63 Lyons RE. Comparative effectiveness of benzoyl peroxide and tretinoin in acne vulgaris. *Int J Dermatol* 1978;**17**:246–51.

64 Bucknall JH, Murdoch PN. Comparison of tretinoin solution and benzoyl peroxide lotion in the treatment of acne vulgaris. *Curr Med Res Opin* 1977;**5**:266–8.

65 Do Nascimento LV, Guedes ACM, Magalhaes GM, De Faria FA, Guerra RM, Almeida FDC. Single-blind and comparative clinical study of the efficacy and safety of benzoyl peroxide 4% gel (BID) and adapalene 0.1% Gel (QD) in the treatment of acne vulgaris for 11 weeks. *J Dermatolog Treat* 2003;**14**:166–71.

66 Christiansen JV, Gadborg E, Ludvigsen K, et al. Topical tretinoin, vitamin A acid (Airol) in acne vulgaris: a controlled clinical trial. *Dermatologica* 1974;**148**:82–9.

67 Van Hoogdalem EJ, Baven TL, Spiegel-Melsen I, Terpstra IJ. Transdermal absorption of clindamycin and tretinoin from topically applied anti-acne formulations in man. *Biopharm Drug Dispos* 1998;**19**:563–9.

68 Mills OH Jr, Kligman AM, Pochi P, Comite H. Comparing 2.5%, 5%, and 10% benzoyl peroxide on inflammatory acne vulgaris. *Int J Dermatol* 1986;**25**:664–7.

69 Smith EB, Padilla RS, McCabe JM, Becker LE. Benzoyl peroxide lotion (20%) in acne. *Cutis* 1980;**25**:90–2.

70 Hunt MJ, Barnetson RS. A comparative study of gluconolactone versus benzoyl peroxide in the treatment of acne. *Australas J Dermatol* 1992;**33**:131–4.

71 Jaffe GV, Grimshaw JJ, Constad D. Benzoyl peroxide in the treatment of acne vulgaris: a double-blind, multi-centre comparative study of "Quinoderm" cream and "Quinoderm" cream with hydrocortisone versus their base vehicle alone and a benzoyl peroxide only gel preparation. *Curr Med Res Opin* 1989;**11**:453–62.

72 Ede M. A double-blind, comparative study of benzoyl peroxide, benzoyl peroxide–chlorhydroxyquinoline, benzoyl peroxide-chlorhydroxyquinoline–hydrocortisone, and placebo lotions in acne. *Curr Ther Res Clin Exp* 1973;**15**:624–9.

73 Lookingbill DP, Chalker DK, Lindholm JS, et al. Treatment of acne with a combination clindamycin/benzoyl peroxide gel compared with clindamycin gel, benzoyl peroxide gel and vehicle gel: combined results of two double-blind investigations. *J Am Acad Dermatol* 1997;**37**:590–5.

74 Yong CC. Benzoyl peroxide gel therapy in acne in Singapore. *Int J Dermatol* 1979;**18**:485–8.

75 Handojo I. Retinoic acid cream (Airol cream) and benzoyl-peroxide in the treatment of acne vulgaris. *Southeast Asian J Trop Med Public Health* 1979;**10**:548–51.

76 Cavicchini S, Caputo R. Long-term treatment of acne with 20% azelaic acid cream. *Acta Derm Venereol Suppl* 1989;**143**:40–4.

77 Shalita AR, Rafal ES, Anderson DN, Yavel R, Landow S, Lee WL. Compared efficacy and safety of tretinoin 0.1% microsphere gel alone and in combination with benzoyl peroxide 6% cleanser for the treatment of acne vulgaris. *Cutis* 2003;**72**:167–72.

78 Cartwright RA, Hughes BR, Cunliffe WJ. Malignant melanoma, benzoyl peroxide and acne: a pilot epidemiological case-control investigation. *Br J Dermatol* 1988;**118**:239–42.

79 Liden S, Lindelof B, Sparen P. Is benzoyl peroxide carcinogenic? *Br J Dermatol* 1990;**123**:129.

80 Kraus AL, Munro IC, Orr JC, Binder RL, LeBoeuf RA, Williams GM. Benzoyl peroxide: an integrated human safety assessment for carcinogenicity. *Regul Toxicol Pharmacol* 1995;**21**:87–107.

81 Eady EA, Jones CE, Tipper JL, et al. Antibiotic resistant propionibacteria in acne: need for policies to modify antibiotic usage. *BMJ* 1993;**306**:555–6.

82 Eady EA, Bojar RA, Jones CE, Cove JH, Holland KT, Cunliffe WJ. The effects of acne treatment with a combination of benzoyl peroxide and erythromycin on skin carriage of erythromycin-resistant propionibacteria. *Br J Dermatol* 1996;**134**:107–13.

83 Shalita AR. Treatment of mild and moderate acne vulgaris with salicylic acid in an alcohol-detergent vehicle. *Cutis* 1981;**28**:556–8.

84 Roth HL. Acne vulgaris: evaluation of a medicated cleansing pad. *Calif Med* 1964;**100**:167.

85 Gibson JR. Azelaic acid 20% cream (Azelex) and the medical management of acne vulgaris. *Dermatol Nurs* 1997;**9**:339–44.

86 Kurokawa I, Akamatsu H, Nishijima S, Asada Y, Kawabata S. Clinical and bacteriologic evaluation of OPC-7251 in patients with acne: a double-blind group comparison study versus cream base. *J Am Acad Dermatol* 1991;**25**:674–81.

87 Cunliffe WJ, Holland KT. Clinical and laboratory studies on treatment with 20% azelaic acid cream for acne. *Acta Derm Venereol Suppl* 1989;**143**:31–4.

88 Katsambas A, Graupe K, Stratigos J. Clinical studies of 20% azelaic acid cream in the treatment of acne vulgaris: comparison with vehicle and topical tretinoin. *Acta Derm Venereol Suppl* 1989;**143**:35–9.

89 Bladon PT, Burke BM, Cunliffe WJ, Forster RA, Holland KT, King K. Topical azelaic acid and the treatment of acne: a clinical and laboratory comparison with oral tetracycline. *Br J Dermatol* 1986;**114**:493–9.

90 Hjorth N, Graupe K. Azelaic acid for the treatment of acne: a clinical comparison with oral tetracycline. *Acta Derm Venereol Suppl* 1989;**143**:45–8.

91 Spellman MC, Pincus SH. Efficacy and safety of azelaic acid and glycolic acid combination therapy compared with tretinoin therapy for acne. *Clin Ther* 1998;**20**:711–21.

92 Graupe K, Zaumseil RP. Skinoren: a new local therapeutic agent for the treatment of acne vulgaris. In: Macher E, Kolde G, Bröcker EB, eds. *Jahrbuch der Dermatologie*. Zülpich: Biermann, 1991:159–69.

93 Graupe K, Cunliffe WJ, Gollnick HP, Zaumseil RP. Efficacy and safety of topical azelaic acid (20 percent cream): an overview of results from European clinical trials and experimental reports. *Cutis* 1996;**57**(Suppl 1):S20–35.

94 Holland KT, Bojar RA. The effect of azelaic acid on cutaneous bacteria. *J Dermatolog Treat* 1989;**1**:17–19.

95 Breathnach AS. Melanin hyperpigmentation of skin: melasma, topical treatment with azelaic acid and other therapies. *Cutis* 1996;**57**(Suppl 1):36–45.

96 Eady EA, Ingham E, Walters CE, Cove JH, Cunliffe WJ. Modulation of comedonal levels of interleukin-1 in acne patients treated with tetracyclines. *J Invest Dermatol* 1993;**101**:86–91.

97 Garner SE, Eady EA, Popescu C, Newton J, Li WA. Minocycline for acne vulgaris: efficacy and safety. *Cochrane Database Syst Rev* 2003;(1):CD002086.

98 Simonart, T, Dramaix. Treatment of acne with topical antibiotics: lessons from clinical studies. *Br J Dermatol* 2005;**153**:395–403.

99 Plewig G, Petrozzi JW, Berendes U. Double-blind study of doxycycline in acne vulgaris. *Arch Dermatol* 1970;**101**:435–8.

100 Hersle K, Gisslen H. Minocycline in acne vulgaris: a double-blind study. *Curr Ther Res Clin Exp* 1976;**19**:339–42.

101 Crounse RG. The response of acne to placebos and antibiotics. *JAMA* 1965;**193**:906–10.

102 Lane P, Williamson DM. Treatment of acne vulgaris with tetracycline hydrochloride: a double-blind trial with 51 patients. *BMJ* 1969;**2**:76–9.

103 Wong RC, Kang S, Heezen JL. Oral ibuprofen and tetracycline for the treatment of acne vulgaris. *J Am Acad Dermatol* 1984;**11**:1076–81.

104 Anderson RL, Cook CH, Smith DE. The effect of oral and topical tetracycline on acne severity and on surface lipid composition. *J Invest Dermatol* 1976;**66**:172–7.

105 Blaney DJ, Cook CH. Topical use of tetracycline in the treatment of acne: a double-blind study comparing topical and oral tetracycline therapy and placebo. *Arch Dermatol* 1976;**112**:971–3.

106 Smith JG Jr, Chalker DK, Wehr RF. The effectiveness of topical and oral tetracycline for acne. *South Med J* 1976;**69**:695–7.

107 Braathen LR. Topical clindamycin versus oral tetracycline and placebo in acne vulgaris. *Scand J Infect Dis* 1984;**16**(Suppl 43):71–5.

108 Gratton D, Raymond GP, Guertin-Larochelle S, *et al.* Topical clindamycin versus systemic tetracycline in the treatment of acne: results of a multiclinic trial. *J Am Acad Dermatol* 1982;**7**:50–3.

109 Feucht CL, Allen BS, Chalker DK, Smith JG, Jr. Topical erythromycin with zinc in acne: a double-blind controlled study. *J Am Acad Dermatol* 1980;**3**:483–91.

110 Stewart WD, Maddin SW, Nelson AJ, *et al.* Therapeutic agents in acne vulgaris, 1: tetracycline. *Can Med Assoc J* 1963;**89**:1096–7.

111 Ashurst PJ. Tetracycline in acne vulgaris. *Practitioner* 1968;**200**:539–41.

112 Ferahbas A, Utas S, Aykol D, Borlu M, Uksal U. Clinical evaluation of roxithromycin: a double-blind, placebo-controlled and crossover trial in patients with acne vulgaris. *J Dermatol* 2004;**31**:6–9.

113 Dubertret L, Alirezai M, Rostain G, *et al.* The use of lymecycline in the treatment of moderate to severe acne vulgaris: a comparison of the efficacy and safety of two dosing regimens. *Eur J Dermatol* 2003;**13**:44–8.

114 Skidmore R, Kovach R, Walker C, *et al.* Effects of subantimicrobial-dose doxycycline in the treatment of moderate acne. *Arch Dermatol* 2003;**139**:459–64.

115 Plewig G. Vitamin A acid: topical treatment in acne vulgaris. *Pennsylvania Med* 1969;**72**:33–5.

116 Al Mishari MA. Clinical and bacteriological evaluation of tetracycline and erythromycin in acne vulgaris. *Clin Ther* 1987;**9**:273–80.

117 Bleeker J. Tolerance and efficacy of erythromycin stearate tablets versus enteric-coated erythromycin base capsules in the treatment of patients with acne vulgaris. *J Int Med Res* 1983;**11**:38–41.

118 Brandt H, Attila P, Ahokas T, *et al.* Erythromycin acistrate: an alternative oral treatment for acne. *J Dermatolog Treat* 1994;**5**:3–5.

119 Cullen SI, Cohan RH. Minocycline therapy in acne vulgaris. *Cutis* 1976;**17**:1208–10.

120 Gammon WR, Meyer C, Lantis S, Shenefelt P, Reizner G, Cripps DJ. Comparative efficacy of oral erythromycin versus oral tetracycline in the treatment of acne vulgaris: a double-blind study. *J Am Acad Dermatol* 1986;**14** (2 Pt 1):183–6.

121 Gibson JR, Darley CR, Harvey SG, Barth J. Oral trimethoprim versus oxytetracycline in the treatment of inflammatory acne vulgaris. *Br J Dermatol* 1982;**107**:221–4.

122 Hubbell CG, Hobbs ER, Rist T, White JW Jr. Efficacy of minocycline compared with tetracycline in treatment of acne vulgaris. *Arch Dermatol* 1982;**118**:989–92.

123 Olafsson JH, Gudgeirsson J, Eggertsdottir GE, Kristjansson F. Doxycycline versus minocycline in the treatment of acne vulgaris: a double-blind study. *J Dermatolog Treat* 1989;**1**:15–17.

124 Samuelson JS. An accurate photographic method for grading acne: initial use in a double-blind clinical comparison of minocycline and tetracycline. *J Am Acad Dermatol* 1985;**12**:461–7.

125 Blechschmidt J, Engst R, Hoting E, *et al*. Behandlung der Acne papulopustulosa: Vergleich der Wirksamkeit und Verträglichkeit von Minocyclin und Oxytetracyclin. *Münch Med Wochenschr* 1987;**129**:562–4.

126 Cunliffe WJ, Grosshans E, Belaich S, Meynadier J, Alirezai M, Thomas L. A comparison of the efficacy and safety of lymecycline and minocycline in patients with moderately severe acne vulgaris. *Eur J Dermatol* 1998;**8**:161–6.

127 Fallica L, Vignini M, Rodeghiero R, *et al*. La minociclina e la tetracicline chloridrato nel trattamento del'acne vogare. *Dermatol Clin* 1985;**5**:145–50.

128 Khanna N. Treatment of acne vulgaris with oral tetracyclines. *Indian J Dermatol Venereol Leprol* 1993;**59**:74–6.

129 Laux B. [Treatment of acne vulgaris: a comparison of doxycycline versus minocycline; in German.] *Hautarzt* 1989;**40**:577–81.

130 Lorette G, Belaich S, Beylot MC, Ortonne JP. [Doxycycline (Tolexine) 50 mg/day versus minocycline 100 mg/day in the treatment of acne vulgaris: evaluation of four months of treatment; in French.] *Nouv Dermatol* 1994;**13**:662–5.

131 Ruping KW, Tronnier H. *Acne Therapy: Results of a Multicentre Study with Minocycline*. London: Royal Society of Medicine Services, 1985: 103–8. (International Congress and Symposium Series.)

132 Schollhammer M, Alirezai M. Etude comparative de la lymecycline, de la minocycline et de la doxycycline dans la traitement de l'acne vulgaire. *Real Ther Derm Venerol* 1994;**42**:24–6.

133 Waskiewicz W, Grosshans E. Traitement de l'acne juvenile par les cyclines de deuxième génération. *Nouv Dermatol* 1982;**11**: 8–11.

134 Kus S, Yucelten D, Aytug A. Comparison of efficacy of azithromycin vs. doxycycline in the treatment of acne vulgaris. *Clin Exp Dermatol* 2005;**30**:215–20.

135 Bossuyt L, Bosschaert J, Richert B, *et al*. Lymecycline in the treatment of acne: an efficacious, safe and cost-effective alternative to minocycline. *Eur J Dermatol* 2003;**13**:130–5.

136 Christian GL, Krueger GG. Clindamycin vs. placebo as adjunctive therapy in moderately severe acne. *Arch Dermatol* 1975;**111**: 997–1000.

137 Lucchina LC, Kollias N, Gillies R, *et al*. Fluorescence photography in the evaluation of acne. *J Am Acad Dermatol* 1996;**35**:58–63.

138 Thomsen RJ, Stranieri A, Knutson D, Strauss JS. Topical clindamycin treatment of acne: clinical, surface lipid composition, and quantitative surface microbiology response. *Arch Dermatol* 1980;**116**:1031–4.

139 Becker LE, Bergstresser PR, Whiting DA, *et al*. Topical clindamycin therapy for acne vulgaris: a cooperative clinical study. *Arch Dermatol* 1981;**117**:482–5.

140 Guin JD. Treatment of acne vulgaris with topical clindamycin phosphate: a double-blind study. *Int J Dermatol* 1981;**20**:286–8.

141 Kuhlman DS, Callen JP. A comparison of clindamycin phosphate 1 percent topical lotion and placebo in the treatment of acne vulgaris. *Cutis* 1986;**38**:203–6.

142 Petersen MJ, Krusinski PA, Krueger GG. Evaluation of 1% clindamycin phosphate lotion in the treatment of acne. *Curr Ther Res* 1986;**40**:232–8.

143 Ellis CN, Gammon WR, Stone DZ, Heezen-Wehner JL. A comparison of Cleocin T solution, Cleocin T gel, and placebo in the treatment of acne vulgaris. *Cutis* 1988;**42**:245–7.

144 McKenzie MW, Beck DC, Popovich NG. Topical clindamycin formulations for the treatment of acne vulgaris: an evaluation. *Arch Dermatol* 1981;**117**:630–4.

145 Shalita A, Myers J, Krochmal L, Yaroshinsky A. The safety and efficacy of clindamycin phosphate foam 1% versus clindamycin phosphate topical gel 1% for the treatment of acne vulgaris. *J Drugs Dermatol* 2005;**4**:48–56.

146 Jones EL, Crumley AF. Topical erythromycin vs. blank vehicle in a multiclinic acne study. *Arch Dermatol* 1981;**117**:551–3.

147 Hellgren L, Vincent J. [Suppression of inflammation in acne vulgaris by topical erythromycin in alcoholic solution; in German.] *Dermatol Monatsschr* 1983;**169**:702–5.

148 Lesher JL Jr, Chalker DK, Smith JG Jr. An evaluation of a 2% erythromycin ointment in the topical therapy of acne vulgaris. *J Am Acad Dermatol* 1985;**12**:526–31.

149 LLorca M, Hernandez-Gill A, Ramos M, *et al*. Erythromycin lauryl sulfate in the topical treatment of acne vulgaris. *Curr Ther Res* 1982;**32**:14–20.

150 Perez M, Aspiolea F, De Moragas JM. [Comparative double-blind study of topical clindamycin phosphate and oral tetracycline in the treatment of acne; in Spanish]. *Med Cutan Ibero Lat Am* 1987;**15**:173–7.

151 Pochi PE, Bagatell FK, Ellis CN, *et al*. Erythromycin 2 percent gel in the treatment of acne vulgaris. *Cutis* 1988;**41**:132–6.

152 Prince RA, Busch DA, Hepler CD, Feldick HG. Clinical trial of topical erythromycin in inflammatory acne. *Drug Intell Clin Pharm* 1981;**15**:372–6.

153 Chalker DK, Shalita A, Smith JG Jr, Swann RW. A double-blind study of the effectiveness of a 3% erythromycin and 5% benzoyl peroxide combination in the treatment of acne vulgaris. *J Am Acad Dermatol* 1983;**9**:933–6.

154 Mills O Jr, Thornsberry C, Cardin CW, Smiles KA, Leyden JJ. Bacterial resistance and therapeutic outcome following three months of topical acne therapy with 2% erythromycin gel versus its vehicle. *Acta Derm Venereol* 2002;**82**(4):260–5.

155 Schachner L, Pestana A, Kittles C. A clinical trial comparing the safety and efficacy of a topical erythromycin-zinc formulation with a topical clindamycin formulation. *J Am Acad Dermatol* 1990;**22**:489–95.

156 Strauss JS, Stranieri AM. Acne treatment with topical erythromycin and zinc: effect of *Propionibacterium acnes* and free fatty acid composition. *J Am Acad Dermatol* 1984;**11**:86–9.

157 Hansted B, Jorgensen J, Reymann F, Christiansen J. Fucidin cream for topical treatment of acne vulgaris. *Curr Ther Res Clin Exp* 1985;**37**:249–53.

158 Sommer S, Bojar R, Cunliffe WJ, Holland D, Holland KT, Naags H. Investigation of the mechanism of action of 2% fusidic acid lotion in the treatment of acne vulgaris. *Clin Exp Dermatol* 1997;**22**:211–5.

159 Knutson DD, Swinyer LJ, Smoot WH. Meclocycline sulfosalicylate: topical antibiotic agent for the treatment of acne vulgaris. *Cutis* 1981;**27**:203–4.

160 Tong D, Peters W, Barnetson RSC. Evaluation of 0.75% metronidazole gel in acne: a double-blind study. *Clin Exp Dermatol* 1994;**19**:221–3.

161 Franz E, Weidner-Strahl S. The effectiveness of topical anti-bacterials in acne: a double-blind clinical study. *J Int Med Res* 1978;**6**:72–7.

162 Parker F. A comparison of clindamycin 1% solution versus clindamycin 1% gel in the treatment of acne vulgaris. *Int J Dermatol* 1987;**26**:121–2.

163 Goltz RW, Coryell GM, Schnieders JR, Neidert GL. A comparison of Cleocin T 1 percent solution and Cleocin T 1 percent lotion in the treatment of acne vulgaris. *Cutis* 1985;**36**:265–8.

164 Cunliffe SJ, Fernandez C, Bojar R, Kanis R, West F, Zindaclin Clinical Study Group. An observer-blind parallel-group, randomized, multicentre clinical and microbiological study of a topical clindamycin/zinc gel and a topical clindamycin lotion in patients with mild/moderate acne. *J Dermatolog Treat* 2005;**16**: 213–8.

165 Alirezai M, Gerlach B, Horvath A, Forsea D, Briantais P, Guyomar M. Results of a randomised, multicentre study comparing a new water-based gel of clindamycin 1% versus clindamycin 1% topical solution in the treatment of acne vulgaris. *Eur J Dermatol* 2005;**15**:274–8.

166 Henderson TA, Olson WH, Leach AD. A single-blind, randomized comparison of erythromycin pledgets and clindamycin lotion in the treatment of mild-to-moderate facial acne vulgaris. *Adv Ther* 1995;**12**:172–7.

167 Leyden JJ, Shalita AR, Saatjian GD, Sefton J. Erythromycin 2% gel in comparison with clindamycin phosphate 1% solution in acne vulgaris. *J Am Acad Dermatol* 1987;**16**:822–7.

168 Mills OH, Berger RS, Kligman AM, McElroy JA, Di Matteo J. A comparative study of Erycette vs. Cleocin-T. *Adv Ther* 1992;**9**: 14–20.

169 Thomas DR, Raimer S, Smith EB. Comparison of topical erythromycin 1.5 percent solution versus topical clindamycin phosphate 1.0 percent solution in the treatment of acne vulgaris. *Cutis* 1982;**29**:624–5.

170 Padilla RS, McCabe JM, Becker LE. Topical tetracycline hydrochloride vs. topical clindamycin phosphate in the treatment of acne: a comparative study. *Int J Dermatol* 1981;**20**:445–8.

171 Robledo AA, Lopez BE, del Pino GJ, *et al.* Multicentric comparative study of the efficacy and tolerance of clindamycin phosphate 1% topical solution and tetracycline topical solution for the treatment of acne vulgaris. *Curr Ther Res Clin Exp* 1988; **43**:21–6.

172 Shalita AR, Smith JG, Parish LC, Sofman MS, Chalker DK. Topical nicotinamide compared with clindamycin gel in the treatment of inflammatory acne vulgaris. *Int J Dermatol* 1995; **34**:434–7.

173 McHugh RC, Sangha ND, McCarty MA, *et al.* A topical azithromycin preparation for the treatment of acne vulgaris and rosacea. *J Dermatolog Treat* 2004;**15**:295–302.

174 Borglund E, Hagermark O, Nord CE. Impact of topical clindamycin and systemic tetracycline on the skin and colon microflora in patients with acne vulgaris. *Scand J Infect Dis* 1984;**16** (Suppl 43):76–81.

175 Stoughton RB, Cornell RC, Gange RW, Walter JF. Double-blind comparison of topical 1 percent clindamycin phosphate (Cleocin T) and oral tetracycline 500 mg/day in the treatment of acne vulgaris. *Cutis* 1980;**26**:424–5.

176 Katsambas A, Towarky AA, Stratigos J. Topical clindamycin phosphate compared with oral tetracycline in the treatment of acne vulgaris. *Br J Dermatol* 1987;**116**:387–91.

177 Cornbleet HA. Long-term therapy of acne with tetracycline. *Arch Dermatol* 1961;**83**:414–16.

178 Hjorth N, Schmidt H, Thomsen K, Dela K. Meclosorb, a new topical antibiotic agent in the treatment of acne vulgaris: a double-blind clinical study. *Acta Derm Venereol* 1984;**64**:354–7.

179 Rapaport M, Puhvel SM, Reisner RM. Evaluation of topical erythromycin and oral tetracycline in acne vulgaris. *Cutis* 1982;**30**: 122–6.

180 Drake LA. Comparative efficacy and tolerance of Cleocin T topical gel (clindamycin phosphate topical gel) versus oral minocycline in the treatment of acne vulgaris. 1980 unpublished data [Pharmacia and Upjohn, Ltd.]

181 Peacock CE, Price C, Ryan BE, Mitchell AD. Topical clindamycin (Dalacin T) compared to oral minocycline (Minocin 50) in treatment of acne vulgaris: a randomized observer-blind controlled trial in three university student health centres. *Clin Trials J* 1990;**27**:219–28.

182 Sheehan-Dare RA, Papworth-Smith J, Cunliffe WJ. A double-blind comparison of topical clindamycin and oral minocycline in the treatment of acne vulgaris. *Acta Derm Venereol* 1990;**70**: 534–7.

183 Wethered R. Sodium fusidate in acne. *Practitioner* 1964;**193**:802–4.

184 Darrah AJ, Gray PL. An open multicentre study to compare fusidic acid lotion and oral minocycline in the treatment of mild-to-moderate acne vulgaris of the face. *Eur J Clin Res* 1996;**8**:97–107.

185 Norris JFB, Hughes BR, Basey AJ, Cunliffe WJ. A comparison of the effectiveness of topical tetracycline, benzoyl-peroxide gel and oral oxytetracycline in the treatment of acne. *Clin Exp Dermatol* 1991;**16**:31–3.

186 Stainforth J, Macdonald-Hull S, Papworth-Smith JW, *et al.* A single-blind comparison of topical erythromycin/zinc lotion and oral minocycline in the treatment of acne vulgaris. *J Dermatolog Treat* 1993;**4**:119–22.

187 Ozolins M, Eady E, Avery A, *et al.* Comparison of five antimicrobial regimens for treatment of mild to moderate inflammatory facial acne vulgaris in the community: randomised controlled trial. *Lancet* 2004;**364**:2188–95.

188 Gollnick H. A new therapeutic agent: azelaic acid in acne treatment. *J Dermatolog Treat* 1990;**1**(Suppl 3):S23–8.

189 Tucker SB, Tausend R, Cochran R, Flannigan SA. Comparison of topical clindamycin phosphate, benzoyl peroxide, and a combination of the two for the treatment of acne vulgaris. *Br J Dermatol* 1984;**110**:487–92.

190 Swinyer LJS, Baker MD, Swinyer TA, Mills OH Jr. A comparative study of benzoyl peroxide and clindamycin phosphate for treating acne vulgaris. *Br J Dermatol* 1988;**119**:615–22.

191 Burke B, Eady EA, Cunliffe WJ. Benzoyl peroxide versus topical erythromycin in the treatment of acne vulgaris. *Br J Dermatol* 1983;**108**:199–204.

192 Borglund E, Kristensen B, Larsson-Stymne B, Strand A, Veien NK, Jakobsen HB. Topical meclocycline sulfosalicylate, benzoyl peroxide, and a combination of the two in the treatment of acne vulgaris. *Acta Derm Venereol* 1991;**71**:175–8.

193 Gamborg NP. Topical metronidazole gel: use in acne vulgaris. *Int J Dermatol* 1991;**30**:662–6.

194 Cambazard F. Clinical efficacy of Velac, a new tretinoin and clindamycin phosphate gel in acne vulgaris. *J Eur Acad Dermatol Venereol* 1998;**11**(Suppl 1):S20–7.

195 Zouboulis C, Derumeaux L, Decroix J, Maciejewska-Udziela B, Cambazard F, Stuhlert A. A multicentre, single-blind, randomized comparison of a fixed clindamycin phosphate/tretinoin gel formulation (Velac) applied once daily and a clindamycin lotion formulation (Dalacin T) applied twice daily in the topical treatment of acne vulgaris. *Br J Dermatol* 2000;**143**:498–505.

196 Rietschel RL, Duncan SH. Clindamycin phosphate used in combination with tretinoin in the treatment of acne. *Int J Dermatol* 1983;**22**:41–3.

197 Richter JR, Bousema MT, De Boulle KLV, Degreef HJ, Poli F. Efficacy of a fixed clindamycin phosphate 1.2%, tretinoin 0.025% gel formulation (Velac) in the topical control of facial acne lesions. *J Dermatolog Treat* 1998;**9**:81–90.

198 Bowman S, Gold M, Nasir A, Vamvakias G. Comparison of clindamycin/benzoyl peroxide, tretinoin plus clindamycin, and the combination of clindamycin/benzoyl peroxide and tretinoin plus clindamycin in the treatment of acne vulgaris: a randomized, blinded study. *J Drugs Dermatol* 2005;**4**:611–8.

199 Mills OH Jr, Kligman AM. Treatment of acne vulgaris with topically applied erythromycin and tretinoin. *Acta Derm Venereol* 1978;**58**:555–7.

200 Cunliffe WJ, Meynadier J, Alirezai M, *et al.* Is combined oral and topical therapy better than oral therapy alone in patients with moderate to moderately severe acne vulgaris? A comparison of the efficacy and safety of lymecycline plus adapalene gel 0.1%, versus lymecycline plus gel vehicle. *J Am Acad Dermatol* 2003; **49**(3 Suppl):S218–26.

201 Thiboutot DM, Shalita AR, Yamauchi PS, *et al.* Combination therapy with adapalene gel 0.1% and doxycycline for severe acne vulgaris: a multicenter, investigator-blind, randomized, controlled study. *Skinmed* 2005;**4**:138–46.

202 Wolf JE Jr, Kaplan D, Kraus SJ, *et al.* Efficacy and tolerability of combined topical treatment of acne vulgaris with adapalene and clindamycin: a multicenter, randomized, investigator-blinded study. *J Am Acad Dermatol* 2003;**49**(3 Suppl):S211–7.

203 Zhang JZ, Li LF, Tu YT, Zheng J. A successful maintenance approach in inflammatory acne with adapalene gel 0.1% after an initial treatment in combination with clindamycin topical solution 1% or after monotherapy with clindamycin topical solution 1%. *J Dermatolog Treat* 2004;**15**:372–8.

204 Marazzi P, Boorman GC, Donald AE, Davies HD. Clinical evaluation of double strength Isotrexin versus Benzamycin in the topical treatment of mild to moderate acne vulgaris. *J Dermatolog Treat* 2002;**13**:111–7.

205 Capizzi R, Landi F, Milani M, Amerio P. Skin tolerability and efficacy of combination therapy with hydrogen peroxide stabilized cream and adapalene gel in comparison with benzoyl peroxide cream and adapalene gel in common acne: a randomized, investigator-masked, controlled trial. *Br J Dermatol* 2004; **151**:481–4.

206 Cunliffe WJ, Holland KT, Bojar R, Levy SF. A randomized, double-blind comparison of a clindamycin phosphate/benzoyl peroxide gel formulation and a matching clindamycin gel with respect to microbiologic activity and clinical efficacy in the topical treatment of acne vulgaris. *Clin Ther* 2002;**24**:1117–33.

207 Packman AM, Brown RH, Dunlap FE, Kraus SJ, Webster GF. Treatment of acne vulgaris: combination of 3% erythromycin and 5% benzoyl peroxide in a gel compared to clindamycin phosphate lotion. *Int J Dermatol* 1996;**35**:209–11.

208 Chu A, Huber FJ, Plott RT. The comparative efficacy of benzoyl peroxide 5%/erythromycin 3% gel and erythromycin 4%/zinc 1.2% solution in the treatment of acne vulgaris. *Br J Dermatol* 1997;**136**:235–8.

209 Sklar JL, Jacobson C, Rizer R, Gans EH. Evaluation of Triaz 10% gel and Benzamycin in acne vulgaris. *J Dermatolog Treat* 1996; **7**:147–52.

210 Basak PY, Gultekin F, Kilinc I, Delibas N. The effect of benzoyl peroxide and benzoyl peroxide/erythromycin combination on the antioxidative defence system in papulopustular acne. *Eur J Dermatol* 2002;**12**:53–7.

211 Thiboutot D, Jarratt M, Rich P, Rist T, Rodriguez D, Levy S. A randomized, parallel, vehicle-controlled comparison of two erythromycin/benzoyl peroxide preparations for acne vulgaris. *Clin Ther* 2002;**24**:773–85.

212 Marsden J. Evidence that the method of use, dose and duration of treatment with benzoyl peroxide and tetracycline determines response of acne. *J R Soc Med* 1985;**78**(Suppl 10):25–8.

213 Brooks JS. The use of acmed in acne. *Australas J Dermatol* 1968; **9**:256–7.

214 Noble W, Naidoo J. Evolution of antibiotic resistance in *Staphylococcus aureus*: the role of the skin. *Br J Dermatol* 1978; **98**:481–9.

215 Eady EA, Holland KT, Cunliffe WJ. Should topical antibiotics be used for the treatment of acne vulgaris? *Br J Dermatol* 1982; **107**:235–46.

216 Wise R, Hart T, Cars O, *et al.* Antimicrobial resistance is a major threat to public health [editorial]. *BMJ* 1998;**317**:609–10.

217 Cooper A. Systematic review of *Propionibacterium acnes* resistance to systemic antibiotics. *Med J Aust* 1998;**169**:259–61.

218 Eady EA, Cove JH, Blake J, Holland KT, Cunliffe WJ. Recalcitrant acne vulgaris: clinical, biochemical and microbiological investigation of patients not responding to antibiotic treatment. *Br J Dermatol* 1988;**118**:415–23.

219 Hughes BR, Murphy CE, Barnett J, Cunliffe WJ. Strategy of acne therapy with long-term antibiotics. *Br J Dermatol* 1989;**121**:623–8.

220 Greenwood R, Burke B, Cunliffe WJ. Evaluation of a therapeutic strategy for the treatment of acne vulgaris with conventional therapy. *Br J Dermatol* 1986;**114**:353–8.

221 Mandy S. Chest and back acne: a retrospective review. *Adv Ther* 1995;**12**:321–32.

222 Layton AM, Hughes BR, Hull SM, Eady EA, Cunliffe WJ. Seborrhoea: an indicator for poor clinical response in acne patients treated with antibiotics. *Clin Exp Dermatol* 1992;**17**:173–5.

223 Leyden JJ, Marples RR, Mills OH Jr, Kligman AM. Gram-negative folliculitis: a complication of antibiotic therapy in acne vulgaris. *Br J Dermatol* 1973;**88**:533–8.

224 Chopra I, Hawkey P, Hinton M. Tetracyclines: molecular and clinical aspects. *J Antimicrob Chemother* 1992;**29**:245–77.

225 Meyer FP. Minocycline for acne: food reduces minocycline's availability. *BMJ* 1996;**312**:1101.

226 Lleyden JJ. Absorption of minocycline hydrochloride and tetracycline hydrochloride: effect of food, milk and iron. *J Am Acad Dermatol* 1985;**12**:308–12.

227 Eady EA, Farmery MR, Ross JI, Cove JH, Cunliffe WJ. Effects of benzoyl peroxide and erythromycin alone and in combination against antibiotic-sensitive and -resistant skin bacteria from acne patients. *Br J Dermatol* 1994;**131**:331–6.

228 Becker FT. The acne problem. *Arch Dermatol Syphiol* 1953;**67**:173.

229 Robinson H. Role of antibiotics in therapy of acne. *Arch Dermatol Syphiol* 1954;**69**:414–7.

230 Smith E, Mortimer PS. Tetracycline in acne vulgaris. *Br J Dermatol* 1967;**79**:78–84.

231 Aulzberger M, Witten V, Steagall R. Treatment of acne vulgaris. *JAMA* 1960;**173**:1911–5.

232 Plewig G, Kligman AM. *Acne: Morphogenesis and Treatment.* Berlin: Springer, 1975.

233 Dreno B, Bodokh I, Chivot M, *et al.* [ECLA grading: a system of acne classification for every day dermatological practice; in French.] *Ann Dermatol Venereol* 1999;**126**:136–41.

234 Gardner KJ, Eady EA, Cove JH, Taylor JP, Cunliffe WJ. Comparison of serum antibiotic levels in acne patients receiving the standard or a modified release formulation of minocycline hydrochloride. *Clin Exp Dermatol* 1997;**22**:72–6.

235 Akamatsu H, Nishijima S, Akamatsu M, Kurokawa I, Asada Y. Clinical evaluation of roxithromycin in patients with acne. *J Int Med Res* 1996;**24**:109–14.

236 Baer RL, Leshaw SM, Shalita AR. High-dose tetracycline therapy in severe acne. *Arch Dermatol* 1976;**112**:479–81.

237 Friedman-Kien A, Shalita AR, Baer RL. Tetracycline therapy in acne vulgaris. *Arch Dermatol* 1972;**105**:608.

238 Burke BM, Cunliffe WJ. The assessment of acne vulgaris: the Leeds technique. *Br J Dermatol* 1984;**111**:83–92.

239 Goolamali S. Management of acne vulgaris. *Prescribers J* 1990;**30**:78–84.

240 Milikan LE, Ameln R. Use of Buf-Puf and benzoyl peroxide in the treatment of acne. *Cutis* 1981;**28**:201–5.

241 Fyrand O, Jakobsen HB. Water-based versus alcohol-based benzoyl peroxide preparations in the treatment of acne vulgaris. *Dermatologica* 1986;**172**:263–7.

Papulopustular rosacea

Alfredo Rebora

Background

Definition

In papulopustular rosacea, papulopustules appear on the nose and cheeks, more rarely on the forehead and chin, and exceptionally on the neck and other body areas, such as the bare skull or the back. In some cases, papules show a granulomatous infiltrate, which is clinically identified from the yellowish color of the lesions and their duration (Figure 16.1).

Lymphedematous rosacea is more rare and is characterized by chronic and persistent edema in the periocular and perinasal areas. The edema persists even when inflammation has abated and is probably linked to inflammatory damage to the region's lymphatic vessels. A hyperacute episode, with most of the face invaded by papulopustules (facial pyoderma), has also been described as rosacea fulminans.

Incidence/prevalence

Rosacea is a very common disease. In the US, it is the fifth most frequently diagnosed skin condition. It affects 10% of the general population in Sweden.

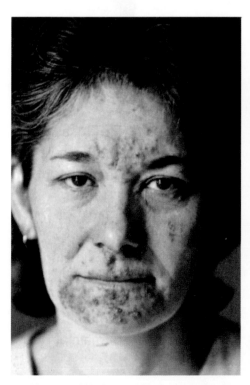 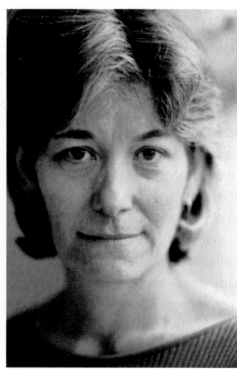

Figure 16.1 A patient with rosacea (a) before and (b) after treatment. (Figures provided by Andrew Herxheimer.)

Etiology/risk factors

Heredity is important. It has been recently shown that 20% of the children with steroid rosacea had at least one close blood relative with rosacea. Fair complexion, blond hair, and green/blue eyes are characteristic of patients with rosacea. About 0.1% of colored people are also affected by rosacea, as reported by an old American observation. Rosacea occurs more frequently in women than in men (3 : 1).

Typically, rosacea is a multistage disease, and the prevalence may vary depending on the stage at which the diagnosis is made. The stages are: the flushing stage, or transitory congestive redness; the erythrosis stage, or persistent telangiectatic redness; the papulopustular stage; and the phyma stage. Only a minority of patients with the first two stages of the disease progress to the papulopustular stage, and even fewer to the phyma stage. The condition appears more often in middle age, although erythrosis develops earlier (mean age 34 years), and phymas later (mean age 66 years).

The etiopathogenesis of papulopustular rosacea is controversial, and it is unclear why a patient proceeds from stages that are mainly functional to those that are inflammatory. Both cell-mediated and humoral immunity may be involved. Antibodies directed against collagen VII, elastotic tissue, and the *Demodex folliculorum* mite have been detected. However, the production of antibodies may be a secondary event, or elastotic tissue and *D. folliculorum* may simply represent structures in which antibodies accumulate spontaneously ("beach effect"). In addition, it has recently been hypothesized that *Helicobacter pylori*, a Gram-negative bacterium, may play a role. Opinions diverge on its association with rosacea, but drugs that eradicate *H. pylori* were used to treat papulopustular rosacea long before the issue of *H. pylori* arose.

Prognosis

No long-term prognostic studies are available.

Aims

The aims of treatment are to suppress the symptoms and to maintain such suppression over time.

Outcomes

The following outcome measures are used: state of lesions over time; use of routine treatments; duration of remission; patient satisfaction; adverse effects of treatments; and clinical activity scores. According to the Cochrane review,[1] one of the primary outcome measures, "quality of life," was not assessed in any of the studies. In a recent randomized controlled trial (RCT) of azelaic acid gel, efficacy was measured using a rosacea-related quality-of-life instrument.[2]

Methods

The Cochrane Library, PubMed, and Isitrial were searched and appraised in March 2006. The search identified one Cochrane review including 29 studies,[1] one systematic review, and one partial review. The data in these reviews were checked and some of the papers quoted were examined.

Papers dealing with granulomatous rosacea and rosacea fulminans were excluded in order to maintain homogeneity. Similarly, papers examining erythema and/or telangiectasia, steroid-induced rosacea, rosacea-like demodicidosis, rosacea conglobata, and rhinophyma were not taken into account.

Questions

What are the effects of systemic treatments?

Tetracyclines

Efficacy

One Cochrane review on cutaneous and ocular rosacea and one systematic review on ocular rosacea were found.[3] In the Cochrane review, data pooled from three studies of oral tetracycline versus placebo, including 152 participants, showed that tetracycline was effective (OR 6.06; 95% CI, 2.96 to 12.42).[1]

The systematic review of ocular rosacea examined 11 papers, only three of which were RCTs. The proportion of patients with improvement ranged from 20% to 100%. It was concluded that there is a moderate benefit with oxytetracycline, whilst the efficacy of tetracyclines and doxycycline could not be established.[3]

Drawbacks

Diarrhea at 750 mg/day was reported in one study.

Comment

In one RCT, a very minor placebo effect contrasted with all of the other trials, in which there was a very marked placebo effect.

Doxycycline

Doxycycline is perhaps the most popular medication for papulopustular rosacea, but the Cochrane review did not identify any RCTs on the topic.

Efficacy

In one controlled clinical trial (CCT), 17 patients received doxycycline 200 mg/day for 4 weeks and then 100 mg/day for 4 weeks. The lesions cleared in 90% of patients in 8 weeks. Comparison with clarithromycin favored the latter.[4] An anecdotal report of two cases stated that 100 mg/day for 9 weeks and 50 mg/day for 1 month were sufficient to clear the lesions.[5]

Drawbacks
No side effects have been reported.

Comment
Doxycycline is a photosensitizing agent in fewer than 1% of patients, but this characteristic needs to be taken into account in patients with rosacea.

Subantimicrobial-dose doxycycline
In one RCT, 20 mg doxycycline was administered to 20 patients with rosacea for 3 months, in comparison with 20 patients treated with a placebo. In both groups, 0.75% metronidazole lotion was added twice daily. The inflammatory lesions were reduced significantly by week 4 in the doxycycline group, and changes from the baseline increased over time and were maintained during doxycycline monotherapy for 1 month.[6]

Comment
Bacterial resistance to doxycycline might arise after such low-dose treatment.

Ampicillin
Ampicillin is rarely used.

Efficacy
In the only RCT, 17 patients were treated with ampicillin 750 mg/day for 6 weeks. There was a 55% improvement in the lesions, compared with 10% with the placebo.[7]

Drawbacks
Two patients developed diarrhea within a few days and withdrew from the study.

Comment
The benefit–harm ratio appears to be low.

Clarithromycin
No systematic reviews and no RCTs were found.

Efficacy
In the only CCT, 23 patients received clarithromycin 500 mg/day for 1 month and then 250 mg/day for a further month. Ninety percent of the lesions cleared in 8 weeks; the comparison with doxycycline was in favor of clarithromycin.[4]

Drawbacks
Clarithromycin was significantly better tolerated than doxycycline.

Comment
Clarithromycin is almost four times more expensive than doxycycline.

Azithromycin
There are no systematic reviews or RCTs.

Efficacy
An uncontrolled study reported that clearing occurred in nine of 10 patients treated with azithromycin 500 mg/day for 4 weeks followed by 250 mg/day for 3 months.[8] Another uncontrolled study reported that 10 adults treated with azithromycin (250 mg three times/week) had moderate or marked improvement within 4 weeks.[9] Another open-labeled study included 18 patients who received azithromycin for 12 weeks, in decreasing doses. In the 14 patients who completed the study, the total scores significantly decreased in 75%, and the improvement continued during the month after treatment.[10]

Drawbacks
Nausea in one patient resolved without the treatment having to be interrupted.

Comment
A once-daily pulse-dosing regimen may improve compliance.

Metronidazole
Oral metronidazole appears to be effective in papulopustular rosacea.

Efficacy
In the first of two RCTs, 29 patients received metronidazole 400 mg/day for 6 weeks. The benefit was significantly superior to placebo.[11] In the second trial, 40 patients received 400 mg/day for 12 weeks. The improvement was similar to that obtained with oxytetracycline.[12] An uncontrolled trial treated 59 patients with 500 mg/day for no more than 6 months, obtaining a 90% success rate.[13] Further trials have been published in German.[14]

Drawbacks
Headache and furred tongue have been noted occasionally.

Comment
The cost of metronidazole is half that of doxycycline.

Eradication of *H. pylori*
It is still a matter of controversy whether *H. pylori* is involved in the pathogenesis of rosacea. However, eradication of *H. pylori* appears to clear rosacea.

Efficacy
Only one RCT was found, in which 44 patients were treated with omeprazole 40 mg/day plus clarithromycin 1500 mg/day for 2 weeks. The lesions cleared in almost all of the patients, but there were no differences from the untreated controls.[15] In one CCT, 37 patients received omeprazole

40 mg/day for 1 month, plus clarithromycin 100 mg/day, plus metronidazole 2000 mg/day for 2 weeks. At the twelfth week, 76% of the patients experienced improvement, compared with no improvement in the 26 untreated patients.[16] In another CCT, 53 patients received omeprazole 20 mg/day, clarithromycin 1 g/day, and metronidazole 1 g/day for 1 week. Ninety-six percent cleared in 2–4 weeks.[17] In an uncontrolled study, 13 patients improved on bismuth 1200 mg/day, amoxicillin 500 mg/day, and metronidazole 1.5 g/day.[18]

Drawbacks
Surprisingly, no information is provided regarding any side effects of such a complex therapy.

Comment
The results are homogeneous, with the exception of the RCT. It is very difficult to believe, however, that the placebo-treated patients improved as much as those who received the eradication therapy.[15] The RCT did not use metronidazole.

Isotretinoin
Isotretinoin is a drug for very severe cases, such as pyoderma faciale.

Efficacy
No systematic reviews were found, but one RCT in which eight patients received isotretinoin 10 mg/day for 4 months. They improved significantly by 70%.[19] In an uncontrolled study, 22 patients received isotretinoin 10 mg/day for 4 months. They improved by 50% in 9 weeks.[20] Two anecdotal reports described clearance in 3–6 months.[21,22]

Drawbacks
Most patients experienced dry lips and facial xerosis, and 25% a mild to moderate increase in serum triglyceride levels.

Comment
Long-term side effects have not been reported.

Octreotide
Efficacy
In an anecdotal observational study, the lesions cleared in three of four patients.[23]

What are the effects of topical drugs?

Topical drugs are less likely to cause systemic adverse effects than systemically administered drugs, and compliance may be better. The drug that has been most widely tested is metronidazole.

Metronidazole
Metronidazole, formulated as either a 1% cream or a 0.75% gel, has proved effective in papulopustular rosacea.

Efficacy
The Cochrane review found nine trials investigating the efficacy of metronidazole versus placebo. Most studies used 0.75% metronidazole applied twice a day. Different formulations, such as gel, cream, and lotion are deemed to be equivalent. The treatment period varied from 8 to 9 weeks in eight of the trials, but was 6 months in one study.[24] The Cochrane review documented improvement over placebo in both "self-assessment by the patient" (three studies, OR 5.96; 95% CI, 2.95 to 12.06) and physician global evaluation (three studies, OR 7.01; 95% CI, 3.56 to 13.81). The data on continuous outcome measures, such as the number of lesions, could not be pooled because of the lack of relevant information such as standard deviation. However, these data supported the positive treatment effect. In an RCT, 88 patients successfully treated with oral tetracycline and topical metronidazole were treated with either 0.76% metronidazole gel or a vehicle. Relapses after 6 months of treatment were significantly fewer (23%) with metronidazole than with the vehicle (42%).[24]

Two studies compared metronidazole with oral tetracyclines.[25,26] Neither study could demonstrate a statistical difference between the drugs analyzed. However, the studies were too small (n = 25 and n = 26) to document a clinically significant difference. Two studies compared topical metronidazole with topical azelaic acid.[27,28] One study (n = 251)[27] was not able to document any difference (OR 1.32; 95% CI, 0.79 to 2.21) in patient self-assessment, but both the physician assessment and count of inflammatory lesions were in favor of azelaic acid (inflammatory lesions 12.9 vs. 10.7; $P = 0.003$). The other study (n = 40)[28] involved a within-patient comparison, and again found that azelaic acid was slightly superior to metronidazole. The clinical significance of the difference documented is difficult to define. In one study in which topical metronidazole was compared with permethrin (n = 63),[29] no difference was documented in the erythema score or papule count, but there was a reduced number of pustular lesions in the permethrin group.

Drawbacks
Side effects occurred in 2–4% of patients and included dryness, burning, and stinging. One paper reported "moderate tolerability."[30]

Comment
The majority of papers were RCTs (some even multicenter), mostly comparing the drug with a vehicle, and were sponsored by manufacturers.

Azelaic acid

Azelaic acid has been found to be effective in rosacea. The Cochrane review found four RCTs comparing azelaic acid with placebo and one RCT comparing the drug with topical metronidazole.

Efficacy

Both 15% and 20% azelaic acid concentrations have been used in placebo-controlled RCTs, and the treatment period ranged from 12 to 13 weeks. It was estimated that about five patients had to be treated to obtain one experiencing complete remission or marked improvement (number needed to treat = 5; 95% CI, 4 to 7). Two RCTs reported comparisons with topical metronidazole (see above).[27,28] Azelaic acid 15% gel proved to be more irritant than metronidazole 0.75% gel in a series of 33 patients.[31]

Drawbacks

Burning and stinging have been noted.

Sulfur

Sulfur appears to be effective in rosacea. Two RCTs were found.[32,33]

Efficacy

In the first RCT, 20 patients were treated for 1 month with a 10% sulfur cream plus placebo tablets and compared with 20 patients treated with lymecycline 150 mg/day plus placebo cream. Ninety-two per cent of the lesions cleared with both treatments.[32] In the second study, a total of 94 patients were treated with a combination of 10% sodium sulfacetamide and 5% sulfur in a lotion for 8 weeks. Inflammatory lesions decreased by 78%, in comparison with 36% in the vehicle group.[33]

Drawbacks

Reactions at the application site decreased in frequency over time.

Permethrin

Efficacy

An RCT has been carried out, including 63 patients randomly assigned to permethrin 5% gel, metronidazole 0.75% gel, or placebo. Permethrin was as effective as metronidazole gel and significantly superior to placebo (see above).[29]

Tretinoin/isotretinoin

Isotretinoin may be effective in rosacea.

Efficacy

In one small RCT, six patients were treated with 0.025% tretinoin cream for 16 weeks. Lesion counts decreased by 42%. No additional benefit was noted if the patients were also treated with oral isotretinoin.[34] In an uncontrolled small trial, four patients were treated with 0.2% isotretinoin cream for 16 days. Inflammatory lesions responded better than noninflammatory lesions.[35]

Drawbacks

No side effects were noted.

Comment

It is well known that isotretinoin irritates normal skin, but surprisingly it does not irritate the sensitive rosacea skin.

Clindamycin

Efficacy

In the only RCT, 43 patients were randomly assigned to treatment with either 1% clindamycin phosphate lotion for 12 weeks or tetracycline 1000 mg for 3 weeks and then 500 mg for 9 weeks. All inflammatory lesions decreased significantly (by about 60%) in the clindamycin arm, while only papules and nodules decreased significantly in the tetracycline arm.[36]

Drawbacks

No side effects were noted with clindamycin.

Benzoyl peroxide

Efficacy

In the only CCT, patients were treated with 5% benzoyl peroxide acetone gel for 1 month and with 10% gel for a further month. Benzoyl peroxide was superior to placebo.[37]

Drawbacks

Twenty-three percent of the patients treated with benzoyl peroxide dropped out of the study.

Key points

- Only a few RCTs have been conducted on systemic agents. In particular, no RCTs have tested doxycycline, clarithromycin, or azithromycin.
- Many RCTs have been performed with topical drugs. In particular, metronidazole has been extensively and thoroughly studied.
- All of the drugs examined except rilmenidine (data not shown) were found to be effective, and this is surprising given the profound chemical diversity of the drugs used and the poor explanation provided for their activity.
- Side effects were surprisingly minimal, even for drugs such as tretinoin and benzoyl peroxide, which are well-known irritants.
- In most studies, a high rate of response to placebos was observed.
- The majority of RCTs have been directly supported by the manufacturer.

Photodynamic therapy
Efficacy
In one open study, three patients experienced improvement; one had a 9-month remission and two had a 3-month remission.[38]

References

1 Van Zuuren EJ, Graber MA, Hollis S, Chaudhry M, Gupta AK, Gover M. Interventions for rosacea. *Cochrane Database Syst Rev* 2005;(**3**):CD003262.

2 Fleischer A, Suephy C. The face and mind evaluation study: an examination of the efficacy of rosacea treatment using physician ratings and patients' self-reported quality of life. *J Drugs Dermatol* 2005;**4**:585–90.

3 Stone DU, Chodosh J. Oral tetracyclines for ocular rosacea: an evidence-based review of the literature. *Cornea* 2004;**23**:106–9.

4 Torresani C, Pavesi A, Manara GC. Clarithromycin versus doxycycline in the treatment of rosacea. *Int J Dermatol* 1997;**36**:942–6.

5 Bikowski JB. Treatment of rosacea with doxycycline monohydrate. *Cutis* 2000;**66**:149–52.

6 Sanchez J, Somolinos AL, Almodovar PI, Webster G, Bradshaw M, Powala C. A randomized, double-blind, placebo-controlled trial of the combined effect of doxycycline hyclate 20-mg tablets and metronidazole 0.75% topical lotion in the treatment of rosacea. *J Am Acad Dermatol* 2005;**53**:791–7.

7 Marks R, Ellis J. Comparative effectiveness of tetracycline and ampicillin in rosacea: a controlled trial. *Lancet* 1971;**ii**:1049–52.

8 Elewski BE. A novel treatment for acne vulgaris and rosacea. *J Eur Acad Dermatol* 2000;**14**:423–4.

9 Fernandez-Obregon A. Oral use of azithromycin for the treatment of acne rosacea. *Arch Dermatol* 2004;**140**:489–90.

10 Bakar O, Demircay Z, Gurbuz O. Therapeutic potential of azithromycin in rosacea. *Int J Dermatol* 2004;**43**:151–4.

11 Pye RJ, Burton JL. Treatment of rosacea by metronidazole. *Lancet* 1976;**i**:1211–2.

12 Saihan EM, Burton JL. A double-blind trial of metronidazole versus oxytetracycline therapy for rosacea. *Br J Dermatol* 1980;**102**:443–5.

13 Guilhou JJ, Guilhou E, Malbos S, *et al.* Traitement de la rosacée par le métronidazole. *Ann Dermatol Venereol* 1979;**106**:127–9.

14 Gamborg-Nielsen P. Metronidazole treatment in rosacea. *Int J Dermatol* 1988;**27**:1–5.

15 Bamford JTM, Tilden RL, Blankush JL, *et al.* Effect of treatment of *Helicobacter pylori* infection on rosacea. *Arch Dermatol* 1999;**135**:659–63.

16 Hergueta-Delgado P, Rojo JM, Martin-Guerrero JM, *et al.* *Helicobacter pylori* in relation with rosacea and chronic urticaria. *Gastroenterology* 1999;**116**:G0808.

17 Szlachcic A, Sliwowski Z, Karczewska E, *et al. Helicobacter pylori* and its eradication in rosacea. *J Physiol Pharmacol* 1999;**50**:777–86.

18 Utas S, Ozbakir O, Turasan A, *et al. Helicobacter pylori* eradication treatment reduces the severity of rosacea. *J Am Acad Dermatol* 1999;**40**:433–5.

19 Ertl GA, Levine N, Kligman AM. A comparison of the efficacy of topical tretinoin and low-dose oral isotretinoin in rosacea. *Arch Dermatol* 1994;**130**:319–24.

20 Erdogan FG, Yurtsever P, Aksoy D, *et al.* Efficacy of low-dose isotretinoin in patients with treatment-resistant rosacea. *Arch Dermatol* 1998;**134**:884–5.

21 Gajardo J. Treatment of severe rosacea with oral isotretinoin. *Rev Med Chile* 1994;**122**:177–9.

22 Mazzatenta C, Giorgino G, Rubegni P, de Aloe G, Fimiani M. Solid persistent facial oedema (Morbihan's disease) following rosacea, successfully treated with isotretinoin and ketotifen. *Br J Dermatol* 1997;**137**:1020–1.

23 Pierard-Franchimont C, Quatresooz P, Pierard GE. Incidental control of rosacea by somatostatin. *Dermatology* 2003;**206**:249–51.

24 Dahl MV, Katz HI, Krueger GG, *et al.* Topical metronidazole maintains remissions of rosacea. *Arch Dermatol* 1998;**134**:679–83.

25 Nielsen PG. A double-blind study of 1% metronidazole cream versus systemic oxytetracycline therapy for rosacea. *Br J Dermatol* 1983;**109**:63–5.

26 Veien NK, Christiansen JV, Hjorth N, Schmidt H. Topical metronidazole in the treatment of rosacea. *Cutis* 1986;**38**:209–10.

27 Elewski BE, Fleischer AB Jr, Pariser DM. A comparison of 15% azelaic acid gel and 0.75% metronidazole gel in the topical treatment of papulopustular rosacea: results of a randomized trial. *Arch Dermatol* 2003;**139**:1444–50.

28 Maddin S. A comparison of topical azelaic acid 20% cream and topical metronidazole 0.75% cream in the treatment of patients with papulopustular rosacea. *J Am Acad Dermatol* 1999;**40**:961–5.

29 Signore RJ. A pilot study of 5 percent permethrin cream versus 0.75 percent metronidazole gel in acne rosacea. *Cutis* 1995;**56**:177–9.

30 Espagne E, Guillaume JC, Archimbaud A, *et al.* Étude en double insu contre excipient du métronidazole gel à 0.75 p. 100 dans le traitement de la rosacé. *Ann Dermatol Venereol* 1993;**120**:129–33.

31 Czernielewski J, Liu Y. Comparison of 15% azelaic acid gel and 0.75% metronidazole gel for the topical treatment of papulopustular rosacea. *Arch Dermatol* 2004;**140**:1282–3.

32 Blom I, Hornmark AM. Topical treatment with sulfur 10 per cent for rosacea. *Acta Dermatol Venereol* 1984;**64**:358–9.

33 Sauder DN, Miller R, Gratton D, *et al.* The treatment of rosacea: the safety and efficacy of sodium sulfacetamide 10% and sulfur 5% lotion (Novacet) is demonstrated in a double-blind study. *J Dermatol Treat* 1997;**8**:79–85.

34 Ertl GA, Levine N, Kligman AM. A comparison of the efficacy of topical tretinoin and low-dose oral isotretinoin in rosacea. *Arch Dermatol* 1994;**130**:319–24.

35 Plewig G, Braun-Falco O, Klovekorn W, Luderschmidt C. [Isotretinoin in local treatment of acne and rosacea and animal experiment studies on isotretinoin and arotinoid; in German.] *Hautarzt* 1986;**37**:138–41.

36 Wilkin JK, Dewitt S. Treatment of rosacea: topical clindamycin versus oral tetracycline. *Int J Dermatol* 1993;**32**:65–7.

37 Montes LF, Cordero AA, Kriner J, *et al.* Topical treatment of acne rosacea with benzoyl peroxide acetone gel. *Cutis* 1983;**32**:185–90.

38 Nybaek H, Jemec GB. Photodynamic therapy in the treatment of rosacea. *Dermatology* 2005;**211**:135–8.

17 Perioral dermatitis

Aditya K. Gupta

Background

Definition

Perioral dermatitis is a symmetrical eruption involving the area bounded by the alae of the nose and the chin, consisting of grouped glistening micropapules, microvesicles, or papulopustules of less than 2 mm in diameter, which occur on a diffuse or patchy erythematous base (Figure 17.1). Some degree of scaling may be present, and cropping of the micropapules is usual. A striking and characteristic feature is the sparing of a narrow border around the vermilion of the lips.[1]

Incidence/prevalence

The exact incidence and prevalence is unknown. Perioral dermatitis predominantly affects women in the 15–40 age group. The peak incidence is between 25 and 35 years. The condition is occasionally seen in men and children.[1]

Etiology

The cause of perioral dermatitis is unknown, but some possible etiologic factors include hormonal or emotional factors, cosmetic sensitivity, fluoride dentifrices, infective agents, and use of potent topical steroids.[1]

Prognosis

Following withdrawal of the offending etiologic factor, and with the appropriate treatment, perioral dermatitis generally resolves within a number of weeks. Perioral dermatitis is therefore associated with an excellent prognosis.

Aims of treatment

When treating patients with perioral dermatitis, physicians aim to achieve clinical clearance and prevent recurrence, while minimizing the adverse effects of treatment.

Outcomes

The standard outcomes of treatment include clinical clearance, recurrence rates, and adverse effects of treatment. We found no standard scales of severity in perioral dermatitis.

Methods of search

To identify studies on the treatment of perioral dermatitis, we searched Medline (1966–2006) for publications in English. Since few randomized controlled trials (RCTs) were identified, case series studies were included. Evidence was graded using the quality of evidence scale system reported by Cox *et al.*[2] All evidence derived from the literature is presented.

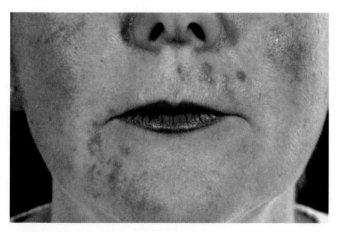

Figure 17.1 A patient with perioral dermatitis.

Questions

What are the effects of metronidazole?

Metronidazole 1% cream
Quality of evidence: I

We found no studies comparing metronidazole 1% cream with placebo. One prospective, double-blind, double-dummy, multicenter RCT was conducted, which evaluated the efficacy of metronidazole 1% cream in comparison with oral tetracycline in the treatment of perioral dermatitis.[3] Tetracycline was statistically more effective in reducing the number of papules associated with perioral dermatitis.

Efficacy
We found one large RCT in which 109 patients were randomly assigned to receive either 1% metronidazole cream plus placebo tablets twice daily, or placebo cream and tetracycline tablets (250 mg twice daily).[3] Patients treated with antibiotics or other medications in the 4 weeks before initiation of the trial were excluded. In the metronidazole group, the median number of papules was reduced to 33% of the original number after 4 weeks and to 8% after 8 weeks. The median number of papule reductions in patients treated with tetracycline was reduced to 4% after 4 weeks, and 0% at 8 weeks. Tetracycline was significantly more effective in reducing the number of papules after 4 and 8 weeks of treatment ($P < 0.01$). No significant differences were noted in any of the other categories evaluated, including erythema and patient and physician assessments.

Drawbacks
Seven patients in the metronidazole group and nine patients in the tetracycline group complained of adverse effects, the most common of which included abdominal discomfort, pruritus, and dryness of the face.

Comment
One RCT was carried out to compare the efficacy of metronidazole 1% cream with that of oral tetracycline. Multiple criteria were evaluated, including papule counts, erythema grading, and patient and physician assessments. Tetracycline was more effective than metronidazole 1% cream in reducing the number of papules. No other significant differences were noted.

Metronidazole 0.75% gel
Quality of evidence: III

We found no reliable evidence on the effects of treatment of perioral dermatitis with metronidazole 0.75% gel. Only case reports were available, and only involved children under

the age of 9 years.[4,5] Studies on adults with perioral dermatitis need to be conducted in order to justify the use of metronidazole 0.75% gel in older patients.

Efficacy
We found no systematic reviews or RCTs. We found two case reports on children in which 17 cases of perioral dermatitis were studied in children between the ages of 9 months and 9 years.[4,5] Eleven of the 17 patients were treated with monotherapy consisting of metronidazole gel 0.75% either once or twice daily. The remaining patients were given combination therapy of metronidazole gel with topical corticosteroids or erythromycin (topical or oral). All patients improved within 8 weeks of therapy. Fourteen patients who were followed up remained lesion-free for up to 16 months.[4]

Drawbacks
None reported.

Comment
All children included in these case reports had used topical steroids prior to treatment with metronidazole. The treatment regimens differed—some patients were treated once daily, whereas most had twice-daily applications. In the small number of patients who have been studied, metronidazole 0.75% gel appeared to be effective. Larger studies would help confirm these preliminary data. We could find no studies that were conducted on adults.

What are the effects of oral antibiotics?

Tetracycline
Quality of evidence: I

We found no good evidence evaluating tetracycline versus placebo. The search found one published RCT evaluating the efficacy of tetracycline (250 mg twice daily) in comparison with metronidazole 1% cream in the treatment of perioral dermatitis.[3] In this study, oral tetracycline was found to be significantly more effective than metronidazole cream with 8 weeks of treatment ($P < 0.01$). After 4 weeks, the number of papules in the tetracycline group was 4% of the original number, in comparison with 33% in the metronidazole group. At 8 weeks, the figures were 0% and 4%, respectively.

We also found some case series reporting the efficacy of oral tetracycline. The follow-up periods for many of the case series ranged from 3 months to 2 years. Tetracycline was shown to be effective, although relapse was common after discontinuation of treatment.[6–10]

Efficacy
No systematic reviews were identified.

Tetracycline versus placebo. We found no placebo-controlled RCTs. We found one case series involving 29 patients with perioral dermatitis, observed over 3 years.[6] The criterion for inclusion was a diagnosis of perioral dermatitis, based on a clinical appearance of papular erythema involving most of the area bordered by the nasolabial folds and the sides of the chin, and a duration of the rash of 3 months or more. Patients were instructed to apply topical 0.5% or 0.25% ichthammol (Ichthyol) in water, or 0.5% or 1% sulfur in calamine lotion at night, alternating with 1% hydrocortisone cream by day. If a favorable response was not seen after 1 or 2 weeks, oral tetracycline was prescribed at a dose of 250 mg three times daily for 1 week and, thereafter, twice daily. Four patients responded to topical therapy alone and did not require treatment with oral tetracycline. Patients treated with tetracycline usually improved within 10–14 days, and had a mean treatment duration of 2–3 months. Relapse occurred when treatment was stopped; however, the tendency to relapse diminished with longer periods of treatment.

Tetracycline plus topical treatments. No placebo-controlled RCTs were found. One trial followed 95 patients with perioral dermatitis for a period of 42 months.[7] Fifty-six patients were treated with oral tetracycline (250 mg q.i.d.), together with a topical sulfacetamide–sulfur–hydrocortisone lotion. Twenty-five patients were treated with sodium sulfacetamide–sulfur–hydrocortisone lotion alone. Of the 56 patients treated with oral tetracycline plus sodium sulfacetamide–sulfur–hydrocortisone lotion, 48 (86%) had complete clearing, with a mean treatment duration of 1 month. Fourteen patients (56%) treated with topical sulfacetamide–sulfur–hydrocortisone lotion only had clearing, with a mean treatment duration of 1 month.

In a small subsidiary study, 37 patients received 1 g of tetracycline daily and 9 patients received 1 g erythromycin daily. Clearing did not occur in 10 patients, even after 10 weeks of treatment. Patients who did achieve complete clearing needed a mean treatment duration of 4.6 weeks.

In one 6-year case series, 39 patients were treated with either tetracycline or erythromycin orally (250 mg twice daily) and with 1% hydrocortisone cream or 0.05% desonide cream, topically twice a day.[8] The mean duration of treatment was 3 months. Twenty-nine (74%) of 39 patients cleared after 2–3 months of therapy and stayed clear. Nine (23%) cleared, but relapsed following discontinuation of therapy. One patient did not achieve remission with therapy.

In a separate study, 43 patients previously given potent local steroids were treated with oral tetracycline at a dose of 250 mg either once or twice daily, combined with either 1% hydrocortisone ointment or Alphaderm ointment.[9] All of the patients experienced improvement after 3 months of treatment, and most had improvement as early as 6 weeks.

Tetracycline with other oral agents. Nine patients with a 3-year history of perioral dermatitis were treated with oral tetracycline or doxycycline administered for 2–3 months.[10] Patients with severe disease were treated with prednisolone 5–15 mg/day given concurrently for 2–3 weeks. Topical therapy included precipitated sulfur lotion and methyl-prednisolone acetate ointment. Seven of the nine patients were reported as being cured after 2 months; the remaining two patients experienced symptomatic relief.

Drawbacks
None reported.

Comment
Most studies did not evaluate the effectiveness of tetracycline alone, but rather in combination with other topical and oral preparations. Much of the available evidence was methodologically flawed. For example, none of the studies adequately defined the term "complete clearing" nor evaluated the results statistically. Prior to consultation, many of the patients included in the case series had been treated unsuccessfully with potent topical steroids, consequently not allowing for a wash-out period. In addition, some studies did not focus only on perioral dermatitis, but included other conditions such as rosacea and rosacea-like dermatitis. Only one double-blind RCT compared oral tetracycline 250 mg twice daily with metronidazole 1% cream.

Oxytetracycline
Quality of evidence: III
The only evidence for the treatment of perioral dermatitis with oxytetracycline was a series of case reports. None of the reports were placebo-controlled, and many used multiple oral and topical agents in combination with oxytetracycline. For this reason, it is very difficult to compare the results of different case series.

Efficacy
No systematic reviews were found.

Oxytetracycline versus placebo. We found no placebo-controlled RCTs. The only evidence available was from case series. One series included 116 patients treated with 250 mg of oxytetracycline twice daily for 3 weeks, then once daily for a similar period.[11] Five patients needed two courses and three patients required three courses of treatment. Eighty patients were seen at the end of their course of treatment, 62 patients at 1–3 months after treatment, nine patients at 6–12 months, and nine patients 2–5 years later. Only five of the returning patients relapsed.

Oxytetracycline plus topical steroids. Another case-series study evaluated 73 patients (5 men, 68 women) using a combination of 1% hydrocortisone cream and oxytetracycline 250 mg twice daily.[12] Seventy-one of the patients had used fluorinated topical steroids previously, and after aggravation of the eruption upon discontinuation of the steroids, virtually all of the patients recovered on the regimen of oxytetracycline and 1% hydrocortisone cream. A 6–14-month follow-up after the study, carried out using a mailed questionnaire, revealed that 11 of 13 respondents remained clear without any further treatment. One patient had experienced a slight recurrence and one had a severe recurrence.

In a separate series, 40 patients were assigned to one of three different groups:

• Group 1: 15 patients treated with topical hydrocortisone and oral oxytetracycline (250 mg twice daily).
• Group 2: 12 patients treated with topical desonide and oxytetracycline (250 mg twice daily).
• Group 3: seven patients treated with desonide and six with hydrocortisone.[13]

Groups 1 and 2 were assigned randomly. Patients in group 3 were selected according to the mildness of their condition, and one patient was included in this group because she was pregnant. In group 1, 14 of the 15 patients improved within 6 weeks and cleared within 3 months. In group 2, improvement within 6 weeks and clearance within 3 months occurred in 11 of the 12 patients. In group 3, 12 of 13 patients responded completely. The pregnant patient experienced no improvement initially and later dropped out. Additionally, there was one drop-out in each of groups 1 and 2.

Drawbacks
None reported.

Comment
We found no RCTs for the treatment of perioral dermatitis with oxytetracycline. Similarly, we found no placebo-controlled trials using oxytetracyclines to treat perioral dermatitis. All studies investigating the treatment of perioral dermatitis with oxytetracyclines were methodologically flawed. For example, in one study patients were randomized to three groups of treatment, but only mild cases were assigned to one treatment group. With the lack of high-quality evidence available, it is difficult to determine the efficacy of oxytetracycline in the treatment of perioral dermatitis.

What are the effects of topical antibiotics?

Topical tetracycline
Quality of evidence: IV
The effects of topical tetracycline were evaluated in the treatment of perioral dermatitis. As the source of this topical preparation was not disclosed, the dose, potency, and efficacy of this type of tetracycline preparation must be questioned.

Efficacy
A case series of 30 patients (26 female, 4 male) with clinically typical perioral dermatitis has been reported.[14] Patients were asked to apply topical tetracycline twice daily to all affected areas after gently washing the face. No other treatment was allowed. Twenty-four patients (80%) experienced complete clearing of their condition in 5–28 days; three patients (10%) were at least 50% clear, but not totally clear, within 28 days; and three patients (10%) discontinued the medication. All patients whose condition cleared were able to maintain clearing with the topical product used on an as-needed basis.

Drawbacks
Two patients discontinued therapy due to stinging, and one patient discontinued because of worsening of the dermatitis.

Comment
We found no RCTs on the treatment of perioral dermatitis with topical tetracycline.

Topical erythromycin
Quality of evidence: IV
We found no good evidence for the effective treatment of perioral dermatitis with topical erythromycin.

Efficacy
Six patients in a case series were treated with 1.5% erythromycin topical solution twice daily in combination with hydrocortisone valerate cream.[15] Topical 1.5% erythromycin was effective in the treatment of perioral dermatitis, with a mean treatment duration of 4.5 weeks.

Drawbacks
None reported.

Comment
No RCTs have evaluated the use of topical erythromycin in the treatment of perioral dermatitis.

What are the effects of nonfluorinated corticosteroids?

Hydrocortisone butyrate
Quality of evidence: IV
We found insufficient evidence on the effects of nonfluorinated corticosteroids in patients with perioral dermatitis. We found one study, a split-face randomized trial, that evaluated rosacea and atopic dermatitis in addition to perioral dermatitis.

Efficacy
We found no systematic reviews.

Hydrocortisone butyrate versus 1% hydrocortisone alcohol cream. In a double-blind, split-face randomized trial, 28 patients with perioral dermatitis (eight patients), rosacea (18 patients), or atopic dermatitis (two patients) randomly treated one side of their face with hydrocortisone alcohol 1% cream and the other side with 0.1% hydrocortisone butyrate.[16] Only patients with severe disease were selected. The participants were instructed to apply the creams twice daily to the appropriate side of the face. Six of the eight patients with perioral dermatitis also received oxytetracycline 250 mg twice daily. The patients were reexamined weekly by the same physician until more improvement was noted on one side of the face in comparison with the opposite side. If no difference was detected, treatment continued for up to 3 months. In addition, the patients were reexamined 1 week after treatment was withdrawn to determine whether any rebound occurred. Two patients with perioral dermatitis achieved better results with hydrocortisone alcohol 1% cream (mean duration of therapy 3.5 weeks, range 3–4 weeks), four patients improved with hydrocortisone butyrate (mean duration: 3–5 weeks, range 2–5 weeks), and two patients found both treatments equally effective.

Drawbacks
Two patients with perioral dermatitis showed a moderate rebound of the eruption after withdrawal of topical treatment, in each case on the hydroxybutyrate-treated side of the face.

Comment
In view of the study design and the small numbers of patients, it is difficult to draw conclusions.

Other treatment modalities

Photodynamic therapy (PDT) with 5-aminolevulinic acid (ALA)
Quality of evidence: IV
We found no placebo-controlled RCTs. The only evidence for the treatment of perioral dermatitis with ALA-PDT was one prospective, split-face trial performed without randomization (in most cases, the side with the highest number of lesions was treated with ALA-PDT).[17] The concentration of the comparator, clindamycin gel applied once daily, was not disclosed. In addition, the results were reported in terms of the per-protocol population (n = 14) instead of the intention-to-treat population (n = 21).

Efficacy
In a split-face study including 21 patients (19 women and 2 men), perioral dermatitis was treated with unoccluded ALA followed by treatment with 410-nm blue light for 8 min on one side of the face and with topical clindamycin phosphate gel applied daily on the other side.[17] The patients had to have at least three facial lesions (as identified by clinical observation) on each side of the face. Patients who completed the study received an average of three weekly treatments (range 1–4) each over 1 month. The responses were considered complete if no lesion was seen at the treatment site. Patient-graded satisfaction was reported using a 5-point scale (where 5 was complete satisfaction).[17]

Fourteen patients (66.7%) completed the study, all of whom received four treatments to achieve complete or nearly complete clearance by either treatment modality. Seven patients did not complete the study due to skin photosensitivity irritation brought on by a failure to avoid sun exposure for the recommended 48 hours after treatment. The mean post-treatment lesion counts—1.4 for ALA-PDT and 2.3 for clindamycin gel—did not differ significantly ($P = 0.1140$). However, the mean lesion counts after treatment were significantly greater than the mean lesion count at baseline for both ALA-PDT ($P < 0.0001$) and clindamycin gel ($P = 0.0001$). The sides treated with ALA-PDT achieved a mean clearance of 92.1% and the clindamycin side had a mean clearance of 80.9%, which was significantly different ($P = 0.0227$). In nine of the 14 patients, the greater level of clearance was on the ALA-PDT side. The mean patient satisfaction level for the side treated with ALA-PDT was 4.4; the level of satisfaction for the clindamycin gel side was not reported.[17]

Drawbacks
Mild postinflammatory hyperpigmentation occurred in three patients in the study. In addition, skin photosensitivity irritation reactions can occur in those who do not avoid sun exposure for 48 hours after treatment.[17]

Comment
In the absence of large-scale, well-designed RCTs, it is difficult to fully assess the impact of ALA-PDT in the treatment of perioral dermatitis. In addition, this seems to be the only published trial incorporating topical clindamycin into a treatment regimen for perioral dermatitis, but again, it is difficult to draw conclusions concerning this treatment modality due to the small number of patients and the overall study design.

Azelaic acid
Quality of evidence: IV
We found no placebo-controlled RCTs involving azelaic acid in the treatment of perioral dermatitis. One open clinical trial investigating the efficacy and tolerability of 20% azelaic acid cream in the treatment of perioral dermatitis in 10 patients (9 women and 1 man) has not yielded sufficient evidence.[18]

Efficacy

Ten patients with perioral dermatitis were treated with 20% azelaic acid cream applied twice daily (overall duration of use not specified). All patients responded to treatment within 2–3 weeks, with clearing of all lesions within 2–6 weeks. There were no reported recurrences of the disease after 4–10 months of follow-up.[18]

Drawbacks

Two of the ten patients reported erythema, itching, and dryness of the face. These were observed mainly in the initial 2 weeks of treatment.[18]

Comment

There is a definite need for placebo-controlled and comparative RCTs before there can be any comment on the effectiveness of azelaic acid in the treatment of perioral dermatitis.[18]

Key points

- Very few RCTs have been conducted to determine appropriate therapies for the treatment of perioral dermatitis.
- It appears that tetracyclines and other oral antibiotics have been used as a standard treatment with some efficacy, but only one RCT has been reported.
- Topical 1% metronidazole cream has been shown to be effective in one RCT.
- Most of the available evidence for these and other treatments comes from case reports.

References

1 Wilkinson D. What is perioral dermatitis? *Int J Dermatol* 1981;**20**:485–6.
2 Cox NH, Eedy DJ, Morton CA. Guidelines for management of Bowen's disease. *Br J Dermatol* 1999;**141**:633–41.
3 Veien NK, Munkvad JM, Nielsen AO. Topical metronidazole in the treatment of perioral dermatitis. *J Am Acad Dermatol* 1991;**24**:258–60.
4 Manders SM, Lucky AW. Perioral dermatitis in childhood. *J Am Acad Dermatol* 1992;**27**:688–92.
5 Miller SR, Shalita AR. Topical metronidazole gel (0.75%) for the treatment of perioral dermatitis in children. *J Am Acad Dermatol* 1994;**31**:847–8.
6 Macdonald A, Feiwel M. Perioral dermatitis: aetiology and treatment with tetracycline. *Br J Dermatol* 1972;**87**:315–9.
7 Bendl BJ. Perioral dermatitis: etiology and treatment. *Cutis* 1976;**17**:903–8.
8 Coskey RJ. Perioral dermatitis. *Cutis* 1984;**34**:55–7.
9 Cotterill JA. Perioral dermatitis. *Br J Dermatol* 1979;**101**:259–62.
10 Urabe H, Koda H. Perioral dermatitis and rosacea-like dermatitis: clinical features and treatment. *Dermatologica* 1976;**152**(Suppl 1):155–60.
11 Wilkinson DS, Kirton V, Wilkinson JD. Perioral dermatitis: a 12-year review. *Br J Dermatol* 1979;**101**:245–7.
12 Sneddon I. Perioral dermatitis. *Br J Dermatol* 1972;**87**:430–4.
13 Cochran REI, Thomson J. Perioral dermatitis: a reappraisal. *Clin Exp Dermatol* 1979;**4**:75–80.
14 Wilson RG. Topical tetracycline in the treatment of perioral dermatitis. *Arch Dermatol* 1979;**115**:637.
15 Bikowski JB. Topical therapy for perioral dermatitis. *Cutis* 1983;**31**:678–82.
16 Sneddon I. A trial of hydrocortisone butyrate in the treatment of rosacea and perioral dermatitis. *Br J Dermatol* 1973;**89**:505–8.
17 Richey DF, Hopson B. Photodynamic therapy for perioral dermatitis. *J Drugs Dermatol* 2006;**5**(2 Suppl):12–6.
18 Jansen T. Azelaic acid as a new treatment for perioral dermatitis: results from an open study. *Br J Dermatol* 2004;**151**:933–4.

Hand eczema

A.M. van Coevorden, Thomas Diepgen, Pieter-Jan Coenraads

Introduction

Definition

The term "hand eczema" implies an inflammation of the skin (dermatitis) that is confined to the hands. Clinically, the condition is characterized by signs of redness, vesicles (tiny blisters), papules, scaling, cracks and hyperkeratosis (callus-like thickening), all of which may be present at different points in time (Figures 18.1, 18.2). Itch, sometimes severe, is a common feature. Microscopically, the disease is characterized by spongiosis with varying degrees of acanthosis, and a superficial perivascular infiltrate of lymphocytes and histiocytes.

Incidence and prevalence

Hand eczema is considered a common condition, with a point prevalence of 1–5% among adults in the general population, and a 1-year prevalence of up to 10%, depend-

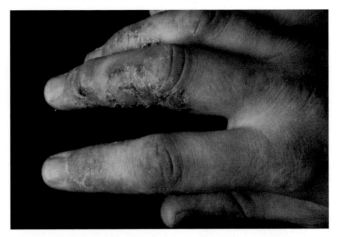

Figure 18.2 Hand eczema: redness, erosions and tiny blisters, accompanied by severe itching.

ing on whether the disease definition includes more pronounced or mild cases. The prevalence may be higher in some countries. Recently, a decreased prevalence has been noted, attributed to decreased occupational exposure to irritants. Hand eczema is twice as common in women as in men, with the highest prevalence in young women. The reasons for this sex difference are unknown, although greater exposure of women to wet work is probably contributory. Reliable data on the incidence are scarce, and are mainly confined to estimates in particular occupational groups. Estimates vary from 0.5 per 1000 in the general population to seven per 1000 per year in high-risk occupations such as bakers and hairdressers.

Etiology

The etiology is multifactorial. Contact irritants are the commonest external causes. Hand eczema caused by such irritants, or mild toxic agents, is known as irritant contact dermatitis. Causal factors that are less common than irritants are contact allergens. Hand eczema caused by skin

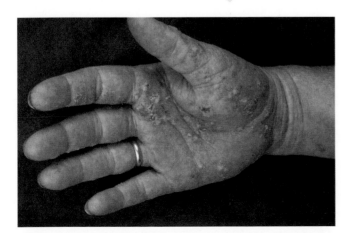

Figure 18.1 Hand eczema: the sides of the fingers are often involved. The yellow crusts indicate secondary infection.

contact with allergens is called allergic contact dermatitis. Ingested allergens (for example, nickel) may also provoke hand eczema. Water is a contact irritant and thus an external causal or contributing factor. Being atopic (with a tendency to develop asthma, hay fever, or eczema) is the major predisposing factor responsible for hand eczema. There are several types of hand eczema for which the cause or predisposing factor is unknown. These (partly overlapping) types are not precisely defined and are commonly described as: hyperkeratotic, tylotic, endogenous, dyshidrotic, pompholyx, and nummular. In particular, dyshidrotic eczema is a subject of debate: a hallmark of this is recurrent vesiculation, which may or may not be associated with factors such as nickel allergy, atopy, and other factors. A combination of the above-mentioned factors appears to play a role in many patients. The relevance of psychosomatic factors remains speculative.

Prognosis

When there is a single, easily avoidable contact allergic factor, the prognosis is good. Several studies, however, have suggested that hand eczema tends to run a long-lasting and chronic relapsing course, probably because of the multifactorial origin.

Diagnostic tests

The diagnosis is mainly based on history and clinical signs; there are no standardized diagnostic criteria. Patients are patch-tested to detect or rule out a contact allergy. In addition, prick tests are performed to detect atopy, and skin scrapings are performed to rule out a mycotic infection. In the majority of cases, no relevant contact allergy can be detected. Specific prick tests are of additional value only in very special cases (such as eczematized urticarial reactions).

Treatment

The treatment of hand eczema is aimed at reducing clinical symptoms (including the disabling itch), preventing relapses, and reducing the burden of disease by allowing the resumption of everyday manual tasks. The outcome of the treatment can be assessed in different ways. Relevant outcome parameters include:
• The percentage of patients reporting a good/excellent response
• The percentage of patients with an investigator-reported good/excellent response
• Reduction in severity (patient-rated and physician-rated scoring systems)
• Dose reduction
• Time until relapse.

Objectives

In everyday clinical practice, we often ask ourselves what treatment would be best for the patient with hand eczema who is sitting in front of us. These questions usually involve a comparison between two treatment modalities. Against this background, we formulated 14 clinically relevant questions.

Because of the tendency of hand eczema to develop a chronic or relapsing course, all of the questions are concerned with chronic hand eczema. In the context of this chapter, chronicity can arbitrarily be defined as a duration of more than 6 months. As prescription of topical corticosteroids is the most common treatment at present, these are the major comparator in the questions below.

Methods of search

Controlled trials dating back to 1977 were located by searching the Cochrane Library, Medline, Embase, Pascal, and Jicst-Eplus. In addition, a hand-search was performed for any trial in major English, German, French, Italian and Dutch dermatology journals. Uncontrolled trials were discarded, unless systematic reviews and controlled trials were lacking on a specific subject. Also, papers studying different dermatoses and not specifically stating the results for the patients with hand eczema were ignored. The questions were formulated before the search, and only papers pertaining to these questions were included.

The content of this chapter relies on an ongoing systematic review of interventions for hand eczema.[1] An overview and quality appraisal of all trials on hand eczema between 1997 and 2003 has been published by the authors.[2]

Questions

Because of the tendency of hand eczema to develop a chronic or relapsing course, all of the questions considered below deal with chronic hand eczema. In the context of this chapter, chronicity can arbitrarily be defined as a duration of more than 6 months. As prescription of topical corticosteroids is at present the most common treatment, it is the major comparator in the questions listed below.
• In adults with chronic hand eczema, do topical corticosteroids lead to a better patient-rated or physician-rated reduction in symptom scores than topical coal-tar preparations?
• In adults with chronic hand eczema, do short bursts of potent topical corticosteroids (class 3 or 4) lead to better patient-rated or physician-rated symptom scores than continuous mild (class 1 or 2) topical steroids?
• In adults with chronic hand eczema, are oral immunosuppressive agents (cyclosporin, methotrexate, mycophenolate

mofetil) better in maintaining a long-term (more than 6 months) reduction of patient-rated or physician-rated symptom scores than topical corticosteroids?

• In adults with chronic hand eczema, does treatment with ionizing radiation lengthen the time until relapse in comparison with topical corticosteroids?

• Does the daily application of a bland emollient lead to dose reduction and/or frequency reduction of topical corticosteroids in adults with chronic hand eczema?

• Is the treatment of chronic hand eczema with local psoralen–ultraviolet A (PUVA) or ultraviolet B (UVB) irradiation better in reducing patient-rated and physician-rated symptom scores than topical corticosteroids?

• In adults with chronic hand eczema, does treatment with PUVA irradiation (oral or topical psoralen) lead to a better reduction in patient-rated and physician-rated symptom scores and remission periods than UVB irradiation?

• In adults with chronic hand eczema, is oral treatment with retinoids better in terms of patient-rated and physician-rated symptom scores than topical corticosteroids?

• In adults with dyshidrotic hand eczema, do iontophoresis or botulinum toxin injections lead to an improvement in patient-rated and physician-rated symptom scores in comparison with topical steroids or UVB/PUVA irradiation?

• In adults with hyperkeratotic hand eczema, does dithranol lead to an improvement in patient-rated and physician-rated symptom scores and longer remission periods after clearance in comparison with topical corticosteroids?

• In adults with relapsing vesicular hand eczema based on contact allergy to nickel, does dietary intervention or oral therapy with chelating agents lead to an improvement in patient-rated and physician-rated symptom scores in comparison with topical corticosteroids?

• In adults with chronic clinically active hand eczema, do protective or occlusive gloves, barrier creams, avoidance of allergens and irritants, and other nonpharmacologic interventions lead to better patient-rated or physician-rated symptom scores than topical steroids?

• Does the addition of a topical antibacterial agent to topical corticosteroids result in better patient-rated or physician-rated symptom scores than topical corticosteroids alone?

• Is the treatment of chronic hand eczema with calcineurin inhibitors better in reducing patient-rated and physician-rated symptom scores than topical corticosteroids?

In adults with chronic hand eczema, do topical corticosteroids lead to a better patient-rated or physician-rated reduction in symptom scores than topical coal-tar preparations?

No systematic review was found, and no trials (controlled or uncontrolled) were identified. Trials may be found in the older literature (pre-1977).

In adults with chronic hand eczema, do short bursts of potent topical corticosteroids (class 3 or 4) lead to better patient-rated or physician-rated symptom scores than continuous mild (class 1 or 2) topical steroids?

We found no studies comparing the effect of short bursts of strong (class 3 or 4) topical corticosteroids (for example, twice weekly, or at weekends only) with continuous application of milder (class 1 or 2) topical corticosteroids. One randomized controlled trial (RCT) compared thrice-weekly application versus weekend application of the same steroid, with limited evidence that the thrice-weekly application was better.

Efficacy
No systematic reviews were found.

Thrice-weekly versus weekend application
There is limited evidence of a preferential effect of thrice-weekly application of mometasone in an RCT of a 30-week maintenance phase (i.e., after induction of remission).[3] The primary outcome variable was the number of recurrences of hand eczema.

Once-daily versus twice-daily application
Once-daily halcinonide 0.1% versus twice-daily betamethasone dipropionate 0.05% showed good efficacy in both groups. In half of the patients, once-daily halcinonide 0.1% was superior.[4]

Two different concentrations
One left–right RCT of 2 weeks' duration comparing different concentrations of the same corticosteroid applied twice daily detected no difference.[5]

Class 2 versus class 3 corticosteroids
One RCT compared short-term (3 weeks) application of fluprednidene acetate 0.1% cream (class 2) with betamethasone valerate 0.1% cream (class 3), both in a once-daily regimen.[6] There were no differences in the time to onset of effect or clinical efficacy.

Class 2 versus class 4 corticosteroids
In a double-blind left–right RCT, more patients remained free of relapses with clobetasol propionate than with fluprednidene acetate.[7] In addition, the time to relapse was longer with clobetasol propionate. Treatment initially and in case of recurrence was twice daily; in the maintenance phase, the application was twice weekly. The side effects were comparable between the two groups.

Drawbacks
Mild skin atrophy was reported in two studies.[3,7]

Comment

With the exception of the study on thrice-weekly versus weekend application, all of the studies were of short duration. None of the studies used tachyphylaxis or atrophy as outcome parameters. No uncontrolled trials were found. Earlier reports (pre-1977) may provide some insight into this issue.

Implications for clinical practice

The appropriate choice of an optimal topical steroid treatment schedule cannot be derived from the current literature on hand eczema trials. Evidence from studies on other eczematous diseases may have to be considered.

In adults with chronic hand eczema, are oral immunosuppressive agents (cyclosporin, methotrexate, mycophenolate mofetil) better in maintaining a long-term (more than 6 months) reduction of patient-rated or physician-rated symptom scores than topical corticosteroids?

Two RCTs were identified, one of which showed that ciclosporin was effective, but not better in terms of clinical signs. The other RCT, studying the same patients, also showed no comparative advantage for ciclosporin over topical corticosteroids in terms of quality of life.

Efficacy

No systematic review was found.

Ciclosporin versus topical betamethasone

One RCT compared ciclosporin with betamethasone dipropionate 0.05% twice daily.[8] The study had three phases, none of which showed a comparative advantage in terms of clinical signs, global assessment, or cumulative relapse rate. The first treatment phase was 6 weeks; the second and third amounted to 30 weeks.

Quality of life was the outcome parameter in a study with the same design and the same patients;[9] this parameter showed no comparative advantage.

Methotrexate

We identified no controlled trials.

Mycophenolate mofetil

We identified no controlled trials.

Drawbacks

Paresthesia ('tingling'), dizziness, insomnia and increase in serum creatinine were reported.

Comment

The comparator in the ciclosporin studies was a relatively strong corticosteroid.

Implications for clinical practice

Ciclosporin may be useful for achieving short-term control, but cannot be recommended for maintenance therapy.

In adults with chronic hand eczema, does treatment with ionizing radiation lengthen the time until relapse in comparison with topical corticosteroids?

We identified six RCTs, all of which had a left–right design (i.e., each patient's contralateral hand served as the control). Two RCTs found no evidence that roentgen rays were superior to conventional topical medication. None of the trials had a follow-up period longer than 6 months; there was therefore no evidence that ionizing radiation induced a longer remission period than conventional topical medication.

Efficacy

No systematic reviews were found.

Versus topical medication

One 18-week study of grenz rays using a grading system as the outcome parameter,[10] and one study of superficial radiotherapy using (near) clearing as the outcome parameter,[11] found no beneficial effect. One 10-week RCT of grenz rays[12] and one 18-week RCT of superficial roentgen rays observed a beneficial effect.[13]

Versus topical PUVA

One trial found a superior effect of radiotherapy at 6 weeks, but after 18 weeks' follow-up there was no difference in the reduction of severity scores.[14]

Superficial roentgen rays versus grenz rays

One study of 18 weeks' duration found a superior effect of conventional roentgen rays from the doctor's point of view, although the patients' rating showed no difference.[15]

Drawbacks

Three trials mentioned an absence of adverse reactions during treatment.[12,13,15] None of the studies was able to assess potentially harmful long-term effects of the radiotherapy.

Comment

None of the trials used the time until relapse as an outcome variable. None of the studies provided any rationale for their sample sizes; the sizes varied between 15 and 30 patients. None of the trials stated explicitly which conventional topical therapy was the comparator; at best, it was described as corticosteroids and/or tar. Overall, the studies did not explicitly describe the types of hand eczema which the patients had: four studies specified the type of eczema as constitutional,[10,13,15] while the other two gave only very partial results among some types of hand eczema.[11,12] Earlier literature reports may provide indications regarding potential long-term harmful effects.

Implications for clinical practice

Given the uncertainties regarding the long-term effects of this treatment modality and the very limited evidence of a short-term effect, radiotherapy cannot be recommended.

Does the daily application of a bland emollient lead to dose reduction and/or frequency reduction of topical corticosteroids in adults with chronic hand eczema?

No RCTs addressing this issue were identified. Only one controlled study compared an emollient with two different topical corticosteroids.

Efficacy

No systematic review was found.

Emollient versus topical corticosteroids

One controlled trial indicated a beneficial effect of a cream containing a camomile extract in comparison with a cream with 0.25% hydrocortisone, but not in comparison with 0.75% fluocortin butyl ester cream.[16] Uncontrolled studies noted a reduction in steroid use in patients treated with a moisturizing cream and in patients treated with a protective foam.[17,18]

Versus each other

In one left–right RCT, using patient preference as the outcome parameter, there was limited evidence in favor of Aquacare-HP over Calmurid, both of which contain 10% urea.[19]

One controlled clinical trial (CCT) with a left–right design did not detect any advantage for a urea cream over an aqueous cream.[20]

An RCT confirmed that the frequent application of emollients resulted in better hand eczema scores.[21] However, a superior effect of emollient with ceramides was not demonstrated. This RCT showed that an emollient with ceramides was able to reduce the use of topical corticosteroids.

The beneficial effect of emollients on hand eczema was also seen in a CCT comparing two bland emollients.[22] There was a decrease in transepidermal water loss, as well as an improvement in physician-rated and patient-rated severity scores.

Drawbacks

No major side effects were reported. Burning and worsening of the preexisting hand eczema were reported.[19] Patients were concerned about greasiness of their hands and with staining of objects they handled.

Comments

Several poor-quality uncontrolled studies were also identified, none of which had steroid dose reduction as the outcome parameter.

Implications for clinical practice

Despite the widespread use of emollients, there is only little evidence of any steroid-sparing or additive effect in the treatment of hand eczema. In general, there seems to be no harm either, apart from occasional contact allergy against an ingredient.

Is the treatment of chronic hand eczema with local PUVA or UVB irradiation better in reducing patient-rated and physician-rated symptom scores than topical corticosteroids?

We identified no trial explicitly comparing PUVA or UVB therapy with topical corticosteroids; only one RCT had ordinary topical treatment with emollients as the comparator. A further six controlled trials were identified that compared the efficacy of PUVA, UVB, or UVA1 therapy with a control group or using a left–right design. There is insufficient evidence that PUVA or UVB therapy is more effective than conventional topical corticosteroid therapy.

Efficacy

No systematic reviews were found.

Topical PUVA

In a double-blind randomized within-patient trial of 15 patients with chronically relapsing vesicular hand eczema, topical PUVA and UVA treatment showed improvement of the severity score over the 8-week treatment period, but no statistical difference between the treated hands at any stage.[23]

In a CCT with a left–right design, topical cream PUVA was compared with UVA1.[24] The study comprised 27 patients with bilateral dyshidrotic hand eczema. Almost all patients showed a good response to both treatments, with a reduction of physician-rated scores of 50%. There were no statistically significant differences between the left and the right hand.

In a left–right design, there was little difference between topical 8-methoxypsoralen (8-MOP) bath PUVA and topical 8-MOP lotion PUVA therapy in 24 patients with chronic hand or foot eczema; there was greater than 80% clearing with both modalities.[25] After 1 month, the most successful treatment was continued on both sides until the lesions cleared; there were no differences in the length of the relapse-free period.

An open-label RCT showed that oral PUVA at home was equally effective as topical bath PUVA in the hospital.[26] In addition, it appeared to result in lower costs and less time off work for the 158 patients.

UVA1

In a double-blind RCT with 28 patients with dyshidrotic hand eczema, five times weekly irradiation with UVA1 was compared with placebo.[27] After 1 week of treatment, a significant difference was seen between the two groups, with greater efficacy for UVA1. Minor erythema was the only side effect observed.

UVB

Eighteen patients with chronic hand eczema resistant to conventional topical therapy with potent corticosteroids were randomly divided into three treatment groups: UVB of the hands only, placebo irradiation, and whole-body UVB irradiation.[28] Local UVB irradiation of the hands was significantly better than placebo; whole-body UVB irradiation with additional irradiation of the hands significantly better than continuing the local treatment alone (not specified), according to a simple clinical grading (cleared, improved, unchanged/worse). A 3-month follow-up period demonstrated fast relapse of the hand eczema.

In an RCT with 48 patients with occupational hand eczema, UVB at home was compared with emollients alone.[29] Physician-rated scores and transepidermal water loss improved in both groups, although the improvement did not reach statistical significance for most parameters.

Drawbacks

PUVA treatment can cause side effects such as burning episodes, subacute eczema, and acute exacerbation of eczema. Ultraviolet therapy may also induce skin cancer as a long-term effect.

Comment

In some studies, patients continued their topical medication or emollients. There are no studies comparing PUVA, UVA1, or UVB therapy with the conventional topical corticosteroid therapy. There is also no evidence that ultraviolet therapy is the most effective for hand eczema (see the next question).

Implications for clinical practice

PUVA and UVB are effective; UVA1 also appears to be effective. The choice of these treatment options is guided by considerations other than proven clinical superiority over other modalities.

In adults with chronic hand eczema, does treatment with PUVA irradiation (oral or topical psoralen) lead to a better reduction in patient-rated and physician-rated symptom scores and remission periods than UVB irradiation?

We identified one RCT on oral PUVA and two CCTs on oral/topical PUVA. The controlled trial on topical bath PUVA demonstrated no comparative advantage, whereas the RCT on oral PUVA showed an effect in favor of PUVA.

Efficacy

No systematic review was found.

Topical bath PUVA versus UVB

A 6-week left–right design CCT including 13 patients showed that, although effective, topical bath PUVA was not better than UVB.[30]

Oral PUVA versus UVB

The only RCT we found, a 3-month study of 35 patients, showed an effect in favor of oral PUVA.[31] In this study, only one hand was treated, but in most patients the untreated hand also improved.

A CCT comparing UVB used at home with PUVA at the clinic showed no comparative advantage.[32]

Drawbacks

Nausea caused by the oral psoralen was reported. Pain, burning, itching, and redness were reported with both therapies, but slightly more from PUVA irradiation.

Comment

Long-term adverse effects could not be assessed. Improvement of the untreated hand may be the result of compliance with topical emollients. More than 17 uncontrolled studies were identified, claiming a beneficial effect of ultraviolet treatment (PUVA or UVB), but there was no comparator in any of the studies.

Implications for clinical practice

PUVA or UVB is effective in treating hand eczema. The question of which modality is better is unsolved.

In adults with chronic hand eczema, is oral treatment with retinoids better in terms of patient-rated and physician-rated symptom scores than topical corticosteroids?

We identified four trials on the use of retinoids in hand eczema; there were no trials comparing oral retinoids with corticosteroids. Both topical and oral treatment with retinoids appeared to be effective.

Efficacy

No systematic reviews were found.

Topical retinoid versus topical corticosteroids

In a symmetrical double-blind nonrandomized study, the efficacy of triamcinolone acetonide 0.1% cream was compared with the same cream containing, in addition, 0.25% retinoic acid.[33] The study included 18 patients with different types of eczema (12 with atopic dermatitis, four with allergic contact dermatitis, one with nummular eczema, and one with dyshidrosis); the palms and soles were involved in only five patients. The duration of treatment was planned for 2 weeks, with the option of extending the treatment to 3 weeks. No statistically significant differences were observed between the treatments.

An open-label RCT with 55 patients compared bexarotene gel monotherapy (ligand for retinoid X receptors) with the same gel in combination with either mometasone furoate 0.1% ointment or with hydrocortisone acetonide 1% ointment.[34] The steroids were applied twice daily, whereas bexarotene gel was applied in an increasing regimen, starting at once every other day up to three times daily, unless adjustment was needed because of irritation. All groups showed a meaningful decrease in physician-rated scores, without significant differences between the groups. Side effects were reported in half the patients in all three groups, without significant differences between the groups, with the exception of stinging and burning, which were more frequent in the combination-treatment arms.

Oral retinoids
An RCT with 29 patients compared once-daily 30 mg acitretin with placebo.[35] A significant improvement in comparison with the placebo group was seen in relation to hyperkeratosis, fissures, and scaling, but not in relation to itch, redness, or vesicles. The improvement occurred in the first 4 weeks, with no additional effect seen in the following 4 weeks. No information was provided on subjective side effects.

A large multicenter double-blind RCT assessed the efficacy of three different dosages of 9-*cis*-retinoic acid (alitretinoin) and placebo.[36] The 319 patients were equally randomized over four groups: oral alitretinoin 10 mg/day, 20 mg/day, 40 mg/day, and placebo. Alitretinoin led to a significant and dose-dependent improvement in the physician-rated score.

Drawbacks
Topical use of retinoic acid plus corticosteroids is reported to cause significantly more subjective irritation than topical corticosteroids without retinoic acid.[33]

Side effects of oral acitretin are common, and almost all patients experience dry lips. The side effects of 9-*cis*-retinoic acid (alitretinoin) were dose-dependent; the most frequently reported were headache (14%, but this was also reported in the placebo group), dry lips (5%), and flushing (3%). Clinically insignificant increases in serum triglyceride, cholesterol, and creatine kinase were reported in the trial on alitretinoin.

Comment
Oral 9-*cis*-retinioic acid appears to be a promising treatment

option, but evidence of an advantage in comparison with conventional therapy is absent. It remains to be demonstrated that this new drug is more effective than conventional topical corticosteroids or UVB/PUVA therapy.

Implications for clinical practice
Oral retinoids appear to be effective in hand eczema. However, as there is no comparison with conventional therapy, it is unclear whether it should be a therapy of first choice.

In adults with dyshidrotic hand eczema, do iontophoresis or botulinum toxin injections lead to an improvement in patient-rated and physician-rated symptom scores in comparison with topical steroids or UVB/PUVA irradiation?

We identified only one RCT using iontophoresis in patients with dyshidrotic hand eczema. This trial showed a significant improvement on the iontophoresis-treated side in comparison with the untreated side. There are no trials comparing iontophoresis with topical corticosteroids or UVB/PUVA therapy. We identified two CCTs dealing with the successful treatment of hand eczema with botulinum toxin injections.

Efficacy
No systematic reviews were found.

Iontophoresis versus no treatment
In a randomized one-sided comparison, the effects of tap-water iontophoresis in addition to steroid-free topical therapy were investigated in 20 patients with dyshidrotic hand eczema.[37] After 3 weeks (20 iontophoresis applications), the parameters "itching" and "vesicle formations" scored significantly better on the iontophoresis-treated side than on the untreated side, but redness and desquamation did not differ significantly.

In an open study of 54 patients with hyperhidrosis, 20 patients with palmoplantar eczema who continued the iontophoresis treatment at home for at least 6 months were compared with a historical sex-matched and age-matched control group of eczema patients without iontophoresis.[38] The relapse-free interval, but not the time needed for clearing, was significantly improved in the iontophoresis-treated group.

Botulinum toxin
One CCT compared the additive effect of botulinum toxin in patients with dyshidrotic hand eczema.[39] The study, with eight patients, had a left–right comparison design, with topical corticosteroids on both hands, and botulinum toxin on the more severely affected hand. It showed an improvement in the physician-rated score, with a reduction of itch and relapses.

Another CCT, including 10 patients, also used an intra-personal comparison.[40] However, one hand was treated with botulinum injections, while the other was left untreated. No topical corticosteroids were used. Both physician-rated and patient-rated scores improved.

Drawbacks

Tap-water iontophoresis was always associated with subjective sensations such as stinging and discrete paresthesia ("tingling"). No severe side effects or possible harmful effects were reported.

Injection with botulinum toxin is painful and has only a temporary effect; repeated injections every few months are needed.

Comment

None of the trials showed sufficient evidence for the benefit of additional iontophoresis therapy in comparison with conventional corticosteroid or UVB/PUVA therapy. The open study that compared the long-term effects of iontophoresis in patients with unspecified hand eczema with historical controls had insufficient evidence to show whether iontophoresis prolongs the relapse-free interval in dyshidrotic hand eczema.[38] Only one study describes the types of dyshidrotic hand eczema which the patients had.[37]

Botulinum toxin appears to be effective as an adjuvant to topical corticosteroids in patients with hand eczema. However, the two CCTs included only 18 patients in total. There were no studies on the effect of iontophoresis.

Implications for clinical practice

Iontophoresis and botulinum toxin injections appear to be harmless, but have not been proved to be effective.

In adults with hyperkeratotic hand eczema, does dithranol lead to an improvement in patient-rated and physician-rated symptom scores and longer remission periods after clearance in comparison with topical corticosteroids?

No systematic reviews were found, and no trials (controlled or uncontrolled) of dithranol for any type of hand eczema were identified. Trials may be found in the earlier literature (pre-1977).

In adults with relapsing vesicular hand eczema based on contact allergy to nickel, does dietary intervention or oral therapy with chelating agents lead to an improvement in patient-rated and physician-rated symptom scores in comparison with topical corticosteroids?

We identified three trials: two RCTs and one CCT. All of the studies were small, conducted in nickel-sensitive patients with hand eczema. Two studies used a nickel-chelating compound and one a low-nickel diet. None of the studies compared the intervention with topical corticosteroids. One multicenter RCT on triethylenetetramine found no significant improvement of hand eczema. The other RCT, on tetraethylthiuram disulfide (disulfiram), found only very limited evidence in favor of this treatment. One controlled trial found no evidence that a low-nickel diet improves dyshidrotic hand eczema.

Efficacy

No systematic reviews were found.

Oral therapy with a nickel-chelating compound

In a multicenter, randomized, double-blind, crossover study, oral treatment with triethylenetetramine 300 mg daily for a 6-week period or a lactose-containing placebo were given to 23 nickel-positive patients with chronic hand eczema after a 4-week rest period before crossover.[41] No significant improvement occurred in hand eczema on the basis of either the patients' or the doctors' evaluations.

In a double-blind, placebo-controlled RCT, tetraethylthiuram disulfide at a gradually increased dosage was given for at least 6 weeks after the full dosage of 200 mg had been reached.[42] Hand eczema was graded according to a semi-quantitative scoring system. During the treatment period, the hand eczema healed in five of the 11 patients treated with tetraethylthiuram disulfide in comparison with two of 13 in the placebo group (not significant). Using the semi-quantitative scoring system, the results in favor of tetra-ethylthiuram disulfide were statistically significant for scaling and frequency of flares, but not for the sum of the parameters.

Low-nickel diet

In a nonrandomized trial including 24 patients with dyshidrotic hand eczema caused by nickel, the effects of a low-nickel diet for 3 months (eight patients) were compared with oral disodium cromoglycate for 3 months (nine patients) and with seven patients who did not give consent to the study and did not receive any treatment.[43] All 24 patients were evaluated blindly for itching and number of vesicles. The low-nickel diet did not lead to improvement in these patients, but those treated with disodium cromoglycate improved significantly and had significantly fewer vesicles than the controls and the patients treated by diet.

Drawbacks

In one RCT, one patient treated with disulfiram had toxic hepatitis after 8 weeks of treatment and two of 30 patients showed signs of hepatic toxicity.[42] One RCT mentioned an absence of adverse reactions during treatment with tri-ethylenetetramine 300 mg daily for a 6-week period.[41] No studies using a low-nickel diet assessed possible harmful effects.

Comment

None of the trials showed sufficient evidence for the benefit of either a low-nickel diet or a nickel-chelating compound. Only two RCTs with small numbers of patients (23 and 11) were carried out. On the basis of the harm and possible side effects, oral treatment with a nickel-chelating compound cannot be recommended. None of the trials compared treatments with conventional topical medication (for example, corticosteroids).

Implications for clinical practice

Given the side effects and the lack of efficacy, oral therapy with a nickel-chelating compound cannot be recommended. There is no evidence that a low-nickel diet improves pompholyx-type hand eczema.

In adults with chronic clinically active hand eczema, do protective or occlusive gloves, barrier creams, avoidance of allergens and irritants, and other nonpharmacologic interventions lead to better patient-rated or physician-rated symptom scores than topical steroids?

Information on avoidance of allergens or irritants on a case-by-case basis can be found in the major textbooks on contact dermatitis. The effect of emollients is covered in the fifth question above.

Efficacy

No systematic reviews were found. There is, however, one systematic review being prepared on interventions to prevent occupational hand dermatitis.[44] A number of issues in connection with this question will be dealt with in this review.

No controlled trials on gloves or protective creams were found. We found a few uncontrolled, rather descriptive studies indicating some benefit of gloves and/or barrier creams, and one study used a within-patient left–right design.[45,46]

Does the addition of a topical antibacterial agent to topical corticosteroids result in better patient-rated or physician-rated symptom scores than topical corticosteroids alone?

No trials compared the additional effect of topical antibacterial agents to topical corticosteroids alone. Only one RCT comparing betamethasone cream with the addition of either fusidic acid or clioquinol was found, showing a similar effect on clinical severity.

Efficacy

No systematic reviews were found.

Addition of fusidic acid or clioquinol to betamethasone

In a multicenter open-label RCT with 120 patients, 4 weeks twice daily application of betamethasone 0.1% clioquinol 3% cream was compared with betamethasone 0.1% fusidic acid 2% cream.[47] The two preparations were equally effective in reducing the observer-rated score. However, the combination of betamethasone cream and fusidic acid produced a better bacteriological response.

Drawbacks

Betamethasone 0.1% fusidic acid 2% cream was considered more cosmetically acceptable than the preparation with clioquinol. The difference was highly significant statistically. Staining of the skin and clothing were the major problems.

Comment

Staphylococcal superantigens in infected areas elsewhere on the body, although the study protocol allowed them to be treated, might have had an effect on the hands.

Implications for clinical practice

There were no comparisons of a corticosteroid with a combination of corticosteroid and antibacterial agents. Evidence of an additional effect of antibacterial agents in patients with hand eczema is still lacking.

Is the treatment of chronic hand eczema with calcineurin inhibitors better in reducing patient-rated and physician-rated symptom scores than topical corticosteroids?

Only one RCT was found that compared the efficacy of topical tacrolimus with mometasone furoate, which appeared to be equivalent. One RCT compared topical pimecrolimus with vehicle.

Efficacy

No systematic reviews were found.

Tacrolimus

Sixteen patients were included in an RCT with intrapersonal comparisons, comparing topical tacrolimus 0.1% ointment with mometasone furoate 0.1% ointment (a class III corticosteroid).[48] The treatment period was 4 weeks, with a follow-up period of up to 8 weeks. Both treatments led to a statistically significant decrease in clinical severity, with no significant differences between the two groups. There was also equivalent efficacy during the follow-up period.

Pimecrolimus

In a multicenter RCT, 294 patients with hand eczema were allocated to up to 3 weeks' treatment with pimecrolimus 1%

cream or to vehicle.[49] Twice-daily application of the study creams (evening application under occlusion) was continued until clearance or completion of 3 weeks' treatment. The efficacy of pimecrolimus 1% cream increased over time, while that of the vehicle plateaued after the second week. There were no statistically significant differences between the two groups, except for those patients in whom palmar involvement was present; pimecrolimus 1% cream was superior in these patients.

Drawbacks
Tacrolimus 0.1% ointment produced stinging upon application; with pimecrolimus 1% cream, however, this was uncommon (0.7% vs. 2.1% in the vehicle group).

Comment
The effect of pimecrolimus 1% cream in comparison with the vehicle might have reached significance if the follow-up period had been longer, as the efficacy of pimecrolimus 1% cream increased over time. Neither study included patient-rated scores.

Implications for clinical practice
Topical calcineurin inhibitors are at best equally effective as topical corticosteroids. With the present evidence, they may be used for rotational therapy with topical corticosteroids, with potent corticosteroids for (severe) exacerbations and topical calcineurin inhibitors in the maintenance phase and for mild exacerbations.

Key points

- There is insufficient evidence on which to base a choice between short bursts of potent topical corticosteroids in comparison with continuous application of mild corticosteroids.
- There is insufficient evidence for oral immunosuppressants as maintenance therapy.
- There is insufficient evidence for a comparative advantage of radiotherapy.
- There is little evidence of a steroid-sparing effect of emollients, although these are widely prescribed.
- PUVA and UVB are effective, but there is no evidence of a clinical advantage of one modality over the other.
- Oral retinoids appear to be effective in hand eczema.
- There is insufficient evidence of an additive effect of iontophoresis or botulinum injections.
- There is insufficient evidence for a low-nickel diet or chelating agents in hand eczema accompanied by nickel allergy.
- There is insufficient evidence of an additive effect of topical antibacterial agents.
- There is insufficient evidence of the superiority of topical calcineurin inhibitors to topical corticosteroids.

Acknowledgment

The authors wish to thank the European Dermato-Epidemiology Network (EDEN) for help in assembling the database of trials and for the evaluation of these trials.

References

1 Van Coevorden AM, Williams HC, Svensson Å, Diepgen TL, Elsner P, Coenraads PJ. Interventions for hand eczema [protocol]. Cochrane Database Syst Rev 2002;(3):CD004055.
2 Van Coevorden AM, Coenraads PJ, Svensson Å, et al. Overview of studies of treatments for hand eczema—the EDEN hand-eczema survey. Br J Dermatol 2004;151:446–51.
3 Veien NK, Larsen PØ, Thestrup-Pedersen K, Schou G. Long-term, intermittent treatment of chronic hand eczema with mometasone furoate. Br J Dermatol 1999;140:882–6.
4 Levy A. Comparison of 0.1% halcinonide with 0.05% betamethasone dipropionate in the treatment of acute and chronic dermatoses. Curr Med Res Opin 1978;5:328–32.
5 Uggeldahl PE, Kero M, Ulshagen K, Solberg VM. Comparative effects of desonide cream 0.1% and 0.05% in patients with hand eczema. Curr Therap Res 1986;40:969–73.
6 Bleeker J, Anagrius C, Iversen N, Stenberg B, Cullberg Valentin K. Double-blind comparative study of Corticoderm cream + Unguentum Merck and Betnovate cream + Unguentum Merck in hand dermatitis. J Dermatol Treat 1989;1:87–90.
7 Möller H, Svartholm H, Dahl G. Intermittent maintenance therapy in chronic hand eczema with clobetasol propionate and flupredniden acetate. Curr Med Res Opin 1983;8:640–4.
8 Granlund H, Erkko P, Eriksson E, Reitamo S. Comparison of cyclosporine and topical betamethasone-17,21-dipropionate in the treatment of severe chronic hand eczema. Acta Derm Venereol (Stockh) 1996;76:371–6.
9 Granlund H, Erkko P, Reitamo S. Comparison of the influence of cyclosporin and topical betamethasone-17,21-dipropionate treatment on quality of life in chronic hand eczema. Acta Derm Venereol (Stockh) 1997;77:54–8.
10 Cartwright PH, Rowell NR. Comparison of Grenz rays versus placebo in the treatment of chronic hand eczema. Br J Dermatol 1987;117:73–6.
11 King CM, Chalmers RJG. A double-blind study of superficial radiotherapy in chronic palmar eczema. Br J Dermatol 1984;111:451–4.
12 Lindelöf B, Wrangsjö K, Lidén S. A double-blind study of Grenz ray therapy in chronic eczema of the hands. Br J Dermatol 1987;117:77–80.
13 Fairris GM, Mack DP, Rowell NR. Superficial X-ray therapy in the treatment of constitutional eczema of the hands. Br J Dermatol 1984;111:445–9.
14 Sheehan-Dare RA, Goodfield MJ, Rowell NR. Topical psoralen photochemotherapy (PUVA) and superficial radiotherapy in the treatment of chronic hand eczema. Br J Dermatol 1989;121:65–9.
15 Fairris GM, Jones DH, Mack DP, Rowell NR. Conventional superficial X-ray versus Grenz ray therapy in the treatment of constitutional eczema of the hands. Br J Dermatol 1985;112:339–41.

16 Aertgeerts P, Albring M, Klaschka F, *et al.* [Comparative testing of Kamillosan cream and steroidal (0.25% hydrocortisone, 0.75% fluocortin butyl ester) and non-steroidal (5% bufexamac) dermatologic agents in maintenance therapy of eczematous diseases; in German.] *Z Hautkr* 1985;**60**: 270–7.

17 Fowler JF. A skin moisturizing cream containing quaternium-18-bentonite effectively improves chronic hand eczema. *J Cutan Med Surg* 2001;**5**: 201–5.

18 Fowler JF. Efficacy of a skin-protective foam in the treatment of chronic hand dermatitis. *Am J Contact Dermat* 2000;**11**:165–9.

19 Fredriksson T, Gip L. Urea creams in the treatment of dry skin and hand dermatitis. *Int J Dermatol* 1975;**14**:442–4.

20 [No authors listed.] Carbamide in hyperkeratosis. *Practitioner* 1973;**210**:294–6.

21 Kucharekova M, Van de Kerkhof PC, Van der Valk PG. A randomized comparison of an emollient containing skin-related lipids with a petrolatum-based emollient as adjunct in the treatment of chronic hand dermatitis. *Contact Dermatitis* 2003;**48**: 293–9.

22 Bock M, Wulfhorst B, Gabard B, Schwanitz HJ. Effektivität von Hautschutzcremes zur Behandlung irritativer Kontaktekzeme bei Friseurauszubildenden. *Dermatol Beruf Umwelt* 2001;**49**:73–6.

23 Grattan CEH, Carmichael AJ, Shuttleworth GJ, Foulds IS. Comparison of topical PUVA with UVA for chronic vesicular hand eczema. *Acta Derm Venereol (Stockh)* 1991;**71**:118–22.

24 Petering H, Breuer C, Herbst R, Kapp A, Werfel T. Comparison of localized high-dose UVA1 irradiation versus topical cream psoralen-UVA for treatment of chronic vesicular dyshidrotic eczema. *J Am Acad Dermatol* 2004;**50**:68–72.

25 Shephard SE, Schregenberger N, Dummer R, Panizzon RG. Comparison of 8-MOP aqueous bath and 8-MOP ethanolic lotion (Meladinine) in local PUVA therapy. *Dermatology* 1998;**197**:25–30.

26 Van Coevorden AM, Kamphof WG, Van Sonderen E, Bruynzeel DP, Coenraads PJ. Comparison of oral psoralen–UV-A with a portable tanning unit at home vs hospital-administered bath psoralen–UV-A in patients with chronic hand eczema: an open-label randomized controlled trial of efficacy. *Arch Dermatol* 2004; **140**:1463–6.

27 Polderman MCA, Govaert JCM, Le Cessie S, Pavel S. A double-blind placebo-controlled trial of UVA-1 in the treatment of dyshidrotic eczema. *Clin Exp Dermatol* 2003;**28**:584–7.

28 Sjövall P, Christensen OB. Treatment of chronic hand eczema with UV-B Handylux in the clinic and at home. *Contact Dermatitis* 1994;**31**:5–8.

29 Bayerl C, Garbea A, Peiler D, *et al.* Pilotstudie zur Therapie des beruflich bedingten Handekzems mit einer neuen tragbaren UVB-Bestrahlungseinheit. *Akt Dermatol* 1999;**25**:302–5.

30 Simons JR, Bohnen IJWE, Van der Valk PGM. A left–right comparison of UV-B photochemotherapy in bilateral chronic hand dermatitis after 6 weeks' treatment. *Clin Exp Dermatol* 1997;**22**:7–10.

31 Rosén K, Mobacken H, Swanbeck G. Chronic eczematous dermatitis of the hands: a comparison of PUVA and UVB treatment. *Acta Derm Venereol (Stockh)* 1987;**67**:48–54.

32 Sjövall P, Christensen OB. Local and systemic effect of UVB irradiation in patients with chronic hand eczema. *Acta Derm Venereol (Stockh)* 1987;**67**:538–41.

33 Schmied C, Piletta PA, Saurat JH. Treatment of eczema with a mixture of triamcinolone acetonide and retinoic acid: a double blind study. *Dermatology* 1993;**187**:263–7.

34 Hanifin JM, Stevens V, Sheth P, Breneman D. Novel treatment of chronic severe hand dermatitis with bexarotene gel. *Br J Dermatol* 2004;**150**:545–53.

35 Thestrup-Pedersen K, Andersen KE, Menné T, Veien NK. Treatment of hyperkeratotic dermatitis of the palms (eczema keratoticum) with oral acitretin. A single-blind placebo-controlled study. *Acta Derm Venereol (Stockh)* 2001;**81**:353–5.

36 Ruzicka T, Larsen FG, Galewicz D, *et al.* Oral alitretinoin (9-cis-retinoic acid) therapy for chronic hand dermatitis in patients refractory to standard therapy. Results of a randomized, double-blind, placebo-controlled, multicenter trial. *Arch Dermatol* 2004; **140**:1453–9.

37 Odia S, Vocks E, Rakoski J, Ring J. Successful treatment of dyshidrotic hand eczema using tap water iontophoresis with pulsed direct current. *Acta Derm Venereol (Stockh)* 1996;**76**:472–4.

38 Wollina U, Uhlemann C, Elstermann D, Köber L, Barta U. [Therapy of hyperhidrosis with tap water iontophoresis. Positive effect on healing time and lack of recurrence in hand-foot eczema; in German.] *Hautarzt* 1998;**49**:109–13.

39 Wollina U, Karamfilov T. Adjuvant botulinum toxin A in dyshidrotic hand eczema: a controlled prospective pilot study with left–right comparison. *J Eur Acad Dermatol Venereol* 2002;**16**:40–2.

40 Swartling C, Naver H, Lindberg M, Anveden I. Treatment of dyshidrotic hand dermatitis with intradermal botulinum toxin. *J Am Acad Dermatol* 2002;**47**:667–71.

41 Burrows D, Rogers S, Beck M, *et al.* Treatment of nickel dermatitis with trientine. *Contact Dermatitis* 1986;**15**:55–7.

42 Kaaber K, Menné T, Veien N, Hougaard P. Treatment of nickel dermatitis with Antabuse: a double blind study. *Contact Dermatitis* 1983;**9**:297–9.

43 Pigatto PD, Gibelli E, Fumagalli M, Bigardi A, Morelli M, Altomare GF. Disodium cromoglycate versus diet in the treatment and prevention of nickel-positive pompholyx. *Contact Dermatitis* 1990;**22**:27–31.

44 Bauer A, Bong J, Coenraads PJ, Elsner P, English J, Williams HC. Interventions for preventing occupational irritant hand dermatitis [protocol]. *Cochrane Database Syst Rev* 2003;(**3**):CD004414.

45 Schleicher SM, Milstein HJ, Ilowite R, Meyer P. Response of hand dermatitis to a new skin barrier protectant cream. *Cutis* 1998;**61**: 233–4.

46 Baack BR, Holguin TA, Holmes HS, Prawer SE, Scheman AJ. Use of a semipermeable glove during treatment of hand dermatitis. *Cutis* 1996;**58**:423–4.

47 Hill VA, Wong E, Corbett MF, Menday AP. Comparative efficacy of betamethasone/clioquinol (Betnovate-C) cream and betamethasone/fusidic acid (Fucibet) cream in the treatment of infected hand eczema. *J Dermatol Treat* 1998;**9**:15–9.

48 Schnopp C, Remling R, Mohrenschlager M, Weigl L, Ring J, Abeck D. Topical tacrolimus (FK506) and mometasone furoate in treatment of dyshidrotic palmar eczema: a randomized, observer-blinded trial. *J Am Acad Dermatol* 2002;**46**:73–7.

49 Belsito DV, Fowler JF, Marks JG, *et al.* Pimecrolimus cream 1%: a potential new treatment for chronic hand dermatitis. *Cutis* 2004; **73**:31–8.

19 Atopic eczema

Kim Thomas, Fiona Bath-Hextall, Jane Ravenscroft, Carolyn Charman, Hywel Williams

Web tables referred to in this chapter are published on the book's web site (http://www.evidbasedderm.com).

Since over 50 types of interventions have been tried in atopic eczema (synonymous with atopic dermatitis), complete coverage of all therapy-related issues for atopic eczema is not possible, even in a chapter of this size. Instead, we have opted to introduce the evidence base for treating atopic eczema by means of three common clinical scenarios:
- Case scenario 1: a child with moderately severe atopic eczema
- Case scenario 2: a person with clinically infected atopic eczema
- Case scenario 3: an adult with severe atopic eczema

Much of the background work and methodology within the sections has been based (with appropriate updates) on the results of the United Kingdom National Health Service (NHS) systematic review of atopic eczema treatments, which was published at the end of 2000. For a more comprehensive and detailed assessment of important areas such as disease prevention that are not covered in this chapter, readers are recommended to read the relevant sections of this report, which is available free in the public domain (http://www.ncchta.org). Additional information on topical tacrolimus and pimecrolimus and on the frequency of use of topical corticosteroids has been identified in three substantial technology reviews produced by the UK National Institute for Health and Clinical Excellence (NICE; www.nice.org.uk). Further extensive accounts of the evidence base for eczema treatments can be found in the technical report of the American Academy of Dermatology guidelines for the care of atopic dermatitis (www.aad.org) and for the 2007 NICE guidelines for managing atopic eczema in children (http://guidance.nice.org.uk). Given the large amount of data described in this chapter, the references are provided at the end of each therapy section, rather than at the end of the chapter. Detailed data tables are provided on the web site accompanying this book.

Background

Definition and diagnostic criteria

Atopic eczema is a chronic inflammatory skin condition characterized by an itchy red rash that favors the skin creases, such as the folds of the elbows, behind the knees, and around the neck. The morphology of the eczema lesions varies in appearance from vesicles to gross lichenification on a background of poorly demarcated redness. Other features such as crusting, scaling, cracking, and swelling of the skin can occur.[1] Atopic eczema is associated with other atopic diseases such as hay fever and asthma, although such associations may reflect shared environmental causes, as opposed to genetics. People with atopic eczema also have a tendency to have a dry skin, which increases their vulnerability to the irritant effects of soaps. Much of the dry skin tendency might be secondary to deficiencies in filaggrin expression, which is genetically determined and important in white European populations.[2]

Atopic eczema typically starts in early life, with about 80% of cases starting before 5 years of age.[3] Although the word "atopic" is used when describing atopic eczema, it should be noted that anything from 20% to 100% of people with otherwise typical atopic eczema are not atopic as defined by the presence of positive skin-prick test reactions to common environmental allergens or through blood tests that detect specific circulating immunoglobulin E (IgE) antibodies.[4] The role of atopy in atopic eczema has been systematically reviewed elsewhere.[5] The word "atopic" in the term "atopic eczema" is simply an indicator of the frequent association with atopy and the need to separate this clinical phenotype from other forms of eczema such as irritant or allergic contact eczema, which have other causes and distinct patterns. The terms "atopic eczema" and "atopic dermatitis" are synonymous. The term "atopic eczema" or just "eczema" is frequently used in the United Kingdom, whereas the term "atopic dermatitis" is used more in the United States. Much scientific energy has been wasted in debating which term should be used, culminating in the World Allergy Organization proposal for a revised nomenclature.[6]

Very often, no definition of atopic eczema is given in clinical studies such as clinical trials. This leaves the reader guessing as to what sort of people were studied. Atopic eczema is a difficult disease to define, as the clinical features are highly variable with regard to morphology, body site, and time. There is no specific diagnostic test encompassing all people with typical eczema that can serve as a reference standard. The diagnosis is, therefore, essentially a clinical one.

At least 10 synonyms for atopic eczema were in common usage in the dermatology literature in the 1970s, and it is doubtful whether physicians were all referring to the same disease. A major development in describing the main clinical features of atopic eczema was the Hanifin and Rajka diagnostic criteria (1980).[7] These criteria are frequently cited in clinical trial articles, and they at least provide some degree of confidence that researchers are referring to a similar disease when using these features. It should be borne in mind, however, that these criteria were developed on the basis of consensus, and their validity and repeatability are unknown in relation to physicians' diagnoses.[4] Some of the minor features have since been shown not to be associated with atopic eczema, and many of the terms, which are poorly defined, probably mean something only to dermatologists. Scientifically developed refinements of the Hanifin and Rajka diagnostic criteria, mainly for epidemiological studies, have been developed by a UK working party, and these criteria have been widely used throughout the world and in clinical trials (Box 19.1).[8,9]

It is quite possible that there are distinct subsets of atopic eczema—for example, those cases associated with atopy, those forms associated with early wheezing,[10] those associated with defective filaggrin expression,[2] and patients who have severe disease with recurrent infections. Until the exact genetic and causative agents are known, it is prudent to consider the clinical disease as one condition. Perhaps prespecified sensitivity analyses should be done within clinical trials, if large enough, for those who are thought to represent distinct subsets—for example, those who are definitely atopic, with raised circulating IgE to allergens, and those with severe disease and associated asthma—especially for trials of certain interventions, such as reducing house dust mites or food exclusions, where the presence of prior sensitization might be key.[4]

Incidence/prevalence

Atopic eczema is a very common problem. European prevalence studies conducted during the last 10 years suggest an overall prevalence of 15–20% in children aged 7–18 years.[11] Standardized questionnaire data from half a million children aged 13–14 years in the International Study of Asthma and Allergies in Childhood (ISAAC) suggest that atopic eczema is not just a problem confined to western Europe, with high prevalences being found in many developing cities undergoing rapid demographic change.[12] There is reasonable evidence to suggest that the prevalence of atopic eczema has increased two- to threefold over the last 30 years, although the reasons for this are unclear.[13] No reliable estimates of the incidence are available for atopic eczema.

Atopic eczema is more frequent in childhood, especially in the first 5 years of life. One study of 2365 patients in Livingston, Scotland, who were examined by a dermatologist for atopic eczema, suggested that atopic eczema is relatively rare over 40 years of age, with a 1-year period prevalence of 0.2%.[14] Yet, because there are many more adults than children, they may make up over 38% of all atopic eczema cases in that community. Adults also tend to represent a more persistent and severe subset of cases.

Most cases of childhood eczema in any given community are mild. One study found that 84% of 1760 children aged 1–5 years from four urban and semi-urban family practitioners around Nottingham, England, were mild, as defined globally by the examining physician, with 14% of cases in the moderate category and 2% in the severe category[15]—a severity distribution that was very similar to that in another population survey in Norway.[16]

Morbidity and costs

Atopic eczema usually accounts for the worst disturbance in quality of life in comparison with other dermatological diseases. Specific aspects of a child's life affected by atopic eczema are:[11]
- Itch and its associated sleep loss (which can also cause considerable family disturbance)
- Social stigmatization from other children and parents

BOX 19.1 In order to qualify as having a case of atopic eczema, the person must have the following:[9]

- An itchy skin condition, plus three or more of:
- Past involvement of the skin creases, such as bends of elbows or behind the knees
- A personal or immediate family history of asthma or hay fever
- A tendency towards a generally dry skin
- Onset under the age of 2 years
- Visible flexural dermatitis, as defined by a photographic protocol

- The need for special clothing and bedding
- Avoidance of activities such as swimming
- The need for frequent applications of topical treatments and visits to health-care professionals.

In financial terms, the cost of atopic eczema is potentially very large. One study of an entire community in Scotland in 1995 estimated that the annual personal costs to patients with atopic eczema was £297 million ($606 million), if extrapolated to the entire UK.[17] The cost to the National Health Service was £125 million, and the annual cost to society through lost working days was £43 million, making the total expenditure on atopic eczema £465 million per year ($949 million). This figure is likely to be an underestimate, since the prevalence of atopic eczema is lower in Scotland in comparison with the rest of the UK. Another study from Australia found that the annual personal financial cost of managing mild, moderate, and severe eczema was A$ 330, A$ 818, and A$ 1255, respectively, which was greater than the costs associated with asthma in that study.[18]

Etiology

Genetics

There is good evidence to suggest that genetic factors are important in the predisposition to atopic eczema. Twin studies have shown a much higher concordance for monozygotic (85%) than for dizygotic twins (21%),[19] although no single gene has yet emerged as a consistent marker for atopic eczema, apart from genes coding for filaggrin protein in some populations.[2] Several genes coding for immune response, skin dryness, and the ability to deal with *Staphylococcus aureus* may be important, and it is possible that the tendency to atopic eczema might be inherited independently from atopy.[20]

Environment

There are several general and specific clues that point strongly to a role of the environment in disease expression.[21] It is difficult to explain the large increase in the prevalence of atopic eczema over the past 30 years in terms of genetics.[13] It has been shown that atopic eczema is more frequent in wealthy families.[22] It is unclear whether this positive social class gradient reflects exposure to indoor allergens or whether it reflects a whole constellation of other factors associated with social "development." Other studies have shown an inverse association between the prevalence of eczema and family size.[23] This observation led to the "hygiene hypothesis"—that children in larger families were "protected" from expressing atopy because of frequent exposure to infections.[24] Some evidence for this "protective" effect of infections on atopic eczema has been shown in relation to measles infection.[25] The link between fewer infections (bacterial or helminthic) and increased eczema has been reviewed comprehensively elsewhere.[26]

Migrant studies also point strongly to the role of environmental factors in atopic eczema. For example, 14.9% of black Caribbean children living in London develop atopic eczema (according to the UK diagnostic criteria), in comparison with only 5.6% of similar children living in Kingston, Jamaica.[27]

Further work has suggested that the tendency to atopy may be programmed at birth and could be related to factors such as maternal age.[28] The observation that many cases of atopic eczema improve spontaneously around puberty is also difficult to explain in genetic terms alone.[3] Specific environmental risk factors for the expression of eczema are still not fully elucidated. Allergic factors such as exposure to house dust mite may be important, but nonallergic factors such as exposure to irritants, bacteria, and hard water may also be equally important.[29]

Pathophysiology

There appears to be a failure to switch off the natural predominance of T-helper 2 (Th2) lymphocytes that occurs in infancy, which leads to an abnormal response of chemical messengers called cytokines to a variety of stimuli.[1,30] The underlying mechanism of disease may be abnormalities in cyclic nucleotide regulation of marrow-derived cells or allergenic overstimulation, causing secondary abnormalities. Some studies have demonstrated a defect in lipid composition and barrier function in people with atopic eczema—a defect that is thought to underlie the tendency to dry skin and possibly the enhanced penetration of environmental allergens and irritants, leading to chronic inflammation.

Prognosis

The majority of children with atopic eczema appear to "grow out" of their disease—at least to the point where the condition becomes a problem no longer in need of medical care. A detailed review of prognostic studies reported elsewhere[3] concluded that most large studies of well-defined and representative cases suggest that about 60% of childhood patients are clear or free of disease symptoms in early adolescence. However, many such apparently clear cases are likely to recur in adulthood, often as hand eczema. The most consistent factors that appear to predict persistent atopic eczema are early onset, severe widespread disease in infancy, concomitant asthma or hay fever, and a family history of atopic eczema.

Aims of treatment

Cure is an unrealistic option for the majority of sufferers, as it is so unusual for there to be a single, treatable cause for atopic eczema, such as a specific food allergy. In addition, the effect of conventional treatment on the long-term natural history of the disease is simply not known. Treatment is thus aimed at relieving troublesome symptoms such as itch and soreness and its associated sleep loss, in order to improve the person's quality of life. Improvement in skin appearance may also be important, as is self-esteem, social confidence, and the ability to participate freely in recreational activities such as swimming.

Relevant outcomes

Outcome measures used in trials have been reviewed by Finlay.[31] Most outcome measures have incorporated some measure of itch, as assessed by a doctor at periodic reviews or patient self-completed diaries. Other more sophisticated methods of objectively recording itch have been tried. Finlay drew attention to the profusion of composite scales used in evaluating atopic eczema outcomes. These usually incorporate measures of the extent of atopic eczema and several physical signs such as redness, scratch marks, thickening of the skin, scaling, and dryness. Such signs are typically mixed with symptoms of sleep loss and itching, and variable weighting systems are used. It has been shown that measuring surface area involvement in atopic eczema is fraught with difficulty[32]—which is not surprising, considering that eczema is, by definition, "poorly defined erythema." Charman et al. carried out a systematic review of named outcome measure scales for atopic eczema and found that of the 13 named scales in current use, only one (*Sco*ring *A*topic *D*ermatitis, SCORAD) had been fully tested for validity, repeatability, and responsiveness.[33] Quality-of-life measures specific to dermatology include the Dermatology Quality of Life Index[34] and Skindex.[35] The Children's Dermatology Life Quality Index (CDLQI) has been used in atopic eczema trials in children. Subsequent work by Charman has resulted in the development of a patient-oriented outcome measure known as the Patient-Orientated Eczema Measure (POEM)—an outcome that measures items that are deemed to be important for patients and which can also be used for rapid monitoring in routine clinical practice.[36]

Most clinical trials of atopic eczema have been very short (i.e., about 6 weeks), which seems inappropriate in a chronic relapsing condition.[37] Few studies have considered measuring the number and duration of disease-free periods, apart from a few exceptions in the use of topical calcineurin inhibitors and "weekend" treatment for topical corticosteroids. In the absence of such long-term studies, it is impossible to say whether modern treatments have increased chronicity at the expense of short-term control. The definition of a "flare" of atopic eczema is problematic and has been reviewed by Langan et al., who also propose a series of long-term outcomes such as the number of "well-controlled weeks," analogous to long-term asthma outcomes.[38]

References: background

1 Archer CB. The pathophysiology and clinical features of atopic dermatitis. In: Williams HC, ed. *Atopic Dermatitis*. Cambridge: Cambridge University Press, 2000: 25–40.

2 Irvine AD. Fleshing out filaggrin phenotypes. *J Invest Dermatol* 2007;**127**:504–7.

3 Williams HC, Wüthrich B. The natural history of atopic dermatitis. In: Williams HC, ed. *Atopic Dermatitis*. Cambridge: Cambridge University Press, 2000: 41–59.

4 Williams HC. What is atopic dermatitis and how should it be defined in epidemiological studies? In: Williams HC, ed. *Atopic Dermatitis*. Cambridge: Cambridge University Press, 2000: 3–24.

5 Flohr C, Johansson SGO, Wahlgren CF, Williams HC. How "atopic" is atopic dermatitis? *J Allergy Clin Immunol* 2004; **114**:150–8.

6 Johansson SG, Bieber T, Dahl R, *et al.* Revised nomenclature for allergy for global use: Report of the Nomenclature Review Committee of the World Allergy Organization, October 2003. *J Allergy Clin Immunol* 2004;**113**:832–6.

7 Hanifin JM, Rajka G. Diagnostic features of atopic eczema. *Acta Derm Venereol (Stockh)* 1980;**92**:44–7.

8 Williams HC. The future research agenda. In: Williams HC, ed. *Atopic Dermatitis*. Cambridge: Cambridge University Press, 2000: 247–61.

9 Williams HC, Forsdyke H, Boodoo G, Hay RJ, Burney PGF. A protocol for recording the sign of visible flexural dermatitis. *Br J Dermatol* 1995;**133**:941–9.

10 Illi S, von Mutius E, Lau S, *et al.* The natural course of atopic dermatitis from birth to age 7 years and the association with asthma. *J Allergy Clin Immunol* 2004;**113**:925–31.

11 Herd RM. The morbidity and cost of atopic dermatitis. In: Williams HC, ed. *Atopic Dermatitis*. Cambridge: Cambridge University Press, 2000: 85–95.

12 Williams HC, Robertson CF, Stewart AW, ISAAC Steering Committee. Worldwide variations in the prevalence of atopic eczema symptoms. *J Allergy Clin Immunol* 1999;**103**:125–38.

13 Williams HC. Is the prevalence of atopic dermatitis increasing? *Clin Exp Dermatol* 1992;**17**:385–91.

14 Herd RM, Tidman MJ, Prescott RJ, Hunter JAA. Prevalence of atopic eczema in the community: the Lothian atopic dermatitis study. *Br J Dermatol* 1996;**135**:18–9.

15 Emerson RM, Williams HC, Allen BR. Severity distribution of atopic dermatitis in the community and its relationship to secondary referral. *Br J Dermatol* 1998;**139**:73–6.

16 Dotterud LK, Kvammen B, Lund E, Falk ES. Prevalence and some clinical aspects of atopic dermatitis in the community of Sør-Varanger. *Acta Derm Venereol* 1995;**75**:50–3.

17 Herd RM, Tidman MJ, Prescott RJ, Hunter JAA. The cost of atopic eczema. Br J Dermatol 1996;**135**:20–3.

18 Su JC, Kemp AS, Varigos GA, Nolan TM. Atopic eczema: its impact on the family and financial cost. *Arch Dis Child* 1997; **76**:159–62.

19 Schultz-Larsen F, Holm NV, Henningsen K. Atopic dermatitis. A genetic-epidemiological study in a population-based twin sample. *J Am Acad Dermatol* 1986;**15**:487–94.

20 Morar N, Williswen SA, Moffatt MF, Cookson WO. The genetics of atopic dermatitis. *J Allergy Clin Immunol* 2006;**118**:24–34.

21 Williams HC. Atopic eczema—why we should look to the environment. *BMJ* 1995;**311**:1241–2.

22 Williams HC, Strachan DP, Hay RJ. Childhood eczema: disease of the advantaged? *BMJ* 1994;**308**:1132–5.

23 McNally N, Phillips D. Social factors and atopic dermatitis. In: Williams HC, ed. *Atopic Dermatitis*. Cambridge: Cambridge University Press, 2000: 139–47.

24 Strachan DP. Hayfever, hygiene, and household size. *BMJ* 1989;**299**:1259–60.

25 Shaheen S. Discovering the causes of atopy. *BMJ* 1997;**314**:987–8.

26 Flohr C, Pascoe D, Williams HC. Atopic dermatitis and the "hygiene hypothesis": too clean to be true? *Br J Dermatol* 2005; **152**:202–16.

27 Burrell-Morris C, Williams HC. Atopic dermatitis in migrant populations. In: Williams HC, ed. *Atopic Dermatitis*. Cambridge: Cambridge University Press, 2000: 169–82.

28 Olesen AB, Ellingsen AR, Olesen H, Juul S, Thestrup-Pedersen K. Atopic dermatitis and birth factors: historical follow up by record linkage. *BMJ* 1997;**314**:1003–8.

29 Hanifin JM. Atopic eczema. In: Marks RM, ed. *Eczema*. London: Dunitz, 1992: 77–101.

30 Hanifin JM, Chan S. Biochemical and immunologic mechanisms in atopic dermatitis: new targets for emerging therapies. *J Am Acad Dermatol* 1999;**41**:72–7.

31 Finlay AY. Measurement of disease activity and outcome in atopic dermatitis. *Br J Dermatol* 1996;**135**:509–15.

32 Charman CR, Venn AJ, Williams HC. Measurement of body surface involvement in atopic eczema: an impossible task? *Br J Dermatol* 1999;**140**:109–11.

33 Charman CR, Williams HC. Outcome measures of disease severity in atopic eczema. *Arch Dermatol* 2000;**136**:763–9.

34 Finlay AY, Khan GK. Dermatology Life Quality Index (DLQI): a simple practical measure for routine clinical use. *Clin Exp Dermatol* 1994;**19**:210–6.

35 Chren MM, Lasek RJ, Flocke SA, Zyzanski SJ. Improved discriminative and evaluative capability of a refined version of Skindex, a quality-of-life instrument for patients with skin diseases. *Arch Dermatol* 1997;**133**:1433–40.

36 Charman CR, Venn AJ, Williams HC. The Patient-Orientated Eczema Measure (POEM): development and initial validation of a new tool for measuring atopic eczema severity from the patients' perspective. *Arch Dermatol* 2004;**140**:1513–9.

37 Hoare C, Li Wan Po A, Williams H. Systematic review of treatments for atopic eczema. *Health Technol Assess* 2000;**4**(37) (see also http://www.ncchta.org).

38 Langan SM, Thomas K, Williams HC. What is meant by a "flare" in atopic dermatitis? A systematic review and proposal. *Arch Dermatol* 2006;**142**:1190–6.

Questions

Case scenario 1: a child with atopic eczema of moderate severity (Figure 19.1)

What is the role of emollients?

Efficacy

We found no systematic reviews on emollients in atopic eczema. Seven randomized controlled trials (RCTs) are reported here.[39–45] Other studies were excluded because we

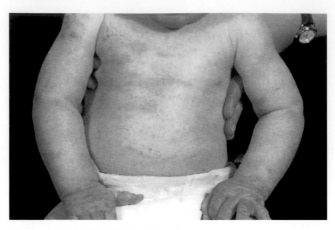

Figure 19.1 A child with flexural atopic eczema.

could not ascertain whether they were properly randomized (for example, Al-Waili[46]); they included conditions other than atopic eczema (for example, Newbold[47], Kucharekova et al.[48]); they presented only biometric data, the clinical relevance of which was difficult to ascertain (for example, Pigatto et al.[49], Hagströmer et al.[50,51]); or they were conducted using healthy volunteers (for example, Wynne et al.[52]).

Kantor et al.[39] compared the use of an oil-in-water emollient (Moisturel) versus a water-in-oil emollient (Eucerin), using a left–right comparison design in 50 patients with symmetrical atopic eczema treated for 3 weeks. Test limbs affected by atopic eczema were treated once daily with the emollients and once daily with 2.5% hydrocortisone cream. Global severity showed a statistically significant reduction with both emollients in comparison with baseline.

The study by Andersson et al.[40] compared a "new" cream containing 5% urea as the active substance against an established licensed cream containing 4% urea and 4% sodium chloride. Forty-eight adults with atopic eczema were enrolled in a parallel-group double-blind study. Patients were asked to apply the creams at least once daily for 30 days. Clinical disease severity showed a significant benefit for both creams, and there were no statistically significant differences between the preparations.

The 1998 study by Hanifin et al.[41] compared the effects of adding an emollient called Cetaphil (manufactured by the study sponsor), applied three times daily, to twice-daily application of 0.05% desonide lotion (a topical steroid) versus twice-daily topical desonide alone. Eighty patients with atopic eczema were enrolled for a 3-week period. Outcomes were recorded by an investigator who was blinded to treatment allocation. At the end of 3 weeks, the relative reduction in disease severity was 70% for desonide alone, in comparison with 80% for the desonide/emollient side ($P < 0.01$).

The studies by Wilhelm *et al.*[42] and Andersson *et al.*[40] both evaluated the benefit of emollients containing urea preparations—a substance intended to improve the water-binding capacity of the outer layer of skin. In the study by Wilhelm *et al.*,[42] 80 patients were randomly assigned to apply a topical formulation containing 10% urea (manufactured by the study sponsors) versus the vehicle base as "placebo" for 4 weeks in a right–left forearm comparison. Skin redness was improved at 70% of the sites on which 10% urea was applied, in comparison with 30% for the sites where the vehicle was applied.

Larregue and colleagues[43] compared 6% ammonium lactate (another substance designed to improve the water-binding capacity of the skin) against its cream base in 46 children aged 6 months to 12 years with atopic dermatitis. The study was a within-person comparison of two symmetrical sites. Lichenification, hyperkeratosis, and dryness were reduced in both groups, but slightly more so in the ammonium lactate group. This was reported to be statistically significant at day 15 for lichenification and for erythema at day 30 (the final evaluation point of the study). Tolerability, as evaluated by the patients, was very similar in both groups.

In a three-arm, parallel-group study, Lodén and colleagues[44] compared 20% glycerine with a placebo preparation and a standard emollient containing 4% urea and 4% sodium chloride. A total of 110 participants were randomly assigned to the three groups, and treatment was applied twice a day for 30 days. Skin dryness was assessed by a dermatologist using a clinical scoring system (including scaling, roughness, redness, and cracks). The cream containing urea and sodium chloride was significantly better than the cream containing glycerine (which was no better than placebo). Patient-assessed outcomes were not captured in this study.

The study by Giordano-Labadie and colleagues[45] is a multicenter study evaluating Exomega milk (a product containing evening primrose oil, Rhealba oat extract, chlorphenesin, phenoxyethanol, butyl hydroxyl toluene, glycols, paraffin jelly, paraffin oil, and Shea butter). Children aged 6 months to 12 years with mild/moderate eczema were randomly assigned to receive either Exomega milk twice a day (plus a cleansing bar), or normal care (plus a cleansing bar). Participants were able to continue their use of topical corticosteroids as per normal care, and the amounts used were documented. Outcomes for eczema severity (SCORAD), tolerance, and quality of life (CDLQI) were reported at 2 months. Interpretation of the results is difficult from this study, and appropriate between-group comparisons were not made. Tolerance for the product was reported to be good to excellent in 97% of cases.

Drawbacks

No drawbacks were reported in the first two studies, with the exception of one patient who experienced a burning sensation when the oil-in-water emollient was applied.[39] In the study by Hanifin *et al.*,[41] 14% of the patients reported stinging or burning on the side treated with desonide, in comparison with 12% on the side treated with the combination at week 1. Most patients (96% versus 4%) preferred the combination treatment. Transient burning was noticed in four patients treated with urea and in five patients treated with vehicle creams in the study by Wilhelm *et al.*[42] No adverse effects were described by Andersson *et al.*[40] Other possible side effects of emollients include occlusion folliculitis on hair-bearing skin and accidents from slipping whilst climbing into the bath when using emollient bath additives.

Comments

The first two studies were of very short duration, and the quality of reporting was generally poor, with little description of the randomization method, limited blinding, and no intention-to-treat (ITT) analysis. The study by Kantor *et al.*[39] failed to show any benefit of one emollient preparation over another (in the presence of a moderate-potency topical steroid), and the study by Hanifin *et al.*[41] suggested that regular use of an emollient with a topical steroid may result in a small increase in treatment response compared with a topical steroid alone. Neither study showed a steroid-sparing effect for emollients.

The first of the two studies on urea preparations[42] showed a possible benefit of a urea-containing preparation in comparison with vehicle. This was confirmed in the study by Lodén *et al.*,[44] in which the preparation containing urea and sodium chloride was better than placebo and better than a preparation containing glycerine. Comparison of two preparations containing urea in different concentrations failed to show any additional benefit of higher concentrations of urea. The quality of reporting on randomization, blinding, and ITT analysis was poor in both studies. Similar findings were found in the study by Larregue *et al.*[43]

It is extremely disappointing to see a virtual absence of clinically useful RCT data on the use of emollients in atopic eczema. In addition to measuring the efficacy of emollients in treating mild atopic eczema, it is important that future RCTs of emollients should measure long-term tolerability, patient preferences, and cosmetic acceptability, since these are probably key determinants for successful long-term use. There is an urgent need to answer several basic questions, preferably through industry-independent randomized controlled trials. Possible questions that require an answer are:

• Do emollients have a useful therapeutic effect (with or without wet wraps) for treating minor flares of atopic eczema in comparison with mild topical steroids?
• Does intensive use of emollients help prevent the onset of eczema in children at high risk of developing atopic eczema?

• Do emollients have a topical steroid–sparing effect without loss of efficacy in the long-term management of atopic eczema?

• For children with atopic eczema, do expensive bath emollients provide any additional benefit over the application of a cheap emollient directly to the skin after a bath?

• Does the regular use of emollients reduce the incidence and severity of secondary infection in atopic eczema?

• Do educational interventions designed to teach the appropriate use of emollients improve the symptoms of atopic eczema?

• How common is clinically relevant contact sensitization to emollient constituents such as lanolin?

• How frequently do emollients need to be applied?

Implications for clinical practice

There is currently no evidence to doubt the belief that regular emollient use is beneficial for the treatment of the dry skin associated with atopic eczema. Equally, there is no clear RCT evidence of their benefit. Whether bath additives provide benefits additional to those of topically applied emollients is particularly unclear.

Key points: emollients

• Seven RCTs have been summarized. Two examined the possible steroid-sparing effects of emollients, two assessed the benefits of using emollients containing urea, one assessed the benefits of emollients containing ammonium lactate, and one assessed the benefits for a product containing evening primrose oil and oat extract.

• The paucity of good clinical trial evidence does not reflect the importance of emollient therapy for the treatment of atopic eczema, and some suggestions for possible future trials have been included.

References: emollients

39 Kantor I, Milbauer J, Posner M, Weinstock IM, Simon A, Thormahlen S. Efficacy and safety of emollients as adjunctive agents in topical corticosteroid therapy for atopic dermatitis. *Today Ther Trends* 1993;**11**:157–66.

40 Andersson AC, Lindberg M, Loden M. The effect of two urea-containing creams on dry, eczematous skin in atopic patients. I. Expert, patient and instrumental evaluation. *J Dermatol Treat* 1999;**10**:165–9.

41 Hanifin JM, Hebert AA, Mays SR, *et al.* Effects of a low-potency corticosteroid lotion plus a moisturizing regimen in the treatment of atopic dermatitis. *Curr Ther Res Clin Exp* 1998;**59**:227–33.

42 Wilhelm KP, Scholermann A. Efficacy and tolerability of a topical preparation containing 10% urea in patients with atopic dermatitis. *Aktuelle Dermatol* 1998;**24**:26–30.

43 Larregue M, Devaux J, Audebert C, Gelmetti DR. A double-blind controlled study on the efficacy and tolerability of 6% ammonium lactate cream in children with atopic dermatitis. *Nouv Dermatol* 1996;**15**:720–1.

44 Lodén M, Andersson AC, Andersson C, Frodin T, Oman H, Lindberg M. Instrumental and dermatologist evaluation of the effect of glycerine and urea on dry skin in atopic dermatitis. *Skin Res Technol* 2001;**7**:209–13.

45 Giordano-Labadie F, Cambazard F, Guillet G, Combemale P, Mengeaud V. Evaluation of a new moisturizer (Exomega milk) in children with atopic dermatitis. *J Dermatol Treat* 2006;**17**:78–81.

46 Al-Waili NS. Topical application of natural honey, beeswax and olive oil mixture for atopic dermatitis os psoriasis: partially controlled, single blinded study. *Complement Ther Med* 2003;**11**:226–34.

47 Newbold PC. Comparison of four emollients in the treatment of various skin conditions. *Practitioner* 1980;**224**:205–6.

48 Kucharekova M, Van De Kerkhof PCM, Van der Valk PGM. A randomized comparison of an emollient containing skin-related lipids with a petroleum-based emollient as adjunct in the treatment of chronic hand dermatitis. *Contact Dermatitis* 2003;**48**:293–9.

49 Pigatto PD, Bigardi AS, Cannistraci C, Picardo M. 10% urea cream (Laceran) for atopic dermatitis: a clinical and laboratory evaluation. *J Dermatol Treat* 1996;**7**:171–5.

50 Hagstromer L, Nyren M, Emtestam L. Do urea and sodium chloride together increase the efficacy of moisturisers for atopic dermatitis skin? A comparative, double-blind and randomised study. *Skin Pharmacol Appl Skin Physiol* 2001;**14**:27–33.

51 Hagströmer L, Kuzmina N, Lapins J, Talme T, Emtestam L. Biophysical assessment of atopic dermatitis skin and effects of a moisturizer. *Clin Exp Dermatol* 2006;**31**:272–7.

52 Wynne A, Whitefield M, Dixon AJ, Anderson S. An effective, cosmetically acceptable, novel hydro-gel emollient for the management of dry skin conditions. *J Dermatol Treat* 2002;**13**:61–6.

Do topical steroids help?

Efficacy

Versus placebo. The effectiveness of topical corticosteroids in comparison with placebo has been demonstrated in one systematic review (search date 1999, 13 RCTs)[53] and four further RCTs[54–57] comparing topical steroids with placebo (vehicle) applied for up to 6 weeks in patients with atopic eczema (Web Table 19.1). Fourteen studies found significant improvement with topical steroid in comparison with placebo.[55–67] Lebwohl[65] includes two RCTs (Web Table 19.1). The three remaining studies were unable to demonstrate a significant difference between steroid and placebo.[54,68,69] No long-term studies were identified.

Versus each other. One systematic review (including 40 RCTs)[53] and three further RCTs (including 495 patients) were identified that compare a variety of topical steroids with each other (Kirkup *et al.*[70] includes two RCTs).[57,70] These studies showed significant improvements in 13–100% of patients after 1–12 weeks of treatment.

Prevention of relapse. Three RCTs have demonstrated that intermittent treatment with a potent topical steroid can reduce the number of flare-ups of atopic eczema.[71–73] In the first two RCTs, adults (n = 430) with atopic eczema were stabilized with a 4-week course of a potent topical steroid (fluticasone propionate), followed by subsequent application of the steroid on two consecutive days a week for 16 weeks. "Weekend" steroid therapy was significantly more effective in maintaining an improvement in comparison with placebo.[71,72] In the third RCT (including 372 adults and children), patients were stabilized with a 4-week course of fluticasone propionate followed by subsequent application on 4 days a week for 4 weeks then on two consecutive days a week for 16 weeks, again showing a significant reduction in the relapse rate in comparison with placebo.[73]

Application under wet wraps. Three RCTs[74–76] and two further small randomized within-patient comparison studies[77,78] have examined the use of wet-wrap bandaging (wet cotton tubular dressings) applied over topical steroids. In the first RCT, 40 children (aged 1–15 years) with moderate to severe eczema were treated once daily with either one-tenth strength mometasone furoate 0.005% ointment or one-tenth strength fluticasone propionate 0.005% ointment unoccluded for 2 weeks, and then randomly assigned to receive the same treatment with or without wet-wrap bandaging for a further 2 weeks. Patients treated with wet wraps finished the study with significantly less extensive and less severe disease, and with a significant improvement in subjective scores.[74] In the second RCT, 50 infants (aged 4–27 months) with moderate to severe eczema were treated with emollients and 1% hydrocortisone, with or without additional wet-wrap bandages, for 4 weeks. In both groups, there was a greater than 50% improvement in the overall eczema score (SCORAD), with no statistically significant differences between the two groups, although the group receiving wet wraps suffered more skin infections.[75] The third RCT was a small randomized controlled pilot study (19 infants < 5 years), which found no benefit with 1% hydrocortisone plus wet wraps versus 1% hydrocortisone alone after 2 weeks.[76] In the first within-patient comparison study, 20 children (aged 2–17 years) were treated with twice-daily wet wraps over 0.1% mometasone furoate or vehicle for 5 days (left–right design), with a statistically significant improvement in the side treated with steroid plus wet wraps versus vehicle plus wet wraps.[77] In the second within-patient comparison study, 24 adults and children with an acute exacerbation of eczema were treated with prednicarbate with or without wet wraps (left–right design) for up to 3 days. This study showed a significantly greater improvement on the side treated with topical steroid and wet wraps in comparison with topical steroid alone.[78]

A recent critical literature review of the use of wet wraps in children includes nine additional observational studies on the use of wet-wrap dressings in children with atopic eczema; it concluded that large prospective RCTs evaluating wet wraps are lacking.[79]

Frequency of application

One systematic review (including 10 RCTs and one earlier systematic review[53]) has addressed this issue.[80] The review found no clear evidence to support twice-daily over once-daily administration of topical corticosteroids, suggesting once-daily treatment as a first step in all patients with atopic eczema.

Pulsed or continuous treatment

One RCT (207 children with mild to moderate atopic dermatitis, aged 1–15 years) has compared 3-day bursts of a potent topical steroid (betamethasone valerate 0.1% ointment) followed by a 4-day rest period versus continuous use of a mild preparation (hydrocortisone 1% ointment) for 7 days. Participants used the preparations as required over an 18-week trial period. No significant differences in patient symptoms or clinical disease severity were demonstrated between the two treatment groups.[81] Another RCT study including 40 children (published in abstract form) concluded that pulsed clobetasone butyrate 0.05% is more effective than continuous treatment.[82]

Drawbacks

No serious systemic effects or cases of skin atrophy were reported in the short-term RCTs described above. Minor adverse effects such as burning, stinging, irritation, folliculitis, hypertrichosis, contact dermatitis, and changes in skin pigmentation occurred in less than 10% of patients. No cases of skin atrophy were seen in two longer RCTs (of 20 and 18 weeks' duration) using histological examination and pulsed ultrasound, respectively.[71,81] No visible signs of skin atrophy were detected in RCTs of children and adults after 4 weeks of twice-daily potent topical steroid followed by intermittent application for 12–20 weeks.[70,73] In a further RCT including 376 adults, one patient developed visible signs of skin atrophy (telangiectasia) during 4 weeks of daily potent topical steroid reatment.[72] No serious systemic effects or cases of skin atrophy were reported with regular topical steroids of mild to moderate potency in a longer cohort study in 14 prepubertal children (median treatment period 6.5 years).[83] Enhanced topical steroid absorption and temporary suppression of the hypothalamic–pituitary–adrenal axis have been demonstrated with wet-wrap dressings in patients with severe widespread eczema.[79]

Four very small RCTs in healthy volunteers (12 adults) have used ultrasound to evaluate skin thickness after topical steroid application.[84–87] Significant skin thinning occurred after 1 week with twice-daily 0.05% clobetasol 17-propionate and after 3 weeks with twice-daily 0.1% triamcinolone acetate and 0.1% betamethasone 17-valerate. All preparations were used for up to 6 weeks, and skin thinning reversed within 4 weeks of stopping treatment. No significant thinning was reported with twice-daily hydrocortisone prednicarbate or once-daily mometasone furoate after 6 weeks.

Comments

The majority of trials of topical steroids for atopic eczema have been of short duration, even though atopic eczema is a chronic relapsing disease in which topical steroids may be required for months or years. Trials have used a wide variety of clinical scoring systems, making it difficult to compare results, and many trials have studied adults only. It is not possible to recommend a "best" topical steroid, as most trials have only compared one against another, but seldom against the same one and never all together. In the only trial comparing short bursts of potent steroid versus a longer duration of mild topical steroids, the majority of patients were recruited from primary care and had mild eczema only. Further trials involving patients with more severe disease are needed in order to define the most effective method of using topical steroids in the long-term management of the disease and prevention of relapse. The majority of RCTs have not specifically addressed skin atrophy and have been of too short a duration to adequately assess risk with long-term use of topical steroids. The clinical significance of skin thinning, as detected by statistically significant changes in total skin thickness when measured by ultrasound, is unclear. Only one RCT has addressed the risks of skin atrophy in children objectively using ultrasound,[81] and further trials using a range of topical steroids of different strengths are needed in order to guide safe prescribing.

Implications for practice

Although topical steroids have been used for the treatment of atopic eczema for over 40 years, surprisingly little work has been done to understand how best to use them for the long-term control of atopic eczema. Most RCTs have compared "me-too" products in studies lasting only a few weeks, instead of addressing important questions such as the optimum duration of application and whether one should use short bursts of potent steroids followed by milder preparations, or vice versa. The short-term studies have failed to evaluate the speed of onset of one type of steroid in comparison with another—an important consideration when trying to control the symptoms quickly in the child depicted in the case scenario. Despite widespread concern about skin thinning with topical steroids, which has arisen from occasional horror stories of people using very potent preparations continuously at sensitive sites such as the face or groin area for inappropriate periods, RCT evidence does not suggest that clinically significant skin thinning is a problem.

In relation to the child portrayed in the case scenario, a possible evidence-based treatment approach could involve the use of a potent topical steroid (for example, an inexpensive preparation such as betamethasone valerate once daily) for 2–3 weeks to gain remission, followed by emollient-only "steroid holidays" to allow any skin thinning to recover.

Future flares could then be treated with 3-day bursts of the same potent preparation. If this should fail to achieve sufficient overall control in terms of frequency and duration of remission, another approach would be to use the same preparation every weekend on active and previously healed sites.

Key points: topical steroids

- RCTs of topical steroids versus placebo suggest a large treatment effect in atopic eczema.
- It is not possible to make recommendations about the "best" topical steroid, as no RCT has compared all the available preparations of similar potency.
- There is no clear RCT evidence to support the use of twice-daily over once-daily topical steroid administration.
- There is good RCT evidence that application of twice weekly potent topical steroid to stabilized eczema can reduce the number of flare-ups in adults and children, although further RCTs are needed to confirm the long-term safety profile of this approach in infants.
- There is no RCT evidence that skin thinning is a problem with correct use of topical steroids, although most RCTs have been of short duration and other non-RCT evidence should be considered before firm conclusions are drawn.

References: topical steroids

53 Hoare C, Li Wan Po A, Williams H. Systematic review of treatments of atopic eczema. *Health Technol Assess* 2000;**4**(37).

54 Cato A, Swinehart JM, Griffin EI, Sutton L, Kaplan AS. Azone enhances clinical effectiveness of an optimized formulation of triamcinolone acetonide in atopic dermatitis. *Int J Dermatol* 2001; **40**:232–6.

55 Lawlor F, Black AK, Greaves M. Prednicarbate 0.25% ointment in the treatment of atopic dermatitis: a vehicle-controlled double-blind study. *J Dermatol Treat* 1995;**6**:233–5.

56 Paller AS, Nimmagadda S, Schachner L, *et al.* Fluocinolone acetonide 0.01% in peanut oil: therapy for childhood atopic dermatitis, even in patients who are peanut sensitive. *J Am Acad Dermatol* 2003;**48**:569–77.

57 Breneman D, Fleischer AB Jr, Kaplan D, *et al.* Clobetasol propionate 0.05% lotion in the treatment of moderate to severe atopic dermatitis: a randomized evaluation versus clobetasol propionate emollient cream. *J Drugs Dermatol* 2005;**4**:330–6.

58 Vanderploeg DE. Betamethasone dipropionate ointment in the treatment of psoriasis and atopic dermatitis: a double-blind study. *South Med J* 1976;**69**:862–3.

59 Roth HL, Brown EP. Hydrocortisone valerate. Double-blind comparison with two other topical steroids. *Cutis* 1978;**21**:695–8.

60 Sudilovsky A, Muir JG, Bocobo FC. A comparison of single and multiple applications of halcinonide cream. *Int J Dermatol* 1981; **20**:609–13.

61 Lupton ES, Abbrecht MM, Brandon ML. Short-term topical corticosteroid therapy (halcinonide ointment) in the management of atopic dermatitis. *Cutis* 1982;**30**:671–5.

62 Sefton J, Loder JS, Kyriakopoulos AA. Clinical evaluation of hydrocortisone valerate 0.2% ointment. *Clin Ther* 1984;**6**:282–93.

63 Wahlgren CF, Hagermark O, Bergstrom R, Hedin B. Evaluation of a new method of assessing pruritus and antipruritic drugs. *Skin Pharmacol* 1988;**1**:3–13.

64 Stalder JF, Fleury M, Sourisse M, Rostin M, Pheline F, Litoux P. Local steroid therapy and bacterial skin flora in atopic dermatitis. *Br J Dermatol* 1994;**131**:536–40.

65 Lebwohl M. Efficacy and safety of fluticasone propionate ointment 0.005% in the treatment of eczema. *Cutis* 1996;**57**(Suppl 2):62–8.

66 Sears HW, Bailer JW, Yeadon A. Efficacy and safety of hydrocortisone buteprate 0.1% cream in patients with atopic dermatitis. *Clin Ther* 1997;**19**:710–9.

67 Maloney JM, Morman MR, Stewart DM, Tharp MD, Brown JJ, Rajagopalan R. Clobetasol propionate emollient 0.05% in the treatment of atopic dermatitis. *Int J Dermatol* 1998;**37**:142–4.

68 Brock W, Cullen SI. Triamcinolone acetonide in flexible collodion for dermatologic therapy. *Arch Dermatol* 1967;**96**:193–4.

69 Gehring W, Gloor M. Treatment of atopic dermatitis with a water-in-oil emulsion with or without the addition of hydrocortisone—results of a controlled double-blind randomized study using clinical evaluation and bioengineering methods. *Z Hautkrankh* 1996;**71**:554–60.

70 Kirkup ME, Birchall NM, Weinberg EG, *et al.* Acute and maintenance treatment of atopic dermatitis in children—two comparative studies with fluticasone propionate (0.05%) cream. *J Dermatolog Treat* 2003;**14**:141–8.

71 Van der Meer JB, Glazenburg EJ, Mulder PGH et al. The management of moderate to severe atopic dermatitis in adults with topical fluticasone propionate. *Br J Dermatol* 1999;**140**:1114–21.

72 Berth-Jones J, Damstra RJ, Golsch S, *et al.* Twice weekly fluticasone propionate added to emollient maintenance treatment to reduce risk of relapse in atopic dermatitis: randomised, double blind, parallel group study. *BMJ* 2003;**326**:1367.

73 Hanifin J, Gupta AK, Rajagopalan R. Intermittent dosing of fluticasone propionate cream for reducing the risk of relapse in atopic dermatitis patients. *Br J Dermatol* 2002;**147**:528–37.

74 Pei AYS, Chan HHL, Ho KM. The effectiveness of wet wrap dressings using 0.1% mometasone furoate and 0.005% fluticasone propionate ointments in the treatment of moderate to severe atopic dermatitis in children. *Pediatr Dermatol* 2001;**18**:343–8.

75 Hindley D, Galloway G, Murray J, Gardener L. A randomised study of "wet wraps" versus conventional treatment for atopic eczema. *Arch Dis Child* 2006;**91**:164–8.

76 Beattie PE, Lewis-Jones MS. A pilot study on the use of wet wraps in infants with moderate atopic eczema. *Clin Exp Dermatol* 2004;**29**:348–53.

77 Schnopp C, Holtmann C, Stock S, *et al.* Topical steroids under wet-wrap dressings in atopic dermatitis—a vehicle-controlled trial. *Dermatology* 2002;**204**:56–9.

78 Foelster HR, Nagel F, Zoellner P, Spaeth D. Efficacy of crisis intervention treatment with topical corticosteroid prednicarbate with and without partial wet-wrap dressing in atopic dermatitis. *Dermatology* 2006;**212**:66–9.

79 Devillers ACA, Oranje AP. Efficacy and safety of "wet wrap" dressings as an intervention treatment in children with severe and/or refractory atopic dermatitis: a critical review of the literature. *Br J Dermatol* 2006;**154**:579–85.

80 Green C, Colquitt JL, Kirby J, Davidson P. Topical corticosteroids for atopic eczema: clinical and cost effectiveness of once-daily vs. more frequent use. *Br J Dermatol* 2005;**152**:130–41.

81 Thomas K, Williams HC, Avery A, *et al.* Randomised controlled trial of short bursts of a potent topical corticosteroid versus prolonged use of a mild preparation for children with mild or moderate atopic eczema. *BMJ* 2002;**324**:768–75.

82 Smitt S, Spuls P, Van Leent EJM, *et al.* Randomized double blind comparison of continuous versus pulsed topical treatment with clobetasone butyrate in 40 children with atopic dermatitis. *Proceedings of the International Symposium on Atopic Dermatitis.* Portland, OR: National Eczema Association for Science and Education, 2001: 24.

83 Patel L, Clayton PE, Addison GM, Price DA, David TJ. Adrenal function following topical steroid treatment in children with atopic dermatitis. *Br J Dermatol* 1995;**132**:950–5.

84 Kerscher MJ, Hart H, Korting HC, *et al.* In vivo assessment of the atrophogenic potency of mometasone furoate, a newly developed chlorinated potent topical glucocorticoid as compared to other topical glucocorticoids old and new. *Int J Clin Pharmacol Ther* 1995;**33**:187–9.

85 Kerscher MJ, Korting HC. Comparative atrophogenicity potential of medium and highly potent topical glucocorticoids in cream and ointment according to ultrasound analysis. *Skin Pharmacol* 1992;**5**:77–80.

86 Korting HC, Vieluf D, Kerscher M. 0.25% Prednicarbate cream and the corresponding vehicle induce less skin atrophy than 0.1% betamethasone-17-valerate cream and 0.05% clobetasol-17-propionate cream. *Clin Pharmacol* 1992;**42**:159–61.

87 Kerscher MJ, Korting HC. Topical glucocorticoids of the non-fluorinated double-ester type. *Acta Derm Venereol* 1992;**72**:214–6.

Do oral antihistamines help?

Only oral antihistamine agents are considered here. For the purposes of answering the question, we have included studies whose outcome measures were global indices such as quality of life (which may actually be enhanced in the context of a sedative drug used nocturnally, but is normally decreased in conventional studies, where daytime sedation is a side effect). We also considered trials in which specific indices such as disease severity scores or itch assessments were assessed irrespective of the systemic side effect profile.

Efficacy

One systematic review was identified, 21 RCTs, and two subsequent RCTs. The studies are summarized in Web Table 19.2.[88–110] Tabulation and systematic analysis of these trials revealed no clear or powerful effect of administering antihistamines to children or adults. Six of the trials used physician-assessed global severity and five used patient-assessed global severity. The most commonly reported outcome was patient-assessed itch. The largest and longest clinical trial to date (conducted over 18 months) found no significant difference in atopic eczema severity, as measured using SCORAD, when cetirizine (a nonsedating antihistamine) was compared with placebo.[109] Another subsequent study suggests that chlorpheniramine (a sedating antihistamine) may help reduce the duration and amount of moderate to strong topical corticosteroid use.[110]

Comments

The lack of emergent clarity in these trials reflects the way many dermatology studies are powered: low patient numbers in trials intrinsically demand large treatment effects to be statistically significant. It is therefore likely, from an intuitive point of view, that no large effects will be derived from the use of antihistamines, as the everyday experience of dermatologists will already attest. The individual merits of antihistamine treatments cannot be covered by such a review, and in particular, the patient-specificity of drug effects is necessarily lost when considering aggregated cohorts and statistical means, not to mention the differences in "utility" that occur for the same drug in differing contexts. The impact of a specific context of drug administration is nowhere better seen than when comparing the sedative and nonsedative antihistamines across daytime and nighttime administrations.

Implications for practice

Collectively, RCTs conducted to date fail to show convincing evidence of a clear benefit for oral antihistamines, regardless of whether sedative or nonsedating treatments are used. An ongoing systematic review of these trials conducted by individuals within the Cochrane Skin Group may reveal more precise conclusions if data from similar studies can be combined. In relation to the child described in the case scenario, we would not recommend the use of oral antihistamines except for very occasional use as a sedative (in which case other sedatives might be just as good).

Key points: oral antihistamines

- Oral antihistamines have been extensively studied.
- Over 20 randomized controlled trials on antihistamines for atopic eczema have been conducted to date, with no clear evidence of benefit, especially in the largest and longest study.
- The individuality of effect of an antihistamine on any one person or given situation is variable enough to allow us to ignore pooled studies and to go on to recommend antihistamines in those contexts, or for those patients, where a potential benefit is obvious or already noted by either the patient, physician, or carer.

References: oral antihistamines

88 Berth-Jones J, Graham-Brown RA. Failure of terfenadine in relieving the pruritus of atopic dermatitis. *Br J Dermatol* 1989;**121**:635–7.

89 Doherty V, Sylvester DG, Kennedy CT, Harvey SG, Calthrop JG, Gibson JR. Treatment of itching in atopic eczema with antihistamines with a low sedative profile. *BMJ* 1989;**298**:96.

90 Foulds IS, MacKie RM. A double-blind trial of the h2 receptor antagonist cimetidine, and the h1 receptor antagonist prome-

thazine hydrochloride in the treatment of atopic dermatitis. *Clin Allergy* 1981;**11**:319–23.

91 Frosch PJ, Schwanitz HJ, Macher E. A double blind trial of h1 and h2 receptor antagonists in the treatment of atopic dermatitis. *Arch Dermatol Res* 1984;**276**:36–40.

92 Hamada T, Ishii M, Nakagawa K, *et al.* Evaluation of the clinical effect of terfenadine in patients with atopic dermatitis. A comparison of strong corticosteroid therapy to mild topical corticosteroid combined with terfenadine administration therapy. *Skin Res* 1996;**38**:97–103.

93 Hannuksela M, Kalimo K, Lammintausta K et al. Dose ranging study: cetirizine in the treatment of atopic dermatitis in adults. *Ann Allergy* 1993;**70**:127–33.

94 Henz BM, Metzenauer P, O'Keefe E, Zuberbier T. Differential effects of new-generation h1-receptor antagonists in pruritic dermatoses. *Allergy* 1998;**53**:180–3.

95 Hjorth N. Terfenadine in the treatment of chronic idiopathic urticaria and atopic dermatitis. *Cutis* 1988;**42**:29–30.

96 Ishibashi Y, Ueda H, Niimura M, *et al.* Clinical evaluation of E-0659 in atopic dermatitis in infants and children. Dose-finding multicenter study by the double-blind method. *Skin Res* 1989;**31**:458–71.

97 Ishibashi Y, Tamaki K, Yoshida H, *et al.* Clinical evaluation of E-0659 on atopic dermatitis. Multicenter double-blind study in comparison with ketotifen. *Rinsho Hyoka (Clinical Evaluation)* 1989;**17**:77–115.

98 Klein GL, Galant SP. A comparison of the antipruritic efficacy of hydroxyzine and cyproheptadine in children with atopic dermatitis. *Ann Allergy* 1980;**44**:142–5.

99 Langeland T, Fagertun HE, Larsen S. Therapeutic effect of loratadine on pruritus in patients with atopic dermatitis. A multi-crossover-designed study. *Allergy* 1994;**49**:22–6.

100 La Rosa M, Ranno C, Musarra I, Guglielmo F, Corrias A, Bellanti JA. Double-blind study of cetirizine in atopic eczema in children. *Ann Allergy* 1994;**73**:117–22.

101 Monroe EW. Relative efficacy and safety of loratadine, hydroxyzine, and placebo in chronic idiopathic urticaria and atopic dermatitis. *Clin Ther* 1992;**14**:17–21.

102 Patel P, Gratton D, Eckstein G, *et al.* A double-blind study of loratadine and cetirizine in atopic dermatitis. *J Dermatol Treat* 1997;**8**:249–53.

103 Savin JA, Paterson WD, Adam K, Oswald I. Effects of trimeprazine and trimipramine on nocturnal scratching in patients with atopic eczema. *Arch Dermatol* 1979;**115**:313–5.

104 Savin JA, Dow R, Harlow BJ, Massey H, Yee KF. The effect of new non-sedative h1-receptor antagonist (In 2974) on the itching and scratching of patients with ectopic eczema. *Clin Exp Dermatol* 1986;**11**:600–2.

105 Simons R, Estelle F, Simons KJ, Becker AB, Haydey RP. Pharmacokinetics and antipruritic effects of hydroxyzine in children with atopic dermatitis. *J Pediatr* 1984;**104**:123–7.

106 Simons R, Estelle F. Prospective long term safety evaluation of the H1-receptor antagonist cetirizine in very young children with atopic dermatitis. *J Allergy Clin Immunol* 1999;**104**:433–40.

107 Wahlgren CF, Hagermark O, Bergstrom R. The antipruritic effect of a sedative and a non-sedative antihistamine in atopic dermatitis. *Br J Dermatol* 1990;**122**:545–51.

108 Zuluaga de Cadena A, Ochoa de VA, Donado JH, Mejia JI, Chamah HM, Montoya de Restrepo F. Comparative study of

the effect of the hidroxicina, the terfenadina and the astemizol in children with atopic dermatitis. Hospital General de Medellin-Centro de Especialistas C.E.S. 1986–1988. *CES Med* 1989;**3**:7–13.

109 Diepgen TL, ETAC Study Group. Long-term treatment with cetirizine of infants with atopic dermatitis: A multi-country, double-blind, randomized, placebo-controlled trial (the ETAC trial) over 18 months. *Pediatr Allerg Immunol* 2002;**13**:278–86.

110 Munday J, Bloomfield R, Goldman M, *et al.* Chlorpheniramine is no more effective than placebo in relieving the symptoms of childhood atopic dermatitis with a nocturnal itching and scratching component. *Dermatology* 2002;**205**:40–5.

What about topical tacrolimus?

Tacrolimus is a powerful immunosuppressant drug used to prevent the rejection of organ transplants. Chemically, it is a macrolide lactone isolated from the bacterium *Streptomyces tsukabaensis*. A topical form of tacrolimus (FK-506) was developed to treat atopic eczema. Topical tacrolimus is thought to benefit atopic eczema by inhibiting phosphatase activity of calcineurin and thereby the dephosphorylation of the nuclear factor for activated T-cell protein, which is necessary for the expression of inflammatory cytokines. Downregulation of the high-affinity IgE receptor on Langerhans cells and inhibition of release of inflammatory mediators from mast cells and basophils may also partly explain the beneficial effect of tacrolimus in atopic eczema.[111,112]

Efficacy

The systematic review highlighted in the first edition of this textbook[113] has been superseded by another high-quality systematic review of topical tacrolimus and pimecrolimus published in the *British Medical Journal* in 2005, based on an extensive literature search up to December 2004.[114] That review identified three placebo-controlled studies, and the results of the rate ratio of the proportion of patients achieving good or excellent improvement according to the investigators' global assessment are shown in Figure 19.2. All show that tacrolimus (0.1% and 0.03%) works better than placebo at 12 weeks. Five further trials have compared 0.03% tacrolimus versus 0.1% tacrolimus, and not surprisingly, these suggest that the stronger preparation is more effective than the weaker one at 12 weeks (Figure 19.2). Additional placebo controlled or dose-finding studies published since 2004 will not be discussed further here, as they add little to clinical decision-making. In terms of active comparators, the systematic review identified two RCTs that compared topical tacrolimus 0.03% with hydrocortisone acetate 1% (a weak topical corticosteroid), which showed that both concentrations of tacrolimus (0.1% and 0.03%) were superior to hydrocortisone acetate at 3 weeks (Figure 19.2). Two RCTs have compared tacrolimus 0.03% and 0.1% with hydrocortisone butyrate 0.1% (a stronger topical corticosteroid), showing that 0.03% tacrolimus was less

effective than the topical corticosteroid, whereas the 0.1% tacrolimus was as effective (rate ratio 0.95, 0.78 to 1.17). In another RCT, topical 0.1% tacrolimus was more effective that hydrocortisone butyrate 0.1% applied to the body and hydrocortisone acetate 1% applied to the face at 12 weeks. One RCT of 141 children compared 1% tacrolimus against 0.03% pimecrolimus and found no significant difference in the proportion of children clear or almost clear at 6 weeks (0.71, 0.45 to 1.12).[115]

Since the systematic review was published, a further RCT including 972 adults with atopic eczema by Reitamo *et al.* has compared twice-daily 0.1% topical tacrolimus up to 6 months against hydrocortisone butyrate 0.1% to the body and hydrocortisone acetate 1% to the face.[116] "Success" was defined as greater than 60% improvement from baseline in modified Eczema and Severity Index score. At 3 months, 73% of patients achieved success in the tacrolimus arm, in comparison with 14% in the corticosteroid group. Two further RCTs were reported by Nakagawa in 2006. The first was a comparison of 0.1% topical tacrolimus versus mid-potency 0.12% betamethasone valerate for moderate to severe eczema on the trunk and limbs, which showed that both groups achieved 90% "at least moderate" improvement at 3 weeks.[117] Another RCT reported in the same paper compared 0.1% tacrolimus against alclometasone dipropionate 0.1% (mild potency) for head and neck eczema for 1 week, with greater improvement in symptom scores in favor of tacrolimus 0.1%.[117] A further RCT (n = 82) compared monotherapy with 0.1% tacrolimus against combined therapy of topical tacrolimus 0.1% with desoximetasone 0.25% for 3 weeks and found superior responses in the combined group in terms of a summary score of physical signs.[118] A review of three RCTs comparing tacrolimus to pimecrolimus in 2005 concluded that tacrolimus was more effective than pimecrolimus, but with a similar safety profile.[119]

All studies were sponsored by the manufacturer, and none was specifically conducted in individuals in whom topical steroids had failed.

Drawbacks

The RCTs and various safety studies published to date suggest that topical tacrolimus is a safe drug, at least in the short term. Very little of the drug is absorbed systemically. Transient burning at the site of application is a common phenomenon, occurring in about half of adults. Topical irritation increases to 80% for 0.1% tacrolimus when applied to the head and neck area.[120] Topical irritation may be diminished with simultaneous application of a topical corticosteroid.[118] The incidence of skin infections was not significantly different from control groups in the systematic review.[114] Apart from case reports, which are prone to selection bias, there is no clear evidence of an increased risk of skin or internal malignancy with topical tacrolimus.[114,121]

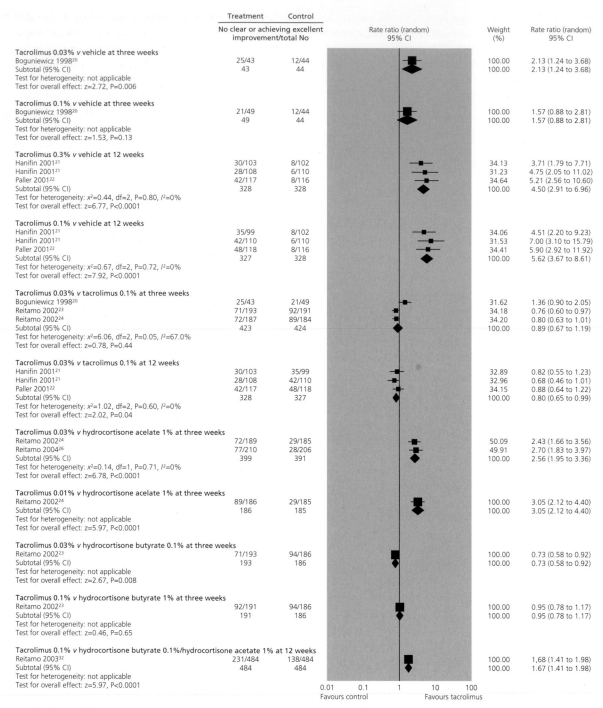

Figure 19.2 The investigators' global assessment of response (clear or excellent improvement) in trials comparing tacrolimus (0.03% and 0.1%) and control. (Reproduced with kind permission of BMJ Publishing Group.)

None of the trials reported key adverse events such as skin thinning or adrenal gland suppression.

Comments

There is little doubt that topical tacrolimus is an effective drug for atopic eczema in comparison with vehicle, with some gains in efficacy for the stronger 0.1% preparation.

The drug appears to be safe in the short term, although it should be borne in mind that tacrolimus is a potent immunosuppressive, and more data will be needed on skin infections such as herpes simplex and eczema herpeticum. Longer-term surveillance data will also be needed on the subsequent risk of internal malignancies. Given that topical tacrolimus is likely to be applied frequently to facial skin—a frequent site for atopic eczema involvement—there is a need to carefully evaluate the risk of excess skin cancer on areas of the skin exposed to the sun.

It is always helpful to have a few alternatives for treating a chronic disease like eczema. What is less clear for the practicing physician is where exactly topical tacrolimus fits in with the other currently available therapies, such as topical corticosteroids.[122]

Studies summarized in the systematic review suggest that 0.1% topical tacrolimus is superior to weak topical corticosteroids, and approximately equivalent to potent topical corticosteroids.[114] A further study has suggested additional efficacy in combination with a topical corticosteroid, and many clinicians are probably using tacrolimus in combination with topical corticosteroids simultaneously at the same and different body sites.

Topical tacrolimus has been licensed in the USA and UK for the treatment of people with moderate to severe atopic eczema that is not adequately responsive, or who are intolerant of conventional therapies. Yet—rather oddly, however—none of the RCTs has been conducted specifically in people in whom topical steroids have failed. In other words, the evidence base is completely absent for the very group of people in whom it is recommended for use. This raises the question of why product licenses were granted for such second-line use, given the lack of relevant evidence to inform such a decision. The percentage of atopic eczema sufferers who are truly "unresponsive" to topical steroids is probably very small (around 10% of patients with *severe* cases seen in secondary care).[123] It is likely, therefore, that the drug will be used in a much wider group of topic eczema patients as an alternative to topical corticosteroids—a prediction that is likely to be fulfilled, given existing widespread and often unjustified public fear of using topical steroids.[124]

The lack of skin thinning with prolonged use of topical tacrolimus is a distinct advantage over topical steroids when the latter have to be used in excessive quantities for sites that are prone to skin thinning, such as the face. Even so, clinically significant skin thinning with intermittent use of topical steroids is rare in modern clinical practice,[125] and it is odd that none of the trials to date has demonstrated a clear reduction in clinical skin thinning with topical tacrolimus in comparison with optimum use of topical corticosteroids—given that lack of skin thinning is one of its main selling points. Some case series have suggested that there is a good response of facial atopic eczema and atopic blepharitis to topical tacrolimus,[126–128] and these may be two scenarios in which the drug will prove to be particularly useful.

One detailed cost-effectiveness technology appraisal using Markov modeling of chronic eczema conducted for the UK Health Technology Assessment Programme in 2005 found wide uncertainty in estimating the cost-effectiveness of tacrolimus in comparison with standard treatment,[129] although another more recent cost-effectiveness study from Sweden suggested that topical tacrolimus was cost-effective in comparison with standard therapy.[130]

Implications for clinical practice

Given the lack of crucial comparisons surrounding the introduction of topical tacrolimus, physicians and patients are left guessing as to how and when it should be used. The lack of a skin thinning effect may point to it being particularly useful when patients with moderate to severe disease are "stuck" on their topical steroid preparations and have to use such preparations almost continuously. Topical tacrolimus may be particularly useful for resistant facial atopic eczema, for similar reasons. Physicians should resist using such a preparation as a "steroid alternative" until more relevant RCT and safety data become available.

Key points: topical tacrolimus

- It is good to see a new effective topical treatment for people with moderate to severe atopic eczema becoming available.
- Topical tacrolimus (0.03% and 0.1%) works much better than vehicle only.
- Topical tacrolimus 0.1% and 0.03% has been shown to be superior to a very weak topical corticosteroid (1% hydrocortisone) in children with moderate to severe atopic eczema.
- Topical tacrolimus 0.1% appears to be equivalent in efficacy to a potent topical steroid (hydrocortisone butyrate), although the 0.03% preparation is inferior to both these preparations.
- Although 0.1% topical tacrolimus is of similar potency to betamethasone valerate, it is much more expensive.
- Topical tacrolimus appears to be safe in the short term.
- Transient burning occurs in about half of adults, but is rarely severe enough to warrant stopping the preparation.
- Long-term data are needed on local and systemic infection, skin cancer rates, and internal cancers such as lymphoma.
- Paradoxically, none of the studies to date has tested topical tacrolimus for its suggested use as a second-line treatment for atopic eczema.
- There is a need for a head-to-head comparison of the cost-effectiveness of topical tacrolimus against topical pimecrolimus and intermittent use of potent modern topical steroids.
- In relation to the child described in the case scenario, we would use topical tacrolimus only when standard therapy with short bursts of once-daily potent topical steroids (or very mild preparations for the face), emollients, and educational support had failed.

References: topical tacrolimus

111 Reitamo S. Tacrolimus: a new topical immunomodulatory therapy for atopic dermatitis. *J Allergy Clin Immunol* 2001;**107**:445–8.
112 Nghiem P, Pearson G, Langley RG. Tacrolimus and pimecrolimus: from clever prokaryotes to inhibiting calcineurin and treating atopic dermatitis. *J Am Acad Dermatol* 2002;**46**:228–41.

113 Hoare C, Li Wan Po A, Williams H. Systematic review of treatments for atopic eczema. *Health Technol Assess* 2000;**4**(37).

114 Ashcroft D, Dimmock P, Garside R, Stein K. Williams HC. Systematic review of the efficacy and tolerability of topical pimecrolimus and tacrolimus in the treatment of atopic dermatitis. *BMJ* 2005;**330**:516–22.

115 Kempers S, Bouguniewicz M, Carter E, *et al.* Comparison of pimecrolimus cream 1% and tacrolimus ointment 0.03% in pediatric patients with atopic eczema. *J Eur Acad Dermatol Venereol* 2003;**17**:P2–41.

116 Reitamo S, Ortonne JP, Sand C, *et al.* A multicentre, randomized, double-blind, controlled study of long-term treatment with 0.1% tacrolimus ointment in adults with moderate to severe atopic dermatitis. *Br J Dermatol* 2005;**152**:1282–9.

117 Nakagawa H. Comparison of the efficacy and safety of 0.1% tacrolimus ointment with topical corticosteroids in adult patients with atopic dermatitis: review of randomised, double-blind clinical studies conducted in Japan. *Clin Drug Investig* 2006;**26**:235–46.

118 Hebert AA, Koo J, Fowler J, Berman B, Rosenberg C, Levitt J. Desoximetasone 0.25% and tacrolimus 0.1% ointments versus tacrolimus alone in the treatment of atopic dermatitis. *Cutis* 2006;**78**:357–63.

119 Paller AS, Lebwohl M, Fleischer AB Jr, *et al.* Tacrolimus ointment is more effective than pimecrolimus cream with a similar safety profile in the treatment of atopic dermatitis: results from 3 randomized, comparative studies. *J Am Acad Dermatol* 2005;**52**:810–22.

120 FK506 Ointment Study Group. [Phase III comparative study of FK506 ointment versus alclometasone dipropionate ointment in atopic dermatitis (face/neck); in Japanese.] *Hihuka Kiyo (Dermatol Bull)* 1997;**92**:277–82.

121 Berger TG, Duvic M, Van Voorhees AS, VanBeek MJ, Frieden IJ, American Academy of Dermatology Association Task Force. The use of topical calcineurin inhibitors in dermatology: safety concerns. Report of the American Academy of Dermatology Association Task Force. *J Am Acad Dermatol* 2006;**54**:818–23.

122 Boucher M. Tacrolimus ointment for the treatment of atopic dermatitis. *Issues Emerg Health Technol* 2001;**19**:1–4.

123 Furue M, Terao H, Rikihisa W, *et al.* Clinical dose and adverse effects of topical steroids in daily management of atopic dermatitis. *Br J Dermatol* 2003;**148**:128–33.

124 Charman CR, Morris AD, Williams HC. Topical corticosteroid phobia in patients with atopic eczema. *Br J Dermatol* 2000;**142**:931–6.

125 Williams HC. Atopic dermatitis. *N Engl J Med* 2005;**352**:2314–24.

126 Sugiura H, Uehara M, Hoshino N, Yamaji A. Long-term efficacy of tacrolimus ointment for recalcitrant facial erythema resistant to topical corticosteroids in adult patients with atopic dermatitis. *Arch Dermatol* 2000;**136**:1062–3.

127 Kawakami T, Soma Y, Morita E, *et al.* Safe and effective treatment of refractory facial lesions in atopic dermatitis using topical tacrolimus following corticosteroid discontinuation. *Dermatology* 2001;**203**:32–7.

128 Mayer K, Reinhard T, Reis A, Bohringer D, Sundmacher R. [FK 506 ointment 0.1%: a new therapeutic option for atopic blepharitis. Clinical trial with 14 patients; in German.] *Klin Monatsbl Augenheilkd* 2001;**218**:733–6.

129 Garside R, Stein K, Castelnuovo E, *et al.* The effectiveness and cost-effectiveness of pimecrolimus and tacrolimus for atopic eczema: a systematic review and economic evaluation. *Health Technol Assess* 2005;**9**:1–230.

130 Hjelmgren J, Svensson A, Jorgensen ET, Lindemalm-Lundstam B, Ragnarson Tennvall G. Cost-effectiveness of tacrolimus ointment vs. standard treatment in patients with moderate and severe atopic dermatitis: a health-economic model simulation based on a patient survey and clinical trial data. *Br J Dermatol* 2007;**156**:913–21.

How might topical pimecrolimus be used?

Like tacrolimus, pimecrolimus is a macrolide immunosuppressive drug.[131] It is currently available in many countries worldwide for "short-term intermittent long-term therapy in the treatment of *mild to moderate* atopic dermatitis in non-immunocompromised patients 2 years of age and older, in whom the use of alternative, conventional therapies is deemed inadvisable because of potential risks, or in the treatment of patients who are not adequately responsive to or are intolerant to conventional therapies."[132] The primary indication of use is almost identical to that described for topical tacrolimus, except that pimecrolimus is aimed at mild to moderate atopic dermatitis and tacrolimus for moderate to severe atopic dermatitis. Given that mild atopic eczema is about ten times more frequent than moderate to severe disease,[133] the market could be a lot larger for pimecrolimus. Pimecrolimus has also been used to prevent disease flares.

The mode of action of pimecrolimus is thought to be similar to that of tacrolimus and ciclosporin in preventing the release of calcineurin-mediated cytokine and pro-inflammatory mediators from mast cells and T cells.[134]

Efficacy

The 2005 systematic review (Figure 19.3) identified four RCTs that show a clear benefit with pimecrolimus 1% in comparison with vehicle at 3 and 6 weeks in terms of the percentage clear or almost clear according to the investigators' global response.[135] In comparison with betamethasone valerate 0.1%, pimecrolimus was markedly inferior (rate ratio of "success" for pimecrolimus 0.22; 95% CI, 0.09 to 0.54). A further trial comparing pimecrolimus 1% to tacrolimus 0.03% failed to show any significant difference (rate ratio of success 0.71; 95% CI, 0.45 to 1.12 in favor of tacrolimus).[136] The systematic review also reported a large study of 658 adults with moderate to severe atopic eczema, which compared pimecrolimus with a combined treatment of triamcinolone acetate 0.1% to the limbs and trunk and 1% hydrocortisone acetate to the face. Combination topical corticosteroids were more effective than pimecrolimus in terms of the proportion of patients who were moderately clear or clear up to 6 months, but not at 12 months. Only 41% of those receiving pimecrolimus 1% completed the study.

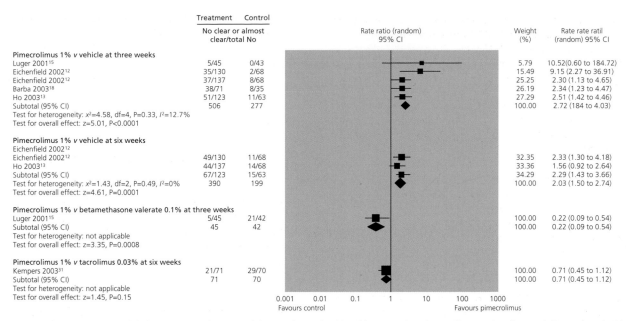

	Treatment	Control		Weight	Rate rate ratil
	No clear or almost clear/total No		Rate ratio (random) 95% CI	(%)	(random) 95% CI
Pimecrolimus 1% v vehicle at three weeks					
Luger 2001[15]	5/45	0/43		5.79	10.52(0.60 to 184.72)
Eichenfield 2002[12]	35/130	2/68		15.49	9.15 (2.27 to 36.91)
Eichenfield 2002[12]	37/137	8/68		25.25	2.30 (1.13 to 4.65)
Barba 2003[18]	38/71	8/35		26.19	2.34 (1.23 to 4.47)
Ho 2003[13]	51/123	11/63		27.29	2.51 (1.42 to 4.46)
Subtotal (95% CI)	506	277		100.00	2.72 (184 to 4.03)
Test for heterogeneity: x^2=4.58, df=4, P=0.33, I^2=12.7%					
Test for overall effect: z=5.01, P<0.0001					
Pimecrolimus 1% v vehicle at six weeks					
Eichenfield 2002[12]					
Eichenfield 2002[12]	49/130	11/68		32.35	2.33 (1.30 to 4.18)
Ho 2003[13]	44/137	14/68		33.36	1.56 (0.92 to 2.64)
Subtotal (95% CI)	67/123	15/63		34.29	2.29 (1.43 to 3.66)
Test for heterogeneity: x^2=1.43, df=2, P=0.49, I^2=0%	390	199		100.00	2.03 (1.50 to 2.74)
Test for overall effect: z=4.61, P=0.0001					
Pimecrolimus 1% v betamethasone valerate 0.1% at three weeks					
Luger 2001[15]	5/45	21/42		100.00	0.22 (0.09 to 0.54)
Subtotal (95% CI)	45	42		100.00	0.22 (0.09 to 0.54)
Test for heterogeneity: not applicable					
Test for overall effect: z=3.35, P=0.0008					
Pimecrolimus 1% v tacrolimus 0.03% at six weeks					
Kempers 2003[31]	21/71	29/70		100.00	0.71 (0.45 to 1.12)
Subtotal (95% CI)	71	70		100.00	0.71 (0.45 to 1.12)
Test for heterogeneity: not applicable					
Test for overall effect: z=1.45, P=0.15					

0.001 0.01 0.1 1 10 100 1000
Favours control ——— Favours pimecrolimus

Figure 19.3 The investigators' global assessment of response (clear or almost clear) in trials comparing pimecrolimus 1% and control. (Reproduced with kind permission of BMJ Publishing Group.)

Since the 2005 systematic review was published, many further vehicle-controlled studies have been published, the purpose of which is unclear. Another RCT suggested that increasing pimecrolimus 1% from twice daily to four times daily for 3 weeks in people with moderate to severe eczema does not increase efficacy.[137]

One interesting RCT published in 2005 evaluated the role of pimecrolimus 1% in preventing flares of eczema in 961 children and infants from two identical RCTs.[138] All patients used emollients for dry skin, but at the first sign of a relapse, randomly allocated participants either used pimecrolimus 1% or vehicle to try and prevent progression of flares. If the flare progressed to severe, then moderate topical cortico-steroids were used as rescue medication. The primary end point was the incidence of flares at 6 and 12 months. The proportion of children not experiencing a flare was around twice as high in the pimecrolimus group in comparison with the vehicle group (51% vs. 28% at 12 months in the children's study and 57% and 29% in the infant study, respectively). A further study by Siegfried et al. using a similar design in 275 children found that pimecrolimus 1% applied twice daily at the first sign of a flare resulted in fewer flares in comparison with vehicle (52% compared with 34% at 6 months).[139]

Drawbacks

Data from RCTs do not suggest any serious adverse effects to date.[135] Application reactions of burning, warmth, sting-ing, and soreness have been consistently reported in the RCTs and are dose-related. Pimecrolimus 1% skin irritation and burning was not significantly different from vehicle in the 2005 systematic review (pooled rate from six trials 0.87; 95% CI, 0.70 to 1.09), but skin burning was higher with pimecrolimus than with topical corticosteroids.[135] The systematic review did not show any increase in skin infec-tions with pimecrolimus 1%. Systemic absorption does occur with pimecrolimus, but this is very small in the majority of people.[140,141] No skin atrophy has been observed in a detailed study comparing topical pimecrolimus with 0.1% betamethasone valerate cream when applied to the forearms of healthy volunteers continuously for 4 weeks.[142] However, this type of study is difficult to interpret, as potent topical steroids are not used in this way and the effects of disease on skin thickness cannot be assessed.

As pimecrolimus is an immunosuppressive agent, the theoretical long-term risk of cancer needs to be monitored, given that the drug is likely to be prescribed in large quantit-ies to millions of children with mild forms of this common disease.

Comments

The quality of reporting in the pimecrolimus studies was generally good. There is no doubt from the many vehicle-controlled studies that pimecrolimus is effective in treating atopic eczema in terms of reducing symptoms, improving physical signs of eczema, and improving the quality of life. Yet despite the profusion of vehicle-controlled studies (which some might consider unethical, given that several early studies established efficacy),[143] numerous open-label studies, and consensus statements produced by physicians with conflicts of interest, the really key comparisons between pimecrolimus and current commonly used treatments for mild to moderate conditions—i.e., mild to moderate topical corticosteroids—appear to be completely missing. The early study that compared pimecrolimus with betamethasone showed that betamethasone was much more effective. Also missing are trials of pimecrolimus 1% in people with atopic eczema in whom topical corticosteroid therapy has failed—i.e., for the precise indication for which it is licensed. Also missing is a demonstration that topical pimecrolimus is useful for eczema in sensitive sites such as the face, or that it is has distinct advantages over topical corticosteroids in terms of less clinically significant skin thinning at such sites. The two studies that evaluated the use of pimecrolimus applied at the first sign of a flare to reduce the flare severity and frequency appear interesting (and at least they address the chronic relapsing nature of atopic eczema[144])—until, that is, one realizes that they are effectively placebo-controlled studies. It could have been the case that early treatment with very mild and safe 1% hydrocortisone acetate ointment would have averted the development of flares equally well. Others have pointed out that it is normal to wait until a flare becomes moderate to severe before initiating treatment with a topical corticosteroid, and in that sense the prevention-of-flare studies are unrealistic.[145] As a result of missing studies, the physician and patient are left guessing about how pimecrolimus compares with the best standard therapy.[146]

One detailed economic assessment concluded that there was too much uncertainty in assessing the cost-effectiveness of pimecrolimus,[135] although a later study suggested that pimecrolimus was cost-effective in comparison with standard therapy in a United States setting.[147]

Implications for practice

In relation to the child described in the case scenario, the lack of key comparisons in published trials makes it difficult to decide with the child's parents when and how to use topical pimecrolimus. We would consider pimecrolimus if the child needed to use potent topical steroids almost continuously in order to obtain a reasonable quality of life, although we would not be too optimistic about the ability of pimecrolimus to work where potent topical corticosteroids had failed. We might use topical pimecrolimus for persistent sensitive-site eczema (such as on the face) if topical corticosteroids or topical 0.03% tacrolimus had failed or caused too much burning or stinging. We would also consider trying pimecrolimus if the child's parents were letting the child suffer terribly from uncontrolled eczema because of an irrational fear of using any form of topical steroids, although we would probably use tacrolimus 0.1% first. We would also consider trying topical pimecrolimus to prevent flares in children with brittle disease if early use of a topical corticosteroid was ineffective.

Key points: topical pimecrolimus

- One percent pimecrolimus cream works better than vehicle cream in children and adults with mild to moderate atopic eczema. There is no need for any more vehicle-controlled studies of pimecrolimus.
- Like topical tacrolimus, pimecrolimus 1% could be useful for eczema in sensitive sites such as the face if topical corticosteroid use is no longer effective or use is excessive.
- There is no evidence to support the view that pimecrolimus is more effective than tacrolimus.
- One percent pimecrolimus cream is much less effective than topical betamethasone valerate in atopic eczema.
- Pimecrolimus 1% has not been compared with 1% hydrocortisone or other mild to moderate topical corticosteroids.
- It is not known whether pimecrolimus is effective in people with atopic eczema who are not well controlled with topical steroids.
- One percent pimecrolimus does not cause skin thinning.
- Local application-site reactions such as burning are mild and transient.
- Topical pimecrolimus appears to be safe in the short term, although its long-term safety is unknown.
- It is not known whether early treatment with topical tacrolimus is any better than early treatment with a weak topical steroid such as 1% hydrocortisone in preventing more severe flares that require potent steroids.
- Independent studies are needed in order to compare the cost-effectiveness of pimecrolimus with standard bursts of topical steroids in the short-term control of mild atopic eczema in children, and to see whether early use of either treatment approach improves disease control over a longer period.

References: topical pimecrolimus

131 Wellington K, Jarvis B. Topical pimecrolimus: a review of its clinical potential in the management of atopic dermatitis. *Drugs* 2002;**62**:817–40.

132 Anon. FDA licensing review of pimecrolimus. www.fda.gov/cder/foi/nda/2001/21-302_Elidel.htm (accessed 27th August, 2002).

133 Emerson RM, Williams HC, Allen BR. Severity distribution of atopic dermatitis in the community and its relationship to secondary referral. *Br J Dermatol* 1998;**139**:73–6.

134 Nghiem P, Pearson G, Langley RG. Tacrolimus and pimecrolimus: from clever prokaryotes to inhibiting calcineurin and treating atopic dermatitis. *J Am Acad Dermatol* 2002;**46**:228–41.

135 Garside R, Stein K, Castelnuovo E, *et al.* The effectiveness and cost-effectiveness of pimecrolimus and tacrolimus for atopic eczema: a systematic review and economic evaluation. *Health Technol Assess* 2005;**9**:1–230.

136 Kempers S, Boguniewicz M, Carter E, *et al.* Comparison of pimecrolimus cream 1% and tacrolimus ointment 0.03% in pediatric patients with atopic eczema. *J Eur Acad Dermatol Venereol* 2003; **17**:P2–41.

137 Ling M, Gottlieb A, Pariser D, *et al.* A randomized study of the safety, absorption and efficacy of pimecrolimus cream 1% applied

twice or four times daily in patients with atopic dermatitis. *J Dermatolog Treat* 2005;**16**:142–8.

138 Papp K, Staab D, Harper J, *et al*. Effect of pimecrolimus cream 1% on the long-term course of pediatric atopic dermatitis. *Int J Dermatol* 2004;**43**:978–83.

139 Siegfried E, Korman N, Molina C, Kianifard F, Abrams K. Safety and efficacy of early intervention with pimecrolimus cream 1% combined with corticosteroids for major flares in infants and children with atopic dermatitis. *J Dermatolog Treat* 2006;**17**:143–50.

140 Van Leent EJ, Ebelin ME, Burtin P, Dorobek B, Spuls PI, Bos JD. Low systemic exposure after repeated topical application of pimecrolimus (Elidel), SDZ ASM 981, in patients with atopic dermatitis. *Dermatology* 2002;**204**:63–8.

141 Robinson N, Singri P, Gordon KB. Safety of the new macrolide immunomodulators. *Semin Cutan Med Surg* 2001;**20**:242–9.

142 Queille-Roussel C, Paul C, Duteil L, *et al*. The new topical ascomycin derivative SDZ ASM 981 does not induce skin atrophy when applied to normal skin for 4 weeks: a randomized, double-blind controlled study. *Br J Dermatol* 2001;**144**:507–13.

143 Freeman SR, Williams HC, Dellavalle RP. The increasing importance of systematic reviews in clinical dermatology research and publication. *J Invest Dermatol* 2006;**126**:2357–60.

144 Hoare C, Li Wan Po A, Williams H. Systematic review of treatments for atopic eczema. *Health Technol Assess* 2000;**4**(37).

145 Anonymous. Pimecrolimus cream for atopic dermatitis. *Drugs Ther Bull* 2003;**41**:33–6.

146 Williams H. New treatments for atopic dermatitis. *BMJ* 2002;**324**: 1533–4.

147 Ellis CN, Kahler KH, Grueger J, Chang J. Cost effectiveness of management of mild-to-moderate atopic dermatitis with 1% pimecrolimus cream in children and adolescents 2–17 years of age. *Am J Clin Dermatol* 2006;**7**:133–9.

Will interventions to reduce house dust mite improve this child's eczema?

Efficacy

This section deals with house dust mite (HDM) eradication for cases of established atopic eczema. No systematic review was found for house dust mite reduction in atopic eczema. However, a recent Cochrane systematic review of house dust mite reduction for the treatment of asthma reported no improvement in the symptoms of asthma.[148] The authors concluded that "It is doubtful whether further studies, similar to the ones in our meta-analysis, are worthwhile."

Seven RCTs[149–155] evaluating the role of house dust mite reduction in the treatment of *established* atopic eczema were identified and are summarized in Web Table 19.3. Trials were excluded if they looked at the prevention of atopic eczema in newborn children (for example, Koopman *et al.*,[156] Horak *et al.*[157]), because the results were not presented for atopic eczema in a disaggregated form (for example, Terreehorst *et al.*[158]), or because data were not presented on the clinical impact of the interventions (for example, Nishioka *et al.*[159]). In general, the evidence to support the efficacy of house dust mite eradication for the treatment of atopic eczema is of poor quality. Interventions such as vacuuming and the use of synthetic mattress covers appear to be most effective in reducing the house dust mite load, but how this impacts on disease severity is still unclear.

The first small RCT by Colloff and colleagues[149] evaluated the daily use of natamycin (a spray used to kill house dust mites) versus a matched placebo spray with and without vacuum cleaning in a parallel-group study for 4 months in 20 young adults with atopic eczema. The authors demonstrated that it was the vacuum cleaning and not the natamycin spray that had a significant impact on reducing house dust mite numbers. There was no significant clinical improvement in those who had been allocated to natamycin versus placebo. The mean symptom score (maximum score 288) in the natamycin and vacuum group changed from 55.2 at baseline to 38.6 at 4 months, in comparison with 45.2 to 35.8 in the group with no natamycin and no daily vacuuming.

A second small, but important, RCT was conducted by Tan and colleagues in 1996,[150] with duplicated publication in 1998 and again in 1999. Tan and colleagues randomly assigned 60 patients (30 adults and 30 children) for a total of 6 months to an intensive dust mite eradication regimen involving Gore-Tex (Intervent, UK) bedding covers, benzyl tannate spray to kill mites and denature their allergens, and a high-filtration vacuum cleaner, or to a control group with plain cotton bedcovers, placebo spray, and a standard upright vacuum cleaner with poor filtration performance. One trained nurse applied the bedcovers and spray each week, and participants were encouraged to vacuum their bedrooms daily. There was a dramatic and very similar reduction in the concentration of house dust mite major allergen (*Der p1*) in bedroom carpets in both the active and placebo treatment groups at the end of 6 months. Disease activity—as recorded in terms of surface area involvement and with a composite severity score (maximum score 108) measured at one point at the end of the 6 months—was reduced by a small amount in both groups, but more so in the active group. The mean reduction in scores for the active and placebo groups were 12.6 and 4.2 units, respectively. Those in the active treatment group had more severe conditions to begin with, and so an analysis of covariance was conducted to allow for baseline scores and initial house dust mite antigen levels. This showed a mean difference of 4.2 in the change of score (95% CI, 1.7 to 6.7 units; $P = 0.008$) between the two treatments. Further analysis also suggested that it was changes in the mattress and carpet dust in the bedroom that mediated much of the treatment effect. Subgroup analysis suggested that only children had a clinically and statistically significant benefit, and that there was no correlation between clinical improvement and positive skin prick tests at the study outset.

Another small study in Japan by Endo and colleagues[151] evaluated the potential benefit of intensive vacuum cleaning in the rooms of 30 children with atopic eczema for a total of 12 months. Both groups were visited every 3 weeks by a team of mite specialists, who either cleaned room floors, mattresses, and quilts very thoroughly and encouraged parents to clean in the same way in between visits, versus a less intensive clean (vacuum suction power reduced to 50%) with similar cleaning between visits. Parents were thus unblinded to the intervention. A statistically significant decrease in mite numbers in favor of the intensive cleaning group was only noted for the room floors. Clinical scores, as evaluated by a physician blind to treatment allocation, were significantly improved in the active group in comparison with baseline, but not in the control group. Clinical scores were given in graphic form only, and the appropriate statistical test of mean difference between the two treatments was not reported.

Oosting et al.[152] compared Gore-Tex mattress, duvet, and pillow covers with placebo covers made from cotton for a period of 12 months. Eighty-six children and adults took part, all of whom had atopic eczema and were allergic to HDM. Whilst the mattress covers resulted in a significant reduction in the HDM load, no significant between-group differences were observed in clinical features or self-reported itch and sleep loss.

The remaining studies were all very small (41 participants,[153] 20 participants,[154] and 43 participants,[155] respectively), making conclusions difficult.

Drawbacks

None of the studies reported any adverse events of the house dust mite removal treatments. This does not necessarily imply that none occurred. The imposition of daily vacuuming for a long period has a cost in terms of time for parents and sufferers, as does the purchase of a high-filtration vacuum cleaner, impermeable mattress covers, and mite sprays.

Comments

Given the strong circumstantial evidence to suggest that house dust mite allergens may play a part in atopic eczema, it is a pity that so few studies on house dust mite avoidance have been performed. Those that have been done tend to be small, and it is difficult to generalize in the absence of more pragmatic studies. The method of randomization and concealment was not reported adequately in any of the studies, and no ITT analyses were performed (although drop-out rates were quite low).

Further studies that separate the different interventions for reducing house dust mite are needed. It is important that such trials should be as pragmatic as possible to determine which groups respond best, which interventions are the most cost-effective, and whether the laborious interventions are sustainable in less motivated people.

Implications for clinical practice

In the absence of strong clinical trial data to support the use of house dust mite avoidance measures, the decision as to whether the cost and effort of implementing such procedures is warranted probably lies with the individual families. In the future, specific immunotherapy with a house dust mite preparation may be possible, and early tests have shown promising results.[160]

Key points: house dust mite

- Seven randomized controlled trials have been reported, although methodological difficulties and small sample sizes limit the interpretation of the results.
- Future, large-scale pragmatic trials are needed if this issue is to be resolved.
- In the meantime, the use of allergen-impermeable mattress and pillow covers, coupled with regular vacuuming of the room, appear to be the best way of reducing house dust mite if such changes are truly beneficial.

References: house dust mite

148 Gøtzsche PC, Johansen HK, Schmidt LM, Burr ML. House dust mite control measures for asthma. *Cochrane Database Syst Rev* 2004;(**4**):CD001187.

149 Colloff MJ, Lever RS, McSharry C. A controlled trial of house dust mite eradication using natamycin in homes of patients with atopic dermatitis: effect on clinical status and mite populations. *Br J Dermatol* 1989;**121**:199–208.

150 Tan BB, Weald D, Strickland I, Friedmann PS. Double-blind controlled trial of effect of housedust-mite allergen avoidance on atopic dermatitis. *Lancet* 1996;**347**:15–8.

151 Endo K, Fukuzumi T, Adachi J, et al. Effect of vacuum cleaning of room floors and bed clothes of patients on house dust mites counts and clinical scores of atopic dermatitis. A double blind control trial. *Arerugi (Jpn J Allergol)* 1997;**46**:1013–24.

152 Oosting AJ, de Bruin-Weller MS, Terreehorst I, et al. Effect of mattress encasings on atopic dermatitis outcome measures in a double-blind, placebo-controlled study: the Dutch mite avoidance study. *J Allergy Clin Immunol* 2002;**110**:500–6.

153 Ricci G, Patrizi A, Specchia F, et al. Effect of house dust mite avoidance measures in children with atopic dermatitis. *Br J Dermatol* 2000;**143**:379–84.

154 Gutgesell C, Heise S, Seubert S, et al. Double-blind placebo-controlled house dust mite control measures in adult patients with atopic dermatitis. *Br J Dermatol* 2001;**145**:70–4.

155 Holm L, Ohman S, Bengtsson A, van Hage-Hamsten M, Scheynius A. Effectiveness of occlusive bedding in the treatment of atopic dermatitis—a placebo-controlled trial of 12 months duration. *Allergy* 2001;**56**:152–8.

156 Koopman LP, van Strien RT, Kerkhof M, et al. Placebo-controlled trial of house dust mite-impermeable mattress covers. *Am J Respir Crit Care Med* 2002;**166**:307–13.

157 Horak F, Matthews S, Ihorst G, et al. Effect of mite-impermeable mattress encasing and an educational package on the development of allergies in a multinational randomized, controlled

birth-cohort study—24 months result of the Study of Prevention of Allergy in Children in Europe. *Clin Exp Allergy* 2004;**34**:1220–5.

158 Terreehorst I, Duienvoorden HJ, Tempels-Pavlica Z, *et al*. The effect of encasings on quality of life in adult house dust mite allergic patients with rhinitis, asthma and/or atopic dermatitis. *Allergy* 2005;**60**:888–93.

159 Nishioka K, Yasueda H, Saito H. Preventive effect of bedding encasement with microfine fibers on mite sensitization. *J Allergy Clin Immunol* 1998;**101**:28–32.

160 Werfel T, Breuer K, Ruéff F, *et al*. Usefulness of specific immunotherapy in patients with atopic dermatitis and allergic sensitization to house dust mites: a multi-centre, randomized, dose-response study. *Allergy* 2006;**61**:202–5.

Will an exclusion diet (such as a milk- or egg-free diet) alone help reduce the symptoms of this child's atopic eczema?

Efficacy

This section deals with exclusion diets for cases of established atopic eczema. One systematic review published in 2001 was found,[161] which described seven RCTs. Since then, two further RCTs have been published in full.[162,163] The nine RCTs examining the role of elimination diets in established atopic eczema are summarized in Web Table 19.4.[162–170]

Drawbacks

Calcium, protein, and calorie deficiency are risks associated with the use of dairy-free diets in children. Such diets should only be used under medical supervision. Three RCTs used soya-based milk substitute, which itself can be allergenic in atopic eczema.

Comments

Methodological difficulties mean that interpretation of these trials is difficult. RCTs that employ a parallel design with an unblinded normal control diet may introduce bias in favor of the active group. In addition, those trials that place all participants on exclusion diets and then reintroduce the suspected offending food, in comparison with a control, risk introducing another allergen (for example, soya) or introducing the suspected allergen (for example, cows' milk) in a way that does not mimic real life. Poor concealment of randomization allocation, lack of blinding, and high dropout rates without an ITT analysis all mean that the above studies should be interpreted with great caution. Future studies should ideally be longer-term and more pragmatic and should ensure that randomization is concealed.

Uncontrolled elimination diets followed by double-blind, placebo-controlled challenges with foods suspected to aggravate symptoms have also been tried in atopic eczema.[171–175] These studies are not the same as RCTs of food elimination. Instead, they try to answer the question: "Does food X make a particular child's atopic eczema worse?" The

precise relationship between such food challenge studies and long-term benefits of exclusion of the suspected foods to atopic eczema sufferers is not clear. Blood and skin-prick tests are usually only helpful in predicting clinical response if they are negative.[176,177] It should also be borne in mind that a high negative predictive value has only been shown in relation to the provocation of symptoms after a double-blind challenge, and not the clinical response following food elimination, which is not necessarily the same thing. The relationship between atopic eczema and food sensitivity is a complex one, and readers are referred to a clear evidence-based work by David for further information.[178]

Implications for clinical practice

Elimination diets are difficult for families and patients to follow, even in the highly motivated environment of a clinical trial. In the absence of clear evidence of the involvement of a particular food substance, the possible harms may outweigh the benefits. In cases in which exclusion diets are indicated, appropriate dietary advice and support should be made available.

Key points: exclusion diet

- There is little evidence to support a diet free of eggs and milk in unselected patients with atopic eczema.
- There is no evidence to support the use of an elemental or few-foods diet in atopic eczema.
- There is some evidence to support the use of an egg-free diet in infants with suspected egg allergy who have positive specific IgE to eggs.
- The most common diets used are those free of milk or eggs.
- The possible risks of impaired growth and development in children should be recognized.

References: exclusion diet

161 Charman C. Atopic eczema. In: Godley F, ed. *Clinical Evidence*, issue 5. London: BMJ Publishing Group, 2001: 1133–45.

162 Niggemann B, Binder C, Dupont C, Hadji S, Arvola T, Isolauri E. Prospective, controlled, multi-center study on the effect of an amino-acid-based formula in infants with cow's milk allergy/intolerance and atopic dermatitis. *Pediatr Allergy Immunol* 2001;**12**:78–82.

163 Leung TF, Ma KC, Cheung LTF, *et al*. A randomized, single-blind and crossover study of an amino acid-based milk formula in treating young children with atopic dermatitis. *Pediatr Allergy Immunol* 2004;**15**:558–61.

164 Atherton DJ, Sewell M, Soothill JF, Wells RS, Chilvers CE. A double-blind controlled crossover trial of an antigen-avoidance diet in atopic eczema. *Lancet* 1978;**1**:401–3.

165 Munkvad M, Danielsen L, Hoj L, *et al*. Antigen-free diet in adult patients with atopic dermatitis. A double-blind controlled study. *Acta Derm Venereol* 1984;**64**:524–8.

166 Cant AJ, Bailes JA, Marsden RA, Hewitt D. Effect of maternal dietary exclusion on breast fed infants with eczema: two controlled studies. *BMJ Clin Res Ed* 1986;**293**:231–3.

167 Neild VS, Marsden RA, Bailes JA, Bland JM. Egg and milk exclusion diets in atopic eczema. *Br J Dermatol* 1986;**114**:117–23.

168 Mabin DC, Sykes AE, David TJ. Controlled trial of a few foods diet in severe atopic dermatitis. *Arch Dis Child* 1995;**73**:202–7.

169 Isolauri E, Sütas Y, Mäkinen-Kiljunen S, Oja SS, Isosomppi R, Turjanmaa K. Efficacy and safety of hydrolyzed cow milk and amino acid-derived formulas in infants with cow milk allergy. *J Pediatr* 1995;**127**:550–7.

170 Lever R, MacDonald C, Waugh P, Aitchison T. Randomised controlled trial of advice on an egg exclusion diet in young children with atopic eczema and sensitivity to eggs. *Pediatr Allergy Immunol* 1998;**9**:13–9.

171 Sloper KS, Wadsworth J, Brostoff J. Children with atopic eczema, I: clinical response to food elimination and subsequent double-blind food challenge. *Q J Med* 1991;**80**:677–93.

172 Devlin J, David TJ. Tartrazine in atopic eczema. *Arch Dis Child* 1992;**67**:709–11.

173 James JM, Bernhisel-Broadbent J, Sampson HA. Respiratory reactions provoked by double-blind food challenges in children. *Am J Respir Crit Care Med* 1994;**149**:59–64.

174 Fuglsang G, Madsen G, Halken S, Jorgensen S, Ostergaard PA, Osterballe O. Adverse reactions to food additives in children with atopic symptoms. *Allergy* 1994;**49**:31–7.

175 Kanny G, Hatahet R, Moneret-Vautrin DA, Kohler C, Bellut A. Allergy and intolerance to flavouring agents in atopic dermatitis in young children. *Allerg Immunol (Paris)* 1994;**26**:204–6.

176 Sampson HA. Comparative study of commercial food antigen extracts for the diagnosis of food hypersensitivity. *J Allergy Clin Immunol* 1988;**82**:718–26.

177 Sampson HA, Ho DG. Relationship between food-specific IgE concentrations and the risk of positive food challenges in children and adolescents. *J Allergy Clin Immunol* 1997;**100**:444–51.

178 David TJ. *Food and Food Additive Intolerance in Childhood*. Oxford: Blackwell Scientific Publications, 1993.

Do probiotics help reduce the symptoms of this child's atopic eczema?

It has been suggested that probiotics (commonly referred to as "good" bacteria that have the ability to modify immune responses) might help prevent and treat atopic eczema by way of altering the intestinal microflora.[179]

This section deals with probiotics used to help reduce the symptoms of atopic eczema. No systematic review was found, although one Cochrane review is in preparation. Twelve RCTs evaluated the role of probiotics in the treatment of *established* atopic eczema and are summarized in Web Table 19.5.[179–190] Six of the 12 studies use extensively hydrolyzed formula (EHF) milk to avoid cows' milk.[179–181,183,185,187]

Efficacy

The six studies looking at elimination diets together with probiotics showed no significant differences in eczema severity between the probiotic groups and placebo. One of these studies[183] conducted an exploratory analysis and found a statistically significant difference between probiotic

and placebo groups in a subset of infants who tested positive for IgE.

One study comparing two probiotic *Lactobacillus* strains, given in combination, with placebo in 58 children (aged 1–13) found no significant difference in the total eczema severity (SCORAD) at 6 weeks.[182] However, in a subset of allergic children (at least one positive skin-prick test response and elevated IgE levels), eczema severity decreased significantly in the probiotic group in comparison with the placebo. Another study comparing two probiotics (*Lactobacillus rhamnosus* and *Bifidobacteria lactis*) to placebo in 60 children found improvement in atopic dermatitis only in food-sensitized children.[190]

Another study compared *Lactobacillus fermentum* VRI-033 PCC to placebo in 56 children (6–18 months) for 8 weeks and found no significant difference between the two groups with regard to the severity of atopic dermatitis, as assessed by SCORAD.[184] However, no adjustments were made for the greater number of severe cases in the placebo group in comparison with the probiotic group at baseline. One study compared a probiotic plus a prebiotic preparation with a probiotic preparation alone and found no significant difference in SCORAD at the end of the study.[189]

Comments

A previous review of four RCTs concluded that there was no convincing evidence that probiotics are helpful in patients with established atopic eczema.[191] Eight further studies have been published since then, and still there is no convincing evidence that probiotics are helpful in established atopic eczema, although two of the studies claim beneficial effects of probiotics for the treatment of atopic eczema. The first study suggests that the use of elimination diets overwhelmed the modest effect from probiotics, and therefore a clear benefit from probiotics was not shown.[183] The second study did not use an elimination diet, and although it did not show a statistically significant difference between the probiotic and placebo groups, it did come close to the 5% significance level.[184]

Drawbacks

Recruitment in one study[181] was prematurely terminated due to concerning adverse gastrointestinal symptoms, which were limited to the group receiving heat-inactivated *Lactobacillus rhamnosus* GG.

Key points: probiotics

- There is little convincing evidence that probiotics produce a clinically useful effect for the treatment of atopic eczema.
- There is some evidence to suggest that a subset of patients who test positive for IgE might benefit from the use of probiotics.
- Trials are needed in these specific subsets of eczema patients before probiotic treatment can be recommended.

References: probiotics

179 Kirjavainen PV, Salminen SJ, Isolauri E. Probiotic bacteria in the management of atopic disease: underscoring the importance of viability. *J Pediatr Gastroenterol Nutr* 2003;**36**:223–7.

180 Majama H, Isolauri E. Probiotics: a novel approach in the management of food allergy. *J Allergy Clin Immunol* 1997;**99**:179–85.

181 Isolauri E, Arvola T, Sutas Y, Moilanen E, Salminen S. Probiotics in the management of atopic eczema. *Clin Exp Allergy* 2000;**30**: 1604–10.

182 Rosenfeldt V, Benfeldt E, Nielsen SD, *et al*. Effect of probiotic *Lactobacillus* strains in children with atopic dermatitis. *J Allergy Clin Immunol* 2003;**111**:389–95.

183 Viljanen M, Savilahti E, Haahtela T, *et al*. Probiotics in the treatment of atopic eczema/dermatitis syndrome in infants: a double-blind placebo-controlled trial. *Allergy* 2005;**60**:494–500.

184 Weston S, Halbert A, Richmond P, Prescott SL. Effects of probiotics on atopic dermatitis: a randomised controlled trial. *Arch Dis Child* 2005;**90**:892–7.

185 Brouwer ML, Wolt-Plompen SAA, Dubois AEJ, *et al*. No effects of probiotics on atopic dermatitis in infancy: a randomised placebo-controlled trial. *Clin Exp Allergy* 2006;**36**:899–906.

186 Folster-Holst R, Muller F, Schnopp N, *et al*. Prospective, randomised controlled trial on *Lactobacillus rhamnosus* in infants with moderate to severe atopic dermatitis. *Br J Dermatol* 2006; **155**:1256–61.

187 Taniuchi S, Hattori K, Yamamoto A, *et al*. Administration of *Bifidobacterium* to infants with atopic dermatitis: changes in fecal microflora and clinical symptoms. *J Appl Res* 2005;**5**:387–96.

188 Grüber C, Wendt M, Sulser C, *et al*. Randomized, placebo-controlled trial of *Lactobacillus rhamnosus* GG as treatment of atopic dermatitis in infancy. *Allergy* 2007;**62**:1270–6.

189 Passeron T, Lacour JP, Fontas E, Ortonne JP. Prebiotics and synbiotics: two promising approaches for the treatment of atopic dermatitis in children above 2 years. *Allergy* 2006;**61**:431–7.

190 Sistek D, Kelly R, Wickens K, Stanley T, Fitzharris P, Crane J. Is the effect of probiotics on atopic dermatitis confined to food sensitized children? *Clin Exp Allergy* 2006;**36**:629–33.

191 [Anon.] Probiotics for atopic disease. *Drug Ther Bull* 2005;**43**: 6–8.

Do Chinese herbal medicines improve the symptoms of atopic eczema?

Efficacy

We located two systematic reviews of Chinese herbal medicines for atopic eczema.[192,193] These reviews reported four randomized trials of atopic eczema.[194–197] All four trials evaluated a commercial preparation of 10 traditional Chinese herbs (Zemaphyte). This preparation is no longer being manufactured.

Sheehan and Atherton compared Chinese herbs (as above) in a decoction and a placebo comprising of a mixture of "inert" plant materials, once daily for 8 weeks, in 47 children with atopic eczema.[194] Median percentage changes in the clinical scores for erythema in comparison with baseline were 51% for Chinese herbs and 6.1% for placebo. Change

in surface damage was 63.1% and 6.2% in the Chinese herb and placebo groups, respectively. A 1-year follow-up study of the children concluded that Chinese herbal medicine, in the medium term, was helpful for approximately half the children who originally took part in the RCT.[198]

Sheehan *et al*. also compared the Chinese herbs (as above) in a decoction and an "inert plant" placebo, once daily, in 40 adult patients with atopic dermatitis.[195] Significant improvements were reported for erythema ($P < 0.001$) and surface damage ($P < 0.001$) with the herbs in comparison with the placebo.

The study by Latchman *et al*.[196] evaluated the same combination of Chinese herbs finely ground and in a more palatable form of freeze-dried granules over an 8-week period in 18 patients with atopic eczema. There was a significant reduction in erythema and surface damage in comparison with baseline ($P < 0.001$). There were no differences between the formulations with regard to the clinical outcome.

The study by Fung *et al*.[197] evaluated the same combination of Chinese herbs in comparison with "inert plant" placebo over an 8-week period in 40 patients with atopic eczema. There was a general trend toward clinical improvement with both the Chinese herbs and the placebo.

Drawbacks

Both active and placebo herbs were reported to be unpalatable and caused 10 and eight drop-outs, respectively, in the studies by Sheehan *et al*.[195,198] Other adverse effects included abdominal distension, headaches, transient dizziness, gastrointestinal upsets, one case of lichenoid eruption, and one case of facial herpes. The potential for hepatotoxicity is a concern with Chinese herbs. However, the three studies that carried out pretreatment and post-treatment liver function tests found no abnormalities.[194,195,197]

Comments

All studies were randomized, but the method and concealment of allocation were not described. All were described as double-blind except for the study by Latchman *et al*.,[196] in which no blinding was mentioned. No ITT analysis was carried out. It is also questionable whether the placebo plants were truly inert. The study by Sheehan and Atherton[194] reported large effects in children, highlighting a promising treatment on atopic eczema. This has not been replicated in the other studies, although they are all quite similar. Clearly, larger-scale RCTs of longer duration are needed.

Implications for clinical practice

There is currently little convincing evidence to support the use of Chinese herbal medicines for the treatment of atopic eczema, although some studies have reported large effects. Further research is needed to address the long-term safety implications.

Key points: Chinese herbal medicines

- Four randomized controlled trials of modest size are reported, all of which used the same herbs for the active intervention group.
- The results are conflicting, and further large-scale studies are needed.
- A number of side effects were identified, the true implications of which cannot be addressed without long-term studies.

References: Chinese herbal medicines

192 Armstrong NC, Ernst E. The treatment of eczema with Chinese herbs: a systematic review of randomised clinical trials. *Br J Clin Pharmacol* 1999;**48**:262–4.

193 Zhang W, Leonard T, Bath-Hextall F, *et al.* Chinese herbal medicine for atopic eczema. *Cochrane Database Syst Rev* 2005;(**2**): CD002291.

194 Sheehan MP, Atherton DJ. A controlled trial of traditional Chinese medicinal plants in widespread non-exudative atopic eczema. *Br J Dermatol* 1992;**126**:179–84.

195 Sheehan MP, Rustin MH, Atherton DJ, *et al.* Efficacy of traditional Chinese herbal therapy in adult atopic dermatitis. *Lancet* 1992;**340**:13–7.

196 Latchman Y, Banerjee P, Poulter LW, Rustin M, Brostoff J. Association of immunological changes with clinical efficacy in atopic eczema patients treated with traditional Chinese herbal therapy (Zemaphyte). *Int Arch Allergy Immunol* 1996;**109**:243–9.

197 Fung AY, Look PC, Chong LY, But PP, Wong E. A controlled trial of traditional Chinese herbal medicine in Chinese patients with recalcitrant atopic dermatitis. *Int J Dermatol* 1999;**38**:387–92.

198 Sheehan MP, Atherton DJ. One year follow-up of children treated with Chinese medicinal herbs for atopic eczema. *Br J Dermatol* 1994;**130**:488–93.

Do washing powders exacerbate the symptoms of atopic eczema?

Efficacy

Detergent enzymes may cause skin irritation, leading some physicians to advise patients with atopic eczema to avoid the use of such detergents in favor of alternative "nonbiological" detergents.[199] We located one RCT testing the hypothesis that enzyme-containing detergents are more likely to aggravate atopic eczema than a nonbiological detergent,[200] and one that looked at the impact of using fabric softeners in adults with atopic dermatitis.[201]

In the first study,[199] 26 adults with mild to moderate atopic eczema (mean age 25 years) were randomly assigned in a double-blind crossover study to use either a trial detergent containing enzymes or a visually identical detergent without enzymes for 1 month. There was a 1-month washout period before randomization, when participants used their usual washing powder. Topical steroids were permitted during the study and were weighed. In the 25 patients who completed the trial, there was no difference between the two groups in terms of disease severity (SCORAD scores of 29 in each group; 95% CI for mean difference, 4 to 5). Similar results were found for the use of topical steroids, patient-reported itch, and eczema activity.

The study looking at fabric softeners[201] was a single-blind randomized trial using a left–right comparison design for a period of 12 days. Twenty volunteers with a history of atopic dermatitis were enrolled in the study (none had active lesions at the time of enrolment). In order to simulate realistic conditions of skin damage, sodium lauryl sulfate was applied to each volar forearm under occlusion 3 days before the start of the study. A control patch using water was also applied to each arm. Repetitive wash tests were performed three times a day using softened or unsoftened fabric in random order to each arm. The investigator was blinded to the fabric used at each site. Both for the control and pre-irritated skin, all measured parameters indicated that "softened" fabric was less aggressive to the skin than "unsoftened" fabric.

Drawbacks

No patients had contact dermatitis to enzymes when patch-tested at the end of the study, and there was no evidence of specific blood IgE against any of the enzymes.[201]

Comment

Although the study by Andersen *et al.*[200] was small, the virtual absence of any differences between the enzyme and nonenzyme detergents and the corresponding narrow confidence intervals provide convincing evidence of a lack of harmful effect. The study was not sponsored by industry. Further long-term studies using a pragmatic design may be helpful in determining any potential benefit from using fabric softeners for patients with atopic eczema.

Implications for clinical practice

There is currently no evidence to suggest that parents should switch from a biological to a nonbiological washing powder.

Key points: washing powders

- Although the parents of children with atopic eczema commonly avoid washing powders that contain enzymes (biological powders), evidence from a small RCT did not support the belief that washing detergents containing enzymes have a provoking effect on eczema severity in comparison with washing detergents without enzymes.
- There is limited evidence to suggest that fabric softeners may be less likely to exacerbate the symptoms of eczema; further pragmatic studies are needed.
- We found no studies looking at the effect of avoiding all contact with washing detergents.

References: washing powders

199 Rothe MJ, Grant-Kels JM. Diagnostic criteria for atopic dermatitis. *Lancet* 1996;**348**:1391–2.

200 Andersen PH, Bindslev-Jensen C, Mosbech H, Zachariae H, Andersen KE. Skin symptoms in patients with atopic dermatitis using enzyme-containing detergents. A placebo-controlled study. *Acta Derm Venereol* 1998;**78**:60–2.

201 Hermanns J, Goffin V, Arrese J, Rodriguez C. Beneficial effects of softened fabrics on atopic skin. *Dermatology* 2001;**202**:167–70.

Can specialized clothing help reduce the symptoms of atopic eczema?

Efficacy

We found no systematic reviews, but found three RCTs evaluating clothing material in atopic eczema.[202–204] Diepgen *et al.*, in 1990[202] and 1995,[203] evaluated the irritative capacity of shirts made of four different materials (cotton and synthetics of different fiber structure). The other RCT, by Seymour *et al.*,[204] evaluated the clinical effects of different types of nappies on the skin of normal infants and infants with atopic eczema.

In the 1990 study by Diepgen *et al.*,[202] 55 patients with atopic eczema were compared with 31 control patients without atopic eczema and were randomly assigned to wear shirts of one of four different types of fiber. At the end of week 2 of the study, those wearing cotton shirts reported better comfort in comparison with the other textile shirts, in increasing order of weight and fiber roughness.

The 1995 study by Diepgen *et al.*[203] (published in a German textile journal) evaluated seven different garments on 20 patients with mild to moderate atopic eczema. The garments were either cotton or polyester, with different fiber roughness, yarn roughness, and fabric weaves. The study was a randomized crossover study (T. Diepgen, personal communication, January 2000), with each garment worn under standardized conditions on four consecutive days. Comfort was statistically significantly higher for warp-knit shirts in comparison with jersey-knit shirts, but was no different for cotton and polyester of fine fiber construction (assessed by scanning electron microscopy).

In the study by Seymour *et al.*,[204] cloth nappies were compared with cellulose-core nappies and cellulose-core nappies containing absorbent gelling material. Eighty-five babies with atopic eczema who were less than 20 months of age were included. Eczema severity and the degree of diaper rash were scored by an independent dermatologist. At the end of the 26-week period, there was no clinical or statistical difference between the different diaper types for the overall grade of atopic eczema. However, diaper rash was significantly less in the group using cellulose nappies with absorbent gelling material in comparison with the others at 26 weeks and throughout the trial ($P < 0.05$).

Drawbacks

None were reported, although specialized cotton clothing for atopic eczema sufferers is more expensive than other synthetic fibers. No adverse events were reported in the trial of different nappies.

Comment

The success of blinding in both of the trials conducted by Diepgen and colleagues[202,203] is questionable because of the different roughness of the various shirt fibers. The magnitude of effects was not stated in the 1995 paper, and it is possible that small differences in comfort between cotton and polyester fabrics were missed. Both RCTs suggest that the smoothness of the fabric is more important than the type of fabric used. Synthetic fibers that are just as comfortable for people with atopic eczema can be manufactured with smooth fibers using yarns and fabric construction.

From the study by Seymour *et al.*,[204] it was unclear if the group with atopic eczema who wore cloth nappies were randomized in the same way as the other two groups and whether statistical comparisons were made with the control population who were not part of the same randomized group. The study nevertheless suggests that diaper rash is less severe in atopic infants who wear diapers with absorbent gelling material. There was no evidence to support any benefit of conventional disposable diapers over cloth diapers, although the study may have lacked power to demonstrate small differences. The environmental implications of the different types of diaper were not discussed.

Implications for clinical practice

There is no need for parents of children to buy expensive cotton clothes if their child finds that other fine-weave synthetics are just as comfortable. The type of diaper used may affect the severity of atopic eczema.

Key points: specialized clothing

- Two small randomized controlled trials found that, in people with atopic eczema, the roughness of clothing textiles is a more important factor for skin irritation than the type of textile fiber (synthetic or natural).
- Polyester and cotton of similar textile fineness seem to be equally well tolerated.
- We found no evidence on the long-term effect of different textiles on the severity of atopic eczema.
- It is possible that diaper rash may be less severe in babies wearing diapers with an absorbent gel.

References: specialized clothing

202 Diepgen TL, Stabler A, Hornstein OP. Irritation from textiles in atopic eczema and controls. Textile intolerance in atopic eczema: a controlled clinical study. *Z Hautkr* 1990;**65**:907–10.

203 Diepgen TL, Salzer B, Tepe A, Hornstein OP. A study of skin irritations by textiles under standardized sweating conditions in patients with atopic eczema. *Melliand English* 1995;**12**:268.
204 Seymour JL, Keswick BH, Hanifin JM, Jordan WP, Milligan MC. Clinical effects of diaper types on the skin of normal infants and infants with atopic dermatitis. *J Am Acad Dermatol* 1987;**17**:988–97.

What is the role of psychological interventions for the treatment of atopic eczema?

Efficacy

The search found one systematic review[205] and one protocol for a Cochrane systematic review dealing with psychological and educational interventions for atopic eczema in children.[206] We found four RCTs[207–210] for psychological interventions. However, the term "psychological intervention" is very broad, and alternative search strategies may be required in order to capture all possible treatment options.

It has been postulated that scratching becomes a habit in atopic eczema, and that it is detrimental because it damages the skin further. Habit reversal is a modified behavioral technique that teaches patients to recognize the habit and then to progressively train them to develop a "competing response practice" such as simply touching, squeezing, or tapping the itching area, or to develop other ways of moving their hands away from the itching area.[211] The technique has been described in two RCTs[207,208] conducted by the same team in Sweden and compared with topical corticosteroids. A further RCT evaluated the potential benefit of three psychological approaches versus dermatological education in the prevention of relapse in atopic eczema.[209]

In the first habit-reversal study,[207] 17 patients with atopic eczema aged 19–41 years were randomly assigned to two groups. The interventions consisted of hydrocortisone cream plus two sessions of habit-reversal treatment, received during week 1 (active-treatment group), or hydrocortisone cream alone (comparator group). The study was unblinded and of 28 days' duration. At the end of the assessment period, the mean reduction in the global eczema score was 67% in the active-treatment group, in comparison with 37% in the comparator group (P < 0.05). The total score for self-assessed annoyance was also markedly reduced in the active group in comparison with the other group. The mean percentage reduction of scratching episodes per day was 79% in the active-treatment group, in comparison with 49% in the comparator group (P < 0.01).

In the later study conducted by the same team,[208] 45 patients were randomly assigned to four groups for a period of 5 weeks. One group applied hydrocortisone cream for the entire 5-week period; another group applied betamethasone valerate (a strong topical steroid) for 3 weeks, followed by hydrocortisone for the remaining 2 weeks. Another group applied hydrocortisone plus habit-reversal for the 5-week period; and another group had betamethasone plus

habit-reversal for the first 3 weeks, followed by hydrocortisone plus habit-reversal for the remaining 2 weeks. The study was unblinded. Significant differences were reported between the behavioral-therapy groups and those taking steroids alone for total skin status. Scratching was reduced by 65% in the hydrocortisone-only group, 74% in the betamethasone followed by hydrocortisone group, 88% in the hydrocortisone plus habit-reversal group, and 90% in the betamethasone plus hydrocortisone plus habit-reversal group.

The study by Ehlers and colleagues in 1995 evaluated the use of an autogenic training program (ATP) as a form of relaxation therapy versus a cognitive-behavioral treatment (BT), versus a standard dermatological educational (DE) program versus combined DE and BT (DEBT).[209] A total of 113 secondary-care patients were randomly assigned to these four groups and were also compared with an additional standard medical treatment group who were not part of the random assignment. The investigators were blinded to the group allocation. The intervention was for 3 months, and the patients were followed up for 1 year. At the end of 1 year, the mean skin severity lesion score dropped from 29.5 to 28.8 in the DE group, from 33.7 to 19.8 in the ATP group, from 31.0 to 20.7 in the BT group, and from 35.4 to 25.8 in the DEBT group. There were no significant differences in the mean severity of itching between the four groups. The DEBT treatment led to significantly greater improvement in global skin severity than intensive education (DE) alone, and this was also accompanied by significant reductions in topical steroid use.

The study by Linnet and colleagues looked at a 6-month intervention of brief dynamic psychotherapy in patients with mild to severe atopic eczema, in comparison with waiting-list controls.[210] The nature of the intervention was poorly described, but it included areas such as illness perception and illness-related conflicts (e.g., disfigurement/body image issues, bodily sensations, feelings of rejection, anxiety, itch–scratch patterns, and depressive feelings). Sixteen participants were randomly assigned to each of the treatment groups, but only 23 participants were included in the analysis (there was no intention-to-treat analysis). No significant differences were found between the two groups, although post-hoc analysis suggested that those with high anxiety levels at the beginning of the study were more likely to benefit from the intervention, or to drop out of the study if they had been allocated to no intervention.

Drawbacks

In the study by Ehlers and colleagues,[209] the behavioral approaches required 12 weekly group sessions of 1.5–2 hours, each with five to seven patients. No adverse events were reported in any of the trials, although some of the drop-outs could possibly be related to the fact that extra visits were needed for the behavioral technique.

Comments

The study by Ehlers *et al.*[5] was clearly reported, and although no ITT analysis was performed, the drop-out rate was low (nine of 113 at 3 months). However, over 14 outcome measures were reported, which introduces the possibility of multiple hypothesis testing. The authors also performed statistical comparisons against a nonrandomized control group, which may not be justified. Nevertheless, the magnitude of improvement for those receiving behavioral techniques in addition to their standard dermatological care (which included topical corticosteroids) was moderately large, and carried more weight than the other two studies,[3,4] as the assessments were made by an investigator blinded to the treatment allocation.

Implications for clinical practice

The combination of habit reversal plus judicious use of topical corticosteroids seems an attractive one, and evidence from two RCTs supports its use. However, the lack of suitably qualified personnel may limit the ability to deliver this intervention in many settings. The role of psychotherapy in the treatment of atopic eczema has yet to be clarified.

Key points: psychological interventions

- Three RCTs suggested that psychological interventions such as habit-reversal techniques are a useful adjunct to dermatological treatment in atopic eczema.
- One RCT looked at brief dynamic psychotherapy, but the study was too small for firm conclusions to be drawn.
- Further studies are required to assess how these findings can be generalized to other settings and patient groups.

References: psychological interventions

205 Chida Y, Steptoe A, Hirakawa N, Sudo N, Kubo C. The effects of psychological intervention on atopic dermatitis. A systematic review and meta-analysis. *Int Arch Allergy Immunol* 2007;**144**:1–9.

206 Ersser SJ, Latter S, Sibley A, Satherley PA, Welbourne S. Psychological and educational interventions for atopic eczema in children. *Cochrane Database Syst Rev* 2007;(**3**):CD004054.

207 Melin L, Frederiksen T, Noren P, Swebilius BG. Behavioural treatment of scratching in patients with atopic dermatitis. *Br J Dermatol* 1986;**115**:467–74.

208 Noren P, Melin L. The effect of combined topical steroids and habit-reversal treatment in patients with atopic dermatitis. *Br J Dermatol* 1989;**121**:359–66.

209 Ehlers A, Stangier U, Gieler U. Treatment of atopic dermatitis: a comparison of psychological and dermatological approaches to relapse prevention. *J Consult Clin Psychol* 1995;**63**:624–35.

210 Linnet J, Psych C, Jemec G. Anxiety level and severity of skin condition predicts outcome of psychotherapy in atopic dermatitis patients. *Int J Dermatol* 2001;**40**:632–6.

211 Noren P. Habit reversal: a turning point in the treatment of atopic dermatitis. *Clin Exp Dermatol* 1995;**20**:2–5.

What is the role of patient education in controlling the symptoms of atopic eczema?

Efficacy

This section deals with patient education as delivered to patients and their families. It does not explicitly deal with studies examining the impact of changes to service delivery. The search found no systematic reviews, but one protocol for a Cochrane systematic review dealing with psychological and educational interventions for atopic eczema in children.[212]

A further eight RCTs are described below;[213–219] one study[220] was excluded, as it included participants with both eczema and psoriasis (and did not present data in a disaggregated form); one study was excluded because it only presented trial methodology and preliminary results.[221]

The trials can be roughly divided into those that deliver education to groups of patients/family and those that provide education on a one-to-one basis. Whilst the content of the training programs varied, information was generally covered relating to the nature of the disease; treatment options (including practical advice and treatment expectations); coping strategies/psychosocial support; and avoidance of allergens and irritants.

Group therapy. Staab *et al.*[213] randomly assigned 992 families of children aged 3 months to 18 years with moderate or severe atopic eczema. The participants received either six group education sessions or no intervention. The education package was multidisciplinary, involving dermatologists, pediatricians, psychologists, and dietitians. Each session lasted for approximately 2 hours. The primary outcome was change in disease severity (as measured by SCORAD) and change in quality of life at 12 months. Significant improvements in disease severity were observed for all age groups, and parental quality of life was significantly improved.

An earlier study by the same group randomly assigned 204 families of children with moderate to severe atopic eczema to a similar education program, in comparison a waiting-list control group.[214] Outcomes were assessed at baseline and 12 months. There were no significant differences between the two groups with regard to disease severity (SCORAD), but significant differences were observed in terms of treatment behavior (e.g., regular use of emollients, use of antiseptics for infected eczema, and a reduction in the use of unconventional medicine). Significant differences between the two groups were also observed with regard to treatment costs, quality of life, and coping strategies.

Coenraads *et al.*[215] provided a 2-week multidisciplinary training and treatment course in small groups (n = 31) in comparison with normal care (n = 20). The participants were aged 18–35 years, with moderate to severe atopic eczema, and outcomes were assessed at baseline, at 10 weeks, and at

9 months. The investigators reported significant improvements in eczema severity and self-care parameters; the participants needed less time for medical consultations and used emollients in a steroid-sparing way.

Niebel et al.[216] allocated patients to one of three groups: parental education (n = 18); standardized video education for parents, plus a handbook (n = 15); or standard eczema therapy and follow-up (n = 14). However, it is unclear how randomization was performed, and there were significant differences between the groups at baseline in terms of disease severity and maternal education. These differences were not adjusted for in the analysis. Significant improvements were seen for the education groups in comparison with the control group in relation to disease severity, sleep, itch, and quality of life, although multiple hypothesis testing meant that the implications of these findings were difficult to assess.

Grillo et al.[217] assessed the impact of a 2-hour workshop on eczema severity and quality of life. It is not entirely clear from the publication whether the intervention was delivered as individual or group therapy, but in either case, the workshop included both parents and their children with atopic eczema. A total of 61 children were randomly assigned to either an educational workshop (plus normal care), or normal care (followed by education upon completion of the trial). The workshops covered a range of topics and practical demonstrations. An ITT analysis showed significant differences between the two groups in eczema severity at 4 and 12 weeks. Improvements were also seen on the Children's Dermatology Life Quality Index (ages 5–16 years), but not on the Infants' Dermatitis Quality of Life Index or the Dermatitis Family Impact questionnaire.

Individualized therapy. Two studies reported educational therapy as delivered by a nurse. Chinn et al.[218] enrolled 235 children in a study comparing a 30-minute consultation with a trained dermatology nurse (working in primary care) with a "normal care" control group. Outcomes were assessed at 4 and 12 weeks post-intervention. The quality of life for the family was assessed using the Family Dermatology Index (FDI), and for the child using either the Infant's Dermatology Quality of Life (IDQOL) questionnaire or the Children's Dermatology Life Quality Index (CDLQI) questionnaire, depending on the child's age. This study failed to show any significant differences between the two groups with regard to improvement in the quality of life. This may have been due to the limited educational input given during the 30-minute session, or because the participants selected for recruitment were based in primary care and therefore had less severe disease than those seen in other studies.

Broberg et al.[219] evaluated the use of an "eczema school" for parents in an open study. The families of 50 consecutive children seen in an outpatient setting (aged 4 months to 6 years) were randomly assigned to receive either routine information from the treating physician, or to receive a visit with a trained dermatology nurse in addition to the physician visit. The 2-hour session with the nurse provided further information on eczema treatment and practical training in controlling eczema. Outcomes were assessed monthly for 3 months, and included eczema severity, itch, and quantity of topical steroid use. There was generally a trend towards improved outcomes for the group that had received the additional education sessions, but the results were poorly reported and are difficult to interpret. Improvements in disease severity were judged to be largely a result of better treatment compliance.

Kardoff et al.[220] randomly assigned 30 children aged 3–6 years, with moderate to severe atopic eczema, to either verbal instructions of the same duration as a standard consultation (control group) or a 10-minute demonstration with a Kardoff–Schnelle-Parker skin model (active group). This model is made of chamois leather and allows the children to experience for themselves the difference between well-moisturized and neglected skin. The sessions took place at baseline and again at 14 days. The main outcome (SCORAD) was assessed blindly at 0, 14, and 42 days. Children allocated to the active group showed significant improvements in their SCORAD scores at 42 days ($P <$ 0.006).

Drawbacks

No drawbacks were identified in any of the reported trials. Health professionals and participants were generally enthusiastic about the value of the education programs on offer. However, care should be taken to ensure that the quality of education provided in the education programs is based on the best evidence available at the time.

Comments

The methodological quality of the trials reported is varied. Most were not blinded (or the blinding could have been compromised), and only two reported an ITT analysis. Nevertheless, the two studies by Staab and colleagues were relatively well-powered and suggest some real patient benefit.[213,214] Several studies looked at long-term outcomes (up to 1 year), and this should be applauded. In the absence of a large cost-effectiveness study, it remains to be seen whether possible improvements in disease severity will result in a reduction in treatment costs.

Implications for practice

There is growing evidence that patients with atopic eczema, as with other chronic conditions, benefit from the provision of formal education relating to the condition and its treatment. It is possible that multidisciplinary training is most beneficial, but this can be expensive and time-consuming to provide.

The provision of group training sessions in a supportive environment may also deliver additional nonspecific benefits for the families.

Key points: patient education

- Seven randomized controlled trials have been reported that broadly support the role of education in the treatment of atopic eczema (although some lacked power to show an effect).
- Most trials included children or adults with moderate or severe disease.
- The evidence to support the use of multidisciplinary education packages in group therapy sessions is better than that for individualized therapy.
- Trials of individual therapy based on a single consultation with a health professional were less conclusive and require further investigation.
- Positive results have been observed up to 1 year following delivery of the education intervention.

References: patient education

212 Ersser S, Latter S, Surridge H, Buchanan P, Satherley P, Welbourne S. Psychological and educational interventions for atopic eczema in children. *Cochrane Database Syst Rev* 2003;(**1**):CD004054.

213 Staab D, Diepgen TL, Fartasch M, *et al.* Age related, structured educational programmes for the management of atopic dermatitis in children and adolescents: multicentre, randomised controlled trial. *BMJ* 2006;**332**:933–8.

214 Staab D, von Rueden U, Kehrt R, *et al.* Evaluation of a parental training program for the management of childhood atopic dermatitis. *Pediatr Allergy Immunol* 2002;**13**:84–90.

215 Coenraads PJ, Span L, Jaspers JP, Fidler V. [Intensive patient education and treatment program for young adults with atopic eczema; in German.] *Hautarzt* 2001;**52**:428–33.

216 Niebel G, Kallweit C, Lange I, Fölster-Holst R. [Direct versus video-aided parent education in atopic eczema in childhood as a supplement to specialty physician treatment. A controlled pilot study; in German.] *Hautarzt* 2000;**51**:401–11.

217 Grillo M, Gassner L, Marshman G, Dunn S, Hudson P. Pediatric atopic eczema: the impact of an educational intervention. *Pediatr Dermatol* 2006;**23**:428–36.

218 Chinn DJ, Poyner T, Sibley G. Randomized controlled trial of a single dermatology nurse consultation in primary care on the quality of life of children with atopic eczema. *Br J Dermatol* 2002; **146**:432–9.

219 Broberg A, Kalimo K, Lindblad B, Swanbeck G. Parental education in the treatment of childhood atopic eczema. *Acta Derm Venereol* 1990;**70**:495–9.

220 Kardoff B, Schelle-Parker G, Kardoff M, Wahlen M, Hönig d'Orville I, Dorittke P. [Successful reduction of the SCORAD score by a short-time teaching method using a simplified skin model in children with atopic eczema in a 6-week comparison; in German.] *J Dtsch Dermatol Ges* 2003;**1**:451–6.

221 Gradwell C, Thomas KS, English JSC, Williams HC. A randomized controlled trial of nurse follow-up clinics: do they help patients and do they free up consultants' time? *Br J Derm* 2002;**147**:513–7.

222 Diepgen TL, Fartasch M, Ring J, *et al.* [Education programs on atopic eczema. Design and first results of the German Randomized Intervention Multicenter Study; in German.] *Hautarzt* 2003;**54**:946–51.

Case scenario 2: How should infected atopic eczema be treated? (Figure 19.4)

Bacterial, viral, and fungal infections may be associated with atopic eczema. Infection needs to be promptly identified and treated. This section will focus on bacterial infection, which is the most common secondary infection.

The relationship between *Staphylococcus aureus* and atopic eczema disease activity has been debated for many years. Most physicians recognize clinically infected eczema as recent onset of weeping, oozing, and serous crusting or overt pus overlying the eczematous lesions. In this situation, *S. aureus* is isolated in 90–100% of cases, usually in high numbers.[223,224] In around 30% of cases, β-hemolytic streptococci are also isolated.[223] Clinical infection is undoubtedly a major problem for some atopic eczema sufferers.[225]

S. aureus is also isolated from the lesions of atopic eczema in 50–90% of patients without overt signs of infection.[226,227] Here, the role that *S. aureus* plays is much less clear. The idea that it may contribute to disease activity has led to the development of many antimicrobial compounds and their widespread use in the management of clinically noninfected atopic eczema. This section evaluates the possible benefit of these agents.

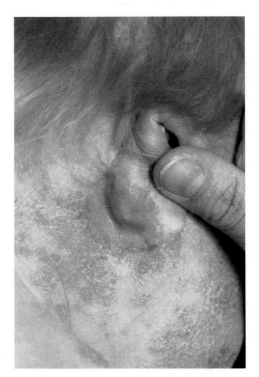

Figure 19.4 Infected atopic eczema.

One systematic review was located,[228] which was the source of much of the data in the last edition of the present book. This has been updated for this edition from searches carried out for a Cochrane systematic review of antistaphylococcal interventions in atopic eczema (in process).

A total of 11 RCTs evaluating the possible benefit of oral or topical antimicrobials in clinically infected atopic eczema were located and are summarized in Web Table 19.6. Additional RCTs evaluating the possible benefit of antiseptics in atopic eczema are presented in Web Table 19.7.

How useful are systemic antibiotics?

Efficacy
Two RCTs evaluating systemic antibiotics for clinically infected eczema were located.[224,229]

Versus placebo. Oral cefadroxil showed significant benefit over placebo for all clinical and microbiological outcomes.[224]

Versus each other. Erythromycin acetate and erythromycin stearate both improved clinical and microbiological outcomes. There was no significant difference between the preparations.[229]

For noninfected eczema. Two further important RCTs have compared systemic antibiotics with placebo in the treatment of nonclinically infected atopic eczema. In the first,[230] oral flucloxacillin 250 mg four times daily for 4 weeks showed no benefit over placebo in terms of clinical efficacy, despite significantly reducing *S. aureus* counts. The second study[231] showed a similar absence of benefit for 2 weeks' oral cefuroxime. Rapid recolonization occurred in both groups after cessation of treatment.

Possible drawbacks
Gastrointestinal side effects occurred in 50% of patients in each group taking erythromycin, one patient on cefuroxime, and 6.5% of patients on cephalexin. Emergence of methicillin-resistant *S. aureus*, which persisted for 2 weeks after completion of treatment, was noted in the flucloxacillin study.

Comments and clinical implications
The quality of reporting in studies was generally poor, with small numbers of patients and a lack of detail regarding concurrent treatments and clinical outcomes. It is common practice to prescribe a short course of oral antibiotics in acute infected eczema. There is some evidence that this improves clinical signs of infection, and there is no evidence of a detrimental effect. In contrast, there is no evidence to support the use of longer-term antibiotics in people with atopic eczema whose skin is colonized with *S. aureus*, and

there is some evidence that use of such antibiotics may promote antibiotic resistance.

Do topical steroids help in clinically infected atopic eczema?

Efficacy
We found no RCTs that addressed this question in clinically infected atopic eczema.

Noninfected eczema. We located three RCTs that have demonstrated the effectiveness of topical steroids in reducing *S. aureus* in clinically noninfected atopic eczema. In the study by Stalder *et al.*,[232] topical desonide was significantly better than its excipient alone in reducing *S. aureus* and the global clinical score. In the second study, group A compared a moderate-strength steroid with an alternative similar steroid in a propylene glycol (antiseptic) base; group B compared a potent steroid alone with potent steroid plus neomycin. In both groups, the addition of the antimicrobial did not improve the clinical outcome.[233] In the third study, 1% hydrocortisone was as effective as 1% hydrocortisone/ 2% fusidic acid in terms of clinical outcome, although the combination treatment was more effective at reducing *S. aureus*.[234]

Possible drawbacks
Minor skin irritation or flare of eczema occurred in 1% of patients.

Comments and implications
No studies have evaluated the efficacy of topical steroids alone for clinically infected atopic eczema. There is evidence that topical steroids alone are effective in reducing bacterial counts in clinically noninfected eczema.

How effective are topical antibiotics in clinically infected atopic eczema?

Efficacy
One RCT has evaluated topical antibiotics in the treatment of clinically infected atopic eczema (Web Table 19.6).

Gentamicin cream was significantly less effective at reducing dermatitis activity than betamethasone valerate/ gentamicin or betamethasone alone.[235]

Noninfected eczema. Three RCTs have looked at topical antibiotics in people with clinically noninfected atopic eczema. In the first, which compared mupirocin ointment with placebo ointment (both with concurrent steroid), mupirocin (but not placebo) significantly reduced *S. aureus* in comparison with baseline, and clinical scores were significantly better in the mupirocin group than the placebo group. However, recolonization occurred during the 4-week follow-up period.[236] Schempp *et al.* compared 1% hyperformin cream with placebo in a half-side comparison study, and showed a significantly greater reduction in modified SCORAD on the treatment side. However, the study only included 18 patients, and there were no significant differences in skin colonization between the groups at the end of treatment, so that it is not possible to draw meaningful conclusions from this study.[237] Ramsay *et al.*[234] showed that fusidic acid 2% cream resulted in more treatment failures than hydrocortisone/fusidic acid.

Possible drawbacks

Minor skin irritation or eczema flare occurred in 18% of patients in the fusidic acid group, in comparison with only 3% in the steroid/fusidic acid group.[234]

Comments and implications

These studies are in keeping with current clinical practice, which recognizes the need for topical steroids in addition to antibiotics in the treatment of clinically infected eczema. There is concern about the emergence of resistant organisms resulting from the use of topical antibiotics.

What is the role of topical steroid/antibiotic combinations?

Efficacy

We found six RCTs evaluating topical steroid/antibiotic combinations for clinically infected atopic eczema (Web Table 19.6). We also located several other studies, which have not been included because the results for atopic eczema could not been separated from other dermatoses.

Versus vehicle. The study by Thaci *et al.*[238] showed superior benefit of both betamethasone/fusidic acid ointment and cream over vehicle alone, with no significant difference between cream and ointment.

Versus topical steroid. Two RCTs found no significant difference in clinical signs or symptoms when betamethasone valerate/fusidic acid[239] or betamethasone/gentamicin[235] were compared with topical steroid alone.

Leyden and Kligman found greater clinical improvement and greater reduction in *S. aureus* with 0.5% neomycin/0.025% fluocinolone than with 0.025% fluocinolone alone.[240]

Most recently, Gong *et al.* compared mupirocin plus hydrocortisone butyrate with vehicle plus hydrocortisone butyrate in a mixed group including 119 patients with atopic dermatitis, infected and noninfected. There was no difference in the global severity scores (Eczema Area and Severity Index, EASI) between the groups at days 7, 14, or 28.[241]

Versus each other. There were no significant differences between 0.1% betamethasone/2% fusidic acid and 0.1%

betamethasone/0.5% neomycin in terms of clinical efficacy or ability to eradicate *S. aureus*.[242]

Noninfected eczema. Four further RCTs were located that have evaluated topical steroid/antibiotic treatment for non-clinically infected atopic eczema.

In the first study, clobetasol propionate 0.05% cream was as effective as betamethasone valerate 0.1% cream in combination with neomycin at reducing *S. aureus* and clearing moderate to severe atopic eczema.[233]

In the second study, 2% fusidic acid/1% hydrocortisone showed no clear benefit over 1% hydrocortisone alone in reducing atopic eczema activity, but it was significantly better at reducing *S. aureus*.[234]

In the third study, four ointments were applied sequentially in random order to each patient: petrolatum base, 1% hydrocortisone in petrolatum, 0.5% prednisolone in petrolatum, and 0.5% prednisolone/0.5% neomycin in petrolatum. The steroid/antibiotic combination of 0.5% prednisolone/0.5% neomycin in petrolatum was more effective at clearing eczema than each of the other treatments.[243]

The fourth study compared 2% fusidic acid/0.1% betamethasone cream with 2% mupirocin ointment plus 0.1% betamethasone cream. There were no differences in clinical improvement or *S. aureus* reduction between the groups.[244]

Possible drawbacks

Minor skin irritation, flare of dermatitis, and possible hypersensitivity reactions occurred in 1–3% of patients across the groups. Despite concerns about the emergence of resistant organisms resulting from the use of topical antibiotics, this was not recorded in any of the studies.

Comments and implications

There is evidence that topical steroid/antibiotic combinations are effective in the treatment of clinically infected atopic eczema. There are conflicting results and there is a lack of good studies to determine whether these combinations are more effective than topical steroid alone in clinically non-infected eczema.

Studies that compared different antibiotic/steroid combinations showed no difference between fusidic acid and neomycin, on the one hand, and fusidic acid and mupirocin on the other, in terms of efficacy.

In noninfected eczema, there is a lack of evidence to show additional benefit of topical antibiotic/steroid combinations over topical steroid alone.

The risk of hypersensitivity and bacterial resistance must be taken into account when topical antibiotic/steroid combinations are used.

The evidence is in keeping with current recommendations that topical steroid/antibiotic combinations should only be used for infected eczema, and for a maximum of 2 weeks at a time.

How useful are topical steroid/antiseptic combinations?

Efficacy

We found two RCTs that evaluated topical steroid/antiseptic combinations in the treatment of clinically infected atopic eczema. In the study by Zienicke, a topical steroid/antiseptic was compared with topical steroid alone; 0.25% prednicarbate/didecyldimethyl ammonium chloride cream and 0.25% prednicarbate cream were both effective at reducing clinical scores and bacterial counts, with no significant differences between them.[23]

In the second study, by Meenan, Tri-Adcortyl cream (steroid/antibiotic/antifungal) and Locoid C (steroid/antiseptic) were equally effective.[24]

Possible drawbacks

Minor skin irritation was reported in one patient.

Comments and implications

There is no evidence to support a benefit from topical steroid/antiseptic combinations over topical steroid alone.

How effective are topical antifungals?

Efficacy

One RCT evaluated a combination of topical steroid/antibiotic/antifungal (Tri-Adcortyl cream) versus topical steroid/antiseptic (Locoid C) in clinically infected atopic eczema (Web Table 19.6).[246] Both combinations produced a highly significant reduction in clinical scores and bacterial counts, with no significant differences between the treatments.

Noninfected eczema. We located two further RCTs evaluating topical antifungals in nonclinically infected atopic eczema.[247,248] The first small study compared topical steroid/antibiotic/antifungal against topical steroid/antibiotic, and showed a significant improvement in the four patients treated with 0.1% triamcinolone acetonide/0.35% neomycin/undecylenic acid, in comparison with the six receiving the same steroid/antibiotic combination but without undecylenic acid.[247] In the second study, Broberg and Faergemann[248] attempted to evaluate the role of antifungals in atopic eczema of the head and neck area. All patients received oral antibiotics, followed by random assignment to either miconazole–hydrocortisone cream plus ketoconazole shampoo or hydrocortisone cream plus placebo shampoo. There were no significant differences between the groups with regard to the clinical outcome.

Possible drawbacks

When side effects were documented, minor skin irritation and possible hypersensitivity reactions were seen in up to 5% of patients across the groups.

Comments and implications

It is difficult to draw conclusions about the role of antifungals from these small and disparate studies. There is no current evidence to support the routine use of antifungals in the treatment of clinically infected atopic eczema.

How useful are antiseptic agents in clinically infected atopic eczema?

This section includes antiseptic emollients, bath additives, and other antiseptic treatments.

Efficacy

There are no RCTs of antiseptics in clinically infected atopic eczema. We located six RCTs of antiseptics in nonclinically infected eczema,[249–254] summarized in Web Table 19.7.

Antiseptic versus standard bath emollient. Two RCTs have compared a standard bath emollient, Oilatum (acetylated wool alcohols 5%, liquid paraffin 63.4%) with an emollient plus antiseptic, Oilatum Plus (benzalkonium chloride 6%, triclosan 2%, light liquid paraffin 52.5%). No significant differences were demonstrated in terms of clinical or microbiological outcomes.[249,250]

Antiseptic soap versus placebo soap. This study compared a soap containing 1.5% triclocarban with an identical placebo soap. The authors state that the global change in atopic eczema severity was significantly greater in the treatment than the placebo group, but the actual data are missing. Graphic data suggest a similar degree of improvement in both groups.[251]

Topical antiseptic versus no topical antiseptic. Two RCTs were identified. The first study reported improvement on the arm treated with daily povidone iodine solution, but not on the untreated side, in comparison with baseline.[252] In the second study, acid electrolytic water sprayed onto infants significantly reduced clinical scores and *S. aureus* counts in comparison with baseline.[253] Neither study reported a comparison of treatments.

Comparison of two topical antiseptics. This study compared a proprietary brand of chlorhexidine with a 1 : 20 000 dilution of potassium permanganate, in addition to topical steroid in both groups, and found no significant differences in the clinical or bacteriological outcomes.[254]

Drawbacks

Skin irritation, pruritus, and worsening of dermatitis were the main side effects reported in the studies in which adverse events were documented. These were reported more frequently overall in the antiseptic-treated groups.

Comments and clinical implications

Antiseptic-containing preparations are in common use in the management of atopic eczema. There are no RCTs of many of the commonly used preparations. The current evidence base for the use of such preparations in infected or clinically noninfected atopic eczema does not provide any clear support for their use. Further large studies with appropriate comparators are required in order to assess the role of antiseptics in preventing secondary infection.

References: case scenario 2

223 Hauser C, Wuethrich B, Matter L, *et al. Staphylococcus aureus* skin colonisation in atopic dermatitis patients. *Dermatologica* 1985; **170**:35–9.

224 Weinberg E, Fourie B, Allmann B, Toerien A. The use of cefadroxil in superinfected atopic dermatitis. *Curr Ther Res Clin Exp* 1992;**52**:671–6.

225 David TJ, Cambridge GC. Bacterial infection and atopic eczema. *Arch Dis Child* 1986;**61**:20–3.

226 Leyden JE, Marples RR, Kligman AM. *Staphylococcus aureus* in the lesions of atopic dermatitis. *Br J Dermatol* 1974;**90**:525–30.

227 Goh CL, Wong JS, Yoke CG. Skin colonisation of *Staphylococcus aureus* in atopic dermatitis patients seen at the National Skin Centre, Singapore. *Int J Dermatol* 1997;**36**:653–7.

228 Hoare C, Li Wan Po A, Williams H. Systematic review of treatments for atopic eczema. *Health Technol Assess* 2000;**4**(37).

229 Salo OP, Gordin A, Brandt H, Antikainen R. Efficacy and tolerability of erythromycin acistrate and erythromycin stearate in acute skin infections of patients with atopic eczema. *J Antimicrob Chemother* 1988;**21**(Suppl D):D101–6.

230 Ewing CI, Ashcroft C, Gibbs AC, Jones GA, Connor PJ, David TJ. Flucloxacillin in the treatment of atopic dermatitis. *Br J Dermatol* 1998;**138**:1022–9.

231 Boguniewicz M, Sampson H, Leung S, Harbeck R, Leung DYM. Effects of cefuroxime axetil on *Staphylococcus aureus* colonisation and superantigen production in atopic dermatitis. *J All Clin Immunol* 2001;**108**:651–2.

232 Stalder JF, Fleury M, Sourisse M, *et al.* Local steroid therapy and bacterial skin flora in atopic dermatitis. *Br J Dermatol* 1994;**131**:536–40.

233 Nilsson EJ, Henning CG, Magnusson J. Topical corticosteroids and *Staphylococcus aureus* in atopic dermatitis. *J Am Acad Dermatol* 1992;**27**:29–34.

234 Ramsay CA, Savoie JM, Gilbert M, Gidon M, Kidson P. The treatment of atopic dermatitis with topical fusidic acid and hydrocortisone acetate. *J Eur Acad Dermatol Venereol* 1996;**7**(Suppl I):S15–22.

235 Wachs GN, Maibach HI. Co-operative double-blind trial of an antibiotic/corticoid combination in impetiginized atopic dermatitis. *Br J Dermatol* 1976;**95**:323–8.

236 Lever R, Hadley K, Downey D, Mackie R. Staphylococcal colonization in atopic dermatitis and the effect of topical mupirocin therapy. *Br J Dermatol* 1988;**119**:189–98.

237 Schempp CM, Hezel S, Simon JC. [Topical treatment of atopic dermatitis with *Hypericum* cream. A randomized, placebo-controlled, double-blind half-side comparison study; in German.] *Hautarzt* 2003;**54**:248–53.

238 Thaci D, Kokorsch J, Kaufmann R. Fusidic acid/betamethasone 17-valerate in potentially infected atopic dermatitis. *J Eur Acad Dermatol Venereol* 1999;**12**(Suppl 2):S163.

239 Hjorth N, Schmidt H, Thomsen K. Fusidic acid plus betamethasone in infected or potentially infected eczema. *Pharmatherapeutica* 1985;**4**:126–31.

240 Leyden JJ, Kligman AM. The case for steroid-antibiotic combinations. *Br J Dermatol* 1977;**96**:179–87.

241 Gong JQ, Lin L, Lin T, *et al.* Skin colonization by *Staphylococcus aureus* in patients with eczema and atopic dermatitis and relevant combined topical therapy: a double-blind multicentre randomized controlled trial. *Br J Dermatol* 2006;**155**:680–7.

242 Wilkinson RD, Leigh DA. Comparative efficacy of betamethasone and either fusidic acid or neomycin in infected or potentially infected eczema. *Curr Ther Res* 1985;**38**:177–82.

243 Polano MK, De Vries HR. Analysis of the results obtained in the treatment of atopic dermatitis with corticosteroid and neomycin containing ointments. *Dermatologica* 1960;**120**:191–9.

244 Ravenscroft JC, Layton AM, Eady EA, *et al.* Short term effects of topical fusidic acid or mupirocin on the prevalence of fusidic acid resistant (FusR) *Staphylococcus aureus* in atopic eczema. *Br J Dermatol* 2003;**148**:1010–7.

245 Zienicke H. Topical glucocorticoids and anti-infectives: a rational combination? *Curr Probl Dermatol* 1993;**21**:186–91.

246 Meenan FO. A double-blind comparative study to compare the efficacy of Locoid C with Tri-Adcortyl in children with infected eczema. *Br J Clin Pract* 1988;**42**:200–2.

247 [Anon.] Treatment of eczemas and infected eczemas. *Br J Clin Pract* 1967;**21**:505–7.

248 Broberg A, Faergemann J. Topical antimycotic treatment of atopic dermatitis in the head/neck area. A double-blind randomised study. *Acta Derm Venereol* 1995;**75**:46–9.

249 Harper J. Double-blind comparison of an antiseptic oil-based bath additive (Oilatum Plus) with regular Oilatum (Oilatum Emollient) for the treatment of atopic eczema. In: Lever R, Levy J, eds. *The Bacteriology of Eczema.* London: Royal Society of Medicine Press, 1995: 42–7.

250 Holland KT, Bojar RA, Cunliffe WJ. A comparison of the effect of treatment of atopic eczema with and without antimicrobial compounds. In: Lever R, Levy J, eds. *The Bacteriology of Eczema.* London: Royal Society of Medicine Press, 1995: 1–5.

251 Breneman DL, Hanifin JM, Berge CA, Keswick BH, Neumann PB. The effect of antibacterial soap with 1.5% triclocarban on *Staphylococcus aureus* in patients with atopic dermatitis. *Cutis* 2000;**66**:296–300.

252 Hizawa T, Sano H, Endo K, Fukuzumi T, Kataoka Y, Aoki T. Is povidone-iodine effective to the lesions of atopic dermatitis? *Skin Res* 1998;**40**(Suppl 20):134–9.

253 Sasai-Takedatsu M, Kojima T, Yamamoto A, *et al.* Reduction of *Staphylococcus aureus* in atopic skin lesions with acid electrolytic water—a new therapeutic strategy for atopic dermatitis. *Allergy* 1997;**52**:1012–6.

254 Stalder JF, Fleury M, Sourisse M, *et al.* Comparative effects of two topical antiseptics (chlorhexidine vs KMn04) on bacterial skin flora in atopic dermatitis. *Acta Derm Venereol Suppl (Stockh)* 1992;**176**:132–4.

Case scenario 3: an adult with severe atopic eczema (Figure 19.5)

What is the role of systemic immunosuppressive therapy?

The systematic review by Hoare *et al.* published in 2000 described several older and experimental immunomodulatory therapies for atopic eczema, including platelet activating factor, immunoglobulins, interferon gamma, and levamisole.[255] Some showed promising results in small studies, but they were not developed further or tested in larger trials. This section concentrates on systemic immunosuppressive agents that are commonly used in dermatology, such as ciclosporin, systemic steroids, azathioprine, and methotrexate, as well as phototherapy and photochemotherapy. A further systematic review of systemic treatments for atopic eczema based on 27 studies including 979 participants was published in 2007.[256]

Efficacy

Systemic steroids. Systemic prednisolone is commonly used in short bursts (a few weeks) in order to get severe atopic eczema into remission. Three randomized controlled trials have suggested that the short-term effect of oral steroids is large in comparison with placebo (Web Table 19.8).[257–259] Relapse rates were not reported in these studies. Oral steroids have not been evaluated for more than 4 weeks in atopic eczema—for example, using them with a high initial

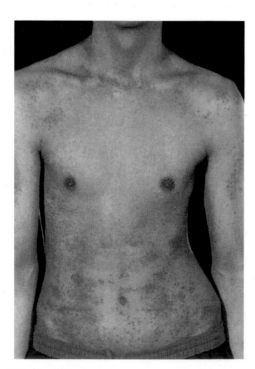

Figure 19.5 Severe atopic eczema.

dose to induce remission, followed by a reducing dose to maintain remission until topical treatments are able to control the disease again. Oral steroids have not been compared with other active immunosuppressive treatments.

Ciclosporin. The systematic review by Schmitt and colleagues identified 11 studies evaluating the efficacy of ciclosporin in atopic eczema,[256] although another systematic review published around the same time by the same team identified another four studies.[260] Of the 15 studies in the review, which included 602 participants, eight were RCTs (two dose-finding, three double-blind parallel studies, and three crossover studies). Only one trial used an active control—a trial of 30 participants that compared oral ciclosporin against topical tacrolimus, which was inconclusive and confounded by topical corticosteroid use.[261] The general quality of the reporting was poor, except in two studies. The review showed some evidence of publication bias—i.e., larger treatment effects in smaller studies—and the authors suggested caution in interpreting the summary results.[260] The systematic review considered that 12 of the studies were sufficiently similar to allow quantitative pooling of data, and found a clear dose–response effect. At 2 weeks, the overall mean decrease in disease severity was 22% (95% CI, 8% to 36%) at a dose of 3 mg/kg and 40% (95% CI, 29% to 51%) for doses of 4 mg/kg and above. After 6–8 weeks of therapy, the mean pooled decrease in severity was 55% (95% CI, 48% to 62%). Effectiveness appeared to be similar in children and adults, although tolerability might be better in children.

Azathioprine. One crossover RCT of azathioprine (2.5 mg/kg) versus placebo in 37 adults with severe atopic eczema was reported by Berth-Jones *et al.* in 2002.[262] After 3 months' treatment, those receiving azathioprine had a 26% reduction in disease severity, in comparison with 3% of those on placebo, in an intention-to-treat analysis.

Oral pimecrolimus. One RCT examined the use of three different doses of oral pimecrolimus versus placebo in 103 patients with moderate to severe atopic eczema, and found good treatment responses (67% at 7 weeks for the 30-mg twice-daily group) and no signs of nephrotoxicity or hypertension.[263]

Methotrexate, mycophenolate, and infliximab. One prospective, open-label study suggested that oral methotrexate is well tolerated and is associated with a sustained reduction in disease activity (55% at 24 weeks) in severe atopic eczema, and suggested that a randomized controlled trial is now warranted.[264] The systematic review of systemic therapies describes two uncontrolled studies of mycophenolate mofetil in 20 patients with severe eczema, with a mean decrease in disease activity of 55% and 68% at 8 and

12 weeks, respectively.[256] The authors also reported another small uncontrolled study of infliximab (5 mg/kg) infusions in nine patients, and found that only two patients experienced greater than 50% improvement at 10 weeks.[256] Such uncontrolled studies are difficult to interpret, due to assessment bias and regression to the mean, especially when patients with severe disease are recruited.

Phototherapy and photochemotherapy. A total of 11 RCTs were identified, and these are summarized in detail in Web Table 19.9. All but four[265–268] were described in the systematic review by Hoare *et al.*[255] The quality of reporting in most of the studies was poor. Most studies were underpowered to exclude clinically important differences between different forms of ultraviolet light, with overlapping confidence intervals between the effect estimates of the different groups. It is also unclear to what extent systemic effects may obscure comparisons of two different types of ultraviolet light used in the same individual—i.e., designs that irradiate one half of the body with one type of light and the other half with another type of irradiating light.[269] Broadly speaking, light therapy appears to be very effective in comparison with placebo (using ordinary fluorescent light) for atopic eczema, although it should be noted that tanning compromises blinding in such placebo studies. For acute eczema, ultraviolet A1 (UVA1) appears to be fast and effective, and there does not seem to be a clear advantage to using a high as opposed to a medium dose. In chronic eczema, ultraviolet B (UVB) may be more effective, especially for narrowband UVB.

A further interesting Norwegian study indirectly assessed the role of ultraviolet light by randomly assigning 30 children to a holiday in the semitropical Canary Islands and 27 at home in cooler Norway.[270] Not surprisingly, the children randomly assigned to the Canary Islands improved more in terms of reduction in eczema scores and quality of life during the holiday, and such an effect was sustained for 3 months after the intervention. It is difficult to separate the effect of ultraviolet light from temperature or sea-water effects, as well as other differences such as diet and psychological effects, between the holiday locations. Nevertheless, the study suggests that a sunny holiday may have a sustained benefit on children with chronic eczema.

Drawbacks

All of the immunosuppressants currently available carry potentially serious side effects such as kidney damage (ciclosporin), bone-marrow suppression (azathioprine), osteoporosis (systemic steroids), and skin cancer (photochemotherapy).[255,256] Long-term effects of oral prednisolone are well known and include hypertension, weight gain, osteoporoses, fat redistribution, diabetes, and acne, although the frequency of such complications when the treatments are used for a few weeks or months to gain control in severe atopic eczema is unknown.[255] The systematic review of ciclosporin found that adverse effects such as gastrointestinal upset occurred in around 40% of patient-months described in 15 studies.[260] An increase in baseline serum creatinine over 30% was found in 115 of patients, hypertension in 6%, and infections in 12% of patients. Treatment appeared to be better tolerated in children, although this may be partly due to larger doses being used in adults. For azathioprine, bone-marrow toxicity may be minimized by assessing blood thiomethylpurine transferase activity beforehand, although the test may not be widely available. In the RCT of azathioprine, 16 of the 37 participants withdrew (12 when on azathioprine and two on placebo), 14 developed gastrointestinal disturbance, two developed leukopenia, and eight had abnormal liver function tests.[262]

Although the one RCT of oral pimecrolimus did not reveal any serious adverse effects,[263] concerns associated with carcinogenicity in animals have prevented this form of therapy from becoming more widely available.[271] More data are needed on methotrexate, mycophenolate, and infliximab in atopic eczema, as the numbers treated so far with these agents are far too small for it to be claimed that they are safe in either the short term or long term.

The short-term drawbacks of ultraviolet therapy include burning and itching, and they can usually be overcome by light testing before therapy and the use of emollients after treatment. Some people find ultraviolet cabinets claustrophobic, and some very young children find the experience frightening. The long-term effects of giving ultraviolet light to young children with atopic eczema in terms of melanoma and nonmelanoma skin cancer is unknown,[255] and caution should be taken when extrapolating guidance based on adults receiving photochemotherapy for psoriasis, especially since susceptibility to melanoma may be enhanced in childhood.

Clinical implications

Both ultraviolet light and systemic treatments such as short courses of oral steroids and ciclosporin are probably useful and safe in the person depicted in the case scenario. The choice of treatment would be largely determined by the person's preferences and local availability of treatment. Safety is a factor limiting the long-term use of all of these agents. Planned short-term use (2–3 months) to try to obtain a remission or give the person a "holiday" from severe symptoms seems a reasonable option, resorting to topical treatments such as intermittent use of potent topical steroids or tacrolimus once control is achieved. It is unclear at this stage whether different genetic subtypes of atopic eczema (e.g., those with a major barrier defect as determined by mutations in the filaggrin gene[272]) respond differently to different systemic treatments. Future trials should consider measuring such genetic markers as possible predictors of treatment response in their study participants.

Key points: systemic immunosuppressive therapy

- There is reasonable RCT evidence to support the use of some systemic immunosuppressive therapies such as oral corticosteroids and ciclosporin.

- Both of these therapies are associated with significant side effects, which limit their use for short-term to medium-term periods during major disease flares, with a return to conventional topical treatment once control is maintained.

- One trial has shown that oral azathioprine is beneficial in patients with eczema, in comparison with placebo, but the effects were not large and side effects were common.

- One trial has shown that oral pimecrolimus was beneficial in moderate to severe atopic eczema, but oral pimecrolimus is not licensed because of concerns about the possible long-term development of lymphomas.

- No randomized controlled studies have yet been conducted on methotrexate, mycophenolate, or biological therapies in patients with atopic eczema.

- Phototherapy (e.g., UVA1 for acute eczema and narrowband UVB for chronic eczema) has consistently been shown to be beneficial in atopic dermatitis, but it is limited by the long-term risk of skin cancer after many treatments.

- There is an urgent need for studies that compare systemic therapies against each other rather than against placebo for people with severe atopic eczema, using oral ciclosporin or oral prednisolone as the standard active comparator.

- There is a need for longer-term studies of systemic immunosuppressive treatment for atopic eczema, in order to evaluate long-term safety and whether the use of these agents alters the natural history of the disease.

References: case scenario 3

255 Hoare C, Li Wan Po A, Williams H. Systematic review of treatments for atopic eczema. *Health Technol Assess* 2000;**4**(37).

256 Schmitt J, Schmitt N, Meurer M. Cyclosporin in the treatment of patients with atopic eczema—a systematic review and meta-analysis. *J Eur Acad Dermatol Venereol* 2007;**21**:606–19.

257 Dickey RF. Parenteral short-term corticosteroid therapy in moderate to severe dermatoses. A comparative multiclinic study. *Cutis* 1976;**17**:179–83.

258 Heddle RJ, Soothill JF, Bulpitt CJ, Atherton DJ. Combined oral and nasal beclomethasone dipropionate in children with atopic eczema: a randomised controlled trial. *BMJ Clin Res Ed* 1984;**289**:651–4.

259 La Rosa M, Musarra I, Ranno C, *et al.* A randomized, double-blind, placebo-controlled crossover trial of systemic flunisolide in the treatment of children with severe atopic dermatitis. *Curr Ther Res Clin Exp* 1995;**56**:720–6.

260 Schmitt J, Schakel K, Schmitt N, Meurer M. Systemic treatment of severe atopic eczema: a systematic review. *Acta Derm Venereol* 2007;**87**:100–11.

261 Pacor ML, Di Lorenzo G, Martinelli N, *et al.* Comparing tacrolimus ointment and oral cyclosporine in adult patients affected by atopic dermatitis: a randomized study. *Clin Exp Allergy* 2004;**34**:639–45.

262 Berth-Jones J, Takwale A, Tan E, *et al.* Azathioprine in severe adult atopic dermatitis: a double-blind, placebo-controlled, crossover trial. *Br J Dermatol* 2002;**147**:324–30.

263 Wolff K, Fleming C, Hanifin J, *et al.* Efficacy and tolerability of three different doses of oral pimecrolimus in the treatment of moderate to severe atopic dermatitis: a randomized controlled trial. *Br J Dermatol* 2005;**152**:1296–303.

264 Weatherhead SC, Wahie S, Reynolds NJ, Meggitt SJ. An open-label, dose-ranging study of methotrexate for moderate-to-severe adult atopic eczema. *Br J Dermatol* 2007;**156**:346–51.

265 Reynolds NJ, Franklin V, Gray JC, Diffey BL, Farr PM. Narrow-band ultraviolet B and broad-band ultraviolet A phototherapy in adult atopic eczema: a randomised controlled trial. *Lancet* 2001;**357**:2012–6.

266 Von Kobyletzki G, Pieck C, Hoffmann K, Freitag M, Altmeyer P. Medium-dose UVA1 cold-light phototherapy in the treatment of severe atopic dermatitis. *J Am Acad Dermatol* 1999;**41**:931–7.

267 Tzaneva S, Seeber A, Schwaiger M, Honigsmann H, Tanew A. High-dose versus medium-dose UVA1 phototherapy for patients with severe generalized atopic dermatitis. *J Am Acad Dermatol* 2001;**45**:503–7.

268 Legat FJ, Hofer A, Brabek E, Quehenberger F, Kerl H, Wolf P. Narrowband UV-B vs medium-dose UV-A1 phototherapy in chronic atopic dermatitis. *Arch Dermatol* 2003;**139**:223–4.

269 Yule S, Dawe RS, Cameron H, Ferguson J, Ibbotson SH. Does narrow-band ultraviolet B phototherapy work in atopic dermatitis through a local or a systemic effect? *Photodermatol Photoimmunol Photomed* 2005;**21**:333–5.

270 Byremo G, Rod G, Carlsen KH. Effect of climatic change in children with atopic eczema. *Allergy* 2006;**61**:1403–10.

271 Arellano FM, Wentworth CE, Arana A, Fernandez C, Paul CF. Risk of lymphoma following exposure to calcineurin inhibitors and topical steroids in patients with atopic dermatitis. *J Invest Dermatol* 2007;**127**:808–16.

272 Sandilands A, Smith FJ, Irvine AD, McLean WH. Filaggrin's fuller figure: a glimpse into the genetic architecture of atopic dermatitis. *J Invest Dermatol* 2007;**127**:1282–4.

General summary observations on the evidence base for atopic eczema

- Although around 400 RCTs have been conducted for atopic eczema, their ability to inform us about the everyday management of patients is limited.

- Many people with atopic eczema are treated in the community, yet community-based trials are very rare in this field.

- Most of the trials of people with atopic eczema have reflected the agenda of the drug industry.

- New drugs have often been only compared against placebo in trials, rather than being compared against existing active treatments, which makes it difficult for clinicians and patients to decide which is best. Independent trials are needed in order to make head-to-head comparisons.

- Some of the limitations of the atopic eczema evidence base are due to a generally poor quality of study reporting.

All dermatology journals have a role to play by insisting on the basic standard of clinical trial reporting, as outlined in the Consolidated Standards of Reporting Trials (CONSORT) statement (http://www.consort-statement.org).

• Outcome measures used in atopic eczema trials are a bit of a mess, characterized by a profusion of poorly developed and unvalidated scales, making comparisons across studies difficult. Investigators should stick to using just one scale common to all studies, such as SCORAD. Quality of life also needs to be reported in all studies.

• Some interventions (for example, topical steroids and topical calcineurin inhibitors) are well supported by RCT evidence.

• For other interventions (such as Chinese herbs and house dust mite reduction), there is simply insufficient evidence to decide whether they are effective; better research is needed.

• In some areas (for example, topical steroid/antibiotic combinations or bath antiseptics), the RCT evidence does not support a clinically useful effect—providing dermatologists and patients with an opportunity to disinvest in such treatments.

• In most people with mild to moderate atopic eczema, the condition can be easily controlled with a combination of emollients and topical corticosteroids for inflammatory flares.

• Cheap and well-tried systemic agents such as oral steroids and azathioprine need to be compared against each other and against the more expensive agents such as ciclosporin that have found their way onto the market through mainly placebo-controlled studies.

• There is still a need for a safe and effective treatment for severe atopic eczema.

• Trials exploring disease prevention need to be conducted for atopic eczema.

• Larger studies need to be conducted in order to explore subgroup differences for different subtypes of eczema—e.g., patients who are atopic, those with associated asthma, and those with filaggrin gene mutations.

Acknowledgments

Hywel Williams was responsible for writing the background section and the evidence summaries on tacrolimus and pimecrolimus, as well as case scenario 3 summarizing systemic treatments, and for editing the other contributions in this chapter. Kim Thomas wrote the sections on emollients and nonpharmacological treatments, and Jane Ravenscroft wrote the section on infected eczema. Carolyn Charman wrote the section on topical steroids, and Fiona Bath-Hextall wrote the section on dietary interventions, antihistamines, and probiotics. Literature searches of the Cochrane Controlled Trials register and Medline were conducted up to April 2007.

20 Seborrheic dermatitis

Mauro Picardo, Norma Cameli

Background

Definition

Seborrheic dermatitis is a chronic inflammatory skin disease characterized by erythematous and scaling plaques, with a distinctive distribution in areas rich in sebaceous glands, such as the scalp, eyebrows, nasolabial folds, retro-auricular regions, sternum, and between the shoulder blades (Figure 20.1).[1]

The relationship between seborrheic dermatitis of the scalp and "dandruff" is unclear; some authors suggest that dandruff is a more generic term that refers to scalp flaking, regardless of etiology.[2] Pruritus of the scalp is often associated with the condition.

Incidence/prevalence

There are two forms of seborrheic dermatitis, an infantile form and an adult form. The former is self-limited and confined to the first 3 months of life, and the latter is chronic, peaking between the ages of 30 and 50. The prevalence of adult seborrheic dermatitis is estimated at 5%.[3]

In patients with acquired immunodeficiency syndrome (AIDS), the incidence increases (30–80%), probably related to CD4 levels (altered immune surveillance).[4]

Oble *et al.* have characterized a novel animal model of seborrheic dermatitis. This model implicates a fungal organism, and CD4+ T cell lymphopenia may mimic the seborrheic dermatitis in acquired immunodeficiency syndrome.[5]

Etiology/risk factors

The etiology of seborrheic dermatitis is not clear. Several factors, such as sebaceous output, androgenic hormones, mycological infection, and neurological disturbances can have a major effect on the development of the condition. In particular, qualitative and quantitative abnormalities in the composition of sebum have been suggested, but not clearly defined. Dandruff and seborrheic dermatitis are chronic scalp manifestations with similar etiology, differing only in severity. The etiology is a convergence of three factors: sebaceous gland secretions, individual susceptibility, and microfloral metabolism. These manifestations are superficial stratum corneum disorders, including alterations of the epidermis with hyperproliferation, excess lipids, interdigitation of the corneal envelope, and parakeratosis.[6] The nonpathogenic fungus *Malassezia furfur* (*Pityrosporum ovale* and *P. orbiculare*) may play a role,[7] but the mechanism has not been completely clarified.

Investigations on the role of these pathogens have focused on their lipid metabolism. *Malassezia restricta* and *Malassezia*

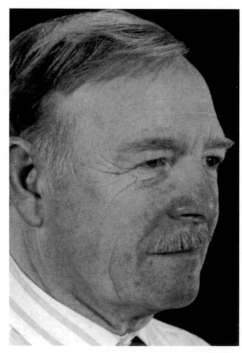

Figure 20.1 A patient with seborrheic dermatitis.

globosa require lipids. The treatment is capable of degrading sebum, releasing free fatty acids from triglycerides, consuming specific saturated fatty acids, and leaving behind the unsaturates. Penetration of the modified short fatty acids results in inflammation and irritation. Some studies have hypothesized that seborrheic dermatitis is caused by an altered immune response to *Malassezia furfur*, which has also been associated with the pathogenesis of the disease. Increased keratinocyte and sebocyte turnover has been reported in association with altered keratinization. Systemic lipid metabolism and antioxidants may play a role in modulating the disease onset and the inflammatory reaction. A few studies have linked the onset or relapses with the patient's psychological condition, alcohol intake, psychotropic drugs, and a deficiency of micronutrients (lithium, zinc, magnesium, biotin).

Prognosis

Although there are many treatments for seborrheic dermatitis, recurrences are very common, with the disease typically relapsing for years. Although the prognostic studies identified were not long-term ones, preventive regimens have been developed and can help reduce the severity of the disease. These include improvement in lifestyle, intake of supplements, and sun exposure.

Aims

The aims of the treatment are to reduce symptoms and relapses and to improve the disease cosmetically with short-term treatment.

Outcomes

No standard scales were found for the assessment of the severity of seborrheic dermatitis. Outcomes include the severity of symptoms (erythema, desquamation, itching), the rate of recurrence, the number of *P. orbiculare* colonies, patient satisfaction, and cosmetic acceptability.

Search methods

Since few RCTs were found that met the criteria for clinical evidence, observational studies were included (Medline, 1981 to May 2006).

Questions

What are the effects of topical treatment?

Antifungal agents

Topical antifungals are well established in the treatment of seborrheic dermatitis. We found several clinical trials showing that different topical antifungal agents improve seborrheic dermatitis.

Efficacy

No systematic reviews were found.

Ketoconazole. We found seven double-blind placebo-controlled trials using cream or shampoo.[8–14] The largest trial, using 2% ketoconazole shampoo (n = 575) reported an excellent response in 88% of the patients treated. The treatment was effective in preventing relapses when used prophylactically once a week.[8] A randomized controlled trial (RCT) comparing 2% ketoconazole shampoo with 2.5% selenium sulfide shampoo found that both treatments were better than placebo; ketoconazole was statistically superior to selenium sulfide ($P = 0.0026$) and was better tolerated.[9] In two double-blind crossover studies (n = 20 and n = 35), the change in the clinical score with ketoconazole shampoo was significant ($P < 0.01$).[10,11] Two RCTs demonstrated the clinical efficacy of 2% cream in comparison with a placebo in 37 and 20 patients, respectively.[12,13] In a double-blind placebo-controlled trial, 18 patients were treated either with a gel containing a combination of 2% ketoconazole and 0.05% desonide or with the unmedicated gel.[14] After 3 weeks, the clinical signs had completely subsided in six of nine patients treated with the medicated gel and one out of nine patients treated with the placebo gel.

One open, randomized, parallel study including a total of 66 patients showed that a 2% formulation was significantly more effective than a 1% formulation ($P < 0.001$) and that intermittent application of 2% ketoconazole shampoo can successfully prevent relapse.[15]

Long-term prophylactic treatment needs to meet a high standard with regard to patient safety. The safety of 2% ketoconazole shampoo is supported by absorption studies and by local irritancy and contact sensitivity studies. Ketoconazole shampoo does not influence sebum production, but improves its delivery onto the skin surface.[16]

Bifonazole. We found three double-blind controlled trials and two open studies.[17–19] The largest, involving 100 patients, reported that 1% bifonazole cream was significantly better than placebo ($P < 0.05$).[17]

Ciclopiroxolamine. One placebo-controlled double-blind study of ciclopiroxolamine 1% cream in facial seborrheic dermatitis (57 patients in the ciclopiroxolamine group and 72 in the vehicle group) found a statistically significant difference ($P < 0.01$) between the two treatment groups at the end of the initial phase (twice daily for 28 days) and in the maintenance phases (once daily for 28 days).[20]

We found five randomized, double-blind, vehicle-controlled trials of ciclopirox shampoo. In one study (n = 203), the most pronounced improvement in the treatment of seborrheic dermatitis of the scalp was seen with ciclopirox 1% shampoo, in comparison with the lowest concentrations (0.1% and 0.3%) and the vehicle.[21] A trial (n = 183) compared different application frequencies of 1% ciclopirox shampoo.[22] The most pronounced improvement was seen in the group treated three times a week and twice a week, in comparison with once a week and vehicle shampoo. Another study (n = 499) reported that an effective treatment response was achieved in 26% of patients treated with ciclopirox in comparison with 12.9% of patients treated with the vehicle.[23] Vardy *et al.* (n = 102) showed that the improvement of seborrheic dermatitis was significantly greater in a group treated with ciclopirox than in a group treated with placebo (93% and 41%, respectively).[24]

In a large study, 949 patients were randomly assigned to receive 1% ciclopirox shampoo once or twice weekly or vehicle for 4 weeks.[25] Ciclopirox once and twice weekly produced response rates of 57.9% and 45.4%, respectively, in comparison with 31.6% for the vehicle.

Terbinafine. We found two RCTs: in one, the lesions cleared in 11 of 18 eligible patients after treatment with 1% terbinafine solution once daily for 4 weeks,[26] while the other study reported complete remission in 10 of 35 patients treated with 1% terbinafine cream.[27]

Other antifungals. Beneficial effects have been reported in open studies with fluconazole[28] and fenticonazole.[29] One study in a group of 30 men demonstrated that 0.2% octopirox in a shampoo vehicle was superior to the same level in the simple shampoo base and equivalent in activity to a much higher level (0.5%) in the base only.[30]

Drawbacks
The few adverse effects reported include erythema, dryness, and pruritus.

Comment
The various antifungal drugs have not been compared. The possible mechanisms of action of these compounds include antifungal and anti-inflammatory effects.

Corticosteroids
Recently, little information has been published on the use of topical steroids. The drugs, applied for 1–4 weeks, improve seborrheic dermatitis and do not cause systemic effects, but relapses are more frequent than with topical antifungals.

Efficacy
No systematic reviews were found. In one RCT, a 1% hydrocortisone solution was compared with miconazole and a combination of miconazole and hydrocortisone in 70 patients;[31] the combination was most effective. Recurrences were seen most frequently in the hydrocortisone group. We found one randomized double-blind controlled trial of 2% ketoconazole cream versus 0.05% clobetasol 17-butyrate cream,[32] and one trial comparing topical application of 0.02% flumethasone pivalate with 2% eosin in 30 infants with seborrheic dermatitis; in the latter study, the two treatments were found to have comparable effects.[33]

Drawbacks
Long-term corticosteroid therapy may induce adverse effects such as skin atrophy and telangiectasia.

Comment
No recent RCTs have demonstrated the efficacy of corticosteroids, although they are used as comparative drugs.

Lithium succinate
RCTs have found that lithium succinate improves seborrheic dermatitis in comparison with placebos.

Efficacy
We found two randomized, double-blind, placebo-controlled trials and one open trial with 8% lithium succinate ointment.[34–36] One crossover trial in nine centers (200 patients) and a parallel-group study in two centers (27 patients) showed that the symptom score improved significantly in the lithium group ($P < 0.0001$).[34] The other double-blind trial, conducted in 12 patients with AIDS-associated seborrheic dermatitis, reported rapid (2–5 days) and significant ($P < 0.01$) clinical improvement in patients treated with lithium succinate.[35]

Drawbacks
Adverse effects consisted of skin and eyelid irritation in a few patients.

Comment
Lithium inhibits growth in small colony strains of *Pityrosporum* and blocks the release of free fatty acids from tissue. Lithium also has potentially anti-inflammatory actions.

Antibacterials
We found only a few studies of metronidazole.

Efficacy
No systematic reviews were found. A double-blind study (n = 44) described significant improvement after the use of 1% metronidazole gel in comparison with a placebo for 8 weeks. Fourteen patients in the metronidazole group and two in the placebo group had complete improvement.[37]

Drawbacks
Metronidazole gel was well tolerated and did not produce adverse effects.

Comment

The mechanism of action of metronidazole is not known.

Benzoyl peroxide

Two controlled studies have reported on the efficacy of benzoyl peroxide.

Efficacy

Of the two studies, one open trial noted improvement in 28 of 30 patients treated for several months with 2.5% benzoyl peroxide.[38] The second, a double-blind RCT including 59 patients, compared 5% benzoyl peroxide with placebo for 4 weeks and reported a significant improvement in erythema, pruritus, and scaling in the group treated with benzoyl peroxide ($P < 0.05$).[39]

Drawbacks

Skin irritation was reported as a side effect.

Propylene glycol

We found one double-blind controlled study, in which 39 patients with seborrheic dermatitis of the scalp were treated with a solution containing 15% propylene glycol.[40] The lesions improved in 89% of the patients treated with propylene glycol, in comparison with 32% in the placebo group. *In vitro*, the *P. orbiculare* counts were reduced significantly after treatment with propylene glycol, but not in the placebo group.

Pimecrolimus

RCTs have found that pimecrolimus cream 1% improves seborrheic dermatitis.

Efficacy

In one study (n = 19), 1% pimecrolimus cream was applied as monotherapy twice daily for 7 days and for an additional period of 7 days until complete clearance was achieved.[41] At the end of the treatment, the percentages of complete clearance were 52%.

We found one open-label clinical trial conducted in 20 patients—11 patients in the 1% pimecrolimus cream group and nine patients in the betamethasone 17-valerate 0.1% cream.[42] Both agents were highly effective in the treatment of seborrheic dermatitis. More severe and frequent relapses were observed with betamethasone than with pimecrolimus.

Drawbacks

Rosaceiform dermatitis is an adverse side effect complicating treatment with 1% pimecrolimus cream.[43]

Comment

Pimecrolimus is a calcineurin inhibitor that has been successfully used in inflammatory skin diseases. It selectively targets T cells and mast cells and inhibits T cell proliferation and the production and release of interleukin-2, interleukin-4, interferon gamma, and tumor necrosis factor-α. In contrast to corticosteroids, pimecrolimus does not induce skin atrophy.

Miscellaneous

Several treatments have been claimed to be effective in uncontrolled studies. A blind, randomized, parallel-group study in 80 patients found that 1% Ichthyol (ichthammol) was superior to 4% coal tar in seborrheic dermatitis of the scalp.[44]

Tacalcitol (1a,24-dihydroxycholecalciferol) was used in four patients, with good results;[45] crude honey (30 patients),[46] borage oil, 40% urea ointment,[47] dithranol (18 patients),[48] pyridoxine, and cystine[49] have been reported to be beneficial in uncontrolled studies.

Ultraviolet light. RCTs have found that phototherapy improves seborrheic dermatitis.

Efficacy

No systematic reviews were found. Limited evidence suggests that natural sunlight has a significant effect on seborrheic dermatitis.[50,51] One RCT (n = 48) found improvement in 85% of patients receiving selective ultraviolet phototherapy, and in 76% of patients treated with psoralen ultraviolet A (PUVA) after a mean of 26 treatments.[52] In an open study, 18 patients with severe seborrheic dermatitis were treated with narrow-band UVB (TL-01) phototherapy, three times weekly, starting with 70% of the minimal erythema dose up to a maximum of 8 weeks. All patients responded to narrow-band UVB. Twelve completed the study; six had complete remission and six had marked improvement.[53]

Drawbacks

No side effects were reported, except for rare episodes of moderate erythema.

Comment

The trials of phototherapy were too few for its effectiveness to be evaluated.

What are the effects of systemic treatments?

Antifungal drugs

We found limited evidence that oral antifungals are beneficial.

Efficacy

We found no systematic reviews.

Ketoconazole. One double-blind placebo-controlled crossover study in 19 patients compared ketoconazole 200 mg/day for 4 weeks with placebo. Seventy percent of the patients showed significantly greater improvement with ketoconazole, particularly on the scalp, in comparison with 10% with placebo ($P < 0.01$).[54]

Terbinafine. In one placebo-controlled trial (n = 60), oral terbinafine 250 mg once daily for 4 weeks significantly reduced scores $(P < 0.0001)$ in comparison with the baseline and with control groups.[55]

In a randomized, double-blind, placebo-controlled study (n = 174) in patients with lesions in nonexposed sites and in patients with lesions in exposed skin areas, oral terbinafine (250 mg/day) or a placebo were each administered for 6 weeks.[56] In patients with lesions in nonexposed sites, the response rate was significantly higher with terbinafine (70% vs. 45.4%; $P = 0.03$). No significant differences were reported in patients in exposed skin areas.

Itraconazole. We found two RCTs of oral itraconazole. In one (n = 32), the treatment was given in two different periods. In the first period, 1% hydrocortisone cream was administered for 4 weeks and 200 mg itraconazole daily during the first week; in the second period, the cream was discontinued and itraconazole was given on the first 2 days of every month for 11 months.[57] Nineteen patients showed significant improvement or complete recovery, six had moderate improvement, and three had slight improvement. In an open, noncomparative trial (n = 29), itraconazole 100 mg was given twice a day for 1 week and then, after a 3-week interval, for the first 2 days of the following 2 months.[58] Clinical improvement was observed in 23 patients.

Drawbacks
Ketoconazole damages the liver and interferes with testosterone metabolism. No side effects were reported during the terbinafine studies.

Comment
Seborrheic dermatitis relapses when the drugs are stopped, so that prolonged treatment is often needed. Systemic antifungal drugs are not suitable for this.

What are the effects of nutrients?

We found no controlled studies of the effects of nutrients, vitamins, and trace elements on seborrheic dermatitis. On the basis of limited observational evidence, seborrheic dermatitis is said to have improved after administration of vitamins A, E, D, B_1, B_2, B_6, and C, niacin, biotin, selenium, zinc, or iron.[59,60]

Do treatments that reduce sebaceous secretions improve the symptoms?

Retinoids and antiandrogens
We found that few drugs interfere with sebum secretion, and there is insufficient evidence that controlling sebum production leads to improvement of seborrheic dermatitis.

Efficacy
Oral retinoids reduce sebaceous gland size, suppress sebum production, and inhibit sebocyte differentiation; they also have anti-inflammatory activity.[61] Antiandrogen and 5-alpha-reductase inhibitors reduce the size of the sebaceous glandular lobules and ducts.[62]

We found no evidence to support the hypothesis that reducing sebum production decreases the probability of developing seborrheic dermatitis.

Key points
- RCTs show that topical antifungal treatment and metronidazole are effective.
- Limited evidence suggests that systemic antifungal therapy can be useful in controlling the disease.
- Few RCTs have examined the efficacy of topical steroids.
- We found limited or no evidence on the effect of natural sunlight and/or systemic nutrients.

References

1 Plewig G, Jansen T. Seborrheic dermatitis. In: Freedberg IM, Eisen AZ, Wolff K, *et al.*, eds. *Fitzpatrick's Dermatology in General Medicine,* 5th ed., vol. 1. New York: McGraw-Hill, 1999: 1482–9.
2 Gupta AK, Bluhm R. Seborrheic dermatitis. *J Eur Acad Dermatol Venereol* 2004;**18**:13–26.
3 Fritsch PO, Reider N. Other eczematous eruptions. In : Bolognia JL, Jorizzo JL, Rapini RP, eds. *Dermatology,* vol. 1. New York: Mosby, 2003: 215–8.
4 Schaub NA, Drewe J, Sponagel L, *et al.* Is there a relation between risk groups or initial CD4T cell counts and prevalence of seborrheic dermatitis in HIV-infected patients? *Dermatology* 1999;**198**: 126–9.
5 Oble DA, Collett E, Hsieh M, *et al.* A novel T cell receptor transgenic animal model of seborrheic dermatitis-like skin disease. *J Invest Dermatol* 2005;**124**:151–9.
6 Ro BI, Dawson TL. The role of sebaceous gland activity and scalp microfloral metabolism in the etiology of seborrheic dermatitis and dandruff. *J Investig Dermatol Symp Proc* 2005;**10**:194–7.
7 Faergemann J, Bergbrant IM, Dohse M, Scott A, Westgate G. Seborrhoeic dermatitis and *Pityrosporum (Malassezia)* folliculitis: characterization of inflammatory cells and mediators in the skin by immunohistochemistry. *Br J Dermatol* 2001;**144**:549–56.
8 Peter RU, Richarz-Barthauer U. Successful treatment and prophylaxis of scalp seborrhoeic dermatitis and dandruff with 2% ketoconazole shampoo: results of a multicentre, double blind, placebo-controlled trial. *Br J Dermatol* 1995;**132**:441–5.
9 Danby FW, Maddin WS, Margesson LJ, Rosenthal D. A randomized, double-blind, placebo-controlled trial of ketoconazole 2% shampoo versus selenium sulfide 2.5% shampoo in the treatment of moderate to severe dandruff. *J Am Acad Dermatol* 1993;**29**:1008–12.
10 Carr MM, Pryce DM, Ive FA. Treatment of seborrhoeic dermatitis with ketoconazole, 1: response of the scalp to topical ketoconazole. *Br J Dermatol* 1987;**116**:213–6.

11 Faergemann J. Treatment of seborrhoeic dermatitis of the scalp with ketoconazole shampoo: a double-blind study. *Acta Derm Venereol* 1990;**70**:171–2.

12 Skinner RB, Noah PW, Taylor RM, *et al.* Double-blind treatment of seborrheic dermatitis with 2% ketoconazole cream. *J Am Acad Dermatol* 1985;**12**:852–6.

13 Green CA, Farr PM, Shuster S. Treatment of seborrhoeic dermatitis with ketoconazole, 2: response of seborrhoeic dermatitis of the face, scalp and trunk to topical ketoconazole. *Br J Dermatol* 1987;**116**:217–21.

14 Pierard-Franchimont C, Pierard GE. A double-blind placebo-controlled study of ketoconazole + desonide gel combination in the treatment of facial seborrheic dermatitis. *Dermatology* 2002;**204**; 344–7.

15 Pierard-Franchimont C, Pierard GE, Arrese JE, De Doncker P. Effect of ketoconazole 1% and 2% shampoos on severe dandruff and seborrhoeic dermatitis: clinical, squamometric and mycological assessments. *Dermatology* 2001;**202**:171–6.

16 Dobrev H, Zissova L. Effect of ketoconazole 2% shampoo on scalp sebum level in patients with seborrhoeic dermatitis. *Acta Derm Venereol* 1997;**77**:132–4.

17 Zienicke H, Korting HC, Braun-Falco O, *et al.* Comparative efficacy and safety of bifonazole 1% cream and the corresponding base preparation in the treatment of seborrhoeic dermatitis. *Mycoses* 1993;**36**:325–31.

18 Segal R, David M, Ingber A, Lurie R, Sandbank M. Treatment with bifonazole shampoo for seborrhea and seborrheic dermatitis: a randomized, double-blind study. *Acta Derm Venereol* 1992;**72**: 454–5.

19 Massone L, Borghi S, Pestarono A, *et al.* Seborrheic dermatitis in otherwise healthy patients and in patients with lymphadenopathy syndrome/AIDS-related complex: treatment with 1% bifonazole cream. *Chemioterapia* 1988;**7**:109–12.

20 Dupuy P, Maurette C, Amoric JC, Chosidow O; Study Investigator Group. Randomized, placebo-controlled, double-blind study on clinical efficacy of ciclopiroxolamine 1% cream in facial seborrhoeic dermatitis. *Br J Dermatol* 2001;**144**:1033–7.

21 Altmeyer P, Hoffmann K. Efficacy of different concentrations of ciclopirox shampoo for the treatment of seborrheic dermatitis of the scalp: results of a randomized, double-blind, vehicle-controlled trial. *Int J Dermatol* 2004;**43**(Suppl 1):9–12.

22 Abeck D. Rationale of frequency of use of ciclopirox 1% shampoo in the treatment of seborrheic dermatitis: results of a double-blind, placebo-controlled study comparing the efficacy of once, twice, and three times weekly usage. *Int J Dermatol* 2004;**43**(Suppl 1):13–6.

23 Lebwohl M, Plott T. Safety and efficacy of ciclopirox 1% shampoo for the treatment of seborrheic dermatitis of the scalp in the US population: results of a double-blind, vehicle-controlled trial. *Int J Dermatol* 2004;**43**(Suppl 1):17–20.

24 Vardy DA, Zvulunov A, Tchetov T, *et al.* A double-blind, placebo-controlled trial of a ciclopiroxolamine 1% shampoo for the treatment of scalp seborrheic dermatitis. *J Dermatol Treat* 2000;**11**:73–7.

25 Shuster S, Meynadier J, Kerl H, *et al.* Treatment and prophylaxis of seborrheic dermatitis of the scalp with antipityrosporal 1% ciclopirox shampoo. *Arch Dermatol* 2005;**141**: 47–52.

26 Faergemann J, Jones TC, Hettler O, *et al. Pityrosporum ovale* (*Malassezia furfur*) as the causative agent of seborrhoeic dermatitis: new treatments. *Br J Dermatol* 1996;**134**(Suppl 46):12–5.

27 Gunduz K, Inanir I, Sacar H. Efficacy of terbinafine 1% cream on seborrhoeic dermatitis. *J Dermatol* 2005;**32**: 22–5.

28 Rigopoulos D, Katsambas A, Antoniou C, *et al.* Facial seborrheic dermatitis treated with fluconazole 2% shampoo. *Int J Dermatol* 1994;**33**:136–7.

29 Merlino A, Malvano L, Cervetti O, Forte M. [Role of *Malassezia furfur* in seborrheic dermatitis in adults and therapeutic efficacy of fenticonazole; in Italian.] *G Ital Dermatol Venereol* 1988;**123**): xxxvii–xxxix.

30 Georgalas A. Enhanced delivery of an anti-dandruff active in a shampoo vehicle. *J Cosmet Sci* 2004;**55**(Suppl):207–14.

31 Faergemann J. Seborrhoeic dermatitis and *Pityrosporum orbiculare*: treatment of seborrhoeic dermatitis of the scalp with miconazole-hydrocortisone (Daktacort), miconazole and hydrocortisone. *Br J Dermatol* 1986;**114**:695–700.

32 Pari T, Pulimood S, Jacob M, *et al.* Randomised double blind controlled trial of 2% ketoconazole cream versus 0.05% clobetasol 17-butyrate cream in seborrheic dermatitis. *J Eur Acad Dermatol Venereol* 1998;**10**:89–90.

33 Shohat M, Mimouni M, Varsano I. Efficacy of topical application of glucocorticosteroids compared with eosin in infant with seborrheic dermatitis. *Cutis* 1987;**40**:67–8.

34 Efalith Multicenter Trial Group. A double-blind, placebo-controlled, multicenter trial of lithium succinate ointment in the treatment of seborrheic dermatitis. *J Am Acad Dermatol* 1992;**26**: 452–7.

35 Langtry JA, Rowland Payne CM, Staughton RC, *et al.* Topical lithium succinate ointment (Efalith) in the treatment of AIDS-related seborrheic dermatitis. *Clin Exp Dermatol* 1997;**22**:216–9.

36 Cuelenaere C, De Bersaques J, Kint A. Use of topical lithium succinate ointment in the treatment of seborrheic dermatitis. *Dermatology* 1992;**184**:194–7.

37 Parsad D, Pandhi R, Negri KS, *et al.* Topical metronidazole in seborrhoeic dermatitis : a double-blind study. *Dermatology* 2001; **202**:35–7.

38 Bonnetblanc JM, Bernard P. Benzoyl peroxide in seborrheic dermatitis. *Arch Dermatol* 1986;**122**:752.

39 Bonnetblanc JM, De Prost Y, Bazex J, *et al.* Treatment of seborrheic dermatitis with benzoyl peroxide. *Ann Dermatol Venereol* 1990; **117**:123–5.

40 Faergemann J. Propylene glycol in the treatment of seborrhoeic dermatitis of the scalp: a double-blind study. *Cutis* 1988;**42**:69–71.

41 Rallis E, Nasiopoulou A, Kouskoukis C. Pimecrolimus cream 1% can be an effective treatment for seborrheic dermatitis of the face and trunk. *Drugs Exp Clin Res* 2004;**30**:191–5.

42 Rigopoulos D, Ioannides D, Kalogeromitros D, *et al.* Pimecrolimus cream 1% vs. betamethasone 17-valerate 0.1% cream in the treatment of seborrheic dermatitis: a randomized open-label clinical trial. *Br J Dermatol* 2004;**151**:1071–5.

43 Gorman CR, White SW. Rosaceiform dermatitis as a complication of treatment of facial seborrheic dermatitis with 1% pimecrolimus cream. *Arch Dermatol* 2005;**141**:1168.

44 Michel V, Reygagne P, Dupuy P. Results of a clinical study comparing 1% Ichthyol with 4% coal tar in seborrhoeic dermatitis of the scalp. *J Eur Acad Dermatol Venereol* 1997;**9**:186.

45 Nakayama J. Four cases of sebopsoriasis or seborrhoeic dermatitis of the face and scalp successfully treated with 1a-24-R-dihydroxy-cholecalciferol (tacalcitol) cream. *Eur J Dermatol* 2000;**10**:528–32.

46 Al Walli NS. Therapeutic and prophylactic effects of crude honey on chronic seborrhoeic dermatitis and dandruff. *Eur J Med Res* 2001;**6**:306–8.

47 Shemer A, Nathansohn N, Kaplan B, *et al.* Treatment of scalp seborrheic dermatitis and psoriasis with an ointment of 40% urea and 1% bifonazole. *Int J Dermatol* 2000;**39**:532–4.

48 Wolbling RH, Schofer H, Milbradt R. [Treatment of seborrhoeic dermatitis with low-dosage dithranol ; in German.] *Hautarzt* 1985;**36**:529–30.

49 Melli MC, Giorgini S. [Clinical evaluation of the efficacy of a topical preparation containing pyridoxine and cystine in seborrheic dermatitis and in seborrheic condition of the face; in Italian.] *G Ital Dermatol Venereol* 1986;**121**:li–liii.

50 Berg M. Epidemiological studies of the influence of sunlight on the skin. *Photodermatology* 1989;**6**:80–4.

51 Maietta G, Rongioletti F, Rebora A. Seborrheic dermatitis and daylight. *Acta Derm Venereol* 1991;**71**:538–9.

52 Salo O, Lassus A, Juvakoski T, Kanerva L, Lauharanta J. [Treatment of atopic dermatitis and seborrheic dermatitis with selective UV-phototherapy and PUVA: a comparative study; in German.] *Dermatol Monatsschr* 1983;**169**:371–5.

53 Pirkhammer D, Seeber A, Honigsmann H, Tanew A. Narrow-band ultraviolet B (ATL-01) phototherapy is an effective and safe treatment for patients with severe seborrhoeic dermatitis. *Br J Dermatol* 2000;**143**:964–8.

54 Ford GP, Farr PM, Ive FA, Shuster S. The response of seborrhoeic dermatitis to ketoconazole. *Br J Dermatol* 1984;**111**:603–7.

55 Scaparro E, Quadri G, Virno G, Orifici C, Milani M. Evaluation of the efficacy and tolerability of oral terbinafine (Daskil) in patients with seborrheic dermatitis: a multicentre, randomized, investigator-blinded, placebo-controlled trial. Br J Dermatol 2001; **144**:854–7.

56 Vena GA, Micali G, Santoianni P, Cassano N, Peruzzi E. Oral terbinafine in the treatment of multi-site seborrheic dermatitis: a multicenter, double-blind placebo-controlled study. *Int J Immunopathol Pharmacol* 2005;**18**:745–53.

57 Baysal V, Yildirim M, Ozcanli C. Itraconazole in the treatment of seborrheic dermatitis: a new treatment modality. *Int J Dermatol* 2004;**43**:63–6.

58 Kose O, Erbil H, Gur AR. Oral itraconazole for the treatment of seborrhoeic dermatitis: an open, noncomparative trial. *J Eur Acad Dermatol Venereol* 2005;**19**:172–5.

59 Brenner S, Horwitz C. Possible nutrient mediators in psoriasis and seborrheic dermatitis. *World Rev Nutr Diet* 1988;**55**:165–82.

60 Passi S, Morrone A, De Luca C, *et al.* Blood levels of vitamin E, polyunsaturated fatty acids of phospholipids, lipoperoxides and glutathione peroxidase in patients affected with seborrheic dermatitis. *J Dermatol Sci* 1991;**2**:171–8.

61 Orfanos CE, Zouboulis CC. Oral retinoids in the treatment of seborrhoea and acne. *Dermatology* 1998;**196**:140–7.

62 Ye F, Imamura K, Imanishi N, *et al.* Effects of topical antiandrogen and 5-alpha-reductase inhibitors on sebaceous glands in male fuzzy rats. *Skin Pharmacol* 1997;**10**:288–97.

21 Psoriasis

Luigi Naldi, Robert J.G. Chalmers

Background

Definition

Psoriasis is an inflammatory disease of the skin characterized by an accelerated rate of epidermal turnover, with hyperproliferation and defective maturation of epidermal keratinocytes. In the majority of cases, psoriasis is a chronic disease, which in its most common form—chronic plaque psoriasis—manifests as well-demarcated, often symmetrically distributed, thickened, red, scaly plaques (Figure 21.1). These may vary considerably both in size and in number and may involve any part of the skin, although they are found most typically on the extensor surfaces of the knees and elbows, in the sacral area, and in the scalp. Appear-

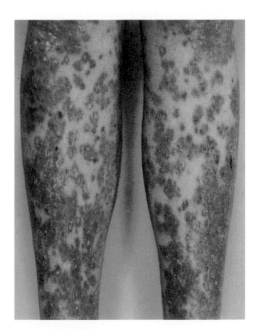

Figure 21.1 Chronic plaque psoriasis.

ances may be modified by the site of involvement, with flexural areas showing beef-red shiny plaques without scale (flexural or inverse psoriasis), palms and soles showing marked hyperkeratosis and fissuring, and nails becoming distorted by thimble-pits, thickening, and nail-plate detachment. Up to 8% of individuals with psoriasis may have an associated inflammatory arthropathy,[1] which in severe cases may be the dominant cause of morbidity.

Acute inflammatory forms of psoriasis may develop *de novo*, or may complicate existing chronic plaque psoriasis. Acute guttate psoriasis characteristically affects children and young adults following streptococcal infection.[2] Typically, showers of tiny red papules (likened to raindrops or guttae) erupt over large areas of the skin surface 1–2 weeks after an episode of acute streptococcal pharyngitis or tonsillitis. Erythrodermic and generalized pustular psoriasis are uncommon but severe and potentially life-threatening forms of psoriasis, which may be complicated by high-output cardiac failure, temperature dysregulation, and septicemia, particularly in the elderly.

Psoriasis is associated with two relatively uncommon conditions that may cause long-lasting disability as a result of severe inflammation and pustulation affecting the hands and feet. The first is now more commonly referred to as palmoplantar pustulosis, but is still widely known as chronic palmoplantar pustular psoriasis. Although associated with psoriasis elsewhere in about one-fifth of cases, it is now considered to be a genetically separate entity.[3] Acropustulosis (acrodermatitis continua of Hallopeau), on the other hand, may be associated with generalized pustular psoriasis.[3] The relationship of these two conditions to psoriasis vulgaris remains poorly understood.

Prevalence

Psoriasis affects 1–3% of the general population. It is believed to be less frequent in some ethnic groups (e.g., in people from West Africa and China), but we have found no reliable epidemiological data to support this.[4]

Etiology

Epidermal turnover is greatly accelerated in psoriasis, such that keratinocytes within active psoriatic plaques may travel from the basal layer of the epidermis to the stratum corneum in as little as 4 days, rather than the normal 28 days. Exactly what drives this process is incompletely understood, but it is agreed that it is mediated by activated T lymphocytes and that there is a strong genetic component.[5] Physical trauma, acute infection, and some medications (e.g., lithium and beta-blockers) are believed to trigger the condition. A few observational studies have linked the onset or relapse of psoriasis with stressful life events and personal habits, including cigarette smoking and, less consistently, alcohol consumption. An association of psoriasis with body mass index is also well documented.[4]

Prognosis

Psoriasis is known to last years or decades and to be subject to periods of remission and relapse. We did not, however, find any long-term studies examining the prognosis. There is growing evidence that moderate to severe psoriasis is associated with a significantly increased risk of cardiovascular morbidity,[6,7] with at least double the prevalence of obesity, type 2 diabetes, arterial hypertension, hyperlipidemia, and coronary heart disease.[7] The odds of having the metabolic syndrome, a defined combination of these conditions, were found to be more than five times higher amongst 581 adult patients hospitalized for severe psoriasis than in a control group of hospitalized patients (OR 5.29).[7] Psoriasis may substantially affect quality of life, by influencing a negative body image and self-image and limiting daily activities, social contacts, and work. One systematic review (search date 2000, 17 cohort studies) confirmed that severe psoriasis is associated with lower levels of quality of life than mild psoriasis.[8] At present, there is no cure for psoriasis. However, in many people it can be well controlled with treatment, at least in the short term.

Aims of treatment

Until there is a safe and effective cure for psoriasis, a balance needs to be struck between patients' individual perceptions of disability from psoriasis, their willingness to devote time and effort to managing the disease, and their preparedness to accept risks from treatment. Successful management may therefore range from reassurance and provision of simple emollients to the use of powerful and potentially hazardous systemic agents.

Relevant outcomes

Outcomes should reflect the aims stated above: clearance or improvement of psoriasis over time; acceptability to patients of treatment regimens; duration of remission; patient satisfaction and autonomy; disease-related quality of life; adverse effects of treatment. We found no documented evidence that clinical activity scores, such as the Psoriasis Area and Severity Index (PASI), are reliable proxies for these outcomes. Recently, the PASI score has been converted into categories of response deemed to be clinically important—for example, at least a 75% reduction in score from baseline (PASI 75) or at least a 90% reduction in score from baseline (PASI 90).

Methods of search

The search strategy "psoria* or 'acrodermatitis continua of Hallopeau' or (impetigo and herpetiformis) or ((palm* or plant* or sole* or bacterid) and (pustul* or psoria*)) or acropustulosis" was used to search the Cochrane Controlled Trials Register (2006, issue 3) and the European Dermatoepidemiology Network (EDEN) database of psoriasis trials, and filtered using the Cochrane Optimal Search Strategy for randomized controlled trials, Medline, and Embase (both to June 2006). The results were cross-checked against the Salford Database of Psoriasis Trials, which was developed for a systematic review of treatments for severe psoriasis published in 2000.[9]

Questions

How effective are treatments for limited stable chronic plaque psoriasis?

Emollients and occlusive dressings

Psoriatic plaques are dry, scaly, and frequently itchy. Emollients may help soften psoriatic scale by increasing its water content, either by forming an occlusive layer on the skin surface (e.g., white soft paraffin) or by an osmotic effect (e.g., urea-containing creams). Most topically applied therapies for psoriasis are formulated in emollient bases, but emollients on their own are frequently advocated for psoriasis. There is little published evidence documenting the benefits of emollient therapy alone in the management of psoriasis.

Occlusive dressings have also been used for treating psoriatic plaques. These have frequently been used to enhance the penetration of applied pharmacological agents such as topical corticosteroids, but have also been examined on their own. Hydrocolloid gel dressings may be useful on their own for selected recalcitrant psoriatic plaques and may enhance the response to topical corticosteroids.

Benefits
Emollients. In a limited number of studies, an improvement

over baseline has been demonstrated after regular application of emollient creams or ointments. In one open-label study in which within-patient comparisons were undertaken in two separate cohorts of 48 patients with chronic plaque psoriasis, the combination of a once-daily application of a water-in-oil cream or lotion with once-daily betamethasone dipropionate cream was shown to be more effective than once-daily, and of equal efficacy to twice-daily, betamethasone dipropionate cream.[10] In another within-patient study (n = 43), the authors found that the rate of psoriasis improvement with ultraviolet B (UVB) phototherapy was significantly enhanced by the application of an oil-in-water emollient cream applied prior to UVB exposure. It was argued that this may have altered the optical properties of the epidermis. In another small within-patient study comparing a 10% urea ointment with its base or with no therapy (n = 10), 2 weeks' therapy with the urea ointment produced a more than 50% reduction in the clinical score in comparison with the untreated side; however, the ointment base alone also produced a significant improvement in the clinical score.[11] In another randomized controlled trial (RCT; n = 40), a 12% urea and 12% sodium chloride cream was shown to be superior to its cream base and to have comparable efficacy to salicylic acid ointment in removing scale from psoriatic plaque.[12]

Hydrocolloid dressings. In a small, open, prospective, bilateral comparison study including 26 patients with stable symmetrical plaque psoriasis, 47% of the treated plaques resolved with weekly applications of an adhesive hydrocolloid occlusive dressing for 10 weeks; furthermore, the dressing was found to be therapeutically superior to twice-daily applications of a potent topical corticosteroid cream (fluocinolone acetonide) for 10 weeks (12% resolution rate), though less effective than erythemogenic ultraviolet B phototherapy administered five times weekly for the same duration (67% resolution rate).[13] The results from another small RCT suggest that 3 weeks' therapy with a hydrocolloid dressing or with a potent topical corticosteroid cream (0.1% triamcinolone acetonide) is insufficient to induce resolution, but that a combination of the two is significantly more efficacious.[14]

Harms

Local irritation and, rarely, allergic contact dermatitis may result from use of emollients or occlusive dressings.

Comments

Patients with mild psoriasis may choose to use emollients alone, because of their convenience and lack of adverse effects. Usually, however, they are used as adjuncts to other therapies. Hydrocolloid gel dressings may be useful on their own for selected recalcitrant psoriatic plaques and may enhance the response to topical corticosteroids.

Keratolytics

Salicylic acid is the most commonly used keratolytic agent in dermatological practice and is often advocated for removing psoriatic scale. This is considered to be beneficial not only because of the obvious effects on reducing scaling and skin shedding, but also because it thereby removes a barrier to the penetration of more active compounds into the skin. It is usually dispensed in an ointment base in concentrations of between 2% and 10%. It is often used in combination with coal tar or corticosteroids. There is little information from RCTs on the efficacy of salicylic acid monotherapy as a descaling agent.

Benefits

We found one systematic review (search date 1999), which identified one small RCT comparing salicylic acid versus placebo.[15] The RCT found no significant difference in psoriasis severity scores between the groups after 3 weeks. One further RCT (n = 408) found that the addition of salicylic acid to a topical corticosteroid preparation enhances efficacy in psoriasis.[16]

Harms

Topical salicylic acid may be absorbed through the skin and thus has the potential to cause systemic toxicity (salicylism). In practice, however, this seems to be rare. It may cause skin irritation and inflammation. Salicylic acid has been shown to interfere with ultraviolet B absorption into the skin and, in one RCT, the addition of salicylic acid to an emollient applied before ultraviolet B phototherapy was shown to decrease the rate of clearance of psoriasis.[17]

Comment

Topical salicylic acid is widely accepted as an effective keratolytic agent.

Tars

Small RCTs, some identified by a systematic review, provide insufficient evidence on the effects of topical coal tar preparations in comparison with placebo or other options.

Benefits

We found one systematic review (search date 1999; one RCT, 18 patients, severity of psoriasis not reported).[15] The RCT found no significant differences between coal tar and placebo in psoriasis severity scores after 4 weeks, but was probably too small to detect a clinically important difference.

Harms

Smell, staining, and burning are the main adverse effects of coal tar.

Comment

In the absence of convincing evidence, tars are often used as adjuncts to other treatments.

Dithranol

One systematic review of small RCTs found that topical dithranol (anthralin) improved chronic plaque psoriasis significantly more than placebo after 4–8 weeks. One systematic review of small RCTs found no significant difference between conventional and short-contact dithranol treatment, but the RCTs may have lacked power to detect clinically relevant differences.

Benefits

Dithranol versus placebo. We found one systematic review of topical preparations for the treatment of psoriasis (search date 1999, three small RCTs, number of patients and severity of psoriasis not reported).[15] It found that dithranol reduced psoriasis severity scores at 4–8 weeks significantly more than placebo.

Conventional versus short-contact treatment with dithranol. We found one systematic review, which assessed the quality of the methods used in published studies (search date 1989, 22 small RCTs) comparing conventional dithranol treatment with dithranol short-contact treatment (a shorter contact time at higher concentrations).[18] It reported no significant difference in outcomes between the groups, but stated that the trials were too small to detect clinically important differences (data not reported in the review, because its focus was on assessing study methods).

Harms

Staining and burning are the main reported adverse effects of dithranol.

Corticosteroids (topical)

We found evidence from a systematic review and additional RCTs that topical corticosteroids, especially "potent" and "very potent" ones, improved psoriasis in the short term in comparison with placebo. The evidence is limited to short-term effects, with a lack of information on maintenance, although it is well known that prolonged use of topical corticosteroids may cause striae and atrophy; steroid potency and occlusive dressings increase these risks.

Benefits

We found one systematic review of topical corticosteroid preparations for the treatment of psoriasis (search date 1999, 17 RCTs, 1686 patients, severity of psoriasis not reported)[15] and several subsequent RCTs. The subsequent RCTs did not offer any substantial new evidence about the role of topical steroids in people with psoriasis.

Clearance. The review found that "potent" and "very potent" topical corticosteroids significantly improved psoriasis sever-

ity scores in comparison with placebo.[15] The study duration was usually no longer than 4 weeks.

Topical corticosteroids plus occlusive dressings. Small RCTs found limited evidence that occlusive polyethylene or hydrocolloid dressings enhanced the clinical activity of topical corticosteroids.[19–21]

Combination therapies. We found evidence from RCTs that combination therapies were more effective than monotherapy: topical corticosteroids plus oral retinoids worked better than either treatment alone; "potent" topical corticosteroids plus vitamin D derivatives improved psoriasis and decreased irritation in the short term in comparison with either treatment alone or with placebo. Adding topical corticosteroids to tazarotene treatment improved the response rate in comparison with tazarotene alone.

Versus vitamin D derivatives. We found evidence of no significant difference in effectiveness between "potent" topical corticosteroids and vitamin D derivatives, although corticosteroids caused less perilesional and lesional irritation than calcipotriol.

Harms

Topical corticosteroids can cause striae and atrophy, which increase with clinical potency and use of occlusive dressings. Continuous use may lead to adrenocortical suppression.[22] Diminishing clinical response with repeated use of corticosteroids (tachyphylaxis) has been suggested, but not documented in a controlled study.

Comment

Topical corticosteroids are a treatment option for psoriasis of limited extent.

Vitamin D derivatives

One systematic review found that topical vitamin D derivatives improved plaque psoriasis in comparison with placebo. One systematic review found no significant difference in effectiveness between topical vitamin D derivatives (calcipotriol) and "potent" topical corticosteroids, but found that calcipotriol caused more perilesional and lesional irritation. In the short term, the combination of vitamin D derivatives plus topical corticosteroids decreased irritation in comparison with monotherapy. Insufficient evidence was available to assess other combination treatments.

Benefits

We found one systematic review (search date 1999, severity of psoriasis not reported).[15]

Vitamin D derivatives versus placebo. We found one systematic review (search date 1999, 14 RCTs, 1537 patients, severity of psoriasis not reported).[15] It found that both calcipotriol (vitamin D) and tacalcitol (a vitamin D derivative) were significantly more effective in improving psoriasis severity scores than placebo at 3–8 weeks.

Maintenance. We found one RCT (97 patients), which compared maintenance treatment with calcipotriol versus placebo in people who had stopped taking methotrexate.[23] The RCT found that calcipotriol significantly prolonged the time to relapse in comparison with placebo (relapse defined as doubling of baseline modified psoriasis severity score; median time to relapse 113 days with calcipotriol versus 35 days with placebo).

Different types of vitamin D derivatives versus each other. The systematic review[15] and subsequent RCTs provided evidence that calcipotriol twice daily was more effective than tacalcitol once daily or calcitriol.

Vitamin D derivatives versus topical corticosteroids. The systematic review found no significant difference in psoriasis severity scores between vitamin D derivatives and "potent" topical corticosteroids (nine RCTs, 1875 patients).

Vitamin D derivatives versus dithranol. The systematic review[15] and additional RCTs found that vitamin D derivatives reduced psoriasis severity scores significantly more than dithranol short-contact therapy at 4–12 weeks.

Vitamin D derivatives versus coal tar. The systematic review[15] found that calcipotriol improved psoriasis significantly more than either coal tar alone or a combination of coal tar, allantoin, and hydrocortisone at 6–8 weeks.

Vitamin D derivatives plus topical corticosteroids versus vitamin D derivatives alone. The systematic review[15] and additional RCTs found that calcipotriol plus "potent" topical corticosteroids reduced psoriasis severity scores significantly more than calcipotriol alone (three RCTs).

Harms
Perilesional irritation from calcipotriol has been reported in as many as 25% of patients, with the face and flexures being the most susceptible areas. Hypercalciuria is a dose-related side effect of therapy, and hypercalcemia may occur when large amounts of calcipotriol are applied to the skin.

Comments
Vitamin D derivatives are an option for the treatment of psoriasis of limited extension. There is a consensus that the dosage of calcipotriol cream 0.005% should be limited to 100 g a week.

Tazarotene
RCTs found that tazarotene, a topical retinoid, improved mild to moderate chronic plaque psoriasis in the short term in comparison with placebo. Four RCTs found that adding topical corticosteroids to tazarotene treatment improved the response rate in comparison with tazarotene alone. Tazarotene is contraindicated in women who are or intend to become pregnant, as it is potentially teratogenic.

Benefits
We found one systematic review[15] of tazarotene for treating psoriasis and nine additional RCTs (published in six papers).

Tazarotene versus placebo. Three RCTs (total of 1672 people with mild to moderate psoriasis) compared tazarotene versus placebo.[22,24,25] All found that tazarotene improved plaque psoriasis in comparison with placebo.

Tazarotene versus topical corticosteroids. One RCT found no significant difference between tazarotene and the potent topical corticosteroid fluocinonide in the reduction of lesion severity at 12 weeks.

Tazarotene plus topical corticosteroids versus tazarotene plus placebo. Three RCTs (including a total of 1198 patients with mild to moderate psoriasis) found that adding topical mid- or high-potency corticosteroids to tazarotene treatment significantly increased the response rate in comparison with tazarotene plus placebo.[26–28]

Tazarotene plus topical corticosteroids versus vitamin D analogues. One RCT (120 patients) found that once-daily treatment with tazarotene 0.1% plus topical mometasone furoate 0.1% significantly improved psoriasis symptoms after 2 weeks in comparison with twice-daily treatment with calcipotriol 0.005%.[29]

Harms
Some perilesional irritation is reported in most people using tazarotene.

Comment
Tazarotene is contraindicated in women who are or intend to become pregnant, as it is potentially teratogenic.

Heliotherapy
One RCT provided insufficient evidence on the effects of heliotherapy for chronic plaque psoriasis. Although we found limited evidence, there is a consensus that heliotherapy is an effective option for most people with chronic plaque psoriasis.

Benefit
We found one crossover RCT (95 patients with mild, moderate, or severe psoriasis), which compared 4 weeks of

supervised heliotherapy versus no intervention.[30] The pre-crossover results showed that heliotherapy significantly improved psoriasis in comparison with no intervention at 1 year.

Harms

Exposure to natural ultraviolet radiation is associated with photoaging and with skin cancer. In a 25-year follow-up of 1738 Danish patients with psoriasis who were treated with heliotherapy at the Dead Sea during 1972–73, the risks of basal cell and squamous cell carcinoma of the skin were 4.2 and 10.7 times higher, respectively, than those expected in the general population.[31] The authors point out that such patients will have had many other exposures to ultraviolet radiation, but there is clearly increased risk from exposure to sunlight.

Comments

Although we found limited evidence, there is a consensus that heliotherapy is an effective option for most people with chronic plaque psoriasis.

How effective are treatments for moderate and severe chronic plaque psoriasis?

Ultraviolet B (UVB)

RCTs provided insufficient evidence on the effects of ultraviolet B in comparison with placebo, other treatments, or on the effects of narrowband in comparison with broadband UVB for either clearance or maintenance treatment. One RCT found limited evidence that UVB given three times weekly cleared psoriasis faster than twice-weekly treatment, with high clearance rates in both groups. RCTs provided insufficient evidence to assess combination treatments using ultraviolet B plus emollients, dithranol, vitamin D analogues, or oral retinoids.

Benefit

UVB versus placebo or no treatment. We found no RCTs.

Narrowband UVB versus broad band UVB. We found one systematic review of patients with severe psoriasis (search date 1999, three small crossover RCTs, 146 people) of narrowband UVB versus broadband UVB.[9] It was not possible to calculate response rates from the results reported by the RCTs.

Twice-weekly versus three times weekly narrowband UVB. We found one RCT (including 113 patients with mild to moderate psoriasis).[32] It found no significant difference in clearance rates between twice-weekly and three times weekly UVB, but found that twice-weekly treatment significantly increased the time to reach clearance in comparison with three times weekly treatment (mean time to clearance: 88 days with twice-weekly *versus* 58 days with three times weekly treatment).

Maintenance treatment versus no maintenance treatment. One RCT (including 104 patients with initial clearance of symptoms) found that significantly more people were still clear of symptoms after 181 days with weekly UVB in comparison with no maintenance treatment (> 50% with UVB vs. 28% with no UVB).[33]

UVB (broadband or narrowband) versus psoralen ultraviolet A (PUVA). We found two RCTs.[34,35] The first RCT (183 patients with moderate to severe psoriasis) found no significant difference in clearance rates between PUVA and broadband UVB (clearance: 88% with PUVA vs. 80% with ultraviolet B). Subgroup analysis showed that broadband ultraviolet B radiation was significantly less effective in people with more than 50% body involvement. The second RCT (including 100 patients) found that more patients achieved clearance with PUVA in comparison with narrowband UVB (clearance: 84% with PUVA vs. 63% with UVB).

Harms

UVB radiation may increase photoaging and the risk of skin cancer. One systematic review (search date 1996) estimated that the excess annual risk of nonmelanoma skin cancer associated with UVB radiation was likely to be less than 2%.[36] Another systematic review (search date 2002, 11 prospective and retrospective cohort or case–control studies, 3400 people, most with psoriasis) also found limited evidence that UVB treatment increases the risk of skin cancer during a follow-up period of around 25 years.[37] There is as yet little evidence on whether narrowband UVB may be more or less harmful than broadband UVB.

Comments

Phototherapy is suitable for inducing remission of psoriasis, but not for long-term maintenance of remission. Exposure to ultraviolet radiation may increase the risks of developing skin cancer.

Psoralen ultraviolet A (PUVA)

There is a consensus that PUVA is effective for clearance of psoriasis. One systematic review identified no RCTs that compared PUVA with no treatment. The systematic review found that higher doses of psoralen improved psoriasis clearance more than lower doses of psoralen. One large RCT found that maintenance treatment with PUVA reduced relapse rates in comparison with no maintenance treatment. RCTs provided insufficient evidence to compare PUVA with other treatments or to assess PUVA combined with other modalities. Long-term adverse effects of PUVA treatment include photoaging and skin cancer (mainly squamous cell carcinoma).

Benefit
We found one systematic review of phototherapy and photochemotherapy in people with severe psoriasis (search date 1999, 51 RCTs).[9] The results could not be pooled due to the heterogeneity of the trials.

PUVA versus no treatment. The systematic review found no RCTs.

Comparison of different doses of psoralen in PUVA regimens. The systematic review (two RCTs, 167 people) concluded that higher-dose psoralen significantly increased success (major improvement or full remission) in comparison with lower-dose psoralen.

Comparison of different oral psoralens in PUVA regimens. The systematic review included two RCTs that compared different oral psoralens. One RCT (including 169 patients) found no significant difference between 5-methoxsalen 1.2 mg/kg and 8-methoxsalen 0.6 mg/kg in the mean cumulative ultraviolet A dose needed for clearance. The other RCT (including 38 patients) found that patients treated with 8-methoxsalen 0.6 mg/kg required a lower mean cumulative ultraviolet A dose to achieve success than those treated with 1.2 mg/kg 5-methoxsalen.

Comparison of different topical psoralens in PUVA regimens. The systematic review included one RCT (38 people), which found no significant difference between 5-methoxsalen and 8-methoxsalen in the mean total dose of ultraviolet A required for clearance.

Comparison of oral versus bath psoralen formulations in PUVA regimen. The systematic review identified two RCTs (137 people), which found no significant difference in the success rate, but found a significantly greater mean cumulative ultraviolet A dose for clearance with oral in comparison with topical psoralens.

Comparison of dose setting strategies in PUVA regimens. The systematic review included two RCTs (157 patients), which compared the routine use of the minimal phototoxic dose of ultraviolet A at each treatment versus a strategy of setting the ultraviolet A dose according to skin type.[38] Neither study found any significant difference in relation to the success rate (clearance).

PUVA versus psoralen plus UVB. The systematic review included five RCTs (285 people). The largest RCT (100 people) found no significant difference between PUVA twice weekly and psoralen plus narrowband ultraviolet B twice weekly (absolute risk reduction for clearance +12%; 95% CI, −4% to +28%).

PUVA or UVB versus topical or systemic treatments (dithranol, tar, vitamin D analogues, corticosteroids, and fish oil). The systematic review included 25 RCTs (1268 patients), which compared different combinations of ultraviolet radiation with systemic or topical treatments, including dithranol, tar, vitamin D analogues, corticosteroids, and fish oil. The RCTs were mostly small and underpowered to detect clinically important differences. The largest of the RCTs (224 patients) found that PUVA cleared psoriasis significantly more often than dithranol.

Maintenance. One large RCT (1005 patients whose psoriasis had been cleared by PUVA) found that maintenance treatment with PUVA reduced relapse rates at 18 months in comparison with no maintenance (rate of flares 27% with treatment once a week *versus* 34% with treatment once every 3 weeks versus 62% with no treatment).[39]

Harms
The best evidence on chronic toxicity comes from an ongoing study of more than 1300 patients who first received PUVA treatment in 1975.[40] The study found a dose-dependent increased risk of squamous cell carcinoma, basal cell carcinoma, and possibly malignant melanoma in comparison with the risk in the general population. After less than 15 years, about a quarter of people exposed to 300 or more treatments of PUVA had at least one squamous cell carcinoma of the skin, with particularly high risk in people with skin phototypes I and II. A systematic review (search date 1998) of eight additional studies has confirmed the findings concerning squamous cell carcinoma.[41] A combined analysis of two cohort studies (944 people treated with bath PUVA) found no increase in the risk of squamous cell carcinoma after a mean follow up of 14.7 years (standardized incidence ratio 1.1; 95% CI, 0.2 to 3.2), suggesting that bath PUVA is possibly safer than conventional PUVA.[42] Premature photoaging is another expected adverse effect. In people who wear ultraviolet A–opaque glasses for 24 hours after psoralen ingestion, the risk of cataract development appears to be negligible.

Comments
There is a consensus that PUVA is effective for clearance of psoriasis, but that the risks of skin cancer limit the number of lifetime exposures that may safely be offered to people with psoriasis. People receiving PUVA need close monitoring for long-term cutaneous carcinogenic effects.

Retinoids (oral etretinate, acitretin)
One systematic review of people with severe psoriasis found limited evidence that clearance rates with oral retinoids were higher than with placebo but lower than with ciclosporin. RCTs provided insufficient evidence on the effects of oral retinoids as maintenance treatment. Adverse effects

frequently led to discontinuation of oral retinoid treatment. Teratogenicity is a problem in women of childbearing age. Etretinate is no longer available in many countries.

Benefit

We found one systematic review of patients with severe psoriasis (search date 1999, 32 RCTs; 13 of etretinate, 11 of acitretin, eight of acitretin versus etretinate).[9]

Etretinate versus placebo. The review included four RCTs. Three RCTs found that etretinate 1 mg/kg significantly increased response rates in comparison with placebo.

Acitretin versus placebo. Results were extractable for only two of the RCTs comparing acitretin with placebo. One RCT (including 38 patients) was underpowered and found no significant difference between acitretin and placebo. The other RCT (including 80 patients) found that higher doses of acitretin (25 mg or 50 mg) significantly increased the proportion of people who achieved a 75% or greater decrease in PASI (60% with 25 mg acitretin versus 25% with placebo).[38]

Acitretin versus etretinate. The review identified six RCTs (598 patients), which found no significant difference between acitretin and etretinate in the proportion of patients achieving marked improvement or total clearance.

Etretinate versus ciclosporin. The review included two RCTs (286 people) comparing higher or lower doses of etretinate versus ciclosporin, and the results could not be pooled. The RCT using the higher dose of etretinate (0.7 mg/kg) found that significantly fewer people treated with etretinate than with ciclosporin 5 mg/kg achieved a marked response (people with = 75% decrease in PASI: 97% with ciclosporin vs. 73% with etretinate).

Maintenance therapy versus placebo. The review identified two RCTs. One of the RCTs (36 patients achieving clearance with PUVA plus etretinate) found that low-dose etretinate (half of the maximum dose tolerated) significantly reduced relapse rates over 1 year in comparison with placebo: absence of relapse in nine of 16 (56%) with etretinate versus three of 20 (5%) with placebo. The second RCT (80 patients) found no significant difference in percentage changes to PASI scores between three dosages of acitretin (10 vs. 25 vs. 50 mg daily) and placebo at 6 months.

Harms

Adverse effects led to discontinuation of oral retinoid treatment in 10–20% of people.[9] Most people experience mucocutaneous adverse effects, such as dry skin, cheilitis, and conjunctivitis. Mucocutaneous effects are generally mild. Increased serum cholesterol and triglyceride concentrations occurred in about half of the people. Low-grade hepatotoxicity was observed in about 1% of people treated with etretinate.[43] Occasionally, acute hepatitis occurred, possibly as an idiosyncratic hypersensitivity reaction. Radiographic evidence of extraspinal tendon and ligament calcifications has been documented. In one cohort study, a quarter of 956 patients treated with etretinate attributed a joint problem or its worsening to the drug.[43] Etretinate is a known teratogen and may be detected in the plasma for up to 2–3 years after treatment stops. Acitretin can undergo esterification to etretinate.

Comments

Women of childbearing age should be given effective contraception for 1 month before starting etretinate or acitretin, throughout treatment, for 2 years after stopping acitretin treatment, and for 3 years after stopping etretinate treatment. Etretinate is no longer available in many countries.

Methotrexate

One small RCT provided insufficient evidence about the effects of methotrexate in comparison with placebo. One RCT found no significant difference between methotrexate and ciclosporin in complete or partial remission, duration of remission of psoriasis, or adverse effects. Long-term methotrexate treatment carries a risk of hepatic fibrosis and cirrhosis, which is related to the dose regimen employed.

Benefit

Methotrexate versus placebo. We found one systematic review (search date 2000).[44] It identified one small RCT (randomization method and concealment not stated; 37 patients with psoriatic arthritis), which found that oral methotrexate 7.5–15.0 mg/week significantly reduced the surface area of psoriasis after 12 weeks in comparison with placebo.

Methotrexate versus ciclosporin. We found one single-blinded RCT (88 patients), which compared oral methotrexate (up to 22.5 mg per week) versus ciclosporin (up to 5 mg/kg per day).[45] It found no significant difference between methotrexate and ciclosporin with regard to complete remission: the rate of complete remission was 17 of 43 (40%) with methotrexate versus 14 of 42 (33%) with ciclosporin. It also found no significant difference between the groups with regard to the duration of either complete or partial remission. However, it is likely to have been underpowered to detect clinically important differences between groups.

Harms

The commonest symptomatic side effect of low-dose methotrexate therapy is nausea, which may affect up to one-third of treated patients. Its most important potential side effect is acute myelosuppression, which is the cause of most of the rare deaths attributable to it when used as a therapy for psoriasis.[46] Methotrexate is eliminated largely via the kidneys, and toxic levels may build up rapidly in the presence of renal impairment. Particular care is required in the elderly, in whom renal function may deteriorate rapidly in response to acute illness; dietary folate deficiency may add to the toxicity. Recent work has shown that circulating homocysteine levels are elevated in psoriasis patients receiving methotrexate, but that folate supplementation can reverse this abnormality; since raised homocysteine levels have been associated with atherothrombotic vascular disease, it may therefore be advisable for all patients on methotrexate to receive folate supplementation.[47] Certain drugs, particularly nonsteroidal anti-inflammatory agents, aspirin, trimethoprim, and sulfonamides, may interfere with methotrexate pharmacokinetics and thus increase the risk of toxicity, particularly in the presence of impaired renal function. Long-term methotrexate treatment carries with it a risk of hepatic fibrosis and cirrhosis, which is related to the dosage regimen employed. The original method of administering methotrexate in small daily doses was shown to be much more hepatotoxic than the same overall amount given as a single weekly dose. One systematic review (search date not reported) found that about 28% (95% CI, 24% to 32%) of people taking long-term methotrexate for psoriasis and rheumatoid arthritis developed liver fibrosis of histological grade I or higher on liver biopsy, whereas 5% developed advanced liver disease (histological grade IIIB or IV).[48] The risk was dose-related and was higher with increased alcohol consumption. A limitation of the systematic review was the lack of untreated control groups. The Psoriasis Task Force of the American Academy of Dermatology recommends that liver biopsy should be carried out in psoriasis patients after treatment has been established and then after each cumulative dose of 1.5 g methotrexate—in practice about every 18 months to 2 years for the average patient.[49] Others have argued that the morbidity and potential hazards of performing regular liver biopsy in patients receiving long-term low-dose methotrexate for psoriasis are difficult to justify when measured against the low yield of information resulting in a change of management.[50] A number of researchers have recommended that a serological marker of hepatic fibrosis, the aminoterminal peptide of type III procollagen, can be used to screen for underlying hepatic damage and that liver biopsy may then be reserved for those with consistently abnormal results.[51]

Pulmonary disease associated with methotrexate has been described as an acute or chronic interstitial pneumonitis.[38] Adverse pulmonary effects of treatment are considered much rarer in psoriasis than in rheumatoid arthritis, but we found no published evidence to support this claim. Methotrexate appears to double the risk of developing squamous cell carcinoma in patients exposed to psoralen plus ultraviolet A and may be an independent risk factor for this type of cancer in patients with psoriatic arthritis.[52] A higher risk of lymphoproliferative diseases in long-term users has been suggested by a few case reports. On the basis of data from a large case series (248 patients), the cumulative incidence of lymphoma is not expected to be much higher than 1%.[53]

Comments
Methotrexate continues to play an important role in the management of severe psoriasis, despite the advent of newer agents. It would appear to be particularly valuable for patients with concomitant arthritis. It is probably safer overall for long-term use than other therapies such as ciclosporin and PUVA. Patients using methotrexate should be closely monitored for liver toxicity and should be advised to limit their consumption of alcohol. The most reliable test of liver damage is still needle biopsy of the liver. It is rare for life-threatening liver disease to develop with the first 1.0–1.5 g of methotrexate.

Hydroxyurea
Hydroxyurea is a systemic therapy for severe psoriasis, which is mainly used in place of more commonly used systemic agents such as ciclosporin or methotrexate when these are contraindicated. Hydroxyurea has not been directly compared with other systemic therapies. Side effects include bone-marrow suppression and teratogenicity.

Benefits
One systematic review (search date 1999, one RCT, 10 patients) identified only one RCT.[9] This compared hydroxyurea 1.0 g daily with matching placebo, each given for 4 weeks in a crossover study including 10 patients. Improvement was noted by the investigators in seven of the 10, and by the participants in nine of 10 periods of active therapy as opposed to only one of 10 periods of placebo therapy.

Harms
The doses of hydroxyurea that have been advocated for psoriasis are close to those that may cause marrow suppression. There is little information on long-term toxicity.

Comment
There is a need for better-quality RCTs of hydroxyurea both in comparison with placebo and in comparison with other systemic agents.

Azathioprine
Oral azathioprine has been used to a limited extent for treating severe psoriasis for many years, but there is little evidence to support its use. It may cause catastrophic myelosuppression. Its efficacy has not been compared in RCTs with either placebo or other systemic therapies.

Benefit

One systematic review[9] and an additional search failed to identify any RCTs of azathioprine treatment in psoriasis.

Harms

In people who are unable to metabolize the drug normally due to a deficiency in thiopurine methyltransferase, there is a high risk of catastrophic bone-marrow suppression. Nausea and vomiting are common. Drug-induced hepatitis may occur.

Comment

There are no data to support a role for azathioprine in psoriasis.

Sulfasalazine

Sulfasalazine is an anti-inflammatory agent that is widely used for the treatment of inflammatory polyarthritides. The findings in one RCT suggest that it is a moderately effective treatment for severe psoriasis.

Benefit

A systematic review (search date 1999)[9] identified one RCT comparing sulfasalazine 3–4 g daily for 8 weeks with placebo. The drug produced a marked improvement (> 60% improvement) in seven of 23 patients (30%), in comparison with none of the 27 who received placebo.

Harms

The most common side effects are headache, nausea, and vomiting. In general, these are dose-related.

Comment

Further RCTs are justified to assess the place of sulfasalazine in the management of psoriasis.

Ciclosporin

One systematic review of patients with severe psoriasis found that ciclosporin improved clearance in comparison with placebo and increased the proportion of people who remained in remission. Dose-related increases in hypertension and renal failure are the main adverse effects of its use in psoriasis.

Benefit

We found one systematic review of patients with severe psoriasis (search date 1999, 18 RCTs; 13 on induction of remission, five on maintenance of remission).[9] Success was defined mostly as a reduction in the Psoriasis Area and Severity Index (PASI) score, or clinical criteria such as "clearance."

Ciclosporin versus placebo for clearance. The review included six RCTs (289 patients). It found that there was signific-

antly greater success with ciclosporin treatment than with placebo. The dosages of ciclosporin ranged from 1.25 to 14 mg/kg daily. The duration of treatment ranged from 4 to 12 weeks. The data could not be pooled.

Ciclosporin versus placebo for maintenance. The review included five RCTs of treatment to maintain remission. Two RCTs compared two doses of ciclosporin (1.5 mg/kg or 3.0 mg/kg daily) versus placebo. Both RCTs found that 3.0 mg/kg daily ciclosporin was better than placebo for maintaining remission. The third RCT compared two different ciclosporin formulations and found no significant difference in the response after 24 weeks between an oil-based and microemulsion preconcentrate formulation. The fourth RCT (400 patients) found that tapering the ciclosporin dose marginally increased the time to relapse in comparison with abrupt stopping of ciclosporin (time to relapse 113 days with tapered ciclosporin versus 109 days with abrupt stopping; $P = 0.038$). The fifth RCT (37 patients) found that, over the 36 months of treatment, continuous ciclosporin was more effective for maintaining remission than intermittent ciclosporin (remission maintained for 69% of the observation period with continuous ciclosporin versus 32% with intermittent treatment).

Comparison of different ciclosporin formulations. The review identified two RCTs (345 patients, 12 weeks, one with a crossover design). They found no significant difference in the proportion of people achieving a marked response (≥ 75% decrease in PASI) between the conventional oil-based ciclosporin formulation and the microemulsion preconcentrate formulation.

Ciclosporin versus etretinate. See benefits of retinoids versus ciclosporin.

Ciclosporin versus methotrexate. See benefits of methotrexate versus ciclosporin.

Harms

The review found that ciclosporin was associated with dose-related increases in hypertension and reduced renal function.[9] Observational evidence suggests that the incidence of these adverse events increases over time. In a case-series follow-up study of 122 consecutive patients treated continuously with ciclosporin for 3–76 months at dosages not exceeding 5 mg/kg daily, 104 patients discontinued treatment.[54] The mean percentage of patients who discontinued treatment due to adverse effects (mostly renal dysfunction and hypertension) rose from 14% at 12 months to 41% at 48 months. One prospective cohort study documented an increased risk of malignancies in 152 people with psoriasis treated with ciclosporin for up to 5 years. Malignancies were diagnosed in 3.8% of patients, with a standardized incidence ratio of 2.1 in comparison with the general population. There was a sixfold increase in the incidence of skin cancer in comparison with the general population, while non-skin malignancies did not show a significantly increased risk.[55]

Comments

Ciclosporin is an established treatment option for moderate to severe psoriasis. Relapses are often seen on withdrawal, and long-term treatment is limited by adverse effects (mainly renal dysfunction and hypertension).

Leflunomide

One RCT in patients with psoriatic arthritis found limited evidence that leflunomide improved cutaneous psoriasis in comparison with placebo.

Benefit

We found one RCT (190 patients with active psoriatic arthritis and psoriasis with at least 3% involvement) comparing oral leflunomide (100 mg/day loading dose followed by 20 mg/day) with placebo for 24 weeks.[56] It found that leflunomide significantly increased the proportion of people with at least a 75% improvement in PASI score in comparison with placebo (17% with leflunomide versus 8% with placebo; $P < 0.05$).

Harms

More people taking leflunomide had increased liver enzymes (alanine transaminase increase of two or more times the upper limit of normal: 12% with leflunomide versus 5% with placebo).

Comments

Leflunomide is currently primarily used in people with psoriatic arthritis; the effects of treatment in people with psoriasis remain unclear, but response rates appear to be low.

Etanercept

Etanercept is a recombinant molecule comprising the human tumor necrosis factor-α p75 receptor fused to the Fc portion of the human immunoglobulin G1 molecule. RCTs found that the proportion of responders at 12–24 weeks was greater with etanercept than with placebo. Etanercept is a relatively new drug for the treatment of psoriasis, and there is limited evidence about the risks of long-term or rare but severe adverse events.

Benefit

Etanercept versus placebo. We found no systematic reviews and four RCTs, reported in six publications.[57–62] A 75% improvement in the Psoriasis Area and Severity Index (PASI) score at 12–24 weeks was seen in a significantly greater proportion of patients receiving etanercept than in those receiving placebo. Quality-of-life scores also improved significantly more in the etanercept groups than in the placebo groups.

Harms

Most of the evidence on the safety of etanercept is from studies in people with rheumatoid arthritis or Crohn's disease. Cutaneous reactions to etanercept have been reported with a frequency of up to 5%, including reactions at the injection site and urticarial manifestations. Severe infections have been reported with etanercept.

Comments

The amount of good evidence on the effects of etanercept in people with plaque psoriasis is still limited. Further comparative studies are needed in order to predict precisely how this drug will fit into current psoriasis management.

Infliximab

Infliximab is a monoclonal antibody that binds to and inhibits the activity of tumor necrosis factor alpha. RCTs in people with severe psoriasis found that infliximab improved response rates after a few weeks in comparison with placebo. Infliximab is a relatively new drug for the treatment of psoriasis, and there is limited evidence regarding the possibility of long-term or rare but severe adverse events.

Benefit

Infliximab versus placebo. We found no systematic reviews and three RCTs, reported in five publications.[63–67] Infliximab at a dose of 3–5 mg/kg at 0, 2, and 6 weeks followed by maintenance therapy every 8 weeks produced higher rates of response in comparison with placebo.

Harms

Most of the evidence on the safety of infliximab is from studies in people with rheumatoid arthritis or Crohn's disease. We found one systematic review (search date 2005; nine RCTs, 3493 patients receiving active treatment, 1512 people receiving placebo) on adverse events with anti-tumor necrosis factor antibodies, infliximab, and adalimumab, in patients with rheumatoid arthritis.[68] Pooled analysis for infliximab and adalimumab suggested an increased risk of malignancies (OR 3.3; 95% CI, 1.2 to 9.1; numbers needed to harm 154, 95% CI, 91 to 500 for one additional malignancy with a treatment period of 6–12 months; absolute data not reported) and severe infections (OR 2.0; 95% CI, 1.3 to 3.1; NNH 59, 95% CI, 39 to 125 for one additional severe infection over a treatment period of 3–12 months). A few cases of lupus-like syndrome have been reported with infliximab treatment.

Comments
The amount of good evidence on the effects of infliximab in people with plaque psoriasis is still limited. Further comparative studies are needed to predict precisely how this drug will fit into current psoriasis management.

Alefacept
Alefacept is a recombinant protein that binds to the CD2 receptor on memory effector T lymphocytes. RCTs found that alefacept improved psoriasis in a greater proportion of recipients than did placebo. Alefacept is a relatively new drug for the treatment of psoriasis, and there is limited evidence regarding the possibility of long-term or rare severe adverse effects.

Benefit
Alefacept versus placebo. We found no systematic reviews and three RCTs, described in at least six publications.[69–74] Intramuscular or intravenous alefacept at a dose of 10–15 mg once weekly significantly improved psoriasis in comparison with placebo.

Harms
One integrated analysis of 13 clinical trials (including six double-blind RCTs and five open-label studies) found that the most commonly reported adverse events during alefacept treatment were headache (≥ 14%), nasopharyngitis (7–25%), influenza (up to 8%), upper respiratory tract infection (≥ 12.5%), and pruritus. Fewer than 1% of patients developed serious infections, and the analysis found no clear relation with CD4+ T-lymphocyte counts.[75]

Comments
Alefacept is a new drug for the treatment of psoriasis. Further comparative studies are needed in order to predict precisely how this drug will fit into current psoriasis management. The response rates appear to be low.

Efalizumab
Efalizumab is a humanized monoclonal antibody that targets the CD11a component of lymphocyte function–associated antigen-1. RCTs found that efalizumab was more effective than placebo at 12 weeks.

Benefit
Efalizumab versus placebo. We found no systematic reviews and five RCTs, published in seven papers.[76–82] The RCTs showed that subcutaneous efalizumab 1–2 mg/kg weekly for 12 weeks significantly improved psoriasis in a greater proportion of recipients than did placebo. The effects were maintained on extended treatment after 24 weeks; however, only a subset of patients completed the treatment period.

Harms
The most common acute adverse events were headache, rigor, pyrexia, and myalgia. Rebound flares of psoriasis have been also reported. There are reports of immune-mediated hemolytic anemia, thrombocytopenia, serious infections, and polyneuropathy.

Comments
Efalizumab is a relatively new drug for the treatment of psoriasis. Further comparative studies are needed in order to predict precisely how these drugs will fit into current psoriasis management.

Fumaric acid derivatives
One systematic review in people with severe psoriasis found limited evidence that oral fumaric acid esters reduced the severity of psoriasis in comparison with placebo. Acute adverse effects were common and included flushing and gastrointestinal symptoms.

Benefit
Fumaric acid derivatives versus placebo. We found one systematic review of people with severe psoriasis (search date 1999, four placebo-controlled RCTs, 203 patients).[9] Two of the RCTs (123 people) compared a mixture of dimethylfumaric and monoethylfumaric acid esters versus placebo. Pooled analysis found that this mixture of fumaric acid derivatives reduced severity significantly more than placebo at 16 weeks. The remaining RCTs published in a single paper documented that the response to dimethylfumaric acid ester was significantly greater than placebo at 16 weeks, whereas the response to monoethylfumaric acid ester was no greater than to placebo.

Harms
All of the RCTs had high withdrawal rates. Acute adverse effects, including flushing and gastrointestinal symptoms, were reported in up to 75% of the patients. Additional adverse effects include diarrhea, stomach cramps, flushing, and skin burning. There have been a few case reports of renal failure associated with high starting doses.

Comments
Fumaric acid derivatives are not available in many European countries or in the USA.

Ingram regimen
The Ingram regimen consists of a daily application of dithranol paste (sometimes in combination with coal tar bath) plus ultraviolet B irradiation. One systematic review suggested that its efficacy in clearing psoriasis is similar to that of psoralen photochemotherapy (PUVA).

Benefit

Ingram regimen versus placebo or no treatment. We found no RCTs.

Ingram regimen versus PUVA. We found one systematic review (search date 1999) examining treatment for severe psoriasis, which identified one RCT comparing the Ingram regimen with psoralen photochemotherapy (PUVA) in 224 people with psoriasis.[9] The difference in success rates was not significant, but the time required for clearance was significantly greater in the PUVA-treated group (34.4 ± 1.8 days) than in the Ingram group (20.4 ± 0.9 days).

Harms

Local irritation and staining of the skin often occur.

Comments

In spite of the limited evidence, there is a consensus that the Ingram regimen is an efficacious treatment for psoriasis.

Goeckerman treatment

Goeckerman treatment consists of a daily application of coal tar followed by ultraviolet B irradiation. Two small RCTs provided insufficient evidence on Goeckerman treatment in chronic plaque psoriasis.

Benefit

Goeckerman treatment versus placebo or no treatment. We found no RCTs.

Goeckerman treatment versus UVB alone. We found one systematic review (search date 1999, one RCT, 49 patients with severe psoriasis)[9] and one additional RCT[83] (22 patients) comparing Goeckerman treatment with UVB alone. The two RCTs found no evidence that adding coal tar to UVB improved the response rates in comparison with UVB alone.

Harms

Local irritation often occurs.

Comments

We found no good evidence to support the use of Goeckerman treatment for psoriasis.

How effective are treatments for guttate psoriasis?

We found two systematic reviews from the same group of investigators; one examined antistreptococcal interventions for both guttate and chronic plaque psoriasis (search date 2000, one RCT, 20 patients) whilst the second examined other interventions for guttate psoriasis (search date 2000, one RCT, 21 patients).[84,85]

Antistreptococcal interventions
Benefits

Antibiotic therapy. Despite recommendations in many standard texts that antibiotics should be given to patients with recurrent guttate psoriasis, the only RCT examining their use found no evidence of benefit in any patient receiving either of two antibiotic regimens.[86]

Tonsillectomy. No RCTs examining the effects of tonsillectomy on the recurrence or persistence of guttate psoriasis were found.

Harms

There is insufficient information. Tonsillectomy carries with it a small risk of a serious adverse outcome.

Comments

There is no available evidence that antistreptococcal interventions improve guttate psoriasis.

Other interventions
Benefits

The reviews identified no trials of standard therapies (tar, topical corticosteroids, vitamin D analogues, phototherapy) for guttate psoriasis, but one study with omega-3 fatty acids.

Omega-3 fatty acids. One RCT (n = 21) compared the effects of daily intravenous infusions of lipid-rich emulsions containing either fish-oil derived omega-3 fatty acids or placebo (omega-6 fatty acids) in hospitalized patients with acute guttate psoriasis. The former produced a rapid beneficial effect (improvement in severity scores of between 45% and 76% over 10 days) not seen in patients receiving omega-6 supplementation (16% to 25% over 10 days).[87] It is not known whether oral supplementation with omega-3 fatty acids would have similar effects.

Harms

There is insufficient information.

Comments

There is very little information to guide practice, particularly with regard to the place of and optimal regimen for phototherapy in guttate psoriasis.

How effective are treatments for chronic palmoplantar pustulosis?

We found one systematic review examining interventions for chronic palmoplantar pustulosis (search date 2006, 23 RCTs, 724 patients).[88]

Topical corticosteroids, with and without occlusion

Moderately potent corticosteroids under hydrocolloid occlusion may induce rapid clearance of chronic palmoplantar pustulosis; such therapy is more effective than superpotent corticosteroids without occlusion.

Benefits
In one RCT (n = 19) identified in the review, 12 of 19 sides receiving medium-strength corticosteroid under hydrocolloid occlusion for 4 weeks cleared, in comparison with three of 19 sides receiving highly potent corticosteroid twice daily. Relapse to pretreatment severity occurred within 4 weeks of discontinuing therapy.

Harms
Prolonged use of potent corticosteroids results in skin atrophy.

Comments
Because of side effects and the rapid relapse seen after interruption of therapy, topical corticosteroids are likely to be helpful mainly as an adjunct to other interventions.

Systemic retinoid monotherapy
Systemic retinoids are widely used for treating chronic palmoplantar pustulosis. Most of the available studies were carried out when etretinate was available, but this has now been replaced by acitretin.

Benefits
High-dose retinoid versus placebo for induction of remission. The review identified four RCTs including 127 patients.[88] They found that about two in five patients achieve a good or excellent response on etretinate or acitretin.

Low-dose retinoid versus placebo for maintenance of remission. The review identified two RCTs including 45 people. Thirteen of 21 patients (62%) who had responded to initial high-dose etretinate therapy (1.0 mg/kg body weight/day) maintained clinical remission for 3 months with low-dose etretinate (20–30 mg daily), in comparison with five of 24 (21%) who received placebo.

Acitretin versus etretinate. One RCT (n = 60) found no difference in the efficacy of the two retinoids, as judged by the reduction in pustule counts.

Versus PUVA. Two RCTs including 121 patients compared etretinate with PUVA (both topical and systemic) and documented that etretinate is more effective than PUVA.

Harms
Systemic retinoids have well-known mucocutaneous side effects that limit their acceptability to many patients. They are teratogenic.

Comments
Both etretinate and acitretin are unsuitable for use in women at risk of pregnancy.

Photochemotherapy alone
The review[88] found little evidence concerning both topical psoralen and systemic photochemotherapy.

Benefit
Versus placebo. Four RCTs including 90 patients compared either topical or systemic PUVA with placebo. Fifteen of 36 patients (42%) receiving oral PUVA cleared, in comparison with none of 36 (0%) receiving placebo. One of 54 patients (2%) receiving topical PUVA cleared, in comparison with none of 54 (0%) receiving placebo.

Topical PUVA versus systemic PUVA. In the one RCT identified (n = 64), four of 51 patients (8%) cleared with topical PUVA, in comparison with none of 13 (0%) who received systemic PUVA: success rate difference 0.08 (95% CI, −0.05 to 0.21).

Versus retinoids. See above.

Harms
Topical PUVA was found to cause blistering and irritation of the skin in a minority of treated patients.

Comments
Photochemotherapy has limited effects in palmoplantar pustulosis.

Combined retinoid and photochemotherapy (RePUVA)
The review[88] identified three RCTs examining the combination of PUVA and retinoid treatment.

Benefits
The combination was more effective than either PUVA or retinoids alone.

Harms
Although patients are exposed to the risks of both retinoids and PUVA, there is some evidence that lower doses of UVA are required than when PUVA monotherapy is used.

Comments
This modality is the most effective treatment available for achieving remission of palmoplantar pustulosis.

Ciclosporin
The review found two RCTs that provided limited evidence of a short-term effect of ciclosporin.

Benefits

Two RCTs (n = 98) of short duration (4 weeks) using low doses of ciclosporin (1 and 2.5 mg/kg b.w./day respectively) were found. Thirty of 47 patients (64%) receiving ciclosporin improved, in comparison with 10 of 51 (20%) receiving placebo.

Harms

Ciclosporin has well-known side effects, including hypertension and renal impairment.

Comments

Further studies are required in order to establish the place of this drug in the management of chronic palmoplantar pustulosis. Uncontrolled studies have reported good to excellent results in patients treated for longer periods at higher doses if required (e.g., more than two-thirds with a good or excellent response at 1 year in 58 patients receiving up to 4 mg/kg b.w./day for a year).[89]

Tetracycline antibiotics

There is evidence from RCTs that oral tetracyclines induce limited improvement in chronic palmoplantar pustulosis.

Benefits

Two RCTs with a crossover design (240 treatment courses in 100 patients) were identified in the review.[88] Overall, improvement was seen in 58 of 120 tetracycline treatment courses (48%) in comparison with 23 of 120 placebo courses (19%).

Harms

Tetracyclines are normally well tolerated, but may cause gastrointestinal upset.

Other therapies that have been advocated for chronic palmoplantar pustulosis psoriasis

The review[88] identified limited benefit from grenz ray therapy and little to support the use of tar, anthralin, colchicine, or methotrexate.

How effective are treatments for acropustulosis (acrodermatitis continua of Hallopeau)?

We found no RCTs of treatments for this uncommon but disabling pustular form of psoriasis, which can cause marked destruction of fingernails, toenails, and surrounding tissues. The largest number of published case reports in which a successful response to treatment is claimed is for ciclosporin, although in individual case reports acitretin, methotrexate, and dapsone have been reported to produce resolution.

Key points

The main limitation of the available evidence is the lack of trials comparing different therapeutic options and the short-term duration of most studies.

Chronic plaque psoriasis

- There is firm RCT evidence of short-term effectiveness of a range of treatments for chronic plaque psoriasis, specifically:
  —Calcipotriol
  —Topical steroids
  —Tazarotene
  —Ciclosporin
  —Systemic retinoids (acitretin and etretinate), especially in combination with phototherapy
  —Phototherapy, including broadband ultraviolet B (UVB), narrowband UVB, and psoralen photochemotherapy (PUVA)
  —Fumaric acid esters
  —Methotrexate, although the effectiveness of this widely accepted drug has been examined specifically in chronic plaque psoriasis in only one RCT.
- A number of new treatment options have been added in recent years, collectively grouped as "biological treatments" or "biologics," as opposed to "conventional treatment." These include: alefacept, efalizumab, etanercept, and infliximab. Additional new options are expected in the near future (e.g., adalimumab). There is a lack of evidence on the comparative value of these new options and limited data on safety.
- There is a lack of firm RCT evidence of the effectiveness of other therapies for chronic plaque psoriasis, including coal tar, tacalcitol, azathioprine, hydroxyurea, and sulfasalazine (although one small RCT has shown moderate efficacy with sulfasalazine).
- There is good evidence of a risk of serious harm from the major treatment modalities used for treating severe psoriasis, including skin cancer with PUVA and heliotherapy, hypertension and renal impairment with ciclosporin, myelosuppression and hepatic fibrosis with methotrexate, and teratogenicity with systemic retinoids.

Guttate psoriasis

- There is virtually no guidance from controlled trials on how to manage guttate psoriasis.

Palmoplantar pustular psoriasis

- There is no ideal treatment for chronic palmoplantar pustular psoriasis, but there is RCT evidence to support the use of topical corticosteroid under hydrocolloid occlusion, systemic retinoids, systemic PUVA, and systemic retinoids in combination with systemic PUVA. Of these, the last appears to provide the greatest chance of disease control.
- There is some evidence that modest improvements may be attained with low-dose ciclosporin or tetracycline.
- There is little evidence to support the use of colchicine, topical PUVA, hydroxyurea, or methotrexate.

References

1 Franssen MJAM, van den Hoogen FHJ, van de Putte LBA. Psoriatic arthropathy. In: van de Kerkhof PCM, editor. *Textbook of Psoriasis*. Oxford: Blackwell Science, 1999:30–42.

2 Telfer NR, Chalmers RJ, Whale K, Colman G. The role of streptococcal infection in the initiation of guttate psoriasis. *Arch Dermatol* 1992;**128**:39–42.

3 Asumalahti K, Ameen M, Suomela S, *et al.* Genetic analysis of PSORS1 distinguishes guttate psoriasis and palmoplantar pustulosis. *J Invest Dermatol* 2003;**120**:627–32.

4 Naldi L. Epidemiology of psoriasis. *Curr Drug Targets Inflamm Allergy* 2004;**3**:121–8.

5 Giardina E, Sinibaldi C, Novelli G. The psoriasis genetics as a model of complex disease. *Curr Drug Targets Inflamm Allergy* 2004;**3**:129–36.

6 Mallbris L, Akre O, Granath F, *et al.* Increased risk for cardiovascular mortality in psoriasis inpatients but not in outpatients. *Eur J Epidemiol* 2004;**19**:225–30.

7 Sommer D, Jenisch S, Suchan M, Christophers E, Weichenthal M. Increased prevalence of the metabolic syndrome in patients with moderate to severe psoriasis. *Arch Dermatol Res* 2006;**298**:321–8.

8 De Korte J, Sprangers MAG, Mombers FMC, *et al.* Quality of life in patients with psoriasis: a systematic literature review. *J Invest Dermatol Symp Proc* 2004;**9**:140–7.

9 Griffiths CEM, Clark CM, Chalmers RJG, Li Wan Po A, Williams HC. A systematic review of treatments for severe psoriasis. *Health Technol Assess* 2000;**4**:1–125.

10 Watsky KL, Freije L, Leneveu MC, Wenck HA, Leffell DJ. Water-in-oil emollients as steroid-sparing adjunctive therapy in the treatment of psoriasis. *Cutis* 1992;**50**:383–6.

11 Hagemann I, Proksch E. Topical treatment by urea reduces epidermal hyperproliferation and induces differentiation in psoriasis. *Acta Dermatovenereol* 1996;**76**:353–6.

12 Fredriksson TLM. A blind controlled comparison between a new cream ("12 + 12"), its vehicle, and salicylic acid in petrolatum on psoriatic plaques. *Curr Ther Res* 1985;**37**:805–9.

13 Friedman SJ. Management of psoriasis vulgaris with a hydrocolloid occlusive dressing. *Arch Dermatol* 1987;**123**:1046–52.

14 David M, Lowe NJ. Psoriasis therapy: comparative studies with a hydrocolloid dressing, plastic film occlusion, and triamcinolone acetonide cream. *J Am Acad Dermatol* 1989;**21**:511–4.

15 Mason J, Mason AR, Cork MJ. Topical preparations for the treatment of psoriasis: a systematic review. *Br J Dermatol* 2002;**146**:351–64.

16 Koo J, Cuffie CA, Tanner DJ, *et al.* Mometasone furoate 0.1%-salicylic acid 5% ointment versus mometasone furoate 0.1% ointment in the treatment of moderate-to-severe psoriasis: a multicenter study. *Clin Ther* 1998;**20**:283–91.

17 Kristensen B, Kristensen O. Topical salicylic acid interferes with UVB therapy for psoriasis. *Acta Dermatovenereol* 1991;**71**:37–40.

18 Naldi L, Carrel CF, Parazzini F, *et al.* Development of anthralin short-contact therapy in psoriasis: survey of published clinical trials. *Int J Dermatol* 1992;**31**:126–30.

19 van de Kerkhof PC, Chang A, van der Walle HB, *et al.* Weekly treatment of psoriasis with a hydrocolloid dressing in combination with triamcinolone acetonide. A controlled comparative study. *Acta Derm Venereol* 1994;**74**:143–6.

20 Dezfoulian B, De la Brassinne M, Rosillon D. A new generation of hydrocolloid dressings in combination with topical corticosteroids in the treatment of psoriasis vulgaris. *J Eur Acad Dermatol Venereol* 1997;**9**:50–3.

21 Volden G, Kragballe K, van de Kerkhof PC, *et al.* Remission and relapse of chronic plaque psoriasis treated once a week with clobetasol propionate occluded with a hydrocolloid dressing versus twice daily treatment with clobetasol propionate alone. *J Dermatol Treat* 2001;**12**:141–4.

22 Krueger GG, Drake LA, Elias PM, *et al.* The safety and efficacy of tazarotene gel, a topical acetylenic retinoid, in the treatment of psoriasis. *Arch Dermatol* 1998;**134**:57–60.

23 de Jong EM, Mork NJ, Seijger MM, *et al.* The combination of calcipotriol and methotrexate compared with methotrexate and vehicle in psoriasis: results of a multicentre placebo-controlled randomized trial. *Br J Dermatol* 2003;**148**:318–25.

24 Weinstein GD, Koo JY, Krueger GG, *et al.* Tazarotene cream in the treatment of psoriasis: two multicenter, double-blind, randomized, vehicle-controlled studies of the safety and efficacy of tazarotene creams 0.05% and 0.1% applied once daily for 12 weeks. *J Am Acad Dermatol* 2003;**48**:760–7.

25 Weinstein GD, Krueger GG, Lowe NJ, *et al.* Tazarotene gel, a new retinoid, for topical therapy of psoriasis: vehicle-controlled study of safety, efficacy, and duration of therapeutic effect. *J Am Acad Dermatol* 1997;**37**:85–92.

26 Green L, Sadoff W. A clinical evaluation of tazarotene 0.1% gel, with and without a high- or mid-high-potency corticosteroid, in patients with stable plaque psoriasis. *J Cutan Med Surg* 2002;**6**:95–102.

27 Gollnick H, Menter A. Combination therapy with tazarotene plus a topical corticosteroid for the treatment of plaque psoriasis. *Br J Dermatol* 1999;**140**(Suppl):18–23.

28 Lebwohl MG, Breneman DL, Goffe BS, *et al.* Tazarotene 0.1% gel plus corticosteroid cream in the treatment of plaque psoriasis. *J Am Acad Dermatol* 1998;**39**:590–6.

29 Guenther LC, Poulin YP, Pariser DM. A comparison of tazarotene 0.1% gel once daily plus mometasone furoate 0.1% cream once daily versus calcipotriene 0.005% ointment twice daily in the treatment of plaque psoriasis. *Clin Ther* 2000;**22**:1225–38.

30 Snellman E, Aromaa A, Jansen CT, *et al.* Supervised four-week heliotherapy alleviates the long-term course of psoriasis. *Acta Derm Venereol* 1993;**73**:388–92.

31 Frentz G, Olsen JH, Avrach WW. Malignant tumours and psoriasis: climatotherapy at the Dead Sea. *Br J Dermatol* 1999;**141**:1088–91.

32 Cameron H, Dawe RS, Yule S, *et al.* A randomized, observer-blinded trial of twice vs. three times weekly narrowband ultraviolet B phototherapy for chronic plaque psoriasis. *Br J Dermatol* 2002;**147**:973–8.

33 Stern RS, Armstrong RB, Anderson TF, *et al.* Effect of continued ultraviolet B phototherapy on the duration of remission of psoriasis. A randomized study. *J Am Acad Dermatol* 1986;**15**:546–52.

34 Boer J, Hermans J, Schothorst AA, *et al.* Comparison of phototherapy (UVB) and photochemotherapy (PUVA) for clearing and maintenance therapy of psoriasis. *Arch Dermatol* 1984;**120**:52–7.

35 Gordon PM, Diffey BL, Mathews JN, *et al.* A randomised comparison of narrow-band TL-01 phototherapy for psoriasis. *J Am Acad Dermatol* 1999;**41**:728–32.

36 Pieternel CM, Pasker-de-Jong M, Wielink G, *et al.* Treatment with UV-B for psoriasis and nonmelanoma skin cancer. A systematic review of the literature. *Arch Dermatol* 1999;**135**:834–40.

37 Lee E, Koo J, Berger T. UVB phototherapy and skin cancer risk: a review of the literature. *Int J Dermatol* 2005;**44**:355–60.

38 Cottin V, Tebib J, Souquet PJ, *et al.* Pulmonary function in patients receiving long-term low-dose methotrexate. *Chest* 1996;**109**:933–8.

39 Melski JW, Tanenbaum L, Parrish JA, *et al.* Oral methoxsalen photochemotherapy for the treatment of psoriasis. A cooperative clinical trial. *J Invest Dermatol* 1977;**68**:328–35.

40 Stern RS, Laird N. The carcinogenic risk of treatments for severe psoriasis. Photochemotherapy follow-up study. *Cancer* 1994;**73**:2759–64.

41 Stern RS, Lunder EJ. Risk of squamous cell carcinoma and methoxsalen (psoralen) and UV-A radiation (PUVA). A meta-analysis. *Arch Dermatol* 1998;**134**:1582–5.

42 Hannuksela-Svahn A, Sigurgeirsson B, Pukkala E, *et al.* Trioxsalen bath PUVA did not increase the risk of squamous cell skin carcinoma and cutaneous malignant melanoma in a joint analysis of 944 Swedish and Finnish patients with psoriasis. *Br J Dermatol* 1999;**141**:497–501.

43 Stern RS, Fitzgerald E, Ellis CN, *et al.* The safety of etretinate as long-term therapy for psoriasis. Results of the etretinate follow-up study. *J Am Acad Dermatol* 1995;**33**:44–52.

44 Jones G, Crotty M, Brooks P. Interventions for psoriatic arthritis. *Cochrane Database Syst Rev* 2000;**(3)**:CD000212.

45 Heydendael VM, Spuls PI, Opmeer BC, *et al.* Methotrexate versus ciclosporine in moderate-to-severe chronic plaque psoriasis. *N Engl J Med* 2003;**349**:658–65.

46 Boffa MJ, Chalmers RJ. Methotrexate for psoriasis. *Clin Exp Dermatol* 1996;**21**:399–408.

47 Malerba M, Gisondi P, Radaeli A, Sala R, Calzavara Pinton PG, Girolomoni G. Plasma homocysteine and folate levels in patients with chronic plaque psoriasis. *Br J Dermatol* 2006;**155**:1165–9.

48 Whiting-O'Keefe QE, Fye KH, Sack KD. Methotrexate and histologic hepatic abnormalities: a meta-analysis. *Am J Med* 1991;**90**:711–6.

49 Roenigk HH, Auerbach R, Maibach HI, Weinstein GD. Methotrexate in psoriasis: consensus conference. *J Am Acad Dermatol* 1998;**38**:478–85.

50 Boffa MJ, Chalmers RJG, Haboubi NY, Shomaf M, Mitchell DM. Sequential liver biopsies during long-term methotrexate treatment for psoriasis: a reappraisal. *Br J Dermatol* 1995;**133**:774–8.

51 Zachariae H, Heickendorff L, Soegaard H. The value of aminoterminal propeptide of type III procollagen in routine screening for methotrexate-induced liver fibrosis: a 10-year follow-up. *Br J Dermatol* 2001;**143**:100–3.

52 Stern RS, Laird N. The carcinogenic risk of treatments for severe psoriasis. Photochemotherapy follow-up study. *Cancer* 1994;**73**:2759–64.

53 Nyfors A, Jensen H. Frequency of malignant neoplasms in 248 long-term methotrexate-treated psoriatics. A preliminary study. *Dermatologica* 1983;**167**:260–61.

54 Grossman RM, Chevret S, Abi-Rached J, *et al.* Long-term safety of ciclosporin in the treatment of psoriasis. *Arch Dermatol* 1996;**132**:623–9.

55 Paul CE, Ho VC, McGeown C, *et al.* Risk of malignancies in psoriasis patients treated with cyclosporine: a 5 y cohort study. *J Invest Dermatol* 2003;**120**:211–6.

56 Kaltwasser JP, Nash P, Gladman D, *et al.* Efficacy and safety of leflunomide in the treatment of psoriatic arthritis and psoriasis: a multinational, double-blind, randomized, placebo-controlled clinical trial. *Arthritis Rheum* 2004;**50**:1939–50.

57 Gottlieb AB, Matheson RT, Lowe N, *et al.* A randomized trial of etanercept as monotherapy for psoriasis. *Arch Dermatol* 2003;**139**:1627–32.

58 Leonardi CL, Powers JL, Matheson RT, *et al.* Etanercept as monotherapy in patients with psoriasis. *N Engl J Med* 2003;**349**:2014–22.

59 Feldman SR, Boer Kimball A, Krueger GG, *et al.* Etanercept improves the health-related quality of life of patients with psoriasis: results of a phase III randomized clinical trial. *J Am Acad Dermatol* 2005;**53**:887–9.

60 Papp KA, Tyring S, Lahfa M, *et al.* A global phase III randomised controlled trial of etanercept in psoriasis: safety, efficacy, and effect of dose reduction. *Br J Dermatol* 2005;**152**:1304–12.

61 Krueger GG, Langley RG, Finlay AY, *et al.* Patient-reported outcomes of psoriasis improvement with etanercept therapy: results of a randomised phase III trial. *Br J Dermatol* 2005;**153**:1192–9.

62 Tyring S, Gottlieb A, Papp K, *et al.* Etanercept and clinical outcomes, fatigue, and depression in psoriasis: double-blind placebo-controlled randomised phase III trial. *Lancet* 2006;**367**:29–35.

63 Chaudhari U, Romano P, Mulcahy LD, *et al.* Efficacy and safety of infliximab monotherapy for plaque-type psoriasis: a randomised trial. *Lancet* 2001;**357**:1842–7.

64 Gottlieb AB, Evans R, Li S, *et al.* Infliximab induction therapy for patients with severe plaque-type psoriasis: a randomized, double-blind, placebo-controlled trial. *J Am Acad Dermatol* 2004;**51**:534–42.

65 Feldman SR, Gordon KB, Bala M, *et al.* Infliximab treatment results in significant improvement in the quality of life of patients with severe psoriasis: a double-blind placebo-controlled trial. *Br J Dermatol* 2005;**152**:954–60.

66 Reich K, Nestle FO, Papp K, *et al.* Infliximab induction and maintenance therapy for moderate-to-severe psoriasis: a phase III, multicentre, double-blind trial. *Lancet* 2005;**366**:1367–74.

67 Reich K, Nestle FO, Papp K, *et al.* Improvement in quality of life with infliximab induction and maintenance therapy in patients with moderate-to-severe psoriasis: a randomised controlled trial. *Br J Dermatol* 2006;**154**:1161–8.

68 Bongartz T, Sutton AJ, Sweeting MJ, *et al.* Anti-TNF antibody therapy in rheumatoid arthritis and the risk of serious infections and malignancies. *JAMA* 2006;**295**:2275–85.

69 Ellis CN, Krueger GG, Alefacept Clinical Study Group. Treatment of chronic plaque psoriasis by selective targeting of memory effector T lymphocytes. *N Engl J Med* 2001;**345**:248–55.

70 Ellis CN, Mordin MM, Adler EY, *et al.* Effects of alefacept on health-related quality of life in patients with psoriasis: results from a randomised, placebo-controlled phase II study. *Am J Clin Dermatol* 2003;**4**:131–9.

71 Krueger GG, Papp KA, Stough DB, *et al.* Randomized, double-blind, placebo-controlled phase III study evaluating efficacy and tolerability of 2 courses of alefacept in patients with chronic plaque psoriasis. *J Am Acad Dermatol* 2002;**47**:821–33.

72 Feldman SR, Menter A, Koo JY. Improved health-related quality of life following a randomized controlled trial of alefacept treatment in patients with chronic plaque psoriasis. *Br J Dermatol* 2004;**150**:317–26.

73 Lebwohl M, Christophers E, Langley R, *et al.* An international, randomized, double-blind, placebo-controlled phase 3 trial of

intramuscular alefacept in patients with chronic plaque psoriasis. *Arch Dermatol* 2003;**139**:719–27.

74 Finlay AY, Salek MS, Haney J. Intramuscular alefacept improves health-related quality of life in patients with chronic plaque psoriasis. *Dermatology* 2003;**206**:307–15.

75 Goffe B, Papp K, Gratton D, *et al*. An integrated analysis of thirteen trials summarizing the long term safety of alefacept in psoriasis patients who have received up to nine courses of therapy. *Clin Ther* 2005;**27**:1912–21.

76 Lebwohl M, Tyring SK, Hamilton TK, *et al*. A novel targeted T-cell modulator, efalizumab, for plaque psoriasis. *N Engl J Med* 2003; **349**:2004–13.

77 Gordon KB, Papp KA, Hamilton TK, *et al*. Efalizumab for patients with moderate to severe plaque psoriasis: a randomized controlled trial. *JAMA* 2003;**290**:3073–80.

78 Leonardi CL, Papp KA, Gordon KB, *et al*. Extended efalizumab therapy improves chronic plaque psoriasis: results from a randomized phase III trial. *J Am Acad Dermatol* 2005;**52**:425–33.

79 Menter A, Gordon K, Carey W, *et al*. Efficacy and safety during 24 weeks of efalizumab therapy in patients with moderate to severe plaque psoriasis. *Arch Dermatol* 2005;**141**:31–8.

80 Dubertret L, Sterry W, Bos JD, *et al*. Clinical experience acquired with the efalizumab (Raptiva) (CLEAR) trial in patients with moderate-to-severe plaque psoriasis: results from a phase III international randomized, placebo-controlled trial. *Br J Dermatol* 2006;**155**:170–81.

81 Ortonne JP, Shear N, Shumack S, Henninger E; CLEAR Multinational Study Group. Impact of efalizumab on patient-reported outcomes in high-need psoriasis patients: results of the international, randomized, placebo-controlled phase III Clinical Experience Acquired with Raptiva (CLEAR) trial [NCT00256139]. *BMC Dermatol* 2005;**5**:13.

82 Papp KA, Bressinck R, Fretzin S, *et al*. Safety of efalizumab in adults with chronic moderate to severe plaque psoriasis: a phase IIIb randomised controlled trial. *Int J Dermatol* 2006;**45**:605–14.

83 Stern RS, Gange RW, Parrish JA, *et al*. Contribution of topical tar oil to ultraviolet B phototherapy for psoriasis. *J Am Acad Dermatol* 1986;**14**:742–7.

84 Owen CM, Chalmers RJG, O'Sullivan T, Griffiths CEM. Antistreptococcal interventions for guttate and chronic plaque psoriasis. *Cochrane Database Syst Rev* 2000;(**2**):CD001976.

85 Chalmers RJG, O'Sullivan T, Owen CM, Griffiths CEM. Interventions for guttate psoriasis. *Cochrane Database Syst Rev* 2000; (**2**):CD001213.

86 Vincent F, Ross JB, Dalton M, Wort AJ. A therapeutic trial of the use of penicillin V or erythromycin with or without rifampin in the treatment of psoriasis. *J Am Acad Dermatol* 1992;**26**:458–61.

87 Grimminger F, Mayser P, Papavassilis C, *et al*. A double-blind, randomized, placebo-controlled trial of n-3 fatty acid based lipid infusion in acute, extended guttate psoriasis. Rapid improvement of clinical manifestations and changes in neutrophil leukotriene profile. *Clin Investig* 1993;**71**:634–43.

88 Marsland AM, Chalmers RJG, Hollis S, Leonardi-Bee J, Griffiths CEM. Interventions for chronic palmoplantar pustulosis. *Cochrane Database Syst Rev* 2006;(**1**):CD001433.

89 Erkko P, Granlund H, Remitz A, *et al*. Double-blind placebo-controlled study of long-term low-dose cyclosporin in the treatment of palmoplantar pustulosis. *Br J Dermatol* 1998;**139**:997–1004.

22 Lichen planus

Laurence Le Cleach, Olivier Chosidow, Bernard Cribier

Background

Definition

Lichen planus (LP) is a chronic inflammatory disease affecting the skin, the oral or genital mucosae, the nails, and/or the scalp. Cutaneous LP is typically a pruritic eruption of shiny, violaceous, flat, polygonal papules, mainly localized on the front of the wrists, the lumbar region, and around the ankles. The most frequent oral presentation is asymptomatic reticular LP, but painful erosive or ulcerative areas may appear.

Incidence/prevalence

The prevalence of oral LP is 0.5–1.5% of the general population. The oral mucosa is the most frequently affected site.

Etiology

The pathogenesis of LP remains unclear. There is some evidence that T lymphocytes infiltrating the epidermis and dermis act as effector agents against keratinocytes, but the target antigens are unknown.

Prognosis

Spontaneous remission of cutaneous LP after 1 year occurs in two-thirds of cases.[1] Patients mainly complain of pruritus. Spontaneous remission of oral LP is much rarer, and may occur in approximately 5% of patients. The reported mean duration of oral LP is about 5 years, but the erosive form does not resolve spontaneously.[2] The erosive form can be extremely painful, leading to major weight loss due to dysphagia. Malignant transformation of oral LP has occasionally been described. Nail or scalp involvement may result in irreversible scars.

Diagnostic tests

Whatever the clinical presentation, histopathological analysis confirms the diagnosis of LP, showing a dermoepidermal papule with hyperkeratosis, hypergranulosis, and acanthosis, basal cell vacuolization, and a band-like inflammatory infiltrate in the superficial dermis.

Aims of treatment

The aim of treatment depends on the clinical form, severity, and response to treatment of LP. In the cutaneous form, the aim of treatment is to reduce pruritus and time to resolution, without inducing severe side effects. The asymptomatic form of oral LP does not usually require treatment. Symptomatic oral LP may need aggressive treatment to stop the pain and to obtain a remission. The aim of the treatment when there is nail or scalp involvement is to stop the inflammatory process as soon as possible, in order to avoid scars.

Relevant outcomes

The expected relevant outcomes in cutaneous LP are the reduction of pruritus and the time to resolution. In oral LP, the relevant outcomes are reduction of erosive lesions, improved quality of life, and reduction of pain. In oral LP, the rate of recurrence is high after withdrawal of treatment. The recurrence rate and the tolerance of long-term treatment should be considered. These relevant outcomes were mostly not evaluated in the studies reviewed, which used imprecise global evaluation scores.

Methods of search

We searched the Medline and Biosis databases to identify articles published before March 1998,[3] and Medline, Embase, and the Cochrane Database of Systematic Reviews between March 1998 and January 2006. We used the key

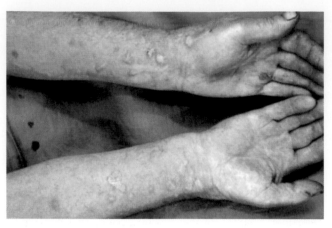

Figure 22.1 Cutaneous lichen planus.

words "lichen" and "treatment or therapy," and we combined each treatment modality with "lichen." Because of the small number of controlled studies, we also reviewed open studies and case reports using the treatments usually recommended in textbooks (Figure 22.1).

Questions

Do corticosteroids improve cutaneous LP?

Efficacy

One randomized controlled study (RCT) compared the efficacy of prednisolone, 30 mg/day, and placebo administered for 10 days in 38 patients.[4] The median time for LP to clear was 18 weeks in the prednisolone group and 29 weeks in the placebo group ($P = 0.02$). Five patients in the corticosteroid group relapsed after treatment withdrawal.

One randomized but not blinded study compared the efficacy of calcipotriol 50 μg/g ointment and betamethasone valerate 0.1% ointment in 31 patients. At week 12, significant clearance (50% or more) was observed in only one patient. No differences were observed between the treatments.[5]

Drawbacks

The side effects of oral prednisolone were minimal. One patient had mild heartburn, and another experienced euphoria.[4]

Comment

Evidence on corticosteroids is scant, although they have been widely used in practice. In the only available RCT that evaluated systemic corticosteroids, topical corticosteroids were allowed, but were not quantified. The absence of blind evaluation in the calcipotriol trial does not allow any conclusions to be drawn regarding the efficacy of this treatment.

Implications for practice

Short courses of systemic corticosteroid therapy are usually recommended as first-line treatment for moderate to severe cutaneous LP, although this is not based on relevant clinical trials and recurrences are possible after treatment withdrawal. Topical corticosteroids are recommended as first-line treatment in mild to moderate cutaneous LP. Topical calcipotriol is not recommended.

Do retinoids improve cutaneous LP?

Efficacy

We found only one RCT evaluating the efficacy of oral retinoids in cutaneous LP.[6] This double-blind study compared acitretin and placebo in 65 patients with cutaneous LP. Treatment consisted of acitretin 30 mg/day for 8 weeks. Of the patients receiving acitretin, 64% (18 of 28) improved significantly or had remissions, in comparison with 13% in the placebo group. Papules persisted in the majority of patients. Nevertheless, the intensity of pruritus, papulosis, and erythema was significantly lower in the acitretin group.

Drawbacks

Tolerability was considered to be good or very good in 73% of the patients.[6] Side effects noted in this study were mainly cheilitis and dry mouth. Side effects are not exceptional with systemic retinoids. The most severe side effect of retinoids is teratogenicity.

Comment

In the RCT evaluating acitretin in cutaneous LP,[6] neither the duration of the disease before inclusion nor the extent of the lesions were detailed. The criteria for remission and marked improvement were not detailed. The level of evidence of acitretin efficacy is therefore of average quality.

Implications for practice

Because of potential side effects, acitretin can only be recommended as a second-line treatment for cutaneous LP. Acitretin may also be combined with psoralen ultraviolet A (PUVA) therapy (see photochemotherapy, below).

Does photochemotherapy improve cutaneous LP?

Efficacy

We found a small controlled trial in which 10 patients with cutaneous LP were treated with hemicorporeal ultraviolet (UV) irradiation after ingestion of psoralen.[7] Eight showed partial improvement, and three were completely cured. The absence of any observed contralateral effect of the PUVA therapy supports the local efficacy of the treatment.

We found six open studies of bath PUVA therapy.[3] The largest included 75 patients, and found that two cycles of

PUVA therapy cured 65% and improved 15% of patients.[8] The relapse rate after a follow-up period of 2–5 years was 25%.

We found three open studies in which five, 10, and 20 patients, respectively, with cutaneous LP were treated with UVB TL-01. The complete remission rates were 100%, 50%, and 55%, respectively, with cumulative doses of 82.7, 17.7 ± 1.6, and 36 J/cm, respectively.[9–11]

Drawbacks
No adverse effects were described in the PUVA or UVB trials. There is probably no major risk of photoaging and/or skin cancer if the treatment is limited to one or two cycles.

Comment
In view of the high rate of spontaneous remission, the evidence for the efficacy of PUVA and UVB TL-01 therapy is weak. Combined treatment with retinoids and PUVA is occasionally recommended, but the efficacy of this has not yet been evaluated.

Implications for practice
PUVA therapy and UVB TL-01 could be an alternative to oral corticosteroids in moderate to severe cutaneous LP.

Does ciclosporin improve cutaneous LP?

Efficacy
We found small uncontrolled series and one case report.[12–16] A total of 21 patients with severe cutaneous LP resistant to retinoids or systemic corticosteroids therapy were treated. A complete response occurred in all patients, with doses ranging from 1 to 6 mg/kg/day, and without relapse during several months of follow up in the majority of patients. Pruritus disappeared after 1–2 weeks of treatment, and clearance of the rash was noted in a mean of 6 weeks.

Drawbacks
In these trials, two of the 21 patients had increased triglyceride and/or creatinine levels (both received 3 mg/kg/day). In long-term treatment for psoriasis (more than 6 months), 6–18% of patients interrupted the treatment because of side effects. The most serious side effects were high blood pressure, renal toxicity, and a potential increase in the risk of cancer. High blood pressure was reported in 5–26% of patients in short-term trials.

Comment
In the absence of controlled studies, the level of evidence for the efficacy of ciclosporin is low. The risk of serious side effects is high.

Implications for practice
The benefit–harm ratio of ciclosporin is too low in LP. Its use for cutaneous LP is therefore not recommended.

Does thalidomide improve lichen planopilaris?

Efficacy
We found three case reports describing four patients with lichen planopilaris, which improved after treatment with thalidomide 100–150 mg/d for 1–6 months.[17–19] We also found a small series reporting failure of thalidomide treatment with 100–200 mg/d for 6 months in six patients with lichen planopilaris.[20] In cutaneous LP, we found only two case reports.

Drawbacks
One patient developed depression and another developed reversible sensory neuropathy. Constipation, mood changes, drowsiness, xerostomia, sensory neuropathy, and headaches are common side effects of thalidomide. The most serious adverse effect is teratogenicity.

Comments
The number of patients treated is low, and the results are contradictory. The risk of side effects is high.

Implication for practice
The benefit–harm ratio of thalidomide is low in lichen planopilaris and very low in cutaneous LP. It is administered rarely, for very severe forms of lichen planus or lichen planopilaris in which all other treatments have failed (Figure 22.2).

Do topical corticosteroids improve oral LP?

Efficacy
Fluocinonide. We found one RCT,[21] in which fluocinonide in an adhesive base, applied six times per day for 9 weeks, was compared with its vehicle in 40 patients with oral LP. The study included 12 patients with erosive LP, 13 with reticular LP, and 15 with a combination. Thirteen of the 20 patients treated achieved complete remission or had a

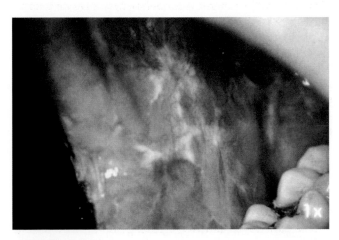

Figure 22.2 Oral lichen planus.

good response, compared with four good responses in the placebo group.

Betamethasone valerate. One RCT[22] compared betamethasone valerate aerosol, four sprays per day for 2 months, with placebo in 23 patients with oral LP, 18 of whom had erosive lesions. After 2 months of therapy, eight of 11 patients had a "good or moderate" response (six of them had erosive LP) in comparison with two moderate responses in the placebo group.

Clobetasol propionate. One study, which was controlled but without randomization or blinding,[23] compared clobetasol propionate ointment 0.05% twice daily for the first 4 months and then once daily for 2 months with fluocinonide ointment 0.05% three times daily for 2 months, then twice daily for 2 months, then once daily for 2 months and with a placebo in 25, 24, and 11 patients, respectively. All of the patients received miconazole and chlorhexidine as prophylaxis against oropharyngeal candidiasis. At 6 months, 75% of the patients treated with clobetasol had complete remission, in comparison with 25% in the group treated with fluocinonide and none in the placebo group. The difference between clobetasol and the placebo was significant, but not the difference between fluocinonide and the placebo.

Drawbacks

In the two RCTs, one with fluocinonide and one with betamethasone valerate, the only adverse effect observed was a case of oral candidiasis. In the clobetasol study, all of the patients reported extrinsic staining of the teeth, and 82% an alteration in the sense of taste. In this study, blood cortisol levels remained stable.

Comments

These three studies included patients with oral LP of varying degrees of severity. The study of fluocinonide gel included only a few patients and used a subjective overall evaluation of responses. A higher complete resolution rate was observed with clobetasol, but the level of evidence from an unrandomized, unblinded study is weak. These studies provide an average level of evidence for the efficacy of topical corticosteroids in oral LP.

Implication for practice

Topical corticosteroids are the first-line treatment for oral LP.

Do systemic corticosteroids improve oral LP?

Efficacy

One RCT compared the efficacy of the addition of a 6-month period of treatment with 0.05% clobetasol propionate ointment after treatment with oral prednisone 50 mg/day (maximum 60 days). Twenty-six patients received prednisone and clobetasol, and 23 patients received clobetasol alone.[24] No differences in the improvement of signs and symptoms were observed between the two groups.

Drawbacks

Seven patients in the group treated with oral prednisone developed systemic side effects.

Comment

This RCT only allows the conclusion that systemic corticosteroids do not increase the efficacy of topical corticosteroids. No controlled studies have evaluated the efficacy of oral corticosteroids versus placebo in oral LP.

Implication for practice

Although systemic corticosteroids are widely used in oral LP, their efficacy has not been documented. Oral corticosteroids are recommended in patients with severe oral lichen planus that is resistant to local treatment.

Do retinoids improve oral LP?

Efficacy

Topical retinoic acid. We found one RCT comparing 0.1% retinoic acid with placebo. The study included 10 patients in each group, all with plaque-like LP lesions.[25] After 4 months of therapy, nine patients in the tretinoin group had improved or were cured, in comparison with four in the placebo group.

Isotretinoin gel. One RCT compared isotretinoin gel with excipient alone for 2 months in 20 patients.[26] The improvement in scores was 90% and 10%, respectively.

Tazarotene. One RCT compared tazarotene gel 0.1% versus placebo in 12 patients with hyperkeratotic oral LP. The clinical score was significantly reduced in the treated group.[27]

Etretinate. We found one RCT[28] including 28 patients with severe oral LP who were treated with etretinate, 75 mg/day, or placebo for 2 months. Improvement (reduction of more than 50% of the erosions and infiltration) was observed in 93% of lesions in the etretinate group, in comparison with 5% of controls. Three months after the end of treatment, 66% of the patients had relapsed.

Oral tretinoin and oral isotretinoin. We found only three open studies of different dosages of oral tretinoin and anecdotal reports of oral isotretinoin.[3]

Drawbacks

Only mild local side effects were observed in the three RCTs on topical retinoic acid, isotretinoin gel, and tazarotene. In the etretinate RCT, severe dermatological side effects and headache led to four withdrawals.

Comments

Both RCTs of topical retinoids were of poor methodological quality, particularly due to incomplete clinical data and the small numbers of patients included. The RCT concerning tazarotene included a small group of patients with a nonerosive form of lichen.

Implications for practice

Topical 0.1% tretinoin gel and 0.1% isotretinoin gel both improve oral LP, but recurrences after withdrawal are frequent. This treatment can be recommended as first-line treatment for oral LP.

Do topical ciclosporin tacrolimus and pimecrolimus improve oral LP?

Efficacy

Topical ciclosporin. We found three RCTs comparing the efficacy of different dosages and methods of application of ciclosporin with placebo in 16, 14, and 20 patients, respectively.[29–31] These RCTs were included in the Cochrane Library review.[32] Two RCTs[29,30] were pooled for symptomatic outcomes. There were statistically significant improvements in both the individual and pooled analyses for ciclosporin. The three studies were pooled for improvement as measured by signs. There was also a statistical advantage for ciclosporin.

Tacrolimus. We found eight series[33–40] and one single case report[41] describing the effect of topical tacrolimus in oral LP in 141 patients. Tacrolimus 0.03% or 0.1% or 0.3% was applied one to four times daily for at least 4 weeks. Complete resolution or good improvement was observed in about 90% of the patients treated, but a relapse was noted a few weeks after withdrawal.

Pimecrolimus. One RCT compared the efficacy of pimecrolimus 1% cream with placebo in 20 patients for 4 weeks.[42] No significant differences were observed between the final and baseline evaluations. No statistical comparisons between the groups were reported.

Drawbacks

The only side effect reported in the RCT with topical ciclosporin was a local burning sensation. No elevated serum ciclosporin levels were observed.[43] The most common adverse effect observed after application of tacrolimus was a burning sensation.

Comments

The dosages, treatment durations, and methods of application of ciclosporin were different in the three RCTs, and the level of evidence is therefore low. Despite the good rate of response in treated patients, in the absence of RCTs the level of evidence of efficacy of tacrolimus is low.

Implications for practice

No formulation of topical ciclosporin is commercially available. The level of evidence for the efficacy of ciclosporin and tacrolimus is low, with few adverse effects. Topical ciclosporin and tacrolimus may represent a second-line treatment for severe oral LP.

Are other topical treatments more effective than topical corticosteroids for treating oral LP?

Efficacy

An RCT compared 0.05% tretinoin with fluocinonide in 33 patients with atrophic and erosive LP.[44] The reduction in the severity score was significantly higher with fluocinonide.

An RCT compared 0.05% retinoic acid with fluocinolone acetonide 0.1%, with four applications per day, in 15 and 18 patients, respectively.[45] At week 4, the improvement in the clinical score was significantly greater in the fluocinolone acetonide group.

An RCT compared topical ciclosporin, with three washes per day (1500 mg/day), with triamcinolone paste in 13 patients.[46] Another controlled trial compared oil-based ciclosporin solution, 50 mg three times daily, with aqueous 1% triamcinolone acetonide solution in 20 patients.[47] No differences were observed in these two RCTs.

An RCT compared ciclosporin 1.5% and clobetasol propionate ointment 0.025% applied twice daily for 2 months in 20 and 19 patients, respectively.[48] Clobetasol was more effective than ciclosporin in inducing clinical improvement (95% vs. 65% of the patients). The two drugs have comparable effects on symptoms. Clobetasol provides less stable results than ciclosporin.

Comment

There was only a small decrease in the severity score in the two tretinoin RCTs, but the 0.05% concentration may have been too low.

Implication for practice

There is no evidence that topical ciclosporin is more effective than corticosteroids in oral LP.

Does thalidomide improve oral LP?

Efficacy

We found one series including six patients[49] with severe erosive lichen planus resistant to oral corticosteroids who were treated with thalidomide 50–100 mg for 4 months.

Complete remission was observed in four patients and improvement in one. Relapse of the lesions was observed after the withdrawal of treatment.

Drawbacks
One patient experienced phlebitis and one had severe axonal neuropathy.

Comments
The observation of complete remissions with thalidomide in patients with very severe LP argues in favor of the efficacy of the drug; however, oral corticosteroids were maintained in three patients (at lower doses), and there are no controlled trials. Severe side effects are observed with thalidomide.

Implications for practice
Patients with very severe oral LP resistant to oral corticosteroids can be treated with thalidomide.

Does photochemotherapy improve oral LP?

Efficacy
Oral photochemotherapy. We found four open studies and one RCT.[3] A controlled study of oral PUVA therapy was conducted on 18 patients with erosive or ulcerative oral LP, after ingestion of psoralen, 0.6 mg/kg, and randomized unilateral irradiation.[50] The end point was a comparison of the treated and nontreated sides. After 12 sessions (total dose 16.5 J/cm^2), the treated side showed marked or slight improvement in 13 patients and the control side improved in six patients.

Extracorporeal photochemotherapy. We found a small series of seven patients with severe resistant erosive oral LP who were treated with extracorporeal photochemotherapy.[51] Complete remission was obtained in all patients.

Drawbacks
In the study of extracorporeal photochemotherapy, a progressive decrease in blood lymphocytes was observed in all patients, but without significant consequences.

Comments
One small RCT suggested that oral photochemotherapy is moderately effective in oral LP.

Implications for practice
In oral photochemotherapy, irradiation is provided by an apparatus designed for light-cured dental fillings, which is not easily available; the level of evidence of efficacy is low. Because of its cost, extracorporeal photochemotherapy must be reserved for very severe oral LP. No comparative studies have yet been conducted.

Summary

This review of the literature shows that many drugs and physical treatments have been used in the treatment of LP, but comparative studies are rare. In almost all studies, the reported efficacy of the treatments was based on imprecise global evaluation scores, and many studies lack precise inclusion criteria. It is impossible to compare the balance of benefit–harm for these treatments in each clinical form of LP.

Nevertheless, the studies contain sufficient preliminary data to encourage the planning of larger RCTs. These future RCTs will need to evaluate cutaneous LP, nonerosive oral LP, and erosive oral LP separately, and use specific objective criteria in each clinical type of LP.

Key points

- Lichen planus is a chronic inflammatory disease mainly affecting the skin and oral mucosae. The aims of the treatment vary depending on the clinical forms. There is a lack of large trials comparing the usually recommended treatments with a placebo.
- We found no evidence for the efficacy of systemic or topical corticosteroids, although this treatment is usually recommended as the first-line treatment for cutaneous LP.
- We found limited evidence of the efficacy of acitretin and PUVA therapy in cutaneous LP.
- We found that the benefit–harm ratio of ciclosporin in cutaneous LP was too low for this treatment to be recommended.
- We found limited evidence for the efficacy of topical corticosteroids, topical 0.1% tretinoin gel, and 0.1% isotretinoin gel in oral LP.
- We found no evidence that topical ciclosporin is more effective than topical corticosteroid in oral LP.

References

1 Irvine C, Irvine F, Champion RH. Long-term follow-up of lichen planus. *Acta Derm Venereol* 1991;**71**:242–4.
2 Scully C, El-Kom M. Lichen planus: review and update on pathogenesis. *J Oral Pathol* 1985;**14**:431–58.
3 Cribier B, Frances C, Chosidow O. Treatment of lichen planus. *Arch Dermatol* 1998;**134**:1521–30.
4 Kelett JK, Ead RD. Treatment of lichen planus with a short course of oral prednisolone. *Br J Dermatol* 1990;**123**:550–1.
5 Theng CT, Tan SH, Goh CL, Suresh S, Wong HB, Machin D. A randomized controlled trial to compare calcipotriol with betamethasone valerate for treatment of cutaneous lichen planus. *J Dermatolog Treat* 2004;**15**:141–5.
6 Laurberg G, Geiger JM, Hjorth N, *et al.* Treatment of lichen planus with acitretin: a double blind, placebo-controlled study in 65 patients. *J Am Acad Dermatol* 1991;**24**:434–7.

7 Gonzales E, Khosrow MT, Freedman S. Bilateral comparison of generalized lichen planus treated with psoralens and ultraviolet A. *J Am Acad Dermatol* 1984;**10**:958–61.

8 Karvonen J, Hannuksela M. Long term results of topical trioxsalen PUVA in lichen planus and nodular prurigo. *Acta Derm Venereol Suppl (Stockh)* 1985;**120**:53–5.

9 Taneja A, Taylor CR. Narrow-band UVB for lichen planus treatment. *Int J Dermatol* 2002;**41**:282–3.

10 Saricaoglu H, Karadogan SK, Baskan EB, Tunali S. Narrowband UVB therapy in the treatment of lichen planus. *Photodermatol Photoimmunol Photomed* 2003;**19**:265–7.

11 Habib F, Stoebner PE, Picot E, Peyron JL, Meynadier J, Meunier L. [Narrow-band UVB phototherapy in the treatment of widespread lichen planus; in French.] *Ann Dermatol Venereol* 2005;**132**:17–20.

12 Higgins EM, Munro CS, Friedmann PS, Marks JM. Cyclosporin A in the treatment of lichen planus. *Arch Dermatol* 1989;**125**:1436.

13 Ho VC, Gupta AK, Nickoloff BJ, Vorhees JJ. Treatment of severe lichen planus with cyclosporine. *J Am Acad Dermatol* 1990;**22**:64–8.

14 Pigatto PD, Chiapino G, Bigardi A, Mozzanica N, Finzi AF. Cyclosporin A for treatment of severe lichen planus. *Br J Dermatol* 1990;**122**:121–3.

15 Levell NJ, Munro CS, Marks JM. Severe lichen planus clears with very low-dose cyclosporin. *Br J Dermatol* 1992;**127**:66–7.

16 Reiffers-Mettelock J. Acute lichen planus treated by Sandimmun (ciclosporin). *Dermatology* 1992;**184**:84.

17 Dereure O, Basset-Seguin N, Guilhou JJ. Erosive lichen planus: dramatic response to thalidomide. *Arch Dermatol* 1996;**132**:1392–3.

18 George SJ, Hsu S. Lichen planopilaris treated with thalidomide. *J Am Acad Dermatol* 2001;**45**:965–6.

19 Boyd AS, King LE Jr. Thalidomide-induced remission of lichen planopilaris. *J Am Acad Dermatol* 2002;**47**:967–8.

20 Jouanique C, Reygagne P, Bachelez H, Dubertret L. Thalidomide is ineffective in the treatment of lichen planopilaris. *J Am Acad Dermatol* 2004;**51**:480–1.

21 Voute AB, Schulten EA, Langendijk PNJ, Kostense PJ, van der Waal I. Fluocinonide in an adhesive base for the treatment of oral lichen planus: a double-blind, placebo-controlled clinical study. *Oral Surg Oral Med Oral Pathol* 1993;**75**:181–5.

22 Tyldesley WR, Harding SM. Betamethasone valerate aerosol in the treatment of oral lichen planus. *Br J Dermatol* 1977;**96**:659–62.

23 Carbone M, Conrotto D, Carrozzo M, Broccoletti R, Gandolfo S, Scully C. Topical corticosteroids in association with miconazole and chlorhexidine in the long-term management of atrophic-erosive oral lichen planus: a placebo-controlled and comparative study between clobetasol and fluocinonide. *Oral Dis* 1999;**5**:44–9.

24 Carbone M, Goss E, Carrozzo M, *et al*. Systemic and topical corticosteroid treatment of oral lichen planus: a comparative study with long-term follow up. *J Oral Pathol Med* 2003;**32**:323–9.

25 Boisnic S, Branchet MC, Pascal F, Ben Slama L, Rostin M, Szpirglas H. [Topical tretinoin in the treatment of lichen planus and leukoplakia of the mouth mucosa: a clinical evaluation; in French.] *Ann Dermatol Venereol* 1994;**121**:459–63.

26 Giustina TA, Stewart JCB, Ellis CN, *et al*. Topical application of isotretinoin gel improves oral lichen planus. *Arch Dermatol* 1986;**122**:534–6.

27 Petruzzi M, De Benedittis M, Grassi R, Cassano N, Vena G, Serpico R. Oral lichen planus: a preliminary clinical study on treatment with tazarotene. *Oral Dis* 2002;**8**:291–5.

28 Hersle K, Mobacken H, Sloberg K, Thilander H. Severe oral lichen planus: treatment with an aromatic retinoid (etretinate). *Br J Dermatol* 1982;**106**:77–80.

29 Eisen D, Ellis CN, Duell EA, Griffiths CEM, Voorhees JJ. Effect of topical cyclosporine rinse on oral lichen planus: a double-blind analysis. *N Engl J Med* 1990;**323**:290–4.

30 Harpenau LA, Plemons JM, Rees TD. Effectiveness of low dose of cyclosporin in the management of patients with oral erosive lichen planus. *Oral Surg Oral Med Oral Pathol Oral Radiol Endod* 1995;**80**:161–7.

31 Gaeta GM, Serpico R, Femiano F, La Rotonda MI, Cappello B, Gombos F. Cyclosporin bioadhesive gel in the topical treatment of erosive oral lichen planus. *Int J Immunopathol Pharmacol* 1994;**7**:125–32.

32 Chan ES, Thornhill M, Zakrzewska J. Interventions for treating oral lichen planus. *Cochrane Database Syst Rev* 2000;(**2**):CD001168.

33 Vente C, Reich K, Rupprecht R, Neumann C. Erosive mucosal lichen planus: response to topical treatment with tacrolimus. *Br J Dermatol* 1999;**140**:338–42.

34 Olivier V, Lacour JP, Mousnier A, Garraffo R, Monteil RA, Ortonne JP. Treatment of chronic erosive oral lichen planus with low concentrations of topical tacrolimus. *Arch Dermatol* 2002;**138**:1335–8.

35 Morrison L, Kratochvil J, Gorman A. An open trial of topical tacrolimus for erosive oral lichen planus. *J Am Acad Dermatol* 2002;**47**:617–20.

36 Kaliakatsou F, Hodgson TA, Lewsey JD, Hegarty AM, Murphy AG, Porter SR. Management of recalcitrant ulcerative oral lichen planus with topical tacrolimus. *J Am Acad Dermatol* 2002;**46**:35–41.

37 Rozycki TW, Rogers RS, Pittelkow MR, *et al*. Topical tacrolimus in the treatment of symptomatic oral lichen planus: a series of 13 patients. *J Am Acad Dermatol* 2002;**46**:27–34.

38 Hogdson TA, Sahni N, Kaliakatsou F, Buchanan JAG, Porter SR. Long-term efficacy and safety of topical tacrolimus in the management of ulcerative/erosive oral lichen planus. *Eur J Dermatol* 2003;**13**:466–70.

39 Byrd JA, Davis MDP, Bruce AJ, Drage LA, Rogers RS. Response of oral lichen planus to topical tacrolimus in 37 patients. *Arch Dermatol* 2004;**140**:1508–12.

40 Thomson MA, Hamburger J, Stewart DG, Lewis HM. Treatment of erosive lichen planus with topical tacrolimus. *J Dermatol Treat* 2004;**15**:308–14.

41 Lener EV, Brieva J, Schachter M, West LE, West DP, El-Azhary RA. Successful treatment of erosive lichen planus with topical tacrolimus. *Arch Dermatol* 2001;**137**:419–22.

42 Swift JC, Rees TD, Plemons JM, Hallmon WW, Wright JC. The effectiveness of 1% pimecrolimus in the treatment of oral erosive lichen planus. *J Periodontol* 2005;**76**:627–35.

43 Becherel PA, Chosidow O, Boisnic S, *et al*. Topical cyclosporine in the treatment of oral and vulvar erosive lichen planus: a blood level monitoring study. *Arch Dermatol* 1995;**131**:495–6.

44 Vigliola PA. Therapeutic evaluation of oral retinoid RO 10-9359 in severe nonpsoriatic dermatoses. *Br J Dermatol* 1980;**103**:483–7.

45 Buajeeb W, Kraivaphan P, Pobrurksa C. Efficacy of topical retinoic acid compared with topical fluocinolone acetonide in the treatment of oral lichen planus. *Oral Surg Oral Med Oral Pathol Oral Radiol Endod* 1997;**83**:21–5.

46 Sieg P, von Domarus H, von Zitzewitz V, Iven H, Färber L. Topical cyclosporin in oral lichen planus: a controlled, randomized, prospective trial. *Br J Dermatol* 1995;**132**: 790–4.

47 Lopez Lopez J, Rosello Llabres XR. Cyclosporine A, an alternative to the oral lichen planus erosive treatment. *Bull Group Int Rech Sci Stomatol Odontol* 1995;**38**:33–8.

48 Conrotto D, Carbone M, Carrozzo M, *et al.* Ciclosporin vs. clobetasol in the topical management of atrophic and erosive lichen planus: a double-blind, randomized controlled trial. *Br J Dermatol* 2006;**154**:139–45.

49 Macario-Barrel A, Balguerie X, Joly P. [Treatment of erosive oral lichen planus with thalidomide; in French.] *Ann Dermatol Venereol* 2003;**130**:1109–12.

50 Lundquist G, Forsgren H, Gajecki M, Emstetam L. Photochemotherapy of oral lichen planus: a controlled study. *Oral Surg Oral Med Oral Pathol Oral Radiol Endod* 1995;**79**:554–8.

51 Bécherel PA, Bussel A, Chosidow O, Rabian C, Piette JC, Francès C. Extracorporeal photochemotherapy in the treatment of multiresistant mucosal lichen planus. *Lancet* 1998;**351**:805.

23 Acute urticaria

Torsten Schäfer

This chapter deals with the management of a single isolated episode of urticaria (acute urticaria), rather than the recurrent episodes observed in chronic urticaria. The discussion is restricted to randomized controlled trials (RCTs). The majority of the RCTs deal with the most recently developed drugs. Earlier experimental work with the first antihistamines is not taken into account, as they were not assessed formally in RCTs. It should be noted that many of the reported RCTs have been conducted in emergency departments. It is unclear whether such results also apply to ordinary practice.

Background

Definition

Common synonyms for urticaria are "hives" and "nettle rash"; the latter term (like the German word for the condition, *Nesselsucht*) focuses on the typical reactions following skin contact with the stinging nettle (*Urtica dioica*).

The primary lesions in this monomorphic exanthematous disease are hives or wheals, which are defined as circumscribed, white to pink-colored, compressible skin elevations produced by dermal edema (Figure 23.1). Accompanying erythemas in the surrounding area are typical. Pathophysiologically, the wheal can be characterized by local vasodilation and an increase in the permeability of capillaries and small venules, followed by transudation of plasma constituents into the papillary and upper reticular dermis. Among a large number of substances, such as kinins, leukotrienes, prostaglandins, and proteolytic enzymes, histamine is the best known elicitor of typical wheal-and-flare reactions. Eruptions of urticarial lesions are usually associated with intense pruritus.

Although the disease is easily diagnosed from the clinical point of view, there are no standardized or validated diagnostic criteria for urticaria. The disease is classified according to its etiology or course.

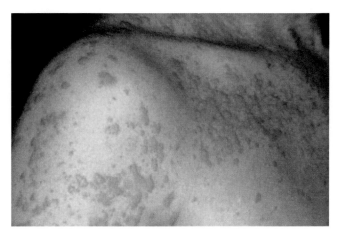

Figure 23.1 A patient with acute urticaria.

Incidence/prevalence

Valid population-based estimates of the incidence of acute urticaria are lacking. Approximately 20–30% of the general population experience at least one episode of urticaria in their life. There is some validity in the assumption that acute urticaria is more common in children. Females predominate in acute and chronic forms of the disease.[1]

Etiology

In principle, the same etiological considerations apply as for chronic urticaria. Corresponding to the course of the disease, acute infections—alone or in combination with concomitant drug intake—have been found to be associated with acute urticaria in 30–50% of cases.[2]

Prognosis

By definition, acute urticaria is restricted to an occurrence lasting no longer than 6 weeks; otherwise it is classified as chronic urticaria. The disease is therefore considered to be self-limiting.

Diagnostic tests

In principle, the same diagnostic considerations apply as for chronic urticaria. However, a full diagnostic work-up is rarely indicated in acute cases. A carefully taken history will provide important etiological hints (e.g., regarding infection or drugs).

Aims of treatment

The aims of treatment are to reduce the symptoms and to shorten the course of the disease.

Relevant outcomes

- Intensity of subjective symptoms (pruritus, sedation)
- Disease/wheal intensity
- General physicians' and patients' assessment as assessed by numeric or visual analogue scales (VAS)
- Surface area (rule of nine)
- Cessation rate

Methods of search

A search was made for all RCTs, meta-analyses, systematic reviews, and Cochrane reviews in the electronic databases PubMed, Cochrane Central Register of Controlled Trials (Central), and the Cochrane Database of Systematic Reviews up to March 2006, using the search terms "acute" and "urticaria," or "hive" or "wheal" or "nettle and rash." We did not include studies with healthy volunteers or studies on experimentally induced histamine reactions.

Questions

Which drugs are effective and safe in the treatment of acute urticaria?

The search of the Cochrane Library and other electronic databases did not identify any systematic reviews or meta-analyses on acute urticaria. A consensus report on the management of urticaria was published following a panel discussion during the clinically oriented European Society for Dermatological Research's symposium "Urticaria 2000."[3] In addition to eliminating the eliciting stimuli, nonsedating H[1] antihistamines were recommended as standard and initial treatment, with prednisolone 50 mg/day for 3 days as an alternative treatment. A further review, published in 2001, presents an evidence-based evaluation of antihistamines in the treatment of urticaria.[4] The section on acute urticaria discusses two studies, which will also be presented in this chapter.[2,5] Other reviews published in 2002,

2003, and 2004 do not refer to any RCTs other than those mentioned below.[6–8]

Recently, European consensus guidelines on urticaria were published, which also applied the methods of evidence-based medicine (a systematic literature search, standardized critical appraisal, levels of evidence, and grades of recommendation).[9] With regard to acute urticaria, nonsedating second-generation H[1] antagonists were recommended (grade of recommendation D) on the basis of two publications on loratadine[2] and cetirizine[10] (both with a level of evidence of 2– and poor methodological quality). The latter trial was designed to assess the prevention, rather than treatment, of acute urticaria.

Nonresponsive patients should receive either oral corticosteroids such as prednisone 2×20 mg/day for 4 days[11] or prednisolone (50 mg/day for 3 days),[2] or alternatively H[2]-blockers (single dose or 5 days).[5,12,13] On the basis of levels of evidence of 2– and 2+ and a poor methodological quality in one study,[2] these therapeutic alternatives have received a grade D recommendation.

With regard to single RCTs, the Cochrane Library lists seven such trials that have acute urticaria as the primary end point of the intervention and not as a reported side effect. Three further trials were identified in PubMed (Table 23.1).

Antihistamines (first-generation H[1] antagonists and H[2] antagonists)

Four studies compared the use of H[1] and H[2] antagonists, or a combination of the two. None of the studies had a placebo arm. Two studies compared diphenhydramine with an H[2] antagonist (famotidine or cimetidine).

Moscati and Moore investigated the efficacy of a single dose of intramuscular cimetidine 300 mg in comparison with intramuscular diphenhydramine 50 mg in 93 young adults.[5] Both treatments let to significant reductions in itching, wheal intensity, and extent after 30 minutes, with no differences between the treatments. A significant increase in sedation was reported by patients in both groups, but was significantly higher in patients treated with diphenhydramine. Absolute changes in the three-point and four-point scoring scales appeared to be clinically significant. The study is limited by flaws in the process of randomization and blinding.

Watson *et al.* compared single-dose intramuscular diphenhydramine 50 mg with intramuscular famotidine 20 mg in 25 adults.[12] After 30 minutes, pruritus was reduced significantly by both treatments, with diphenhydramine appearing to be more effective. Famotidine also significantly reduced the body surface area affected. The physician-rated intensity of urticaria was reduced equally and significantly by both drugs. A nonsignificant increase in sedation was reported by patients receiving diphenhydramine. The small sample size and unbalanced group

Table 23.1 Summary of data from randomized controlled trials on the treatment of acute urticaria

First author, ref.	Intervention	Outcome measures	Patients (n)	Results
Moscati and Moore[5]	Single-dose cimetidine 300 mg i.m. *or* diphenhydramine 50 mg i.m.	Itching, wheal intensity, sedation, wheal extent, overall improvement on a 3–4 point numerical scale; validity and reliability not known	93 No dropouts	No difference for clinical response Diphenhydramine significantly more sedation
Watson et al.[12]	Single-dose H$_2$-receptor antagonist famotidine 20 mg i.m. vs. H$_1$-receptor antagonist diphenhydramine 50 mg i.m. in the treatment of acute urticaria	Pruritus (patient, VAS) Intensity of urticaria (physician, VAS) Surface area (physician, rule of nine) Sedation (patient, VAS)	25 No dropouts	Only within-group comparisons (before/after comparison)
Lin et al.[14]	Diphenhydramine 50 mg + ranitidine 50 mg vs. diphenhydramine 50 mg + placebo	Presence of urticaria at baseline and after 1 and 2 h Extent (number of involved areas)	Unclear	Presence of urticaria after 2 h: 16.2% vs 8.3% (+ ranitidine); P = 0.02
Runge et al.[15]	Single-dose diphenhydramine 50 mg + placebo i.v. *or* cimetidine 300 mg + placebo i.v. *or* diphenhydramine 50 mg + cimetidine 300 mg i.v.	VAS (110 mm) to assess: Pruritus, throat tightness, and facial swelling (patient) Urticaria, pharyngeal tissue swelling and facial swelling (physician) Change of 25 mm considered clinically significant Adverse effects	39	More urticaria patients receiving diphenhydramine + cimetidine (11/12) experienced relief in comparison with those receiving diphenhydramine (5/11, P = 0.027) or cimetidine (8/10, n.s.) alone
Simons[10]	Oral cetirizine 0.25 mg/kg twice daily vs. placebo over 18 months in children with atopic eczema	Incidence of diary-reported symptoms typical for acute urticaria	795	Cumulative incidence of urticaria 16.2% vs. 5.8% during 18-month treatment (P < 0.001); 4.6% vs. 3.0% during 6-month follow-up (n.s.)
Pollack and Romano[11]	Single-dose diphenhydramine 50 mg i.m., followed by oral hydroxyzine 25 mg every 4–8 h plus oral prednisone 20 mg twice daily for 4 days or placebo	Pruritus (VAS 10 cm) Adverse effects	43	Significantly more improvement with the addition of steroid
Zuberbier et al.[2]	Loratadine 10 mg/day until remission vs. prednisolone 50 mg/day for 3 days, followed by loratadine 10 mg/day until remission	Cessation of whealing	109	Percentage cessation at five time points Significant differences only after 3 days (when the intervention arm had so far received prednisolone alone; 93.8% vs. 65.9%)

I.m., intramuscular; i.v., intravenous; n.s., not significant; VAS, visual analogue scale.

size (diphenhydramine n = 10, famotidine n = 15; no block randomization) does not allow meaningful comparison of the groups.

Lin *et al.* compared the efficacy of single-dose intravenous diphenhydramine 50 mg alone or in combination with intravenous ranitidine 50 mg in 91 adults.[14] Significantly more patients receiving the combination therapy (91.7%) were free of symptoms after 2 hours in comparison with those who received diphenhydramine alone (73.8%). After control for the baseline extent, the combination therapy was found to be able to reduce the number of involved areas significantly within 2 hours. Significantly more additional antihistamines were administered in the diphenhydramine group, however, which may have shifted the effect towards the zero-effect level.

Runge *et al.* studied 39 adults with acute allergic reactions, including urticaria.[15] Fourteen patients received a single dose of intravenous diphenhydramine 50 mg, 12 received intravenous cimetidine 300 mg, and 13 received both preparations. After 30 minutes, the combination therapy led to a significantly greater reduction in the urticaria (evaluated using a VAS) in comparison with diphenhydramine alone. The latter, however, achieved the best results in reduction of pruritus, and the differences were significant in comparison with cimetidine. The study is limited by the small sample size and significant differences in the mean treatment scores for urticaria between the study groups, which were not adjusted for in later analyses.

Pontasch et al. compared three oral medications in the treatment of acute urticaria in adults.[13] Seven patients received diphenhydramine, six received famotidine, and another seven received cromolyn sodium (sodium cromoglicate). Patient satisfaction was highest with diphenhydramine (six of seven), followed by famotidine (three of six), and cromolyn sodium (three of seven). Adverse effects were reported by three of the seven patients treated with diphenhydramine, by three of the six in the famotidine group, and by one patient who received cromolyn sodium.

Corticosteroids

The addition of oral prednisone 20 mg twice daily for 4 days to the standard treatment with H_1 antagonists was investigated in 43 adults by Pollack and Romano.[11] The intensity of itching, as scored on a VAS, was significantly reduced by both regimens after 2 and 5 days of follow-up. However, the addition of prednisone reduced the symptom score significantly more than the standard therapy. Although the standard therapy with antihistamines is generally considered sufficient, the addition of prednisone appears to be helpful in selected cases (in relation to the severity of the condition and the need to shorten the period of antihistamine treatment).

Similarly, Zuberbier et al. showed that prednisolone 50 mg/day for 3 days led to a significantly higher clearing rate (93.8%) after 3 days than therapy with loratadine 10 mg/day in 109 patients.[2] The study may be limited by aspects of its design (an open study with pseudorandomization by consecutive time periods and differential allocation of possibly pregnant women).

A best-evidence report dating from 2004 summarizes the two studies mentioned above.[16]

Other treatments and nonrandomized trials

A case series including five patients with acute urticaria following insect stings reported good therapeutic effects with intravenous cimetidine 300 mg initially followed by 300 mg orally four times daily after ineffective administration of epinephrine, H_1 antagonists, and corticosteroids.[17]

A further report investigated the effect of flunarizine, a calcium antagonist, in the treatment of acute urticaria. In this uncontrolled trial, 20 patients received a single 10-mg sublingual dose of flunarizine. After 3 hours, 16 patients had experienced improvement, with the effects being more pronounced for itching than for the reduction of wheals. Four patients remained unresponsive and five other patients reported drowsiness as a major side effect.[18]

A Chinese publication describes the therapeutic effect of the added ingredient of Angelica sinensis root in 106 patients with acute urticaria. Unfortunately, the lack of an abstract in English makes it difficult to draw conclusions.[19]

Prevention

A European multicenter study entitled Early Treatment of the Atopic Child (ETAC) investigated the preventive effect of long-term (18 months) administration of cetirizine 0.25 mg/kg twice daily in 1–2-year-old children with atopic eczema and a positive family history of allergies.[10] In addition to the primary end point (asthma), symptoms typical of acute urticaria were recorded in a diary during the intervention period and a 6-month follow-up period. During the intervention period, significantly fewer episodes of acute urticaria (5.8%) were reported in the intervention group in comparison with the placebo arm (16.2%). This effect did not persist after medication was stopped (3.0% versus 4.6%).

Harms

On the basis of the available studies on acute urticaria, the major side effect is sedation associated with first-generation H_1 antagonists. The next chapter, on chronic urticaria (Chapter 24), discusses the newer antihistamines.

Comment: implications for clinical practice

Generally, the therapeutic evidence available on acute urticaria is quantitatively and qualitatively weak. RCTs of the therapeutic efficacy of the second-generation antihistamines are lacking, although one would like to regard these as the first choice for treatment on the basis of studies on chronic urticaria. There is some evidence that a combination of H_1 and H_2 antagonists has additional beneficial effects. A short-term intervention with corticosteroids appears to be superior to treatment with antihistamines alone, but should be considered in the context of individual needs.

Key points

- Acute urticaria is a common disease.
- It appears to predominate in children and females.
- The etiology remains largely unclear, but there is evidence that acute infections and concomitant drugs, as well as food hypersensitivity, are important elicitors.
- Evidence on the effects of treatment for acute urticaria is qualitatively and quantitatively poor.
- There is evidence that first- and second-generation antihistamines are effective and that a combination with H_2 antagonists may have additional beneficial effects.
- A short-term intervention with corticosteroids appears to be superior to treatment with antihistamines alone, but should be considered in the context of individual needs.

References

1 Schäfer T, Ring J. Epidemiology of urticaria. In: Burr ML, ed. *Epidemiology of Clinical Allergy*. Basle: Karger, 1993: 49–60. (Monographs in allergy, vol. 31.)

2 Zuberbier T, Ifflander J, Semmler C, Henz B. Acute urticaria: clinical aspects and therapeutic responsiveness. *Acta Derm Venereol* 1996;**76**:296–7.

3 Zuberbier T, Greaves M, Juhlin L, Merk H, Stingl G, Henz B. Management of urticaria: a consensus report. *J Investig Dermatol Symp Proc* 2001;**6**:128–31.

4 Lee E, Maibach H. Treatment of urticaria: an evidence-based evaluation of antihistamines. *Am J Clin Dermatol* 2001;**2**:27–32.

5 Moscati R, Moore G. Comparison of cimetidine and diphenhydramine in the treatment of acute urticaria. *Ann Emerg Med* 1990;**19**:12–5.

6 Kaplan AP. Clinical practice. Chronic urticaria and angioedema. *N Engl J Med* 2002;**346**:175–9.

7 Zuberbier T. Urticaria. *Allergy* 2003;**58**:1224–34.

8 Muller BA. Urticaria and angioedema: a practical approach. *Am Fam Physician* 2004;**69**:1123–8.

9 Zuberbier T, Bindslev-Jensen C, Canonica W, *et al.* EAACI/GA2LEN/EDF guideline: management of urticaria. *Allergy* 2006; **61**:321–31.

10 Simons FE. Prevention of acute urticaria in young children with atopic dermatitis. *J Allergy Clin Immunol* 2001;**107**:703–6.

11 Pollack CJ, Romano T. Outpatient management of acute urticaria: the role of prednisone. *Ann Emerg Med* 1995;**26**:547–51.

12 Watson N, Weiss E, Harter P. Famotidine in the treatment of acute urticaria. *Clin Exp Dermatol* 2000;**25**:186–9.

13 Pontasch M, White L, Bradford J. Oral agents in the management of urticaria: patient perception of effectiveness and level of satisfaction with treatment. *Ann Pharmacother* 1993;**27**:730–1.

14 Lin R, Curry A, Pesola G, *et al.* Improved outcomes in patients with acute allergic syndromes who are treated with combined H₁ and H₂ antagonists. *Ann Emerg Med* 2000;**36**:462–8.

15 Runge J, Martinez J, Caravati E, Williamson S, Hartsell S. Histamine antagonists in the treatment of acute allergic reactions. *Ann Emerg Med* 1992;**21**:237–42.

16 Poon M, Reid C. Best evidence topic reports: oral corticosteroids in acute urticaria. *Emerg Med J* 2004;**21**:76–7.

17 Rusli M. Cimetidine treatment of recalcitrant acute allergic urticaria. *Ann Emerg Med* 1986;**15**:1363–5.

18 Allegue F, Martin M, Harto A, Ledo A. Treatment of acute urticaria with sublingual flunarizine. *Int J Dermatol* 1988;**27**:265–6.

19 Wang C, Zhang Z, Wang Q. Therapeutic effect of 106 acute urticaria patients with the added ingredient of radix angelicae sinesis. *J Shanxi Coll Trad Chin Med* 1997;**20**:25.

24 Chronic urticaria

Conrad Hauser, Philip Taramarcaz

Background

Definition

Urticaria is a skin eruption consisting of erythematous or anemic (blanched) papules (hives, wheals) with surrounding erythema due to circumscribed vascular edema of the upper dermis (Figure 24.1). Chronic urticaria (CU) is defined as recurrent or permanently appearing lesions of more than 6 weeks' duration. The size, number, and shape of the lesions vary considerably. Angioedema (acute localized swelling of subcutaneous or submucosal tissue) can be associated with chronic urticaria. Pressure urticaria—localized whealing induced by application of pressure to the skin—is frequently associated with CU (in up to 37% of cases).[1] Concomitant urticarial dermographism is also observed. CU compromises the quality of life.[2,3] In one study, the

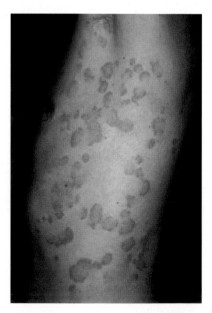

Figure 24.1 Urticarial lesions on the thorax of a young man.

degree of suffering in patients with CU was found to be greater, in relation to numerous parameters, in comparison with that in patients with upper allergic respiratory allergies such as hay fever.[4] In another study, the physical discomfort in patients with CU was found to be more significant than in patients with psoriasis.[5]

Incidence/prevalence

CU is frequent. One report speculated that the incidence is 1.3% in the general population.[6] A recent population-based survey in Spain reported a prevalence of 0.6%, with the rate being 3.8 times higher in females than in males.[7]

Etiology

The etiology of CU is heterogeneous. The relative number of patients in whom the etiology and/or an underlying disease can be identified varies considerably in different reports, but appears to be small. In a subset of patients with CU, mast cell and basophil-degranulating serum antibodies have been found. Many of these sera contain autoantibodies to FcεRI,[8–10] suggesting an autoimmune mechanism of pathogenic significance (Figure 24.2). Complement and complement-fixing isotypes (IgG1 and IgG3) appear to be required for histamine release by these antibodies.[11,12] This group is sometimes referred to as autoimmune CU, and patients may suffer from more severe and longer-lasting disease.[13–16] In some patients, anti-IgE antibodies and antibodies to the low-affinity IgE receptor (FcεRII, CD23), releasing mediators from eosinophils that induce mast cell degranulation, have been identified.[17] Aspirin and other nonsteroidal anti-inflammatory drugs can aggravate CU in one-third to two-thirds of patients. Angiotensin-converting enzyme inhibitors can aggravate angioedema and urticaria.

Numerous foods and food additives have been reported to aggravate or provoke urticaria. Their role in CU remains controversial, because only in a minority of cases does urticaria appear reproducible in double-blind placebo-

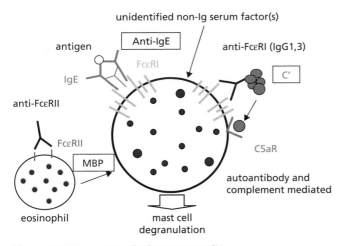

Figure 24.2 How autoantibodies may cause CU. When fixed by IgE antibodies bound to the surface of mast cells via the high-affinity receptor for IgE (FcεRI), antigens can induce mediator release in disorders such as allergic urticaria or allergic rhinitis. Autoantibodies (IgG1 and 3) binding to the FcεRI (α-chain), activating complement (C) and releasing C5a may contribute to mast cell release in CU. Autoantibodies to IgE may also contribute to mast cell release. Autoantibodies to the low affinity IgE receptor (FcεRII) on eosinophils may induce release of mediators including major basic protein (MBP) that contribute to mast cell release. Additional nonantibody serum factors may induce release of mediators from mast cell.

controlled oral challenge tests.[18–21] Foods and drugs usually induce acute urticaria and/or angioedema as well as other symptoms of anaphylaxis, rather than CU. A role of food or food additives in recurrent CU should only be suspected if there is a close temporal relation between uptake and whealing. Some foods containing vasoactive amines (including histamine) and mast cell degranulating compounds may aggravate CU.

CU may be aggravated by nonspecific infections such as upper respiratory tract infections. The role of specific infections is controversial. The remission rate in patients with CU and chronic dental infections did not differ after dental treatment compared with nontreated patients with chronic urticaria.[22] This also appears to be the case for sinusitis, urinary tract infections, and gallbladder infections.[23] Similarly, the dental status in patients with CU did not differ from that in controls.[24] The remission rate of CU after dental intervention was low. Although high prevalence rates were reported in uncontrolled studies, *Helicobacter pylori* infection is no more frequent in patients with chronic urticaria than in controls.[25] Various remission rates in patients with CU who receive eradication treatment after positive *H. pylori* tests have been reported in open studies, but there is a lack of high-quality controlled studies. Hepatitis C was not significantly associated with urticaria in a recent European study.[26] Hepatitis B serology was frequently positive in patients with CU, but there have been no controlled studies. *Candida* is unlikely to cause chronic urticaria. The role of

Campylobacter jejuni and *Blastocystis hominis* remains controversial. Parasites may occasionally cause chronic urticaria.

Exposure to inhalant allergens may rarely induce CU. CU or urticarial vasculitis may be found in a large spectrum of systemic immune disorders and syndromes, including collagen vascular diseases (Box 24.1), but these disorders are

> **BOX 24.1** CU and urticaria-like skin lesions as a symptom in systemic diseases and syndromes
>
> **Genetic diseases**
> - Muckle–Wells syndrome (MIM 191900)
> - Familial cold autoinflammatory syndrome (MIM 120100)
> - Familial Mediterranean fever (MIM 249100)
> - Familial Hibernian fever/tumor necrosis factor receptor-associated periodic syndrome (TRAPS) (MIM 19190)
> - Hyper-IgD syndrome (MIM 251170)
> - Chronic infantile neurological cutaneous and auricular (CINCA) syndrome, neonatal-onset multisystem inflammatory disease (NOMID), Prieur–Griscelli syndrome (MIM 607115)
> - Canale–Smith syndrome, autoimmune lymphoproliferative syndrome (ALPS1a; MIM 601859)
> - Immune dysregulation, polyendocrinopathy, and enteropathy, x-linked (IPEX), x-linked autoimmunity-allergic dysregulation (XLAAD) syndrome (MIM 304790)
>
> **Immune disorders**
> - Systemic lupus erythematosus
> - Sjögren syndrome
> - Dermatomyositis
> - Mixed connective-tissue disease (Sharp syndrome)
> - Juvenile rheumatoid arthritis (Still disease)
> - Cogan syndrome
> - Serum sickness
> - Relapsing polychondritis
> - Hypocomplementemic urticaria vasculitis (McDuffy syndrome)
> - Acquired C1 inhibitor deficiency
> - Cryoglobulinemia (as precursor of palpable purpura)
> - Presence of thyroid autoantibodies/thyroid function abnormalities
>
> **Vasculitides**
> - Urticarial vasculitis
> - Eosinophilic vasculitis of skin
> - Wegener granulomatosis
> - Churg–Strauss syndrome
> - Takayasu arteritis
>
> **Hematologic diseases**
> - Systemic mastocytosis, including forms without cutaneous infiltration
> - Polycythemia vera (Vaquez disease)
> - Hypereosinophilic syndrome and other hematologic conditions with highly elevated eosinophil blood counts
> - Episodic angioedema with eosinophilia (Gleich syndrome)
> - Schnitzler syndrome

rare in patients with CU. In such cases, urticarial lesions may be atypical (burning/pain rather than pruritus, persistence of skin lesions for more than 24 hours at the same site, purpura), the skin biopsy may show signs of urticarial vasculitis (leukocytoclastic vasculitis), and other signs and symptoms of systemic disease may appear. CU appears to be frequent in cystic fibrosis.[27] The association of CU and celiac disease remains controversial.[28,29] There is a lack of association between CU and cancer.[30] Anecdotal reports suggest that metallic implants may cause CU.

CU may flare premenstrually and during pregnancy. In anecdotal cases, the eruption was reproducible by administration of progesterone and, more rarely, of estrogen.

Prognosis

In one of the largest studies, urticaria cleared within 6 months in about 50% of patients.[23] After 10 years, about 80% of patients with CU and about half of those with CU and angioedema were free of symptoms. A more recent study reported a complete remission rate of 35% and a partial remission rate of 29% within 1 year.[31] Another study reported 5-year and 10-year remission rates of 29% and 44%, respectively.[32] The association with angioedema did not affect the remission rate in this study. A third recent study reported 1-year and 5-year remission rates of 30% and 86%, respectively.[15] In this study, disease duration was associated with angioedema. Referral bias and a lack of distinction between acute and CU in all studies may have influenced the outcome.

Diagnostic tests

Opinions regarding the number of laboratory tests that should be conducted vary considerably, ranging from those who decline any investigation to those who carry out a comprehensive work-up. Many experts agree that the work-up for CU should include measurement of the erythrocyte sedimentation rate and red and white blood counts, including a differential white cell count.[33] Similar recommendations were made at a French consensus development conference[34] and in the recent guidelines published by the European Academy of Allergy and Clinical Immunology (EAACI).[35] Physical urticaria should be considered and tested accordingly if suspected. In case of blood eosinophilia, a parasite work-up should be included. In cases in which it is thought that food or drugs are involved, a double-blind placebo-controlled food challenge test should be performed after elimination of the suspected food item or drug. If there are associated systemic symptoms, an elevated erythrocyte sedimentation rate or abnormal blood count underlying systemic disease should be considered. A search for paraprotein may identify patients with Schnitzler syndrome, in which there is a combination of paraprotein

(usually IgM, rarely IgG) and CU, sometimes associated with osteosclerosis and bone or joint pain.[36] The intradermal autologous serum test correlates fairly well with the occurrence of basophil-degranulating antibodies. Tests to determine basophil-degranulating antibodies based on the expression of CD63 are currently being used for this purpose.[37,38] However, it has not yet been shown that the test results have any impact on the treatment. Autoantibodies to thyroid and thyroid function abnormalities were found to be significantly more frequent in patients with CU in several studies.[39] Autoimmune CU was significantly and selectively associated with thyroid abnormalities (autoantibodies and function) in one study.[40] It is currently not clear whether a search for thyroid abnormalities should only be carried out in patients with a positive autologous serum test or in all patients with chronic urticaria. Skin biopsies are not routinely taken, but should be performed in order to exclude vasculitis if the lesions are purpuric, and may be helpful in case of other atypical features (e.g., persistence of skin lesions for more than 24 hours at the same site, burning or pain, and other signs and symptoms of systemic disease). Three studies report a very low incidence of urticarial (leukocytoclastic) vasculitis in CU,[41–43] whereas this histologic pattern was found in 12% in one study including 100 patients.[44] If urticarial vasculitis is diagnosed histologically, there is a greater likelihood of an underlying systemic disease.[45,46] Figure 24.3 presents a general diagnostic algorithm.

The differential diagnosis of CU includes scabies, arthropod bite reactions, and insect sting reactions (sometimes referred to as papular urticaria), cutaneous mastocytosis, the urticarial stages of autoimmune bullous skin diseases, including bullous pemphigoid and dermatitis herpetiformis, and the early stages of vasculitis and erythema multiforme (see also Box 24.1). In case of annular lesions, the various forms of annular erythema may need to be considered. Annular or reticulate erythema can sometimes precede attacks of hereditary angioedema.

Aims of treatment

The aims of treatment are to reduce pruritus, wheal size, wheal number and whealing frequency, sleep disturbance, and the total symptom score and to achieve an overall improvement in the patient's condition (including quality of life) and permanent remission of the disease.

Relevant outcomes

- Pruritus
- Wheal size, number, and frequency
- Loss of wakening
- Overall physician assessment
- Overall patient assessment

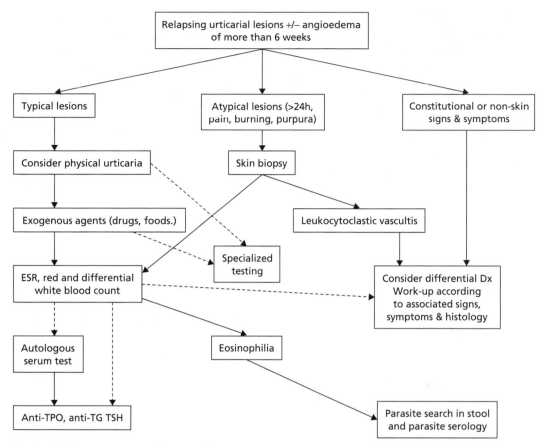

Figure 24.3 Algorithm for the investigation and diagnosis of CU. When angioedema is not associated with urticaria different diagnostic considerations need to be included (such as congenital and acquired C1 esterase deficiency, converting enzyme inhibitors, vibratory angioedema) in addition to those presented in this chapter. Dx, diagnosis.

- Quality of life
- Permanent remission of disease

Methods of search

A search was carried out for "urticaria" using the National Library of Medicine Gateway for the period 2000–2006.

Questions

Which drugs are effective in CU?

Efficacy

Newer-generation oral antihistamines. The newer-generation antihistamines are all H_1 receptor antagonists, with good evidence for clinical efficacy in CU. The currently available newer-generation antihistamines are among the most frequently taken drugs and are generally very safe. In particular, they are less sedative and are free of anticholinergic effects in comparison with the first-generation antihistamines. Some clinically relevant details on pharmacology, pharmacotherapy, and efficacy in CU can be found in Table 24.1,[47–89] and several reviews have been published recently.[90–93] The dosage in children over 12 years is the same as that for adults; the manufacturers' recommendations should be followed for children aged up to 12 years.

Many newer-generation antihistamines have additional anti-inflammatory properties, but their effect on clinically relevant parameters has not been demonstrated. In many trials, pruritus, wheal size, wheal number, total clinical scores, and overall patient and physician assessment were studied as relevant outcomes. Quality of life has only been studied rarely. A systematic review of the newer-generation antihistamines is not currently available, but there is one forthcoming from the Cochrane Collaboration, which will provide further details.

The evidence for their efficacy seems to be well established, on the basis of 25 randomized controlled trials (RCTs) that we identified. There are no studies on the

Table 24.1 Pharmacologic and pharmacotherapeutic details of newer-generation antihistamines (H1 blockers)

Drug (general references)	Elimination half-life (h)	Dose	Central nervous system impairment at				Clinically relevant cardiotoxicity	Dose adjustment			Trials (references)
			Standard dose	High dose	With alcohol	Clinically relevant		Elderly	Renal impairment	Hepatic impairmen	
Acrivastine[47]	1.4–2.1	8 mg three times daily	Possible	+	+	+	–	Not known	NA	NA	RTC[48–50] CCT[51–54]
Azelastine[55]	22–36	1–2 mg twice daily	Possible	+	+	+	–	No	NA	NA	RCT[56]
Cetirizine[57]	7–10	10 mg daily	–	+	Possible	–	–	No	Yes	Yes	RTC[58–63] CCT[64,65]
Desloratadine[66,67]	17	5 mg daily	–	Probably not	Probably not	–	–	No	NA	NA	RCT[68,69]
Ebastine[70]	10–16 (AM)	10 mg daily	–	Possible	–	–	Unlikely	No	No	No	RCT[71]
Fexofenadine[72]	14	180 mg daily/ 60 mg twice daily	–	–	–	–	Unlikely	No	No	No	RCT[73–76] CCT[77,78]
Levocetirizine[79,80]	7.9	5 mg daily	–	Possible	Possible	–	–	No	Yes	Yes	RCT[81]
Loratadine[82]	27 (AM)	10 mg daily	–	–	+	–	–	Yes	+	Yes	RCT[61,83,84] CCT[85]
Mizolastine[86]	8–10	10 mg daily	–	–	–	–	Unlikely	No	–	No	RCT[87,88] CCT[89]

AM, active metabolite; CCT, controlled clinical trial; RCT, randomized controlled trial; NA, not applicable.

long-term relapse rate of CU after discontinuation of the drug. Most studies are placebo-controlled. Some involve comparisons with older-generation antihistamines, to demonstrate the superior side-effect profile, and a minority are comparisons with other newer nonsedating antihistamines. Most, if not all, of the clinical studies were probably sponsored by pharmaceutical companies. Some studies are published in journals that are hard to obtain. The number of patients included in the studies varies between approximately 20 and 400. The duration of the studies varied generally between 4 and 12 weeks. Topical antihistamines should not be prescribed, because of their irritant and sensitizing potential.[94]

Older-generation antihistamines, with pronounced sedative effects. Sedative antihistamines are also effective in treating CU. The sedative effects may be welcome to prevent awakening at night. Many controlled data about the effectiveness of sedative antihistamines in CU originate from studies in which they were compared with newer-generation antihistamines. The individual drugs are listed in Table 24.2.[53,64,95–102] All references cited in the table are from studies with newer-generation antihistamines.

Combination treatments. A combination of H_1 and H_2 blockers was found to be superior to H_1 blockers alone in four RCTs.[103–106] It appears that H_2 blockers increase the plasma concentration of H_1 blockers.[107,108] H_1 plus H_2 blockers in combination with nifedipine, a calcium-channel blocker, was found to be better than H_1 blockers alone in one small CCT.[109] The combination of newer H_1 blockers and leukotriene receptor antagonist has been recently investigated. In three out of four of these studies, the combination therapy was found to be more effective in the treatment of CU than anti-H_1 alone, despite the fact that the additional benefit of antileukotrienes appears to be modest.[77,110–112] An unusual combination of cetirizine and slow release theophylline over a period of 6 months was reported to improve various effectiveness and visual analogue scale scores after 2 to 3 months of treatment.[113]

Other drug treatments
- Very few controlled trials with other than H_1/H_2 blockers have been published.
- Doxepin, used as an antidepressant, has been shown to have a high affinity for the H_1 receptor[114] and is an effective H_1 blocker. Doxepin has been shown to be effective in CU in one RCT and three CCTs.[115–117]
- After the identification of autoantibodies to FcεRI, immunomodulators were studied. Ciclosporin was found to be effective in two RCTs.[118,119] The autologous serum test was found not to be predictive of a response to ciclosporin in one study,[120] although *in vitro* histamine release from basophils stimulated with sera from patients with functional anti-FcεRI antibodies was inhibited by ciclosporin in another report.[121]
- Thyroid hormone substitution in individuals with thyroid abnormalities induced an unusually high remission rate in several open studies.[122–128] Unfortunately, controlled studies are lacking.
- Stanozolol was found to be better in combination with an H_1 blocker than the H_1 blocker alone in one RCT including 50 patients.[129]
- Hydroxychloroquine was added to conventional CU therapy for 12 weeks. It significantly improved the quality of life, but not the symptom scores.[130]

Other drugs that are sometimes used for CU, but for which no controlled studies have been conducted, include warfarin, colchicine, danazol, dapsone (diaminodiphenylsulfone), sulfasalazine, methotrexate, azathioprine, thalidomide, intravenous immunoglobulin, rofecoxib in combination with desloratadine, cyclophosphamide, nortriptyline, and mirtazapine. The European Academy of Allergy and Clinical Immunology (EAACI) has recently published management guidelines for urticaria, including CU.[131]

Ultraviolet A or B light (UVA, UVB), including narrowband UVB, has been used in CU. Treatment-resistant patients have undergone plasmapheresis.

Drawbacks
Newer-generation antihistamines are generally very safe and free of cardiotoxicity (Table 24.1). Rarely, they induce urticaria as a side effect. Although included in the B or C lists, they should generally not be prescribed during pregnancy. Nonetheless, some B list drugs such as loratadine appear to be safe.[132]

Older-generation antihistamines are sedating. They should not be prescribed (even at night) to individuals who have to

Table 24.2 Selected randomized controlled trials (RCTs) and controlled clinical trials (CCTs) with older-generation antihistamines

Drug	Type of trial	References
Brompheniramine	RCT	95
Clemastine	RCT	95,96
	CCT	97
Cyproheptadine	CCT	53
Dimetindene	RCT	98,99
Hydroxyzine	RCT	100
	CCT	64
Ketotifen	CCT	97
Oxatomide	RCT	101
	CCT	102

carry out demanding tasks (the following day), including driving. Paradoxical central nervous system stimulation may occur, particularly in children. Older-generation antihistamines may have pronounced anticholinergic effects, including urinary difficulty and retention, dry mouth, palpitations, chest tightness, decreased intestinal tone and motility, blurred vision, and thickened respiratory tract secretions. Some of the older antihistamines may also increase appetite and lead to weight gain.

Skin prick and intradermal skin tests are inhibited by all antihistamines and should not be carried out until a week after discontinuation of the drug.

A review of the potential harms of all other drugs used in CU is beyond the scope of this chapter; the reader is referred to the specialized literature.

Comment

Cetirizine, levocetirizine, loratadine, desloratadine, fexofenadine, and mizolastine are generally equivalent in the treatment of CU, with the exception of the points listed in Table 24.1. Some patients who respond poorly to fexofenadine may respond better to cetirizine. The shorter delay in the onset of action of acrivastine in comparison with other newer-generation antihistamines is more of a promotional than a clinically relevant argument. Some authors have recommended various forms of diet, but controlled clinical trials are lacking.

Implications for clinical practice

The search for underlying conditions in CU has a notoriously poor outcome. In individual patients, it can sometimes be difficult to distinguish between a random association with other conditions and a real cause–effect relationship. Newer-generation antihistamines have the best evidence for clinical efficacy, are remarkably low in adverse effects, and are the first choice in the management of CU. Most of the newer-generation antihistamines are administered once daily, but the recommended daily dose can be increased up to four times.[131] The requirement for three times daily administration of acrivastine is a relative disadvantage in the treatment of CU. Combination treatments and doxepin have the next-best evidence of efficacy. If loss of sleep is a problem, sedating older-generation antihistamines may be used, with the restrictions mentioned. The leukotriene receptor antagonist montelukast may become the second choice in add-on therapy, but should not be used in monotherapy. Ciclosporin and other similar immunosuppressants may be considered in cases resistant to the drugs above. Potential long-term adverse effects are still not yet fully known. Prolonged treatment of CU with oral corticosteroids, although apparently often successful, is not advisable because of the harmful long-term effects of this class of drugs. The effectiveness of elimination diets is a matter of controversy.

Key points

- CU is a common disorder.
- CU significantly impairs the patient's quality of life.
- CU is often associated with physical urticaria, but rarely with systemic inflammatory and/or autoimmune disorders.
- Many suspected etiological factors are still matters of controversy.
- Extensive work-up not directed by associated symptoms should not be carried out.
- One-third or more of patients with so-called "idiopathic" CU have autoimmune abnormalities; many have functional autoantibodies to the high-affinity receptor for IgE, and fewer have thyroid abnormalities. The autologous serum injection test, which can reproduce an urticaria lesion, is easy to perform. Its usefulness in clinical practice still needs to be better defined.
- Newer-generation antihistamines are safe and represent the first choice in the symptomatic treatment of CU.
- CU is sometimes managed with unproven methods or drugs for which the evidence of efficacy is poor or absent.

References

1 Barlow RJ, Warburton F, Watson K, Black AK, Greaves MW. Diagnosis and incidence of delayed pressure urticaria in patients with chronic urticaria. *J Am Acad Dermatol* 1993;**29**:954–8.
2 Poon E, Seed PT, Greaves MW, Kobza-Black A. The extent and nature of disability in different urticarial conditions. *Br J Dermatol* 1999;**140**:667–71.
3 O'Donnell BF, Lawlor F, Simpson J, Morgan M, Greaves MW. The impact of chronic urticaria on the quality of life. *Br J Dermatol* 1997;**136**:197–201.
4 Baiardini I, Giardini A, Pasquali M, *et al.* Quality of life and patients' satisfaction in chronic urticaria and respiratory allergy. *Allergy* 2003;**58**:621–3.
5 Grob JJ, Revuz J, Ortonne JP, Auquier P, Lorette G. Comparative study of the impact of chronic urticaria, psoriasis and atopic dermatitis on the quality of life. *Br J Dermatol* 2005;**152**:289–95.
6 Paul E, Greilich KD. [Epidemiology of urticaria diseases; in German.] *Hautarzt* 1991;**42**:366–75.
7 Gaig P, Olona M, Munoz LD, *et al.* Epidemiology of urticaria in Spain. *J Investig Allergol Clin Immunol* 2004;**14**:214–20.
8 Ferrer M, Kinet JP, Kaplan AP. Comparative studies of functional and binding assays for IgG anti-Fc(epsilon)RIalpha (alpha-subunit) in chronic urticaria. *J Allergy Clin Immunol* 1998;**101**:672–6.
9 Fiebiger E, Maurer D, Holub H, *et al.* Serum IgG autoantibodies directed against the alpha chain of Fc epsilon RI: a selective marker and pathogenetic factor for a distinct subset of chronic urticaria patients? *J Clin Invest* 1995;**96**:2606–12.
10 Hide M, Francis DM, Grattan CE, Hakimi J, Kochan JP, Greaves MW. Autoantibodies against the high-affinity IgE receptor as a cause of histamine release in chronic urticaria. *N Engl J Med* 1993;**328**:1599–604.
11 Fiebiger E, Hammerschmid F, Stingl G, Maurer D. Anti-FcepsilonRIalpha autoantibodies in autoimmune-mediated dis-

orders: identification of a structure–function relationship. *J Clin Invest* 1998;**101**:243–51.

12 Ferrer M, Nakazawa K, Kaplan AP. Complement dependence of histamine release in chronic urticaria. *J Allergy Clin Immunol* 1999;**104**:169–172.

13 Sabroe RA, Fiebiger E, Francis DM, *et al.* Classification of anti-FcepsilonRI and anti-IgE autoantibodies in chronic idiopathic urticaria and correlation with disease severity. *J Allergy Clin Immunol* 2002;**110**:492–9.

14 Staubach P, Onnen K, Vonend A, *et al.* Autologous whole blood injections to patients with chronic urticaria and a positive autologous serum skin test: a placebo-controlled trial. *Dermatology* 2006;**212**:150–9.

15 Toubi E, Kessel A, Avshovich N, *et al.* Clinical and laboratory parameters in predicting chronic urticaria duration: a prospective study of 139 patients. Allergy 2004;**59**:869–73.

16 Caproni M, Volpi W, Giomi B, *et al.* Chronic idiopathic and chronic autoimmune urticaria: clinical and immunopathological features of 68 subjects. *Acta Derm Venereol* 2004;**84**:288–90.

17 Puccetti A, Bason C, Simeoni S, *et al.* In chronic idiopathic urticaria autoantibodies against Fc epsilonRII/CD23 induce histamine release via eosinophil activation. *Clin Exp Allergy* 2005;**35**:1599–607.

18 Di Lorenzo G, Pacor ML, Mansueto P, *et al.* Food-additive-induced urticaria: a survey of 838 patients with recurrent chronic idiopathic urticaria. *Int Arch Allergy Immunol* 2005;**138**:235–42.

19 Hernandez Garcia J, Garcia Selles J, Negro Alvarez JM, Pagan Aleman JA, Lopez Sanchez JD. [Incidence of adverse reactions to additives: our experience over 10 years; in Spanish.] *Allergol Immunopathol (Madr)* 1994;**22**:233–42.

20 Simon RA. Additive-induced urticaria: experience with monosodium glutamate (MSG). *J Nutr* 2000;**130**:1063S–1066S.

21 Nettis E, Colanardi MC, Ferrannini A, Tursi A. Sodium benzoate-induced repeated episodes of acute urticaria/angio-oedema: randomized controlled trial. *Br J Dermatol* 2004;**151**:898–902.

22 Goga D, Vaillant L, Pandraud L, Mateu J, Ballon G, Beutter P. [The elimination of dental and sinusal infectious foci in dermatologic pathology: a double-blind study in 27 cases confined to chronic urticaria; in French.] *Rev Stomatol Chir Maxillofac* 1988;**89**:273–5.

23 Champion RH, Roberts SO, Carpenter RG, Roger JH. Urticaria and angio-oedema: a review of 554 patients. *Br J Dermatol* 1969;**81**:588–97.

24 Buchter A, Kruse-Losler B, Joos U, Kleinheinz J. [Odontogenic foci: possible etiology of urticaria? In German]. *Mund Kiefer Gesichtschir* 2003;**7**:335–8.

25 De Koster E, De Bruyne I, Langlet P, Deltenre M. Evidence based medicine and extradigestive manifestations of *Helicobacter pylori. Acta Gastroenterol Belg* 2000;**63**:388–92.

26 Cribier BJ, Santinelli F, Schmitt C, Stoll-Keller F, Grosshans E. Chronic urticaria is not significantly associated with hepatitis C or hepatitis G infection: a case–control study. *Arch Dermatol* 1999;**135**:1335–9.

27 Laufer P, Laufer R. Contact dermatitis in cystic fibrosis. *Cutis* 1985;**35**:557.

28 Caminiti L, Passalacqua G, Magazzu G, *et al.* Chronic urticaria and associated coeliac disease in children: a case-control study. *Pediatr Allergy Immunol* 2005;**16**:428–32.

29 Gabrielli M, Candelli M, Cremonini F, *et al.* Idiopathic chronic urticaria and celiac disease. *Dig Dis Sci* 2005;**50**:1702–4.

30 Lindelof B, Sigurgeirsson B, Wahlgren CF, Eklund G. Chronic urticaria and cancer: an epidemiological study of 1155 patients. *Br J Dermatol* 1990;**123**:453–6.

31 Kozel MM, Mekkes JR, Bossuyt PM, Bos JD. Natural course of physical and chronic urticaria and angioedema in 220 patients. *J Am Acad Dermatol* 2001;**45**:387–91.

32 Van Der Valk PG, Moret G, Kiemeney LA. The natural history of chronic urticaria and angioedema in patients visiting a tertiary referral centre. *Br J Dermatol* 2002;**146**:110–3.

33 Bindslev-Lensen C, Finzi A, Greaves M, *et al.* Chronic urticaria: diagnostic recommendations. *J Eur Acad Dermatol Venereol* 2000;**14**:175–80.

34 Agence Nationale d'Accréditation et d'Evaluation en Santé; Société Française de Dermatologie. [Management of chronic urticaria: recommendations (long text). French Society of Dermatology. National Agency for Health Accreditation and Evaluation; in French.] *Ann Dermatol Venereol* 2003;**130**(Spec No 1):1S182–92.

35 Zuberbier T, Bindslev-Jensen C, Canonica W, *et al.* EAACI/GALEN/EDF guideline: definition, classification and diagnosis of urticaria. *Allergy* 2006;**61**:316–20.

36 Lipsker D, Veran Y, Grunenberger F, Cribier B, Heid E, Grosshans E. The Schnitzler syndrome: four new cases and review of the literature. *Medicine (Baltimore)* 2001;**80**:37–44.

37 Gyimesi E, Sipka S, Danko K, *et al.* Basophil CD63 expression assay on highly sensitized atopic donor leucocytes: a useful method in chronic autoimmune urticaria. *Br J Dermatol* 2004; **151**:388–96.

38 De Swerdt A, Van Den Keybus C, Kasran A, *et al.* Detection of basophil-activating IgG autoantibodies in chronic idiopathic urticaria by induction of CD 63. *J Allergy Clin Immunol* 2005; **116**:662–7.

39 Dreskin SC, Andrews KY. The thyroid and urticaria. *Curr Opin Allergy Clin Immunol* 2005;**5**:408–12.

40 O'Donnell BF, Francis DM, Swana GT, Seed PT, Kobza BA, Greaves MW. Thyroid autoimmunity in chronic urticaria. *Br J Dermatol* 2005;**153**:331–5.

41 Natbony SF, Phillips ME, Elias JM, Godfrey HP, Kaplan AP. Histologic studies of chronic idiopathic urticaria. *J Allergy Clin Immunol* 1983;**71**:177–83.

42 Sanchez JL, Benmaman O. Clinicopathological correlation in chronic urticaria. *Am J Dermatopathol* 1992;**14**:220–3.

43 Peters MS, Winkelmann RK. Neutrophilic urticaria. *Br J Dermatol* 1985;**113**:25–30.

44 Peteiro C, Toribio J. Incidence of leukocytoclastic vasculitis in chronic idiopathic urticaria: study of 100 cases. *Am J Dermatopathol* 1989;**11**:528–33.

45 Mehregan DR, Hall MJ, Gibson LE. Urticarial vasculitis: a histopathologic and clinical review of 72 cases. *J Am Acad Dermatol* 1992;**26**:441–8.

46 Doutre MS, Beylot C, Bioulac P, Conte M. [Immunopathology in 35 cases of chronic urticaria; in French.] *Sem Hop* 1984;**60**:1040–2.

47 Brogden RN, McTavish D. Acrivastine: a review of its pharmacological properties and therapeutic efficacy in allergic rhinitis, urticaria and related disorders. Drugs 1991;**41**:927–40.

48 Sussman G, Jancelewicz Z. Controlled trial of H$_1$ antagonists in the treatment of chronic idiopathic urticaria. *Ann Allergy* 1991; **67**:433–9.

49 Van Joost T, Blog FB, Westerhof W, *et al.* A comparison of acrivastine versus terfenadine and placebo in the treatment of

chronic idiopathic urticaria. *J Int Med Res* 1989;**17**(Suppl 2):14B–17B.

50 Juhlin L, Gibson JR, Harvey SG, Huson LW. Acrivastine versus clemastine in the treatment of chronic idiopathic urticaria: a double-blind, placebo-controlled study. *Int J Dermatol* 1987;**26**: 653–4.

51 Gale AE, Harvey SG, Calthrop JG, Gibson JR. A comparison of acrivastine versus chlorpheniramine in the treatment of chronic idiopathic urticaria. *J Int Med Res* 1989;**17**(Suppl 2):25B–27B.

52 Leyh F, Harvey SG, Gibson JR, Manna VK. A comparison of acrivastine versus clemastine and placebo in the treatment of patients with chronic idiopathic urticaria. *J Int Med Res* 1989; **17**(Suppl 2):22B–24B.

53 Neittaanmaki H, Fraki JE, Gibson JR. Comparison of the new antihistamine acrivastine (BW 825C) versus cyproheptadine in the treatment of idiopathic cold urticaria. *Dermatologica* 1988; **177**:98–103.

54 Paul E, Bodeker RH. Comparative study of astemizole and terfenadine in the treatment of chronic idiopathic urticaria: a randomized double-blind study of 40 patients. *Ann Allergy* 1989;**62**:318–20.

55 McTavish D, Sorkin EM. Azelastine: a review of its pharmacodynamic and pharmacokinetic properties, and therapeutic potential. *Drugs* 1989;**38**:778–800.

56 Camarasa JM, Aliaga A, Fernandez-Vozmediano JM, Fonseca E, Iglesias L, Tagarro I. Azelastine tablets in the treatment of chronic idiopathic urticaria: phase III, randomised, double-blind, placebo and active controlled multicentric clinical trial. *Skin Pharmacol Appl Skin Physiol* 2001;**14**:77–86.

57 Spencer CM, Faulds D, Peters DH. Cetirizine. A reappraisal of its pharmacological properties and therapeutic use in selected allergic disorders. Drugs 1993;**46**:1055–80.

58 Breneman DL. Cetirizine versus hydroxyzine and placebo in chronic idiopathic urticaria. *Ann Pharmacother* 1996;**30**:1075–9.

59 Goh CL, Wong WK, Lim J. Cetirizine vs placebo in chronic idiopathic urticaria: a double blind randomised cross-over study. *Ann Acad Med Singapore* 1991;**20**:328–30.

60 Lambert D, Hantzperg M, Danglas P, Bloom M. [Double-blind comparative study of terfenadine and cetirizine in chronic idiopathic urticaria]. *Allerg Immunol (Paris)* 1993;**25**:235–40.

61 Guerra L, Vincenzi C, Marchesi E, *et al.* Loratadine and cetirizine in the treatment of chronic urticaria. *J Eur Acad Dermatol Venereol* 1994;**3**:148–52.

62 Kietzmann H, Macher E, Rihoux JP, Ghys L. Comparison of cetirizine and terfenadine in the treatment of chronic idiopathic urticaria. *Ann Allergy* 1990;**65**:498–500.

63 Juhlin L, Arendt C. Treatment of chronic urticaria with cetirizine dihydrochloride a non-sedating antihistamine. *Br J Dermatol* 1988;**119**:67–71.

64 Kalivas J, Breneman D, Tharp M, Bruce S, Bigby M. Urticaria: clinical efficacy of cetirizine in comparison with hydroxyzine and placebo. *J Allergy Clin Immunol* 1990;**86**:1014–8.

65 Juhlin L. Cetirizine in the treatment of chronic urticaria. *Clin Ther* 1991;**13**:81–6.

66 Henz BM. The pharmacologic profile of desloratadine: a review. Allergy 2001;**56**(Suppl 65):7–13.

67 Geha RS, Meltzer EO. Desloratadine: a new, nonsedating, oral antihistamine. *J Allergy Clin Immunol* 2001;**107**:751–62.

68 Ring J, Hein R, Gauger A, Bronsky E, Miller B. Once-daily desloratadine improves the signs and symptoms of chronic idiopathic urticaria: a randomized, double-blind, placebo-controlled study. *Int J Dermatol* 2001;**40**:72–6.

69 Monroe E, Finn A, Patel P, Guerrero R, Ratner P, Bernstein D. Efficacy and safety of desloratadine 5 mg once daily in the treatment of chronic idiopathic urticaria: a double-blind, randomized, placebo-controlled trial. *J Am Acad Dermatol* 2003; **48**:535–41.

70 Hurst M, Spencer CM. Ebastine: an update of its use in allergic disorders. *Drugs* 2000;**59**:981–1006.

71 Kalis B. Double-blind multicentre comparative study of ebastine, terfenadine and placebo in the treatment of chronic idiopathic urticaria in adults. *Drugs* 1996;**52**(Suppl 1):30–4.

72 Simpson K, Jarvis B. Fexofenadine: a review of its use in the management of seasonal allergic rhinitis and chronic idiopathic urticaria. *Drugs* 2000;**59**:301–21.

73 Nelson HS, Reynolds R, Mason J. Fexofenadine HCl is safe and effective for treatment of chronic idiopathic urticaria. *Ann Allergy Asthma Immunol* 2000;**84**:517–22.

74 Finn AF Jr, Kaplan AP, Fretwell R, Qu R, Long J. A double-blind, placebo-controlled trial of fexofenadine HCl in the treatment of chronic idiopathic urticaria. *J Allergy Clin Immunol* 1999;**104**: 1071–8.

75 Kaplan AP, Spector SL, Meeves S, Liao Y, Varghese ST, Georges G. Once-daily fexofenadine treatment for chronic idiopathic urticaria: a multicenter, randomized, double-blind, placebo-controlled study. *Ann Allergy Asthma Immunol* 2005;**94**:662–9.

76 Degonda M, Pichler WJ, Bircher A, Helbling A. [Chronic idiopathic urticaria: effectiveness of fexofenadine. A double-blind, placebo controlled study with 21 patients; in German.] *Schweiz Rundsch Med Prax* 2002;**91**:637–43.

77 Nettis E, Dambra P, D'Oronzio L, Loria MP, Ferrannini A, Tursi A. Comparison of montelukast and fexofenadine for chronic idiopathic urticaria. *Arch Dermatol* 2001;**137**:99–100.

78 Thompson AK, Finn AF, Schoenwetter WF. Effect of 60 mg twice-daily fexofenadine HCl on quality of life, work and classroom productivity, and regular activity in patients with chronic idiopathic urticaria. *J Am Acad Dermatol* 2000;**43**:24–30.

79 Simons FE, Simons KJ. Levocetirizine: pharmacokinetics and pharmacodynamics in children age 6 to 11 years. *J Allergy Clin Immunol* 2005;**116**:355–61.

80 Day JH, Ellis AK, Rafeiro E. Levocetirizine: a new selective H_1 receptor antagonist for use in allergic disorders. *Drugs Today (Barc)* 2004;**40**:415–21.

81 Nettis E, Colanardi MC, Barra L, Ferrannini A, Vacca A, Tursi A. Levocetirizine in the treatment of chronic idiopathic urticaria: a randomized, double-blind, placebo-controlled study. *Br J Dermatol* 2006;**154**:533–8.

82 Haria M, Fitton A, Peters DH. Loratadine: a reappraisal of its pharmacological properties and therapeutic use in allergic disorders. Drugs 1994;**48**:617–37.

83 Belaich S, Bruttmann G, Degreef H, *et al.* Comparative effects of loratadine and terfenadine in the treatment of chronic idiopathic urticaria. *Ann Allergy* 1990;**64**:191–4.

84 Abu Shareeah AM. Comparative efficacy of loratadine and terfenadine in the treatment of chronic idiopathic urticaria. *Int J Dermatol* 1992;**31**:355–6.

85 Siergiejko Z, Chyrek-Borowska S. [Results of treatment with loratadine in patients with chronic urticaria; in Polish]. *Pol Tyg Lek* 1994;**49**:334–6.

86 Simons FE. Mizolastine: antihistaminic activity from preclinical data to clinical evaluation. *Clin Exp Allergy* 1999;**29**(Suppl 1):3–8.

87 Brostoff J, Fitzharris P, Dunmore C, Theron M, Blondin P. Efficacy of mizolastine, a new antihistamine, compared with placebo in the treatment of chronic idiopathic urticaria. *Allergy* 1996;**51**:320–5.

88 Dubertret L, Murrieta AM, Tonet J. Efficacy and safety of mizolastine 10 mg in a placebo-controlled comparison with loratadine in chronic idiopathic urticaria: results of the MILOR Study. *J Eur Acad Dermatol Venereol* 1999;**12**:16–24.

89 Leynadier F, Duarte-Risselin C, Murrieta M. Comparative therapeutic effect and safety of mizolastine and loratadine in chronic idiopathic urticaria. URTILOR study group. *Eur J Dermatol* 2000;**10**:205–11.

90 Horak F, Stubner UP. Comparative tolerability of second generation antihistamines. *Drug Saf* 1999;**20**:385–401.

91 Slater JW, Zechnich AD, Haxby DG. Second-generation antihistamines: a comparative review. Drugs 1999;**57**:31–47.

92 Walsh GM, Annunziato L, Frossard N, *et al.* New insights into the second generation antihistamines. Drugs 2001;**61**:207–36.

93 Simons, FE. Advances in H_1-antihistamines. *N Engl J Med* 2004; **351**:2203–17.

94 Valsecchi R, di Landro A, Pansera B, Cainelli T. Contact dermatitis from a gel containing dimethindene maleate. *Contact Dermatitis* 1994;**30**:248–9.

95 Jolliffe DS, Sim-Davis D, Templeton JS. A placebo-controlled comparative study of sustained-release brompheniramine maleate against clemastine fumarate in the treatment of chronic urticaria. *Curr Med Res Opin* 1985;**9**:394–9.

96 Fredriksson T, Hersle K, Hjorth N, *et al.* Terfenadine in chronic urticaria: a comparison with clemastine and placebo. *Cutis* 1986;**38**:128–30.

97 Kamide R, Niimura M, Ueda H, *et al.* Clinical evaluation of ketotifen for chronic urticaria: multicenter double-blind comparative study with clemastine. *Ann Allergy* 1989;**62**:322–5.

98 May KL, Nelemans FA. The antipruritic effect of Fenistil (dimethypyrindene) in allergic conditions: double blind clinical study. *Acta Allergol* 1966;**21**:337–42.

99 Sobye P, Ulrich J. Dimethpyrindene and a new antihistamine HS 592 (Sandoz) in the treatment of severe chronic urticaria. *Acta Allergol* 1968;**23**:24–34.

100 Monroe EW. Relative efficacy and safety of loratadine, hydroxyzine, and placebo in chronic idiopathic urticaria and atopic dermatitis. *Clin Ther* 1992;**14**:17–21.

101 Peremans W, Mertens RL, Morias J, Campaert H. Oxatomide in the treatment of chronic urticaria: a double-blind placebo-controlled trial. *Dermatologica* 1981;**162**:42–50.

102 Beck HI, Cramers M, Herlin T, Sondergaard I, Zachariae H. Comparison of oxatomide and clemastine in the treatment of chronic urticaria: a double blind study. Dermatologica 1985;**171**: 49–51.

103 Bleehen SS, Thomas SE, Greaves MW, *et al.* Cimetidine and chlorpheniramine in the treatment of chronic idiopathic urticaria: a multi-centre randomized double-blind study. *Br J Dermatol* 1987;**117**:81–8.

104 Diller G, Orfanos CE. [Management of idiopathic urticaria with $H_1 + H_2$ antagonists: a crossover double blind long-term study; in German.] *Z Hautkr* 1983;**58**:785–93.

105 Paul E, Bodeker RH. Treatment of chronic urticaria with terfenadine and ranitidine: a randomized double-blind study in 45 patients *Eur J Clin Pharmacol* 1986;**31**.277–80.

106 Harvey RP, Wegs J, Schocket AL. A controlled trial of therapy in chronic urticaria. *J Allergy Clin Immunol* 1981;**68**:262–6.

107 Simons FE, Sussman GL, Simons KJ. Effect of the H_2-antagonist cimetidine on the pharmacokinetics and pharmacodynamics of the H_1-antagonists hydroxyzine and cetirizine in patients with chronic urticaria. *J Allergy Clin Immunol* 1995;**95**:685–93.

108 Salo OP, Kauppinen K, Mannisto PT. Cimetidine increases the plasma concentration of hydroxyzine. *Acta Derm Venereol* 1986; **66**:349–50.

109 Bressler RB, Sowell K, Huston DP. Therapy of chronic idiopathic urticaria with nifedipine: demonstration of beneficial effect in a double-blinded, placebo-controlled, crossover trial. *J Allergy Clin Immunol* 1989;**83**:756–63.

110 Erbagci Z. The leukotriene receptor antagonist montelukast in the treatment of chronic idiopathic urticaria: a single-blind, placebo-controlled, crossover clinical study. *J Allergy Clin Immunol* 2002;**110**:484–8.

111 Bagenstose SE, Levin L, Bernstein JA. The addition of zafirlukast to cetirizine improves the treatment of chronic urticaria in patients with positive autologous serum skin test results. *J Allergy Clin Immunol* 2004;**113**:134–40.

112 Di Lorenzo G, Pacor ML, Mansueto P, *et al.* Randomized placebo-controlled trial comparing desloratadine and montelukast in monotherapy and desloratadine plus montelukast in combined therapy for chronic idiopathic urticaria. *J Allergy Clin Immunol* 2004;**114**:619–25.

113 Kalogeromitros D, Kempuraj D, Katsarou-Katsari A, *et al.* Theophylline as "add-on" therapy to cetirizine in patients with chronic idiopathic urticaria: a randomized, double-blind, placebo-controlled pilot study. *Int Arch Allergy Immunol* 2006;**139**:258–64.

114 Figueiredo A, Ribeiro CA, Goncalo M, Almeida L, Poiares-Baptista A, Teixeira F. Mechanism of action of doxepin in the treatment of chronic urticaria. *Fundam Clin Pharmacol* 1990;**4**:147–58.

115 Goldsobel AB, Rohr AS, Siegel SC, *et al.* Efficacy of doxepin in the treatment of chronic idiopathic urticaria. *J Allergy Clin Immunol* 1986;**78**:867–73.

116 Greene SL, Reed CE, Schroeter AL. Double-blind crossover study comparing doxepin with diphenhydramine for the treatment of chronic urticaria. *J Am Acad Dermatol* 1985;**12**:669–75.

117 Harto A, Sendagorta E, Ledo A. Doxepin in the treatment of chronic urticaria. *Dermatologica* 1985;**170**:90–3.

118 Grattan CE, O'Donnell BF, Francis DM, *et al.* Randomized double-blind study of cyclosporin in chronic "idiopathic" urticaria. *Br J Dermatol* 2000;**143**:365–72.

119 Di Gioacchino M, Di Stefano F, Cavallucci E, *et al.* Treatment of chronic idiopathic urticaria and positive autologous serum skin test with cyclosporine: clinical and immunological evaluation. *Allergy Asthma Proc* 2003;**24**:285–90.

120 Toubi E, Blant A, Kessel A, Golan TD. Low-dose cyclosporin A in the treatment of severe chronic idiopathic urticaria. *Allergy* 1997;**52**:312–6.

121 Marsland AM, Soundararajan S, Joseph K, Kaplan AP. Effects of calcineurin inhibitors on an in vitro assay for chronic urticaria. *Clin Exp Allergy* 2005;**35**:554–9.

122 Leznoff A, Sussman GL. Syndrome of idiopathic chronic urticaria and angioedema with thyroid autoimmunity: a study of 90 patients. *J Allergy Clin Immunol* 1989;**84**:66–71.

123 Rumbyrt JS, Katz JL, Schocket AL. Resolution of chronic urticaria in patients with thyroid autoimmunity. *J Allergy Clin Immunol* 1995;**96**:901–5.

124 Heymann WR. Chronic urticaria and angioedema associated with thyroid autoimmunity: review and therapeutic implications. *J Am Acad Dermatol* 1999;**40**:229–32.

125 Koh CK, Hew FL, Chiu CL. Treatment of chronic urticaria with thyroxine in an euthyroid patient with thyroglobulin and microsomal antibodies. *Ann Acad Med Singapore* 2000;**29**:528–30.

126 Gaig P, Garcia-Ortega P, Enrique E, Richart C. Successful treatment of chronic idiopathic urticaria associated with thyroid autoimmunity. *J Investig Allergol Clin Immunol* 2000;**10**:342–5.

127 Palma-Carlos AG, Palma-Carlos ML. Chronic urticaria and thyroid auto-immunity. *Allerg Immunol (Paris)* 2005;**37**:143–6.

128 Aversano M, Caiazzo P, Iorio G, Ponticiello L, Lagana B, Leccese F. Improvement of chronic idiopathic urticaria with L-thyroxine: a new TSH role in immune response? *Allergy* 2005;**60**:489–93.

129 Parsad D, Pandhi R, Juneja A. Stanozolol in chronic urticaria: a double blind, placebo controlled trial. *J Dermatol* 2001;**28**:299–302.

130 Reeves GE, Boyle MJ, Bonfield J, Dobson P, Loewenthal M. Impact of hydroxychloroquine therapy on chronic urticaria: chronic autoimmune urticaria study and evaluation. *Intern Med J* 2004;**34**:182–6.

131 Zuberbier T, Bindslev-Jensen C, Canonica W, *et al.* EAACI/GA2LEN/EDF guideline: management of urticaria. *Allergy* 2006;**61**:321–31.

132 Gilbert C, Mazzotta P, Loebstein R, Koren G. Fetal safety of drugs used in the treatment of allergic rhinitis: a critical review. *Drug Saf* 2005;**28**:707–19.

IIIb Skin cancer, moles, and photoaging

Hywel Williams, Editor

25 Primary prevention of skin cancer

Ros Weston

Background

Incidence, mortality, and morbidity of nonmelanoma skin cancers

Skin cancer is more common than any other type of cancer. Nonmelanoma skin cancers (NMSCs) are the most common. NMSC includes basal cell carcinoma (BCC), also known as rodent ulcer, and squamous cell carcinoma (SCC). Around 600 000 cases of NMSC occur per year—500 000 BCCs and 100 000–150 000 SCCs. In the United Kingdom, the incidence of NMSC is approximately 18 times higher than that of malignant melanoma. The lifetime risk for BCC in a child born in 1994 is estimated at 28–33%.

NMSCs respond well to treatment, and the survival rates for both types are over 95%. While BCCs rarely metastasize, SCCs can.[1] In 2003, there were 514 deaths in the UK from NMSCs. Eighty percent of NMSCs occur in people aged 60 or over. NMSC is a major public health problem, due to the very large numbers of cases each year.

Incidence, mortality, and morbidity of malignant melanoma

Melanoma skin cancer is the most serious form of skin cancer.[1] The incidence in Caucasians is doubling every 10–15 years, probably due to increased ultraviolet exposure from the sun. Melanoma is preventable and curable when it is diagnosed at an early stage (Figure 25.1). As yet, interventions for primary and secondary prevention have had limited success in reducing the incidence. The survival rates for melanoma in Europe improved from 13% to 11% between 1999 and 2002, and differences in the mortality rates between countries decreased. The European and world estimated age-standardized rates of cutaneous melanoma are shown in Figures 25.2 and 25.3. Melanoma is 2.3 times commoner in women than in men. In 2002, melanoma was the sixth most common cancer in women and the twelfth for men.

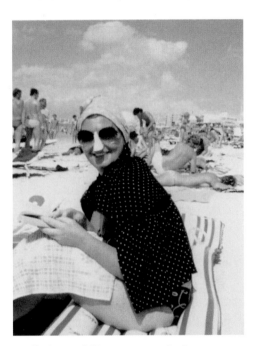

Figure 25.1 The future of skin cancer prevention?

The distribution of cancers on the body also varies by sex: over a third of the lesions arise on the trunk, especially the back, in males, while the most common site in women is on the legs.[1]

Risk factors

Phenotype: skin color and ethnicity

White (Caucasian) populations with fair, red, or light brown hair, blue eyes, and freckles are 80 times more likely to develop basal cell and squamous cell carcinoma and 20 times more likely to develop melanoma than black populations. Racial and ethnic differences in skin cancer rates are probably due to skin color, determined by the levels of melanin produced by melanocytes. These cells protect the

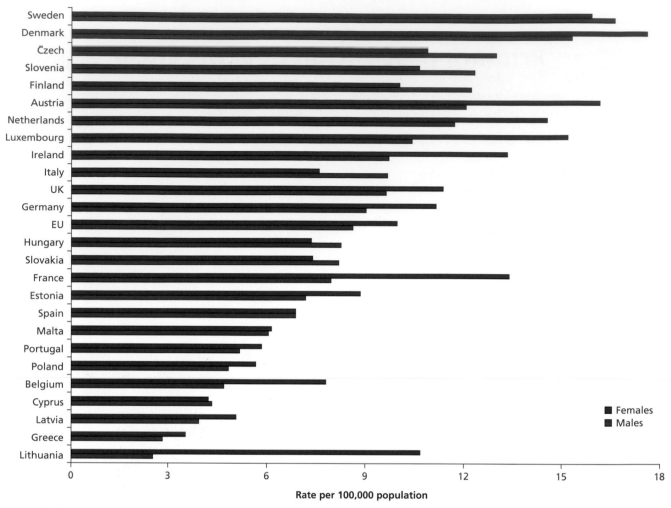

Figure 25.2 European age-standardized incidence rates for malignant melanoma, by sex (European Union estimates, 2002).

skin DNA from damage by ultraviolet radiation (UVR). Dark-skinned people are at risk with incremental exposure to UVR. The risk increases for those who sunburn easily but tan poorly. Exposure to sun for long periods, a history of sunburn, skin type, and exposure to ultraviolet light are the main factors contributing to NMSCs. The depletion of the ozone layer may in the future be an important factor contributing to the incidence rates.[1]

Ultraviolet light and exposure to the sun

Epidemiological evidence suggests that NMSCs and melanoma are caused by exposure to ultraviolet radiation. Repeated episodes of sunburn (erythema) in childhood and adulthood have a role in the development of skin cancers. The type of exposure—such as intermittent (i.e., lying for long periods in the sun on annual foreign vacations) or continuous (i.e., daily exposure over long periods, as in those working outdoors)—may differ between the three

main types of cancer. There is substantial evidence to suggest that the risk increases with increasing intermittency of exposure. The evidence for intermittent exposure supports an increased risk for melanoma, probably for BCC, but not for SCC.

The risk for SCC appears to depend only on the accumulated amount of exposure to the sun. There is as yet no definitive evidence for the relationship between total exposure to UVR and melanoma. Further evidence that UVR causes skin cancer has been provided by the observation that people with the rare genetic condition of xeroderma pigmentosum have a very high risk of melanoma and NMSC.

Environmental factors increase the amount of UVR exposure: proximity to the equator, higher altitudes, and lower-level cloud cover (this can allow up to 80% of ultraviolet rays to penetrate the atmosphere). Reflective materials such as sand, water, snow, and paving stones can also increase the risk.[1]

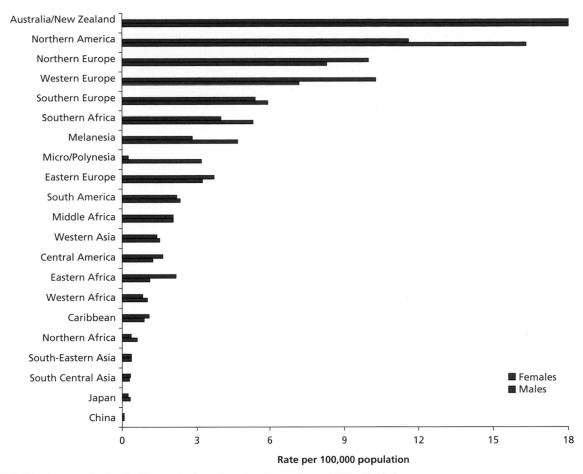

Figure 25.3 World age-standardized incidence rates for malignant melanoma, by sex (2002 estimates).

Age

The incidence of melanoma rises rapidly in Caucasians after the age of 20, and the incidence of NMSCs increases exponentially with age. Older people have absorbed UVR over a lifetime, while the skin's capacity for repair declines with age. Younger people are also at risk, as their total current exposure is high in comparison with those aged 75 or over.[1]

Genetic susceptibility

Those with a family history of melanoma have approximately twice the risk for melanoma in comparison with those who have no family history. There are rare families in which there are more than three cases of melanoma, which may be due to a hereditary susceptibility associated with the *CDKN2A* gene, carriers of which are at considerable lifetime risk.[1]

Mutation in the *TP53* gene appears to be an important step in the development of skin cancers. Exposure to sunlight causes a number of chemical changes in DNA. If these changes are not repaired, mutation begins. DNA damage can produce signature mutations, and it is hypothesized that these are linked to carcinogenesis. Signature mutations

have been found in the *TP53* tumor suppressor gene in normal skin cells, and their presence has been correlated with the extent of exposure. Signature mutations in the *TP53* gene have also been found in BCC and SCC of the skin, whereas they are rare in this gene for other types of cancer. In the general population, there is conflicting evidence regarding excision repair of DNA and the risk for BCC.[1]

Nevi on the skin

Individuals with certain types of pigmented lesion (dysplastic or atypical nevi), several large nondysplastic nevi, many small nevi, or with moderate freckling have a twofold to threefold increase in the risk of developing melanoma. Individuals with familial dysplastic nevus syndrome, or with several dysplastic or atypical nevi, have a greater than fivefold increase in the risk of developing melanoma.[1]

Demographics

Malignant melanoma is positively related to affluence. In Scottish patients diagnosed between 1991 and 1995, the age-standardized incidence rates in the most affluent areas were almost twice as high as those in the most deprived areas

(13.6 vs. 7.4 per 100 000). In England, the age-standardized rates in 1988–93 in deprived areas were 60–70% lower than those in the most affluent areas. The difference is perhaps related to the frequency and destination of vacations. As more people travel abroad for vacations, especially to very sunny destinations, the incidence rates may rise.[1]

Early diagnosis

Early diagnosis is the key to reducing deaths from skin cancers, especially melanoma, as delayed diagnosis increases the risk of mortality. The Scottish Melanoma Group analyzed the data for presentation of patients with thick melanomas over a 20-year period. The findings suggested that the main reason for improved survival rates is that primary and secondary prevention programs have increased the numbers of patients presenting with thin lesions that have a good prognosis. There has been a decrease in the proportion of thick melanomas with a poor prognosis, although the total numbers presenting per year have not significantly altered. The thick melanoma group is an increasingly older age group. Resources currently directed at public and professional education on melanoma appear to be having little effect in this group of patients.[1]

Aims in primary prevention

Primary prevention involves interventions designed to prevent skin cancer from occurring for the first time. Interventions for primary sun protection aim to change risk behavior (as an intermediate measure) in order to reduce the incidence (as a health outcome measure). The main sun-protection strategies are: wearing of wide-brimmed hats and clothes when outdoors, staying out of the sun between 10 a.m. and 4 p.m., and the use of shade. Sunscreens are a popular prevention strategy, but there is limited evidence that they are successful as the sole prevention strategy (this is discussed more fully in Chapter 26).[2,3]

Aims in secondary prevention

Secondary prevention involves interventions aimed at encouraging the recognition of skin changes, so that the patient can seek early diagnosis and treatment (see Chapter 26). The present chapter only discusses primary prevention.

Search strategy

Studies for this review were found by searching the Cochrane Library, PubMed, and Medline. Four searches were made between February and June 2006. The key words used were: meta-analysis, systematic review, randomized controlled studies, prevention, intervention, skin cancer, and

malignant melanoma. One systematic review was located for primary prevention and one for secondary prevention.[3,4]

Review of evidence on primary prevention

A systematic review reported on interventions for preventing skin cancer by reducing exposure to ultraviolet radiation,[3] incorporating studies reviewed in the International Agency for Research on Cancer/World Health Organization meta-analysis[5] and in the review by the Centers for Disease Control and Prevention in Atlanta (CDC).[3] The present author has only reported here on the studies included in each category of the systematic review. The review represents a major advance in methodology and assessment techniques, but readers should check the methodology, results, and discussion on the review team's web site (www.thecommunityguide.org/cancer). It proved impossible to include fully all of the information necessary in the present chapter, which is a summary of the wide-ranging, complex, and comprehensive systematic review.[3]

Four main categories were used to assess studies on the primary prevention and reduction of exposure (intermediate measure) in relation to reducing skin cancers (health outcome):
- Interventions directed at individuals
- Studies aimed at environmental and policy factors
- Media campaigns
- Multiple-component programs

Interventions directed at individuals

Interventions in this category include informational and behavioral interventions aimed at individuals, or small groups, as discrete elements of community interventions across various settings. The main aim of these interventions is to motivate or educate by providing knowledge and skills in order to change attitudes and behavior. Such interventions use small media (printed material), lessons, and skills development, with the aim of changing attitudes in different age groups and occupational groups. For a full discussion of the results, see www.thecommunityguide.org/cancer.

Educational and policy interventions in childcare settings

These are interventions aimed at children aged 5–18. Ultraviolet exposure is estimated in relation to parental behavior, with the responsibility for limiting UVR lying with parents, childcare providers, and teachers. Nine reports met the inclusion criteria, but only two qualified for the report in the category for childcare centers.[6,7] In the studies included, the median relative change was approximately 2% overall (for a comprehensive critical analysis of studies and the results of the meta-analysis, see www.thecommunityguide.org/cancer).

Comment

There is reasonable evidence that interventions in primary schools for "covering up"—i.e., wearing hats and clothes—are effective. There is insufficient evidence for other sun-protection behaviors. There is insufficient evidence for policy development and change. The interventions did, however, report on intermediate outcomes, showing an improvement in knowledge, changes in attitudes, and increased sunscreen use. The evidence regarding reductions in the incidence of sunburn was insufficient. There was poor reporting of relevant outcomes and of changes in children's behavior (as an outcome), changing policies, practices, or caregivers' knowledge and behavior in relation to ways of reducing exposure.

Interventions in secondary schools and colleges

Thirteen interventions in secondary schools and colleges met the inclusion criteria for this important setting. Young people are more likely to be exposed to UVR and less likely to follow parental or expert guidance. Knowledge about UVR is high, but risk activity is also high, and this age group is therefore a challenge for health promoters. Most of the studies reporting intervention arms described multiple outcomes. The interventions were inconsistent and the outcomes were poorly measured, so that their effectiveness is hard to determine. An increase in knowledge was demonstrated in nine intervention arms;[7-19] seven studies included groups in which attitudes were investigated, but the results were inconsistent. Seven studies assessed intentions (mainly with regard to sunscreen use), but the results were again inconsistent (www.thecommunityguide.org/cancer).[8-20]

Comment

There is insufficient evidence to determine the effectiveness of educational and policy interventions in secondary schools and colleges aimed at reducing UVR exposure, since:

• The studies concerned were poorly designed.
• The reported interventions and outcomes varied.
• The studies only had short follow-up periods.
• Few of the studies had a design from which evidence could be determined.

There is evidence that intermediate measures (knowledge and attitudes) were changed by the interventions.

Studies aimed at environmental and policy factors

Educational and policy interventions in recreational and tourist settings

Eleven of 18 studies evaluating behavior outcomes qualified for review.[21-31] Five arms in three studies demonstrated sufficient evidence of effectiveness for protective clothing, with a relative difference of 11.2% (interquartile range 5.1–12.9%) on adult behavior in relation to UVR. For children, two arms demonstrated inconsistent effects for wearing a hat, shirt, or using shade. Two arms in one study demonstrated a desirable effect, with a 41.2% reduction in sunburn. This is deemed insufficient for recommendations, as too few studies are available. Five arms in four studies were related to differences in sunscreen use (median relative difference 15.4%).

Comment

The authors conclude that there is sufficient evidence to demonstrate an increase in sun-protective behavior (covering up) in recreational and tourism settings.

The studies included show inconsistent effectiveness for information seeking, changes in knowledge and attitudes, beliefs, and intentions, sun-protection measures, and environmental support at outdoor recreational centers and swimming pools. There is insufficient evidence of effectiveness for reducing exposure to UVR in adults and children. There was evidence of effectiveness for children's sun-protection behavior, including sunscreen, and for composite behavior (clothes, hats, staying indoors, and use of shade). The evidence was not strong enough for any firm recommendations to be made.

Programs in outdoor occupational settings

Interventions in occupational settings are aimed at promoting sun-protection behaviors among workers, using information activities to improve knowledge and change attitudes and beliefs through role models, demonstrations, and environmental policies such as provision of sunscreen and shade. Fourteen studies were considered, only eight of which qualified (www.thecommunityguide.org/cancer).

Comment

Due to the small number of reports and inconsistent results, the available reports provide insufficient evidence to assess the effectiveness of interventions in occupational settings in reducing UVR exposure or increasing sun-protective behaviors. For a discussion of the individual studies and evidential problems, see www.thecommunityguide.org/cancer.

Health-care system and provider settings (pharmacies, clinics, family practitioners, medical and nursing schools)

Activities include educational and training activities aimed at providers (e.g., pharmacists), to enable them—via information and/or role-modeling—to encourage behavior change by increasing knowledge and changing the beliefs of customers or clients using counseling and advice. Nineteen reports met the inclusion criteria, with 11 qualifying for assessment. Three studies showed effective intermediate outcomes (knowledge, attitudes, behavior).[32–49] Some positive effects (a desirable direction of change) were noted, but the findings were not consistent enough to provide statistical significance. Lack of measurement of key behaviors and health outcomes, as well as inconsistent results, mean that there is insufficient evidence to determine the effectiveness of such interventions.

Comment

The authors report insufficient evidence for or against counseling by primary-care physicians for reducing sun exposure, avoiding sunlamps, using sunscreen or protective clothing, or for skin self-examination. This review builds on the U.S. Preventive Services Task Force recommendations[50] by evaluating more providers. The use of diverse targets was problematic, and the content of the interventions and the media through which they were communicated were unclear.

Media campaigns

Efficacy of media campaigns in reducing UVR exposure in community settings

These campaigns involve interventions intended to reduce UVR exposure in community settings, using various mass media and small media such as television, radio, newspapers and magazines, billboards, letters, brochures, and flyers. They address risk behavior by raising awareness in order to improve knowledge and change attitudes.

Health outcomes for adults and children were assessed in a study including the "SunSmart" and "Slip! Slop! Slap!" programs in Australia.[42] Community programs in the USA were also modeled on the Australian experience. No systematic reviews have reported on such campaigns in either country, although longitudinal surveys from the two-decade Australian program have been published.

The review team included nine studies[51–59] and two reports[43,44] on the effectiveness of mass media campaigns without other activities. It is important to note that the review team did not include any study that did not report on the effect of mass media on behavior change as a discrete element of the campaign. Two of the included reports assessed primary prevention measures.

Comment

There was insufficient evidence to determine the effectiveness of mass media approaches in promoting sun-safe behaviors or a reduction in ultraviolet exposure. The studies included show that some aspects of knowledge were changed by the campaign. The evidence is poor due to limitations in the design of the studies and because there was no clear separation between primary and secondary prevention targets and outcomes. Studies were few, ineffec-

tually implemented, and varied in their intended outcomes. Assessment and evaluation were problematic.

Programs for caregivers

These are interventions that promote the reduction of ultraviolet exposure and protective behaviors among parents or other childcare personnel—anyone caring for children for an extended period. The interventions involved include changes in behavioral outcomes for adults or children in relation to ultraviolet exposure, such as information provided through instruction or small media, or both. The activities involved were intended to change knowledge, attitudes, beliefs, intentions, or behavior among parents or caregivers, and to lead to environmental change and use and scheduling of activities to avoid the midday sun.

Only two reports were included,[52,53] one based on a sun-safe curriculum and one on an interactive classroom project. Both were intended to promote covering-up behavior, seeking shade, and sunscreen use (using various classroom-based and parental/staff activities). Neither showed any significant effects for the influence of safe-sun policies or changes in behavior for any of the categories. The reports did show significant changes in the intermediate outcome —knowledge about safe-sun practices, including covering up, was improved.

Comment

There is insufficient evidence for the effectiveness of interventions on parental sun-protection behavior, parental and children's ultraviolet exposure, and the incidence of sunburn (too few reports). The results were inconsistent in many studies.

The effects of the intervention on parental knowledge, attitudes, beliefs, and parental intentions were inconsistent. Three arms in two reports demonstrated desirable and consistent effects of the intervention on children's attitudes or beliefs, with a median relative value of 67.6%. There is insufficient evidence to determine the effectiveness of interventions for parents or caregivers in preventing ultraviolet exposure or skin cancer. There were too few reports, and the evidence was inconsistent.

Interventions led to improvements in children's attitudes or beliefs, as well as to sun-safety measures and environmental support, at outdoor centers and swimming pools. Changes in policy did not necessarily translate into changes in ultraviolet exposure or behavior.

Community-wide multiple-component interventions

These are defined as interventions that use a combination (integration) of individual directed strategies, mass media campaigns, and environmental policy changes in clearly defined geographic areas with specific targets. They usually have a logo, a theme, a name, and a specific set of messages. The review team included studies that had a clearly defined geographic boundary, at least two components, and included two settings. Comprehensive community-wide interventions are multiple-level approaches that address large numbers in the given population.

The aim in interventions of this type is to change the behavior of the population. As well as providing education, they aim to instigate or improve policy and environmental support. Examples include the 20-year "Slip! Slop! Slap!" and SunSmart campaigns in Victoria, Australia, the Sun-Safe project in New Hampshire, and the Falmouth Safe Skin Project in Massachusetts. Australia has the longest-running and most sustained campaigns. However, the results may not be easily generalizable to other countries, including the USA and Europe, as Australia has the highest skin cancer rate and sun protection is a major public health concern.

Thirty-five reports on the effectiveness of multiple-component and comprehensive community-wide interventions met the inclusion criteria, of which nine qualified for assessment.[51–59] Of these, seven studies measured covering-up or sun-avoidance behaviors. Four showed generally positive outcomes, with three showing no significant change in recommended behaviors (covering up and sun avoidance).

Comment

Community-wide studies showed more positive results for sun-protection behaviors. The results, all from Australia, show promise, but still provide insufficient evidence of effectiveness, as there were too few studies and there were limitations in the design and implementation of the studies. The evidence does not suggest ineffectiveness, but the studies need to be developed further in order to confirm the effectiveness and generalizability of the approaches used.

Studies that evaluated sunscreen use generally demonstrated desirable effects (increased sunscreen use).

There were positive process measures for changes in school and government policy, as well as environmental policy—with increases in safe-sun policies in schools or government, retail outlets offering low-cost sunscreen, and an increase in the information provided. The effects for knowledge, attitudes, and beliefs among adults and children were inconsistent. The findings suggest that there is insufficient evidence to determine the effectiveness of multiple-component programs in reducing ultraviolet exposure or increasing sun-protective behaviors, due to inconsistent results.

Educational and policy interventions in primary schools

Twenty-one reports met the criteria and were therefore assessed.[16,54–73] The studies were assessed for effectiveness in outcome behaviors in the sun: staying in shade, avoiding

the sun during peak UVR hours, and wearing long-sleeved/long-legged clothes—i.e., covering up. Composite behavior was a combination of at least two of these measures plus using sunscreen. The way in which the results were presented meant that differentiation was not possible, especially in relation to the effect of one outcome measure on another. A wide range of intervention activities were used, but few included environmental or policy approaches. The majority of the intervention arms showed a significant increase in knowledge (22 out of 25) and a significant change in attitude (13 out of 17) studies. Only four reports evaluated intentions, and their findings were inconsistent and generally not significant.

One study evaluated policy interventions and reported significant improvements in the adoption of a comprehensive sun-protection policy in primary schools. However, this showed a weak relationship between the adoption of policy and associated sun-protective behavior changes that might have resulted from such a change in policy. One study evaluated the effects of an intervention to reduce sunburn: the results showed a 43% reduction in reported sunburns. The study design (in all of the studies assessed) markedly affected the effect size in the data: for sun-avoidance behaviors; the median relative changes were 4% in studies that had a concurrent comparison group and 16% in studies with a before-and-after design. For "covering-up behaviors," the median relative change ranged from 25% (concurrent comparison) to 70% (before and after). For sunscreen use, the relative change ranged from 17% (concurrent comparison) to 34% (before and after). Composite behaviors were measured in one study with controls; the relative change was 2% (see www.thecommunityguide.org/cancer for all data analysis and results).

Comment on educational and policy interventions in primary schools

In general, there is sufficient evidence to determine the effectiveness of interventions in primary schools in improving covering-up behavior; however, there is insufficient evidence to determine the effectiveness of interventions in improving other sun-protective behaviors, such as avoiding the sun (minimizing UVR exposure, seeking shade, or not going outside), due to inconsistent results.

There is also insufficient evidence to determine the effectiveness of interventions in primary schools in changing policies and practices or health outcomes, due to the small numbers of studies and limitations in their design and execution. These interventions improved knowledge and attitudes related to skin cancer prevention. They also increased sunscreen use, although this was not a recommendation outcome, as stated previously.

The available studies therefore provide reasonable evidence of the effectiveness of interventions in primary schools in improving covering-up behavior. Due to inconsistencies, there was insufficient evidence to determine the effectiveness of the interventions in improving other protective behaviors or decreasing sunburns.

Overall conclusions and comment on the Centers for Disease Control review

Evidence has been established of the effectiveness of interventions in primary schools in improving children's and adults' covering-up behavior, and of the effectiveness of interventions in recreational and tourist settings in reducing skin cancer. There are, however, general research issues that remain problematic; too few studies measure key target behaviors or health outcomes. Significant progress has been made by the Centers for Disease Control and Prevention in Atlanta in evaluating primary prevention sun-protection measures by using behavior in the sun as the surrogate measure for reducing UVR exposure and reduction of the risk of skin cancer. Reviewers assessed randomized controlled trials in conjunction with a cognitive–conceptual framework. This framework made it possible to carry out an analysis of the relationship between reported interventions and relevant intermediate outcomes: knowledge, attitudes, beliefs, intentions, key sun-protection behavior, and assumed relationships between sun-protective behaviors and skin cancer prevention. Surrogate and intermediate measures were not always clearly defined, nor were health outcomes (reduction in skin cancers). Confounding variables were sometimes not accounted for in the study designs and in the implementation of the studies. This has resulted in possible fundamental attribution error, alpha bias (exaggeration of the effect of the intervention) or beta bias (underestimation of the effect), as well as misunderstandings about which target behavior or behaviors changed due to which processes.

The CDC cognitive–conceptual framework clarified interventions in relation to "setting," acknowledging the complexity of primary prevention interventions within various health-promotion settings and populations. The CDC review was a major advance in review methodology, as it enabled reviewers to comment on reliability and validity in relation to the effectiveness of interventions. The CDC reviewers acknowledge that reliability may sometimes have to be sacrificed for validity, especially in community-wide interventions, if they are to be ecologically valid.

Other approaches for primary prevention

Can chemoprevention interventions reduce the risk of cancer?

The International Agency for Research on Cancer reported on three separate meta-analyses: vitamin A intake,[74] carotenoids,[75] and retinoids[76] and their effect on cancers, including skin cancer.

Retinol (vitamin A). The reviewers concluded that there was no association between the dietary intake of retinol and the risk of skin cancer in a small number of observational studies (one case–control and three cohort studies). These studies were conducted among Caucasian populations with a wide range of disease risk. The risk estimates in the individual studies were generally greater than unity, and in every instance the 95% confidence interval (CI) included 1.0. Two prospective studies of prediagnostic levels of retinol and melanoma both reported no significant association, on the basis of 30 and 10 cases, respectively. This is consistent with the findings of a case–control study of melanoma and dietary intake of preformed vitamin A.[74]

Beta-carotene (vitamin B). Beta-carotene does not prevent cancer when used as a high-dose supplement, and there is inadequate evidence with regard to its effect at the usual dietary levels (see Chapter 26). There is inadequate evidence with respect to the possible cancer-preventive activity of other individual carotenoids. This is in contrast with some results from animal studies.[77]

Isotretinoin. A number of randomized studies have evaluated the efficacy of chemoprevention agents such as isotretinoin and beta-carotene for individuals at increased risk of developing NMSC. High-dose isotretinoin was found to prevent new skin cancers in individuals with xeroderma pigmentosum. An RCT of long-term treatment with isotretinoin in individuals previously treated for BCC showed that such treatment did not prevent the recurrence of new BCCs and produced the side effects characteristic of isotretinoin treatment.[78]

Selenium. A multicenter double-blind, randomized, placebo-controlled trial including 1312 patients with a history of BCC or SCC of the skin and a mean follow-up period of 6.4 years showed that 200 µg of selenium (in brewer's yeast tablets) did not have a significant effect on the primary end point of the development of BCC or SCC of the skin.[79]

Comment

The evidence from RCTs suggests that vitamin A and beta-carotene are not effective in preventing skin cancers.

The evidence for the effect of isotretinoin is equivocal, but the agent may be of some use in high-risk groups. There is no evidence that selenium in brewer's yeast tablets has a preventive effect against NMSCs.

Can other medicines reduce the risk of skin cancer and melanoma?

A Cochrane Review reported on medications lowering statins and fibrate lipid on outcomes in patients with melanoma.[4] Sixteen RCTs qualified for assessment (seven on statin and nine on fibrate, n = 62 197). A total of 66 melanomas were reported in groups receiving the experimental drug and 86 in groups receiving a placebo or other control therapies. For the statin trials, this translated into an odds ratio of 0.90 (95% CI, 0.56 to 1.44) and for the fibrate trials into an odds ratio of 0.58 (95% CI, 0.19 to 1.82). Subgroup analysis failed to show statistically significant differences in melanoma outcomes in relation to gender, melanoma occurrence after 2 years of participation in the trial, histology, or trial funding. Subgroup analysis by type of fibrate or statin also failed to show statistically significant differences for the statin subgroup analysis, which showed a reduced melanoma incidence for lovastatin on the basis of only one trial (odds ratio 0.52; 95% CI, 0.27 to 0.99).[4]

Comment

The outcome data do not exclude the possibility that these drugs prevent melanoma. There were 10% and 42% reductions for participants on statins and fibrates, respectively, but the results were not significant. Until further evidence is obtained, limiting exposure to ultraviolet radiation will continue to be the most effective way of reducing the risk of melanoma.

Implications for practice

The CDC review[3] led to systematic sun-protection policies for specific settings as part of the "Healthy People 2010" campaign in the United States (www.healthypeople.gov). The evidence suggests that these policies should also be considered by other countries in the northern hemisphere in order to reduce the incidence of skin cancers. Cultural changes (relative to specific countries and populations) may be required for these policies to be effective, but the suggested policies are provided here as a guide for future research:

• Government and voluntary agency partnerships, combined with joint agency working in the community, should enhance effective sun-protection policy in all settings. Sun-protection policy continues to be a priority for countries in the northern hemisphere, following the lead provided by Australia.

• Melanoma deaths should be reduced to < 2.5 per 100 000 population.

• The proportion of people who use at least one of the following protective measures should be increased to 75%: avoid sun between 10 a.m. and 4 p.m.; wear sun-protective clothing when exposed to the sun; use sunscreen with a sun-protection factor > 15; and avoid artificial sources of sunlight (i.e., sun-beds).

Key points

• There is fair to good evidence that increased sun exposure increases the risk of nonmelanoma skin cancer.

• The relationships between sun exposure and melanoma risk are complex, and observational studies suggest that intermittent or intense sun exposure is a greater risk factor for melanoma than chronic exposure.

• Light-skinned people are at much higher risk for skin cancer than those with darker skin.

• There is good evidence that sunscreens can reduce the risk of squamous cell cancer, but sunscreen use alone is not an effective protection strategy against ultraviolet radiation. Sunscreen use appears to reduce the use of other protective measures such as clothing and shade. There is insufficient evidence to determine the effect of sunscreen use on the risk of melanoma (see Chapter 26).

• There is insufficient evidence to determine whether clinician counseling is effective in changing patient behaviors to reduce the risk of skin cancer.

• Counseling parents may increase their use of sunscreen for children, but there is little evidence to determine the effects of counseling parents on other protective behaviors (clothing, reducing sun exposure, avoiding sun lamps, or practicing skin self examination).

• The evidence regarding the effects of sunlamp use or skin self-examination on the risk of melanoma is poor.

• The benefits of sun-protective measures exceed any potential harm.

References

1 Cancer Research UK. UK malignant melanoma mortality statistics (available at: http://info.cancerresearchuk.org/cancerstats/types/melanoma/mortality/).

2 Scott D, Weston R, eds. *Evaluating Health Promotion*. Cheltenham, UK: Thornes, 1998.

3 Saraiya M, Glanz K, Briss PA, *et al*. Interventions to prevent skin cancer by reducing exposure to ultraviolet radiation: a systematic review. *Am J Prev Med* 2004;**27**:422–66.

4 Dellavalle RP, Drake A, Graber M, *et al*. Statins and fibrates for preventing melanoma. *Cochrane Database Syst Rev* 2005;(**4**): CD003697.

5 International Agency for Research on Cancer/World Health Organization. *IARC Handbooks of Cancer Prevention*, vol. 5: *Sunscreens*. Lyons, France: IARC Press, 2001.

6 Loescher LJ, Emerson J, Taylor A, Christensen DH, McKinney M. Educating preschoolers about sun safety. *Am J Public Health* 1995;**85**:939–43.

7 Crane LA, Schneider LS, Yohn JJ, Morelli JG, Plomer KD. "Block the sun, not the fun": evaluation of a skin cancer prevention program for child care centers. *Am J Prev Med* 1999;**17**:31–7.

8 Schofield MJ, Edwards K, Pearce R. Effectiveness of two strategies for dissemination of sun-protection policy in New South

Wales primary and secondary schools. *Aust N Z J Public Health* 1997;**21**:743–50.

9 Dernhardt JM. Tailoring messages and design in a web-based skin cancer prevention intervention. *Int Electron J Health Educ* 2001; **4**:290–7.

10 Cody R, Lee C. Behaviors, beliefs, and intentions in skin cancer prevention. *J Behav Med* 1990;**13**:373–89.

11 Jones JL, Leary MR. Effects of appearance-based admonitions against sun exposure on tanning intentions in young adults. *Health Psychol* 1994;**13**:86–90.

12 Kamin CS, O'Neill PN, Ahearn MJ. Developing and evaluating a cancer prevention teaching module for secondary education: Project SAFETY (Sun Awareness for Educating Today's Youth). *J Cancer Educ* 1993;**8**:313–8.

13 Katz RC, Jernigan S. Brief report: an empirically derived educational program for detecting and preventing skin cancer. *J Behav Med* 1991;**14**:421–8.

14 Lowe JB, Balander KP, Stanton WR, Gillespie AM. Evaluation of a three-year school-based intervention to increase adolescent sun protection. *Health Educ Behav* 1999;**26**:396–408.

15 Mahler HI, Fitzpatrick B, Parker P, Lapin A. The relative effects of a health-based versus an appearance-based intervention designed to increase sunscreen use. *Am J Health Promot* 1997;**11**:426–9.

16 Mermelstein RJ, Reisenberg LA. Changing knowledge and attitudes about skin cancer risk factors in adolescents. *Health Psychol* 1992;**11**:371–6.

17 Mickler TJ, Rodrigue JR, Lescano CM. A comparison of three methods of teaching skin self examinations. *J Clin Psychol Med Settings* 1999;**6**:273–6.

18 Prentice-Dunn S, Jones JL, Floyd DL. Persuasive appeals and the reduction of skin cancer risk: the roles of appearance concern, perceived benefits of a tan, and efficacy information. *J Appl Soc Psychol* 1997;**27**:1041–7.

19 Rothman AJ, Salovey P, Antone C, Keough K, Martin CD. The influence of message framing on intentions to perform health behaviors. *J Exper Social Psychol* 1993;**29**:408–33.

20 Stephenson MT, Witte K. Fear, threat, and perceptions of efficacy from frightening skin cancer messages. *Public Health Rev* 1998; **26**:147–74.

21 Detweiler JB, Bedell BT, Salovey P, Pronin E, Rothman AJ. Message framing and sunscreen use: gain-framed messages motivate beach-goers. *Health Psychol* 1999;**18**:189–96.

22 Dey P, Collins S, Will S, Woodman CB. Randomised controlled trial assessing effectiveness of health education leaflets in reducing incidence of sunburn. *BMJ* 1995;**311**:1062–3.

23 Glanz K, Chang L, Song V, Silverio R, Muneoka L. Skin cancer prevention for children, parents, and caregivers: a field test of Hawaii's SunSmart program. *J Am Acad Dermatol* 1998;**38**:413–7.

24 Glanz K, Lew RA, Song V, Murakami-Akatsuka L. Skin cancer prevention in outdoor recreation settings: effects of the Hawaii SunSmart Program. *Eff Clin Pract* 2000;**3**:53–61.

25 Glanz K, Geller AC, Shigaki D, Maddock JE, Isnec MR. A randomized trial of skin cancer prevention in aquatics settings: the Pool Cool program. *Health Psychol* 2002;**21**:579–87.

26 Keesling B, Friedman HS. Interventions to prevent skin cancer: experimental evaluation of informational and fear appeals. *Psychol Health* 1995;**10**:477–90.

27 Lombard D, Neubauer TE, Canfield D, Winett RA. Behavioral community intervention to reduce the risk of skin cancer. *J Appl Behav Anal* 1991;**24**:677–86.

28 Mayer J, Slymen DJ, Eckhardt L, *et al.* Reducing ultraviolet radiation exposure in children. *Prev Med* 1997;**26**:516–22.

29 Mayer JA, Lewis EC, Eckhardt L, *et al.* Promoting sun safety among zoo visitors. *Prev Med* 2001;**33**:162–9.

30 Segan C, Borland R, Hill D. Development and evaluation of a brochure on sun protection and sun exposure for tourists. *Health Educ J* 1999;**58**:177–91.

31 Weinstock MA, Rossi JS, Redding CA, Maddock JE. Randomized controlled community trial of the efficacy of a multicomponent stage-matched intervention to increase sun protection among beachgoers. *Prev Med* 2002;**35**:584–92.

32 Gooderham MJ, Guenther L. Impact of a sun awareness curriculum on medical students' knowledge, attitudes, and behaviour. *J Cutan Med Surg* 1999;**3**:182–7.

33 Dolan NC, Ng JS, Martin GJ, Robinson JK, Rademaker AW. Effectiveness of a skin cancer control educational intervention for internal medicine housestaff and attending physicians. *J Gen Intern Med* 1997;**12**:531–6.

34 Gerbert B, Wolff M, Tschann JM, *et al.* Activating patients to practice skin cancer prevention: response to mailed materials from physicians versus HMOs. *Am J Prev Med* 1997;**13**:214–20.

35 Harris JM Jr, Salasche SJ, Harris RB. Using the Internet to teach melanoma management guidelines to primary care physicians. *J Eval Clin Pract* 1999;**5**:199–211.

36 Johnson EY, Lookingbill DP. Sunscreen use and sun exposure. Trends in a white population. *Arch Dermatol* 1984;**120**:727–31.

37 Liu KE, Barankin B, Howard D, Guenther LC. One year follow-up on the impact of a sun awareness curriculum on medical students' knowledge, attitudes and behavior. *J Cutan Med Surg* 2001;**5**:193–200.

38 Mayer JA, Slymen DJ, Eckhardt L, *et al.* Skin cancer prevention counseling by pharmacists: specific outcomes of an intervention trial. *Cancer Detect Prev* 1998;**22**:367–75.

39 McCormick LK, Masse L, Cummings SS, Burke C. Evaluation of a skin cancer prevention module for nurses: change in knowledge, self-efficacy, and attitudes. *Am J Health Promot* 1999;**13**:282–9.

40 Mikkilineni R, Weinstock MA, Goldstein MG, Dube CE, Rossi JS. The impact of the basic skin cancer triage curriculum on provider's skin cancer control practices. *J Gen Intern Med* 2001;**16**:302–7.

41 Palmer RC, Mayer JA, Eckhardt L, Sallis JF. Promoting sunscreen in a community drugstore. *Am J Public Health* 1998;**88**:681.

42 Montague M, Borland R, Sinclair C. Slip! Slop! Slap! and SunSmart, 1980–2000: skin cancer control and 20 years of population-based campaigning. *Health Educ Behav* 2001;**28**:290–305.

43 Geller AC, Hufford D, Miller DR, *et al.* Evaluation of the Ultraviolet Index: media reactions and public response. *J Am Acad Dermatol* 1997;**37**:935–41.

44 Kiekbusch S, Hannich HJ, Isacsson A, *et al.* Impact of a cancer education multimedia device on public knowledge, attitudes, and behaviors: a controlled intervention study in southern Sweden. *J Cancer Educ* 2000;**15**:232–6.

45 Dietrich AJ, Olson AL, Sox CH, *et al.* A community-based randomized trial encouraging sun protection for children. *Pediatrics* 1998;**102**:E64.

46 Dietrich AJ, Olson AL, Sox CH, Tosteson TD, Grant-Petersson J. Persistent increase in children's sun protection in a randomized controlled community trial. *Prev Med* 2000;**31**:569–74.

47 Miller DR, Geller AC, Wood MC, Lew RA, Koh HK. The Falmouth Safe Skin Project: evaluation of a community program to promote sun protection in youth. *Health Educ Behav* 1999;**26**:369–84.

48 English DR, Milne E, Jacoby P, Giles-Corti B, Cross D, Johnston R. The effect of a school-based sun protection intervention on the development of melanocytic nevi in children: 6 year follow up. *Cancer Epidemiology bio markers Prev.* 2005 April;14(4): 977–80.

49 Biger C, Epstein LM, Hagoel L, Tamir A, Robinson E. An evaluation of an education programme for prevention and early diagnosis of malignancy in Israel. *Eur J Cancer Prevention* 1994;**3**:305–12.

50 U.S. Preventive Services Task Force. Counseling to prevent skin cancer: recommendations and rationale of the U.S. Preventive Services Task Force. *MMWR Recomm Rep* 2003;**52**(RR-15):13–7.

51 New South Wales Cancer Council. *Report on the Seymour Snowman Sun Protection Campaign (1997–1998).* North Sydney, New South Wales, Australia: New South Wales Cancer Council, 1998.

52 Rassaby J, Larcombe I, Hill D, Wake R. Slip Slop Slap: health education about skin cancer. *Cancer Forum* 1983;**7**:63–9.

53 Sanson-Fisher R. *Me No Fry 1994/95 Summer Campaign Evaluation Report.* North Sydney, New South Wales, Australia: NSW Department of Health, 1995.

54 Grant-Peterson J, Dietrich AJ, Sox CH, Winchell CW, Stevens MM. Promoting sun protection in elementary schools and child care settings: the Sun Safe Project. *J Sch Health* 1999;**69**:100–6.

55 Bastuji-Garin S, Grob JJ, Grognard C, Grosjean F, Guillaume JC. Melanoma prevention: evaluation of a health education campaign for primary schools. *Arch Dermatol* 1999;**135**:936–40.

56 Buller DB, Buller MK, Beach B, Ertl G. Sunny days, healthy ways: evaluation of a skin cancer prevention curriculum for elementary school-aged children. *J Am Acad Dermatol* 1996;**35**:911–22.

57 Buller DB, Hall JR, Powers PJ, *et al.* Evaluation of the "Sunny Days, Healthy Ways" sun safety CD-ROM program for children in grades 4 and 5. *Cancer Prev Control* 1999;**3**:188–95.

58 Buller MK, Goldberg G, Buller DB. Sun Smart Day: a pilot program for photoprotection education. *Pediatr Dermatol* 1997;**14**:257–63.

59 Buller MK, Loescher LJ, Buller DB. "Sunshine and skin health": a curriculum for skin cancer prevention education. *J Cancer Educ* 1994;**9**:155–62.

60 DeLong M, LaBat K, Gahring S, Nelson N, Leung I. Implications of an educational intervention program designed to increase young adolescents' awareness of hats for sun protection. *Cloth Text Res J* 1999;**17**:73–83.

61 Girgis A, Sanson-Fisher RW, Tripodi DA, Golding T. Evaluation of interventions to improve solar protection in primary schools. *Health Educ Q* 1993;**20**:275–87.

62 Gooderham MJ, Guenther L. Sun and the skin: evaluation of a sun awareness program for elementary school students. *J Cutan Med Surg* 1999;**3**:230–5.

63 Hoffman RG III, Rodrigue JR, Johnson JH. Effectiveness of a school-based program to enhance knowledge of sun exposure: attitudes toward sun exposure and sunscreen use among children. *Child Health Care* 1999;**28**:69–86.

64 Hornung RL, Lennon PA, Garrett JM, DeVellis RF, Weinberg PD, Stretcher VJ. Interactive technology for skin cancer prevention targeting children. *Am J Prev Med* 2000;**18**:69–76.

65 Hughes AS. Sun protection and younger children: lessons from the Living with Sunshine program. *J Sch Health* 1994;**64**:201–4.

66 Labat KI, Delong MR, Gahring S. Evaluation of a skin cancer intervention program for youth. *J Fam Consumer Sci* 1996;**88**:3–10.

67 Milne E, English DR, Johnston R, *et al.* Improved sun protection behaviour in children after two years of the Kidskin intervention. *Aust N Z J Public Health* 2000;**24**:481–7.

68 McWhirter JM, Collins M, Bryant I, Wetton NM, Newton Bishop J. Evaluating "Safe in the Sun," a curriculum programme for primary schools. *Health Educ Res* 2000;**15**:203–17.

69 Ramstack JL, White SE, Hazelkorn KS, Meyskens FL. Sunshine and skin cancer: a school-based skin cancer prevention project. *J Cancer Educ* 1986;**1**:169–76.

70 Reding DJ, Fischer V, Gunderson P, Lappe K, Anderson H, Calvert G. Teens teach skin cancer prevention. *J Rural Health* 1996;**12**(4 Suppl):265–72.

71 Reding DJ, Fischer V, Gunderson P, Lappe K. Skin cancer prevention: a peer education model. *Wis Med J* 1995;**94**:77–81.

72 Thornton C, Piacquadio DJ. Promoting sun awareness: evaluation of an educational children's book. *Pediatrics* 1996;**98**:52–5.

73 Vitols P, Oates RK. Teaching children about skin cancer prevention: why wait for adolescence? *Aust N Z J Public Health* 1997; **21**:602–5.

74 International Agency for Research on Cancer/World Health Organization. *IARC Handbooks of Cancer Prevention*, vol. 3: *Vitamin A.* Lyons, France: IARC Press, 1998.

75 International Agency for Research on Cancer/World Health Organization. *IARC Handbooks of Cancer Prevention*, vol. 2: *Carotenoids.* Lyons, France: IARC Press, 1998.

76 International Agency for Research on Cancer/World Health Organization. *IARC Handbooks of Cancer Prevention*, vol. 4: *Retinoids.* Lyons, France: IARC Press, 2000.

77 Darlington S, Williams G, Neale R, Frost C, Green A. A randomized controlled trial to assess sunscreen application and beta carotene supplementation in the prevention of solar keratoses. *Arch Dermatol* 2003;**139**:451–5.

78 Tangrea JA, Edwards BK, Taylor PR, *et al.* Long-term therapy with low-dose isotretinoin for prevention of basal cell carcinoma: a multicenter clinical trial. Isotretinoin–Basal Cell Carcinoma Study Group. *J Natl Cancer Inst* 1992;**84**:328–32.

79 Clark LC, Combs GF Jr, Turnbull BW, *et al.* Effects of selenium supplementation for cancer prevention in patients with carcinoma of the skin: a randomized controlled trial. Nutritional Prevention of Cancer Study Group. JAMA 1996;**276**:1957–63.

26

Do sunscreens reduce the incidence of skin cancers?

Ros Weston

Background

Historical development and sun protection factor

Sunscreens were first used in 1928 and became popular with those intentionally trying to gain a suntan. They mainly filter out the wavelengths responsible for sunburn—ultraviolet B (UVB, 280–315 nm). Following evidence that longer wavelengths of sunlight—ultraviolet A (UVA, 315–400 nm)—are involved in the sunburn reaction and photocarcinogenesis, UVA absorbers have been added to most sunscreens to widen their absorption spectra. There is good evidence that sunscreens protect against sunburn, but evidence for a role in the prevention of skin cancers is still equivocal and there is some evidence to suggest that they are ineffective as the only protection measure.[1,2] The concept of a sunscreen effectiveness index (ratio) is attributed to Schulze and Greiter, who proposed the specific term "sun protection factor" (SPF) and the associated method for assessing SPF.[3] SPF activity is the ratio of the least amount of UV energy required to produce erythema (reddening of the skin) on sunscreen-protected skin to the amount of energy to produce the same effect on unprotected skin (Figure 26.1).

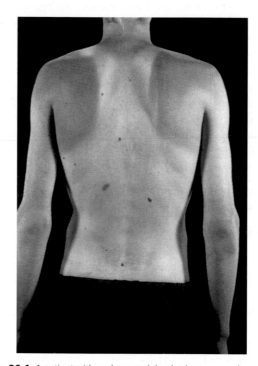

Figure 26.1 A patient with sunburn and dysplastic nevus syndrome.

Testing and regulation of sunscreens

Topical sunscreens applied to the skin act by absorbing and/or scattering incident ultraviolet radiation (UVR). The shape of the absorption spectrum is the fundamental attribute of a topical sunscreen. It is expressed as the extinction coefficient: the measure of the degree to which the sunscreen absorbs individual wavelengths across the terrestrial UVR spectrum (290–400 nm). Absorption is the product of the extinction coefficient, the concentration of the active ingredient, and the effective thickness of application on exposed parts of the body.

Sunscreens are regulated for specific formulations in most countries. In the European Union, Japan, and South Africa they are regulated as cosmetics, and in other countries (Australia, Canada, and New Zealand) as drugs. Testing for toxic effects is mandatory in each country. Control in Europe is by a directive of the European Commission (2000). This mandates that labeling should include a full list of ingredients in decreasing order of concentration, and that this should be displayed on the containers of all cosmetics that include sunscreen formulations.[4–7] Sunscreens are now readily available in most countries during all seasons. In Australia, the availability of sunscreens has been maximized through sales tax exemptions, and they are now available in workplaces and schools; their use by children is actively promoted.[8–10]

Paradoxical findings: problems with use of sunscreen as a primary prevention aim

Protecting against sun damage and reducing the risk of sunburn and skin cancers involves behavioral choices. Studies demonstrate that increased use of sunscreens is often accompanied by a reduction in other photoprotective methods such as wearing of hats and protective clothing and the use of shade (Fig. 26.1), thus increasing net sun exposure. Most sunscreens are made to prevent against sunburn, and most sunburn occurs during intentional exposure to the sun in children and adults.[11–14] The use of sunscreens, including those with high SPFs, during intentional exposure has been found to have little effect on the occurrence of sunburn.[15–17] Results from surveys of beachgoers suggest that increased over-reliance on sunscreens reduces the use of other protective measures. Individuals seem to balance protective behaviors according to personal motivation and characteristics and the desire for a suntan.[18–24]

Intended and actual sun protection from sunscreens

There is some evidence that the numerical measure of protection indicated on the product pack is generally higher than that achieved in practice. The photoprotection of sunscreens (the SPF) is measured by phototesting *in vivo* at internationally agreed levels of thickness of application (2 mg/cm^2). To receive the SPF quoted on sunscreen packaging, an individual would need to use 35 mL of sunscreen for total body surface protection. Studies have demonstrated that individuals are more likely to use $0.5–1.5 \text{ mg/cm}^2$ and that most users get, in protective terms, the benefit of between one-quarter and one-half of the product.[25] Individuals get sunburnt because they use too little sunscreen, spread it unevenly, miss parts of the body surface exposed to the sun, and because sunscreen is rubbed or washed off. Thus, individuals' use of a sunscreen makes a difference in how effective sunscreens are in the prevention of sunburn and explains why sunburn still occurs even with higher SPF sunscreens. If individuals want to be supine in the sun for long periods of time (hours), then it is recommended that SPFs of 20–30 or higher are necessary. Sunscreens need to be applied evenly 30 minutes before the individual goes out into the sun. They need to be reapplied at regular intervals, as much is washed off by swimming and other water sports and by any abrasive action, particularly from sand on the beach.[2]

Possible drawbacks of sunscreens

No published studies have demonstrated toxic effects of sunscreens in humans. Case reports suggest there is an increase in the frequency of photocontact dermatitis among patients who are frequent sunscreen users and who have photodermatoses such as polymorphic light eruption. There is no clear evidence that sunscreen use affects vitamin D levels. Using sunscreen does not cause adverse effects on reproduction or fetal development, although some effects have been seen with high oral doses of sunscreen ingredients in animal models. In some experimental conditions, topically applied sunscreen (in the absence of UVR) affects the immune system, but most toxicity studies have shown that the active ingredients in sunscreens are safe when applied topically at recommended concentrations. DNA damage has been reported in one study.[2]

Search strategies

Searches of Medline, PubMed and the Cochrane Library were carried out up until June 2006 using "sunscreen," "cutaneous melanoma," and "skin cancer" as key words, searching for appropriate meta-analyses, systematic reviews, and randomized controlled trials (RCTs). Health education and promotion journals were also searched.

The search located two systematic reviews,[26,27] one for reducing risk of skin cancers that incorporates sunscreen use as part of multi-strategy community interventions, and one systematic review for effectiveness of sunscreen and risk for cutaneous melanoma. Three randomized controlled trials using a nevi count as a surrogate measure for melanoma risk were also located.[28–32]

Outcome measures

Ideally, the main outcome measure of studies addressing sunscreen use and cancer risk would be numbers of incident cancers in those using sunscreens compared with those not using sunscreens. However, this is very difficult, because of the long latency period for a skin cancer to develop and the relative rarity of such events. Intermediate outcomes such as incidence of actinic keratoses or reduction in nevi are used as short-term surrogates for longer-term skin cancer risk. Other surrogate outcome measures, such as reported protective behavior, are also often used in studies. All of these surrogate measures have their problems. There are many confounding factors when assessing sunscreen use. Many studies use behavior (for example, reported use of sunscreen or sun avoidance) as the outcome measure. Such data may be unreliable, as recall of use is not necessarily accurate and other protective measures are confounding factors. Lack of specificity of outcome measures remains problematic in this field.

Questions

Can the use of sunscreen prevent cutaneous melanoma?

Case–control studies of sunscreen use and melanoma

One systematic review published in 2003 (see www.annals.

org for results) included 18 studies,[26] of which 15 were case–control studies, reported in the first edition of this chapter in 2003 (Table 26.1).[33-47] The review included cohort and case–control studies that measured sunscreen use in relation to melanoma. There were no cohort or cross-sectional studies of sunscreen use and development of melanoma. The authors examined subgroups of studies that reported adjustment for sun sensitivity, sunburns, and other sun exposure. Because of the general heterogeneity of the studies, they were scored for potential confounding factors (sun sensitivity in relationship to sunscreen and

Table 26.1 Case–control studies of sunscreen use and risk for cutaneous melanoma

Population place/date	Type of cases/controls	No. cases/ controls	Exposure	RR[a] (95% CI)	Comments	Reference
Norway 1974–75	Hospital cases Other cancer controls	78 cases 131 controls	Sometimes, often or almost always use sun lotion/oil	M 2.8[b] (1.2–6.7) F 1.0[b] (0.42–2.5) T 2.3[b] (1.3–4.1)	Elevated risks among males only. Sunscreens not differentiated from "sun lotions"	Klepp and Magnus (1979)[26]
USA 1974–80	Hospital cases Other cancer controls	404 cases 521 controls	Used sunscreen Used suntan lotion	M 2.2[b] (1.2–4.1) M 1.7 (1.1–2.7) F "no added risk"	Elevated risks among males only	Graham et al. (1985)[27]
USA 1977–79	Population cases and controls	324 male trunk melanoma cases 415 controls	Always used "suntan lotion"	2.6[b] (1.4–4.7) Not significant after control for "tendency to sunburn and water sports"	"Suntan lotions" and "sunscreens" not differentiated in questionnaire	Herzfeld et al.[28] (1993)
Sweden 1978–83	Hospital cases Population controls	523 cases 505 controls	Often used sun protection agents	1.8[b] (1.2–2.7)		Beitner et al.[29] (1990)
Canada 1979–81	Population cases and controls	369 trunk and lower limb melanomas 369 controls	Used sunscreen almost always	1.1 (0.75–1.6)	Highest risk in those using sunscreen "only for first few hours" RR, 1.62 (1.04–2.52)	Elwood and Gallagher[30] (1999)
Australia 1980–81	Population cases and controls	507 cases 507 controls	Used sunscreens ≤ 10 years	1.1 (0.71–1.6)		Holman et al.[31] (1986)
USA 1981–86	Population cases and controls	452 cases 930 controls	Always used sunscreens	All cutaneous melanoma 0.62[b] (0.49–0.83) Superficial spreading melanoma (SSM) 0.43 (CI not available)	Study involved only women aged 25–59 at diagnosis. CI estimated. RR for SSM adjusted for host factors and sun exposure	Holly et al.[32] (1995)
Denmark 1982–85	Population cases and controls	474 cases 926 controls	Always used sunscreens	1.1[b] (0.8–1.5)		Osterlind et al. (1997)[33]
Australia 1987–94	Population cases Controls from same school	50 cases 156 controls All children < 15	Always used sunscreens	2.2 (0.4–12) on holidays 0.7 (0.1–6.0) at school		Whiteman et al. (1997)[34]
Sweden 1988–90	Population cases and controls	400 cases 640 controls	Almost always used sunscreens	Trunk 1.4 (0.6–3.2) Other sites 2.0 (1.1–3.7)	No information on duration of use	Westerdahl et al. (1995)[35]

Table 26.1 *Cont'd*

Population place/date	Type of cases/controls	No. cases/controls	Exposure	RRª (95% CI)	Comments	Reference
Spain 1989–93	Hospital cases Hospital visitors	105 cases 138 controls	Always used sunscreens	0.2 (0.04–0.79)		Rodenas *et al.* (1996)[36]
Spain 1990–94	Hospital cases and controls	116 cases 235 controls	Used sunscreen	0.48 (0.34–0.71)	Inadequate description of measurement of sunscreen use	Espinoza-Arranz *et al.* (1991)[37]
Europe 1991–92	Hospital cases Neighbourhood controls	418 controls 438 controls	Ever use psoralen sunscreens Ever use sunscreen	2.3 (1.3–4.0) 1.5 (1.1–2.1) M 1.8 (1.1–2.7) F 1.3 (0.87–2.0)	Highest risk for sun-sensitive subjects using sunscreens to tan: RR, 3.7 (1.0–7.6)	Autier *et al.* (1995, 1997b)[38]
Austria 1993–94	Hospital cases and controls	193 cases 319 controls	Often used sunscreen	3.5 (1.8–6.6)		Wolf *et al.* (1998)[39]
Sweden 1995–97	Population cases and controls	571 cases 913 controls	Always used sunscreen Used sunscreens to spend more time sunbathing	1.8 (1.1–2.9) 8.7 (1.0–76)		Westerdahl *et al.* (2000)[40]

ª Relative risk estimates adjusted for phenotype and sun-related factors where possible.
ᵇ Crude relative risk ratio only available.

melanoma according to the method by which sun sensitivity was measured). Higher scores were allocated to studies adjusting for skin color, skin type, ability to tan, and tendency to burn, whereas a lower score was assigned to those that only adjusted for hair color, eye color, or freckling. Credit was given to studies that adjusted for potential confounders such as sunburn, other sun exposure, and to those that partially adjusted for these confounders. A score was awarded for matched sex and age studies, and for those studies that examined sunscreen use: credit was given to those that gave detail other than "ever use"—e.g., those reporting years of use and frequency of use. The maximum score was 19 points (see www.annals.org).

Reliability was measured by using the κ statistic for categorical measures, and total scores were compared by using interclass correlation. The reliability scores varied: the κ value was correlated at 1.0 for whether the survey was completed by an interviewer or was self-administered, selection of control groups, and adjustment for sunburn. All other values had a κ value greater than 0.60. These quality scores have not been validated and were not used in the data analysis for dichotomous factors ("ever use" of sunscreen). The reviewers used fixed-effects and random-effects models to obtain pooled relative risk estimates. To assess heterogeneity, between-study variance was estimated. The sample was stratified by type of controls, adjustment for sun sensitivity, and for studies not reporting odds ratio (OR) and

confidence intervals (CI), as well as an estimate of "ever use" based on case and control distribution for frequency of sunscreen. For multiple ordinal categories (frequency of sunscreen use and years of sunscreen use), the reviewers used a fixed dose–response method to evaluate linear relationships.

The "ever use" of sunscreen category identified five studies (www.annals.org) with a pooled odds ratio and 95% CI for "ever sunscreen use," and for other studies the odds ratio was estimated using frequency of sunscreen use. The pooled odds ratio for melanoma as an outcome in 18 studies on "ever sunscreen use" was 1.0 (95% CI, 0.8 to 1.2; P value for heterogeneity < 0.001). No differences in odds ratios were found between the types of control group. When the five studies that adjusted for hair color were pooled with those for sun sensitivity, no association was found (odds ratio 1.0). The odds ratio for melanoma was smaller when these five studies were excluded. When studies were adjusted for sun sensitivity only, the pooled odds ratio decreased to 0.8 (95% CI, 0.6 to 1.0).

For skin sensitivity, the data were homogeneous; two studies reported null associations (odds ratio 1.14 and 1.17). One study reported a significant protective effect (odds ratio 0.66). The results demonstrated that overall, sun-sensitive persons, who are more likely to use sunscreens, are at higher risk for melanoma. The association for sunscreen use and melanoma was homogeneous and nonsignificantly protective (OR 0.9; 95% CI, 0.7 to 1.2; P value for homogeneity 0.13). For sun-resistant individuals (Fitzpatrick 3 or 4), one study reported a null association between sunscreen use and melanoma (OR 1.17), two reported increased associations (OR 0.6; 95% CI, 1.3 to 1.7), and one study reported a significant protective effect with heterogeneous associations ($P = 0.002$).

In the between-group categories, a linear model that assumed equal distance was used for pooled data on ordered categories from 12 case–control studies. The results showed that the studies were heterogeneous, with no apparent association (OR 1.1; $P = 0.09$) between melanoma and frequency of sunscreen use (84% of 12 studies). There was significant between-study variation. Four studies did not adjust for confounding factors of sun sensitivity, or only adjusted for hair color. When these four studies were excluded, the odds ratio for the relationship decreased to 0.93 (95% CI, 0.81 to 1.07). Three additional studies did not adjust for confounding effects of a history of sunburn. When the five studies adjusted for sunburn and sun sensitivity were pooled, a significant protective effect was observed (OR 0.76; 95% CI, 0.65 to 0.90). The studies remained heterogeneous and study variation remained at 84%, suggesting that the ordered categories for frequency of sunscreen use may not be comparable across studies, but this may also reflect how people quantify their sunscreen use.

The overall results do not support a positive association between sunscreen use and melanoma, or melanoma and "ever use" of sunscreen. However, the heterogeneity limits the validity of the pooled results. No association was found among homogeneous odds ratios for sun-sensitive persons, and the reviewers suggest that further research is necessary, as the risk may be related to prolonged exposure to sun after maximum tanning. Inconsistent findings and heterogeneity in the dose response for frequency of use of sunscreens is unsurprising. Participants were asked how often they used sunscreens, but not about re-application or duration of their use of sunscreens. The data on "years of use" were not heterogeneous, with low odds ratios across increasing categories of use in all four studies. The lack of a dose–response effect for "years of use" supports a null hypothesis between sunscreen use and melanoma risk. Studies that properly adjust for confounding effects of sun sensitivity and sunburn as well as skin type are required to confirm any reduction of melanoma with sunscreen use.

The reviewers conclude that increased melanoma risk with sunscreen use is a misleading conclusion, mainly because sun-sensitive individuals are more likely to use sunscreen and are at higher risk of melanoma. Increased risk for melanoma among sunscreen users may reflect increased risk among sun-sensitive persons rather than an increased risk solely due to sunscreen use. The lack of an overall association does not support an increased melanoma risk with sunscreen.

Sun exposure is a major confounding factor of sunscreen use, because it can be intermittent or chronic: it allows sun-resistant individuals to spend a longer time in the sun, thus absorbing more UVR. The strong correlation between sun exposure and sunscreen use means it is difficult to adjust for and interpret. Differences in these patterns and in the formulation of sunscreens may affect the association between sunscreen use and melanoma development. The UVR protection characteristics of sunscreens have changed during the last quarter of a century. Some differences may be related to such changes, and results should be interpreted cautiously, especially for older people who did not have the benefit of modern sunscreens when they were likely to have maximum exposure. Studies did not control for factor of sunscreen, how it adhered to skin, water resistance, and efficiency and effectiveness of application; these are all major confounding factors. In case–control studies, patients may have increased their sunscreen protection after having a diagnosis of melanoma, and this may also bias results. Individual interpretations of sunscreen use are problematic, and therefore systematic terms and research instruments need to be tested for reliability and validity in future studies.[26]

Comment

The reviewed observational studies do not provide evidence of an increased risk for melanoma with sunscreen use. A few studies suggest a protective effect, but most of these were carried out before other known protective factors were accepted as necessary and sun protection factors were standardized.

The effects of prolonged sun exposure due to the use of sunscreens to prevent sunburn are unclear. Further research including systematic measurement of sunscreen use and control of confounding factors is necessary.

There is general agreement that sunscreens alone are not sufficient protection for reduction of melanoma risk: wearing of clothes, hats, use of shade, and staying out of the sun between 10 a.m. and 4 p.m. remain important protection factors.

Can sunscreen use reduce the size, thickness, and number of nevi?

Three randomized controlled studies using nevi count as a surrogate marker for melanoma risk are reported.

A randomized controlled trial tested the efficacy of educational letters and free sunscreen and reported no additional effect on sun protection for German children (n = 1812) in two German cities randomly assigned to three study arms:

1 The parents were informed about the study purpose and sun protection measures at an initial education meeting.
2 Parents received educational material three times per year.

3 Education and 800 mL free broad-spectrum sunscreen, protection factor 25, on a yearly basis.

The final follow-up after 3 years included 1232 children (68% of the initial sample). There were few changes in sun protection behavior, with no differences attributable to the intervention effects. There were no significant differences between the three study arms for the main outcome measure—the number of melanocytic nevi—after bivariate and multivariate analysis. The authors conclude that education plus sunscreen intervention had no additional effect on sun protection for German children. High preexisting use of sunscreen, social desirability, and inadequate application of sunscreen were confounding variables.[28]

One RCT using a standard interview with parents about their children's sun exposure and sun-protective behavior concludes that sunscreen use encourages sun exposure. Multivariate analysis adjusted for confounders showed no significant protective effects of sunscreen on the nevus count. The authors conclude that protective clothing is more effective. The increased risk is related to both UVA and UVB light.[29]

The North Queensland "Sun-Safe Clothing" study reports a randomized controlled trial aimed at preventing melanocytic nevi by minimizing sun exposure through the use of protective clothing. The study included 652 Caucasian children aged 0–35 months from 25 childcare centers (13 in the intervention arm and 12 in the control arm) living in a high solar irradiation climate. The children in the intervention arm were provided with protective clothing rated as providing good to excellent protection. The trial began in 1999, with follow-up in 2005. At the baseline, the two groups were similar with regard to nevi count, phenotype, age, demographic characteristics, sun protection habits, and history of sun exposure, with more in the control group suffering painful sunburn episodes and blistering ($P = 0.006$). The authors found that higher melanocytic nevus counts were associated with more time outdoors and a history of sunburn, while sunscreen during milder months seemed to have a protective effect. Nevus development in young children, they conclude, is related to levels of sun exposure. The results show only two significant differences (in 393 children) between the controls and the study group: the proportion who had one blistering painful sunburn (0% vs. 2%, $P = 0.0060$) and the proportion who wore legionnaire hats (50.1% vs. 39.3%; $P = 0.0453$).

When hat wearing was examined further, similar proportions in both groups were found to wear hats (79.5% vs. 79.4%; $P = 0.9658$). In the bivariate analysis, increasing age ($P \leq 0.001$), a history of sunburn ($P = 0.019$), and applying sunscreen at home in winter half the time ($P = 0.025$) were found to be significant predictors of higher than median melanocytic nevus counts. The significance of playing outside in the sun almost every day during warmer months

changed from $P = 0.021$ to $P = 0.070$) after adjustment for the confounding variable of the reaction of a child's skin to sun. Red hair had a more protective effect than blond or dark hair ($P = 0.002$) The results table can be viewed at www.aje.oxfordjournals.org.[30]

Comment on randomized controlled trials on nevi count

There were four randomized controlled trials using nevi count or development as a surrogate measure for the risk of cutaneous melanoma. Two of the four suggest there may be a positive correlation between the use of sunscreen and increased exposure to the sun. One suggests that sunscreen is protective for the development of new nevi, but that clothes are a more effective protection. One suggests that nevus are reduced or thinned by the use of protective sunscreen. One study found no protective effect. The evidence on the use of sunscreen for reducing nevi development is equivocal. Three studies provide evidence that increased sun exposure is related to an increased risk of nevi.

Studies using the nevus count as an outcome do not provide any conclusive evidence about the relationship between the use of sunscreen and reduced nevi and thus reduced risk for cutaneous melanoma. There is minimal evidence suggesting that nevi may be increased. In all studies, the confounding variables and lack of reported data are problematic.

Can the use of sunscreen reduce the risk of basal cell carcinoma (BCC) and squamous cell carcinoma (SCC)?

The Nambour Skin Cancer Prevention Trial[46] (an RCT), and the subsequent follow-up data, investigating sunscreen behavior and risk for BCC and SCC in subgroups of the study population is significant. Researchers are continuing to follow up 1300 original residents of Nambour district (in Queensland) who were participants in a field trial of sunscreen use and/or beta-carotene supplementation in the prevention of skin cancer (1992–96). There is intermittent follow-up for documenting new skin cancers and recording sun exposure and protection behaviors using self-administered questionnaires. A number of participants have taken part in discussion groups about their knowledge, attitudes, and behavior in relation to skin cancer prevention.

This study explored the risk of SCC and BCC and the protective effects of sunscreen as well as beta-carotene supplements.[47] The results demonstrate that sunscreen, but not beta-carotene use, could be significant in reducing the risk of SCC.

Participants were invited to use a daily application of SPF 16 sunscreen and use 30 mg of beta-carotene supplement in the prevention of skin cancer; a total of 1647 took part in a baseline assessment that included a cancer risk factor assessment and a full skin examination by a dermatologist. Any detected skin cancers were removed at the start of the study, and 1621 individuals aged 25–74 years were included.

The participants were randomly assigned to one of four study groups: daily sunscreen and use of beta-carotene; daily sunscreen and placebo beta-carotene; discretionary sunscreen use and beta-carotene; and discretionary sunscreen use and placebo beta-carotene. They attended a clinic every 3 months to receive new sunscreen and beta-carotene. The weight of the sunscreen returned to the clinics every 3 months was recorded. A random subgroup of sunscreen users kept a 7-day diary on three occasions to record their frequency of sunscreen application and sun exposure. Dermatologist examinations were given at these visits, and any cancers were removed and recorded.

No protective effect for prevention of SCC was found in the beta-carotene group. Sunscreen use was analyzed for all groups regardless of beta-carotene use, as no interaction was seen between the two interventions (sunscreen and beta-carotene).

A total of 28 new SCCs were detected in 22 people in the group given daily sunscreen and 46 new SCCs in the 25 people using sunscreens at their own discretion (relative risk 0.61; 95% CI, 0.46 to 0.81). The authors concluded that daily sunscreen use could be of significant benefit in protecting against SCC. No placebo sunscreen was used (which may be considered unethical). The comparison group of usual discretionary use of sunscreens was not ideal, reducing the power of the study to detect a major effect of daily sunscreen use.

The authors[47] subsequently reported that the solar exposure of those given sunscreen did not differ from those not given sunscreen. The prevalence of sunburn was lower among those receiving sunscreen than among those not receiving it (tested on a random sample of participants wearing photosensitive badges). The findings suggest that the reduction of the incidence of SCC seen in the group using sunscreens was probably due to the attenuation of the UVR by the sunscreen rather than due to behavioral change (reducing time in the sun). Higher-factor sunscreen use, especially for older people, may not result in them spending a longer time in the sun.

Further data from the 4–5-year follow-up on prevention of skin cancer from a subgroup of the same study population specifically assessed the influence of sunscreen application on the time to first BCC and the time to subsequent BCC.[47] Three different approaches of time to ordered multiple events were applied and compared: the Anderson–Gill, Wei–Lin–Weissfeld, and Prentice–Williams–Peterson models. Robust variance estimation approaches were used for all multifailure survival models. The authors conclude that sunscreen treatment was not associated with time to first

occurrence of a BCC (hazards ratio 1.04; 95% CI, 0.79 to 1.45). Time to subsequent BCC tumors using the Anderson–Gill model resulted in a lower estimate of hazard among daily sunscreen users, and the result was not statistically significant (hazards ratio 0.82; 95% CI, 0.59 to 1.15). Similarly, the Wei–Lin–Weissfeld marginal hazards and the Prentice–Williams gap-time model revealed trends toward a lower risk of subsequent BCC tumors among the sunscreen intervention group. The authors suggest that it is important to conduct multiple event analysis for recurring events, as the risk factors for a single event may differ from those where repeated events are considered.[47]

Comment on the Nambour studies

The Nambour Skin Cancer Prevention Trial continues to be significant for assessing the effectiveness of sunscreen on BCC, SCC, and actinic keratoses. Follow-up data (2006) suggest that the original conclusions in each of the three categories are consistent with previous findings. The outcomes have been adjusted for age, sex, eye and hair color, skin type, occupational sun exposure, smoking, and skin cancer history.

There is limited evidence to suggest that the daily application of SPF > 16 can lead to attenuation of UVR, possibly reducing risk of incidence of SCC. This needs further research.

There is some evidence to suggest that older people do not spend longer in the sun as a result of using sunscreen. It is uncertain at this stage whether sunscreen use prevents subsequent BCCs.

There is no evidence that beta-carotene supplements reduce risk of BCC or SCC or solar keratoses.

Studies with intermediate end points, such as the incidence of solar keratoses, as markers for BCC and SCC risk

Actinic (solar) keratoses are a risk factor for BCC and are precursor lesions for SCC. They are related to solar exposure and phenotype. The rate of development of SCC is low, and many of the lesions regress spontaneously, especially when exposure to UVR is reduced. Actinic keratoses have therefore been used as an intermediate end point in studies on the use of sunscreens in the prevention of SCC.

Nambour skin cancer findings. The Nambour trial assessed the effect of daily sunscreen use and a food supplement of beta-carotene on the development of solar keratoses.[48] The findings were that the daily application of sunscreen retarded the rate of solar keratoses but that the supplement of beta-carotene had no influence on the occurrence of solar keratoses.

The results for the comparison of daily use with intermittent use of sunscreen on solar keratoses in a subgroup of the original Nambour study population provide limited evidence for the protective effect of sunscreens, especially if they are used systematically (appropriate cover regularly) and daily. The authors report an increase of solar keratoses of 20% with daily sunscreen versus 57% with discretionary sunscreen (adjusted ratio of 76%; $P < 0.05$). They acknowledge that this is only one measure and that it needs to be used with appropriate clothing, shade, and exposure time.[48]

Longitudinal follow-up data for 1300 participants from the original Nambour study population, using a self-administered questionnaire, show that daily use of sunscreen compared to discretionary use reduced the incidence of new solar keratoses on the head, neck, arms, and hands after 4.5 years and over the whole body after 2.5 years. Participants who had never or rarely used sunscreen before the trial were more likely to be sustaining regular application to their face ($P < 0.0001$, 20% vs. 11%) and to the forearms (14% vs. 5%) if they had been allocated to daily, not discretionary, use of sunscreen for 5 years. The authors conclude that regular voluntary sunscreen use for skin cancer prevention can be sustained by sun-sensitive people in the long term. Habit formation appears to be an important goal for sun protection interventions among those living or vacationing in sunny places.

In a short-term RCT in a population in Victoria, Australia, daily use of sunscreen compared to with placebo reduced the incidence of new solar keratoses after 7 months for participants over 40 years of age who had had previous solar keratoses (n = 588; mean number of new lesions per person, 1.6 with sunscreen vs. 2.3 with placebo; relative risk 0.62; 95% CI, 0.54 to 0.71) and significantly increased lesion remission (OR 1.5; 95% CI, 1.3 to 1.8).[49]

Comment on sunscreen use and BCC and SCC

There is limited evidence to suggest that the daily use of sunscreen may significantly reduce SCC after 4–5 years and may reduce the incidence of solar keratoses in 7 months compared to discretionary use. Confidence intervals were quite wide and the subgroup analysis may have lacked sufficient power to rule out clinically important differences.[49] Limited evidence, therefore, exists suggesting that daily application of sunscreen protects against the development of new SCCs. Confounding variables in all studies make it difficult to be certain about such evidence.

Do multifaceted interventions increase the intention to use sunscreens as a protective measure for reducing the risk of melanoma and nonmelanocytic skin cancers?

Multifacet interventions for reducing the risk of skin cancer and melanoma by reducing UVR exposure are reviewed in Chapter 25.[50] Policy interventions are recommended as the most effective way to achieve a reduction in UVR exposure. There is some evidence that interventions to reduce UVR exposure in primary schools, recreational settings, and tourist settings are effective when under a sun-protection policy umbrella.

There is very limited evidence that interventions lead to changes in knowledge, attitudes, and beliefs.

There is no evidence for effectiveness in secondary school or college settings, nor in occupational settings, as there are too few reports and inconsistent evidence. There is no evidence that interventions are successful either in healthcare or retail settings. There is no evidence that comprehensive community interventions for reducing UVR exposure, increasing protection in the sun, or changing behavior are successful either, because the studies had limited designs and there were few of them.

Implications for clinical practice

- There is good evidence that sunscreen use alone is not an effective sun-protective measure and that clothes, hats, shade, and staying out of the sun from 10 a.m. to 4 p.m. are important for protection from UVR.
- There is no clear evidence to suggest that sunscreen use may inadvertently increase the skin cancer risk because it may encourage longer periods in the sun. This requires further testing.
- There is no clear evidence that sunscreen use decreases the incidence of new BCCs.
- There is some evidence that sunscreen use can decrease the incidence of actinic keratoses and SCC, especially when it is used daily.

The following educational messages are needed:

- To ensure that sunscreens are not used as the first or only choice for skin cancer prevention.
- To ensure that sunscreens are not used simply as a means of extending total sun exposure (i.e., sunbathing and suntanning).
- To ensure that sunscreens are not used as a substitute for clothes on body sites that are not usually exposed, such as the trunk and buttocks.
- Daily use of sunscreen with a high SPF (> 16) on areas of the body that are not usually exposed is recommended for those who work outdoors or undertake regular outdoor leisure pursuits.
- Daily use of a sunscreen can reduce actinic keratoses and risk of SCC.
- Protecting children against solar exposure during childhood is more important than at any time in life.
- Using photoprotective clothing, hats, and shade is important. Parents, carers, schools, and leisure organizations need to encourage and promote knowledge about sun-protective behavior but not at the risk of increased exposure.

Recommendations for future research

- Future research should seek to understand the role of sunscreens in the prevention of skin cancers and the role of UVR in the causation of these diseases, the dose–response relationship, the dose rate and pattern of delivery on risk, and the action spectrum for each effect.
- RCTs should be conducted in adults to evaluate whether a reduction in late-stage exposure to UVR can reduce the incidence of cutaneous melanoma and precursor lesions such as clinically atypical nevi.
- In children, studies are needed to evaluate whether a reduction in early-stage exposure to UVR can reduce the prevalence of acquired nevi.
- Trials should ideally include a quantitative assessment of solar exposure and an evaluation of the various methods for reducing solar exposure—sunscreens, clothing, and sun avoidance. This remains an important area for future research.
- As sunscreens are increasingly used on children, an evaluation of their safety for long-term use is needed.
- There is a need to evaluate whether the qualitative rating of the potential function of sunscreens against UVR—such as low, medium, high, and ultra-high, rather than SPF—would promote appropriate use of sunscreens.
- There is a need to better understand the role of the mechanisms of skin cancer etiology and how sunscreens might affect this. Intermediate end points (for example, nevi and biochemical markers of carcinogenesis such as DNA damage and *p53* mutations) could be studied to assess their relationship to sunscreen use.
- Researchers in health promotion need to develop qualitative and quantitative methods for measuring sunscreen use in order to identify major confounding variables such as sun sensitivity and sun exposure.
- There is a need to be able to measure, in the field, how much protection is provided by sunscreens at various sites on the skin.
- There is a need to understand how efficiently individuals use sunscreen. This would enable manufacturers to develop sunscreens that achieve adequate protection against UVR when in common use. There is a need for further research and for consistent use of RCTs to test the effectiveness of the daily use of sunscreen, clothes, and optimum vs. minimum exposure time for the reduction of solar keratoses, SCC, and BCC, as well as melanoma.
- There is an urgent need for researchers to systematically identify, define, and reach agreement about the numerous confounding variables affecting the design and results of RCTs, cross-sectional, cohort, and case–control studies. There is a need for standardization of terminology as well as possible confounding effects.

References

1 Shaath NA. Evolution of modern sunscreen chemicals. In: Lowe NJ, Shaath NA, Pathak MA, editors. *Sunscreens: Development, Evaluation and Regulatory Aspects,* 2nd ed. New York: Dekker, 1997: 3–33. (Cosmetic Science and Technology Series, vol. 15.)

2 Bestak R, Barneston RS, Neath MR, Halliday GM. Sunscreen protection of contact hypersensitivity responses from chronic solar-simulated ultra irradiation correlates with the absorption spectrum of the sunscreen. *J Invest Dermatol* 1995;**105**:345–51.

3 Schulze R. [Some tests and remarks regarding the problem of sunscreens that are found on the market; in German]. *Parfum Kosmet* 1956;**37**:310–6.

4 Diffey B. A method for broad spectrum clarification of sunscreens (1994) *Int. Journal Cosmet* **16**:47–52.

5 Lock-Anderson J, Wulf HC Threshold level for measurement of UV sensitivity: reproducibility of phototest. *Photodermatol Photoimmunol Photomed* 1996;**12**:154–61.

6 Janousek A. Regulatory aspects of sunscreens in Europe. In: Lowe NJ, Shaath NA, Pathak MA, editors. *Sunscreens: Development, Evaluation and Regulatory Aspects,* 2nd ed. New York: Dekker, 1997: 215–25. (Cosmetic Science and Technology Series, vol. 15.)

7 Fukuda M, Takata S. The evolution of recent sunscreens. In: Altmeyer P, Hoffmann K, Stücker M, editors. *Skin Cancer and UV Radiation.* Berlin: Springer, 1997: 265–76.

8 Standards Australia/Standards New Zealand. *Sunscreen Products—Evaluation and Classification.* Sydney: Standards Australia/ Wellington: Standards New Zealand, 1998. (AS/NZS 2604:1998.)

9 Health Canada. *Issue Analysis Summary: Regulatory Strategy for Pharmaceutical Products with Photo Co-Carcinogenic Potential.* Ottawa: Therapeutic Products Programme, 1999.

10 European Commission. *Directive 76/78: Guidelines for Testing of Cosmetic Ingredients.* Brussels: European Commission/SCCMF, 1976.

11 Hill D, White V, Marks R, *et al.* Melanoma prevention: behavioral and nonbehavioral factors in sunburn among an Australian urban population. *Prev Med* 1992;**21**:654–69.

12 McGee R, Williams S, Cox B, Elwood M, Bulliard JL. A community survey of sun exposure, sunburn and sun protection. *NZ Med J* 1995;**108**:508–10.

13 Melia J, Bulman A. Sunburn and tanning in a British population. *J Public Health Med* 1995;**17**:223–9.

14 Autier P, Dore JF, Cattaruzza MS, *et al.* Sunscreen use, wearing clothes, and number of nevi in 6- to 7-year-old European children. European Organization for Research and Treatment of Cancer Melanoma Cooperative Group. *J Natl Cancer Inst* 1998;**90**:1873–80.

15 Wulf HC, Stender IM, Lock-Andersen J. Sunscreens used at the beach do not protect against erythema: a new definition of SPF is proposed. *Photoderm Photoimmunol Photomed* 1997;**13**:129–32.

16 Autier P, Dore JF, Negrier S, *et al.* Sunscreen use and duration of sun exposure: a double-blind, randomized trial. *J Natl Cancer Inst* 1999;**91**:1304–9.

17 McCarthy EM, Ethridge KP, Wagner RF Jr. Beach holiday sunburn: the sunscreen paradox and gender differences. *Cutis* 1999; **64**:37–42.

18 Hill D, White V, Marks R, Borland R. Changes in sun-related attitudes and behaviours, and reduced sunburn prevalence in a population at high risk of melanoma. *Eur J Can Prev* 1993;**2**:447–56.

19 Baade PD, Balanda KP, Lowe JB. Changes in sun protection behaviors, attitudes, and sunburn in a population with the highest incidence of skin cancer in the world. *Cancer Detect Prev* 1996;**20**:566–75.

20 Rivers JK, Gallagher RP. Public education projects in skin cancer: experience of the Canadian Dermatology Association. *Cancer* 1995;75(2 Suppl):661–6.

21 Miller RW, Rabkin CS. Merkel cell carcinoma and melanoma: etiological similarities and differences. *Cancer Epidemiol Biomarker Prev* 1999;**8**:153–8.

22 Lombard D, Neubauer TE, Canfield D, Winett RA. Behavioral community intervention to reduce the risk of skin cancer. *J Appl Behav Anal* 1991;**24**:677–86.

23 Gooderham MJ, Guenther L. Sun and the skin: evaluation of a sun awareness program for elementary school students. *J Cutan Med Surg* 1999;**3**:230–5.

24 Cockburn J, Thompson SC, Marks R, Jolley D, Schofield D, Hill D. Behavioural dynamics of a clinical trial of sunscreens for reducing solar keratoses in Victoria, Australia. *J Epidemiol Community Health* 1997;**51**:716–21.

25 International Agency for Research on Cancer/World Health Organization. *IARC Handbooks of Cancer Prevention*, vol. 5: *Sunscreens*. Lyons, France: IARC Press, 2001.

26 Saraiya M, Glanz K, Briss PA, *et al.* Interventions to prevent skin cancer by reducing exposure to ultraviolet radiation: a systematic review. *Am J Prev Med* 2004;**27**:422–66.

27 Dennis LK, Beane Freeman LE, VanBeek MJ. Sunscreen use and the risk of melanoma: a quantitative review. *Ann Intern Med* 2003;**139**:966–78.

28 Bauer J, Buttner P, Wiecker TS, Luther H, Garbe C. Interventional study in 1232 young German children to prevent the development of melanocytic nevi failed to change sun exposure and sun protective behavior. *Int J Cancer* 2005;**116**:755–61.

29 Lee TK, Rivers JK, Gallagher RP. Site-specific protective effect of broad-spectrum sunscreen on nevus development among white schoolchildren in a randomized trial. *J Am Acad Dermatol* 2005;**52**:786–92.

30 Autier P, Boniol M, Severi G, Pedeux R, Grivegnee AR, Dore JF. Sex differences in numbers of nevi on body sites of young European children: implications for the etiology of cutaneous melanoma. *Cancer Epidemiol Biomarkers Prev* 2004;**13**:2003–5.

31 Harrison SL, Buettner PG, Maclennan R. The North Queensland "Sun-Safe Clothing" study: design and baseline results of a randomized trial to determine the effectiveness of sun-protective clothing in preventing melanocytic nevi. *Am J Epidemiol* 2005;**161**:536–45.

32 Herzfeld PM, Fitzgerald EF, Hwang SA, Stark A. A case–control study of malignant melanoma of the trunk among white males in upstate New York. *Cancer Detect Prev* 1993;**17**:601–8.

33 Beitner H, Norell SE, Ringborg U, Wennersten G, Mattson B. Malignant melanoma: aetiological importance of individual pigmentation and sun exposure. *Br J Dermatol* 1990;**122**:43–51.

34 Holman CDJ, Armstrong BK, Heenan PL. Relationship of cutaneous melanoma to individual sunlight-exposure habits. *J Natl Cancer Inst* 1986;**76**:403–14.

35 Holly EA, Kelly JW, Shpall SN, Chin SH. Number of melanocytic nevi as a major risk factor for malignant melanoma. *J Am Acad Dermatol* 1987;**17**:459–68.

36 Osterlind A, Tucker MA, Stone BJ, Jensen OM. The Danish case–control study of cutaneous malignant melanoma. II. Importance of UV-light exposure. *Int J Cancer* 1988;**42**:319–24.

37 Whiteman DC, Valery P, McWhirter W, Green AC. Risk factors for childhood melanoma in Queensland, Australia. *Int J Cancer* 1997;70:**26**–31.

38 Westerdahl J, Olsson H, Masback A, Ingvar C, Jonsson N. Is the use of sunscreens a risk factor for malignant melanoma? *Melanoma Res* 1995;**5**:59–65.

39 Rodenas JM, Delgado-Rodriguez M, Herranz MT, Tercedor J, Serrano S. Sun exposure, pigmentary traits, and risk of cutaneous malignant melanoma: a case–control study in a Mediterranean population. *Cancer Causes Control* 1996;**7**:275–83.

40 Espinosa Arranz J, Sanchez Hernandez JJ, Bravo Fernandez P, *et al.* Cutaneous malignant melanoma and sun exposure in Spain. *Melanoma Res* 1999;**9**:199–205.

41 Autier P, Dore JF, Schifflers E, *et al.* Melanoma and use of sunscreens: an EORTC case–control study in Germany, Belgium and France. The EORTC Melanoma Cooperative Group. *Int J Cancer* 1995;**61**:749–55.

42 Wolf P, Quehenberger F, Mullegger R, Stranz B, Kerl H. Phenotypic markers, sunlight-related factors and sunscreen use in patients with cutaneous melanoma: an Austrian case–control study. *Melanoma Res* 1998;**8**:370–8.

43 Westerdahl J, Ingvar C, Masback A, Olsson H. Sunscreen use and malignant melanoma. *Int J Cancer* 2000;**87**:145–50.

44 Klepp O, Magnus K. Some environmental and bodily characteristics of melanoma patients. A case–control study. *Int J Cancer* 1979;**23**:482–6.

45 Graham S, Marshall J, Haughey B, *et al.* An inquiry into the epidemiology of melanoma. *Am J Epidemiol* 1985;**122**:606–19.

46 Pandeya N, Purdie DM, Green A, Williams G. Repeated occurrence of basal cell carcinoma of the skin and multifailure survival analysis: follow-up data from the Nambour Skin Cancer Prevention Trial. *Am J Epidemiol* 2005;**161**:748–54.

47 Darlington S, Williams G, Neale R, Frost C, Green A. A randomized controlled trial to assess sunscreen application and beta-carotene supplementation in the prevention of solar keratoses. *Arch Dermatol* 2003;**139**:451–5.

48 Green A, Marks R, Squamous cell carcinoma of the skin (nonmetastatic). *Clin Evid* 2006;**15**:1–2.

49 Thompson SC, Jolley D, Marks R, Reduction of solar keratoses by regular sunscreen use. *N Engl J Med* 1993;**329**:1147–51.

50 Weston R. Primary Prevention of Skin Cancer in chapter 25—current chapter 25 in this book in press Current reference 4 in ref list.

27

Cutaneous melanoma

Dafydd Roberts, Thomas Crosby

Localized disease

Background

Malignant melanomas (MMs) of the skin arise from melanocytes within the epidermis. After a variable period of time, the tumor becomes invasive and penetrates the underlying dermis and subcutaneous fat. Once this occurs, the tumor has potential for distant metastatic spread. MMs may also rarely arise from other areas of the body, including the meninges, retina, gastrointestinal tract, nasopharyngeal epithelium, and vagina (Figure 27.1).

Incidence

The incidence of cutaneous MM—particularly thin, curable lesions—has increased steadily over the past 30 years in all Western countries, and this has been accompanied by a similar but less marked increase in mortality.[1] Whilst mortality has continued to rise in most countries, recent reports from Scotland, Canada, Australia, and Wales suggest that

mortality rates may have leveled off or declined in some groups, notably in women.[2–5] This may be the result of intensive public education campaigns leading to earlier detection of thinner lesions, with a better prognosis. The prevention of MM is an important topic and is dealt with along with other skin cancers in Chapter 26. Early recognition of MMs and surgical excision present the best opportunity for cure.

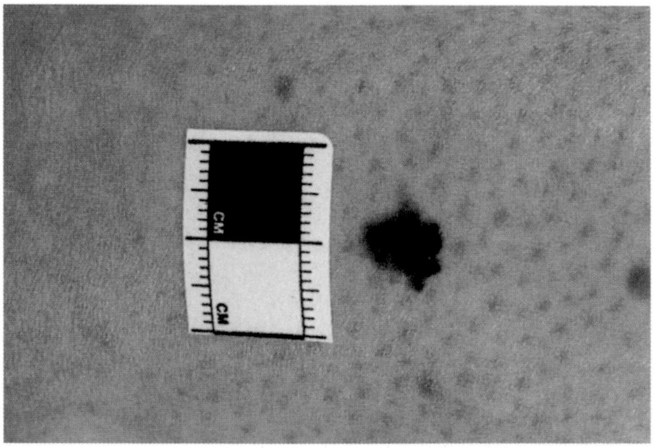

Prognosis

The prognosis of MM is related to a number of factors, including sex, tumor site, and ulceration, but the single most important guide to prognosis is the Breslow thickness.[6] This is a measure of the depth of invasion of the tumor from the granular layer of the epidermis. Lesions that are confined to the epidermis have no metastatic potential. Those that are less than 1 mm in depth have a very good prognosis, with 5-year survival rates of approximately 95%. Tumors deeper than 4 mm are associated with survival rates of about 50%. The involvement of regional lymph nodes with metastases at presentation further reduces survival rates to 25–50%.[7] If a patient has a positive sentinel node biopsy, the prognosis is worsened, regardless of the Breslow thickness.[8]

Diagnosis

The clinical diagnosis of classical MM is straightforward, but early changes may be subtle. Various clinical guides have been developed—such as the ABCDE rule (A, asymmetry; B, irregular border; C, irregular color; D, diameter > 5 mm; and E, elevation) and the seven-point checklist—which may be useful as reminders of the main features of MM on clinical examination and history. The main clinical features are of a pigmented lesion with an irregular edge and irregular pigmentation, over 95% of patients giving a history of change in size, shape, or color, and fewer than 50% describing a change in sensation or bleeding of the lesion.[9,10] Dermatoscopy has gained ground as an aid to diagnosis, but training and experience are required to maximize its usefulness.[11] Several new digital imaging systems

Figure 27.1 Cutaneous melanoma.

are being assessed as aids in the diagnosis of pigmented lesions.[12]

Treatment objectives

The main aims of treatment are to detect the lesion as early as possible and to excise it with adequate margins, but without mutilating the patient unnecessarily. Outcomes measured usually include both disease-free survival (i.e., until the first appearance of recurrence of the primary lesion or distant metastatic spread) and overall survival.

Searches

Medline and CENTRAL were searched for the period 1966 to the end of 2005. Citations found in review articles and other main articles found were also scrutinized for additional evidence.

Questions

What is the place of a diagnostic incisional biopsy?

Occasionally, pigmented lesions that are clinically suspicious of being an MM may be considered to be too large or in a difficult anatomical site for complete immediate excision without extensive surgery. There is therefore a dilemma for the clinician as to whether an incisional biopsy of the lesion may be needed to confirm the diagnosis before more extensive surgery. Also, provided that the biopsy is taken from a representative area of the melanoma, an incisional biopsy provides an indication of the depth of invasion of the lesion, thereby assisting the planning of the next course of appropriate treatment. There is some concern, based on empirical reasoning, that taking a biopsy of part of a malignant lesion might release some malignant cells into the bloodstream and local tissues, thereby worsening the eventual prognosis for that person.

Efficacy

There have been no randomized controlled trials (RCTs) of incisional versus excisional surgery. Retrospective studies of large numbers of patients have reported different results. A large study in 1985 of 472 patients with stage I cutaneous MM reported on the survival rate with different modalities of surgery. A total of 119 patients initially underwent an incisional or punch biopsy, and 353 patients had their lesions excised. Survival in the two groups did not differ, regardless of the depth of invasion. Of 76 patients who had an incisional biopsy of a lesion < 1.7 mm in depth, none died. In the intermediate-thickness group (1.7–3.64 mm), there was a 35% mortality rate compared with 18% in the excision group, and in the thick-lesion group (> 3.65 mm), the mortality rates were 64% and 50%, respectively. Cox regression analysis showed that the best predictors for outcome were tumor thickness and anatomical location, but not biopsy type.[13] In a further study of 1086 patients fol-

lowed up for 5 years, 96 of these underwent an incisional biopsy initially. The mortality was 48.9% in the incisional-biopsy group (mean thickness 3.47 mm) and 39.2% in the wide-excision group (mean thickness 2.77 mm), compared with 33.9% in the narrow-margin group (mean thickness 2.34 mm). After correcting for tumor thickness, there was no statistical difference in survival rates or local recurrence between those having an incisional biopsy and those who had their lesions fully excised initially.[14] A more recent and larger case–control study from Scotland of 5727 patients identified 265 patients who had undergone an incisional biopsy. These were matched with 496 controls. The survival analysis of time to recurrence and time to death revealed no differences between the groups.[15] The most recent study of 2164 patients who had cutaneous MMs with 1 mm or greater Breslow thickness and who had undergone excisional, incisional, or shave biopsies concluded that biopsy type had no influence on disease-free or overall survival.[16]

Drawbacks

Incisional biopsy runs the inherent risk of providing material that is not representative of the whole tumor, and errors may therefore occur in assessing the depth of the tumor. One study reported that 38 of the 96 incisional biopsies on patients with cutaneous melanoma (40%) gave insufficient material to provide a full histological assessment of the lesion.[14] On the other hand, excising all pigmented lesions suspected of being an MM, regardless of their site and size, could lead to inappropriate surgery in some cases. One study reported the results of a retrospective series of patients with cutaneous melanoma limited to the head and neck. A total of 159 patients were followed up for a median period of 38 months, of whom 79 patients had their lesions fully excised and 48 had an incisional biopsy, while other procedures such shave excision or cryotherapy were carried out in a further 32. Thirty-one percent of the patients who underwent an incisional biopsy died, and 25% of the other biopsy group died, compared with 9% of those who had their lesions excised initially. As this was a retrospective study, the initial surface area of the lesions was not known. There were no significant differences between the three groups in the depth of invasion of the tumors or the sex of the patients, but a significantly higher proportion of the patients in the incisional biopsy and other-procedure groups had ulcerated tumors compared with the excision group.[17]

Comment

The evidence on incisional biopsy in MM remains controversial, but the balance of observational evidence suggests that it is unlikely to influence prognosis adversely. Large studies have shown that, in general, incisional biopsies do not affect prognosis, except for the single study of melanoma of the head and neck, where there was a significant worsening in the survival of patients who underwent an incisional biopsy compared with those who had their lesions excised initially.[17] This study was, however, retrospective, and no adjustment was made for ulceration of the tumors, which is known to worsen the prognosis. Any future study should be prospective and the design of the study should ensure that study groups are randomized to balance for the various factors that may influence the prognosis.

What are the surgical recommendations for excision margins for different Breslow thickness tumors?

Breslow thickness represents the depth of invasion of cutaneous melanoma and is the single best indicator of prognosis in primary cutaneous MM.[6] All of the trials so far performed in patients with MM have used the Breslow thickness of the tumor to categorize different patient groups. As a result of these trials, surgical margins for excision of MM have decreased significantly over the past 20 years.

Efficacy

The recommendations for surgical margins are based on four RCTs and have included patients with lesions of Breslow thickness up to 5 mm. A systematic review of excision margins for primary cutaneous melanoma found three RCTs up to 2003, involving 2087 patients. No statistical differences were found between wide surgical margins (3–5 cm) and narrower margins (1–2 cm) with respect to mortality, disease-free survival, or local recurrence.[18] The World Health Organization Melanoma Group randomized 612 patients with melanomas less than 2 mm in depth to surgical excision with either 1 cm or 3 cm margins.[19] The 305 patients who received narrow excision margins had an 8-year actuarial survival rate of 89.6%, compared with 90.3% for those who underwent wide excision, and the difference was not statistically significant ($P = 0.64$). The corresponding figures for disease-free survival were 81.6% and 84.4%, and again the difference was not significant ($P > 0.74$). A U.S. Intergroup Study randomized 486 patients with intermediate-thickness lesions (1–4 mm in depth) to either 2 cm or 4 cm margins.[20] The median follow-up period was 6 years. The local recurrence rate was 0.8% for the 2 cm margin group and 1.7% for the 4 cm group (P = not significant; no confidence intervals are provided in original paper). The overall survival rates over 5 years were 79.5% and 83.7%, respectively (not significant). The Swedish Melanoma Study Group randomized 769 patients with lesions of 0.8–2.0 mm in depth to either 2 cm or 5 cm margins, and have reported long-term results with a median follow-up period of 11 years.[21] The estimated relative hazards ratios for overall survival and relapse-free survival were 0.96 (95% CI, 0.75 to 1.25) and 1.02 (95% CI, 0.8 to 1.30), respectively. There was no statistically significant difference in local recurrence rates or overall survival between the narrower and wider margins of excision in any of the trials. A retrospective observational study of 278 patients with thick lesions (median thickness 6 mm) suggested that 2 cm margins were adequate and that wider margins did not improve local recurrence rates, disease-free survival, or overall survival rates.[22] A European study comparing 2 cm versus 5 cm excision margins for MMs less than 2.1 mm thick concluded that, in 326 patients who were eligible for analysis, the wider margin of 5 cm had no impact on either the overall or disease-free survival compared to 2 cm margins. The disease-free survival rates at 10 years were 85% for the 2 cm group and 83% for the 5 cm group ($P = 0.83$). The corresponding results for overall survival rates at 10 years were 87% and 86% ($P = 0.56$).[23] The most recent RCT of surgical margins in cutaneous melanoma compared 1 cm and 3 cm margins for patients with MMs 2 mm or greater in depth. A total of 900 patients were enrolled; 453 had 1 cm margin excisions and 447 had 3 cm margin excisions, with a median follow-up of 60 months. The 1 cm margin group had a significantly increased risk of locoregional recurrence, with 168 recurrences in the 1 cm group and 142 in the 3 cm group (hazards ratio 1.26; 95% CI, 1 to 1.59; $P = 0.05$). Overall survival was similar in the two groups, with 128 deaths occurring in the 1 cm group and 105 in the 3 cm group (hazards ratio for death 1.07; 95% CI, 0.85 to 1.36; $P = 0.6$).[24]

Drawbacks

Excision with narrow surgical margins can often be performed in an outpatient setting, whereas larger margins may require skin grafting and in-patient treatment. The World Health Organization Study demonstrated that skin grafting could be reduced by 75% with the 1 cm versus the 3 cm margins.[19] Some concern was expressed in the Intergroup Trial, as three patients developed local recurrences as a first sign of relapse, all of whom had received a 1 cm excision margin for primary lesions between 1 mm and 2 mm in thickness.[20] The recent study comparing 1 cm and 3 cm margins in patients with cutaneous MM deeper than 2 mm showed that those who had the narrower margins were significantly more likely to develop locoregional metastases and, although overall survival was the same for both groups, the results suggest that narrow margins in this group of patients should be avoided.

Comment

The evidence that narrow surgical margins are not inferior in comparison with more extensive surgical treatment in terms of local recurrence and survival is reasonably strong for thinner lesions. The studies have suggested that lesions < 1 mm in depth can be safely treated with surgical margins of 1 cm and that lesions equal to or more than 1 mm in depth can be safely treated with margins of 2 cm. There is also evidence from one observational study that 2 cm margins are also sufficient for thicker tumors. A note of caution from the most recent RCT, however, suggests that 1 cm margins are unsafe for patients presenting with Breslow thickness lesions equal to or greater than 2 mm in depth.

MMs < 0.75 mm in depth have not been studied in any controlled trials, nor have lesions > 4 mm in depth. Melanomas *in situ*, where the melanoma cells are confined to the epidermis, appear to have no potential for metastatic spread,[25] and the current consensus based on empirical reasoning is that it is safe to excise such lesions with a margin of 5 mm of clinically normal skin to obtain a clear histological margin.[26]

How should patients with lentigo maligna or lentigo maligna melanoma be managed?

Lentigo maligna (LM) refers to the presence of malignant melanocytes entirely confined to the epidermis, and is the premalignant phase of lentigo maligna melanoma (LMM). Lentigo maligna usually occurs on sun-exposed sites such as the face and neck. There is usually a prolonged premalignant phase before dermal invasion and the development of LMM. The lesions are difficult to manage, for several reasons. Patients with these lesions tend to be elderly, with other comorbidities that may limit extensive surgery. The lesions themselves may be large and occur close to important anatomical structures, and therefore full surgical excision with suitable margins may be difficult or even impossible. In addition, histological changes within the epidermis may occur at some distance from the clinically obvious margins.[27]

Efficacy
LM and LMM are considered separately below.

Lentigo maligna
Surgery. There have been no RCTs of patients in this category. A comparative study of 42 cases of LM showed a recurrence rate of 9% (two of 22) following surgical excision, compared with 35% (seven of 20) with other techniques such as radiotherapy, curettage, and cryotherapy surgery, with a mean follow-up period of 3.5 years (range 1 month to 11 years).[28] A further retrospective report of 38 cases of LM suggested cure rates of 91% (two recurrences) over a time period of 1–12 years (mean 3 years).[29] Mohs micrographic surgery has also been evaluated in small numbers of patients, usually with excellent results. Twenty-six patients with LM were treated in one study, with no recurrences after a median follow-up of 58 months.[30] A recent retrospective follow-up study of a staged excision technique in 55 patients with LM and seven with LMM who were followed up for a median of 54 months reported that 95% were free of recurrences, three had local recurrences, and none had distant metastases.[31]

Cryotherapy. There have been no RCTs of cryotherapy for the treatment of LM. One study of 30 patients reported recurrence rates of 6.6% (two patients) in a follow-up period of 3 years. Eleven patients who were observed for more than 5 years had no recurrences.[32] A further study of 12 patients showed a recurrence rate of 8.3% over a follow-up period of 51 months.[33]

Radiotherapy. There have been no RCTs of radiotherapy for LM. One case series reported two recurrences in 68 patients with a 5-year follow-up.[34] A further study showed an 86% cure rate in 36 patients at 5 years.[35]

Other treatments. There have been a few case reports on the use of various lasers in LM, but the numbers are too small to be conclusive. A study of 5-fluorouracil cream showed a 100% recurrence rate,[36] and a similar study on topical retinoic acid showed no benefit.[37] Azelaic acid was reported to give a recurrence rate of 22% in 50 patients, all of whom subsequently cleared with repeat treatment.[38] Several case reports and small series have been reported on the use of an immune response modifier, 5% topical imiquimod cream, in patients with LM. In one study, 28 patients showed no relapse after a year and another reported six patients successfully treated, with a follow-up of 3–18 months.[39,40]

Lentigo maligna melanoma
Surgery. Patients with LMM have not been included in any of the large randomized trials on surgical margins. However, it has been shown that the prognosis for patients with invasive LMM is the same as that for any other type of melanoma when matched for thickness.[41] Patients with LMM were included in a case series of Mohs micrographic surgery, which found a 100% cure rate after 29 months and a 97% cure rate after 58 months.[30]

Radiotherapy. An uncontrolled follow-up study of fractionated radiotherapy in both LM and LMM showed that of 64 patients with LM, none showed any signs of recurrence. Among 22 patients with LMM who also had the nodular part of the lesion excised, there were two recurrences. The mean follow-up period was 23 months.[38]

Drawbacks
All of the treatment modalities, including surgery, cryotherapy, radiotherapy, and any other destructive treatment, can result in scarring, and no studies have compared the long-term scars with any other methods described. Cryotherapy may lead to inadequate destruction of melanocytes extending down hair follicles, and there have been subsequent reports of recurrences, sometimes amelanotic in type, after cryotherapy of these lesions. No reports have compared the short-term discomfort, pain, or costs of these treatments.

The use of imiquimod has been reported widely as a successful treatment for LM in selected cases. However, nearly all reported a brisk inflammatory response, and the length of follow-up is too short in these reports for an accurate assessment of long-term cure rates to be made.[42]

Comment

In the absence of any controlled trials, it is not surprising that a recent survey of dermatologists has shown a wide variation in treatment modalities for LM and LMM in the UK. An algorithm was devised on the basis of the current treatments for LM, suggesting that surgical resection was the initial treatment of choice if possible, and Mohs surgery when the margins were unclear. For those lesions that are not amenable to surgical resection, radiotherapy or cryotherapy may be suitable choices. Imiquimod treatment may also be a viable alternative, and RCTs with a long follow-up period are needed. There is an absence of information on the rate of progression of LM, and in the very old and infirm, observation only may be considered appropriate.[8] As the prognosis of LMM is the same as any other MM when matched for Breslow thickness, the same surgical margins should be advised whenever possible until better evidence becomes available.

Does elective lymph-node dissection improve outcome?

There is still some uncertainty about the place of elective lymph-node dissection where there are no clinically involved lymph nodes.

Efficacy

Four RCTs have compared elective lymph-node dissection with primary excision of the cutaneous lesion only. In all, 1718 people with no clinical evidence of lymph-node metastases were included in the studies. None of these studies showed an overall survival benefit in patients receiving elective lymph-node dissection. However, an unplanned subgroup analysis found nonsignificant trends in favor of elective lymph-node dissection in those over the age of 60 years with intermediate-thickness tumors.[43-46]

Drawbacks

Lymph-node dissection is not without risk, lymphedema being the most frequent complication, occurring in 20% in one study; temporary seroma occurred in 17%, wound infection in 9%, and wound necrosis in 3%.[47]

Comments

In view of the lack of any clear benefits for elective lymph-node dissection in the RCTs mentioned above, elective lymph-node dissection has been largely abandoned. Sentinel lymph-node biopsy (SLNB) is considered separately below.

What is the role of sentinel lymph-node biopsy?

The technique of SLNB involves the identification and biopsy of the first-station lymph-node draining an affected area. Its use in MM was pioneered by Morton et al.[48]

The sentinel node is found by injecting blue dye and/or radiolabeled colloid into the skin surrounding the primary lesion. The technique allows the identification of patients with micrometastases affecting the regional lymph nodes and can successfully identify the sentinel node in up to 97% of cases. Patients identified as having micrometastases in this way are then submitted to a therapeutic lymph-node dissection.

The technique is well established and is reproducible.[49] It is now regarded as an excellent indicator of prognosis and has therefore been incorporated into the new American staging system for MMs (the American Joint Committee on Cancer staging).[50] Gershenwald et al. demonstrated that of 580 patients who underwent SLNB, 85 patients (15%) were positive and 495 were negative. This study showed that sentinel-node status was the most significant prognostic factor with respect to disease-free and disease-specific survival. Although tumor thickness and ulceration influenced survival in sentinel node–negative patients, they provided no additional prognostic information in sentinel node–positive patients.[51] The psychological benefits of accurate staging for a patient have not been studied extensively, but one small questionnaire study of 110 patients did show a slight psychological benefit in those who underwent SNLB, regardless of the result of the biopsy.[52]

Efficacy

No fully published RCTs of SLNB accompanied by further treatment, such as lymph-node dissection or interferon therapy, as an intervention (as opposed to SLNB as a pure staging procedure) could be found.

Drawbacks

Patients who do not undergo SLNB are treated by wide excision of the primary cutaneous melanoma. The additional surgery therefore entails some risk, because a general anesthetic is usually necessary and there are also additional costs, although these are difficult to quantify. About 3% of patients developed a seroma, and a further 3% developed a wound infection in one report of SLNB.[53] When the SLNB is followed by complete lymph-node dissection, however, the complication rates rise significantly, as 23.2% of 44 patients experienced major or minor complications in a recent report.[54]

Comment

SLNB is generally agreed to be useful as a staging procedure in patients with primary cutaneous melanoma, but no randomized trials have yet shown any therapeutic benefit in patients who have undergone SLNB followed by subsequent therapy. A retrospective study showed no overall survival benefit in 291 patients who had undergone SLNB in comparison with 377 who had not.[55] A randomized multi-center trial is now comparing survival after wide excision alone versus wide excision plus SLNB in patients with cutaneous melanoma (1 mm in depth or Clark level IV). The preliminary results of the trial, known as MSLT1, were discussed at a meeting of the American Society of Clinical Oncology (ASCO) in 2005, and the report is available on the ASCO web site (www.asco.org). The full publication is awaited with interest.

There are additional potential benefits of accurate staging in patients with positive results if adjuvant treatments such as interferon prove to be of value.

Are there any effective adjuvant treatments?

Once patients with MM develop distant metastatic disease, the prognosis is poor. There is therefore a need to investigate additional or adjuvant treatments, which may be given either after primary tumor resection in those with thicker lesions in patients who appear to have nonmetastatic disease, or after regional lymph-node resection in those with established metastatic disease.

The role of adjuvant treatments, mainly in the form of interferon alfa-2b, is still controversial. Several studies have shown that interferon alfa has a biologically modifying effect on MM, but the effect on overall survival has been variable. Side effects are a major problem with patients receiving high-dose interferon alfa.

Efficacy

Trials have studied the role of interferon alfa in high-dose, medium-dose, and low-dose regimens.

High-dose interferon. An early RCT of high-dose treatment (intravenous interferon alfa-2b 20 MU/day for 1 month, followed by 10 MU three times weekly for 11 months), in 287 people with lesions greater than 4 mm in depth at presentation showed a significant improvement in disease-free and overall survival in comparison with those treated with surgery alone. The overall survival in the interferon group was 3.1 years, compared with 2.8 years in those treated with surgery alone.[56] However, in a larger study of 642 patients, there was no difference in the overall survival of patients with either high-dose or low-dose interferon alfa compared with no further therapy.[57] A study from the same authors compared high-dose interferon alfa-2b with vaccine treatment (GM2-KLH/QS-21) in patients with resected stage IIB–III melanoma of the skin.[58] A total of 880 patients were randomized equally between the two interferon alfa and vaccine groups. The trial demonstrated a significant treatment benefit for those receiving interferon alfa-2b in both relapse-free survival (hazards ratio 1.47; 95% CI, 1.14 to 1.90; $P = 0.0015$) and overall survival (hazards ratio 1.52; 95% CI, 1.07 to 2.15; $P = 0.009$). There was no control arm

(with observation only), so a direct comparison with no adjuvant treatment could not be made. However, based on comparisons with the observation arm of previous adjuvant trials, the outcome for patients receiving the vaccine seemed to be no worse than for similar patients receiving observation only. This study therefore seems to have confirmed the relapse-free survival and overall survival benefits of high-dose interferon reported earlier.[56] Recently, the two high-dose trials have been updated with a longer follow-up; the overall survival benefit in one has disappeared and in the other the statistical significance has become borderline.[59]

Intermediate-dose interferon. In an RCT, 1388 patients who had a thick (> 4 mm depth) lesion or regional lymph-node involvement were randomized to receive treatment for either 13 months or 25 months, or observation. The treatment regimen was 4 weeks of 10 million units of interferon alfa followed by either 10 MU of interferon alfa three times a week for a year or 5 MU three times a week for 2 years. After a median follow-up of 4.65 years, the authors concluded that these treatments did not improve the outcome and could not be recommended.[60]

Low-dose interferon. To date, three clinical trials have used low-dose subcutaneous interferon (3 MU three times weekly) in patients presenting with lesions greater than 1.5 mm in depth but with negative lymph nodes. In the first trial of 499 patients, this regimen was continued for 18 months and compared with surgery alone. There was a significant extension of the relapse-free interval and a trend towards extension of overall survival.[61] The second trial randomized 311 patients to receive treatment for 12 months versus observation only, after surgical removal of the melanoma. At 41 months, the relapse-free survival was prolonged, but the overall survival was not.[62] The most recent study compared low-dose treatment with interferon for 2 years or until recurrence with no adjuvant treatment. A total of 674 patients with lesions greater than 4 mm in depth or with locoregional metastases were randomized, and there was no difference in the overall survival or disease-free survival between the two groups.[63] A recent prospective, double-blind RCT compared the combination of isotretinoin plus interferon to low-dose interferon alone in patients with 2A and 2B MM. A total of 407 patients were included in the study, which was study was stopped due to futility, as there was no difference in the overall survival, with the overall 5-year survival rates being 76% (95% CI, 67% to 84%) and 81% (95% CI, 74% to 88%), respectively.[64]

Drawbacks

Toxicity and withdrawal rates have been high in the high-dose interferon studies. In one study,[56] there were two treatment-related deaths. In the latest study,[58] 10% of patients discontinued treatment because of adverse advents, but there were no treatment-related deaths. The most frequent side effects in patients receiving high-dose interferon alfa-2b were fatigue in 20%, granulocytopenia/leukopenia in over 50%, and liver abnormalities and neurological toxicity in about 30%.

In the low-dose interferon trials, about 10% of people suffered significant toxicity as well as the milder nausea and flu-like symptoms experienced by most patients on the day of treatment.

Comments

A comprehensive meta-analysis of the data relating to adjuvant treatment with interferon alfa has demonstrated a dose-dependent effect on recurrence-free survival and a nonsignificant effect of benefit for overall survival.[65] Treatment with interferon is expensive. In an analysis of the high-dose regimen, the estimated cost per life-year gained was $ 13 700 over 35 years and $ 32 600 over 10 years; the estimated cost of low-dose treatment per life-year gained was estimated to be $ 1700 over a lifetime and $ 6600 over 10 years. These costs were thought to be comparable to those of many other oncological treatments.[66,67]

Key points—localized disease

- The incidence of cutaneous malignant melanoma is continuing to rise worldwide, but there is evidence of a leveling of mortality in some groups as patients are presenting earlier.

- Incisional biopsy of a melanoma does not in general alter the prognosis adversely, but may lead to problems in interpreting the histology.

- The main treatment for primary cutaneous melanoma is surgical excision.

- There is good evidence from RCTs that the narrower margins used over the past 20 years are safe.

- All the treatments used for LM and LMM have poor evidence to support them, and well-organized RCTs are needed in this area. Surgical excision probably represents the best treatment on current evidence.

- Elective lymph-node dissection of uninvolved nodes does not improve the prognosis in most patient groups.

- Sentinel lymph-node biopsy is a useful staging tool, but there is no evidence as yet that it improves overall survival.

- Interferons used as adjuvant treatments can benefit some patient groups with MM, but further information is needed to clarify the optimum usage of this treatment.

Metastatic malignant melanoma

Metastatic, or stage IV, MM is a devastating disease. It is defined by dissemination of the cutaneous tumor to other

Table 27.1 Survival of patients with metastatic malignant melanoma

Prognostic factor	Median survival (months)
Number of metastatic sites	
1	7
2	4
3	2
Site of metastatic disease	
Cutaneous nodes	12.5
Lung	11
Brain, liver, bone	2–6

organs or nonregional lymph nodes. The skin, subcutaneous tissues, and lymph nodes are the first site of metastatic disease in 59% of patients. When hematogenous spread to liver, bone, and brain occurs, the natural history is that of one of the most aggressive of all malignant diseases.

For all patients with metastatic disease, the median survival is approximately 7 months; 25% will be alive after 1 year and only 5% of patients will be alive 5 years after diagnosis. Patients with a higher performance status (a numerical measure of physical fitness) and women have a better prognosis ($P = 0.001$ and $P = 0.056$, respectively).[68,69] Survival is also better in patients with a longer duration of remission after primary disease and fewer metastatic sites involved, and in those with nonvisceral disease (Table 27.1).

The intention of treatment remains palliative in all but a few patients. A patient who is fit enough to tolerate systemic therapy will often choose active therapy, despite the modest responses seen with such treatment. The aim of therapy should clearly be to optimize a patient's quality of survival, and must therefore take into account the morbidity and convenience of therapy.

Questions

Is there a preferred systemic therapy in metastatic melanoma?
Efficacy
A systematic review found no RCTs testing systemic therapy against best supportive care.[70] It is doubtful that such a trial will ever be done, given that there is great deal of evidence for (albeit modest) activity in patients with advanced disease.

Dacarbazine (dimethyltriazenoimidazole carboxamide, DTIC) has been the most tested single chemotherapeutic agent. With current antiemetics, it is well tolerated and is considered by many to be the "gold standard" against which other therapies should be tested.[71–74] When used alone, it gives partial response rates of about 20% (> 50% regression for at least 4 weeks), complete responses (complete regression of measurable disease for at least 4 weeks) in 5–10%, and long-term remissions in fewer than 2% of patients. It is usually given intravenously at 850–1000 mg/m^2 on day 1 every 3 weeks or 200 mg/m^2 on days 1–5 every 4 weeks. It is given with intravenous or oral 5-HT3 antagonist and dexamethasone as antiemetics.

Temozolomide is a novel oral alkylating agent with a broad spectrum of antitumor activity. It has 100% oral bioavailability and good penetration of the blood–brain barrier and cerebrospinal fluid. Its efficacy is at least equal to that of dacarbazine in metastatic MM, the median survival being 7.7 months with temozolomide and 6.4 months with dacarbazine (hazards ratio 1.18; 95% CI, 0.92–1.52), and with improvement in some parameters of quality of life.[75] Given its similar mechanism of action to dacarbazine, it is not surprising that response rates are fairly similar, but in a disease with such a poor prognosis, ease of administration and quality of life are clearly very important.

Drawbacks

The dose-limiting toxicities with such regimens are bone-marrow suppression and nausea/vomiting, requiring hospital admission or threatening life in 20% and 5% of patients, respectively.[76,77]

Does combination chemotherapy help?
Efficacy

Many other drugs—such as platinum agents, vinca alkaloids, nitrosoureas, and more recently, taxanes—have been tried alone and in various combination regimens. Higher response rates have been claimed for some of these, but it remains unclear whether they offer significant improvement in quantitative or qualitative outcome over single-agent therapy. An example of the false promise of such combinations was seen when a response rate of 55% was reported for the combination of dacarbazine, cisplatin, carmustine, and tamoxifen,[78] which has become known as the Dartmouth regimen. However, a multicenter randomized trial comparing this regimen with single-agent dacarbazine found no survival advantage and only a small, nonsignificant increase in tumor response in an intention-to-treat analysis (Table 27.2).[76]

Table 27.2 Comparison of single-agent dacarbazine with the Dartmouth regimen of combination chemotherapy

	Dacarbazine	Dartmouth regimen
Response rate (%)	9.9	16.8
Median survival in months (95% CI)	7.7 (5.4–8.7)	6.3 (5.4–8.7)
1-year survival (%)	27	22

Drawbacks

Bone-marrow suppression, nausea/vomiting, and fatigue were significantly more common with the combined therapies.[76]

Comment

Combination therapies should not be used routinely outside the context of clinical trials.

Efficacy

Tamoxifen, an estrogen receptor-blocking agent widely used to treat breast cancer, has also been used, usually together with cytotoxic agents, and may modify the disease response to such drugs. An early study in 117 patients suggested a benefit for the addition of tamoxifen to single-agent dacarbazine (response rates 28% versus 12%; $P = 0.03$, median survival 48 weeks versus 29 weeks, $P = 0.02$).[79] Again, this was not confirmed in a four-arm study in 258 patients with metastatic MM. Response rates were 19% (95% CI, 12 to 26) for patients receiving tamoxifen and 18% in the non-tamoxifen group (95% CI, 12 to 25).[80]

Drawbacks

Antiestrogens can cause hot flushes, thromboembolic events, pulmonary embolism, and endometrial cancer.

Comment

There is no consistent evidence to suggest a benefit for hormonal therapy.

Does immunotherapy help, used either alone or with cytotoxic therapy?

The immune system is important in metastatic MM, as evidenced by lymphoid infiltration into tumor and surrounding tissues, and well-reported spontaneous remissions.[71,72,74,81] This has led to attempts to modulate the immunological environment of tumors, usually by the use of cytokines, particularly interferon alfa[82] and interleukin-2,[83] given directly or by gene therapy. This has improved outcomes in other tumors.[84] Such therapy has single-agent response rates of 15–20%, and it has been suggested that it produces a higher rate of durable remissions.[82]

Efficacy

One meta-analysis compared single-agent dacarbazine and combination chemotherapy with or without immunotherapy in metastatic MM.[85] Twenty RCTs were found, including a total of 3273 patients. Although the addition of interferon alfa increased the response rate by 53% over dacarbazine alone, and dacarbazine combination therapy by 33% over single-agent therapy, there was no overall survival advantage for combination treatment. Two recent RCTs have been published of temozolomide with/without interferon alfa[86] and dacarbazine, cisplatin, and interferon alfa-2b with/without interleukin-2.[87] These studies confirm the results of the previous meta-analysis.

Drawbacks

Interferons commonly cause malaise, fevers, and flu-like symptoms. High-dose interferon alfa caused significant (greater than grade 3) myelosuppression in 24% of people, hepatotoxicity in 15% (including two deaths), and neurotoxicity in 28%.[56] With low-dose interferon, 10% of people suffered significant toxicity.[88]

Comment

Outside clinical trials, it is difficult to justify the additional toxicity with these complex regimens.

Does biological therapy improve outcomes in patients with metastatic malignant melanoma?

Most recently, trials of novel approaches targeting the sensitivity of tumor cells to chemotherapy through modifying apoptosis (induced tumor cell death) and through the use of melanoma vaccines have been tried. Oblimersen, an antisense molecule targeting Bcl-2, a key inhibitor of the mitochondrial apoptosis signaling pathway, showed an encouraging 14% response rate and median survival of 12 months when given with dacarbazine to patients with advanced melanoma expressing Bcl-2.[89] In a subsequent randomized trial, 771 patients were randomized to receive single-agent dacarbazine 1000 mg/m^2 every 3 weeks with or without oblimersen 7 mg/kg/day for 5 days every cycle. Results are available in abstract form only. The response rates were higher in patients receiving oblimersen (12.4% vs 6.8%; $P = 0.007$) and there was a trend towards improved median survival (9 vs. 7.8 months; $P = 0.077$).[90] Cancer vaccines induce tumor cell kill by enhancing presentation of tumor specific antigens to T-cells or the cytotoxicity of lymphocytes cells, inducing an immune response specific for tumor cells. Many trials are underway assessing the efficacy of this approach, but a recent published randomized study of autologous peptide-pulsed dendritic cells failed to demonstrate any survival advantage over single-agent dacarbazine.[91]

Drawbacks

Bcl-2-targeted therapy is associated with neutropenia, thrombocytopenia, fevers, and an increased risk of thrombosis. Further data are awaited on the effect on quality of life and the cost-effectiveness of such therapy. Autologous peptide-pulsed dendritic cells are generally well tolerated.

Comment

Mature data for completed and ongoing studies of targeted therapies are awaited with interest, but will need to be carefully evaluated before such treatment can be recommended.

Implications for clinical practice

Treatment for malignant MM remains unsatisfactory. Response rates often appear encouraging in single-center single-arm studies, but when the treatments have been tested in larger, multicenter randomized trials, the results have to date been very disappointing. Responses are usually partial (10–25% of patients), rarely complete (less than 10%), and are of short duration (median overall survival approximately 6 months).

Outside of clinical trials, standard therapy should remain as single-agent dacarbazine, with temozolomide for selected patients such as those in whom intravenous therapy may particularly interfere with quality of life and possibly those with predominantly cranial metastases.

Key points—metastatic malignant melanoma

- Metastatic malignant melanoma is a devastating disease; only 5% of patients survive for more than 5 years.
- No randomized trials have been performed comparing systemic therapy with no active treatment or placebo.
- Outside of clinical trials, single-agent chemotherapy with dacarbazine should be considered for the majority of these patients.

References

1 Armstrong BK, Kricker A. Cutaneous melanoma. *Cancer Surv* 1994;**19–20**:219–40.

2 Mackie RM, Hole D, Hunter JA, *et al.* Cutaneous malignant melanoma in Scotland: incidence survival and mortality 1979–1994. *BMJ* 1997;**315**:1117–21.

3 Giles GG, Armstrong BK, Burton RC, *et al.* Has mortality from melanoma stopped rising in Australia? Analysis of trends between 1931 and 1994. *BMJ* 1996;**312**:1121–5.

4 National Cancer Institute of Canada. *Canadian Cancer Statistics 1997.* Toronto: National Cancer Institute of Canada, 1997.

5 Holme SA, Malinovsky K, Roberts DL. Malignant melanoma in South Wales: changing trends in presentation (1986–98). *Clin Exp Dermatol* 2001;**26**:484–9.

6 Breslow A. Thickness, cross-sectional areas and depth of invasion in the prognosis of cutaneous melanoma. *Ann Surg* 1970;**172**:902–8.

7 Balch CM, Soong SJ, Shaw HM, *et al.* An analysis of prognostic factors in 8500 patients with cutaneous melanoma. In: Balch CM, Houghton AN, Milton GW, Sober AL, Soong SJ, eds. *Cutaneous Melanoma,* 2nd ed. Philadelphia: Lippincott, 1992: 165–87.

8 Friedmann RJ, Rigel DS, Silverman M, Kopf AW. The continued importance of the early detection of malignant melanoma. *CA Cancer J Clin* 1991;**41**:201–26.

9 Healsmith MF, Bourke JF, Osborne JE, Graham Brown RAC. An evaluation of the revised seven-point checklist for the diagnosis of cutaneous malignant melanoma. *Br J Dermatol* 1994;**130**:48–50.

10 Nachbar F, Stolz W, Merkle T, *et al.* The ABCD rule of dermatoscopy: high prospective value in the diagnosis of doubtful melanocytic skin lesions. *J Am Acad Dermatol* 1994;**30**:551–9.

11 Menzies SW, Bischof L, Talbot H, *et al.* The performance of SolarScan: an automated dermoscopy image analysis instrument for the diagnosis of primary melanoma. *Arch Dermatol* 2005; **141**:1444–6.

12 Lederman JS, Sober AJ. Does biopsy type influence survival in clinical stage I cutaneous melanoma? *J Am Acad Dermatol* 1985; **13**:983–7.

13 Lees VC, Briggs JC. Effect of an initial biopsy on prognosis in stage I invasive cutaneous malignant melanoma; review of 1086 patients. *Br J Surg* 1991;**71**:1108–10.

14 Bong JL, Herd RM, Hunter JAA. Incisional biopsy and melanoma prognosis. *J Am Acad Dermatol* 2002;**46**:690–4.

15 Martin RC 2nd, Scoggins CR, Ross MI, *et al.* Is incisional biopsy harmful? *Am J Surg* 2005;**190**:913–7.

16 Austin JR, Byers RM, Brown WD, Wolf P. Influence on biopsy on the prognosis of cutaneous melanoma of the head and neck. *Head Neck* 1996;**18**:107–17.

17 Haigh PI, DiFronzo LA, McCready DR. Optimal excision margins for primary cutaneous melanoma: a systematic review and meta-analysis. *Can J Surg* 2003;**46**:419–26.

18 Veronesi U, Cascinelli N. Narrow excision (1 cm margin); a safe procedure for thin cutaneous melanoma. *Arch Surg* 1991;**126**:438–41.

19 Balch CM, Urist MM, Karakousis CP, *et al.* Efficacy of 2-cm surgical margins for intermediate-thickness melanomas (1 to 4 mm): result of a multi-institutional randomized surgical trial. *Ann Surg* 1993;**218**:262–7.

20 Cohn-Cedermark G, Rutqvist LE, Andersson R, *et al.* Long term results of a randomized study by the Swedish Melanoma Study Group on 2-cm versus 5-cm resection margins for patients with cutaneous melanoma with a tumour thickness of 0.8–2.0 mm. *Cancer* 2000;**89**: 1495–501.

21 Heaton KM, Sussman JJ, Gershenwald JE, *et al.* Surgical margins and prognostic factors in patients with thick (> 4 mm) primary melanoma. *Ann Surg Oncol* 1998;**5**:322–8.

22 Khayat D, Rixe O, Martin G, *et al.* Surgical margins in cutaneous melanoma (2 cm versus 5 cm for lesions measuring less than 2.1 mm thick). *Cancer* 2003;**97**:1941–6.

23 Thomas JM, Newton-Bishop J, A'Hern R, *et al.* Excision margins in high-risk malignant melanoma. *N Engl J Med* 2004;**350**:757–66.

24 Guerry D 4th, Synnestvedt M, Elder DE, Schultz D. Lessons from tumor progression: the invasive radial growth phase of melanoma is common, incapable of metastasis, and indolent. *J Invest Dermatol* 1993;**100**:342S–345S.

25 Sober AJ, Chuang TY, Duvic M, *et al.* Guidelines of care for primary cutaneous melanoma. *J Am Acad Dermatol* 2001;**45**:579–86.

26 Mackie RM. Melanocytic naevi and malignant melanoma. In: Champion RH, Burton JL, Burns DA, Breathnach SM, eds. *Textbook of Dermatology*, 6th ed. Vol. 2. Oxford: Blackwell Science, 1998: 1741–50.

27 Pitman GH, Kopf AW, Bart RS, *et al.* Treatment of lentigo maligna and lentigo maligna melanoma. *J Dermatol Surg Oncol* 1979;**5**: 727–37.

28 Coleman WP III, Davis RS, Reed RJ, *et al.* Treatment of lentigo maligna and lentigo maligna melanoma. *J Dermatol Surg Oncol* 1980;**6**:476–9.

29 Cohen LM, McCall MW, Zax RH. Mohs micrographic surgery for lentigo maligna and lentigo maligna melanoma: a follow-up study. *Dermatol Surg* 1998:**24**: 673–7.

30 Bub JL, Berg D, Slee A, Odland PB. Management of lentigo maligna and lentigo maligna melanoma with staged excision: a 5-year follow-up. *Arch Dermatol* 2004;**140**:607–8.

31 Kufflik EG, Gage AA. Cryosurgery for lentigo maligna. *J Am Acad Dermatol* 1994;**31**:75–8.

32 Bohler-Sommerregger K, Schuller-Petrovic S, Knobner R, *et al.* Reactive lentiginous hyperpigmentation after cryosurgery for lentigo maligna. *J Am Acad Dermatol* 1992;**27**:523–6.

33 Arma-Szlachcic M, Ott F, Storck H. Zur Strahlentherapie der melanotischen Präcancerosen. *Hautarzt* 1970;**21**:505–8.

34 Tsang RW, Liu F, Wells W, Payne DG. Lentigo maligna of the head and neck: results of treatment by radiotherapy. *Arch Dermatol* 1994;**130**:1008–12.

35 Litwin MS, Kremetz ET, Mansell PW, Reed RJ. Topical treatment of lentigo maligna with 5-fluorouracil. *Cancer* 1995;**3**:721–33.

36 Rivers JK, McCarthy WH. No effect of topical tretinoin in lentigo maligna [letter]. *Arch Dermatol* 1991;**127**:129.

37 Nazzoro-Porro M, Passi S, Zina G, *et al.* Ten years' experience of treating lentigo maligna with topical azelaic acid. *Acta Derm Venereol* 1989;**143**(Suppl):49–57.

38 Naylor MF, Crowson N, Kuwahara R, *et al.* Treatment of lentigo maligna with topical imiquimod. *Br J Dermatol* 2003;**149**(Suppl 66):66–70.

39 Wolf IH, Cerroni L, Kodama K, Kerl H. Treatment of lentigo maligna (melanoma in situ) with the immune response modifier imiquimod. *Arch Dermatol* 2005;**141**:510–4.

40 Cox NH, Aitchison TC, Sirel JM, MacKie RM. Comparison between lentigo maligna melanoma and other histogenic types of malignant melanoma of the head and neck. Scottish Melanoma Group. *Br J Cancer* 1996;**73**:940–4.

41 Schmid-Wendtner MH, Brunner B, Konz B, *et al.* Fractionated radiotherapy of lentigo maligna and lentigo maligna melanoma in 64 patients. *J Am Acad Dermatol* 2000;**43**:477–82.

42 Mahendran R, Newton-Bishop JA. Survey of UK current practice in the treatment of lentigo maligna. *Br J Dermatol* 2001;**144**:71–6.

43 Balch CM, Soong SJ, Bartolucci AA, *et al.* Efficacy of an elective regional lymph node dissection of 1 to 4 mm thick melanomas for patients 60 years of age and younger. *Ann Surg* 1996;**224**:255–63.

44 Cascinelli N, Morabito A, Santinami M, MacKie RM, Belli F. Immediate or delayed dissection of regional nodes in patients with melanoma of the trunk: a randomised trial. WHO Melanoma Programme. *Lancet* 1998;**351**:793–6.

45 Sim FH, Taylor WF, Ivins JC, Pritchard DJ, Soule EH. A prospective randomized study of the efficacy of routine elective lymphadenectomy in management of malignant melanoma: preliminary results. *Cancer* 1978;**41**:948–56.

46 Veronesi U, Adamus J, Bandiera DC, *et al.* Inefficacy of immediate node dissection in stage I melanoma of the limbs. *N Engl J Med* 1977;**297**:627–30.

47 Baas PC, Schraffordt Koops H, Hoekstra HJ, van Bruggen JJ, van der Weele LT, Oldhoff J. Groin dissection in the treatment of lower-extremity melanoma: short-term and long-term morbidity. *Arch Surg* 1992;**127**:281–6.

48 Morton DL, Wen DR, Wong JH, *et al.* Technical details of intra-operative lymphatic mapping for early stage melanoma. *Arch Surg* 1992;**127**:392–9.

49 Morton DL, Thompson JF, Essner R, *et al.* Validation of the accuracy of intraoperative lymphatic mapping and sentinel lymphadenectomy for early-stage melanoma: a multicenter trial. Multicenter Selective Lymphadenectomy Trial Group. *Ann Surg* 1999;**230**:453–65.

50 Balch CM, Buzard AC, Soong SJ, *et al.* Final version of the American Joint Committee on Cancer staging system for cutaneous melanoma. *J Clin Oncol* 2001;**19**:3635–48.

51 Gershenwald JE, Thompson W, Mansfield PF, *et al.* Multi-institutional melanoma lymphatic mapping experience: the prognostic value of sentinel lymph node status in 612 stage I or II melanoma patients. *J Clin Oncol* 1999;**17**:976–83.

52 Rayatt SS, Hettiaratchy SP. Having this biopsy gives psychological benefits [letter]. *BMJ* 2000;**321**:1285.

53 Jansen L, Nieweg OE, Peterse JL, Hoefnagel CA, Ohnos RA, Kroon BBR. Reliability of sentinel lymph node biopsy for staging melanoma. *Br J Surg* 2000;**87**:484–9.

54 Wrightson WR, Wong SL, Edwards MJ, *et al.* Complications associated with lymph node biopsy for melanoma. *Ann Surg Oncol* 2003;**10**:676–80.

55 Gutzmer R, Al-Ghazal M, Geerlings H, Kopp A. Sentinel node biopsy in melanoma delays recurrence but does not change melanoma related survival: a retrospective analysis of 673 patients. *Br J Dermatol* 2005;**153**:1137–41.

56 Kirkwood JM, Strawderman MH, Ernstoff MS, Smith TJ, Borden EC, Blum RH. Interferon alfa-2b adjuvant therapy of high-risk resected cutaneous melanoma: the Eastern Cooperative Oncology Group Trial EST 1684. *J Clin Oncol* 1996;**14**:7–17.

57 Kirkwood JM, Ibrahim JG, Sondak VK, *et al.* High- and low-dose interferon alfa-2b in high-risk melanoma: first analysis of Intergroup trial 1690/S9111/C9190. *J Clin Oncol* 2000;**18**:2444–58.

58 Kirkwood JM, Ibrahim JG, Sosman JA, *et al.* High-dose interferon alfa-2b significantly prolongs relapse-free and overall survival compared with the GM2-KLH/QS-21 vaccine in patients with resected stage IIB–III melanoma: results of Intergroup trial E1694/S9512/C509801. *J Clin Oncol* 2001;**19**:2370–80.

59 Kirkwood JM, Manola J, Ibrahim J, Sondak V, Ernstoff MS, Rao U. A pooled analysis of Eastern Cooperative Oncology Group and Intergroup trials of adjuvant high-dose interferon for melanoma. *Clin Cancer Res* 2004;**10**:1670–7.

60 Eggermont AM, Suciu S, MacKie R, *et al.* Post-surgery adjuvant therapy with intermediate doses of interferon alfa 2b versus observation in patients with stage IIb/III melanoma (EORTC 18952): randomised controlled trial. *Lancet* 2005;**366**:1189–96.

61 Grob JJ, Dreno B, de la Salmoniere P, *et al.* Randomised trial of interferon alpha-2a as adjuvant therapy in resected primary melanoma thicker than 1.5 mm without clinically detectable node metastases. French Cooperative Group on Melanoma. *Lancet* 1998;**351**:1905–10.

62 Pehamberger H, Soyer HP, Steiner A, *et al.* Adjuvant interferon alfa-2a in resected primary stage II cutaneous melanoma. Austrian Malignant Melanoma Cooperative Group. *J Clin Oncol* 1998;**16**:1425–9.

63 Hancock BW, Wheatley K, Harris S, *et al.* Adjuvant interferon in high-risk melanoma: the AIM HIGH Study—United Kingdom Coordinating Committee on Cancer Research randomized study of adjuvant low-dose extended-duration interferon alfa-2a in high-risk resected malignant melanoma. *J Clin Oncol* 2004;**22**:53–61.

64 Richtig E, Soyer HP, Posch M, *et al.* Prospective, randomized, multicenter, double-blind placebo-controlled trial comparing adjuvant interferon alfa and isotretinoin with interferon alfa alone in stage IIA and IIB melanoma: European Cooperative Adjuvant Melanoma Study Group. *J Clin Oncol* 2005;**23**:8655–63.

65 Wheatley K, Ives N, Hancock B, Gore M, Eggermont A, Suciu S. Does adjuvant interferon-alpha for high-risk melanoma provide a worthwhile benefit? A meta-analysis of the randomised trials. *Cancer Treat Rev* 2003;**29**:241–52.

66 Hillner BE, Kirkwood JM, Atkins MB, Johnson ER, Smith TJ. Economic analysis of adjuvant interferon alfa-2b in high-risk melanoma based on projections from Eastern Cooperative Oncology Group 1684. *J Clin Oncol* 1997;**15**:2351–8.

67 Lafuma A, Dreno B, Delauney M, *et al.* Economic analysis of adjuvant therapy with interferon alpha-2a in stage II malignant melanoma. *Eur J Cancer* 2001;**37**:369–75.

68 Balch CM, Reintgen DS, Kirkwood JM, *et al.* Cutaneous melanoma. In: DeVita VT Jr, Hellman S, Rosenberg SA, eds. *Cancer: Principles and Practice of Oncology,* 5th ed. Philadelphia: Lippincott-Raven, 1997: 1947–94.

69 Unger JM, Flaherty LE, Liu PY, *et al.* Gender and other survival predictors in patients with metastatic melanoma on Southwest Oncology Group Trials. *Cancer* 2001;**91**:1148–55.

70 Crosby T, Fish R, Coles B, Mason MD. Systemic treatments for metastatic cutaneous melanoma. *Cochrane Database Syst Rev* 2000;(2):CD001215.

71 Balch CM, Atkins MB, Sober AJ. Cutaneous melanoma. In: DeVita VT Jr, Hellman S, Rosenberg SA, eds. *Cancer: Principles and Practice of Oncology,* 7th ed. Philadelphia: Lippincott, 2004:1754–809.

72 Cascinelli N, Clemente C, Belli F. Cutaneous melanoma. In: Peckham M, Pinedo HM, Veronesi U, eds. *Oxford Textbook of Oncology.* Oxford: Oxford University Press, 1995:902–28.

73 Pritchard KI, Quirt IC, Cowman DH, *et al.* DTIC therapy in metastatic malignant melanoma: a simplified dose schedule. *Cancer Treat Rep* 1980;**64**:1123–6.

74 Taylor A, Gore M. Malignant melanoma. In: Price P, Sikora K, eds. *Treatment of Cancer,* 3rd ed. London: Chapman and Hall Medical, 1995: 763–7.

75 Middleton MR, Grob JJ, Aaronson N, *et al.* Randomized phase III study of temozolomide versus dacarbazine in the treatment of patients with advanced metastatic malignant melanoma. *J Clin Oncol* 2000;**18**:158–66.

76 Chapman PB, Einhorn LH, Meyers ML, *et al.* Phase III multicenter randomized trial of the Dartmouth regimen versus dacarbazine in patients with metastatic melanoma. *J Clin Oncol* 1999;**17**:2745–51.

77 Falkson CI, Falkson G, Falkson HC. Improved results with the addition of interferon alfa-2b to dacarbazine in the treatment of patients with metastatic malignant melanoma. *J Clin Oncol* 1991;**9**:1403–8.

78 Del Prete SA, Maurer LH, O'Donnell J, Forcier RJ, LeMarbre P. Combination chemotherapy with cisplatin, carmustine, dacarbazine, and tamoxifen in metastatic melanoma. *Cancer Treat Rep* 1984;**68**:1403–5.

79 Cocconi G, Bella M, Calabresi F, *et al.* Treatment of metastatic malignant melanoma with dacarbazine plus tamoxifen. *N Engl Med J* 1992;**327**:516–23.

80 Falkson CI, Ibrahim J, Kirkwood JM, Coates AS, Atkins MB, Blum RH. Phase III trial of dacarbazine versus dacarbazine with

interferon alpha-2b versus dacarbazine with tamoxifen versus dacarbazine with interferon alpha-2b and tamoxifen in patients with metastatic malignant melanoma: an Eastern Cooperative Oncology Group Study. *J Clin Oncol* 1998;**16**:1743–51.

81 Rosenberg SA, Yang JC, Topalian SL, *et al.* Treatment of 283 consecutive patients with metastatic melanoma or renal cell cancer using high-dose bolus interleukin-2. *JAMA* 1994;**271**:907–13.

82 Legha SS. The role of interferon alfa in the treatment of metastatic melanoma. *Semin Oncol* 1997;**24**(1 Suppl 4):S24–31.

83 Legha SS, Gianin MA, Plager C, *et al.* Evaluation of interleukin-2 administered by continuous infusion in patients with metastatic melanoma. *Cancer* 1996; **77**:89–96.

84 Atzpodien J, Kirchner H, Franzke A, *et al.* Results of a randomized clinical trial comparing SC interleukin-2, SC alpha-2a-interferon, and IV bolus 5-fluorouracil against oral tamoxifen in progressive metastatic renal cell carcinoma patients. *Proc Am Assoc Clin Oncol* 1997;**16**:326.

85 Huncharek M, Caubet JF, McGarry R. Single-agent DTIC versus combination chemotherapy with or without immunotherapy in metastatic melanoma: a meta-analysis of 3273 patients from 20 randomized trials. *Melanoma Res* 2001;**11**:75–81.

86 Kaufmann R, Spieth K, Leiter U, *et al.* Temozolomide in combination with interferon-alfa versus temozolomide alone in patients with advanced metastatic melanoma: a randomized, phase III,

multicenter study from the Dermatologic Cooperative Oncology Group. *J Clin Oncol* 2005;**23**:9001–7.

87 Keilholz U, Punt CJ, Gore M, *et al.* Dacarbazine, cisplatin, and interferon-alfa-2b with or without interleukin-2 in metastatic melanoma: a randomized phase III trial (18951) of the European Organisation for Research and Treatment of Cancer Melanoma Group. *J Clin Oncol* 2005;**23**:6747–55.

88 Kleeberg UR, Brocker EB, Lejeune F. Adjuvant trial in melanoma patients comparing rIFN-alfa to rIFN-gamma to Iscador to a control group after curative resection high risk primary or regional lymph node metastasis (EORTC 18871). *Eur J Cancer* 1999;**35**(Suppl 4):S82.

89 Jansen B, Wacheck V, Heere-Ress E, *et al.* Chemosensitisation of malignant melanoma by BCL2 antisense therapy. *Lancet* 2000; **356**:1728–33.

90 Kirkwood JM, Bedikian AY, Millward MJ, *et al.* Long-term survival results of a randomized multinational phase 3 trial of dacarbazine (DTIC) with or without Bcl-2 antisense (oblimersen sodium) in patients (pts) with advanced malignant melanoma (MM). *J Clin Oncol* 2005;**23**(Suppl 16):7506.

91 Schadendorf D, Ugurel S, Schuler-Thurner B, *et al.* Dacarbazine (DTIC) versus vaccination with autologous peptide-pulsed dendritic cells (DC) in first-line treatment of patients with metastatic melanoma: a randomized phase III trial of the DC study group of the DeCOG. *Ann Oncol* 2006;**17**:563–70.

28 Squamous cell carcinoma

Nanette J. Liegeois, Su-Jean Seo, Suzanne Olbricht

Background

Definition

Squamous cell carcinoma (SCC) is a form of skin cancer that originates from epithelial keratinocytes.[1] It is thought to arise as a focal intraepidermal proliferation from precancerous lesions, including actinic keratosis, SCC *in situ*, Bowen's disease, bowenoid papulosis, erythroplasia of Queyrat, and arsenical keratoses.[2] Without treatment, SCC may continue to grow, invade deep tissue, or metastasize.[3] This chapter focuses on interventions for localized, nonmetastatic invasive cutaneous SCC. The prevention of SCC is dealt with in Chapter 25. Excluded from this chapter are: SCC of the penis and vulva, Buschke–Löwenstein tumor, and advanced head and neck cancers.

Epidemiology

Since the 1960s, the overall incidence of SCC has been increasing annually.[4,5] In 1997, the Rochester Epidemiology Project in the United States estimated the overall incidence of invasive SCC to be 106 per 100 000 people.[5] Recent data from the same database indicate that the incidence of SCC in people younger than 40 is now 3.9 per 100 000 and that it is continuing to rise.[6] The age-standardized rate of SCC in Australia has also been increasing and was calculated as 387 per 100 000 people in 2006.[7] Similarly, the incidence of nonmelanoma skin cancer, including SCC, doubled or tripled between 1960 and 2000 in Canada.[8]

Sunlight exposure is an established independent risk factor for the development of SCC. SCC arises more commonly in sun-exposed areas of skin, including the head, neck, and arms, but also occurs on the trunk and buttocks, as well as other areas.[9] Several population-based studies support the role of sun exposure in the pathogenesis of SCC. SCC appears to correlate with geographic latitude. The reported incidence of SCC is higher in tropical regions than in temperate climates, with an annual incidence approaching one in 100 in Australia.[10–13] Regional differences related to latitude have also been noted in the United States.[4,14–17] In the Swedish database of familial cohorts, analysis suggested intentional tanning as a contributing factor in the increase in the incidence of SCC in the younger generation.[18]

Other risk factors for SCC include older age, male sex, Celtic ancestry, increased sensitivity to sun exposure, an increased number of precancerous lesions, and immunosuppression.[4,19,20] Exposure to oral psoralens, arsenic, cigarette smoking, coal-tar products, ultraviolet A (UVA) photochemotherapy, and human papillomavirus have also been associated with SCC. Genetic disorders that predispose to SCC include epidermodysplasia verruciformis, albinism, and xeroderma pigmentosum. Stasis ulcers, osteomyelitic sinuses, scarring processes such as lupus vulgaris, and vitiligo have been reported to increase the risk of SCC. In the latter conditions, it is unclear whether the morphology of the underlying process obscures or delays the diagnosis.[15,16]

Pathogenesis

Several studies have shown that sun exposure, photo-irradiation, and ionizing irradiation play a major role in the pathogenesis of SCC. DNA damage is a fundamental process that occurs in the development of cancer. Both ultraviolet light and ionizing radiation are potent mutagens. Specifically, UVB light, a key component of sunlight, has been shown to produce pyrimidine cyclobutane dimers in DNA; these dimers result in DNA point mutations during keratinocyte replication, which lead to abnormal cell function and replication.

In addition to direct DNA damage, genes involved in DNA repair have been implicated in the pathogenesis of SCC. The p53 tumor-suppressor gene is mutated in the majority of SCC tumors; proper p53 function is thought to be critical in suppressing the development of SCC by allowing necessary repair of ultraviolet-damaged DNA.[21–24] Keratinocytes with p53 mutations cannot repair the mutations induced by irradiation and subsequently undergo proliferation, and further mutations ensue and culminate in cancerous growth.[17] Mutations in p53 can also be acquired via exposure to human papillomavirus, carcinogens, or radiation, or may be inherited. People with xeroderma pigmentosum have an inherited defective p53 pathway, so that they cannot repair mutations induced by irradiation, resulting in the development of numerous skin cancers.[25]

Immunological status has also been implicated in the development of SCC. The rate of SCC in transplant recipients is high, particularly in those with a kidney or heart transplant.[26–29] The way in which immunosuppression increases the risk is not fully understood, but in addition to lowering surveillance functions, recent reports suggest a strong association with common viral infections, such that the immunosuppression allows the virally induced disease to degenerate into malignancy.[30] Decreasing the immunosuppressive therapy helps reduce the number of SCCs.[31] Further studies are needed to determine how altered immune responses influence the development of SCC.

Prognosis

The prognosis for the patient with regard to local recurrence, metastases, and survival in SCC depends on the location of the disease and the modality of treatment. Rowe *et al.*[32] analyzed data from more than 200 studies published from the 1930s to the 1990s, including all reports in which there was treatment of more than 20 patients with SCC, specified separately from basal cell carcinoma (BCC), and in which the results were separated by treatment modality. These studies did not have consistent follow-up intervals, and it is doubtful whether the choice of tumor for each modality was similar; however, some features of SCC became clear. The recurrence rate increased as the length of follow-up increased. The overall local recurrence rate after excision of an SCC involving sun-exposed areas was 8%, while the recurrence rates on the ear and lip were 19% and 11%, respectively. The metastatic rate for primary SCC of sun-exposed areas was 5%, while the rates for SCC on the external ear, lip, and areas not exposed to the sun were 9%, 14%, and 38%, respectively. The survival rate associated with metastatic SCC of the skin was 44% in studies with follow-up periods of less than 5 years and 34% in those with longer-term follow-up.

Diagnostic tests

The diagnosis of SCC relies on biopsy of a suspicious lesion. The pathognomonic histopathological findings are cytologically atypical hyperproliferative keratinocytes, cytological and architectural disorganization, decreased differentiation, and atypical mitoses. While precancerous actinic keratosis includes cytologic atypia and some undifferentiated features in the lower third of the epidermis, SCC *in situ* is diagnosed when full-thickness cytologic atypia with a lack of keratinocyte maturation is identified in the epidermal compartment. Invasive SCC is distinguished from SCC *in situ* by invasion of the dermis by epithelioid cells in atypical nests and cords, and rarely as single cells. SCC may also be classified according to the degree of differentiation—a clinically important specification, since less differentiated tumors are associated with poor prognosis.[33]

Aims of treatment and relevant outcomes

The aim of treatment is to remove or destroy the tumor completely and to minimize cosmetic and functional impairment. Success should therefore be measured by rates of recurrence or metastasis at fixed time points, or by survival analyses that document the time to first recurrences in groups of patients. The morbidity of the procedure, as measured by short-term or chronic pain, infection, scarring, skin function, and overall cosmesis should all be considered when choosing the appropriate treatment modality.[34,35] In addition, the cost and tolerance of the specific treatment modalities should be considered.

In general, SCC has not been thoroughly or rigorously studied, and there are very few prospective randomized controlled trials (RCTs). Treatments of BCC, which is a more common tumor, have been more adequately assessed. It is generally assumed that the procedures and outcomes in the treatment of BCC are relevant to the outcomes in SCC, but that may or may not be a correct assumption. Many series of treatments for nonmelanoma skin cancers or BCC include some SCCs (see Chapter 29 for the relevant data).

Methods of search

The following databases were searched:
- Medline, January 1966–December 2006
- Embase, January 1980–December 2006
- The Cochrane Skin Group Trials Register
- The Cochrane Database of Systematic Reviews and Cochrane Central Register of Controlled Trials

Search items included: SCC, squamous cell carcinoma, squamous cell cancer, skin neoplasms, xeroderma pigmentosum, nonmelanoma skin cancers, nonmelanoma skin cancer, and transplant skin cancers.

Questions

The following questions relate to the treatment of a large (> 2 cm) invasive perineural SCC on the temple of a 52-year-old woman (Figure 28.1).

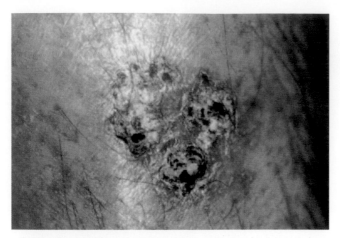

Figure 28.1 A biopsy-proven neurotropic squamous cell carcinoma of the right temple in a 52-year-old woman.

What are the effective therapeutic interventions for localized invasive SCC of the skin? How do the effective therapeutic interventions for SCC compare with each other? How do the cosmetic outcomes for these interventions compare?

Excision

Surgical excision is still the primary treatment for invasive SCC. Surgical excision of SCC is performed in the outpatient setting, usually under local anesthesia. The standard excision technique involves estimation of the clinically obvious tumor, either visually or via curetting. The surgeon marks an area of normal-appearing skin as an additional margin to be taken around the tumor. A steel blade is used to excise the tumor and margins. Closure is performed using primary layered, flap, or graft technique, or sometimes the wound is allowed to heal by secondary intent using appropriate wound-care regimens. The histology of the tumor is examined in formalin-fixed sections, including a sampling of the margins to assess whether the tumor has been completely removed. This report is generally received 2–10 days after the procedure. Examination of the margins is sometimes carried out in frozen sections, which may be immediately available.

Effectiveness

No large RCTs have compared the effectiveness of surgical excision with any other treatment modality. No RCTs have compared predetermined margin widths for the surgical removal of SCC.

Several case series show excellent clearance of SCC lesions with surgical excision. Freeman *et al.*[36] reported 91 surgically excised SCCs, with follow-up periods ranging from 1 to 5 years. Metastases developed in three of the 91 patients. The authors did not note the size or location of the tumors. For SCC with clinically visible tumor less than 2 cm in diameter, surgical excision resulted in a 5-year disease-free survival of 96% (22 of 23 patients). For lesions clinically larger than 2 cm, 83% (10 of 12) of the patients were free of disease 5 years later.

While many authors report low recurrence rates for excision, with variable follow-up, recommendations for the width of the margin of clinically normal skin excised have ranged from 4 mm to 1 cm. In one prospective study, 141 SCC lesions were excised with incremental 1-mm margins, and the subclinical extension of tumors was examined using frozen-tissue sectioning via the technique of Mohs micrographic surgery (MMS).[37] With 4-mm surgical margins, tumors appearing to be less than 2 cm in diameter had a greater than 95% clearance, while tumors clinically larger than 2 cm required at least 6-mm excision margins to achieve a greater than 95% clearance.

Drawbacks

Large tumors, or tumors in cosmetically complex areas such as near the eyelids or ears, often require an involved flap or graft procedure for repair. The subsequent scar from surgical excision usually results in a hypopigmented line, and hypertrophic and keloidal changes may occur. SCC excision and repair also require removal of at least superficial subcutaneous fat, which may disrupt the normal vasculature, lymphatics, or innervation. Since the surgical site is most often closed at the time of surgery and histology is later evaluated on fixed tissues, the discovery of residual tumor may mean that the patient has to return for further surgical interventions.

Comment

Surgical excision is still the major definitive treatment option for SCCs less than 2 cm in diameter. Caution is necessary when using this technique for larger SCCs or lesions in cosmetically complex areas.

Mohs micrographic surgery (MMS)

MMS is a procedure that is carried out in stages over several hours. The surgeon excises the tumor and a small clinically normal margin, processes the specimen as a frozen section, reads the slides to mark margins with residual tumor, re-excises tissue at the positive margin, and processes the new specimen. These steps are followed until all margins are clear of tumor. This differs from excision with frozen-section margin control in four ways. Firstly, the initial specimen is excised as one intact disk with beveled edges, yielding a saucer-shaped specimen. This shape facilitates orientation and preparation for microscopic evaluation. Secondly, the processing of the specimen is different from the processing of specimens as performed by the pathology department. Horizontal sections are prepared in such a way that the entire margin from the epidermis to the deepest portion of the specimen is viewed under the microscope in very few sections. Thirdly, the surgeon is trained to be a histopathologist as well and reads the slides, allowing him or her to orient any residual tumor relative to other structures in the skin, such as the plane of sebaceous glands or a prominent blood vessel. Finally, it is less expensive to do MMS than excision with frozen-section control.[38]

Final closure is performed once the entire margin is clear. MMS is considered to be a highly curative procedure for nonmelanoma skin cancers, since immediate histopathological evaluation of the entire margin is possible. In addition, histopathologically uninvolved skin is spared, as the mapping technique allows specific reexcision of only the involved margins, limiting potential damage to adjacent tissues.

Effectiveness

Although MMS is frequently used in the treatment of SCCs, there have been no RCTs comparing MMS with other treatments for SCC.

Mohs reported a 5-year recurrence rate of 5% for primary SCC.[39] In a case-series analysis, Rowe *et al.* found that MMS resulted in a lower rate of local recurrences in comparison with other treatment modalities.[32] Holmkvist and Roenigk report a recurrence rate for primary SCC of the lip of 5% after MMS for 50 patients, with an average follow-up period of 2–5 years.[40] Lawrence and Cottel[41] reported only three local recurrences of SCC in 44 patients with perineural invasion treated with MMS with a 1-year follow-up, and further noted that the predicted survival was higher than previously published survival rates for surgical excision.[41–43]

Drawbacks

MMS is expensive and is not accessible to all patients. Full extirpation of the tumor may require multiple stages over a period of many hours. Patients who cannot lie down due to a comorbid condition may not tolerate the potentially lengthy procedure. In addition, the processing of the frozen sections is labor-intensive.

Comments

MMS appears to have lower recurrence rates than other treatment modalities. As it involves sequential extirpation of tissue, it is more sparing of adjacent tissue. This provides a cosmetic advantage for tumors located in functionally critical areas. The procedure is performed in an outpatient setting, and most patients tolerate it without difficulty.[29] Two large series have documented the safety of this procedure in an office setting. In 3937 patients, Kimayai-Aasadi and colleagues found only one serious complication, consisting of gastrointestinal hemorrhage due to naproxen prescribed postoperatively for auricular chondritis in one patient.[44] In a prospective study by Cook and Perone of 1052 patients (1358 MMS patients), the overall complication

rate was 1.64%. Significantly, there were no serious complications requiring involvement by another specialist or hospitalization of the patient.[45] The technique avoids the delay associated with formalin-processed tissues and the need for multiple surgical procedures. For low-risk small-diameter SCCs (minimally invasive or in low-risk sites), other treatment modalities should be considered, as there is probably little to be gained in efficacy and much to be lost in terms of cost and time.

Electrodessication and curettage

Electrodessication and curettage (ED&C) is frequently used in the treatment of SCC, particularly for *in situ* or minimally invasive lesions on the trunk or limbs. The tumor is prepared for ED&C, and margins are marked. Taking advantage of the finding that skin tumors are usually more friable than the surrounding normal tissue, the sharp tip of a curette is used to debulk the tumor. Electric current through a fine-tipped needle is used to desiccate the base and destroy any residual tumor. This sequence is repeated several times, and the eschar that remains is left to heal by secondary intention.

Effectiveness

ED&C is frequently used for SCC, but no RCTs have compared ED&C with other treatments. Several case series have examined the recurrence rate after ED&C for SCC lesions. Freeman *et al.*[30] treated 407 SCC lesions using ED&C over a 20-year period, with follow-up periods ranging from 1 year to over 5 years. In patients with more than 5 years of follow-up, no recurrences were observed in 96% (46 of 48) of SCCs less than 2 cm in diameter or in 100% (all of nine) SCCs larger than 2 cm in diameter. Of the 407 SCC lesions treated, 355 were less than 2 cm, suggesting that this is the technique of choice for smaller SCCs. Knox *et al.*[46] noted that only four SCC lesions recurred in 315 tumors treated with a follow-up period of 4 months to 2 years. The SCC lesions in this study were all less than 2 cm and without significant invasion. Honeycutt and Jansen[47] treated 28 invasive SCC lesions with ED&C and reported three recurrences during a follow-up period of up to 4 years. Of the patients who developed recurrences, two had had tumors larger than 2 cm. Whelan and Deckers[48] treated 26 SCC lesions on the trunk and extremities and reported no recurrences in 100% of lesions during a 2–9-year follow-up. It is difficult to make comparisons of ED&C studies with studies of other treatments, as this high success rate probably reflects in part a selection bias for smaller and less invasive lesions.

Drawbacks

Cosmetically, the scar from ED&C is usually a hypopigmented sclerotic circle, rather than the thin line resulting from excision. Although the circular scar often contracts, hypertrophic changes can also occur, making it difficult to recognize recurrent SCC. For SCC lesions on the face, particularly adjacent to critical tissues, contraction of resultant scars may distort or destroy the normal or functional anatomy. In addition, a surgeon performing ED&C at sites adjacent to vital or anatomically complex structures (such as the nose or eye) might limit the margins of destruction or be less aggressive in order to preserve native tissue; this is likely to diminish the effectiveness of this technique. Whelan and Deckers[48] found that the majority (65%) of lesions took 4 weeks to heal after ED&C, while in a separate study they found that the average time for healing was 5.1 weeks.[49] Prolonged healing in comparison with surgical excision should be taken into consideration, particularly for lesions on the lower extremities. Daily wound care is an essential part of ED&C, and diligence is required in order to prevent infection.

With the ED&C technique, no tissue is obtained that can be examined microscopically to determine whether the margins of the treatment are clear of tumor. If curettage develops a deep wound suggestive of deep tumor, it would be reasonable to consider excising the curettage wound with a 3–4-mm margin and sending the specimen to pathology, rather than completing the standard ED&C procedure.

Comment
ED&C appears to be effective for minimally invasive SCC lesions less than 2 cm in diameter. One clear advantage of ED&C over other modalities is that it is rapidly and easily performed by the experienced surgical clinician. Although the healing time may be increased, ED&C is an affordable, effective, and rapid treatment option for SCC and should be considered for small or histologically less invasive tumors. Adequate follow-up is essential to recognize the rare recurrences.

Cryotherapy
Cryotherapy has been used for decades and is highly effective for treating small or minimally invasive SCCs. The standard treatment protocol for cryotherapy consists of two cycles of freezing with liquid nitrogen, lasting 1–5 min per cycle. The technique takes longer than ED&C, but requires less time than surgical excision.

Effectiveness
No RCTs have compared the effectiveness of cryotherapy with other treatments. Several case series have examined use of cryosurgery in SCC. Over an 18-year period, Zacarian[50] treated 4228 skin cancers with cryotherapy, which included 203 SCC lesions. He noted a 97% disease-free survival over follow-up periods ranging from less than 3 months to over 10 years. Most recurrences (87%) occurred during the first 3 years. Zacarian further noted a healing

time that ranged from 4 to 10 weeks. Kuflik and Gage[51] found a 96% 5-year disease free survival rate for 52 SCC lesions. Holt[14] reported on 34 SCC lesions treated with cryotherapy, with a 97% disease-free survival after follow-up periods ranging from 6 months to 5 years.

Drawbacks
Cryotherapy at an effective dosage is always complicated by an initial period of significant edema, followed by formation of a large bulla. After rupture, the wound weeps and then crusts, taking 4–10 weeks to heal.[41] Hypopigmentation is universal, with occasional hypertrophic scarring.[41] Atrophic scars can be seen on the face, and neuropathy has been reported.[41]

With the cryotherapy procedure, no tissue is obtained for histologic examination. Since cryotherapy rarely destroys deep tissues, clinically suspected or biopsy-proven invasion into subcutaneous fat or deeper planes should be considered a relative contraindication.[41]

Patients with abnormal cold tolerance, cryoglobulinemia, autoimmune deficiency, or platelet deficiency should not be treated with cryotherapy.[41]

Comment
Cryotherapy is effective for treating minimally invasive SCC on the trunk or limbs. Caution is warranted when treating SCC on the face, particularly near vital structures that are susceptible to cold injury or distortion from scarring.

Photodynamic therapy
Photodynamic therapy (PDT) is a procedure in which a photosensitive topical compound is applied to the skin and the compound is activated by visible light. Upon activation, the compound releases reactive oxygen species, causing tissue destruction. This form of local treatment has proven effective for actinic keratoses[52] and therefore holds interest in the treatment of SCC *in situ*. While many photosensitizing compounds have been studied, aminolevulinic acid and methyl aminolevulinate (MAL; the ester of aminolevulinic acid) are the two agents currently in use. MAL is not currently approved in the United States. The light sources commonly used for activation include blue light, red light (not approved in the United States), and intense pulsed light (IPL).

Effectiveness
In 40 dermatology centers in 11 European countries, 225 patients with biopsy-proven SCC *in situ* and no evidence of progression to invasive SCC were randomly assigned to treatment with MAL-PDT (red light), placebo cream PDT (red light), cryotherapy, or topical fluorouracil.[53] They were examined 3 and 12 months after treatment for clinical

response as well as cosmetic outcome. At the 12-month clinical follow-up, MAL-PDT was found to be associated with an 80% rate of complete response in comparison with 67% for cryotherapy ($P = 0.047$) and 69% for fluorouracil ($P = 0.19$). In addition, MAL-PDT had a more acceptable cosmetic outcome, which was maintained for 12 months. On the basis of these preliminary data, MAL-PDT appears to be adequate for the treatment of SCC *in situ*, assuming that the patient is being seen regularly in follow-up to monitor for longer-term recurrences.

Drawbacks

Because tissue is not examined during or after treatment to evaluate for clear margins, insufficiently treated tumor is not noticed until the tumor recurs. The presence of foci of invasive SCC in the lesion may not be appreciated in the biopsy specimen, due to sampling error.

Comment

MAL-PDT is an interesting modality that may prove to be beneficial to patients, particularly those with multiple small SCC *in situ* tumors.

Radiotherapy

A wide variety of radioactive modalities and dosages have been used, with irradiation techniques being adapted to tumor characteristics such as location and size. Radiotherapy for SCC generally involves superficial external irradiation of the lesion and its margins. Uninvolved tissue is protected from radiation by the use of specially-fitted lead masks or shields as necessary. Several fractionated doses of radiation are delivered over the course of a few weeks; administration of radiation in a single or a few high-dose fractions is now less commonly used, due to the increased risk of radionecrosis.

Effectiveness

No standard protocols have been tested and generally adopted for radiotherapy for SCC, and no RCTs have examined the effectiveness of radiotherapy in comparison with other treatments for SCC. Several retrospective studies have examined the role of radiotherapy for SCC. Rowe *et al.*[54] analyzed the literature on SCC of the skin from 1940 to 1992 and found an average local recurrence rate of 10.0% after ≥ 5 years in 160 patients who had received radiotherapy for primary SCC. This was a higher recurrence rate than for ED&C (3.7% in 82 patients), surgical excision (8.1% in 124 patients), and MMS (3.1% in 2065 patients) ≥ 5 years after treatment. Several case studies in the radiation oncology literature have noted that increasing tumor size is associated with a progressively decreasing success rate in treating SCC with radiotherapy. Previous treatment is also a poor prognostic factor.[55–59]

Drawbacks

Radiotherapy usually requires multiple treatment sessions, which may make it less convenient for patients. Unlike other standard treatments for SCC, ionizing radiation causes a small increased risk of cutaneous carcinoma within the treatment field.[60] Atrophy, hypopigmentation, alopecia, and telangiectases are also commonly seen late cutaneous sequelae of radiotherapy, yielding an eventual suboptimal cosmetic outcome in spite of excellent early cosmesis.[61] These side effects make this modality of treatment for SCC less desirable for younger patients. Given the risk of radionecrosis, caution should also be exercised when considering radiotherapy for lesions overlying bone or cartilage.[62]

Comment

The main advantages of radiotherapy include preservation of perilesional normal tissue, and the tolerability of the treatment. Radiotherapy does not require anesthesia, and patients who are medically unable to tolerate or who refuse a surgical procedure may be able to undergo radiotherapy. Radiotherapy appears to be an effective treatment for SCC, particularly for small lesions that have not been previously treated. As tumor-free margins are not assessed during treatment, the treatment sites should be closely monitored at follow-up visits for possible recurrences.

Clinical implications

In considering the clinical scenario of a large perineural SCC on the temple of a middle-aged woman, the choice of treatment will largely depend on the geographic medical options for a particular patient, the surgeon's preference, convenience to the patient, and cost. Surgical excision has the advantage of producing a tissue specimen in which the margins can be evaluated histologically using formalin-embedded tissue-processing with special stains, and surgical repair would yield a much less obvious scar. ED&C and cryotherapy are comparatively time-efficient, but there is a lack of data on the disease-free survival in patients with a histologically high-risk SCC; the value of these methods is therefore more likely to involve the treatment of lesions that are less aggressive histologically and smaller in size clinically. MMS has the advantage that it provides horizontal sections that track the tumor along nerve branches, so that tumor can be cleared before surgical closure. Mohs micrographic surgery should be considered for this particular lesion because of its aggressive perineural spread seen on biopsy, its proximity to important functional and cosmetic structures in the face, and the technique's ability to achieve and document clear margins before a complex definitive repair.

Key points

- Risk factors for the recurrence of cutaneous SCCs are the treatment modality, size larger than 2 cm, depth greater than 4 mm, poor histological differentiation, location on the ear or mucosal areas, perineural involvement, location within scars or chronic inflammation, previously failed treatment, and immunosuppression.
- The evidence base for the treatment of cutaneous SCC is poor.
- None of the commonly used procedures has been tested in rigorous RCTs for invasive SCC.
- Case series that have followed up patients with cutaneous SCC treated by surgical excision, Mohs micrographic surgery, electrodesiccation and curettage, cryotherapy and radiotherapy all suggest 3–5-year recurrence rates of 10% or less. SCCs on the lip and ear recur more commonly.
- Comparison of the recurrence rates between the major commonly used treatments is almost impossible, as the choice of treatment is probably based on the likelihood of success (for example, only people with small uncomplicated SCCs are treated with destructive rather than excisional techniques).
- On the basis of the available case series, there is no evidence to suggest that any of the commonly used treatments for SCC are ineffective.
- Small thin tumors less than 2 cm in diameter in noncritical sites can probably be treated equally well by surgical excision with 4-mm margins, electrodesiccation and curettage, or cryotherapy.
- A prospective RCT comparing three destructive modalities in the treatment of SCC *in situ* suggests that photodynamic therapy using methyl aminolevulinate and red light is more effective at 12 months than cryotherapy or the application of topical fluorouracil.
- Larger tumors, especially at sites where tissue sparing becomes vital, or tumors at high risk for recurrence, are probably best treated with Mohs micrographic surgery.
- RCTs with adequate long-term follow-up are needed in order to inform clinicians about the relative merits of the various treatments currently used for people with SCC. Such trials will need to be large in order to exclude small but important differences, and they will need to accurately describe the sorts of people entered in terms of risk factors for recurrences. The follow-up period in such studies needs to be 5 years or longer.

References

1 Kirkham N. Tumors and cysts of the epidermis. In: Elder D, Eleritas R, Jaworsky C, Johnson B Jr, eds. *Lever's Histopathology of the Skin*. Philadelphia: Lippincott-Raven, 1997: 685–746.
2 Lohmann CM, Solomon AR. Clinicopathologic variants of cutaneous squamous cell carcinoma. *Adv Anat Pathol* 2001;**8**:27–36.
3 Barksdale SK, O'Connor N. Barnhill R. Prognostic factors for cutaneous squamous cell and basal cell carcinoma. Determinants of risk of recurrence, metastasis, and development of subsequent skin cancers. *Surg Oncol Clin North Am* 1997;**6**:625–38.
4 Preston DS, Stern RS. Nonmelanoma cancers of the skin. *N Engl J Med* 1992;**327**:1649–62.
5 Gray DT, Suman VJ, Siu WPD, et al. Trends in the population-based incidence of squamous cell carcinoma of the skin first diagnosed between 1984 and 1992. *Arch Dermatol* 1997;**133**:735–40.
6 Christenson LJ, Barrowman TA, Vachon CM, et al. Incidence of basal cell and squamous cell carcinoma in a population younger than 40 years. *JAMA* 2005;**294**: 681–90.
7 Staples MP, Elwood M, Burton RC, et al. Non-melanoma skin cancer in Australia: the 2002 national survey and trends since 1985. *Med J Aust* 2006;**184**:6–10.
8 Demers AA, Nugent Z, Mikhalcioiu C, et al. Trends of non-melanoma skin cancer from 1960 through 2000 in a Canadian population. *J Am Acad Dermatol* 2005;**53**:320–8.
9 Dinehart SM, Pollack SV. Metastases from squamous cell carcinoma of the skin and lip. An analysis of twenty-seven cases. *J Am Acad Dermatol* 1989;**21**:241–8.
10 Stenbeck KD, Balanda KP, Williams MJ, et al. Patterns of treated non-melanoma skin cancer in Queensland – the region with the highest incidence rates in the world. *Med J Aust* 1990;**153**:511–5.
11 Magnus K. The Nordic profile of skin cancer incidence. A comparative epidemiological study of the three main types of skin cancer. *Int J Cancer* 1991;**47**:12–9.
12 Marks R, Staples M, Giles GG. The incidence of non-melanocytic skin cancers in an Australian population: results of a five-year prospective study. *Med J Aust* 1989;**150**:475–8.
13 Giles GG, Marks P, Foley P. Incidence of non-melanocytic skin cancer treated in Australia. *BMJ Clin Res Ed* 1988;**296**:13–17.
14 Holt PJ. Cryotherapy for skin cancer: results over a 5-year period using liquid nitrogen spray cryosurgery. *Br J Dermatol* 1988;**119**: 231–40.
15 Scotto J, Kopf AW, Urbach F. Non-melanoma skin cancer among Caucasians in four areas of the United States. *Cancer* 1974;**34**: 1333–8.
16 Schreiber MM, Shapiro SL, Berry CZ, Dahlen RF, Friedman RP. The incidence of skin cancer in southern Arizona (Tucson). *Arch Dermatol* 1971;**104**:124–7.
17 Serrano H, Scotto J, Shornick G, Fears TR, Greenberg ER. Incidence of nonmelanoma skin cancer in New Hampshire and Vermont. *J Am Acad Dermatol* 1991;**24**:574–9.
18 Hemminki K, Zhang H, Czene K. Time trends and familial risks in squamous cell carcinoma of the skin. *Arch Dermatol* 2003;**139**: 885–9.
19 Johnson TM, Rowe DE, Nelson BR, Swanson NA. Squamous cell carcinoma of the skin (excluding lip and oral mucosa). *J Am Acad Dermatol* 1992;**26**:467–84.
20 Kwa RE, Campana K, Moy RL. Biology of cutaneous squamous cell carcinoma. *J Am Acad Dermatol* 1992;**26**:1–26.
21 Ziegler A, Jonason AS, Leffell DJ, et al. Sunburn and p53 in the onset of skin cancer. *Nature* 1994;**372**:773–6.
22 Taguchi M, Watarabe S, Yashima K, Murakami Y, Sekiya T, Ikeda S. Aberrations of the tumor suppressor p53 gene and p53 protein in solar keratosis in human skin. *J Invest Dermatol* 1994;**103**:500–3.
23 Campbell C, Quinn AG, Ro YS, Angus B, Rees JL. p53 mutations are common and early events that precede tumor invasion in squamous cell neoplasia of the skin. *J Invest Dermatol* 1993;**100**: 746–8.

24 Brash DE, Rudolf JA, Simon JA. A role for sunlight in skin cancer: UV-induced p53 mutations in squamous cell carcinoma. *Proc Natl Acad Sci USA* 1991;**88**:10124–8.

25 Robbins JH. Xeroderma pigmentosum. Defective DNA repair causes skin cancer and neurodegeneration. *JAMA* 1988;**260**:384–8.

26 Hartevelt MM, Bavinck JN, Kootte AM, Vermeer BJ, Vandenbrouke JP. Incidence of skin cancer after renal transplantation in the Netherlands. *Transplantation* 1990;**49**:506–9.

27 Liddington M, Richardson AJ, Higgins RM, *et al.* Skin cancer in renal transplant recipients. *Br J Surg* 1989;**76**:1002–5.

28 Boyle J, Mackie RM, Brigs JD, Junior BS, Aitchison TC. Cancer, warts and sunshine in renal transplant patients. A case–control study. *Lancet* 1984;**i**:702–5.

29 Dinehart SM, Chu DZ, Mahers AW, Pollack SV. Immunosuppression in patients with metastatic squamous cell carcinoma from the skin. *J Dermatol Surg Oncol* 1990;**16**:271–4.

30 Vajdic CM, McDonald SP, McCredie MR, *et al.* Cancer incidence before and after kidney transplantation. *JAMA* 2006;**296**:2823–31.

31 Otley CC, Maragh SL. Reduction of immunosuppression for transplant-associated skin cancer: rationale and evidence of efficacy. *Dermatol Surg* 2005;**31**:163–8.

32 Rowe DE, Carroll RJ, Day CL Jr. Prognostic factors for local recurrence, metastasis, and survival rates in squamous cell carcinoma of the skin, ear, and lip. Implications for treatment modality selection. *J Am Acad Dermatol* 1992;**26**:976–90.

33 Immerman SC, Scanlon EF, Christ M, *et al.* Recurrent squamous cell carcinoma of the skin. *Cancer* 1983;**51**:1537–49.

34 Motley R, Kersey P, Lawrence C. Multiprofessional guidelines for the management of the patient with primary cutaneous squamous cell carcinoma. *Br J Dermatol* 2002;**146**:18–25.

35 Drake LA, Dinehart SM, Goltz RW, *et al.* Guidelines of care for Mohs micrographic surgery. *J Am Acad Dermatol* 1995;**33**:271–8.

36 Freeman RG, Knox JM, Heaton CL. The treatment of skin cancer: a statistical study of 1341 skin tumor comparing results obtained with irradiation, surgery, and curettage followed by electrodesiccation. *Cancer* 1964;**17**:535–8.

37 Brodiand DG, Zitelli JA. Surgical margins for excision of primary cutaneous squamous cell carcinoma. *J Am Acad Dermatol* 1992;**27**:241–8.

38 Cook J, Zitelli JA. Mohs micrographic surgery: a cost analysis. *J Am Acad Dermatol* 1998;**39**:698–703.

39 Mohs FE. Chemosurgery: microscopically controlled surgery for skin cancer. Springfield, IL: Thomas, 1978.

40 Holmkvist KA, Roenigk RK. Squamous cell carcinoma of the lip treated with Mohs micrographic surgery: outcome at 5 years. *J Am Acad Dermatol* 1998;**38**:960–6.

41 Lawrence N, Cottel W. Squamous cell carcinoma of skin with perineural invasion. *J Am Acad Dermatol* 1994;**31**:30–3.

42 Goepfert H, Dichtel WJ, Medina JE, Lindberg RD, Lura MD. Perineural invasion in squamous cell carcinoma of the head and neck. *Am J Surg* 1984;**148**:542–7.

43 Ballantyne AJ, McCarten AB, Ibanez ML. The extension of cancer of the head and neck through peripheral nerves. *Am J Surg* 1963;**106**:651–67.

44 Kimayai-Asadi A, Goldberg LH, Peterson SR, *et al.* The incidence of major complications form Mohs micrographic surgery

performed in office-based and hospital-based settings. *J Am Acad Dermatol* 2005;**53**:628–34.

45 Cook JL, Perone JB. A prospective evaluation of the incidence of complications associated with Mohs micrographic surgery. *Arch Dermatol* 2003;**139**:143–52.

46 Knox JM, Lyles TW, Shapiro EM, Martin RD. Curettage and electrodesiccation in the treatment of skin cancer. *Arch Dermatol* 1960;**82**:197–204.

47 Honeycutt WM, Jansen GT. Treatment of squamous cell carcinoma of the skin. *Arch Dermatol* 1973;**108**:670–2.

48 Whelan CS, Deckers PJ. Electrocoagulation for skin cancer: an old oncologic tool revisited. *Cancer* 1981;**47**:2280–7.

49 Whelan CS, Deckers PJ. Electrocoagulation and curettage for carcinoma involving the skin of the face, nose, eyelids, and ears. *Cancer* 1973;**31**:159–64.

50 Zacarian SA. Cryosurgery of cutaneous carcinomas. An 18-year study of 3022 patients with 4228 carcinomas. *J Am Acad Dermatol* 1983;**9**:947–56.

51 Kuflik EG, Gage AA. The five-year cure rate achieved by cryosurgery for skin cancer. *J Am Acad Dermatol* 1991;**24**:1002–4.

52 Freeman M, Vinciullo C, Francis D, *et al.* A comparison of photodynamic therapy using topical methyl aminolevulinate (Metvix) with single cycle cryotherapy in patients with actinic keratosis: a prospective, randomized study. *J Dermatolog Treat* 2003;**14**:99–106.

53 Morton C, Horn M, Leman J, *et al.* Comparison of topical methyl aminolevulinate photodynamic therapy with +cryotherapy or fluorouracil for treatment of squamous cell carcinoma *in situ*: results of a multicenter randomized trial. *Arch Dermatol* 2006;**142**:729–35.

54 Rowe DE, Carroll RJ, Day CL. Prognostic factors for local recurrence, metastasis, and survival rates in squamous cell carcinoma of the skin, ear, and lip. *J Am Acad Dermatol* 1992;**26**:976–90.

55 Petrovich Z, Parker RG, Luxton G, Kuisk H, Jepson J. Carcinoma of the lip and selected sites of head and neck skin. A clinical study of 896 patients. *Radiother Oncol* 1987;**8**:11–7.

56 Mazeron JJ, Chassagne D, Crook J, *et al.* Radiation therapy of carcinomas of the skin of nose and nasal vestibule: a report of 1676 cases by the Groupe Européen de Curiethérapie. *Radiother Oncol* 1989;**13**;165–73.

57 Lovett RD, Perez CA, Shapiro SJ, Garcia DM. External irradiation of epithelial skin cancer. *Int J Radiation Oncology Biol Phys* 1990;**19**:235–42.

58 Silva JJ, Tsang RW, Panzarella T, Levin W, Wells W. Results of radiotherapy for epithelial skin cancer of the pinna: the Princess Margaret Hospital Experience, 1982–1993. *Int J Radiation Oncology Biol Phys* 2000;**47**:451–9.

59 Locke J, Karimpour S, Young G, Lockett MA, Perez CA. Radiotherapy for epithelial skin cancer. *Int J Radiation Oncology Biol Phys* 2001;**51**:748–55.

60 Karagas MR, McDonald JA, Greenberg R, *et al.* Risk of basal cell and squamous cell skin cancers after ionizing radiation therapy. *J Natl Cancer Inst* 1996;**88**:1848–53.

61 Morrison WH, Garden AS, Ang KK. Radiation therapy for nonmelanoma skin carcinomas. *Clin Plast Surg* 1997;**24**:719–29.

62 Goldman GD. Squamous cell cancer: a practical approach. *Semin Cutan Med Surg* 1998;**17**:80–95.

29 Basal cell carcinoma

Fiona Bath-Hextall, William Perkins

Background

Definition

Basal cell carcinoma (BCC) is defined as a slow-growing, locally invasive malignant epidermal skin tumor, which mainly affects Caucasians.[1]

Incidence/prevalence

BCC (or rodent ulcer) is the most common malignant cutaneous neoplasm found in humans.[1–3] For example, over 30,000 new cases are reported each year in the UK. This is likely to be an underestimate, because of inconsistencies in registration of BCCs at regional cancer registries.[4] Many registries only register a person's first skin cancer, thus further underestimating the real burden of the problem (Figures 29.1–29.3).

The tumor may occur at any age, but the incidence of BCC increases markedly after the age of 40. The incidence of

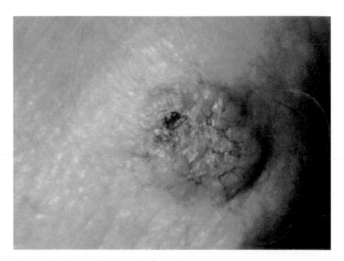

Figure 29.2 A nodular basal cell carcinoma.

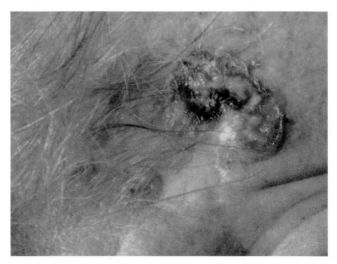

Figure 29.3 A morpheic basal cell carcinoma.

BCC appears to be increasing in younger people, probably as a result of increased sun exposure.[5–7] The incidence rate (standardized using the European standard population) for new BCCs in the Trent Cancer Registry (UK) increased

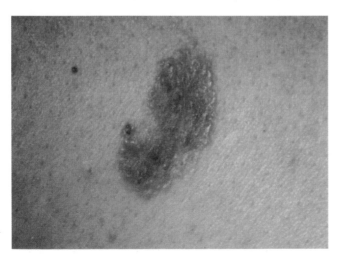

Figure 29.1 Superficial basal cell carcinoma (BCC).

from 41.5 in 1985 to 86.7 in 2003 for men, and from 30.2 to 63.6 in 2003 for women (Trent Cancer Registry, written communication, February 2006). A total of 4812 new BCCs were registered in Trent in 2003 (80% of all nonmelanoma skin cancers). A sustained rise in the incidence of BCC has been documented using a validated register in South Wales, UK.[8] Reliable national figures for BCC incidence are impossible to obtain, because some cancer registries in the UK do not register BCCs. In the USA, the incidence of BCC has doubled approximately every 14 years,[9] and similar changes have occurred in Australia.[10]

Etiology

Eighty-five percent of all BCCs appear on the head and neck region.[11,12] Risk factors are fair skin, tendency to freckle,[13] degree of sun exposure,[14–16] excessive sun-bed use, radiotherapy, phototherapy, male sex, and a genetic predisposition.[17] Nevoid BCC syndrome (Gorlin syndrome) is an autosomal-dominantly inherited condition characterized by developmental abnormalities and the occurrence of multiple BCCs. Mutations in patients with nevoid BCC syndrome have been found on the patched gene located on chromosome 9, which appears to be crucial for proper embryonic development and for tumor suppression.[18]

Clinical patterns

As Figures 29.1–29.3 show, clinical appearances and morphology for BCC are diverse. They include nodular, cystic, ulcerated (rodent ulcer), superficial, morpheic (scarring), keratotic, and pigmented variants. Nodular BCC is the most common type (60%) in the UK. However, in other countries such as Australia, superficial BCC is the most common type.[19] Eighty-five percent of all BCCs appear on the head and neck region,[11,12] visible areas where a good cosmetic and functional result is important.

Prognosis

Growth of BCC is a localized phenomenon in people with a competent immune system. BCCs tend to infiltrate surrounding tissues in a three-dimensional fashion through the irregular extension of finger-like outgrowths, which may not be apparent clinically.[3,20] If left untreated, or if inadequately treated, the BCC can cause extensive local tissue destruction, particularly on the face. Neglected cases may even infiltrate bone and deeper structures such as the brain and cause death.[21] Death from BCC is extremely rare, but may occur in neglected cases and/or those with major underlying immunosuppression. The clinical course of BCC is unpredictable. A BCC can remain small for years with little tendency to grow, it may grow rapidly, or it may proceed by successive spurts of extension of tumor and partial

regression.[22] Histological subtype (infiltrative, micronodular or morpheic patterns), initial diameter, and male sex have been shown to be the best independent predictors of BCC invasion.[23] It is unknown whether the phenotypic characteristics of people who present with clusters of BCCs or those who develop BCCs on truncal sites are also associated with increased growth once a BCC has established.

Diagnostic tests

The diagnosis is usually made clinically, with histological confirmation being made at the time of the intended definitive treatment—often surgical removal. Diagnostic biopsies are usually performed before treatments such as radiotherapy.

Aims of treatment

The three fundamental principles of treatment are to:
- Eradicate the tumor
- Preserve function
- Produce an excellent or acceptable cosmetic result

From a patient's perspective, the treatment should result in as little distress as possible in terms of pain, number of hospital visits, and scarring. From a health provider's perspective, it is important to balance efficacy against cost.

Relevant outcomes

- Clearance of the lesion, as measured by absence of early treatment failure (within 6 months) and absence of long-term recurrence of the lesion measured at 3–5 years
- Adverse effects in terms of atrophy, scarring, changes in pigmentation, and discomfort to the patient in terms of pain during treatment and afterwards

Search methods

The following databases were searched up to the end of February 2006:
- Medline from 1966
- Embase from 1980
- Bath Information and Data Services/Institute for Scientific Information (BIDS-ISI; Science Citation Index from 1981)
- The Cochrane Skin Group Specialized Trials Register
- The Cochrane Library, Cochrane Database of Systematic Reviews, and Cochrane Central Register of Controlled Trials
- Mega Register of Controlled Trials on the Current Controlled Trials web site and the National Research Register's Medical Research Council (MRC) Clinical Trials Directory

The search strategy used to locate randomized controlled trials (RCTs) included search terms 1–29 as given in the *Cochrane Reviewers' Handbook*,[24] Appendix 5b.2. Search terms included: BCC, basal cell carcinoma, basal cell cancer, nodular BCC, nevoid BCC, Gorlin syndrome, rodent ulcer, Jacob's ulcer, basal cell epithelioma, basalioma, and non-melanoma skin cancer (NMSC), including squamous cell carcinoma and BCC.

Pharmaceutical companies were contacted when appropriate for reviews or unpublished trials.

Prevention of skin cancer is discussed in Chapter 25.

Questions: What are the effective therapeutic interventions for BCC of the skin? How do the therapeutic interventions for BCC compare with each other? How do the cosmetic outcomes for these interventions compare? Are these interventions cost-effective?

The first-line treatment of BCC is often surgical excision. Numerous alternatives are available, including: curettage, cryosurgery, laser, excision with predetermined margins, excision under frozen-section control, Mohs micrographic surgery (the use of horizontal frozen sections and mapping to determine tumor clearance), radiotherapy, topical therapy, intralesional therapy, photodynamic therapy (PDT; the application of a cream to induce photodamage to the tumor using various light sources), immunomodulators (agents used to stimulate the immune system and work on eradicating the tumor), and chemotherapy. Surgical treatment requires access to a minor operating room, and most other treatments are carried out in specialist centers. Although there is wide variety in the treatment modalities used in the management of BCC, and the vast majority of the tumors are probably treated successfully, little research is available that accurately compares these different treatment modalities. The evidence cited in the following summaries refers to randomized controlled trials (RCTs) unless specified otherwise.

Surgical excision

Despite the fact that surgical excision is probably the most frequent treatment, only two RCTs were found that compared surgical excision with a predetermined margin with other interventions.[25,26] There are, however, large case series that demonstrate excellent "success" rates for this modality.[27]

No RCTs have investigated the margin of excision that would be effective in the removal of BCC by surgical excision with predetermined margins. Proxy measures based on Mohs micrographic surgical margins required to remove BCCs, and histopathological studies of excised specimens, have suggested that for small nodular or superficial BCC, a 4-mm margin of normal skin will clear 95% of tumors.[20,28]

Larger margins are required for tumors greater than 20 mm and for morpheic tumors.[20]

Surgery versus photodynamic therapy

One RCT of 103 patients compared surgical excision versus methyl aminolevulinate (MAL) PDT in primary nodular BCC of the face.[25] As shown in Table 29.1, the primary outcome was early treatment failure at 3 months. Secondary end points were sustained response rate at 12 months and cosmetic results at 3 and 12 months.

Efficacy

The response at 3 months was 98% for surgery versus 91% for PDT, difference 4.8% (95% CI, −3.4% to 13%). Response at 12 months was 96% for surgery versus 83% for PDT ($P = 0.15$). The cosmetic outcome was significantly better at 12 and 24 months on the patients' assessment and at 3, 12, and 24 months on investigator evaluation ($P < 0.001$).

Potential drawbacks

Significantly more patients treated with MAL PDT compared to those treated with surgery reported adverse events (52% versus 29%; $P = 0.03$). Most of the adverse events were transient local reactions commonly associated with PDT, such as a burning sensation on the skin, pain in the skin, or erythema.

Comments

Concealment of allocation was clear, but the analysis was per-protocol. Lesions with an incomplete response to PDT at 3 months received a second treatment cycle and were evaluated 3 months later.

Implications for clinical practice

There is a trend toward higher recurrence rates with PDT in comparison with surgery, and significantly more patients reported adverse events in the PDT group. However, PDT may be preferred for its cosmetic results.

Surgical excision with frozen-section margin control

One RCT of 347 patients compared surgical excision with frozen-section margin control to radiotherapy in primary BCC less than 40 mm in diameter on the face.[29] As shown in Table 29.1, the main outcome measure was persistent or recurrent disease at 4 years. The secondary end point was the cosmetic result assessed by the patient, the dermatologist, and three persons not involved in the trial.

Efficacy

The 4-year failure rate was 0.7% (95% CI, 0.1% to 3.9%) in the surgery group and 7.5% (95% CI, 4.2% to 13.1%) in the radiotherapy group. Cosmetic outcome as assessed by five observers over the 4 years of the study consistently favored surgery.[30] At 4 years, the 87% of patients assessed

Table 29.1 Randomized controlled trials evaluating surgical excision in the treatment of basal cell carcinoma

Study	Method	Participants	Interventions	Outcomes	Notes
Avril et al. 1997[29] (France)	Single center Randomization by sequential sealed envelopes ITT	HP BCCs T1: 174, T2: 173 patients Histological type T1: 79 N, 52 ulcerated, 36 S and pagetoid, 7 sclerosing; T2: 74 N, 50 ulcerated, 41 S and pagetoid, 8 sclerosing Location T1: 53 nose, 36 eyelids, 36 forehead, 10 chin, 5 ear; T2: 49 nose, 42 cheek, 35 eyelids, 29 forehead, 12 chin, 6 ear	T1: surgery—resection of whole tumor with a free margin of at least 2 mm from visible borders; T2: radiotherapy—interstitial brachytherapy, superficial contract therapy or conventional therapy, chosen by radiotherapist according to tumor parameters and location and patient characteristics	FU: 3, 6, 12 months after end of treatment; then yearly until fourth year Rate of histologically confirmed persistent tumor or recurrence after 4 years Patients examined by dermatologists; photographs of scar taken at three standardized distances	Ex: BCC on scalp or neck, patients who had total removal of BCC at biopsy, with 5 or more BCCs, life expectancy < 3 years
Smeets et al. 2004[26] (Netherlands)	Multicenter, telephone randomization	HP primary or recurrent BCC, 1 cm diameter, high risk or aggressive histo-pathological subtype. Primary T1: 198, T2: 199; recurrent T1: 102, T2: 102 patients	T1: MMS, T2: surgery	FU: recurrence at 18 and 30 months	ITT analysis
Rhodes et al. 2004[25] (UK)	Multicenter, phone/fax randomization	HP, N BCC, T1: 52, T2: 49 patients (110 lesions)	T1: MAL-PDT (75 J/cm^2 red light (570–670 nm), T2: surgery (with 5 mm margin)	FU: clinical clearance at 3, 12 months after treatment. Cosmetic outcome at 3, 12 months. Cosmesis and lesion recurrence at 24 months	Ex: high-risk BCC on face. 24% of lesions were re-treated. Analysis PP.

BCC, basal cell carcinoma; Ex, exclusion; FU, follow-up; HP, histologically proven; ITT, intention to treat; MAL-PDT, methyl aminolevulinate photodynamic therapy; MMS, Mohs micrographic surgery; N, nodular; PP, per protocol; S, superficial.

their cosmetic results as good after surgery and 69% after radiotherapy.

Potential drawbacks
After radiotherapy, dyspigmentations and telangiectasia developed in more than 65% of the patients at 4 years. Radiodystrophy affected 41% of the patients at 4 years.

Comment
Concealment of allocation was clear and the paper showed evidence of an *a priori* sample size calculation; however, the analysis was conducted on a per-protocol basis. Several previous studies have reported good cure rates and cosmetic results with surgery and radiotherapy; however, the above study was the first randomized trial giving an unbiased comparison of the two treatments.

Implications for practice
The trial shows that the failure rate was significantly lower in surgery than in radiotherapy for the treatment of BCC of

the face for lesions less than 4 cm in diameter. Surgery may also be preferred for its cosmetic result.

Mohs micrographic surgery (MMS)
Mohs micrographic surgery is a technique in which 100% of the surgical margin is examined by mapping horizontal frozen sections from successive excision layers until clearance is achieved. A large case series with 5-year follow-up suggested that this modality has the highest cure rates for all types of BCC 0.5–1.3%, depending on site.[31] One RCT compared Mohs micrographic surgery with conventional surgical excision for high-risk BCCs of the face.[26]

Surgical excision versus Mohs micrographic surgery
One RCT[26] of 374 patients with 408 primary lesions and 204 patients with 191 recurrent lesions compared MMS with surgery. As shown in Table 29.1, the primary outcome was recurrence and the secondary outcome was incomplete excision, suboptimal aesthetic results, and excessive costs of treatment.

Efficacy

Primary BCC. Recurrence at 30 months did not differ significantly between the groups—five of 171 (3%) in standard excision versus three of 160 (2%) for MMS (difference 1%, 95% CI, –2.5% to 3.7%; $P = 0.724$).

Recurrent BCC. Recurrence at 18 months did not differ significantly between the groups—three of 93 (3%) in standard excision versus none of 95 after MMS (difference 3.2%, 95% CI, –2.0% to 5%; $P = 0.119$). The overall aesthetic outcome did not differ significantly between MMS and standard excision. Primary BCCs had a significantly better aesthetic outcome than recurrent BCCs ($P = 0.038$), and cosmetic results became significantly poorer with increasing defect size for both primary ($r = 0.383$, $P < 0.001$) and recurrent BCCs ($r = 0.351$, $P = 0.001$). Total operative costs for both primary and recurrent BCCs are higher for MMS than standard excision ($P < 0.001$).

Potential drawbacks

Thirty-one primary BCCs (18%) and 31 recurrent BCCs (32%) were incompletely excised on first excision in the standard excision group. Primary tumors with aggressive histopathology were significantly more likely to be incompletely excised than those of the nonaggressive type. No adverse events were reported.

Comments

Concealment of allocation was clear, and an intention-to-treat analysis was used.

It was suggested that the groups might not have been large enough for a significant difference to be detected. This study used 3-mm margins for both treatments to standardize the two treatment modalities (smaller margins are usually used for MMS). If standard excision was incomplete, a reexcision with a 3-mm margin was done. If the margins remained positive after the second excision, then MMS was undertaken.

Implications for practice

This is the only RCT comparing MMS with surgical excision for patients with high-risk facial BCCs. Treatment with MMS slightly, but not significantly, lowered the recurrence rate for both primary and recurrent BCCs in comparison with surgical excision. Five-year follow-up data are needed to determine definite recurrence rates in both groups. Almost a quarter of all aggressive carcinomas of 1 cm or more in diameter and about a third of all recurrent carcinomas were incompletely excised with a 3-mm margin, and therefore MMS may well be preferable to use for these tumors to avoid larger defects, poor aesthetic outcome, and functional problems.

One further RCT found that preoperative tumor curettage in Mohs was associated with an increase in wound size.[32]

Cryotherapy

Three RCTs were found and are summarized in Table 29.2.

Cryotherapy versus radiotherapy

One study of 93 patients compared radiotherapy with cryotherapy for primary BCC, excluding lesions on the nose or pinna.[33] The aims of the study were to compare the control of the tumors with the two treatments, to assess the final cosmetic result, and to compare the discomfort and inconvenience experienced by the patient. Cryotherapy consisted of two freeze–thaw cycles, freezing for 1 minute each time.

Efficacy

Recurrence rates at 1 year were 4% (two of 49) in the radiotherapy group and 39% (17 of 44) in the cryotherapy group. At 2 years, no further tumors had recurred in either group. The cosmetic results for the two modes of treatment were not significantly different.

Potential drawbacks

The degree of pain, discomfort, discharge, and bleeding from the treated areas was the same in both groups. Only one patient from each group was seriously inconvenienced by the treatment. Hypopigmentation was more common than hyperpigmentation with both modes of treatment (81% of those in the radiotherapy group and 88% of those in the cryotherapy group). Seven patients treated with radiotherapy developed some radiation telangiectasia. Hypopigmentation and telangiectasia tend to be lifelong. Five patients treated with cryotherapy developed milia, which all disappeared by 1 year.

Comments

The concealment of allocation was unclear, and the analysis was conducted on a per-protocol basis. There was no indication of the type of lesion.

Implication for clinical practice

Cryotherapy, although convenient and less expensive than radiotherapy, does not appear to have better cure rates than radiotherapy (especially for lesions > 2 cm). Cosmetic effects for radiotherapy and cryotherapy are comparable. Variations in technique occur between different physicians and may account for differences in outcome. Lesions larger than 2 cm in diameter treated by cryotherapy recurred, but lesions larger than 2 cm and treated with radiotherapy were controlled. It was concluded that cryotherapy does not offer a satisfactory alternative to radiotherapy in the treatment of BCC.

Cryotherapy: varying number of freeze–thaw cycles

In a second RCT of 84 patients, one freeze–thaw cycle of 30 seconds was compared with two freeze–thaw cycles of 30 seconds for low-risk facial BCCs.[34]

Table 29.2 Randomized controlled trials evaluating cryotherapy in the treatment of basal cell carcinoma

Study	Method	Participants	Interventions	Outcomes	Notes
Hall et al. 1986[33] (UK)	Single center Method of randomization not known, PP	105 patients BP BCCs T1: 44, T2: 49 patients Sites: T1: 30 neck and face, 6 eyelids, 8 trunk. T2: 40 neck and face, 3 eyelids, 6 trunk	T1: cryotherapy using a Cry-Owen liquid nitrogen spray gun; all lesions treated with two freeze–thaw cycles, freezing for 1 min each time, with a thaw time of at least 90 s T2: radiotherapy, (130 KV X-rays)	FU: recurrence of tumor and cosmetic appearance at 1, 6, 12, 24 months after treatment Tumor identified histologically	12 excluded: 5 died of other causes, 7 lost to FU Ex: recurrent tumors, lesions on nose or pinna, lesion near eye and vision in eye < 6/18
Mallon and Dawber, 1996[34] (UK)	Single center Method of randomization not known, PP	84 patients Mostly clinically proven BCCs Facial lesions ≤ 1.5 cm not extending > 3 mm below skin were included. T1: 36, T2: 48 patients Mean age T1: 67, T2: 69 years	T1: single 30-s freeze–thaw cycle T2: double 30-s freeze–thaw cycle	FU: T1: 10 months to 7.1 years, T2: 1.2– 6.1 years Lesions assessed clinically	7 lost to FU, T1: 2, T2: 5
Thissen et al. 2000[35] (Netherlands)	Single center Method of randomization not known, PP	103 patients Some BP BCCs Lesions S or N, < 2 cm diameter, localized anywhere on the head and neck	T1: surgery T2: cryosurgery (no. 3 curette used to debulk the tumor; no. 1 used to remove remainder of BCC around the borders. Freezing: two freezing periods, each lasting 20 s)	FU: cosmetic and recurrence at 1 year Recurrence assessed clinically	Lost to FU: 3 in control group did not turn up for visits, 1 died (unrelated to treatment), 3 developed recurrent BCC (all T2)

BCC, basal cell carcinoma; BP, biopsy-proven; Ex, exclusion; FU, follow-up; HP, histologically proven; N, nodular; PP, per protocol; S, superficial.

Efficacy

Recurrence rates were significant: 4.7% with two freeze–thaw cycles and 20.6% with one cycle after a median of 18 months.

Potential drawbacks

No mention was made of adverse effects of the treatment.

Comments

Concealment of allocation was unclear, and the analysis was conducted on a per-protocol basis. Only common facial lesions of 1.5 cm or less were included, and not all of the lesions were biopsied. Variations in technique between different physicians may account for differences in outcome.

Implications for clinical practice

Facial lesions require a double freeze–thaw cycle with liquid nitrogen if the high cure rates in many reports of formal excision or radiotherapy are to be achieved. Although case series suggest that higher clearance rates can be achieved, particularly with low-risk tumors, more prospective evidence is required.

Cryotherapy versus surgical excision

A third RCT of 96 patients[35] compared cryosurgery with surgical excision for BCC of the head and neck. The primary outcome was the cosmetic result, but recurrence rates in both groups were also compared. Recurrences were treated by surgical excision. Cosmetic results were judged by five independent professional observers and by the patients.

Efficacy

The recurrence rate for cryosurgery was three of 48 at 1 year, whereas in the surgery group no recurrences developed at 1 year. The cosmetic results after surgical excision generally received a significantly better evaluation in comparison with cryosurgery for superficial and nodular subtypes localized in the head/neck region.

Comments

Concealment of allocation was unclear. The analysis was conducted on a per-protocol basis, although the paper showed evidence of an *a priori* sample size calculation.

Potential drawbacks

Two patients (4%) developed secondary wound infections in the first and second week after surgery, for which systemic antibiotics were given. Ninety percent of the patients in the cryotherapy group complained of moderate to severe swelling of the treated area, followed by long-lasting leakage of exudates from the defect. After cryotherapy, three patients (6%) had secondary wound infection, for which systemic antibiotics were given.

Implications for clinical practice

Surgical excision for nodular and superficial lesions smaller than 2 cm is cosmetically more acceptable than cryosurgery. Cryotherapy does not appear to be a satisfactory alternative to surgery for superficial or nodular lesions in the head and neck area of less than 2 cm in diameter.

Photodynamic therapy (PDT)

PDT is a nonionizing radiation treatment modality under development. It uses the interaction between visible light and tumor-sensitizing agents to generate cell death.

Comparison of PDT with surgery has already been discussed above in the section on surgical excision.

MAL-PDT versus placebo

Two smaller RCTs and published in abstract form only at the time of writing, with short follow-up periods of just 3 and 6 months, compared MAL-PDT with placebo,[36,37] and these are summarized in Table 29.3. Both studies found that the cosmetic outcome was better for MAL-PDT. Full results are awaited.

PDT versus cryotherapy

One RCT of 88 patients compared PDT with cryotherapy with two freeze–thaw cycles for BCC.[38] There was no significant difference in recurrence rates at 12 months, and both were quite high. Histological recurrence rates at 1 year were 25% (11 of 44) in the PDT group, compared with 15% (six of 39) in the cryotherapy group, despite multiple re-treatments in the PDT group. Scarring and tissue defects scored significantly better following PDT.

A second study (in abstract form only) of 118 patients[39] compared MAL-PDT for superficial BCC. Recurrence at 1 year was 8% (eight of 97) in the PDT group, compared with 16% (15 of 91) in the cryotherapy group. At 36 months, the estimated complete response rate was 74% for both groups. The cosmetic outcome was substantially better for MAL-PDT (89%) than cryotherapy (63%).

Potential drawbacks

In the first study, more patients indicated pain and discomfort during and after treatment with PDT, but the differences were not statistically significant.

Comments

For the first study, concealment of allocation was clear. For both studies, the analysis was conducted on a per-protocol basis and no sample size calculation was given. It was not clear in the second study whether recurrence was histologically verified.

Implications for clinical practice

Although tolerability for patients was greater and cosmetic outcomes were considered better in the PDT group, the published efficacy data to date do not support the introduction of PDT for the treatment of BCC. We could not find any published RCTs comparing PDT with standard therapy (excisional surgery). Further studies demonstrating greater efficacy are needed, and follow-up periods for outcome assessment should be 3–5 years.

Laser versus broadband halogen light

Another RCT[40] of 83 patients compared the clinical and cosmetic outcome of superficial BCCs using either laser or broadband halogen light in PDT with topical 5-aminolevulinic acid (ALA).

Efficacy

At the end of the study (6 months), 86% in the laser group and 82% in the broadband halogen group were evaluated as having complete responses by both investigators. The study showed no significant differences in the cure rate ($P = 0.49$, 95% CI, -7% to 14%) or cosmetic outcome ($P = 0.075$) between light exposure from a simple broad lamp with continuous spectrum (570–740 nm) or from a red-light laser (monochromatic 630 nm).

Potential drawbacks

Eighty-three percent of patients receiving PDT with laser light and 76% of those receiving PDT with broadband halogen light reported some discomfort during and after illumination. Sixty-eight percent of the patients who received laser light and 74% of the patients who received broadband halogen light reported some degree of discomfort (stinging, itching, pain, headache, sensation of warmth, or blushing) during the first week of treatment. No serious adverse events were reported during the 6-month follow-up.

Comments

Although 83 patients were involved, 245 superficial BCCs were included in the study, indicating more than one lesion per patient. Concealment of allocation was clear and analysis

Table 29.3 Randomized controlled trials evaluating photodynamic therapy in the treatment of basal cell carcinoma

Study	Method	Participants	Interventions	Outcomes	Notes
Wang et al. 2001[38] (Sweden)	Single center Randomized according to a stratified randomization pattern in blocks of 10 patients, PP	HP BCC 44 women; 44 men; age range 42–88 years Type: T1: 22 S, 25 N; T2: 17 S, 24 N Distribution: 47 trunk, 25 head and neck, 10 legs, 6 arms	T1: PDT (20% weight-based ALA/water-in-oil cream applied to lesion; irradiation 6 h later. T2: cryosurgery (2 freeze–thaw cycles)	FU: 1, 4, 8 weeks, 3 months after treatment Last FU 12 months after first treatment Punch biopsy at 3 and 12 months	Ex: BCC on nose; M growth; porphyria; abdominal pain of unknown etiology; photosensitivity; treatment of BCC with topical steroids type III or IV within the last month
Soler et al. 2000[40] (Norway)	Single center Randomization numbers in locked envelopes. The patients were randomly allocated on the treatment day to one of the two arms in blocks of four patients, ITT	HP BCC 83 patients 245 lesions	All lesions in both groups topical 20% ALA, removed after 3 h and light source applied: T1: laser light (630 nm); T2: broadband light	FU: 3, 6 months after treatment Outcomes: complete, partial, or no response; cosmetic outcome and pain intensity during treatment and FU	
Foley 2003[37] (Australian)	Method of randomization not given	N BCC, n = 66	T1: MAL-PDT, T2: placebo	FU: 3 months	Abstract
Tope 2005[36] (US)	Multicenter; method of randomization not given	N BCC, 65 patients (80 lesions)	T1: MAL-PDT; T2: placebo	FU: 3, 6 months	Abstract
Lui 2004[42] (Canada)	Multicenter Method of randomization not given	54 patients (421 BP N or S BCC or Bowen disease) Age range 22–79 y, mean 55	Single i.v. infusion of 14 mg/m^2 of verteporfin followed 1–3 h later by 60, 120 or 180 J/cm^2	FU: 6 months (biopsy-proven)	7 patients (51 tumors) lost to FU. Analysis PP
Basset-Seguin 2003[39] (European)	Multicenter, open randomized study. Method of randomization not given. Analysis PP	118 patients (219 lesions) with S BCCs. T1: 60, T2: 58 patients. T1: gentle removal of surface prior to PDT	T1: MAL-PDT; T2: cryo (double freeze–thaw)	FU: 3, 12, 36 months	Abstract

ALA, aminolevulinic acid; BCC, basal cell carcinoma; BP, biopsy-proven; Ex, exclusion; FU, follow-up; HP, histologically proven; ITT, intention to treat; M, morphea-like; MAL-PDT, methyl aminolevulinate photodynamic therapy; MMS, Mohs micrographic surgery; N, nodular; PDT, photodynamic therapy; PP, per protocol; S, superficial.

was carried out on an intention-to-treat basis; however, no sample size calculation was included.

A further ongoing randomized trial aims to compare the efficacy of 5-ALA PDT following minimal debulking curettage with surgery for low-risk nodular BCCs and to compare the pain and morbidity experienced by patients undergoing each procedure.[41]

Implications for practice
The results show that topical ALA-based PDT with a broad-band halogen light source gives short-term (6 months) cure rates and a cosmetic outcome similar to those obtained with a laser light source, although both are considerably inferior to excisional surgery. Reduced costs, increased safety, as well as the possibility of general use by dermatologists, are other elements in favor of the lamp as a suitable light source.

Verteporfin and red light—a dose-ranging study
One RCT[42] compared three different light doses in 54 patients with 421 multiple BCCs and found a dose response for histological clearance 6 months after treatment (nodular BCC 76–100% and superficial BCC 63–97%) (Table 29.3).

Implications for practice
There is a need for long-term follow-up in order to identify the correct light dose, balancing response and cosmetic appearance.

Intralesional interferon therapy

Interferons are naturally occurring glycoproteins that exhibit antiviral, antitumor, and immunomodulatory activities. Four RCTs were found (Table 29.4).

Interferon alfa-2a and/or 2b
Efficacy

In the first trial,[43] 45 patients were randomly assigned to receive 15 or 30 million units of interferon alfa-2a, -2b or both interferon alfa-2a and -2b. The aim of the study was to evaluate the effectiveness of the interferons alone and whether this effect might be increased by their combination.

The complete response at 8 weeks was similar, at 66–73% in each treatment group. No significant differences were found between the groups in this respect.

Potential drawbacks

One drawback is pain at the injection site. All patients had flu-like syndrome (fever, chills, headaches, fatigue, myalgia), especially within the first 2 weeks after the initiation of interferon therapy.

Comments

Concealment of allocation was unclear; however, the analysis was performed on an intention-to-treat basis.

Table 29.4 Randomized controlled trials evaluating intralesional interferon in the treatment of basal cell carcinomas

Study	Method	Participants	Interventions	Outcomes	Notes
Alpsoy *et al.* 1996[43] (Turkey)	Single center Method of randomization not known ITT	45 patients HP BCC: T1: 15, T2: 15, T3: 15 patients Mean age T1: 58.7, T2: 63.6, T3: 60.3 years Histological types T1: 12 N, 1 S, 2 M; T2: 11 N, 2 S, 2 M; T3: 11 N, 2 S, 2 M	T1: INF alfa-2a; T2: INF alfa-2b; T3: INF alfa-2a and-2b	FU: cytologic specimens taken 8 weeks after completion of therapy; all cases evaluated clinically and histologically	Ex: Recurrent lesions, genetic or nevoid conditions, deep tissue involvement
Cornell *et al.* 1990[44] (USA)	Multicenter (4) Randomization by computer-generated PP	T1: 123, T2: 42 patients BP BCC Mean age T1: 56, T2: 57 years Histological type T1: 57 S, 66 N ulcerative; T2: 19 S, 23 N	T1: intralesional injections 1.5 million IU IFN alfa-2b; T2: vehicle for IFN preparation 3 alternate days/week for 3 consecutive weeks	FU: weekly after each of the three treatments. then at 5, 9, 13 weeks after completion of treatment, then every 3 months to 52 weeks	Ex: Previously received therapy to test site, immunosuppressive or cytotoxic therapy (within previous 4 weeks), or exogenous IFN/IFN alfa-2b (Intron A), debilitating illness, lesion in perioral or central area of the face or penetrating to deep tissue
Edwards *et al.* 1990[45] (USA)	Single center Method of randomization not known, PP	T1: 33; T2: 32 patients BP BCC Age range 35–65 y Histological type: T1: 16 S, 17 N, T2: 15 S, 15 N	10 million IU zinc chelate IFN alfa-2b: T1: single injection; T2: one dose per week for 3 weeks	BCC measured, photographed before each treatment and at beginning of weeks 2, 8, 12, and 16 after the first injection Biopsy at week 16	Ex: thromboembolic disease, radiation therapy to the test site area, history of arsenic ingestion, pregnancy, immunosuppression, receiving nonsteroidal anti-inflammatory drugs, M BCC, recurrent cancers, deeply invasive lesions, periorificial tumors, central facial BCC
Rogozinski *et al.* 1997[46] (Poland)	Single center. Method of randomization not known, ITT	T1: 17, T2: 18 patients	T1: recombinant INF beta; T2: placebo	FU: 16 weeks after treatment and 2 years	

BCC, basal cell carcinoma; BP, biopsy-proven; Ex, exclusion; FU, follow-up; HP, histologically proven; IFN, interferon; M, morphea-like; N, nodular; PP, per protocol; S, superficial.

Implications for clinical practice
Combining interferon alfa-2a and -2b does not appear to increase their effectiveness.

Interferon alfa-2b versus vehicle
Another trial of 165 patients[44] compared interferon alfa-2b at 1.5 million units three times weekly for 3 weeks with vehicle in a 3 : 1 ratio of interferon-treated to placebo-treated patients.

Efficacy
Eighty-one percent of interferon-treated patients were clinically and histologically cured at 52 weeks, compared with 20% of the placebo recipients. The cure rate was independent of lesion type or size.

Potential drawbacks
Flu-like symptoms occurred more commonly in the interferon-treated group.

Comments
Concealment of allocation was clear; however, the analysis was conducted on a per-protocol basis. Interestingly, 20% of the patients treated with vehicle appeared to have a histological cure at 1 year. Longer-term studies are needed to determine whether this is genuine.

Implications for clinical practice
Interferon alfa-2b has not been compared with current standards of surgical or radiotherapy cures and so cannot be recommended as a first-line therapy. Interferon alfa-2b could be considered for patients who are not candidates for simple surgery or who desire nonsurgical therapy.

Number of dosages of interferon alfa-2b
A third RCT[45] compared a single dose of 10 million IU protamine zinc chelate interferon alfa-2b (a sustained-release preparation) with the same dose weekly for 3 weeks in 65 patients. Histological cure rates at 16 weeks were 52% and 80% for one and three doses weekly, respectively, and the cosmetic effect was graded as excellent by 51% of the patients. Side effects were similar for both the single-dosage

and repeated-dosage groups, and were those common to interferon (Table 29.4).

Implications for clinical practice
Refinement of the formulation to improve the release of interferon in order to help minimize side effects has not been realized. A trial is needed to compare the sustained-release formulation of interferon alfa-2b with standard interferon alfa-2b.

Interferon beta
Recombinant interferon beta at 1 million units three times weekly for 3 weeks has been compared with placebo in a trial of 35 patients.[46]

Efficacy
After 2 years of follow-up, 47% of patients in the treatment group showed a complete response, compared with none in the placebo group.

Potential drawbacks
Inflammation at the injection site was found in 11 of the 16 patients in the treatment group and four of the 18 receiving placebo.

Comment
The analysis was conducted on a per-protocol basis; concealment of allocation is not known.

Implications for clinical practice
The paper suggests recombinant interferon beta as an alternative treatment for BCC. The response rate at 47% is too low for it to be recommended as a treatment for BCC.

BEC-5 cream
BEC-5 is a mixture of 0.005% solasodine glycosides found in solanaceous plants (aubergine). BEC-5 cream binds to endogenous ectins and shows preferential cytotoxicity to human cancer cells.

In a double-blind randomized trial, BEC-5 cream was compared with matching vehicle[47] (Table 29.5). Biopsy-proven

Table 29.5 Randomized controlled trials evaluating BEC-5 in the treatment of basal cell carcinoma

Study	Method	Participants	Interventions	Outcomes	Notes
Punjabi et al. 2000[47] (UK)	Multicenter Method of randomization not known	94 patients BP BCC Age 32–95 y	T1:BEC-5; T2: vehicle; twice daily under occlusion for 8 weeks	Patients reviewed every 2 weeks Repeat punch biopsy at 8 weeks in 84 patients	10 patients in T1 did not complete the study

BCC, basal cell carcinoma; BP, biopsy-proven.

Table 29.6 Randomized controlled trials evaluating 5-fluorouracil (5-FU) in the treatment of basal cell carcinoma

Study	Method	Participants	Interventions	Outcomes	Notes
Romagosa et al. 2000[49] (USA)	Single center Method of randomization not known ITT	13 patients, 17 BP non-S BCCs ≥ 0.7 cm greatest diameter	T1: 5% 5-FU in PC vehicle T2: 5% 5-FU in petrolatum base Applied a.m. and p.m. for 4 consecutive weeks	FU: every 4 weeks for 16 weeks Final visit was biopsy of site	Ex: systemic disease, women of childbearing age, facial BCCs
Miller et al. 1997[50] (USA)	Multicenter, randomized, open-label Method of randomization not known PP	97 males, 25 females Single BP BCC Mean age 61 years Histological type: 38 S, 85 N Location: 9 head, 9 neck, 38 upper extremities, 11 lower extremities, 55 trunk Lesion area median 80 mm²	6 treatment regimens with 5-FU/epi gel: T1: 1.0 mL once weekly for 6 weeks; T2: 0.5 mL once weekly for 6 weeks; T3: 1.0 mL twice weekly for 3 weeks; T4: 0.5 mL twice weekly for 3 weeks. T5: 0.5 mL twice weekly for 4 weeks, T6: 0.5 mL three times weekly for 2 weeks	FU examinations of patients at 1, 4, 8, 12 weeks after last injection At each visit, patient and investigator gave subjective evaluation of cosmetic appearance of lesion	Ex: high-risk sites. Lesions with deep tissue involvement, basal cell nevus syndrome, hypersensitivities or allergies to 5-FU, sulfites, epinephrine, bovine collagen, history of autoimmune disease, pregnancy. Six patients were lost to follow-up

BCC, basal cell carcinoma; BP, biopsy-proven; Ex, exclusion; FU, follow-up; 5-FU, 5-fluorouracil; ITT, intention to treat; N, nodular; PP, per protocol; S, superficial.

lesions, excluding morpheic BCC, were treated twice daily under occlusion with BEC-5 or vehicle for 8 weeks.

Efficacy

There was a statistically significant difference in histological cure at week 8: 66% (41 of 62) in the BEC-5 group and 25% (eight of 32) in the vehicle group. The cure rates after 1 year of follow-up were also significantly different: 52% (32 of 62) in the BEC-5 group and 16% (five of 32) in the placebo group.

Potential drawbacks

There were no major treatment-related adverse effects.

Comment

Concealment of allocation was unclear, and the analysis was conducted on an intention-to-treat basis. The proportions of nodular and superficial BCCs were not clear from the published abstract.

Implications for clinical practice

Although significant differences were found between the groups, the cure rate is not sufficiently high in comparison with other treatments for this method to be recommended.

5-Fluorouracil (5-FU) applied topically

The primary mechanism of action of 5-FU is thought to be inhibition of DNA synthesis by competitive inhibition of thymidylate synthetase.[48]

5-FU in phosphatidylcholine versus 5-FU in petrolatum

A double-blind randomized pilot study[49] of 5-FU 5% cream in phosphatidylcholine (PC) vehicle was compared with 5-FU 5% in petrolatum. Further details of this study are given in Table 29.6. PC was used as a vehicle to facilitate the penetration of 5-FU.

Efficacy

Histological cure at week 16 was 90% with the PC vehicle and 57% with the petrolatum-based cream. The patients also evaluated the treatment site on each visit for cosmetic appearance. No differences were detected in the clinical appearance or adverse effects between the two therapeutic arms of the study.

Comments

The study was not adequately powered to detect any statistically significant differences in outcome between the groups, and concealment of allocation was unclear; however, the analysis was conducted on an intention-to-treat basis.

Potential drawbacks

Local irritation, erythema, ulceration, and tenderness were common reactions, but were well tolerated by the patients. Minimal itching and discomfort were experienced by some of the patients in both treatment arms.

Implications for clinical practice

The study may indicate an increase in short-term eradication of BCC using a PC-based vehicle in comparison with conventional petrolatum-based formulations of 5-FU. There was an excellent cosmetic outcome in all treatment sites before excision at week 16. Further large-scale double-blind trials with long-term follow-up periods of 3–5 years are needed to establish the efficacy of this treatment modality.

5-FU/epinephrine injectable gel

An open-label randomized study of 122 patients[50] tested the safety, tolerability, and efficacy of six treatment regimens of 5-FU/epinephrine gel. Two doses and four treatment schedules were used (Table 29.6).

Efficacy

Overall, the average response rate for the six regimens was 91%, as defined by the absence of any tumor on the basis of histological analysis of excised specimen. A 100% complete response rate was observed in patients who received 5 mL 5-FU/epinephrine gel twice weekly for 4 weeks—a 92% response rate for superficial lesions and a 91% response rate for nodular lesions.

All regimens appeared to work well and there were no statistically significant differences between them. The various treatment regimens with higher doses and/or treatment frequency resulted in higher complete response rates than obtained in an earlier pilot study.[51] The cosmetic appearance of the lesion site prior to excision at 3 months ranged from good to excellent.

Potential drawbacks

All patients had transient, moderate to severe stinging, burning, or pain at the time of injection. Local tissue reactions were confined to the treatment site and included erythema, swelling, desquamation, erosions, and eschar in most patients. Hyperpigmentation was observed in 83% of the patients, but typically cleared up during the follow-up period. Forty-seven percent of the patients had ulcerations at the treatment site. The lowest incidence and severity of reactions occurred with 0.5 mL 5-FU/epinephrine gel three times weekly for 2 weeks.

Comments

The analysis was per protocol. Concealment of allocation was unclear. No sample size calculation was described.

Implications for clinical practice

High local drug concentrations can be maintained for longer with the epinephrine gel delivery of 5-FU. A trial of 5-FU/epinephrine gel versus surgical excision, monitoring adverse effects, is required to confirm the claim that the response rates are comparable to those with surgery.

Imiquimod

Imiquimod is an immune-response modifier. It induces cytokines that promote a TH1 lymphocyte or cell-mediated immune response.[52–54] These cytokines include interferon alfa and gamma, and interleukin-12 (IL-12). In animal studies, imiquimod has demonstrated broad antiviral and antitumor effects that are largely mediated by interferon alfa.[53] In humans, imiquimod 5% cream is safe and effective in the treatment of external anogenital warts.[55,56] More recently, imiquimod has been licensed in the UK for superficial BCC. We found ten RCTs, which are summarized in Table 29.7.

Efficacy compared to vehicle cream

One study of 35 patients evaluated the safety and efficacy of imiquimod 5% cream in the treatment of superficial and nodular BCC.[57,58] This small trial suggested short-term success rates similar to those of excision surgery, with the added advantage of no scarring.

In a phase II dose–response trial of imiquimod 5% cream applied for 6 weeks in 99 Australian patients with primary superficial BCC,[59] histological clearance rates (defined as patients with no histological evidence of BCC when the site of the treated lesion was excised 6 weeks after imiquimod treatment) were 100% (all of three), 88% (29 of 33), 73% (22 of 30), and 70% (23 of 33) for twice daily, once daily, six times weekly, and three times weekly regimens, respectively.

Another similar multicenter RCT of 128 patients with superficial BCC compared imiquimod twice daily, once daily, 5 days/week and 3 days/week with vehicle using the same end points.[60] The intention-to-treat analysis showed clearance rates of 100% (10 of 10), 87% (27 of 31), 81% (21 of 26), and 52% for the twice daily, once daily, 5 days/week and 3 days/week groups, respectively. Interestingly, there was a small vehicle response rate—19% (six of 32).

Pooled data from two identical industry-funded studies[61] conducted in the U.S. in 724 patients with superficial BCC compared imiquimod daily either five times per week or seven times per week for 6 weeks versus vehicle. The histological clearance rates for the five times weekly and seven times weekly imiquimod groups were 82% and 79%, respectively.

One further industry-sponsored trial conducted in Europe[62] in 166 patients evaluated imiquimod 5% cream for the treatment of superficial BCC. At 12 weeks post-treatment, composite clearance was demonstrated in 77% (95% CI, 67% to 85%) and 6% (95% CI, 3% to 13%) of patients treated with imiquimod and vehicle cream, respectively ($P < 0.001$), and histological clearance was demonstrated in 80% (95% CI, 70% to 87%) and 6% (95% CI, 3% to 13%), respectively ($P < 0.001$).

Two similar studies[63] of 93 and 90 patients with superficial BCC and nodular BCC, respectively, found no significant difference in the treatment failure rate when occlusion was used.

Two further industry-sponsored trials[64] conducted in the U.S. have evaluated imiquimod 5% cream for the treatment of nodular BCC. One study reported histological clearance

Table 29.7 Randomized controlled trials evaluating imiquimod 5% cream in the treatment of basal cell carcinoma

Study	Method	Participants	Interventions	Outcomes
Beutner *et al.* 1999[57] (USA)	Single center Randomization to give 2 : 1 ratio of imiquimod cream to vehicle cream Method of randomization not known ITT	Age range 37–81 years BP BCCs: T1: 7; T2: 4; T3: 4; T5: 5; T6: 11 patients Size: 0.5–2.0 cm^2 Mainly upper body Histological type: T1: 1 N, 2 S; T2: 1 N, 3 S; T3: 4 S; T4: 2 N, 3 S; T5: 2 N, 2 S; T6: 1 N, 10 S	Imiquimod 5% cream: T1: twice/day; T2: once/day; T3: three times/week; T4: twice/week; T5: once/week; T6: vehicle	FU: 6 weeks after treatment. Tumor site excised and examined histologically
Marks *et al.* 2001[59] (Australia, New Zealand)	Multicenter Method of randomization not known ITT	72 male, 27 female HP S BCC; surface area 0.5–2.0 cm^2 Location: 32% upper limbs, 28% trunk, 40% head and neck	% imiquimod: T1: twice/day, T2: once/day, T3: twice/day for 3 days/week, T4: once/day for 2 days/week	FU: 1, 2, 4, 6 weeks Excision at week 6 Lost to FU: T2: 2 (pruritus) T3: 1 (cerebrovascular accident); T4: 1 (excision of nearby tumor)
Geisse *et al.* 2002[52] (USA)	Multicenter, randomized, blinded, vehicle-controlled dose–response Method of randomization not known ITT	128 patients. Single, primary BP S BCC (0.5–2.0 cm^2)	Imiquimod for 12 weeks: T1: twice daily; T2: once daily; T3: Mon–Fri; T4: Mon, Wed, Fri	FU: surgical excision 6 weeks after treatment
Sterry *et al.* 2002[63] (Europe)	Multicenter, randomized open-label, dose–response Method of randomization not known ITT	Two studies. HP BCC. 93 N BCC (0.5–2.0 cm^2), 90 S BCC (0.25–1.5 cm^2)	T1/T2: imiquimod 3 times/week for 6 weeks with (T1) and without (T2) occlusion; T3/T4: twice/week for 6 weeks, with (T3) and without (T4) occlusion	FU: surgical excision 6 weeks after treatment
Shumack *et al.* 2002[64] (USA)	Two studies: Multicenter, randomized, open-label, dose–response and a multicenter, randomized, blinded, vehicle-controlled dose–response Method of randomization not known ITT	Study 1: 99 patients, single, primary, BP N BCC (0.5–2.0 cm^2) Study 2: 92 patients, single, primary BP N BCC (0.5–2.0 cm^2)	Study 1: imiquimod for 6 weeks: T1: twice daily; T2: once daily; T3: twice daily 3 days/week for 6 weeks; T4: 3/week for 6 weeks Study 2: imiquimod for 12 weeks: T1 twice daily; T2: once daily; T3: Mon–Fri; T4: Mon, Wed, Fri	FU: surgical excision 6 weeks after treatment
Schulze *et al.* 2005[62] (Europe)	Multicenter, randomized, double blinded, vehicle-controlled Computer-generated randomization schedule ITT	166 patients, HP S BCC on limbs, trunk, neck or head. Not high-risk areas. Minimum area 0.5 cm^2 and maximum diameter 2.0 cm	Imiquimod 5% cream or vehicle daily, 7 x/week for 6 weeks	FU: excised 12 weeks post-treatment
Geisse *et al.* 2004[61] (USA)	Multicenter, randomized, double-blinded, vehicle-controlled. Computer-generated randomization schedule ITT	724 patients with BP S BCC, (0.5 cm^2 in area with max. diameter of 2 cm)	Imiquimod 5% cream or vehicle, daily either 5 x/week or 7 x/week for 6 weeks	FU: weeks 4 and 12 post-treatment

BCC, basal cell carcinoma; BP, biopsy-proven; FU, follow-up; HP, histologically proven; ITT, intention to treat; N, nodular; S, superficial.

rates of 71% (25 of 35) for once daily treatment for 6 weeks. Another vehicle-controlled RCT of 92 patients with nodular BCC who underwent treatment for 12 weeks using twice daily, once daily, 5 days/week, or 3 days/week reported intention-to-treat histological clearance rates of 75% (three of four), 76% (16 of 21), 70% (16 of 23) and 60% (12 of 20), respectively, with a vehicle response rate of 13% (three of 24).

These studies suggested that longer treatment times (i.e., 12 weeks as opposed to 6 weeks) are needed to treat nodular tumors. This is what one might anticipate from a treatment that relies on percutaneous penetration—tumor depth may be an important predictor of treatment response.

Potential drawbacks

There may be some local skin reaction to the cream, including: redness, edema, skin hardening, vesicles, erosion, ulceration, flaking, and scabbing. These brisk inflammatory reactions, at least clinically, would be consistent with an acute immunologic reconstitution of the sun-damaged skin, resulting in an immunologically mediated elimination of malignant and premalignant cells. In all studies, local reactions were common, mostly mild or moderate, were well tolerated by patients, and declined in incidence and severity with less frequent dosing.[57–60,63,64]

Comment

Concealment of allocation was unclear for all of the imiquimod trials; however, the analysis was on an intention-to-treat basis. There was no long-term follow-up for recurrence, which is very important for assessing treatments. Increasing severity of erythema, erosion, and scabbing/crusting was associated with higher clearance rates. Patients were able to apply the cream themselves in all of the trials—a feature that could reduce the need for attendance at busy hospital departments for low-risk lesions.

Implications for clinical practice

Topical imiquimod could become a useful treatment for superficial and low-risk BCCs and would allow dermatologists to concentrate on the high-risk BCCs, but long-term results comparing topical imiquimod with excisional surgery are essential. A study of this type is being conducted by the authors of this chapter.

Key points

- Despite the enormous amount of work involved in the treatment of BCC, there are still very few good-quality RCTs concerning the efficacy of the treatment modalities used.
- Surgery and radiotherapy appear to be the most effective treatments.
- The majority of studies have been performed on low-risk BCCs, the results of which are probably not applicable to tumors of the morpheic type shown in Figure 29.3.

- Cryotherapy, although convenient and less expensive than surgery or radiotherapy, has poor cure rates in comparison with surgery or radiotherapy (especially for lesions > 2 cm). The cosmetic effect is better with surgery and comparable with radiotherapy.
- If cryosurgery is to be used, two freeze–thaw cycles are recommended for nodular and superficial facial lesions (Figs. 29.1 and 29.2) if cure rates approaching equivalence to those with formal excision or radiotherapy are to be achieved.
- Greater efficacy needs to be demonstrated for PDT and interferon before they can be recommended.
- A broadband halogen light source may give cure rates and cosmetic outcome similar to laser light PDT, with the possible benefits of reduced costs, increased safety, and ease of use, although both are inferior to surgery.
- The efficacy of interferon alfa has not been directly compared with standard surgical treatment; interferons are associated with significant side effects, which may overshadow their usefulness, especially in the elderly. Interferon therapy requires several clinic visits.
- Increased short-term eradication of BCC using 5-FU in a phosphatidylcholine-based vehicle to increase penetration should be compared with surgery, with long-term follow-up.
- Preliminary studies suggest a high success rate (87–88%) for imiquimod in the treatment of superficial BCC using a once-daily regimen for 6 weeks, and a useful (76%) treatment response when treating nodular BCC for 12 weeks. A long-term study is underway with excision surgery as a comparator.
- All future RCTs of BCC treatment should include 3–5-year outcomes, as short-term (less than 1 year) improvement may simply be a temporary phenomenon. This is especially important for topical application, which may appear to improve the surface of the lesion only to leave deeper extensions that the dermatologist may find it difficult to see on clinical examination.

References

1 Telfer N, Colver G, Bowers P. Guidelines for the management of basal cell carcinoma. British Association of Dermatologists. *Br J Dermatol* 1999;**141**: 415–23.

2 Preston DS, Stern RS. Nonmelanoma cancers of the skin. *N Engl J Med* 1992;**327**:1649–62.

3 Miller SJ. Biology of basal cell carcinoma (part 1). *J Am Acad Dermatol* 1991;**24**:1–13.

4 Goodwin R, Roberts D. Skin cancer registration in the United Kingdom. *Br J Dermatol* 2001;**145**(Suppl 59):17.

5 Walberg P, Skog E. The increasing incidence of basal cell carcinoma. *Br J Dermatol* 1994;**131**:914–5.

6 Christenson LJ, Borrowman TA, Vachon CM, *et al.* Incidence of basal cell and squamous cell carcinomas in a population younger than 40 years. *JAMA* 2005;**294**:681–90.

7 de Vries E, van de Poll-Franse LV, Louwman WJ, de Gruijl FR, Coebergh JW. Predictions of skin cancer incidence in the Netherlands up to 2015. *Br J Dermatol* 2005;**152**:481–8.

8 Holme SA, Malinovszky K, Roberts DL. Changing trends in non-melanoma skin cancer in South Wales, 1988–98. *Br J Dermatol* 2000;**143**:124–9.

9 Chuang TY, Popescu A, Su WP, Chute CG. Basal cell carcinoma: a population-based incidence study in Rochester, Minnesota. *J Am Acad Dermatol* 1990;**22**: 413–7.

10 Marks R, Staples M, Giles GG. Trends in non-melanocytic skin cancer treated in Australia: the second national survey. *Int J Cancer* 1993;**53**:585–90.

11 Roenigk RK, Ratz JL, Bailin PL, Wheeland RG. Trends in the presentation and treatment of basal cell carcinomas. *J Dermatol Surg Oncol* 1986;**12**:860–5.

12 McCormack CJ, Kelly JW, Dorevitch AP. Differences in age and body site distribution of the histological subtypes of basal cell carcinoma: a possible indicator of differing causes. *Arch Dermatol* 1997;**133**:593–6.

13 Gilbody JS, Aitken J, Green A. What causes basal cell carcinoma to be the commonest cancer? *Aust J Public Health* 1994;**18**:218–21.

14 Zaynoun S, Ali L, Shaib J. The relationship of sun exposure and solar elastosis to basal cell carcinoma. *J Am Acad Dermatol* 1985;**12**:522–5.

15 Pearl D, Scott E. The anatomical distribution of skin cancers. *Int J Epidemiol* 1986;**15**:502–6.

16 Mackie R, Elwood J, Hawkes J. Links between exposure to ultraviolet radiation and skin cancer: a report of the Royal College of Physicians. *J R Coll Physicians Lond* 1987;**21**:91–6.

17 Schreiber MM, Moon TE, Fox SH, Davidson J. The risk of developing subsequent nonmelanoma skin cancers. *J Am Acad Dermatol* 1990;**23**:1114–8.

18 Johnson R, Rothman A, Xie J. Human homolog of patched, a candidate gene for the basal cell nevus syndrome. *Science* 1996;**272**:1668–71.

19 Staples M, Marks R, Giles G. Trends in the incidence of non-melanocytic skin cancer (NMSC) treated in Australia 1985–1995: are primary prevention programs starting to have an effect? *Int J Cancer* 1998;**78**:144–8.

20 Breuninger H, Dietz K. Prediction of subclinical tumor infiltration in basal cell carcinoma. *J Dermatol Surg Oncol* 1991;**17**:574–8.

21 Gussack GS, Schlitt M, Lushington A, Woods KE. Invasive basal cell carcinoma of the temporal bone. *Ear Nose Throat J* 1989;**68**: 605–6, 609–11.

22 Franchimont C. Episodic progression and regression of basal cell carcinomas. *Br J Dermatol* 1982;**106**:305–10.

23 Takenouchi T, Nomoto S, Ito M. Factors influencing the linear depth of invasion of primary basal cell carcinoma. *Dermatol Surg* 2001;**27**:393–6.

24 Alderson P. Optimal search strategy for RCTs. In: Alderson P, Green S, Higgins J, eds. *Cochrane Reviewers Handbook* 4.2.1 (updated December 2003). Chichester, UK: Wiley, 2004.

25 Rhodes LE, de Rie M, Enstrom Y, *et al.* Photodynamic therapy using topical methyl aminolevulinate vs surgery for nodular basal cell carcinoma: results of a multicenter randomized prospective trial. *Arch Dermatol* 2004;**140**:17–23.

26 Smeets NW, Krekels GA, Ostertag JU, *et al.* Surgical excision vs. Mohs' micrographic surgery for basal-cell carcinoma of the face: randomised controlled trial. *Lancet* 2004;**364**:1766–72.

27 Dubin N, Kopf A. Multivariate risk score for recurrence of cutaneous basal cell carcinoma. *Arch Dermatol* 1983;**119**:373–7.

28 Wolf D, Zitelli J. Surgical margins for basal cell carcinoma. *Arch Dermatol* 1987;**123**.340–4.

29 Avril MF, Auperin A, Margulis A, *et al.* Basal cell carcinoma of the face: surgery or radiotherapy? Results of a randomized study. *Br J Cancer* 1997;**76**:100–6.

30 Petit JY, Avril MF, Margulis A, *et al.* Evaluation of cosmetic results of a randomized trial comparing surgery and radiotherapy in the treatment of basal cell carcinoma of the face. *Plast Reconstr Surg* 2000;**105**:2544–51.

31 Rowe D, Carroll R, Day CJ. Long term recurrence rates in previously untreated (primary) basal cell carcinoma: implications for patient follow up. *J Dermatol Surg Oncol* 1989;**15**:315–28.

32 Huang CC, Boyce S, Northington M, Desmond R, Soong SJ. Randomized, controlled surgical trial of preoperative tumor curettage of basal cell carcinoma in Mohs micrographic surgery. *J Am Acad Dermatol* 2004;**51**:585–91.

33 Hall VL, Leppard BJ, McGill J, Kesseler ME, White JE, Goodwin P. Treatment of basal-cell carcinoma: comparison of radiotherapy and cryotherapy. *Clin Radiol* 1986;**37**:33–4.

34 Mallon E, Dawber R. Cryosurgery in the treatment of basal cell carcinoma. *Dermatol Surg* 1996;**22**:854–8.

35 Thissen MR, Nieman FH, Ideler AH, Berretty PJ, Neumann HA. Cosmetic results of cryosurgery versus surgical excision for primary uncomplicated basal cell carcinomas of the head and neck. *Dermatol Surg* 2000;**26**:759–64.

36 Tope W, Menter A, El-Azhary R. Randomized prospective comparison of topical methyl aminolevulinate photodynamic therapy verus placebo photodynamic therapy in nodular basal cell carcinoma. [Paper presented at 9th World Congress of Cancers of the Skin, Seville, Spain, May 2003.]

37 Foley P. A phase III randomized study comparing photodynamic therapy (PDT) using Metvix or placebo cream in nodular basal cell carcinoma (BCC). *Aust J Dermatol* 2003;**44**:A5.

38 Wang I, Bendsoe N, Klinteberg CA, *et al.* Photodynamic therapy vs. cryosurgery of basal cell carcinomas: results of a phase III clinical trial. *Br J Dermatol* 2001;**144**:832–40.

39 Basset-Seguin N, Ibbotson S, Emtestam L. Photodynamic therapy using methyl aminolevulinate is as efficacious as cryotherapy in basal cell carcinoma, with better cosmetic results. [Paper presented at British Association of Dermatologists 83rd Annual Meeting, Brighton, UK, July 2003.]

40 Soler AM, Angell-Petersen E, Warloe T, *et al.* Photodynamic therapy of superficial basal cell carcinoma with 5-aminlevulinic acid with dimethylsulfoxide and ethylenediaminetetraacetic acid: a comparison of two light sources. *Photochem Photobiol* 2000;**71**: 724–9.

41 Clark C. Randomised trial of minimal curettage and topical 5-aminolaevulinic acid (5-ALA) photodynamic therapy (PDT) compared with excision for the treatment of basal cell carcinomas with low risk. [Ongoing trial, Photobiology Unit, Ninewells Hospital and Medical Schools, Tayside University Hospitals NHS Trust, Dundee, UK.]

42 Lui H, Hobbs L, Tope WD, *et al.* Photodynamic therapy of multiple nonmelanoma skin cancers with verteporfin and red light-emitting diodes: two-year results evaluating tumor response and cosmetic outcomes. *Arch Dermatol* 2004;**140**:26–32.

43 Alpsoy E, Yilmaz E, Basaran E, Yazar S. Comparison of the effects of intralesional interferon alfa-2a, 2b and the combination of 2a

and 2b in the treatment of basal cell carcinoma. *J Dermatol* 1996; **23**:394–6.

44 Cornell R, Greenway H, Tucker S. Intralesional interferon therapy for basal cell carcinoma. *J Am Acad Dermatol* 1990;**23**:694–700.

45 Edwards L, Tucker SB, Perednia D, *et al.* The effect of an intralesional sustained-release formulation of interferon alfa-2b on basal cell carcinomas. *Arch Dermatol* 1990;**126**:1029–32.

46 Rogozinski T, Jablonska S, Brzoska J, Michalska I, Wohr C, Gaus W. Intralesional treatment with recombinant interferon beta is an effective alternative for the treatment of basal cell carcinoma: double-blind, placebo-controlled study. *Przegl Dermatol* 1997;**84**: 259–63.

47 Punjabi S, Cook I, Kersey P, *et al.* A double-blind, multicentre parallel group study of BEC-5 cream in basal cell carcinoma. *J Eur Acad Dermatol Venereol* 2000;**14**(Suppl 1): 47–60.

48 McEvoy GK. Fluorouracil. In: McEvoy GK, ed. *American Hospital Formulary Service—Drug Information 93.* Bethesda, MD: American Society of Hospital Pharmacists, 1993: 573–7.

49 Romagosa R, Saap L, Givens M, *et al.* A pilot study to evaluate the treatment of basal cell carcinoma with 5-flourouracil using phosphatidyl choline as a transepidermal carrier. *Dermatol Surg* 2000; **26**:338–40.

50 Miller BH, Shavin JS, Cognetta A, *et al.* Nonsurgical treatment of basal cell carcinomas with intralesional 5-flourouracil/epinephrine injectable gel. *J Am Acad Dermatol* 1997;**36**:72–7.

51 Orenberg E, Miller B, Greenway H. The effect of intralesional 5-fluorouracil therapeutic implant (MPI 5003) for treatment of basal cell carcinoma. *Acad Dermatol* 1992;**27**:723–8.

52 Testerman T, Gerster J, Imbertson L. Cytokine induction by the immunomodulators imiquimod and S-27609. *J Leukoc Biol* 1995; **58**:365–72.

53 Slade HB, Owens ML, Tomai MA, Miller RL. Imiquimod 5% cream. *Expert Opin Investig Drugs* 1998;**7**:437–49.

54 Imbertson L, Beaurline J, Couture A. Cytokine induction in hairless mouse and rat skin after topical application of the immune response modifiers imiquimod and S-28463. *J Invest Dermatol* 1998;**110**:734–9.

55 Beutner K, Tyring S, Trofatter K. Imiquimod: a patient applied immune response modifier for treatment of external genital warts. *Antimicrob Agents Chemother* 1998;**42**:788–94.

56 Edwards L, Ferenczy A, Eron L. Self-administered topical 5% imiquimod cream for external anogenital warts. *Arch Dermatol* 1998;**134**:25–30.

57 Beutner KR, Geisse JK, Helman D, Fox TL, Ginkel A, Owens ML. Therapeutic response of basal cell carcinoma to the immune response modifier imiquimod 5% cream. *J Am Acad Dermatol* 1999;**41**(6):1002–7.

58 Bavinck J, Biological treatment of basal cell carcinoma. *Arch Dermatol* 2000;**136**:774–5.

59 Marks R, Gebauer K, Shumack S, *et al.* Imiquimod 5% cream in the treatment of superficial basal cell carcinoma: results of a multicentre 6-week dose-response trial. *J Am Acad Dermatol* 2001;**44**: 807–13.

60 Geisse JK, Rich P, Pandya A, *et al.* Imiquimod 5% cream for the treatment of superficial basal cell carcinoma: a double-blind, randomized, vehicle-controlled study. *J Am Acad Dermatol* 2002; **47**:390–8.

61 Geisse J, Caro I, Lindholm J, Golitz L, Stampone P, Owens M. Imiquimod 5% cream for the treatment of superficial basal cell carcinoma: results from two phase III, randomized, vehicle-controlled studies. *J Am Acad Dermatol* 2004;**50**:722–33.

62 Schulze HJ, Cribier B, Requena L, *et al.* Imiquimod 5% cream for the treatment of superficial basal cell carcinoma: results from a randomized vehicle-controlled phase III study in Europe. *Br J Dermatol* 2005;**152**:939–47.

63 Sterry W, Ruzicka T, Herrera E, *et al.* Imiquimod 5% cream for the treatment of superficial and nodular basal cell carcinoma: randomized studies comparing low-frequency dosing with and without occlusion. *Br J Dermatol* 2002;**147**:1227–36.

64 Shumack S, Robinson J, Kossard S, *et al.* Efficacy of topical 5% imiquimod cream for the treatment of nodular basal cell carcinoma. *Arch Dermatol* 2002;**138**:1165–71.

30 Primary cutaneous T-cell lymphoma

Sean Whittaker

Background

Definition

Primary cutaneous T-cell lymphomas (CTCLs) represent a heterogeneous group of extranodal non-Hodgkin's lymphomas, of which mycosis fungoides/Sézary syndrome are the most common clinicopathological subtypes.[1] Mycosis fungoides is characterized by distinct clinical stages of cutaneous disease consisting of patches/plaques, tumors, and erythroderma in which the whole skin is involved. Peripheral adenopathy may or may not be present. Sézary syndrome is defined by the presence of erythroderma, peripheral lymphadenopathy, and a minimum number of Sézary cells within the peripheral blood. These clinico-pathological entities are closely related pathogenetically, but are distinct from other less common types of primary CTCL (Figures 30.1–30.4).

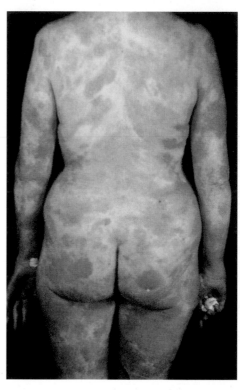

Figure 30.2 Plaque-stage mycosis fungoides (IB/IIA).

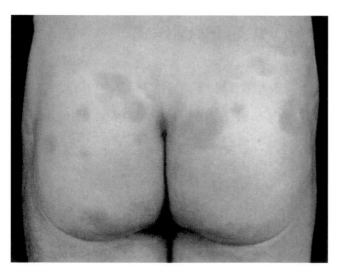

Figure 30.1 Patch-stage mycosis fungoides (IA).

Incidence/prevalence

The overall annual incidence of primary CTCL in the USA in 1988 was 0.5–1.0 per 100 000, based on population data. However, the prevalence is much higher, because most patients have low-grade disease and live long.[2] Males and the black population are affected more commonly.[2,3] The incidence has increased during the past two decades, but this almost certainly partly reflects improved diagnosis of earlier stages and possibly better registration, particularly in the USA.[3]

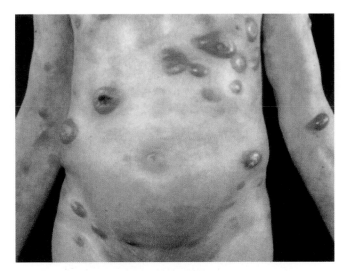

Figure 30.3 Tumor-stage mycosis fungoides (IIB).

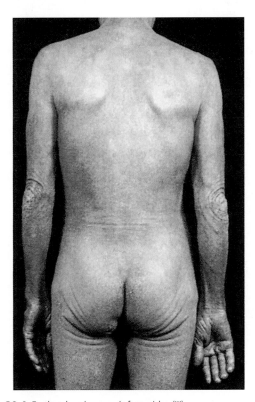

Figure 30.4 Erythrodermic mycosis fungoides (III).

Etiology

The underlying etiology is unknown. There is evidence for inactivation of key tumor suppressor genes and TH2 cytokine production by tumor cells in mycosis fungoides/ Sézary syndrome, but no disease-specific molecular abnormality has yet been identified.[4] Primary CTCL must be distinguished from human T-lymphotropic virus type-1

(HTLV-I)–associated adult T-cell leukemia lymphoma (ATLL), in which skin involvement often closely mimics the clinicopathological features of mycosis fungoides/Sézary syndrome and may be the presenting feature.[1]

Prognosis

Most cases of primary CTCL are not curable. Independent prognostic features in mycosis fungoides include the extent of skin involvement, lymph-node stage, and age of onset (> 60 years). The lymph-node status and tumor burden within peripheral blood determine the prognosis in Sézary syndrome.[5,6] Serum lactate dehydrogenase and the thickness of the infiltrate in plaque-stage mycosis fungoides are also independent markers of prognosis.[7] Multivariate analysis indicates that an initial complete response to various therapies is an independent favorable prognostic feature, particularly in early stages of disease.[8–10] For mycosis fungoides, two staging systems are in regular use, including a TNM (primary tumor, regional nodes, metastasis) system and a clinical staging specifically designed for CTCL (Box 30.1).[5] These staging systems can also be applied to Sézary syndrome, but neither system provides a quantitative method for assessing peripheral blood disease other than an additional B0 and B1 in the TNM system, and this has prompted alternative approaches for Sézary syndrome.[6]

Table 30.1 summarizes recent actuarial survival data for mycosis fungoides.[3,8–12] The 5- and 10-year overall survival rates in mycosis fungoides are 80% and 57%, respectively, with disease-specific survival rates of 89% and 75% at 5 and 10 years, respectively.[8] Patients with very early-stage disease (IA) are highly unlikely to die of their disease, with disease-specific survival rates of 100% and 97–98% at 5 and 10 years, respectively, and risks of disease progression varying from 0% to 10% over 5–20 years.[8–11] In one study of 122 patients with stage IA disease, median survival was not reached at 32.5 years.[9]

Stage IB patients have an overall survival rate of 73–86% at 5 years and 58–67% at 10 years, and disease-specific survival rates of 96% and 83% at 5 and 10 years respectively.[3,8,10] A median survival of 12.1–12.8 years should be expected for stage IB patients, with a risk of disease progression varying from 10% to 39%. The explanation for this marked variation in different studies of stage IB is unclear, but it appears that patients with folliculotropic variants of mycosis fungoides have a worse prognosis than other patients with stage IB disease; this may reflect the depth of infiltrate, which perhaps makes skin-directed therapy less effective.[8]

Accurate data on stage IIA patients (patches/plaques and clinical adenopathy with no histological evidence of lymphoma) are scant, but this stage may be associated with a worse outcome—with overall survival rates of 49%, disease-specific survival rates of 68%, and risks of disease

BOX 30.1 The TNM (primary tumor, regional nodes, metastasis) classification for mycosis fungoides (including a "B" system for cutaneous T-cell lymphoma, to incorporate Sézary syndrome)

Skin
- T1, limited patches/plaques (< 10% of total skin surface)
- T2, extensive patches/plaques (> 10% of total skin surface)
- T3, tumors
- T4, erythroderma

Nodes
- N0, no clinical lymphadenopathy
- N1, clinically enlarged lymph nodes but histologically uninvolved
- N2, lymph nodes not enlarged but histologically involved
- N3, clinically enlarged lymph nodes and histologically involved

Visceral
- M0, no visceral involvement
- M1, visceral involvement

Blood
- B0, no peripheral blood Sézary cells (< 5%)
- B1, peripheral blood Sézary cells (> 5% of total lymphocyte count)

Clinical staging system for cutaneous T-cell lymphoma (mycosis fungoides)

Stage	T	N	M
IA	T1	N0	M0
IB	T2	N0	M0
IIA	T1–2	N1	M0
IIB	T3	N0–1	M0
III	T4	N0–1	M0
IVA	T1–4	N2–3	M0
IVB	T1–4	N0–3	M1

progression of 65% at both 5 and 10 years. The lack of difference in outcome at 5 and 10 years in this study is unreliable, since the data came from only 18 patients.[8] Of the 176 patients reported by Kim et al.,[10] 56 (32%) had peripheral adenopathy (stage IIA), but in 23 of these 56 no histological assessment was made and some of them could therefore have had stage IVA disease. Nevertheless, the overall survival rate is similar to stage IB disease at 5 years (73%), with a slight difference at 10 years (45% versus 58%), associated with a small difference in median survival of 10 years (stage IIA) compared with 12.8 years (stage IB) and an overall risk of disease progression of 34% and 20%, respectively. Further studies of larger numbers of patients with stage IIA disease are needed to compare outcomes with those of stage IB patients.

Patients with tumor-stage disease (stage IIB) have overall survival rates of 40–65% at 5 years and 20–39% at 10 years,[3,8,9] and a median survival of 2.9 years in one study.[9] In one study, disease-specific survival rates of 80% and 42% at 5 and 10 years, respectively, were reported for patients with stage IIB disease.[8] The survival data for patients with erythrodermic mycosis fungoides but no evidence of lymph-node or peripheral blood involvement (stage III) are broadly similar to those for stage IIB disease, although median survival may be better (4.6 versus 3.6 years).[3,9,12] In contrast, the overall survival and disease-specific survival rates at 5 and 10 years for stage IVA and IVB patients is poor (15–40% and 5–20% for stage IVA and 0–15% and 0–5% for stage IVB at 5 and 10 years, respectively), with a median survival of 13 months for both extracutaneous stages.[8,11,12]

The overall survival rates in CTCL, based on the stage of the disease, have led to suggestions that the staging system should be modified using four broad categories:[13]

Table 30.1 Published outcomes according to clinical stage in cutaneous T-cell lymphoma

Overall survival (%)	IA	IB	IIA	IIB	III	IVA	IVB	Overall	Reference	No of patients	Median follow up (years)
5 years	99	86	49	65		40	0	80	Doorn et al. 2000[8a]	309	5.2
	100	84		52	57				Zackheim et al. 1999[3b]	489	4.7
	96	(78)		(40)	(40)				Kim et al. 1996[9c]	122	9.8
		73	73[d]						Kim et al. 1999[10d]	176	8
					45	17			Kim et al. 1995[12e]	106	10.5
						15	15		Coninck et al. 2001[11f]	112	
10 years	84	61	49	27		20	0	57	Doorn et al. 2000[8]	309	5.2
	100	67		39	41				Zackheim et al. 1999[3]	489	4.7
	88	(60)		(20)	(20)				Kim et al. 1996[9]	122	9.8
		58	45[d]						Kim et al. 1999[10]	176	8
						5	5		Coninck et al. 2001[11]	112	

Table 30.1 *Cont'd*

Overall survival (%)	IA	IB	IIA	IIB	III	IVA	IVB	Overall	Reference	No of patients	Median follow up (years)
Disease-free survival (%)											
5 years	100	96	68	80		40	0	89	Doorn *et al.* 2000[8]	309	5.2
10 years	97	83	68	42		20	0	75	Doorn *et al.* 2000[8]	309	5.2
	98								Kim *et al.* 1996[9]	122	9.8
Median survival (years)	NR[c]	12.1		2.9	3.6				Kim *et al.* 1996[9]	556	9.8
		12.8y	10.0						Kim *et al.* 1999[10]	176	8
					4.6	13 mos			Kim *et al.* 1995[12]	106	10.5
						3 mos	13 mos		Coninck *et al.* 2001[11]	546	
Disease progression (%)											
5 years	4	21	65	32		70	100		Doorn *et al.* 2000[8]	309	5.2
10 years	10	39	65	60		70	100		Doorn *et al.* 2000[8]	309	5.2
20 years	0	10		36	41				Coninck *et al.* 2001[11]	546	
Overall	9								Kim *et al.* 1996[9]	122	9.8
		20	34[d]						Kim *et al.* 1999[10]	176	8
FFR (%)											
5 years	50								Kim *et al.* 1996[9]	122	9.8
		36	9						Kim *et al.* 1999[10]	176	8
10 years	25 (50)								Kim *et al.* 1996[9]	122	9.8
		31	3						Kim *et al.* 1999[10]	176	8

All overall (OS) survival curves were calculated using the Kaplan–Meier method.

[a] In the study by Doorn *et al.*[8] the presence of follicular mucinosis was an independent poor prognostic feature possibly related to depth of infiltrate in patients with stage IB disease (disease-free survival of 81% and 36% and OS of 75% and 21% at 5 and 10 years, respectively). A lack of a complete response to initial therapy was also associated with a poor outcome (*P* < 0.001) in a multivariate analysis as well as increasing clinical stage and the presence of extracutaneous disease. A different staging system was used in this study (Hamminga *et al. Br J Dermatol* 1982;**107**:145–155) but for the purposes of this table the staging has been altered to be consistent. This study is the only one to provide comprehensive disease-specific survival (DSS) data for different stages of mycosis fungoides. Only three patients had stage IVB disease and only 18 patients each had stage IIA and IVA disease. Therefore the results for these stages must be interpreted cautiously.

[b] In the study by Zackheim *et al.*,[3] black patients had a relatively more advanced stage of disease than white patients. The TNM classification was used in this study. Lymph node stage had an unfavourable impact on survival but this trend did not reach significance for *each individual* T stage because of a lack of sufficient power (an estimated 1700 subjects required) and IIA/IVA patients were not designated separately. Similar considerations apply to peripheral blood involvement. Similar outcomes for patients with stage IIB (T3) and III (T4) disease is consistent with other studies but this might reflect a lack of lymph node staging data included in this study.

[c] The 1996 study by Kim *et al.*[9] primarily included data on 122 patients with stage IA disease, but survival data on 556 patients with all stages were also included to give the values in parentheses. The free from relapse (FFR) data at 5 and 10 years are confusing because the text states that the FFR at 10 years was 25% but the figure indicates that it remains at approximately 50%, as for FFR at 5 years. The median survival for stage IA patients was not reached at 32.5 years. NR, not reached.

[d] In the 1999 study by Kim *et al.*,[10] OS at 20 years for stage IB and IIA patients was 27%. DSS was better for patients < 58 years of age (*P* < 0.03). In 23 of the 56 patients with palpable lymphadenopathy, no histological assessment was made and these patients were assumed to have reactive/dermatopathic nodes (IIA). This might account for the lack of difference in OS at 5 years between stage IB and IIA patients, although there appears to be a difference in OS at 10 years.

[e] In the 1995 study by Kim *et al.*,[12] the OS and median survival data were calculated from the date of initial treatment, which was usually within 3 months of diagnosis. This study also stratified patients into three groups according to the presence of none, one, or two or three poor prognostic parameters, namely: age at presentation (> 65 years), the presence of clinical adenopathy, and B1 stage, producing varied median survivals of 10.2 years (no factors), 3.7 years (one factor) and 1.5 years (two or three factors); *P* < 0.005.

[f] The study by Coninck *et al.*[11] included 112 patients with extracutaneous disease at presentation or with progression and 434 patients with only cutaneous disease, giving the 546 patients listed in the table for median survival and disease progression.

1 Stage IA patients have a normal life expectancy.

2 Stage IB and IIA disease may have a similar prognosis, although the thickness of the infiltrate is an important prognostic factor in this group.

3 The prognosis is also similar for stage IIB and III disease, which is better than in patients with stage IVA/B.

4 Nodal or visceral disease (IVA/B).

This proposal resembles that suggested by Sausville *et al.* in 1988.[14]

Patients with Sézary syndrome have an 11% 5-year survival, with a median survival of 32 months from diagnosis.[1] In contrast, other clinicopathological variants of CTCL are generally associated with an excellent long-term prognosis (100% 5-year survival in lymphomatoid papulosis and 90% in primary cutaneous CD30+ large-cell anaplastic cutaneous lymphoma), with the exception of patients with subcutaneous panniculitis-like T-cell lymphomas and primary cutaneous natural-killer (NK)-like T-cell/NK cell lymphomas.[1]

Diagnostic tests

The diagnosis of different variants of primary CTCL is based on a critical assessment of the clinicopathological features. Repeated biopsies may be required to establish the diagnosis, and correlation between the histology and clinical features is essential. Immunophenotypic studies are required to identify different CTCL variants, and analysis of T-cell receptor genes in DNA extracted from skin biopsies can identify a T-cell clone, which helps to confirm the diagnosis. However T-cell clones are not always detected in early stages of mycosis fungoides because of a lack of sensitivity. Investigations—including a computed tomography (CT) scan of the chest, abdomen, and pelvis to exclude systemic involvement and assessment of peripheral blood for Sézary cells and lymphocyte subsets—are indicated in all patients, with the exception of those with early stages of mycosis fungoides (IA/IB) and lymphomatoid papulosis.[15] Bone-marrow aspirate/trephine biopsies are indicated in CTCL variants, but rarely in mycosis fungoides and Sézary syndrome.

Aims of treatment

The aim of treatment is to induce complete or partial remission of disease and to prolong the disease-free survival and overall survival, while maintaining the patient's quality of life (Table 30.2).

Relevant outcomes

- Severity of symptoms (pruritus, sleep disturbance, pain) and signs (erythema, scaling, fissuring, excoriation, edema

Table 30.2 Treatment of mycosis fungoides/Sézary syndrome

Stage	First-line treatment	Second-line treatment	Experimental	Not suitable
IA	SDT or no therapy	SDT or no therapy	Bexarotene gel	Chemotherapy
IB	SDT	Interferon alfa + PUVA, TSEB	Denileukin diftitox, bexarotene, antibody therapies	Chemotherapy
IIA	SDT	Interferon alfa + PUVA, TSEB	Denileukin diftitox, bexarotene, antibody therapies	Chemotherapy
IIB	Radiotherapy or TSEB, chemotherapy	Interferon alfa, denileukin diftitox,* bexarotene	Autologous PBSCT, mini-allograft, antibody therapies	Ciclosporin
III	PUVA ± interferon alfa, ECP ± interferon alfa, methotrexate	TSEB, bexarotene, denileukin diftitox,* chemotherapy, alemtuzumab	Autologous PBSCT, mini-allograft, antibody therapies	Ciclosporin
IVA	Radiotherapy or TSEB, chemotherapy	Interferon alfa, denileukin diftitox,* alemtuzumab, bexarotene	Autologous PBSCT, mini-allograft, antibody therapies	Ciclosporin
IVB	Radiotherapy, chemotherapy	Palliative therapy	Autologous PBSCT, mini-allograft	

ECP, extracorporeal photopheresis; PBSCT, peripheral blood stem cell transplant; PUVA, psoralen + ultraviolet A; SDT, skin-directed therapy including topical emollients, steroids, mechlorethamine, carmustine, bexarotene gel, UVB/PUVA, superficial radiotherapy; TSEB, total skin electron beam.
Antibody therapies—other than alemtuzumab.
Stage III includes Sézary syndrome, although some cases of Sézary syndrome will be stage IVA. ECP is ideal for those patients with peripheral blood involvement.
* Not yet licensed in Europe.

and thickness of plaques, presence of nodules, tumors, peripheral lymphadenopathy).
- Body surface area involvement.
- Assessment of overall tumor burden, with histological assessment of skin and lymph nodes, staging CT scans and peripheral blood Sézary cell counts/lymphocyte subsets.
- Establishment of molecular remission using T-cell receptor gene analysis of skin and peripheral blood.
- Quality of life.

Recent trials have used scoring systems involving computed measures of the above, which are broadly based on a severity-weighted assessment toll (SWAT).[16] However, most studies included in this review define responses in terms of simple clinical observation, with complete response defined as complete resolution of clinically apparent disease (based in CTCL usually on cutaneous signs of disease) for at least 4–6 weeks. Partial response is usually defined as > 50% reduction of clinical disease or tumor burden, although some studies in CTCL have defined this as > 25% reduction in tumor burden. More importantly, most studies do not include a validated scoring system, which effectively makes any interpretation of partial response impossible. Similar considerations apply to assessment of stable disease, defined usually as < 50% improvement, and progressive disease, defined as > 25% increase in tumor burden. For most studies in CTCL, progressive disease is defined as a deterioration in the clinical stage of the disease. A quality-of-life assessment for CTCL has been published, although this has rarely been assessed in CTCL studies so far.[17]

Methods of search

Systematic reviews, controlled clinical trials, and clinical trials were located by searching the Cochrane Library (1999–2006) and Medline (1985–2005). Because of a limited number of randomized clinical trials (RCTs) and the overall low incidence of CTCL, some small studies are included, and the limitations of such studies are discussed.

Questions

What are the effects of topical therapy in mycosis fungoides?

Topical corticosteroids
Efficacy
No systematic reviews or RCTs were identified. One large open uncontrolled study of 79 patients with mycosis fungoides (stage T1/T2) who were treated with class I to III (potent/moderate potency) topical corticosteroids twice daily for 3–4 months and under occlusion showed complete clinical remission in 63% and partial response in 31%

of stage T1 patients, and complete response and partial response in 25% and 57%, respectively, for patients with stage T2.[18] Complete response was confirmed histologically in seven patients, but the median duration of the complete response was not documented.

Drawbacks
Reversible depression of serum cortisol levels occurred in 13% of patients, and skin atrophy in one patient.

Comment
The lack of controlled studies and a short median follow-up of 9 months weakens the impact of the results. No evidence of impact on disease-specific survival or overall survival was reported. However, it does appear that topical corticosteroids, especially class 1 (potent) compounds, are effective at temporarily clearing patches and plaques in some patients with early stage IA/IB mycosis fungoides.

Topical mechlorethamine (nitrogen mustard)
Efficacy
No RCTs were found. A retrospective review of 123 patients treated at one institution (1969–85) with whole-body once-daily application of topical mechlorethamine (10–20 mg/mL; aqueous preparation from 1968 to 1980 and ointment base from 1980 to 1985) until maximum response reported complete response rates of 51% in IA, 26% in IB, 0% in IIB, and 22% in stage III disease.[19] There were no differences in outcome with the aqueous or ointment base. Fifty patients had received total skin electron beam (TSEB) therapy before topical mechlorethamine. Relapse occurred in 56% of patients who achieved complete response, despite continued maintenance treatment for 1–2 years.[19]

A study of 117 patients reported complete response in 76% with stage I disease, 45% with stage II and 49% with stage III patients within 2 years of therapy (median response duration of 45 months).[20] Patients in this study were allowed local radiotherapy for tumors and were not excluded as responders. The overall 5-year survival for all patients in this study was 89%.

In a retrospective review of 331 patients (all stages, 1968–82) treated with topical mechlorethamine daily and with maintenance therapy daily or alternate days for at least 3 years for those with a complete response, a complete remission lasting 4–14 years was observed in 20%, but was confined to those with stage IA–IB.[21] However, patients in this series were allowed other therapies, including radiotherapy, TSEB, phototherapy, and methotrexate to achieve a response. Subsequent relapse occurred in only 17% of these patients within 8 years of therapy being withdrawn, suggesting that some patients with very early-stage disease may have achieved a cure. Response rates were highest in the early stages of disease (IA, 80%; IB, 68%; IIA, 61%; IIB,

49%; III, 60%; IVA, 13%; IVB, 11%). The stage-specific 5/10-year survival rates were 94/89% (IA), 85/83% (IB), 82/67% (IIA), 59/31% (IIB), 75/19% (III), 20/13% (IVA), and 11/0% (IVB).[21] In a recent prospective open study, 64 patients with stage IA–IIA mycosis fungoides were treated with twice-weekly mechlorethamine (0.02% aqueous solution) to the whole skin surface (with the exception of the head), followed by immediate topical application of betamethasone cream for 6 months in all patients.[22] Overall, 58% achieved a complete response after a mean treatment duration of 3.6 ± 2.5 months (20 of 33, 61%, with stage IA; 15 of 26, 58%, with stage IB; and two of five, 40%, with stage IIA). Eighteen patients (28%) developed severe cutaneous reactions necessitating treatment withdrawal, and the complete response rates were significantly lower in these patients. Relapse occurred in 17 patients (46%) after a mean duration of 7.7 ± 6.5 months from complete response.

A retrospective study of 203 stage I–III patients treated with topical mechlorethamine (10–20 mg/100 mL to whole skin surface once daily until complete response, as the initial therapy, revealed an overall response rate of 83% and a complete response rate of 50%, with a median time to response of 12 months and a median time to relapse of 12 months despite maintenance therapy.[23] Responses were better for early-stage IA disease (65% complete response) than for stage IB (34% complete response). Only 10% of patients developed contact reactions with the ointment preparation, and only 8% developed secondary malignancies. Pediatric patients (n = 6) were also treated, and there was no significant toxicity. Overall, 68% of the patients were only treated throughout the follow-up period with topical mechlorethamine, and in this group the overall responses were higher (T1, 77% complete response; T2, 53% complete response), with relapse-free rates of 74% and 54% for T1 and 54% and 29% for T2 at 2 and 5 years, respectively.

Drawbacks
Topical mechlorethamine may cause an irritant reaction, and up to 40% of patients develop contact hypersensitivity, which may be less common with reduced frequencies of application. This is less common with the ointment (0.01–0.02%). The aqueous solution (10–20 mg in 40–60 mL water) is less stable than the ointment. Mechlorethamine (nitrogen mustard) is carcinogenic, and secondary cutaneous malignancies (nonmelanoma skin cancer) have been attributed to long-term use of topical mechlorethamine (with an 8.6-fold and 1.8-fold increased risk for squamous cell carcinoma and basal cell carcinoma, respectively). Home use is acceptable, with patients applying topical treatment overnight; however, partners should avoid contact, especially if pregnant. Appropriate protection for staff members applying topical therapy in the hospital setting is required, although no toxic effects have been reported.[24]

Comments
Mechlorethamine is an effective topical therapy for early-stage (patches/thin plaques) mycosis fungoides. However, interpretation of the studies is confounded by the use of other therapeutic modalities for most patients and by the retrospective nature of the studies. Duration of response varies, and the efficacy of maintenance therapy (6–18 months) and whole-body application remains unclear, but some patients with stage IA disease may appear to be cured. The survival data reported for topical mechlorethamine are similar to those previously published for patients with early-stage disease (Table 30.1). Any clinical efficacy of topical mechlorethamine therapy after TSEB therapy has to be confirmed. Almost all patients with stage IA mycosis fungoides have a normal life expectancy, and so controlled trials are required.

Topical carmustine
Efficacy
No RCTs were identified. A retrospective review of therapy in 143 patients revealed complete responses in 86% of stage IA patients, 47% in stage IB patients, 55% in stage IIA patients, 17% in stage IIB patients, 21% in stage III patients and 0% in stage IV patients.[25] Median time to complete response was 11·5 weeks. Alternate day or daily treatment with 10 mg 1,3-*bis*(2-chloroethyl)-1-nitrosourea (BCNU) in dilute (95%) alcohol (60 mL) or 20–40% BCNU ointment can be used.

Drawbacks
Contact hypersensitivity is uncommon (10%), but bone-marrow suppression is common (30%). The risk of secondary cutaneous malignancies may be lower than with mechlorethamine. Total doses should not exceed 600 mg per course, and repeated courses may be required. Maintenance therapy should be avoided. The ointment is more stable than the alcohol solution (3 months).

Comments
Limited data suggest that topical carmustine is clinically effective but is more extensively absorbed than mechlorethamine and therefore has a significant risk of bone-marrow suppression. It may help in patients with early-stage disease who show an irritant or allergic contact reaction to mechlorethamine. Comparative trials are needed.

Topical retinoids
Efficacy
No RCTs were found. A phase I/II open study of 0.1–1% bexarotene (Targretin) gel as incremental doses in 67 patients with stage IA/IB/IIA disease (initially alternate-day treatment, increasing to a maximum of four times daily if tolerated) showed a response rate of 63%, with 21% of patients showing a complete clinical response.[26] The median

time to response and the duration of the response were 20 and 99 weeks, respectively.

Drawbacks
Bexarotene 1% gel twice daily was well tolerated. Mild/moderate pruritus, burning pain, and rash (12% irritant contact dermatitis) were common.

Comment
The lack of a placebo control makes interpretation difficult, but the United States Food and Drug Administration (FDA) has approved 1% Targretin gel for the treatment of patients with stage IA/IB disease. Further controlled studies are required.

Topical peldesine (BCX-34)
Peldesine is an inhibitor of purine nucleoside phosphorylase, an enzyme involved in purine degradation within lymphocytes.

Efficacy
One RCT has compared topical application of peldesine twice daily to the entire skin surface for 24 weeks with a placebo (vehicle control) in 90 patients with stage IA/IB mycosis fungoides.[27] Partial or complete clinical responses occurred in 28% of patients treated with peldesine and 24% of patients treated with placebo ($P = 0.677$).

Drawbacks
A minority of patients noted minor pruritus and rash.

Comment
This is the only published placebo-controlled trial in CTCL. Although no significant efficacy is apparent, the results indicate a high placebo therapeutic response (mostly partial response), which should be considered when interpreting the efficacy of different topical therapies in early-stage mycosis fungoides. This study also emphasizes the importance of developing a validated scoring system to assess partial response.

Other topical therapies (photodynamic therapy and immune-response modifiers)
Efficacy
No RCTs were found. An isolated report of topical use of immune response modifiers has suggested a complete response to 5% imiquimod cream in comparison with placebo in a single patient with stage IA disease after daily application to specific lesions for 4 months. Responses were assessed clinically and with post-treatment biopsies.[28]

Topical photodynamic therapy with 5-aminolevulinic acid (5-ALA) and 100 J/cm² red light has been reported to be effective in isolated cases for patches and plaques, with clinical and/or histological clearance in 50–100% of cases,

which appears to be sustained.[29] In one report, a solitary tumor responded.

Drawbacks
Both these topical therapies can only be used for limited areas, which is a significant limitation for patients with widespread cutaneous disease.

Comments
The current studies are based on limited case reports, and there would have to be comparative studies with other topical therapies and radiotherapy to justify the use of these therapies in CTCL. Furthermore, until there are technical developments of these topical therapies to permit application to large areas, it is unlikely that either will become a standard form of skin-directed therapy for CTCL.

What are the effects of phototherapy in mycosis fungoides/Sézary syndrome?

Efficacy
No RCTs were found. Broadband ultraviolet B (UVB, 290–320 nm) phototherapy with maintenance therapy produced a complete response in 83% of 35 patients with early-stage disease (IA/IB), with a median response time of 5 months and a median response duration of 22 months.[30]

Narrow-band UVB (TL-01; 311–313 nm) also produced a complete response in 75% of patients (six of eight patients with early patch-stage disease, IA), with a mean duration of response of 20 months.[31]

A retrospective study of 24 patients with stage IA/IB disease and patches only showed complete responses in 13 (54%) and partial responses in seven (29%), with a histological response confirmed in nine of 10 patients and a mean time to relapse of 12.5 weeks.[32]

High-dose ultraviolet A1 (UVA1) phototherapy (340–400 nm; 100 J/cm² on a 5 day per week basis) has been used in 13 patients (eight in stage IB, four in stage IIB, and one in stage III) until maximal response. Eleven of the 13 patients showed a complete response, defined as a complete resolution of cutaneous lesions (mean number of sessions 22; cumulative dose 2149 J/cm²) and seven patients remained in complete response after a mean follow-up period of 7.2 months.[33]

Drawbacks
One drawback is UV-induced erythema/pruritus. In addition, high cumulative doses of UVA contribute to an increased risk of nonmelanoma skin cancer.

Comments
UVB phototherapy is an effective short-term therapy for early patch and thin plaques, but the duration of disease-free remission varies and the treatment probably does

not affect long-term survival rates. UVA1 penetrates more deeply than UVB and psoralen ultraviolet A (PUVA), but whether this is clinically relevant has not yet been established. No adequate comparative studies between different forms of phototherapy and PUVA have been published.

PUVA photochemotherapy
Efficacy
No RCTs were found. An open study of 82 patients treated with PUVA and followed for up to 15 years reported an overall complete response rate of 65% (79% for stage IA, 59% for stage IB, and 83% for stage IIA disease) and mean cumulative doses of 134 J/cm^2 (IA), 140 J/cm^2 (IB) and 240 J/cm^2 (IIA), with a median time to complete response of 3 months.[34] Few patients with more advanced disease were treated, making interpretation of the results for patients with stage > IIA difficult. In this study, 67% of stage IA, 41% of stage IB, and 67% of stage IIA patients were free of disease at 2 years, but maintenance PUVA was given to most patients.[34] Survival rates at 5 and 10 years were 89% for stage IA, 78% for stage IB, and—surprisingly—100% for stage IIA.

A further open study of PUVA in 82 patients with CTCL showed a complete response in 62% of patients, with an 88% complete response rate in stage IA (mean cumulative PUVA dose 160 J/cm^2), 52% in stage IB (498J/cm^2), and 46% in stage III disease (178 J/cm^2). No responses were seen in stage IIB patients. The maximum duration of response was 68 months; 38% of the complete responders relapsed despite maintenance PUVA.[35]

Although maintenance therapy has been recommended for responders, a further open study has shown that 56% of stage IA and 39% of stage IB patients with complete response had no recurrence of CTCL during a maximum period of 44 months' follow-up, despite no maintenance therapy.[36]

A retrospective study of the long-term outcome following complete remission from PUVA monotherapy at a single institution, in 66 patients with stage IA and IB/IIA disease, reported that 50% of patients (n = 33) maintained a complete response after a median follow-up of 84 months, while 50% experienced a relapse, with a median disease-free interval of 39 months.[37] Maintenance PUVA was given to almost all patients with a complete response/partial response. The only significant difference between the two groups was a higher cumulative UVA dose and the number of PUVA sessions in those achieving a complete response. There was no significant difference in the overall survival rate for the nonrelapse and relapse cohorts.

Drawbacks
Nausea, phototoxic reactions, and skin carcinogenesis are well-recognized adverse effects. The risk of nonmelanoma skin cancer is directly related to the cumulative dose and total number of sessions.

Comments
Despite the lack of controlled trials, PUVA remains one of the most useful skin-directed therapies for early stages of mycosis fungoides. RCTs comparing PUVA with TL-01 and topical mechlorethamine would be helpful in early-stage disease (IA/IB). Data on the duration of response and disease-free survival/overall survival data are slowly emerging. The role of maintenance therapy is unclear, but high cumulative doses entail a significant risk of squamous cell carcinoma. Disease-free survival and overall survival rates in patients treated with topical chemotherapy, phototherapy and TSEB are difficult to compare without RCTs, but there appears to be little difference in early-stage disease, which emphasizes the urgent need for RCTs.

Combination regimens involving photochemotherapy
Efficacy
An RCT has compared PUVA two to five times weekly, plus interferon alfa, 9 MU three times weekly, with interferon alfa plus acitretin, 25–50 mg/day, in 98 patients (maximum duration of treatment in both groups 48 weeks).[38] In 82 patients with stage I/II disease, complete response rates were 70% in the PUVA/interferon group in comparison with 38% in the interferon/acitretin group ($P < 0.05$). Responses were assessed on the basis of clinical observation only. Time to response was 18.6 weeks in the PUVA/interferon group, compared with 21.8 weeks in the interferon/acitretin group ($P = 0.026$), but no data on the duration of response were reported. The total cumulative doses of interferon alfa were similar in the two groups.

An open study of 69 patients compared PUVA and acitretin with PUVA alone in mycosis fungoides.[39] This showed that the cumulative dose of PUVA needed to achieve a complete response was lower in the combined-treatment group, although the overall complete response was similar in the two groups (73% and 72%, respectively). No data on the duration of response were documented.[39]

Phase I and II studies of PUVA (three times weekly) combined with variable doses of interferon alfa (maximum tolerated dose of 12 MU/m^2 three times weekly) in 39 patients with mycosis fungoides (all stages) and Sézary syndrome have reported an overall response rate of 100%, with 62% showing a complete response and 28% a partial response (the complete response rates were 79% in stage IB patients, 80% in IIA patients, 33% in stage IIB patients, 63% in stage III patients, and 40% in stage IVA patients).[40] PUVA was continued as a maintenance therapy indefinitely, while interferon alfa was continued for 2 years or until disease progression or withdrawal due to adverse effects. The median response duration was 28 months, with a median survival of 62 months.[40]

A prospective phase II study of PUVA (three times weekly with maintenance PUVA after complete response) combined with interferon alfa (escalating dose schedule of 3 MU to 12 × 3 weekly according to tolerability) in 63 patients with all stages (37 in stage IB and 12 in stage III) for 1 year reported a complete response rate of 75%, with a median response duration of 32 months.[41] The overall 5-year disease-free survival rate was 75%. A further recent prospective phase II study assessing the combination of interferon alfa (6–18 MU/week) and PUVA in 89 patients with stage IA–IIA mycosis fungoides treated for 14 months showed an 84% complete response rate, with sustained remission in 20%.[42]

Drawbacks

These were as for PUVA, interferon alfa, and acitretin alone. In the RCT,[38] similar rates of mild/moderate adverse effects were noted in both groups, but more patients discontinued treatment in the interferon/acitretin group because of adverse effects.

Comments

The RCT is one of very few in CTCL, and it shows that combined PUVA and interferon alfa is more effective than interferon alfa or acitretin in early stage I/II disease. Weaknesses of this study are the lack of a validated scoring system to assess tumor burden and a lack of evidence that outcome was assessed blind to allocation status. In addition, data regarding the duration of response and disease-free survival/overall survival are urgently required. The trial comparing PUVA alone with PUVA plus acitretin[39] suggests a reduction in the mean cumulative dose of PUVA to complete response, which would be helpful; disappointingly, however, there is no evidence for increased overall efficacy in the retinoid–PUVA group. The combination of interferon alfa and PUVA appears to be highly effective in all stages of CTCL. It should be noted, however, that the overall remission rate may be similar to that with PUVA alone, and randomized data for duration of remission and cumulative UVA dose are urgently required.

What are the effects of immunotherapy in mycosis fungoides/Sézary syndrome?

Interferon alfa

Efficacy

No RCTs of interferon alfa in CTCL have been reported, except as combination therapy (see above).

In an open study, 20 heavily pretreated patients (stage IB–III) were given maximum tolerated doses of interferon alfa (50 MU/m^2 intramuscularly three times weekly) for 3 months.[43] An overall response rate of 45% was reported, with a median response duration to maximum tolerated doses of interferon alfa of 5 months.

A subsequent nonrandomized study revealed response rates of 64% in 22 patients (stage IA–IVA), with an overall complete response rate of 27%.[44] Objective responses were greater in the group treated with an escalating-dose schedule of interferon alfa (36 MU/day) compared with those on a low-dose regimen (3 MU/day) for 10 weeks (78% versus 37%), but overall numbers were too small for statistical comparison.

An open study of 43 patients treated with escalating doses (3–18 MU daily) of interferon alfa showed an overall response rate of 74%, with a complete response rate of 26%.[45] Responses were more common in those who had not had prior treatment and in those with stage I/II (88%) than in those with stage III/IV (63%) disease. The disease-free survival rate was 21% at 55 months.

A phase II study of intermittent high-dose interferon alfa-2a given on days 1–5 every 3 weeks (mean dose 65.5 MU/m^2/week) showed a response rate of 29%, with only one complete response in 24 patients with advanced (IVA/B) refractory CTCL.[46] Dose reductions were necessary, and no improved responses were seen in those patients receiving dose escalation.

In an open study, 45 patients with CTCL, including 13 patients with Sézary syndrome, received low-dose interferon alfa (6–9 MU daily) for 3 months; those responding were continued on interferon alfa alone, while non-responders were given interferon alfa plus acitretin, 0.5 mg/kg/day.[47] After 12 months' therapy, 62% achieved a partial response or complete response, including 11 patients on combined therapy. However, this study design does not exclude the possibility that the response in the interferon alfa non-responder group was due to a delayed efficacy from continued interferon alfa therapy after 3 months.

Intralesional interferon alfa (1–2 MU three times weekly for 4 weeks) can induce complete regression of individual plaques (10 of 12 sites) compared with placebo-treated sites (one of 12 sites).[48]

Drawbacks

The dose-limiting toxicity of interferon alfa includes reversible hematological abnormalities, hepatitis, weight loss, headache, depression, and flu-like symptoms consisting of fever, myalgia, lethargy, and anorexia.

Comments

The clinical efficacy of interferon alfa in all stages of CTCL is supported by the complete response rates seen in these uncontrolled studies. It appears that higher doses are more effective, but dose-limiting toxicity is a problem. Critical questions remain about the effect on disease-free survival and overall survival and the role of combined therapy with PUVA. RCTs are required to address these issues.

Interferon gamma

Efficacy

No RCTs were found. A phase II trial of intramuscular

gamma interferon in 16 CTCL patients with escalating doses to a maximum of 0.5 mg/m^2 daily reported an objective partial response rate of 31%, with a median duration of 10 months.[49]

Drawbacks
As for interferon alfa.

Comments
The lack of complete response is disappointing. Further studies are required, but are a low priority.

Interleukins
Efficacy
No RCTs were found. Interleukin-2 (IL-2) (20 MU/m^2 every 2 weeks for 6 weeks and then monthly for 5 months) produced responses in five of seven CTCL patients, including a complete response in three.[50]

In a phase I dose-escalation study of subcutaneous IL-12 (50–300 ng/kg) twice weekly for up to 24 weeks, objective responses were noted in five CTCL patients (four of five with stage IB disease; one of three with Sézary syndrome).[51] Two patients with stage IB disease had a complete response within 7–8 weeks, which was confirmed histologically. Intralesional therapy was also effective for individual tumors in two patients with stage IIB disease, but both developed progressive disease.[51]

Drawbacks
Side effects were minor and included flu-like symptoms, mild transient liver function abnormalities, and depression.

Comments
RCTs are required to establish whether IL-2 and IL-12 have any therapeutic role in CTCL.

Extracorporeal photopheresis
Efficacy
No RCTs were reported. A systematic review (1987–98) of response rates and outcomes in open nonrandomized and mostly retrospective studies of extracorporeal photopheresis (ECP) in erythrodermic CTCL (stage III/IVA) showed an overall response rate of 35–71%, with complete response rates of 14–26%.[52] Responses have been assessed mostly using a scoring system similar to that devised for the original study.[53]

A further retrospective study of 34 patients with mostly erythrodermic CTCL (22 stage IV, 10 stage III, and two stage I) reported an overall response rate of 50%, with 18% achieving complete response.[54] Response was restricted to those with erythrodermic disease. This study involved a modified "accelerated" treatment schedule consisting of nine (as opposed to six) collections during each cycle and an increase to twice-monthly treatment if there was a lack of response.

Other studies have reported minor responses (25–50% improvement), but this would not satisfy accepted criteria for partial response. ECP is generally administered on two consecutive days (one cycle) each month, and it is accepted that at least six cycles are required to assess response. Survival data have been reported in four studies of erythrodermic disease, with median survivals of 39–100 months from diagnosis.[55–58]

A randomized crossover study comparing ECP with PUVA in patients with nonerythrodermic (stage IB–IIA) mycosis fungoides has shown no clinical efficacy for ECP in early stages of the disease in comparison with PUVA.[59] In contrast, other uncontrolled studies have reported successful responses in patients with nonerythrodermic disease.

A 9-year retrospective study of ECP alone in 37 patients (68% stage IB, 5% stage IIB, 27% stage III) showed a complete response rate of 14% and a partial response rate of 41%, with an improved response rate in resistant patients with the addition of interferon alfa.[60]

A prospective open nonrandomized study of 14 patients with nonerythrodermic mycosis fungoides (stage IIA/IIB) treated with combined interferon alfa (maximum tolerated dose of 18 MU three times weekly) and ECP for 6 months showed a complete response in four and a partial response in three (overall response 50%), but this design does not exclude responses to interferon alfa alone.[61]

A nonrandomized retrospective study in erythrodermic disease (stage III/IVA) (1991–1996) showed that six of nine patients treated with interferon alfa plus ECP showed a response (with four complete responses), while only one of 10 patients treated with ECP alone achieved a complete response. In the patients achieving a complete response, lymph-node disease also resolved.[62] In contrast, the combination of interferon alfa plus ECP failed to produce significant clinical responses in six patients with Sézary syndrome,[63] although isolated case reports have described patients with Sézary syndrome in whom a complete clinical and molecular remission has been achieved with this combination.[64,65]

A retrospective nonrandomized study (1974–97) has compared disease-specific survival and overall survival in 44 patients with erythrodermic CTCL treated with either TSEB alone or TSEB and adjuvant or neoadjuvant ECP (see below).

A retrospective cohort study of 47 stage III/IVA patients (42 of whom had peripheral blood involvement) treated with ECP for six or more cycles showed an overall response rate of 79%, with a 26% complete response rate, a 53% partial response rate, and a median survival from initiation of therapy of 74 months.[66] A combination of ECP with immunomodulatory therapy (interferon alfa, retinoids, interferon gamma, and/or sargramostim) was employed in 31 patients.

Drawbacks

ECP is well tolerated. Mild lymphopenia and anemia can occur with long-term therapy. High cost and lack of availability means that ECP will remain confined to specialist centers.

Comments

Controlled trials are urgently required to compare ECP with standard single-agent chemotherapy regimens in erythrodermic disease and specifically in Sézary syndrome. Some previous studies have not clearly defined their diagnostic criteria for erythrodermic CTCL, and others have included patients with nonerythrodermic disease. Combination therapy with ECP and interferon alfa is frequently used, but the existing studies do not exclude a beneficial response to interferon alfa alone. An RCT to address this important issue is currently being considered by the European Organization for Research and Treatment of Cancer (EORTC). Studies suggest that ECP requires a minimum tumor burden within peripheral blood,[67] and the only RCT of ECP in nonerythrodermic, early-stage disease suggests that it is not effective.

Thymopentin

Efficacy

In a phase II trial, 20 patients with Sézary syndrome were treated with 50 mg intravenous thymopentin (TP-5), a synthetic pentapeptide, three times weekly for a mean of 16 months. The overall response rate was 75%, with eight complete responses and seven partial responses and a median duration of 22 months. Four-year survival was 54%.[68]

Drawbacks

Thymopentin was well tolerated. Mild hypersensitivity reactions during the infusion were noted.

Comments

The mechanism of action of thymopentin remains unclear. The overall response rate is very high, but the lack of subsequent reports is surprising and further studies are required to confirm this isolated small study.

Ciclosporin

Efficacy

A phase II case series of ciclosporin, 15 mg/kg/day, in 16 patients with refractory T-cell lymphomas, including 11 CTCL (all stage IVA/B), revealed only two responses in CTCL, with eight CTCL patients developing progressive disease; there was one drug-related death.[69] The two

patients showing a partial response had a rapid relapse of disease when treatment was discontinued.

Drawbacks

High doses of ciclosporin are poorly tolerated and frequent dose reductions are required. Hypertension, renal toxicity and infection were common.

Comments

This study suggests that ciclosporin is not effective in CTCL, and anecdotal reports suggest that ciclosporin can actually cause rapid disease progression in CTCL.

What are the effects of systemic retinoids in mycosis fungoides/Sézary syndrome?

Etretinate/acitretin/isotretinoin

Efficacy

A systematic review (1988–94) of open studies of oral retinoids in CTCL (mycosis fungoides and Sézary syndrome) showed an overall mean response rate of 58% and a complete response rate of 19%, with a median duration of response of 3–13 months.[70]

A nonrandomized study of 68 patients with various stages of mycosis fungoides and Sézary syndrome compared 13-cis-retinoic acid with etretinate and found similar efficacy and toxicity (isotretinoin: complete response 21%, partial response 38%; etretinate: complete response 21%, partial response 46%).[71] A phase II study of isotretinoin in 25 patients with mycoses fungoides (IB–III) showed an overall response rate of 44%, with three patients achieving a complete response, and a median response duration of 8 months using high doses (2 mg/kg/day).[72]

An RCT comparing PUVA and interferon alfa with PUVA and acitretin showed a significantly better response rate for PUVA and interferon alfa[38] (see above).

Drawbacks

Adverse events included mucocutaneous erosions and xerosis, hyperlipidemia, hepatotoxicity, and teratogenicity.

Comments

Acitretin and etretinate have some efficacy in the early stages of disease, but are no better and probably less effective than, for example, PUVA and interferon alfa.

Bexarotene

Bexarotene is a new retinoid capable of binding to the retinoid X receptor as opposed to the retinoic acid receptor. This drug has antiproliferative and proapoptotic properties.

Efficacy

No RCTs were found. A phase II open trial compared

two doses (6.5 mg/m^2/day and 650 mg/m^2/day) of oral bexarotene in 58 patients with refractory stage IA–IIA CTCL.[73] The optimal dose was 300 mg/m^2/day in terms of response and tolerability. Objective responses of 20%, 54%, and 67% were noted at the 6.5, 300, and 650 mg/m^2/day doses, respectively. Rates of disease progression were 47%, 21% and 13%, respectively. Median duration of response at the highest dose level was 516 days. In late stages of disease (stage IIB–IVB), overall response rates of 45% (at 300 mg/m^2/day) and 55% (at doses > 300 mg/m^2/day) have been reported, with a relapse rate of 36% and a projected median duration of response of 299 days.[74]

Drawbacks

Reversible adverse effects included hyperlipidemia, central hypothyroidism, leukopenia, headache, and asthenia as well as other retinoid adverse effects.

Comments

These studies suggest a therapeutic efficacy for bexarotene in all stages of CTCL, but comparisons with other therapies and data on effects on disease-free survival and overall survival in later stages of disease are required. An EORTC randomized controlled trial comparing PUVA with PUVA and bexarotene in stage IB is due for completion shortly. Combination with other therapies, including phototherapy and interferon alfa, appears to be well tolerated,[75,76] but controlled data on the clinical benefits of combination therapies are awaited.

What are the effects of antibody and toxin therapies in mycosis fungoides/Sézary syndrome?

Anti-CD4 monoclonal antibody
Efficacy
In a phase I/II trial, seven patients with mycosis fungoides were treated with a chimeric (murine/human) anti-CD4 monoclonal antibody with successive increasing doses (10, 20, 40 and 80 mg) twice weekly for 3 weeks. All patients showed some clinical response, with one complete response and two partial responses, but these were all short-lived (with a median duration of 2 weeks).[77]

A subsequent study from the same group showed a partial response in seven of eight patients given higher doses (50–200 mg), with a median freedom from progression of 28 weeks.[78]

Drawbacks

Treatment was well tolerated, with no acute toxicity. There is a marked but temporary suppression of T-cell proliferative responses to phytohemagglutinin. There is no documented depletion of CD4 counts. The immunogenicity of the antibody is unclear.

Alemtuzumab (Campath-1H)
Efficacy
As part of a phase II trial in advanced low-grade non-Hodgkin's lymphoma, eight patients with mycoses fungoides received 30 mg intravenous Alemtuzumab (Campath-1H) three times weekly for a maximum of 12 weeks.[79] Four CTCL patients achieved a response, with two (25%) showing complete response. No details of the duration of response were provided. An identical regimen was utilized in a phase II study of eight mycosis fungoides/Sézary syndrome patients with refractory and/or advanced disease.[80] Overall, 38% (three partial responses) achieved a response (no complete responses), but the response duration was short (3 months). An additional phase II study of 22 advanced mycosis fungoides/Sézary syndrome patients reported a 32% complete response rate and a 23% partial response rate, with a median time to treatment failure of 12 months.[81]

Drawbacks

Severe neutropenia and opportunistic infections are common, including cytomegalovirus reactivation. Reports of increased cardiac toxicity due to alemtuzumab[82] have not been confirmed in a review of larger cohorts,[83] but might reflect prior use of anthracycline-based chemotherapy.

Comments

Alemtuzumab (Campath-1H) is a humanized anti-CD52 antibody that binds to all lymphocytes. This study suggests that patients with CTCL show the highest response rate, but infectious complications leading to death do occur. Further studies are justified.

Denileukin diftitox (diphtheria IL-2 fusion toxin)
Efficacy
A phase III open uncontrolled study of denileukin diftitox in 71 patients with stage IB–IVA CTCL has shown an overall response rate of 30%, with 10% showing a complete clinical response.[84] Only CTCL cases with biopsies showing > 20% CD25$^+$ (IL-2R) lymphocytes were enrolled. The median duration of response was 6.9 months. No difference in response rates or duration of response was noted between 9 and 18 µg/kg/day. The development of anti-denileukin diftitox antibodies apparently did not affect response rates. A phase I study of combined denileukin diftitox (18 µg/kg/day × 3 days every 21 days) and escalating doses of bexarotene (75–300 mg/day) in 14 patients with relapsed or refractory CTCL showed an overall response rate of 67% (four complete responses, four partial responses) and no increased toxicity.[85]

Drawbacks

Adverse effects include flu-like symptoms, acute infusion-related hypersensitivity effects, a vascular leak syndrome, and transient elevations of hepatic enzymes.

Comments

This uncontrolled study suggests that people with CD25$^+$ CTCL can respond to this new fusion toxin, but the duration of the response is short. However, patients recruited for this trial were heavily pretreated, suggesting that this is likely to be a useful additional therapy for CTCL patients with resistant disease, despite potential adverse effects. A randomized placebo-controlled trial in patients with stage IB/IIB/III mycosis fungoides who have undergone fewer than three previous treatments is ongoing.

Ricin-labelled anti-CD5 immunoconjugate (H65-RTA)

Efficacy

A phase I trial of H65-RTA in 14 patients with resistant CTCL revealed a maximum tolerated dose of 0.33 mg/kg/day and partial response in only four patients of short duration (3–8 months).[86]

Drawbacks

Acute hypersensitivity effects and vascular leak syndrome were noted.

Radioimmunoconjugate (90Y-T101)

Efficacy

A phase I trial of this radioimmunoconjugate (which also targets CD5$^+$ lymphocytes) in 10 patients (CD5$^+$) with hematological malignancies, of whom eight patients had CTCL, showed partial responses in three CTCL patients, with a median response duration of 23 weeks.[87] Biodistribution studies showed good uptake into skin and involved lymph nodes.

Drawbacks

Bone-marrow suppression was observed. T cells recovered within 3 weeks, but B-cell suppression persisted after 5 weeks.

Comments

This is an interesting phase I study, because CTCL is a radiosensitive tumor. Further studies are required.

What are the effects of radiotherapy in mycosis fungoides/Sézary syndrome?

Superficial radiotherapy

Efficacy

No systematic reviews or RCTs were identified. Dose–response studies have clearly established that localized superficial radiotherapy is an effective palliative therapy for individual lesions in mycosis fungoides.[88] A retrospective study of palliative superficial radiotherapy used to treat 191 lesions from 20 patients with mycosis fungoides showed complete responses of 95% for plaques and small (< 3 cm)

tumors and a complete response of 93% for large tumors (> 3 cm), irrespective of dose. However in-field recurrences within 1–2 years were more common for those lesions treated with lower doses (42% for < 1000 cGy, 32% for 1000–2000 cGy, 21% for 2000–3000 cGy, and 0% for > 3000 cGy).

Drawbacks

Superficial radiation is well tolerated. Mild local erythema and occasional erosion have been reported. Use of low-dose/energy (400 cGy in two or three daily fractions at 80–150 kV) is therapeutically effective and allows treatment of overlapping fields and lower limb sites.

Comments

CTCL is a highly radiosensitive malignancy, and localized superficial radiotherapy is an invaluable form of palliative treatment for patients with all stages of mycosis fungoides. Treatment should be palliative except for patients with solitary localized disease, in whom a "cure" is theoretically possible. Although in-field recurrence rates were very low for lesions treated with > 3000 cGy, the number of lesions treated with this dose was very low in comparison with the other groups, and this form of therapy is only palliative in mycosis fungoides, as the disease is multifocal. The use of high-dose fractionation regimens for individual lesions should therefore be avoided in mycosis fungoides, because the complete response rates are similar to those for low-dose regimens (see above) and recurrent disease adjacent to previously treated fields can be treated with overlapping fields if necessary. However, treatment of disease on the lower legs can be difficult, in view of a higher risk of radiation necrosis with repeated treatments.

Total skin electron beam therapy (TSEB)

Efficacy

A systematic review (meta-analysis) of open uncontrolled and mostly retrospective studies of TSEB as monotherapy for 952 patients with all stages of CTCL has established that the rate of complete response is dependent on the stage of disease and the skin surface dose and energy, with complete response rates of 96% in stage IA/IB/IIA disease, 36% in stage IIB disease, and 60% in stage III disease.[89] A greater skin surface dose (32–36 Gy) and higher energy (4–6 MeV) were significantly associated with a higher rate of complete response; 5-year relapse-free survivals of 10–23% were noted.[89]

One small RCT has compared TSEB with topical mechlorethamine in 42 patients, with similar rates of complete response and duration of response in both groups in early stages of disease, but better overall responses in later stages of disease with TSEB.[90]

A retrospective study of TSEB (median dose 32 Gy; median treatment time 21 days) as monotherapy for 45 patients with erythrodermic CTCL (28 stage III, 13 stage IVA, four stage IVB) showed a 60% complete response rate, with 26% disease-free at 5 years.[91] The overall median survival was 3.4 years, which was associated significantly with an absence of peripheral blood involvement (stage III disease). Higher rates of complete response (74%) and disease-free progression (36%) were noted in those patients receiving a more intense regimen (32–40 Gy and 4–6 MeV).

A retrospective study of 66 CTCL patients (1978–96) treated with 30 Gy in far fewer fractions (12 fractions over 40 days) showed a complete response rate of 65%, with progression-free survival of 30% at 5 years and 18% at 10 years.[92] Responses, and specifically the 5-year overall survival, were highest in those with early-stage disease (79–93% for IA/IB/III compared with 44% for IIB/IVA/B).

Although it has been recommended that TSEB can only be given once in a lifetime, several reports have described multiple courses in CTCL.[93,94] A retrospective analysis of 15 patients (1968–90) with mycosis fungoides who received two courses of TSEB reported a mean dose of 32.6 Gy for the first course and 23.4 Gy for the second, with a mean interval of 41.3 months. No additional toxicities were noted, but the complete response rate for the second course was lower (40% compared with 73%).[93] A further retrospective study of 14 patients with CTCL reported a mean dose of 36 Gy for the first (93% complete response) and 18 Gy for the second course (86% complete response).[94] In this series, five patients received a third course (total dose 12–30 Gy). The median duration of response was 20 months for the first and 11.5 months for the second course. No additional toxicities were reported. In both of these studies, the fractionation regimens employed may have been critical for tolerability (1 Gy per day at 6 MeV over 9–12 weeks).

Combination TSEB regimens

An RCT including 103 CTCL patients in which TSEB and multiagent chemotherapy (cyclophosphamide, Adriamycin, vincristine, and etoposide, CAVE) with sequential topical therapy, including superficial radiotherapy and phototherapy, reported a higher complete response rate in the TSEB/chemotherapy group (38% compared with 18%; $P = 0.032$), but after a median follow-up of 75 months, the disease-free survival and overall survival did not differ significantly.[95]

A retrospective nonrandomized study comparing TSEB (32–40 Gy) alone with TSEB followed by ECP (given 2 days monthly for a median of 6 months) in 44 patients with erythrodermic CTCL (57% stage III, 30% stage IVA, 13% stage IVB; overall, 59% had B1 hematological involvement) has reported an overall complete response rate of 73% after TSEB, with a 3-year disease-free survival of 49% for 17 patients who received only TSEB (overall survival 63%) and 81% for 15 patients who received TSEB followed by ECP (overall survival 88%).[96] A multivariate analysis suggested that the combination of TSEB and ECP was significantly

associated with a prolonged disease-free and cause-specific survival when corrected for peripheral blood involvement (B1) and stage of disease.

Drawbacks

Adverse effects of TSEB include radiation-induced secondary cutaneous malignancies, telangiectasia, pigmentation, anhidrosis, pruritus, alopecia, and xerosis. Treatment is generally only given once in a lifetime, but several reports suggest that multiple therapies may be tolerated (see above).

Comments

Although these studies are uncontrolled and mostly retrospective, the response rates indicate that TSEB is highly effective for CTCL. The lack of a long-term response in early-stage disease suggests that TSEB should be reserved for later stages of disease, particularly as an RCT has indicated that responses are similar for TSEB and topical mechlorethamine. Meta-analysis of observational data indicates that higher-dosage regimens are more effective (32–40 Gy with 4–6 MeV). EORTC consensus guidelines for TSEB use in CTCL have been published.[97]

Although an RCT in CTCL indicates that combined TSEB and chemotherapy is no more effective than sequential skin-directed therapy, a further trial comparing TSEB alone with TSEB and chemotherapy in late stages of disease (stage IIB) would be helpful. The current data on long-term disease-free survival and overall survival in erythrodermic CTCL suggest that TSEB is effective, particularly if combined with ECP, but this requires confirmation in an RCT.

What are the effects of single-agent chemotherapy in mycosis fungoides/Sézary syndrome?

Single-agent chemotherapy regimens
Efficacy

No RCTs have been reported. A systematic review of uncontrolled open studies of single-agent regimens in 526 CTCL patients (1988–1994) revealed OR rates of 62%, with a complete response rate of 33% and median response durations of 3–22 months.[70] These therapies included alkylating agents (chlorambucil and cyclophosphamide), antimetabolites (methotrexate), vinca alkaloids, and topoisomerase II inhibitors.

Drawbacks

As with all chemotherapy regimens, infection and myelosuppression are significant risks.

Comments

The lack of controlled studies makes interpretation difficult, but single-agent regimens may have similar efficacy to combination regimens (see below) although with lower toxicity and may therefore be preferable as palliative therapy in the late stages of mycosis fungoides and Sézary syndrome, especially as durable responses and cures are rarely, if ever, achieved. RCTs are urgently required.

Methotrexate/trimetrexate
Efficacy
No RCTs were identified. A retrospective report of low-dose methotrexate in 29 patients with erythrodermic CTCL (III/IVA) has shown a 41% complete remission rate, with an overall response rate of 58%.[98] Median freedom from treatment failure was 31 months and overall survival was 8.4 years. Weekly doses ranged from 5 to 125 mg for a median duration of 23 months. A majority (62%) of patients satisfied the criteria for a diagnosis of Sézary syndrome. Trimetrexate, a lipophilic antifolate which (unlike methotrexate) diffuses passively into cells and is therefore less prone to drug resistance, was assessed in an open trial of 20 patients with refractory/resistant CTCL (three with anaplastic large-cell lymphoma, 15 with mycosis fungoides/Sézary syndrome with large-cell transformation in 14, and two with peripheral T-cell lymphoma) using a schedule of 200 mg/m^2 every 14 days for up to 12 doses. This revealed an overall response rate of 45% (one complete response and eight partial responses), including two patients who had previously been resistant to methotrexate.[99]

Drawbacks
Adverse effects in the methotrexate trial included reversible abnormalities of liver function, mucositis, cutaneous erosions, reversible leukopenia and thrombocytopenia, nausea, diarrhea, and in one case pulmonary fibrosis. Trimetrexate has a similar pattern of adverse effects and appears to be well tolerated.

Comments
Although these data are uncontrolled, the overall survival in the methotrexate study is surprisingly good. A randomized study comparing methotrexate with other single-agent chemotherapies in erythrodermic CTCL would be worthwhile. The use of trimetrexate in CTCL merits further investigation.

Purine analogues
Efficacy
No RCTs were found. A systematic review of purine analogues in CTCL (1988–94) revealed overall and complete response rates, respectively, of 41% and 6% for deoxycoformycin (n = 63), 41% and 19% for 2-chlorodeoxyadenosine (n = 27), and 19% and 3% for fludarabine (n = 31).[70] Most of these studies included some patients with peripheral T-cell lymphomas. No comparative studies were available.

A prospective open study of deoxycoformycin in 28 heavily pretreated patients, of whom 21 had CTCL (14 with Sézary syndrome, seven in stage IIB) revealed an overall response rate of 71%, with 25% complete response and 46% partial response (overall response 10 of 14 patients with Sézary syndrome; four with complete response, and four of seven stage IIB patients; one complete response). The response was short-lived (median duration of 2 months for stage IIB disease and 3.5 months for Sézary syndrome), except in two cases of Sézary syndrome, with remissions for 17 and 19 months. The regimen consisted of starting doses of 3.75–5.0 mg/m^2/day for 3 days every 3 weeks. A dose escalation to 6.25 mg/m^2/day was rarely possible because of toxicity.[100]

Two recent open studies of deoxycoformycin in patients with CTCL (27 mycosis fungoides and 37 Sézary syndrome) have shown overall response rates ranging from 35% to 56%, with complete response rates from 10% to 33% and a reported median disease-free interval of 9 months in one of the studies.[101,102] Interestingly, responses were better in Sézary syndrome than in mycosis fungoides. The usual schedule for deoxycoformycin consists of a once-weekly intravenous dose of 4 mg/m^2 for 4 weeks and then every 14 days for either 6 months or until maximal response.

Combination therapy consisting of deoxycoformycin and interferon alfa in CTCL has shown overall response rates and complete response rates of 41% and 5%, respectively.[103]

A recent phase II trial of 2-chlorodeoxyadenosine in 21 refractory CTCL patients (mycosis fungoides IIB/IV and Sézary syndrome) revealed an overall response rate of 28%, with a 14% complete response rate (median duration of 4.5 months) and a 14% partial response rate (median duration of 2 months).[104]

Drawbacks
Side effects include nausea, infections (especially herpetic), CD4 lymphopenia, renal toxicity, hepatotoxicity, and myelosuppression (especially for 2-chlorodeoxyadenosine and fludarabine).

Comments
Purine analogues are attractive therapeutic candidates for CTCL because they are potent inhibitors of the enzyme adenosine deaminase, which preferentially accumulates in lymphoid cells, such that these drugs are selectively lymphocytotoxic independently of cell division. Although efficacy in CTCL is moderate, most of these patients were heavily pretreated and relatively chemoresistant. Patients with Sézary syndrome appear to respond better than those with late stages of mycosis fungoides. Purine analogues are appropriate as monotherapy, especially in Sézary syndrome, but the response duration may be short. Comparative trials

with other single-agent regimens in Sézary syndrome are required.

Gemcitabine
Efficacy
A phase II prospective trial (1200 mg/m² weekly for 3 weeks each month for a total of three cycles) in 44 previously treated patients with CTCL (30 mycosis fungoides patients with stage IIB or III disease) reported a partial response rate of 59% and a complete response rate of 12%, with median durations of 10 and 15 months, respectively.[105] A recent phase II prospective trial in 32 patients with either CTCL (26 with mycosis fungoides and one with Sézary syndrome) or peripheral T-cell lymphoma (n = 5) treated with 1200 mg/m² on days 1, 8, and 15 of a 28-day cycle for six cycles revealed seven (22%) complete responses and 17 (53%) partial responses, with a median duration of complete response of 10 months. The treatment was well tolerated.[106]

Drawbacks
The treatment was well tolerated and only mild hematological toxicity was noted.

Comments
Gemcitabine is a new pyrimidine analogue that appears to be well tolerated in heavily pretreated patients with advanced stages of mycosis fungoides. Further trials are required.

Doxorubicin
Efficacy
An open study of pegylated liposomal doxorubicin, 20 mg/m² monthly to a maximum of 400 mg or eight cycles, in 10 patients with various stages of mycosis fungoides, revealed a complete response in six and a partial response in two patients, with a median response duration of 15 months.[107,108] A retrospective study of 34 patients with CTCL treated with variable doses of pegylated liposomal doxorubicin, 20–40 mg/m² (26 received 20 mg/m²) every 2–4 weeks for eight cycles, revealed an overall response rate of 88% (15 complete responses and 15 partial responses).

Drawbacks
Mild hematological but no cardiac toxicity was reported. Palmoplantar erythrodysesthesia occurred rarely.

Comments
An EORTC phase II trial assessing a dose of 20 mg/m² every 2 weeks for six cycles in advanced stages of mycosis fungoides (> IIB) is currently open. Pegylated liposomal doxorubicin is an effective and well tolerated chemotherapeutic agent in CTCL.

What are the effects of multiagent chemotherapy regimens in mycosis fungoides/Sézary syndrome?

Combination chemotherapy
Efficacy
An RCT in 103 CTCL patients comparing TSEB and multiagent chemotherapy (CAVE) with sequential topical therapy, including superficial radiotherapy and phototherapy, revealed a higher complete response rate in the TSEB/chemotherapy group (38% compared with 18%; P = 0.032, with overall response rates of 90% and 65%, respectively), but after a median follow-up of 75 months there was no significant difference in the disease-free survival or overall survival.[95]

A systematic review of all systemic therapy in CTCL (mycoses fungoides and Sézary syndrome, 1988–94) showed an overall response rate of 81% in 331 patients treated with various different combination chemotherapeutic regimens, with a complete response rate of 38% and response duration ranging from 5 to 41 months, with no documented cures for patients with late stages of disease (IIB–IVB).[70]

Recent prospective nonrandomized studies of different multiagent chemotherapy regimens have revealed similar overall response rates. A third-generation anthracycline (idarubicin) was used in combination with etoposide, cyclophosphamide, vincristine, prednisolone, and bleomycin (VICOP-B) to treat 25 CTCL patients (eight stage IIB, 13 IVA, four stage IVB) for 12 weeks. Overall response rates of 80%, with 36% complete response, were documented, although 10 patients had not received any previous therapy. The two patients with Sézary syndrome did not respond, and the median duration of response in patients with mycoses fungoides was 8.7 months. Stage IIB patients had a median duration of response of 22 months, but four previously untreated patients received additional TSEB therapy after completion of chemotherapy.[109]

A combination of etoposide, vincristine, doxorubicin, cyclophosphamide, and prednisolone (EPOCH) was used to treat 15 patients with advanced, refractory CTCL (six with Sézary syndrome; four with stage IVB mycoses fungoides, one with adult T-cell lymphoma, and four with large-cell anaplastic lymphoma). After a median of five cycles, 27% had a complete response and 53% achieved a partial response (overall response rate 80%), with an overall median survival of 13.5 months.[110]

Drawbacks
Multiagent chemotherapy regimens are associated with very high rates of toxicity and considerable morbidity, including nausea, anorexia, infection, hepatotoxicity, and myelosuppression. Patients with CTCL are at high risk of septicemia, and therapy-related mortality with combination chemotherapy is a significant risk.

Comments

Patients with late stages of CTCL (IIB–IVB) will require treatment with a chemotherapy regimen, although the response duration is short. In the RCT,[95] overall survival/ disease-free survival was similar to that in those treated with skin-directed therapy, although in this study patients with early-stage disease were also included. The individual patient's quality of life should always be considered before embarking on very toxic regimens with limited efficacy. Single-agent regimens (see above) appear to have similar efficacy, although studies involving a comparison between single-agent and multiagent regimens, with or without TSEB, are required. To date, there have been no studies assessing the use of biochemotherapy in CTCL, although subsequent treatment with immunotherapy for patients achieving a response with chemotherapy should be considered.

Myeloablative chemotherapy with autologous/allogeneic peripheral blood/ bone-marrow stem-cell transplantation
Efficacy

No systematic reviews or RCTs were identified. Most studies were based on small numbers of patients. High-dose chemotherapy with TSEB and total-body irradiation (TBI) in four and three patients with mycosis fungoides (two patients had both TSEB and TBI), followed by autologous bone-marrow transplantation in six patients (three stage IIB, one stage IVA, two stage IVB) produced five complete clinical responses, but disease relapse occurred within 100 days in three patients.[111] The other two patients, who had both received a combination of carmustine, etoposide, and cisplatin chemotherapy, were disease-free at almost 2 years (666 and 631 days post-transplant).

High-dose chemotherapy combined with either TSEB or TBI and followed by autologous peripheral blood stem-cell transplantation in patients with stage IIB/IVA mycosis fungoides revealed complete responses in eight patients and durable clinical responses in four patients (median disease-free survival 11 months).[112]

Isolated case reports of high-dose chemotherapy with TBI/cyclophosphamide conditioning followed by allogeneic bone-marrow or stem-cell transplantation have shown durable complete remissions in five of six patients with stage IIB–IVA mycosis fungoides/Sézary syndrome.[113–116]

Reports of nonmyeloablative allogeneic transplantation (HLA-matched sibling donors) using cyclophosphamide/ fludarabine/TBI conditioning have shown durable complete remissions in two of three patients with refractory mycosis fungoides/Sézary syndrome, with one treatment-related death due to infectious complications.[117] A mini-allogeneic stem-cell transplantation was successful in a patient with a CD30 large-cell lymphoma, using a fludarabine/TBI conditioning regimen with a mismatch-related donor.[118] A recent retrospective study of allogeneic transplantation has shown durable complete clinical and molecular remissions in six of eight patients with refractory CTCL, with a median follow-up of 56 months and a median age of 45.5 years. Four patients (one matched unrelated donor) underwent full allogeneic peripheral blood stem-cell transplantation/bone-marrow transplantation using conditioning with TBI/cyclophosphamide (three patients) and busulphan/cyclophosphamide (one patient). Four patients (three matched unrelated donors) had nonmyeloablative peripheral blood stem-cell transplantation/bone-marrow transplantation with fludarabine/melphalan conditioning.[119] There were two treatment-related deaths due to graft-versus-host disease (full-allo) and respiratory syncytial virus infection (mini-allo).

Drawbacks

Myeloablative therapy is associated with a high incidence of toxicity and systemic infections. Significant mortality —especially with allogeneic transplantation—occurs, but there may be less toxicity with nonmyeloablative stem-cell transplantation.

Comments

Controlled trials comparing autologous/allogeneic transplantation with standard chemotherapy in late stages of mycosis fungoides are required. However, autologous stem-cell transplantation/bone-marrow transplantation appears to be associated with only short-term remission, and although the mortality rate associated with allogeneic transplantation makes this a less attractive approach, the use of nonmyeloablative allogeneic procedures to induce a graft-versus-tumor effect therefore appears to be an important option to be considered in younger patients with advanced refractory CTCL, in view of the potential for long-term complete remission.

Key points

Implications for practice

- Although there are not many well-designed RCTs in CTCL, there is some convincing evidence from uncontrolled studies that several skin-directed therapies have a significant therapeutic effect.
- However, there is a fundamental lack of data on the impact of different therapies on disease-free survival and overall survival, which will only become clearer when the results of key RCTs in different stages of disease become available.
- In addition, patients with early-stage disease can have a normal life expectancy, and so aggressive therapies with a significant mortality and morbidity should be avoided in these patients, especially when the chance of a cure is very low.
- Patients with early-stage disease (IA/IB/IIA) should be offered skin-directed therapies such as topical mechlorethamine,

phototherapy, PUVA, and superficial radiotherapy. Interferon alfa should be considered for patients with persistent or recurrent stage IB/IIA disease. Some patients with stage IA disease may not require any specific therapy.

- Patients with late stages of disease (IIB/IV) should be offered TSEB, single-agent palliative chemotherapy and multiagent chemotherapy, according to performance status.
- Patients with erythrodermic disease should be offered photopheresis, immunotherapy, and single-agent chemotherapy as palliative therapy, aiming to improve the quality of life. TSEB therapy may be indicated for erythrodermic disease when there is a lack of significant peripheral blood tumor burden.

Recommendations for the future

- New topical therapies should be assessed in the context of well-designed clinical trials comparing them with topical mechlorethamine.
- The role of new immunotherapies and retinoids in early stage (IB/IIA) disease should involve comparative RCTs with standard therapies such as PUVA.
- TSEB therapy, with or without adjuvant immunotherapy and chemotherapy, should be reserved for patients with late stages of disease, preferably in the context of clinical trials.
- There is an urgent need for more effective therapy for late-stage disease, and this should be based on appropriate RCTs involving new immunotherapies, adjuvants, single-agent and multiagent chemotherapies, and both (mini)allogeneic and autologous transplants in selected individuals.

References

1 Willemze R, Jaffe ES, Burg G. WHO-EORTC classification for cutaneous lymphomas. *Blood* 2005;**105**:3768–85.
2 Weinstock M, Horm J. Mycosis fungoides in the United States: increasing incidence and descriptive epidemiology. *JAMA* 1988;**260**:42–6.
3 Zackheim H, Amin S, Kashani-Sabet M, McMillan A. Prognosis in cutaneous T-cell lymphoma by skin stage: long term survival in 489 patients. *J Am Acad Dermatol* 1999;**40**:418–25.
4 Siegel R, Pandolfino T, Guitart J, Rosen S, Kuzel T. Primary cutaneous T-cell lymphoma: review and current concepts. *J Clin Oncol* 2000;**18**:2908–25.
5 Bunn P, Lamberg S. Report of the committee on staging and classification of cutaneous T-cell lymphomas. *Cancer Treat Rep* 1979;**63**:725–8.
6 Scarisbrick J, Whittaker S, Evans A, *et al.* Prognostic significance of tumour burden in the blood of patients with erythrodermic primary cutaneous T-cell lymphoma. *Blood* 2001;**97**:624–30.
7 Marti L, Estrach T, Reverter J, Mascaro J. Prognostic clinico-pathologic factors in cutaneous T-cell lymphoma. *Arch Dermatol* 1991;**127**:1511–6.
8 Doorn R, Van Haselan C, Voorst Vader P, *et al.* Mycosis fungoides: disease evolution and prognosis of 309 Dutch patients. *Arch Dermatol* 2000;**136**:504–10.
9 Kim Y, Jensen R, Watanabe G, Varghese A, Hoppe R. Clinical stage IA (limited patch and plaque) mycosis fungoides. *Arch Dermatol* 1996;**132**:1309–13.
10 Kim Y, Chow S, Varghese A, Hoppe R. Clinical characteristics and long-term outcome of patients with generalised patch and/or plaque (T2) mycosis fungoides. *Arch Dermatol* 1999;**135**:26–32.
11 Coninck E, Kim Y, Varghese A, Hoppe R. Clinical characteristics and outcome of patients with extracutaneous mycosis fungoides. *J Clin Oncol* 2001;**19**:779–84.
12 Kim Y, Bishop K, Varghese A, Hoppe R. Prognostic factors in erythrodermic mycosis fungoides and the Sézary syndrome. *Arch Dermatol* 1995;**131**:1003–8.
13 Kashani-Sabet M, McMillan A, Zackheim H. A modified staging classification for cutaneous T-cell lymphoma. *J Am Acad Dermatol* 2001;**45**:700–6.
14 Sausville E, Eddy J, Makuch R, Fischmann A, *et al.* Histopathologic staging at initial diagnosis of mycosis fungoides and the Sézary syndrome: definition of three distinctive prognostic groups. *Ann Intern Med* 1988;**109**:372–82.
15 Bunn P, Huberman M, Whang-Peng J, *et al.* Prospective staging evaluation of patients with cutaneous T-cell lymphomas. *Ann Intern Med* 1980;**93**:223–30.
16 Stevens S, Ke M, Parry E, Mark J, Cooper K. Quantifying skin disease burden in mycosis fungoides-type cutaneous T-cell lymphomas. *Arch Dermatol* 2002;**138**:42–8.
17 Demierre M, Tien A, Miller D. Health related quality of life assessment in patients with cutaneous T-cell lymphoma. *Arch Dermatol* 2005;**141**:325–30.
18 Zackheim H, Kashani-Sabet M, Amin S. Topical corticosteroids for mycosis fungoides. *Arch Dermatol* 1998;**134**:949–54.
19 Hoppe R, Abel E, Deneau D, Price N. Mycosis fungoides: management with topical nitrogen mustard. *J Clin Oncol* 1987;**5**:1796–1803.
20 Ramsey D, Ed M, Halperin P, *et al.* Topical mechlorethamine therapy for early stage mycosis fungoides. *J Am Acad Dermatol* 1988;**19**:684–91.
21 Vonderheid E, Tan E, Kantor A, *et al.* Long term efficacy, curative potential and carcinogenicity of topical mechlorethamine chemotherapy in cutaneous T-cell lymphoma. *J Am Acad Dermatol* 1989;**20**:416–28.
22 De Quatrebarbes J, Esteve E, Bagot M, *et al.* Treatment of early stage mycosis fungoides with twice-weekly applications of mechlorethamine and topical corticosteroids: a prospective study. *Arch Dermatol* 2005;**141**:1117–20.
23 Kim Y, Martinez G, Varhese A, Hoppe R. Topical nitrogen mustard in the management of mycosis fungoides. *Arch Dermatol* 2003;**139**:165–73.
24 Zachariae H, Thestrup-Pedersen K, Sogaard H. Topical nitrogen mustard in early mycosis fungoides. *Acta Derm Venereol* 1985;**65**:53–8.
25 Zackheim H, Epstein E, Crain W. Topical carmustine (BCNU) for cutaneous T-cell lymphoma: a 15-year experience in 143 patients. *J Am Acad Dermatol* 1990;**22**:802–10.
26 Breneman D, Duvic M, Kuzel T, Yocum R, Truglia J, Stevens V. Phase I and I trial of Bexarotene gel for skin directed treatment of patients with cutaneous T-cell lymphoma. *Arch Dermatol* 2002;**138**:325–32.
27 Duvic M, Olsen E, Omura G, *et al.* A phase III, randomized, double-blind, placebo-controlled study of peldesine (BCX-34) cream as topical therapy for cutaneous T-cell lymphoma. *J Am Acad Dermatol* 2001;**44**:940–7.

28 Suchin K, Junkins-Hopkins J, Rook A. Treatment of stage IA cutaneous T-cell lymphoma with topical application of the immune response modifier imiquimod. *Arch Dermatol* 2002;**138**: 1137–9.

29 Leman J, Dick D, Morton C. Topical 5-ALA photodynamic therapy for the treatment of cutaneous T-cell lymphoma. *Exp Dermatol* 2002;**27**:516–8.

30 Ramsey D, Lish K, Yalowitz C, Soter N. Ultraviolet-B phototherapy for early stage cutaneous T-cell lymphoma. *Arch Dermatol* 1992;**128**:931–3.

31 Clark C, Dawe R, Evans A, Lowe G, Ferguson J. Narrowband TL-01 phototherapy for patch-stage mycosis fungoides. *Arch Dermatol* 2000;**136**:748–52.

32 Gathers R, Scherschun L, Malick F, Fivenson D, Lim H. Narrowband UVB phototherapy for early stage mycosis fungoides. *J Am Acad Dermatol* 2002;**47**:191–7.

33 Zane C, Leali C, Airo P, *et al.* "High dose" UVA1 therapy of widespread plaque-type, nodular and erythrodermic mycosis fungoides. *J Am Acad Dermatol* 2001;**44**: 629–33.

34 Hermann J, Roenigk H, Hurria A, *et al.* Treatment of mycosis fungoides with photochemotherapy (PUVA): long term follow-up. *J Am Acad Dermatol* 1995;**33**:234–42.

35 Roenigk HH Jr, Kuzel TM, Skoutelis AP, *et al.* Photochemotherapy alone or combined with interferon alpha-2a in the treatment of cutaneous T-cell lymphoma. *J Invest Dermatol* 1990;95(6 Suppl):198S–205S.

36 Honigsmann Brenner W, Rauschmeier W, Konrad K, Wolff K. Photochemotherapy for cutaneous T cell lymphoma. *J Am Acad Dermatol* 1984;**10**:238–45.

37 Querfeld C, Rosen S, Kuzel T, *et al.* Long term follow-up of patients with early stage cutaneous T-cell lymphoma who achieved complete remission with psoralen plus UV-A monotherapy. *Arch Dermatol* 2005;**141**:305–11.

38 Stadler R, Otte H, Luger T, *et al.* Prospective randomised multicentre clinical trial on the use of interferon alpha-2a plus acitretin versus interferon alpha-2a plus PUVA in patients with cutaneous T-cell lymphoma stages I and II. *Blood* 1998;**10**:3578–81.

39 Thomsen K, Hammar H, Molin L, *et al.* Retinoids plus PUVA (RePUVA) and PUVA in mycosis fungoides plaque stage. *Acta Derm Venereol* 1989;**69**:536–8.

40 Kuzel T, Roenigk H, Samuelson E, *et al.* Effectiveness of interferon alfa-2a combined with phototherapy for mycosis fungoides and the Sézary syndrome. *J Clin Oncol* 1995;**13**:257–63.

41 Chiarion-Sileni V, Bononi A, Fornasa CV, *et al.* Phase II trial of interferon-alpha-2a plus psoralen with ultraviolet light A in patients with cutaneous T-cell lymphoma. *Cancer* 2002;**95**:569–75.

42 Rupoli S, Goteri G, Pulini S, *et al.* Long-term experience with low-dose interferon-alpha and PUVA in the management of early mycosis fungoides. *Eur J Haematol* 2005;**75**:136–45.

43 Bunn P, Ihde D, Foon K. The role of recombinant interferon alpha-2a in the therapy of cutaneous T-cell lymphomas. *Cancer* 1986;**57**:1689–95.

44 Olsen E, Rosen S, Vollmer R, *et al.* Interferon alfa-2a in the treatment of cutaneous T-cell lymphoma. *J Am Acad Dermatol* 1989;**20**:395–407.

45 Papa G, Tura S, Mandelli F, *et al.* Is interferon alpha in cutaneous T-cell lymphoma a treatment of choice? *Br J Haematol* 1991;**79**:48–51.

46 Kohn E, Steis R, Sausville E, Veach S, *et al.* Phase II trial of intermittent high-dose recombinant interferon alfa-2a in mycosis fungoides and the Sézary syndrome. *J Clin Oncol* 1990;**8**:155–60.

47 Dreno B, Claudy A, Meynadier J, *et al.* The treatment of 45 patients with cutaneous T-cell lymphoma with low doses of interferon-alpha 2a and etretinate. *Br J Dermatol* 1991;**125**:456–9.

48 Vonderheid E, Thompson R, Smiles K, Lattanand A. Recombinant interferon alpha-2b in plaque phase mycosis fungoides. Intralesional and low dose intramuscular therapy. *Arch Dermatol* 1987;**123**:757–63.

49 Kaplan E, Rosen S, Norris D, *et al.* Phase II study of recombinant interferon gamma for treatment of cutaneous T-cell lymphoma. *J Natl Cancer Inst* 1990;**82**:208–12.

50 Marolleau J, Baccard M, Flageul B, *et al.* High dose recombinant interleukin-2 in advanced cutaneous T-cell lymphoma. *Arch Dermatol* 1995;**131**:574–9.

51 Rook A, Wood G, Yoo E, *et al.* Interleukin-12 therapy of cutaneous T-cell lymphoma induces lesion regression and cytotoxic T-cell responses. *Blood* 1999;**94**:902–8.

52 Russell Jones R. Extracorporeal photopheresis in cutaneous T-cell lymphoma: inconsistent data underline the need for randomised studies. *Br J Dermatol* 2000;**142**:16–21.

53 Edelson R, Berger C, Gasparro F, *et al.* Treatment of cutaneous T-cell lymphoma by extracorporeal photochemotherapy. *N Engl J Med* 1987;**316**:297–303.

54 Duvic M, Hester J, Lemak N. Photopheresis therapy for cutaneous T-cell lymphoma. *J Am Acad Dermatol* 1996;**35**:573–9.

55 Heald P, Rook A, Perez M, *et al.* Treatment of erythrodermic cutaneous T-cell lymphoma with extracorporeal photopheresis. *J Am Acad Dermatol* 1992;**27**:427–33.

56 Zic J, Stricklin G, Greer J, *et al.* Long term follow up of patients with cutaneous T-cell lymphoma treated with extracorporeal photochemotherapy. *J Am Acad Dermatol* 1996;**35**:935–45.

57 Gottlieb S, Wolfe J, Fox F, *et al.* Treatment of cutaneous T-cell lymphoma with extracorporeal photopheresis monotherapy and in combination with recombinant interferon-alpha: a 10 year experience at a single institution. *J Am Acad Dermatol* 1996;**35**: 946–57.

58 Fraser-Andrews E, Seed P, Whittaker S, Russell-Jones R. Extracorporeal photopheresis in Sézary syndrome: no significant effect in the survival of 44 patients with a peripheral blood T-cell clone. *Arch Dermatol* 1998;**134**:1001–5.

59 Child F, Mitchell T, Whittaker S, Watkins P, Seed P, Russell-Jones R. A randomised cross-over study to compare PUVA and extracorporeal photopheresis (ECP) in the treatment of plaque stage (T2) mycosis fungoides. *Br J Dermatol* 2001;**145**(Suppl 59):16.

60 Bisaccia E, Gonzalez J, Palangio M, Schwartz J, Klainer A. Extracorporeal photochemotherapy alone or with adjuvant therapy in the treatment of cutaneous T-cell lymphoma: a 9 year retrospective study at a single institution. *J Am Acad Dermatol* 2000;**43**:263–71.

61 Wollina U, Looks A, Meyer J, *et al.* Treatment of stage II cutaneous T-cell lymphoma with interferon alfa-2a and extracorporeal photochemotherapy: a prospective controlled trial. *J Am Acad Dermatol* 2001;**44**:253–60.

62 Dippel E, Schrag H, Goerdt S, Orfanos CE. Extracorporeal photopheresis and interferon-alpha in advanced cutaneous T-cell lymphoma. *Lancet* 1997;**350**:32–3.

63 Vonderheid E, Bigler R, Greenberg A, Neukum S, Micaily B. Extracorporeal photopheresis and recombinant interferon alfa-2b in Sézary syndrome. *Am J Clin Oncol* 1994;**17**:255–63.

64 Haley H, Davis D, Sams M. Durable loss of a malignant T-cell clone in a stage IV cutaneous T-cell lymphoma patient treated with high-dose interferon and photopheresis. *J Am Acad Dermatol* 1999;**41**:880–3.

65 Yoo E, Cassin M, Lessin S, Rook A. Complete molecular remission during biologic response modifier therapy for Sézary syndrome is associated with enhanced helper T type I cytokine production and natural killer cell activity. *J Am Acad Dermatol* 2001;**45**:208–16.

66 Suchin K, Cucchiara A, Gottlieb S, et al. Treatment of cutaneous T-cell lymphoma with combined immunomodulatory therapy. *Arch Dermatol* 2002;**138**:1054–60.

67 Evans A, Wood B, Scarisbrick J, et al. Extracorporeal photopheresis in Sézary syndrome: hematologic parameters as predictors of response. *Blood* 2001;**98**:1298–301.

68 Bernengo M, Appino A, Bertero M, et al. Thymopentin in Sézary syndrome. *J Natl Cancer Inst* 1992;**84**:1341–6.

69 Cooper D, Braverman I, Sarris A, et al. Cyclosporine treatment of refractory T-cell lymphomas. *Cancer* 1993;**71**:2335–41.

70 Bunn P, Hoffman S, Norris D, Golitz L, Aeling J. Systemic therapy of cutaneous T-cell lymphomas (mycosis fungoides and the Sézary syndrome). *Ann Intern Med* 1994;**121**:592–602.

71 Molin L, Thomsen K, Volden G, et al. Oral retinoids in mycosis fungoides and Sézary syndrome: a comparison of isotretinoin and etretinate. *Acta Dermatol Venereol* 1987;**67**:232–6.

72 Kessler J, Jones S, Levine N, et al. Isotretinoin and cutaneous helper T-cell lymphoma (mycosis fungoides). *Arch Dermatol* 1987;**123**:201–4.

73 Duvic M, Martin A, Kim Y, et al. Phase 2 and 3 clinical trial of oral bexarotene (Targretin capsules) for the treatment of refractory or persistent early stage cutaneous T-cell lymphoma. *Arch Dermatol* 2001;**137**:581–93.

74 Duvic M, Hymes K, Heald P, et al. Bexarotene is effective and safe for treatment of refractory advanced-stage cutaneous T-cell lymphoma: multinational phase II–III trial results. *J Clin Oncol* 2001;**19**:2456–71.

75 Talpur R, Ward S, Apisarnthanarax N, Breuer-Mcham J, Duvic M. Optimizing bexarotene therapy for cutaneous T-cell lymphoma. *J Am Acad Dermatol* 2002;**47**:672–84.

76 Singh F, Lebwohl M. Cutaneous T-cell lymphoma treatment using bexarotene and PUVA: a case series. *J Am Acad Dermatol* 2004;**51**:570–3.

77 Knox S, Levy R, Hodgkinson S, et al. Observations on the effect of chimeric anti-CD4 monoclonal antibody in patients with mycosis fungoides. *Blood* 1991;**77**:20–30.

78 Knox S, Hoppe R, Maloney D, et al. Treatment of cutaneous T-cell lymphoma with chimeric anti-CD4 monoclonal antibody. *Blood* 1996;**87**:893–9.

79 Lundin J, Osterborg A, Brittinger G, et al. CAMPATH-1H monoclonal antibody in therapy for previously treated low-grade non-Hodgkin's lymphomas: a phase II multicenter study. European Study Group of CAMPATH-1H Treatment In Low-Grade Non-Hodgkin's Lymphoma. *J Clin Oncol* 1998;**16**:3257–63.

80 Kennedy G, Seymour J, Wolf M, et al. Treatment of patients with advanced mycosis fungoides and Sézary syndrome with alemtuzumab. *Eur J Haematol* 2003;**71**:250–6.

81 Lundin J, Hagberg H, Repp R, et al. Phase II study of alemtuzumab (anti-CD52 monoclonal antibody) in patients with advanced mycosis fungoides/Sézary syndrome. *Blood* 2003;**101**:4267–72.

82 Lenihan D, Alencar A, Yang D, et al. Cardiac toxicity of alemtuzumab in patients with mycosis fungoides/Sézary syndrome. *Blood* 2004;**104**:655–8.

83 Lundin J, Kennedy B, Dearden C, Dyer M, Osterborg A. No cardiac toxicity associated with alemtuzumab therapy for mycosis fungoides/Sézary syndrome. *Blood* 2005;**105**:4148–9.

84 Olsen E, Duvic M, Frankel A, et al. Pivotal phase III trial of two dose levels of Denileukin Diftitox for the treatment of cutaneous T-cell lymphoma. *J Clin Oncol* 2001;**19**:376–88.

85 Foss F, Demierre M, Divenuti G. A Phase I trial of bexarotene and denileukin diftitox in patients with relapsed or refractory cutaneous T-cell lymphoma. *Blood* 2005;**106**:454–7.

86 LeMaistre C, Rosen S, Frankel A, et al. Phase I trial of H65-RTA immunoconjugate in patients with cutaneous T-cell lymphoma. *Blood* 1991;**78**:1173–82.

87 Foss F, Raubitscheck A, Mulshine J, et al. Phase I study of the pharmacokinetics of a radioimmunoconjugate, 90Y-T101, in patients with CD5-expressing leukaemia and lymphoma. *Clin Cancer Res* 1998;**4**:2691–700.

88 Cotter GW, Baglan RJ, Wasserman TH, Mill W. Palliative radiation treatment of cutaneous mycosis fungoides: a dose response. *Int J Radiat Oncol Biol Phys* 1983;**9**:1477–80.

89 Jones G, Hoppe R, Glatstein E. Electron beam treatment for cutaneous T-cell lymphoma. *Haematol Oncol Clin North Am* 1995;**9**:1057–76.

90 Hamminga B, Noordijk E, van Vloten W. Treatment of mycosis fungoides: total-skin electron-beam irradiation vs. topical mechlorethamine therapy. *Arch Dermatol* 1982;**118**:150–3.

91 Jones G, Rosenthal D, Wilson L. Total skin electron beam radiation for patients with erythrodermic cutaneous T-cell lymphoma (mycosis fungoides and the Sézary syndrome). *Cancer* 1999;**85**:1985–95.

92 Kirova YM, Piedbois Y, Haddad E, et al. Radiotherapy in the management of mycosis fungoides: indications, results, prognosis. Twenty years experience. *Radiother Oncol* 1999;**51**:147–51.

93 Becker M, Hoppe R, Knox S. Multiple courses of high dose total skin electron beam therapy in the management of mycosis fungoides. *Int J Radiat Oncol Biol Phys* 1995;**30**:1445–9.

94 Wilson L, Quiros P, Kolenik S, et al. Additional courses of total skin electron beam therapy in the treatment of patients with recurrent cutaneous T-cell lymphoma. *J Am Acad Dermatol* 1996;**35**:69–73.

95 Kaye F, Bunn P, Steinberg S, et al. A randomized trial comparing combination electron beam radiation and chemotherapy with topical therapy in the initial treatment of mycosis fungoides. *N Engl J Med* 1989;**321**:1748–90.

96 Wilson L, Jones G, Kim D, et al. Experience with total skin electron beam therapy in combination with extracorporeal photopheresis in the management of patients with erythrodermic (T4) mycosis fungoides. *J Am Acad Dermatol* 2000;**43**:54–60.

97 Jones G, Kacinski B, Wilson L, et al. Total skin electron radiation in the management of mycosis fungoides: consensus of the European Organization for Research and Treatment of Cancer (EORTC) Cutaneous Lymphoma Project Group. *J Am Acad Dermatol* 2002;**47**:364–70.

98 Zackheim H, Kashani-Sabet M, Hwang S. Low dose methotrexate to treat erythrodermic cutaneous T-cell lymphoma: results in twenty-nine patients. *J Am Acad Dermatol* 1996;**34**:626–31.

99 Sarris A, Phan A, Duvic M, *et al.* Trimetrexate in relapsed T-cell lymphoma with skin involvement. *J Clin Oncol* 2002;**20**:2867–80.

100 Kurzrock R, Pilat S, Duvic M. Pentostatin therapy of T-cell lymphomas with cutaneous manifestations. *J Clin Oncol* 1999;**17**:3117–21.

101 Deardon C, Matutes E, Catovsky D. Pentostatin treatment of cutaneous T-cell lymphoma. *Oncology* 2000;**14**:37–40.

102 Ho A, Suciu S, Stryckmans P, *et al.* Pentostatin in T-cell malignancies. Leukaemia Cooperative Group and the European Organisation for Research and Treatment of Cancer. *Semin Oncol* 2000;**27**:52–7.

103 Foss F, Ihde D, Breneman D, *et al.* Phase II study of pentostatin and intermittent high dose recombinant interferon alfa-2a in advanced mycosis fungoides/Sézary syndrome. *J Clin Oncol* 1992;**10**:1907–13.

104 Kuzel T, Hurria A, Samuelson E, *et al.* Phase II trial of 2-chlorodeoxyadenosine for the treatment of cutaneous T-cell lymphoma. *Blood* 1996;**87**:906–11.

105 Zinzani P, Baliva G, Magagnoli M, *et al.* Gemcitabine treatment in pretreated cutaneous T-cell lymphoma: experience in 44 patients. *J Clin Oncol* 2000;**18**:2603–6.

106 Marchi E, Alinari L, Tani M, *et al.* Gemcitabine as frontline treatment for cutaneous T-cell lymphoma. *Cancer* 2005;**104**:2437–41.

107 Wollina U, Graefe T, Kaatz M. Pegylated doxorubicin for primary cutaneous T-cell lymphoma: a report on ten patients with follow-up. *J Cancer Res Clin Oncol* 2001;**127**:128–34.

108 Wollina U, Dummer R, Brockmayer N, *et al.* Multicenter study of pegylated liposomal doxorubicin in patients with cutaneous T-cell lymphoma. *Cancer* 2003;**98**:993–1001.

109 Fierro M, Doveil G, Quaglino P, Savoia P, Verrone A, Bernengo M. Combination of etoposide, idarubicin, cyclophosphamide, vincristine, prednisone and bleomycin (VICOP-B) in the treatment of advanced cutaneous T-cell lymphoma. *Dermatology* 1997;**194**:268–72.

110 Akpek G, Koh H, Bogen S, O'Hara C, Foss F. Chemotherapy with etoposide, vincristine, doxorubicin, bolus cyclophosphamide and oral prednisone in patients with refractory cutaneous T-cell lymphoma. *Cancer* 1999;**86**:1368–76.

111 Bigler R, Crilley P, Micaily B, *et al.* Autologous bone marrow transplantation for advanced stage mycosis fungoides. *Bone Marrow Transplant* 1991;**7**:133–7.

112 Olavarria E, Child F, Woolford A, *et al.* T-cell depletion and autologous stem cell transplantation in the management of tumour stage mycosis fungoides with peripheral blood involvement. *Br J Haematol* 2001;**114**:624–31.

113 Burt R, Guitart J, Traynor A, *et al.* Allogeneic hematopoietic stem cell transplantation for advanced mycosis fungoides: evidence of a graft-versus-tumour effect. *Bone Marrow Transplant* 2000;**25**:111–3.

114 Molina A, Nademanee A, Arber D, Forman S. Remission of refractory Sézary syndrome after bone marrow transplantation from a matched unrelated donor. *Biol Blood Marrow Transplant* 1999;**5**:400–4.

115 Guitart J, Wickless S, Oyama Y, *et al.* Long term remission after allogeneic hematopoietic stem cell transplantation for refractory cutaneous T-cell lymphoma. *Arch Dermatol* 2002;**138**:1359–65.

116 Masood N, Russell K, Olerud J, *et al.* Induction of complete remission of advanced stage mycosis fungoides by allogeneic hematopoietic stem cell transplantation. *J Am Acad Dermatol* 2002;**47**:140–5.

117 Soligo D, Ibatici A, Berti E, *et al.* Treatment of advanced mycosis fungoides by allogeneic stem-cell transplantation with a non-myeloablative regimen. *Bone Marrow Transplant* 2003;**31**:663–6.

118 Fijnheer R, Sanders C, Canninga M, de Weger R, Verdonck L. Complete remission of a radiochemotherapy-resistant cutaneous T-cell lymphoma with allogeneic non-myeloablative stem cell transplantation. *Bone Marrow Transplant* 2003;**32**:345–7.

119 Molina A, Zain J, Arber D, *et al.* Durable clinical, cytogenetic and molecular remissions after allogeneic hematopoietic cell transplantation for refractory Sézary syndrome and mycosis fungoides. *J Clin Oncol* 2005;**23**:6163–71.

31 Actinic keratoses and Bowen's disease

Aditya K. Gupta, Jenna E. Bowen, Elizabeth A. Cooper, Seaver L. Soon, Peterson Pierre, Suephy C. Chen

Background

Definition

Actinic keratoses (AK), also known as solar or senile keratoses, and Bowen's disease (BD) are precursors of invasive squamous cell carcinoma (SCC). Whereas AK is precancerous, BD represents intraepidermal (*in situ*) SCC.[1] AK presentation is characterized by multiple, erythematous, scaly papules that may be pink, red, or brown in color. AK lesions are typically less than 1 cm in diameter.[2,3] AK is termed "actinic cheilitis" if the lips are involved. BD usually presents as a solitary, well-demarcated, erythematous plaque of varying size, with irregular borders and a crusted, scaling, or fissured surface (Figures 31.1, 31.2).[4]

AK arises on areas of intense ultraviolet light exposure, with over 80% developing on the head and neck, forearms, and hands.[5–7] A male predominance is observed.[3,8] Other contributing factors include skin type, age, sun exposure, latitude, and ozone integrity.[2,3] The distribution of BD varies, demonstrating predominance on the lower legs in women and on the head and neck in men in the UK and Australia.[9–11]

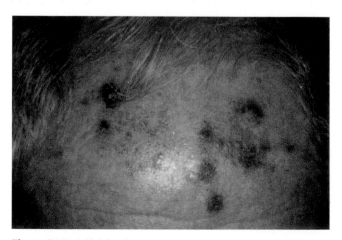

Figure 31.1 Acitinic keratoses.

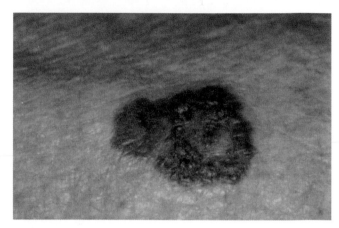

Figure 31.2 Bowen's disease.

Australia and Denmark feature a marginal propensity of BD for women (56%) and occurrence on the head and neck (44–54%).[11,12] Approximately one-third of patients with BD have other nonmelanoma skin cancers at diagnosis.[12]

Incidence/prevalence

The exact incidence and prevalence of AK and BD is unknown. Both increase in prevalence with advancing age.[2,11,13,14] AK may occur in children with albinism and xeroderma pigmentosum.[15]

Etiology

Chronic solar damage is the principal etiological factor in AK and BD.[11,16–18] People with light complexions, blue eyes, and childhood freckling are at highest risk, given their innate lack of protective pigment.[5] Individuals with compromised immunity, such as organ-transplant recipients; with diminished or absent melanin, such as albinos; and with decreased capacity to repair ultraviolet-induced damage, such as persons with xeroderma pigmentosum, all demonstrate an increased risk for AK. Risk factors for BD include arsenic exposure,[19–22] immunosuppression,[23] and human papillomavirus (HPV), particularly HPV-16 in ano-genital lesions.[24,25]

Prognosis

Although the condition is precancerous,[26,27] the probability of a given AK undergoing malignant transformation is unknown.[13] The reported risk of progression to SCC for individual lesions ranges from 0.025% to 16% per year.[28] The 10-year risk of malignant transformation of at least one AK on a given patient is 10.2%.[29] The relative risk of malignant transformation depends ultimately on factors related to the AK itself (for example, thickness), as well as patient characteristics (for example, drug therapy, degree of pigmentation, immune status).[3] However, another aspect that may confound estimation of the prognosis of AK is the spontaneous regression rate. A study from Queensland[30] reported a spontaneous regression rate of 85% (95% CI, 75% to 96%) in people with prevalent AK (AK diagnosed on a person during the first examination) and 84% (95% CI, 72% to 96%) in persons with incident AK (AK appearing for the first time during the study). However, the distribution of lesions per person was highly skewed, with 12% of study participants having 65% of the total number of AKs.

BD is associated with an excellent prognosis, related to the disease's indolent nature and its favorable response to a range of therapies. Although there is no recent literature on the risk of BD progression to invasive SCC, older studies suggest the risk is 3–5% if lesions are left untreated.[31,32] Contrary to the findings of earlier reports,[33–36] a meta-analysis of 12 studies in 1989 determined no significant association between BD and internal malignancy.[37]

Aims of treatment

The aims of treatment are to achieve clinical and histological clearance, prevent progression to invasive SCC, prevent recurrence, achieve cosmetic improvement, and minimize adverse effects of treatment.

Relevant outcomes

- Short-term clinical and histological clearance.
- Recurrence rates (these should be calculated at least 1 year following treatment, in order to assess the recurrence of AK and BD lesions adequately).
- Prevention of SCC.
- Adverse effects of treatment.

Methods of search

To identify studies of 5-fluorouracil (5-FU) and cryotherapy in patients with AK, we reviewed Medline from 1966 to

---

BOX 31.1 The quality-of-evidence scale used in the British Association of Dermatology guidelines, derived from the U.S. Task Force on Preventive Care Guidelines.[23,38]

I   Evidence obtained from at least one properly designed RCT.

II-i   Evidence obtained from well-designed control trials without randomization.

II-ii   Evidence obtained from well-designed cohort or case–control analytical studies, preferably from more than one center or research group.

II-iii   Evidence obtained from multiple time series with or without the intervention. Dramatic results in uncontrolled experiments could also be included.

III   Opinions of respected authorities based on clinical experience, descriptive studies, or reports of expert committees.

IV   Evidence inadequate owing to problems of methodology (for example, sample size, length or comprehensiveness of follow-up, or conflicts in evidence).

---

the end of December 2006. We searched non-5-FU and non-nitrogen therapies by name and type, as well as the term "actinic keratosis treatment." We scrutinized review articles for treatments not detected through database searches.

To locate articles on interventions for BD, we searched Medline (from 1966 to the end of 2006). We limited the topic to nonanogenital BD and to English publications, since we did not have ready access to translation facilities as part of the chapter project. We reported numbers of patients as well as number of lesions treated wherever information was available. Studies that used patients as the unit of randomization (which makes the best clinical sense) were preferred over studies that used lesions as the unit of randomization without adjusting for a person effect.

Since few randomized controlled trials (RCTs) were found, uncontrolled trials were included in this report. Evidence was graded using the quality-of-evidence scale employed in the British Association of Dermatology guidelines, and derived from the U.S. Task Force on Preventive Care guidelines.[23,38] We have only presented data from the best-quality studies; for example, data from comparative studies are presented preferentially over data from case series when both exist for a given intervention. The grading system is shown in Box 31.1.

Questions

What are the effects of non-drug therapy?

Cryotherapy
Cryotherapy involves delivering liquid nitrogen to affected areas with a spray device or cotton tip applicator. Studies of

varying quality investigated the efficacy of cryotherapy for AK and BD.

Actinic keratoses (quality of evidence: I)

We found one systematic review[39] and four RCTs.[40–43] All four RCTs were comparative studies. Three of the four compared cryotherapy with methyl aminolevulinate photodynamic therapy (MAL/PDT; n = 119, 204, and 193).[40–42] The efficacy of MAL/PDT will be discussed later in the chapter. The fourth RCT compared cryotherapy with 0.5% fluorouracil to cryotherapy with a vehicle cream (n = 144).[43] One nonrandomized, uncontrolled study examining the use of cryosurgery for the treatment of AK is also discussed.[44] The systematic review found only one study with quantifiable results.[45]

Benefits

The lesion response rates evaluated by the three RCTs (overall, 516 patients with 2963 lesions) comparing cryotherapy with MAL/PDT were comparable among the studies. Three months after a single cryotherapy session, the lesion response rates were found to be 76.2%, 68%, and 75%, respectively.[40–42] After 6 months, and a second treatment in patients who had not experienced complete clearance, the lesion response rates were at an even higher rate of 86.1%.[40] The lesion response rates were clinically evaluated as the percentage of lesions that disappeared completely. The fourth RCT (n = 144) found significantly higher percentages of patients with complete lesion clearance who were treated with cryotherapy and 0.5% fluorouracil in comparison with those treated with cryotherapy and a vehicle cream (51.4% versus 15.4% 6 months after treatment, $P < 0.001$; 36.8% versus 26.7% 1 year after treatment, $P = 0.028$).[43] It should be noted that in this study, cryotherapy was only administered to lesions that were still remaining at the 4-week assessment after 7 days of treatment with either fluorouracil or a vehicle cream. A nonrandomized, uncontrolled study found that the freeze duration may influence the success of cryotherapy threatment.[44] Complete responses in lesions with freeze times greater than 5 seconds were higher than responses for lesions with freeze times less than 5 seconds (69% compared to 39%). The complete response rate for lesions with freeze times greater than 20 seconds was 83%.[44] The study examined in the systematic review treated a total of 1018 lesions in 70 patients. Clinical follow-up after treatment ranged from 1 to 8.5 years. Twelve recurrences were reported, giving a success rate of 98.8% during a follow-up period of 1–8.5 years. However, not all of the lesions were followed uniformly after 1 year.[45]

Harms

Adverse events associated with cryotherapy treatment include stinging, pain, or a burning sensation, erythema,

edema of the skin, hyperpigmentation or hypopigmentation, blistering, skin infection, crusting, itch, and peeling skin.[41,46] However, the majority of events are of mild to moderate severity, are well tolerated, and are of short duration.[42,46] The percentages of patients who reported local adverse reactions after a single cryotherapy treatment in three of the RCTs were 72.3%, 35%, and 26%, respectively.[40–42] Unfortunately, the longer the duration of freezing, the more likely it is that an adverse event will occur. Very aggressive freezing may lead to a large blister, ulcer, longer healing times, more postoperative pain, and more pigmentary changes.[47]

Comment

Cryotherapy continues to be a popular and relatively effective treatment for isolated AKs. Consideration should be given to the duration of treatment, since longer freeze times result in a greater response. Longer freeze times should particularly be used for larger lesions or those that are more hyperkeratotic. In the studies comparing cryotherapy and PDT, treatment preferences varied. One study reported comparable outcomes with the two treatments, but the cosmetic outcomes and patient and investigator preferences favored MAL/PDT.[40] The two other studies reported conflicting results, with one study reporting higher response rates with MAL/PDT[41] and the other reporting higher response rates with cryotherapy.[42]

Bowen's disease (quality of evidence: I)

We found no systematic reviews and one RCT. The RCT was a comparison of cryotherapy (n = 20 lesions) with photodynamic therapy (n = 20 lesions).[48] One quasi-randomized controlled trial compared the efficacy of MAL/PDT (n = 96), placebo/PDT (n = 17), cryotherapy (n = 82), and fluorouracil (n = 30).[49] The treating investigator chose whether the patient would receive either cryotherapy (n = 82) or fluorouracil (n = 30). One unblinded controlled trial compared cryotherapy (n = 36) with curettage (n = 44),[50] and one retrospective study compared cryotherapy (n = 82) with external beam radiotherapy (n = 59).[51]

Benefits

In the RCT, cryotherapy produced complete clearance in 50% of the lesions after a single treatment and 100% clearance after the second or third treatment with liquid nitrogen maintained for 20 s.[48] The clinical response was determined at 2-monthly intervals for 12 months. Following cryotherapy, 10% of the lesions recurred within the 1-year follow-up period. Lesion size was found to affect the probability that it would be completely cleared after a single treatment. The probability that a lesion would be completely cleared after a single treatment was greater for photodynamic therapy (PDT) than for cryotherapy.[48] PDT was also associated with fewer adverse effects and a lower recurrence rate. In the quasi-randomized study, the complete lesion response for patients treated with cryotherapy was 86% at 3 months following a single treatment. At 12 months post-treatment, 21% of the lesions had recurred.[49] Complete clinical clearance was comparable between cryotherapy (94% with one treatment and 100% with two) and curettage (100% after one treatment) 1 week after treatment. Overall, the average time to healing was 60 days. Healing was significantly prolonged for lower-leg lesions treated by cryotherapy in comparison with curettage (90 versus 30 days, $P < 0.001$). No difference in healing time was observed for other sites. Recurrence rates were lower (12% versus 50%, $P < 0.04$) and the time to recurrence was longer ($P < 0.0087$) for curettage.[50] In comparison with radiotherapy, there was a higher rate of recurrence in the cryotherapy group (6%, one as invasive SCC, versus 0%).[51]

Harms

Complications of cryotherapy include pain, poor healing, and infection, requiring antibiotics.[52] Pain of mild to moderate severity was reported in 19 of 20 lesions during cryotherapy, which was significantly higher than pain reported during PDT ($P < 0.01$).[48] Ulceration occurred in five of the 20 lesions, and two of the five patients concerned were later prescribed antibiotics for cellulitis developing around the lesions. Visible scarring in four of the 20 lesions was observed at 12 months post-treatment.[48] Patients were 10.4 times more likely to report pain with cryotherapy ($P < 0.001$) and were 5.5 times more likely to report pain on the lower leg in comparison with other body sites, irrespective of the treatment method used ($P < 0.016$).[50] Poor healing occurred in 2% of patients who received cryotherapy in this retrospective comparison study.[51] Biopsy of these poorly healing lesions revealed residual tumor. The authors speculate that failure to heal may suggest residual BD and may be an indication for surgical excision.

Comment

These studies report high short-term clearance rates with liquid-nitrogen cryotherapy, although poor healing, as well as discomfort related to the procedure, may limit its utility in BD of such sites as the lower legs. In relation to the study comparing cryotherapy and curettage, methodological limitations include deviation from an intention-to-treat (ITT) analysis and use of nonrandom allocation. The former omission would tend to overestimate the efficacy of the intervention, whereas the latter would tend to weaken the validity of the results, as there is no assurance that known and unknown confounders are homogeneously distributed between the comparison groups.

Laser treatment

Studies investigating laser therapy for AK and BD highlight its capacity to selectively vaporize the epidermis and upper papillary layer, yielding minimal scar formation. We found no systematic reviews for either AK or BD and no RCTs for BD.

Actinic keratoses (quality of evidence: I)

We found no systematic reviews and one RCT. The RCT was a comparison study between laser resurfacing with an erbium–yttrium aluminum garnet (Er:YAG) laser and topical 5-fluorouracil in the treatment of AK (n = 55).[53] Patients were randomly assigned to either treatment group and were followed for 1 year after treatment. Three uncontrolled trials investigated the use of the Er:YAG laser to treat AK using different energy rates.[54–56] The first report treated only eight lesions, with a follow-up period of 12–15 months.[56] The second report provided full-face laser resurfacing for four of five patients (n = 121 lesions), with a follow-up period of 3 months.[55] The third report treated 29 patients, with a follow-up period of 3 months.[54] Two retrospective studies investigated the use of either the Er:YAG laser or the CO_2 laser to treat AK.[57,58] One report followed 24 patients (all with at least 30 lesions) for 2 years.[57] The other study followed 25 patients (with widespread AK on the scalp, forehead, or face) for a follow-up period ranging from 7 to 70 months.[58]

Benefits

One year after treatment, the mean percentages of lesions cleared were 91.1% for patients who underwent laser treatment and 76.6% for patients treated with 5-fluorouracil.[53] The difference between the two treatments was statistically significant ($P = 0.048$). One of the uncontrolled laser studies reported 93%[55] clearance of AK lesions at 3 months, and another reported 100%[56] clearance at 12–15 months. The third uncontrolled trial reported that 89.7% of patients experienced complete lesion clearance 3 months after treatment.[54] One retrospective study also reported high success rates with laser treatment, with an overall reduction in AK lesions of 94%.[57] The other retrospective study reported that 72% of patients with severe actinic damage had a clinical improvement of 75–100%.[58]

Harms

Laser treatment may be associated with erythema, edema, infections, crust formation, pain, irritation, itching, hypopigmentation, acne, milia, and scars.[53] Reepithelialization usually occurs within 7–10 days after treatment, but may take longer for larger lesions. While some studies suggest that most adverse events usually resolve within a few weeks,[54–56] other studies with longer-term follow-ups reported side effects lasting for over a year after treatment.[53,58] On the other hand, one of the retrospective studies did not report any adverse events following laser treatment at all.[57] One year after treatment, a 40.1% recurrence rate for AK lesions was reported in one study,[53] while recurrences were reported in 12.5% of patients in another.[57] In one of the retrospective studies, 56% of patients with widespread AK developed a few new lesions (between one and 15) after treatment.[58] Of these recurrences, 20% occurred within a year of treatment and the other 36% occurred after 1 year.[58] BCC was diagnosed in two of 24 patients in one study,[57] and three of 25 patients developed malignancies in another study.[58]

Comments

Laser treatment appears to be highly effective in the immediate treatment of AK lesions. However, most studies included only short-term follow-up periods (usually 3 months), and those with longer follow-ups reported variable recurrence rates. Side effects associated with this treatment may also produce longer-term, undesirable cosmetic outcomes. In addition, laser therapy is a more expensive treatment in comparison with other treatment modalities such as 5-FU and cryosurgery. Larger studies with longer follow-up periods would be required for confirmation of long-term effects and recurrence rates. Further studies should be performed before Er:YAG or CO_2 laser therapy can become a routine treatment for AK.

Bowen's disease (quality of evidence: II-iii)

Two small uncontrolled trials reported the use of CO_2 laser therapy for BD of the digits.[59,60] The first report[60] described treatment of five lesions with a 36-month follow-up (n = 5); the second report[59] described treatment of six lesions with an 84-month follow-up (n = 6). A third uncontrolled trial reported the use of CO_2 laser therapy for BD on the legs.[61] This study treated 16 patients with 25 lesions with a 6-month follow-up. An update on patient health 12 months after discharge from this study was also published.[62]

Benefits

Both studies in which BD of the digits was treated reported 100% clearance within 10–24 days following the procedure. Determination of clearance in both studies was based on clinical criteria and, in cases deemed necessary by the supervising dermatologist, by histological criteria. Biopsies showed only slightly thinned epidermis and mild superficial fibroplasia of the papillary dermis.[59,60] Recurrence rates varied between 0% at 84 months[59] and 20% (one of five patients) at 5 months. (After re-treatment with electrodesiccation and curettage—i.e., an additional intervention—no recurrence was observed at 20 months.)[60] The disparate recurrence rates may be related to differences in energy settings and in the width of the clinically normal margins included in the treatment area. No impairment in digital function was noted in either study. The study that treated BD on the legs found that eight of the 25 lesions took longer than 4 weeks to heal, but all lesions had healed completely at 8 weeks after treatment. Examination at 6 months found no recurrence of BD lesions.[61]

Harms

Exudation, crusting, and erythema may follow laser treatment. Reepithelialization occurs 7–10 days after treatment, but erythema may persist for 3 weeks or more. One Er:YAG laser study[55] found no post-therapeutic dyspigmentation. The CO_2 laser studies that treated BD on the digits report hypopigmentation, mild cutaneous atrophy, and nail dystrophy.[55,59] Two of the 16 patients receiving CO_2 laser treatment on the legs developed infections requiring dressings and antibiotics.[61] No other adverse events were reported in this study; however, the study was published as an abstract in conference proceedings, and a detailed summary of all of the results was not provided. An update on the condition of patients included in the study revealed that three of the 16 patients (three of 25 lesions, 12%) had returned with lesions that had been identified on biopsy as squamous cell carcinomas.[62] These were all identified within 12 months after discharge from the study. The authors presume that the patients developed SCC due to foci of malignant change that lay more deeply than the original treatment plane, rather than as a result of laser treatment. However, this possibility could not be ruled out.

Comment

CO_2 lasers may be particularly useful in the treatment of digital BD lesions. Clearance rates in the small uncontrolled trials were high, with acceptable recurrence rates during follow up periods of up to 7 years. The suitability of CO_2 laser therapy for digital BD relates principally to two properties. Firstly, CO_2 laser has the ability to vaporize the epidermis and the upper papillary dermis, leading to healing with minimal scar formation. This feature is desirable in mobile areas such as the fingers, where a contracting scar following excision may lead to functional impairment. Secondly, the concern that CO_2 lasers may not penetrate to a depth sufficient to eradicate perifollicular BD is obviated by the paucity of hair on the fingers. The risk of recurrence secondary to perifollicular involvement is therefore less of a concern in digital lesions than in lesions at other body sites. It has been projected that about 3% of patients with BD per annum will proceed to develop invasive malignancy. Given that the progression to invasive malignancy was higher than expected (12%) in patients receiving laser treatment for BD on the legs,[62] careful consideration should be given to the use of laser therapy at body sites other than the digits. CO_2 lasers may thus be helpful for digital lesions, while other treatment options should be explored for lesions at other body sites.

Radiotherapy

We found no systematic reviews or RCTs for either AK or BD.

Actinic keratoses (quality of evidence: IV)
We found only one case report using radiotherapy for AK.[63]

Benefit
One person with a large AK recalcitrant to 5-FU responded to fractionated radiotherapy.[64]

Comment
Given the absence of high-quality evidence for radiotherapy and the availability of other therapeutic modalities, radiotherapy should not be used for the treatment of AK.

Bowen's disease (quality of evidence: II-iii)
We found one study comparing the effect of radiotherapy with cryotherapy on lower-leg lesions,[51] as reported above. We also found a small retrospective study of 11 patients with 16 BD lesions treated with radiotherapy.[65]

Benefits
Radiotherapy was more effective than cryotherapy in terms of recurrence (0% versus 6% at 2 years post-treatment).[51] Skin cosmesis following radiotherapy is reported as "good" to "excellent" in the majority of patients in uncontrolled trials, with only 5–15% of irradiated skin considered "fair" to "unsatisfactory."[64,66] All BD lesions followed in the retrospective study had 100% clearance at the time of last follow-up (the follow-up periods ranged from 17 to 1723 days).[65]

Harms
The 100% clinical clearance and 0% recurrence rate was offset by poor healing in 20% of lesions.[51] Poor healing in this study was defined as a residual ulcer requiring salvage surgery that ceased to show signs of continuing reduction in diameter, or was considered by the dermatologist to be progressing poorly over at least 3 months. The retrospective study also reported poor healing, with 25% of lesions failing to heal due to ulcers, all of which were located on the lower leg.[65] Other reported adverse effects from uncontrolled studies included minor pain and burning during the procedure,[67,68] short-term hypopigmentation,[68] radiation dermatitis, and radionecrosis.[67] Poor healing, including radionecrosis, appears to be associated with older age, an irradiation field diameter > 4 cm, and a total dose > 3000 cGy.[51,67]

Comment
As noted by the authors of the retrospective comparative study of radiotherapy and cryotherapy, the conclusions must be considered in the light of the noncomparability of the groups. This study was retrospective, and shows a selection bias inasmuch as the severity and extent of a lesion often determines its initial therapy. A higher propor-

tion of broad and thick lesions were thus treated in the radiotherapy group. Considering the radiotherapy group alone, however, may be informative in that poor healing was significantly related to age > 90 years, a field irradiation diameter > 4 cm, and a radiotherapy dose > 3000 cGy. In view of the risk for poor healing, the authors suggested that patients meeting these criteria require cautious consideration in determining their candidacy for radiotherapy. Caution should also be used when selecting patients for radiotherapy who have lesions in potentially poorly healing areas such as the lower legs.

Chemical peels
Chemical peels have only been investigated for AK.

Quality of evidence: I
We found no systematic reviews and one RCT. The RCT was a within-patient comparison of 5-fluorouracil combined with a glycolic acid (GA) peel versus the GA peel alone (n = 18).[69] We found two comparative studies[70,71] (with one follow-up study[71]) using trichloroacetic acid (TCA). Pretreatments included topical tretinoin (0.05%, increasing to 0.1%) in the first study[70] and Jessner's solution in the second study.[71,72] The concentrations of TCA varied from 35% to 40%.

The first study[70] was reportedly randomized. However, all of the patients pretreated with tretinoin had previously received topical therapies in addition to cryotherapy, whereas all of the patients without tretinoin pretreatment had previously received only cryotherapy. The study reported a 6-month follow-up. In the second study, a split-face design was used. One side of the face received a TCA chemical peel after pretreatment with Jessner's solution, and the other side received 5% topical 5-FU twice daily for 3 weeks. Despite a small sample size, follow-up was reported at 12 months[71] and 32 months.[72]

Benefits
Six months after eight weekly pulse peels, the combination of 5-FU and GA had cleared significantly more lesions than GA alone (91.94% versus 19.67%; $P < 0.05$).[69] No significant differences were observed for pretreatment with topical tretinoin before 40% TCA; AK was reduced by 20–75% in both groups. The authors used a reduction in the appearance of lesions, which was not necessarily a reduction in the number of lesions. Scores for photodamage decreased and telangiectasias improved with tretinoin pretreatment. Jessner's solution followed by TCA did not differ significantly from topical 5-FU: both yielded a 75% reduction in the number of lesions that persisted for 12 months. Analysis of eight patients at the 32-month follow up showed that three (37%) had more lesions than at baseline, but that three patients maintained a 50% reduction from baseline.

The patients were extremely pleased with the cosmetic results of the TCA facial peels, and scored improvement significantly higher than the clinicians did. Patients preferred the facial peel to 5-FU because of the convenient single application and the shorter duration of adverse effects.

Harms

Few side effects were associated with the combination GA peel and 5-FU or the GA peel alone. Slight facial erythema and mild xerosis were experienced, but resolved with an emollient cream.[69] The medium-depth facial peel procedures were associated with erythema lasting generally 10 days to 2 weeks. Mild desquamation was noted.

Comments

The combination of 5-FU with a GA peel is a better option than a GA peel alone. Facial peel with TCA appears to be a viable option if the patient is not a good candidate for cryotherapy (i.e., with widespread facial AK), or is intolerant to other topicals applied over the long term, such as 5-FU.

Dermabrasion

Dermabrasion was investigated only for AK.

Quality of evidence: II-i

We found one unblinded comparative study[73] comparing recurrence rates for dermabrasion, 50% phenol chemical peels, and 1% topical 5-FU. Methodological problems included a small sample size, varying follow-up periods, lack of data on initial elimination rate, and lack of explicit evaluation criteria for remission or recurrence.

Benefits

Dermabrasion yielded a longer time to recurrence than facial peel, but shorter times than 5-FU. However, no statistical data were presented.[73]

Harms

No information on adverse events was reported in the unblinded study. One case series of dermabrasion of the scalp[74] reported a conspicuous line marking the periphery of abrasion at postoperative week 6–8.

Comments

This small study concluded that topical 5-FU was more effective and easier to use than dermabrasion. Although dermabrasion may produce longer-term clearance than chemical peels, the case series[74] indicated a risk of scarring. Although larger studies are necessary for definitive conclusions to be reached, it would appear that the indication for dermabrasion as a primary therapeutic modality for AK is minimal.

Surgery and electrodesiccation and curettage

Surgery is commonly used for BD, but not for AK.

Quality of evidence: II-iii

We found no systematic reviews or RCTs. We found one small retrospective uncontrolled trial investigating surgical excision (n = 4)[75] and two large retrospective uncontrolled trials for electrodesiccation and curettage (ED&C) (n = 20,[75] n = 83[64]).

Benefits

Although surgical excision appeared to clinically clear all four cases, two cases recurred.[75] The author did not report the time to recurrence. ED&C[64,75] resulted in complete clinical clearance rates ranging from 80% to 90%, with recurrences ranging from 10% to 20% during a follow-up period of up to 18 years. Again, the time to recurrence was not reported in either study.

Harms

No harms were reported with ED&C or with surgical excision, other than the understood risks of bleeding, infection, and local anesthesia associated with minor surgery.

Comment

Surgical excision is commonly reported as the treatment of choice for BD, although no RCTs and only this small series were found to support its use. The unmatched efficacy ascribed to surgical excision probably relates to the notion that excision of an *in situ* neoplasm is, by definition, curative. The predominance of BD in elderly populations and its slow progression to SCC suggest that additional outcomes such as healing, scarring, and patient preferences should be considered in determining the choice of treatment. The large series investigating ED&C suggested high efficacy, with tolerable recurrence rates during a sufficiently long follow-up period. ED&C may thus be a highly useful procedure for patients with small solitary lesions.

Hyperthermia

Quality of evidence: II-iii

One uncontrolled trial[76] examined the use of hyperthermic pocket warmers applied with direct pressure to BD lesions in eight patients every day for 4–5 months. Complete histological clearance was seen in three patients, isolated tumor cells remained in three cases, and two patients showed no change.

Comment

Although noninvasive and innovative, the low efficacy, the troublesome nature of the therapy for the patient, and the poor level of evidence provided by uncontrolled studies suggest that hyperthermic pocket-warmer therapy should be considered only in patients who decline more conventional therapy.

What are the effects of topical therapy?

Topical retinoids
Topical retinoids were reported only for AK.

Actinic keratoses (quality of evidence: I)
We found four double-blind RCTs investigating topical retinoids for AK.[77–80] The first study compared tretinoin cream (n = 25) with Ro 14-9706 (arotinoid methyl sulfone cream; n = 25) using a split-face design.[77] The second study was a parallel-group multicenter trial comparing 0.1% isotretinoin (n = 41) with placebo (n = 47).[78] The third study was a four-arm comparison trial investigating the use of all-*trans*-retinoic acid (ATRA) cream, calcipotriol cream, a combination of the two creams, and a vehicle cream in renal transplant recipients.[79] Thirteen patients with multiple AKs applied each of the four treatments to different lesions, the order of which was randomly assigned. The fourth study compared the efficacy of 0.1% adapalene gel (n = 30), 0.3% adapalene gel (n = 30), and a vehicle gel (n = 30).[80]

Benefit
Reductions in the number of AK lesions by 30% and 38% were reported for tretinoin and Ro 14-9706, respectively. Complete clearance of all lesions occurred in 8% of patients using tretinoin.[77] In comparison with placebo, 0.1% topical isotretinoin significantly reduced the number of facial lesions (65% versus 45%, $P < 0.005$).[78] No differences in the number of AK lesions were found between each of the four treatments used in the third study after 6 weeks of treatment.[79] It was concluded by the authors that neither all-*trans*-retinoic acid, calcipotriol, nor a combination of these two creams should be used to treat AKs in renal transplant recipients. After 9 months of treatment, patients treated with 0.3% adapalene gel had significantly fewer lesions in comparison with the baseline than those treated with vehicle cream ($P < 0.05$).[80] The complete lesion clearance rate for patients in both adapalene treatment groups was only 3%, while an increase in the numbers of lesions was observed in the vehicle group.

Harms
Severe local skin irritation was associated with topical tretinoin, whereas the irritation was mild to moderate with isotretinoin. No significant changes in laboratory parameters were observed. Higher levels of erythema, peeling, dryness, burning, and pruritus were associated with 0.3% and 0.1% adapalene treatment in comparison with the vehicle treatment.[80]

Comments
Although some reduction in AK counts and size has been noted, few patients (8%[77] and 3%[80]) had complete clearance of lesions, which should be the goal of effective AK treatment. The relatively high rate of reduction noted with placebo use indicates either that the study was flawed or that topical retinoids may not enhance the clearance of AK lesions sufficiently to be used as a standard treatment for AK.

5-Fluorouracil
Topical chemotherapy with 5-FU interferes with DNA and RNA synthesis. It is indicated for diffuse, ill-defined AK in which treatment of individual lesions is impractical or impossible. It is also used in BD.

Actinic keratoses (quality of evidence: I)
We found two systematic reviews[39,81] and five RCTs.[43,82–85] One RCT used a split-face trial to compare 0.5% 5-FU with 5% 5-FU (n = 21),[83] while another compared daily applications of 0.5% 5-FU (n = 13) with weekly applications (n = 7).[84] The third RCT compared 0.5% 5-FU (n = 12) with two different forms of photodynamic therapy (n = 12 for both groups).[85] The fourth RCT compared 0.5% 5-FU with cryotherapy (n = 72) to 0.5% 5-FU with a vehicle cream (n = 72),[43] and finally the last RCT compared 5% 5-FU (n = 30) with masoprocol (n = 27).[82] Details of masoprocol and photodynamic therapy are described later in the chapter.

Benefits
One systematic review[39] found marked heterogeneity in the concentration of 5-FU and drug vehicles, ranging from 1% in propylene glycol[86,87] or 1% cream,[88] to 3% ointment,[89] to 5% solution,[69,90] ointment,[91–95] or cream.[71,72,96,97] Combination therapies have also been reported.[69,98] To complicate issues further, variation in treatment sites and outcomes was noted. An attempt to combine studies using meta-analysis techniques[39] revealed that only three studies could be combined.[92–94] This combination showed that the overall efficacy (treatment period of 2–8 weeks and follow-up period of 3–18 months) of 5% 5-FU ointment ranged from 79% (95% CI, 72% to 87%) using patient-level data (by pooling individual participants' data) to 84% (77% to 91%) using study-level data (by using the reported effect size from each study, weighted by the reported variance).[39] The second systematic review combined six studies[71,86,94,99–101] to include in a meta-analysis.[81] The included studies used only 0.5%, 1%, or 5% 5-FU as treatment, treated only the face and/or scalp, and measured the proportion of patients with no visible AKs at follow-up. The proportion of patients with complete clearance ranged from 0% to 100% (with treatment periods of 2–8 weeks and follow-up periods of 1–11 months). The pooled average for patient response was

52.2 + 18%.[81] In the RCT comparing 5-FU with masoprocol, the authors demonstrated a significantly higher percentage reduction in the number of lesions ($P < 0.0001$) and improvement in the investigators' global assessment ($P < 0.001$).[82] In the RCT comparing 5-FU with PDT with blue light and PDT with laser light, lesion response rates were found to be 79%, 80%, and 50%, respectively.[85] Daily application of 5-FU was found to reduce more lesions than weekly application at all time points after week 0 (outcomes measured at 3, 12, 24, and 52 weeks, all $P < 0.05$),[84] and 0.5% 5-FU was found to reduce significantly more lesions than 5% 5-FU at the end of a 4-week follow-up phase ($P = 0.044$).[83] Although both cryotherapy with 5-FU and cryotherapy with a vehicle cream were successful in significantly reducing the number of lesions from baseline, cryotherapy with 5-FU pretreatment was found to be more effective following each treatment cycle.[43]

Harms

5-FU can be associated with pain, inflammation, and erosions.[86,102] In one RCT, 5-FU produced significantly more necrosis ($P < 0.007$), erosions ($P < 0.001$), pain ($P < 0.001$), erythema ($P < 0.016$), and contact dermatitis ($P < 0.016$) than masoprocol.[82] Although both 0.5% 5-FU and 5% 5-FU were found to have comparable degrees of irritation as rated by the investigator, patients preferred the 0.5% cream, which was rated as more tolerable ($P = 0.003$).[83]

Comments

Although 5-FU has a high efficacy rate, one should note that it is associated with a high degree of morbidity, including pain, inflammation, and erosions. Thus, if patients are unable to tolerate these side effects, we would expect the cure rate to drop off dramatically.

Of methodological note, the authors of several of the RCTs did not perform an ITT analysis,[82,84,85] and in the remaining RCTs it is unclear whether or not analysis was carried out on an ITT basis.[43,83] If the participants who dropped out of these studies were included in the denominator, as prescribed in an ITT analysis, the efficacy rate would likely decrease. For example, in the RCT that compares 5-FU with masoprocol, the efficacy rate (by investigator global assessment of cure) of 5-FU falls from 77% to 67%, while that of masoprocol falls from 23% to 20%, if all ITT patients are included in the analysis. Despite the lack of ITT analysis, however, the difference between 67% and 20% undoubtedly reaches statistical significance.

Bowen's disease (quality of evidence: I)

We found no systematic reviews and one RCT. The RCT was a comparison trial between 5% 5-FU (n = 20 patients with 33 lesions) and photodynamic therapy (n = 20 patients with 33 lesions).[103] We found one small unblinded, quasi-randomized controlled trial comparing topical 5% 5-FU cream with intralesional interferon alfa-2b (1 000 000 units/injection) for both BD and AK.[101] The treatment-allocation method was not specified. Ten lesions of BD and AK were allocated to each group, and clinical clearance and histological change were assessed at 1 and 2 months' follow up. We found six uncontrolled trials addressing the therapeutic efficacy of 5-FU.[64,75,104–107]

Benefits

One year after treatment with either PDT or 5-FU, the complete clinical clearance rate of lesions in the PDT group was 88%. This was significantly more effective ($P = 0.006$) than 5-FU, which had a complete clearance rate of 48%.[103] For the quasi-RCT, clinical clearance in the 5-FU group was superior to that in the interferon alfa-2b group (100% versus 90%) at an 8-week assessment. A statistically significant difference in the histological response to treatment was further noted at 4 and 8 weeks in favor of interferon ($P < 0.05$).[101] This trial failed to specify the number of BD lesions in each treatment group; consequently, the reported data do not allow any conclusions for BD independent of AK.

In the uncontrolled trials, clinical clearance rates were generally high, ranging from 87%[104] to 100%.[64] It is noteworthy that among studies with a sufficiently long follow-up period for recurrences to be documented (at least 12 months), one study reported a significantly higher recurrence rate (20%)[105] than other studies (0% and 8%).[64,75,105,107] The largest uncontrolled trial (n = 41) used 5-FU (in 1–3% in propylene glycol) applied twice daily for 2–3 months.[75] The clinical clearance rate in this study was 93%, with an 8% recurrence rate during a median follow-up period of 8 years (range 6–121 months). The authors suggest that at least 2.5% 5-FU in propylene glycol is required for extrafacial sites.

The base in which 5-FU is delivered significantly affects its activity: 20% 5-FU in an ointment base, 5% 5-FU in a cream base, and 1% 5-FU in propylene glycol provide approximately equivalent cytotoxic activity.[94,102,108,109] Several studies investigated ways of enhancing 5-FU activity. Iontophoresis does not appear to improve 5-FU activity in comparison with 5-FU alone.[64,75,105,106] Application under occlusion, pretreatment with keratolytic agents, or deliberate exposure to sunlight (photosensitivity effect of 5-FU) are anecdotally reported as enhancement techniques.[75]

Harms

Expected side effects include pain, pruritus, burning at the site of application, erythema, inflammation, and erosions.[52] Some authors suggest application of the medication four times daily to reduce the duration of treatment,[110] while others advocate pulse therapy once or twice weekly to decrease the intensity of discomfort.[111] Although compliance with the latter regimen is higher, cure rates may be lower.[112] Lower-leg ulceration has been reported with 5%

5-FU cream,[75,103] and an allergic reaction to 5-FU has been reported in conjunction with iontophoretic therapy.[104]

Comment

Although most of the studies have significant methodological limitations, 5-FU appears to be of likely benefit in treating BD. As with AK, if patients are unable to tolerate the side effects of 5-FU, then we would expect the cure rate to drop off dramatically. For example, in the RCT, treatment was discontinued in five of the 33 lesions treated with 5-FU due to widespread dermatitic reactions (compared to none of 33 in the PDT group), which likely explains the low clearance rates for this treatment group (48%).[103]

The quasi-randomized controlled trial comparing 5-FU with interferon suffers from two methodological limitations in addition to the non-randomized allocation. No data are presented regarding the proportion of BD and AK in each treatment group, and conclusions regarding therapeutic efficacy can therefore only be generalized to BD and AK in aggregate and may be distorted by the response of a few patients with lots of lesions. Furthermore, the significant difference in histological response in favor of interferon does not correlate with the higher efficacy of 5-FU in terms of clinical clearance. Thus, the histological response may have been used as a surrogate outcome for clinical response and should be viewed accordingly in clinical decision-making.

It is impossible to draw definitive conclusions from uncontrolled trials. However, it is worth noting that the disparity in recurrence rates may relate to different therapeutic regimens: the study reporting a higher recurrence employed weekly topical pulse therapy for a minimum of 12 weeks, whereas most other studies used once-daily or twice-daily applications for 2–16 weeks.[75,101,104]

Imiquimod

The immunomodulator imiquimod is one of the newest treatments studied for use in AK and BD.

Actinic keratoses (quality of evidence: I)

We found three systematic reviews[81,113,114] and one RCT.[115] The RCT randomly assigned 18 patients in a 2 : 1 ratio to receive either imiquimod cream (n = 12) or a vehicle cream (n = 6).[115] The three systematic reviews performed a meta-analysis of randomized controlled trials,[113,114] or RCTs and other relevant studies,[81] which assessed the efficacy of 5% imiquimod in treating actinic keratosis. The first review[113] included five studies in its meta-analysis,[116–120] the second review[114] included four studies,[116,117,119,121] and the third review[81] also included four studies.[117,119,121,122]

Benefit

A total of 1293 patients clinically or histologically diagnosed with AK were evaluated in the RCTs included in the first systematic review.[113] All of these studies sufficiently

measured both the benefits and harms of imiquimod, but only one study[120] had a long enough follow-up period (≥ 1 year) to effectively assess recurrence rates. Complete clinical clearance of all AK lesions occurred in 50% of patients treated with imiquimod, in comparison with only 5% in those treated with a vehicle cream.[113] The mean clinical response was not calculated in the second systematic review, which included 1266 patients,[114] but complete clearance of lesions was more common in imiquimod-treated patients than in control-treated patients (P < 0.0001). The third systematic review, which included a total of 393 patients, reported slightly higher efficacy rates with imiquimod. The proportion of patients with complete clinical clearance for this review was 70.8% ± 12.3% (mean ± 95% CI).[113] For the RCT, complete clinical clearance was achieved in 45% of the imiquimod-treated patients and in 0% of the patients treated with vehicle cream.[115]

Harms

Many local adverse events are associated with imiquimod treatment, including: erythema, scabbing or crusting, flaking, erosion, edema, and weeping.[113] Several studies noted that better clearance was observed in patients with the most severe adverse events.[116,120] Several authors also reported that the number of AK lesions increased in the initial stages of treatment.[116–118] It was proposed that this was more likely to be an appearance of subclinical lesions rather than formation of new lesions, and considered to be a benefit of imiquimod treatment. A recurrence rate of 10% was reported by the only long-term (≥ 1 year) follow-up study, which treated patients with imiquimod three times a week for a maximum of 12 weeks.[120]

Comment

There is good evidence that imiquimod is an effective short-term treatment for actinic keratosis. Future studies should include longer follow-up periods to assess the long-term effects of this treatment.

Bowen's disease (quality of evidence: I)

We found a single, small RCT and three uncontrolled trials. The double-blinded RCT randomly assigned 31 patients to receive either a placebo cream (n = 16) or imiquimod (n = 15) daily for 16 weeks.[123] The first uncontrolled trial treated 16 lesions of the lower limbs with once-daily application of imiquimod cream for 16 weeks[124] and the second used imiquimod cream and oral sulindac, 200 mg twice daily, for 16 weeks in five immunocompromised patients.[125] The third uncontrolled trial treated five BD lesions with imiquimod once daily, five times a week for a maximum of 16 weeks.[126]

Benefits

The RCT reported that 73% of imiquimod-treated patients achieved complete resolution of BD lesions, which was significantly greater than in the placebo group, in which no resolution was achieved ($P < 0.001$).[123] The first uncontrolled study reported a 93% treatment response (15 of 16 patients), evidenced by no residual tumor on histology, although six patients withdrew prematurely because of local skin reactions and were not included in the final analysis.[124] An ITT analysis showed that 87.5% (14 of 16 patients) had no residual tumor. All immunocompromised patients showed complete clinical responses within 4 weeks of therapy and a histological response at 20 weeks after initiation of therapy.[125] Four of five BD lesions (80%) showed complete clearance after 8–12 weeks of imiquimod treatment.[126]

Harms
In the RCT, imiquimod treatment was generally well-tolerated, and no serious adverse events were reported.[123] Two imiquimod-treated patients withdrew from the study, one due to infection at the treatment site, and the other due to an inflammatory reaction. This reaction was presumed to have been due to treatment application to an area greater than the original lesion. No recurrence of lesions was reported during the 9-month follow-up period. In uncontrolled BD trials, adverse events included marked local skin irritation requiring discontinuation of therapy, superinfection requiring antibiotics, and satellite lesions in adjacent sun-damaged areas.[124]

Comments
Imiquimod 5% cream appears to be an efficacious treatment for BD of the lower limbs, particularly for large lesions on the lower extremity, such as the shin, where poor healing is of particular concern. The dosing schedule and length of treatment require further evaluation in RCTs.

Diclofenac
Diclofenac is a nonsteroidal anti-inflammatory drug formulated as a 3% topical gel in 2.5% hyaluronate sodium.

Actinic keratosis (quality of evidence: I)
We found one systematic review,[127] which conducted a meta-analysis of three RCTs (n = 364).[128–130] All of the RCTs included in the review compared the efficacy of twice-daily applications of diclofenac (treatment durations were between 60 and 90 days) with a placebo gel 30 days after treatment. We also found one RCT for diclofenac (n = 130), but only the abstract was accessible to the authors. Although complete and partial responses were reported, neither was defined; the time of final assessment was not defined.[131] Clearance rates for 90-day treatments are also available from two placebo-controlled trials (n = 117 and n = 108) reported in the package insert for Solaraze (diclofenac), but the trials are unavailable to the authors.[132]

Benefits
The meta-analysis of the three RCTs revealed that 39% of patients experienced complete lesion clearance at 30 days after the end of treatment, in comparison with 12% of patients treated with a placebo gel.[127] This response rate is similar to the response rates reported on the package insert for Solaraze.[132] Complete lesion clearance rates (for two separate trials) 30 days after a 90-day treatment with diclofenac were 47% and 34%, in comparison with 19% and 18% for the placebo groups.[132] Although the time of assessment was not reported, the complete response rates for the RCT were 29% for the diclofenac-treated group and 17% for the control group (24 weeks of twice-daily applications).[131]

Harms
The most common adverse effects reported after treatment with 3% diclofenac in 2.5% hyaluronic acid gel are pruritus, contact dermatitis, dry skin, rash, and scaling. Treatment is generally well-tolerated.[127]

Comments
Treatment of AK using 3% diclofenac in 2.5% hyaluronic gel appears to be well tolerated, but with relatively low efficacy. The lesion clearance rates in all of these studies were clinically assessed, which may lead to overestimation. Future studies should include biopsy confirmation of clearance and long-term follow-up periods in order to determine the long-term efficacy and recurrence rates.

Bowen's disease quality of evidence: IV)
We found no systematic reviews or RCTs. We found one case series, which treated two patients (each with one BD lesion) with 3% diclofenac in 2.5% hyaluronan gel twice daily for 90 days.[133]

Benefits
Both patients were clinically free of Bowen's disease 10–12 months after treatment.

Harms
One patient developed severe dermatitis and had to discontinue treatment after 80 days.

Comments
Insufficient research has been conducted to establish the efficacy of this treatment for BD lesions. Given the high rates of SCC transformation of BD, and the low response rate of AK to diclofenac, it seems questionable and unethical for any further research to be conducted.

Photodynamic therapy (PDT)
PDT involves activation of a photosensitizer, usually a porphyrin derivative, by visible light. A common photosensitizer is topical aminolevulinic acid (ALA).

Actinic keratoses (quality of evidence: I)

We found no systematic reviews and 14 RCTs. These trials are difficult to compare, due to the wide variety of parameters used in this type of treatment (i.e., light source, wavelength, photosensitizing agent, length of incubation, filter range. etc.). Three RCTs used the photosensitizing agent ALA and PDT with blue light exposure for 1000 seconds and an incubation period of 14–18 h, which was compared with placebo/PDT.[134–136] One study compared treatment of hand lesions with ALA/PDT, using red light and a 4-h incubation period, against topical 5% 5-FU.[137] Another study compared ALA/PDT with red light to ALA with pulsed dye laser (PDL).[138] Another study compared ALA/PDT with blue light to ALA with PDL, and to 0.5% 5-FU.[85] A further study compared the use of ALA/PDT at three different dosages of red light.[139] One final study looked at the efficacy of ALA/PDT by comparing four groups, two of which underwent either narrow-filter exposure with various fluence rates while the other two groups underwent broad-filter exposure with various fluence rates.[140] Three other RCTs compared the use of the photosensitizing agent methyl aminolevulinic acid (MAL) and PDT with placebo/PDT.[41,141,142] One of the above-mentioned studies[41] and two other RCTs compared MAL/PDT with cryotherapy.[40,42] The last RCT compared different treatment regimens of MAL/PDT—with one group receiving a single session of MAL/PDT with repeat treatment at 3 months for any remaining lesions, and the other group receiving two treatment sessions 1 week apart.[143]

Benefits

In the three RCTs that compared ALA/PDT using a blue light source with placebo/PDT, the percentages of individual lesions that cleared were 91% (12 weeks after treatment),[134] 88% (8 weeks after treatment)[135] and 83% (8 weeks after treatment)[136] for the ALA/PDT group, in comparison with 25%, 6%, and 33%, respectively, for the placebo/PDT group. Use of ALA/PDT with red light for lesions on the hands was not significantly different from 5-FU (73% versus 70% reduction).[137] Complete clearance was not observed in either group.[137] ALA/PDT induced complete responses in 88.1% of lesions, in comparison with 66.7% of lesions for ALA/PDL at 4 months after treatment.[138] The clearance rates at 4 weeks after treatment for 5-FU, ALA/PDT, and ALA/PDL were 79%, 80%, and 50%, respectively.[85] Both photodynamic therapy treatments were better tolerated than 5-FU.[85] There were no significant differences in clearance rates between patients treated with three different light doses of ALA/PDT at 3 months after treatment (88% for 70 J/cm², 77% for 100 J/cm², and 69% for 140 J/cm²).[139] The percentage of ALA/PDT patients with complete clearance (7 weeks after treatment) who were treated with a narrow filter and the lowest fluence rate was 88.8%, in comparison with 40.0–44.4% of patients in the three other treatment groups, who received either a higher fluence rate or were treated with a broad filter.[140] Complete response rates for MAL/PDT-treated lesions were 91% (3 months after treatment),[41] 89% (3 months after treatment),[141] and 90% (16 weeks after treat-ment),[142] in comparison with 30%, 38%, and 0% for placebo/PDT-treated lesions. In the three RCTs that compared MAL/PDT with cryotherapy, the complete lesion response rates after one or two treatments of MAL/PDT were 89.1% (24 weeks after treatment),[40] 69% (3 months after treatment),[42] and 91% (3 months after treatment, as mentioned above).[41] Patient and investigator preferences, as well as the cosmetic outcome, favored MAL/PDT over cryotherapy.[40] Patients who received a single treatment with MAL/PDT (with a second treatment 3 months later for any remaining lesions) had a complete lesion response rate of 92% in comparison with 86% in patients receiving two MAL/PDT treatments 1 week apart.[143] Lesion response rates were assessed 3 months after the last treatment.

Harms

Most patients experienced a stinging or burning sensation during photoirradiation, which generally ceased on completion of phototherapy. The treated lesions typically became erythematous and edematous after treatment. Healing generally occurs over 2–4 weeks. ALA/PDT was significantly more painful than ALA/PDL ($P < 0.001$).[138]

Comments

Photodynamic therapy, using either aminolevulinic acid or methyl aminolevulinic acid as a photosensitizing agent, has been highly successful in treating AK lesions, especially if they are widespread. PDT with pulsed dye laser may not be as efficient as some of the other treatment modalities. Although the healing process is somewhat lengthy, it is comparable to the events experienced by patients following 5-FU and other topical regimens. As treatment takes place over 2 days, rather than many weeks with topical formulations, PDT may be more convenient for the patient willing to undergo the process; however, long-term efficacy has not been established. Moreover, PDT has not been effective in treating hyperkeratotic lesions. It is an expensive treatment that requires a trained specialist and costly equipment to administer it.

Bowen's disease (quality of evidence: I)

We found no systematic reviews, three RCTs, and one unblinded controlled trial. One RCT compared photodynamic therapy using the photosensitizing agent methyl aminolevulinate (MAL; n = 96) with placebo/PDT (n = 17), or to another standard therapy.[49] The standard therapy involved either cryotherapy or fluorouracil, as chosen by the treating investigator. The second RCT investigated 61 lower leg lesions to compare the efficacy of green light and red light wavelengths after incubation with 20% 5-ALA for 4 h.[144] The follow-up period was 12 months. The third RCT compared PDT using aminolevulinic acid (n = 20) with 5% 5-FU (n = 20).[103] The unblinded, controlled trial investigated 40 lesions to determine the relative efficacy of 20% 5-ALA cream and a modified portable desktop lamp against cryotherapy.[48] The method of randomization in this study was not specified. The follow-up period was 12 months.

Benefits
The complete response rate 3 months after treatment for lesions treated with MAL/PDT was 93% in comparison with 21% for placebo/PDT-treated lesions.[49] The recurrence rates for these treatments (1 year after treatment) were 15% for MAL/PDT and 50% for placebo/PDT.[49] Ninety-four percent of patients who experience pain related to MAL/PDT reported that it was of mild or moderate severity. Lesions receiving red light showed a significantly greater clinical clearance rate, as determined by the dermatologist's examination (94% versus 76%, $P < 0.002$) and a lower recurrence rate (6% versus 38%) in comparison with green light (odds ratio 0.13; 95% CI, 0.04 to 0.48). The authors attribute this difference to the reduced depth of tissue penetration by green light, postulating that periappendageal BDs (which may extend up to 3 mm in depth) may survive ALA-PDT using less penetrating wavelengths. No ulceration, infection, scarring, or photosensitivity reactions were reported in either group. There was no significant difference in pain between the groups, and the majority of patients reported "none" to "moderate" pain. In the third RCT, complete clearance 6 weeks after treatment was reported in 88% of lesions treated with ALA/PDT, in comparison with 67% in lesions treated with 5-FU.[103] After 12 months of follow-up, lesion recurrences reduced these rates to 82% for PDT and 48% for 5-FU (odds ratio 4.78; 95% CI, 1.56 to 14.62). Pain was reported as mild to moderate in 85.7% of patients and severe in 14.3%.[103]

In the unblinded controlled trial, a significant difference —that a lesion of any size would clear after the first treatment with PDT in comparison with the first treatment with cryotherapy—was observed ($P < 0.01$). However, there were no significant differences in the overall clearance rates between treatments following three cryotherapy treatments ($P < 0.08$).[48] The clinical clearance rates at the 12-month follow-up were 90% in the cryotherapy group and 100% in the PDT group.

Harms
Adverse effects of PDT include treatment-induced pain, requiring anesthesia, in up to 25% of lesions,[145–147] skin fragility and dyspigmentation,[147–149] permanent hair loss,[148] toxic reactions to ALA cream,[146] and photosensitivity reactions.[145]

Comments
Photodynamic therapy appears promising for the treatment of Bowen's disease. While the first RCT was double-blinded,[49] investigators in the second RCT were not blinded to the type of light used,[144] thus potentially introducing bias. Blinding was impossible in the third RCT[103] due to the differences in treatment types being compared in the study. Although more objective outcomes, such as clinical clearance and recurrence, are less susceptible to bias related to lack of blinding, the validity of the results concerning treatment-related pain may be improved with blinding. The analyses for the first[49] and second RCTs[144] were not based on an ITT approach, since patients who discontinued treatment or were lost to follow-up were excluded from the final analysis—thus risking overestimation of the efficacy of the treatment and underestimation of recurrences.

Masoprocol
Masoprocol (mesonordihydroguaiaretic acid) is a potent 5-lipoxygenase inhibitor with antitumor properties, investigated for use in AK.[150]

Actinic keratoses (quality of evidence: I)
We found two double-blind RCTs.[82,150] The first study[150] compared masoprocol (n = 113) with topical placebo (n = 41), and the second study[82] compared masoprocol (n = 27) with topical 5% 5-FU (n = 30). Both studies reported a 1-month follow-up after the end of treatment.

Benefits
Masoprocol produced a larger median percentage reduction in the number of AK lesions than placebo (71.4% versus 4.3%, respectively; $P < 0.0003$), and an 11% (12 of 113) cure rate on a per-patient basis.[150] Masoprocol produced a 78% reduction in AK lesions, in comparison with a 98% reduction with 5-FU ($P < 0.0001$). Cure rates with masoprocol and 5-FU on a per-patient basis were 22% (five of 23) and 77% (20 of 26), respectively.

Harms
Erythema occurred at rates of 53% and 22% with masoprocol and placebo, respectively, and flaking occurred at rates of 53% versus 4% with masoprocol and placebo, respectively. Itching, burning, edema, tightness and dryness, and bleeding of the skin were also reported with masoprocol.[150] In comparison with 5-FU, masoprocol caused significantly fewer and less severe adverse effects, including necrosis, erosion, and erythema.[82] One report[151] described a potential for masoprocol to induce potent sensitization (allergic contact dermatitis). The two clinical studies reported here did not exclude the possibility of allergic contact dermatitis with masoprocol.

Comments

Masoprocol produces a significant reduction in AK lesions compared to placebo, but low overall cure rates in relation to patients as the unit of analysis. 5-FU appears to provide higher rates of cure on a per-patient basis. Masoprocol may provide an alternative for those who cannot tolerate 5-FU. The long-term efficacy of masoprocol has yet to be established.

Miscellaneous topical therapies

A variety of other topical therapies have been assessed as treatments for actinic lesions, with varied success. These include Curaderm (0.005% solasodine glycosides, 10% salicylic acid, 5% urea, 0.1% melaleuca oil, 0.05% linolenic acid in cetomacrogol-based cream) and the nucleoside tubercidin (7-deaza-adenosine).

Quality of evidence: IV

We found no systematic reviews for either of these topical therapies. A case series used tubercidin to treat five patients with facial and scalp AK lesions.[152] A single open-label trial treated 56 AK lesions using Curaderm,[153] with follow-up at 3 months post-treatment.

Benefits

Curaderm has been reported to cure AK lesions completely (clinically and histologically) in a mean of 2.9 weeks (range 1–4 weeks), in an open-label Australian trial.[153] However, no recent literature on this treatment was found in any searches, and no North American use has been reported.

The nucleoside tubercidin interferes with glycolysis and inhibits synthesis of DNA, RNA, and proteins. Tubercidin was not effective in a case series of five patients with facial and scalp AK.[104] Four of the patients showed no response of lesions to tubercidin after 4 weeks of treatment.

Harms

The one patient who had complete resolution with tubercidin had marked facial erythema. Curaderm produced itching and burning sensations in lesions during treatment, but no abnormal hematological, biochemical, or urinalysis parameters were noted.

Comments

Topical treatments, which patients can apply in the comfort of the home, are more convenient than treatments that have to be administered by a physician, and in general are more convenient than cryotherapy in treating multiple lesions. None can be recommended at present, in the absence of high-quality studies comparing their efficacy with standard treatments using liquid-nitrogen cryotherapy and 5-FU.

What are the effects of intralesional or oral medication?

Oral retinoids

Actinic keratoses (quality of evidence: I)

We found two double-blind placebo-controlled RCTs investigating the reduction in AK lesion size and overall grade (based on number, diameter, thickness and hyperkeratosis).[154,155] Both studies used a crossover design and followed patients from 2 to 18 months.

Benefits

Both RCTs did not report the relevant outcomes, but instead recorded lesion size, the usefulness of which is dubious. Oral etretinate (Tegison) reduced the lesion size in 82–86% of patients in the first study,[154] both when etretinate was the primary drug (19 of 22, followed by placebo) or when etretinate was used after crossover from placebo (18 of 22). Placebo reduced lesion size in only 4.3% of patients (one of 23) who used placebo before etretinate. Use of placebo following etretinate resulted in no change in lesions in 95% of the participants (18 of 19). In the second study,[155] etretinate improved the overall grading of lesions in 89–100% of patients (eight of nine patients using etretinate before placebo and all of six using etretinate after placebo). Placebo improved lesion gradings in 17% of patients who used placebo before crossing over to etretinate (one of six). In patients who crossed over to placebo from etretinate, only 11% had any further improvement (one of nine).

Harms

Dry lips and mouth may occur in a high proportion of patients using etretinate, although symptoms are alleviated with dose reduction. Transient elevations of serum cholesterol and triglycerides, as well as one case of drug-related hepatitis, were reported.[155]

Comments

The rates of reduction in lesion size and grading appear to be significantly better for etretinate than placebo. However, these results are based on outcome measurements that are limited in their usefulness. One should also be careful of crossover study designs, in which a considerable carry-over effect is likely. If insufficient time is allowed for the etretinate to wash out in the patients in whom etretinate was given before the placebo, then the effects of etretinate were probably confounding the results of the placebo. Long-term efficacy has not been established, but it is unlikely to reflect the efficacy rates reported in the studies, since they reported reductions in AK size. If the AK lesions are not eradicated, they will surely regrow; moreover, even if a particular AK lesion is eradicated, it does not prevent new ones from forming.

Bowen's disease (quality of evidence: IV)

One uncontrolled trial[156] examined the use of aromatic retinoid tablets, 1 mg/kg daily, over a period of 2–7 months in five patients with multiple BD lesions secondary to chronic arsenism.

Comment

Residual tumor cells were found in all patients. Oral retinoids cannot be recommended for treatment of BD.

Interferon

Actinic keratoses (quality of evidence: I)

We found one double-blind, placebo-controlled, parallel-group RCT each for intralesional interferon alfa[157] and topical interferon gel (Intron A; interferon alfa-2b).[158] The studies included 16–23 patients, with a post-treatment follow up period of 1–2 months. No indication of complete cure on a per-patient basis was indicated.

Benefit

High-dose interferon given intralesionally three times weekly for 2–3 weeks produced complete cure in 47–93% of the lesions treated.[157] No complete cures were produced with topical interferon gel, and only 9% of the lesions (n = 35) showed marked improvement (> 75%).[158]

Comment

While high doses of intralesional interferon appear promising, it is unlikely that the topical formulation will be of much benefit. However, intralesional interferon should be reserved for those patients who cannot use more conventional and economical therapies.

Bowen's disease (quality of evidence: II-i)

We found one small unblinded quasi-randomized controlled trial comparing topical 5-FU (5% cream) with intralesional interferon alfa-2b (1 000 000 units/injection) in the treatment of BD and AK, as reported above.[101]

Benefit

The 5-FU group showed 100% clinical clearance, whereas the interferon group showed 90% clinical clearance at the 8-week assessment. The study did not differentiate between BD and AK.

Comment

Intralesional interferon may be a good option for BD in those not responsive to more conventional and economical therapies.

Bleomycin

There is one anecdotal report of the successful use of intralesional bleomycin in the treatment of BD.[159] The risks of publication bias are very high with such a single report.

Clinical scenarios

Scenario 1

An elderly man with recurrent AK has 30 lesions on his sun-damaged head. How would you approach his problem?

The most likely therapy that a dermatologist would offer for such a widespread area is 5-FU, since it has a high success rate, is easy for the clinician, and if the patient has medical insurance, it is relatively inexpensive. If the patient does not respond to this particular treatment, topical therapy with imiquimod is also a good option. However, the elderly patient may not tolerate the side effects of these therapies. The clinician may then offer photodynamic therapy, chemical peels, or topical retinoids. Cryotherapy, which is more commonly used for solitary lesions (up to 10) is also a common therapy with proven efficacy. Masoprocol, while likely to be beneficial according to the evidence, is not yet widely available and has a disappointing magnitude of effect so far. Similarly, while intralesional interferon is likely to be beneficial, injection into the lesions is unlikely to be tolerated by the patient.

Scenario 2

A woman in her 50s presents with a large (diameter > 20 mm) biopsy-proven BD lesion on her ankle. What would you do?

While there are no studies demonstrating strong evidence in favor of one therapy, several therapies are likely to beneficial on the basis of the evidence presented. Cryotherapy and ED&C are both likely to be beneficial, and the patient may feel reassured about these therapies because they are destructive and are performed by the clinician. However, cryotherapy may result in poor and slow healing of the treated area. While PDT is also likely to be beneficial, and is the treatment of choice for such a large lesion, it may not be widely available. Topical imiquimod and 5-FU are also likely to be beneficial and can be used in patients who are either very compliant and/or would not otherwise tolerate a more invasive procedure. Intralesional interferon is also likely to be beneficial, but will probably be a second-line agent because of its cost.

Implications for clinical practice

Spontaneous regression rates

As discussed in the "Background" section above, the prognosis for patients with AKs without treatment is confounded by the spontaneous regression rate. A study in Queensland[30] reported a spontaneous regression rate of 85% (95% CI, 75% to 96%) in people with prevalent AK (AK diagnosed on a person during their first examination) and 84% (95% CI, 72% to 96%) in persons with incident AK (AK appearing for the first time during the study).

We (P.P. and S.C.) compared the efficacy of 5% 5-FU with a range of plausible spontaneous regression rates of AK.[39] While we could not pinpoint the exact threshold of spontaneous regression rate above which 5-FU would be less effective than no therapy, we find it intriguing that the natural regression rate of AK can be such that the efficacy of a therapeutic modality may appear to be less than no therapy, although regression rates may well vary across the world and be much higher in areas such as Australia, where elderly white people may have hundreds of lesions. Assuming the efficacy of 5-FU ointment to be 79%, we calculated that if the spontaneous AK regression rates were above 75%, no therapy may be better than using 5-fluorouracil.

Of note, the standard care is usually to treat AK, because we cannot predict which cases will resolve spontaneously and which will progress to cancers. Given the reported spontaneous regression rates of AK lesions and the lack of evidence suggesting that any treatment reduces the chances of progression to invasive SCC, the decision to treat AKs is largely debatable. To explore this idea more fully, we propose large future studies to directly compare three strategies: 5-FU, cryotherapy, and no therapy to see whether they really reduce the risk of SCC in the long term.

Implications for future studies

General points that future investigators should bear in mind include using a double-blind randomized study design wherever possible, in order to minimize bias and confounding factors. Randomization sequences must be rigorously concealed in order to avoid selection bias. If investigators wish to use a crossover study design, extreme care must be taken because of the potentially long wash-out periods for most AK therapies. Lastly, investigators should report results based on ITT analysis. If patients who drop out of the study are not taken into account, the results can be misleading.

While any given individual AK lesion has a high probability of resolving spontaneously, a patient with extensive involvement most probably has a much lower probability that all of his or her AK lesions will resolve spontaneously—an issue unique to AK. Thus, studies should either take into account the high correlation of multiple AK lesions if they choose to use the number of lesions as their unit of analysis, or results should be stratified by the severity of AK if persons cleared are used as the unit of analysis. The latter outcome is likely to be of more interest, as it is clinically more relevant.

Another precaution unique to AK studies is to ensure that the outcome measure is reliable. Weinstock *et al.*[160] reported their experience in counting numbers of AK lesions, a commonly used technique. They found the outcome measure to be unreliable, most likely because of the spectrum of clinical features. Discussion of discrepancies among investigators enhanced the reliability of the counts, but substantial variation remains. Thus, investigators should test the reliability of their outcome measure before proceeding with the therapeutic part of a study. More attention should be directed toward measuring outcomes that dictate a policy of treatment—i.e., the long-term risk of skin cancer (Table 31.1).

Table 31.1 Summary of therapies for actinic keratosis (AK) and Bowen's disease (BD). Therapies were designated as "beneficial" if they had a quality-of-evidence level of I (see Box 31.1) and an efficacy of at least 75%. Therapies were "likely to be beneficial" if they had quality-of-evidence levels II-i or II-ii and an efficacy of at least 60%. Therapies were of "unknown effectiveness" if their quality-of-evidence level was II-iii, III, or IV. Therapies were "unlikely to be beneficial" if they had a quality-of-evidence level of I and had an efficacy rate of less than 30%. It should be noted that simply categorizing a treatment as "beneficial" does not quantify the magnitude of that benefit.

Beneficial	Likely to be beneficial	Unknown effectiveness	Unlikely to be beneficial
Actinic keratosis			
Topical 5-fluorouracil	Cryotherapy	Laser	Diclofenac
Imiquimod	Chemical peels	Radiotherapy	Topical retinoids
Photodynamic therapy	Oral retinoids	Dermabrasion	Topical interferon
	Masoprocol	Tubercidin	
	Intralesional interferon	Curaderm	
Bowen's disease			
Imiquimod	Cryotherapy	Laser	Diclofenac
Photodynamic therapy	ED&C	Radiotherapy	
	Intralesional interferon	Oral retinoids	
	Topical 5-fluorouracil	Intralesional bleomycin	

ED&C, electrodesiccation and curettage.

Key points

Actinic keratoses

- We found good evidence to suggest that photodynamic therapy, topical 5-fluorouracil (5-FU), and imiquimod may be beneficial in the treatment of AK.
- The evidence supporting the efficacy of most therapies is insufficient or limited.
- It is still unclear whether any of the treatments reduce the incidence of invasive squamous cell carcinoma—the outcome of most importance.
- Studies were not consistent in choosing their units of analysis. Some used the number of lesions, others used persons cleared, and others used both as their units of analysis. Readers should determine which unit is most relevant to their practice.
- Given the high rate of spontaneous resolution of AKs over time, debate still exists on whether all patients need treatment.

Bowen's disease

- Imiquimod and photodynamic therapy (PDT) may be beneficial in the treatment of BD.
- The evidence for treatment of BD is generally of poor quality.
- The choice of therapy in BD should take into account the location of the lesions, particularly the lower legs and the digits, where healing may be complicated.
- Electrodesiccation and curettage (ED&C), 5-FU, imiquimod, PDT, and cryotherapy are acceptable first-line treatments for BD, given the available evidence.
- ED&C may be superior to cryotherapy for lower-leg lesions.
- There appears to be good evidence for the superior efficacy of red light over green light in PDT with aminolevulinic acid.

Other useful resources

For further information on the treatment of AK or BD, the British Association of Dermatologists publications on the management of Bowen's disease[161] and actinic keratosis[162] may also be helpful.

References

1 Bowen J. Precancerous dermatoses: a study of two cases of chronic atypical epithelial proliferation. *J Cutan Dis* 1912;**30**:241–55.
2 Marks R, Staples M, Giles GG. Trends in non-melanocytic skin cancer treated in Australia: the second national survey. *Int J Cancer* 1993;**53**:585–90.
3 Schwartz RA. The actinic keratosis: a perspective and update. *Dermatol Surg* 1997;**23**:1009–19.
4 Lee MM, Wick MM. Bowen's disease. *CA Cancer J Clin* 1990; **40**:237–42.
5 Frost CA, Green AC. Epidemiology of solar keratoses. *Br J Dermatol* 1994;**131**:455–64.
6 Vitasa BC, Taylor HR, Strickland PT, *et al.* Association of non-melanoma skin cancer and actinic keratosis with cumulative solar ultraviolet exposure in Maryland watermen. *Cancer* 1990; **65**:2811–7.
7 Salasche SJ. Epidemiology of actinic keratoses and squamous cell carcinoma. *J Am Acad Dermatol* 2000;**42**:4–7.
8 Marks R, Jolley D, Dorevitch AP, Selwood TS. The incidence of non-melanocytic skin cancers in an Australian population: results of a five-year prospective study. *Med J Aust* 1989;**150**: 475–8.
9 Cox NH. Body site distribution of Bowen's disease. *Br J Dermatol* 1994;**130**:714–6.
10 Eedy DJ, Gavin AT. Thirteen-year retrospective study of Bowen's disease in Northern Ireland. *Br J Dermatol* 1987;**117**:715–20.
11 Kossard S, Rosen R. Cutaneous Bowen's disease: an analysis of 1001 cases according to age, sex, and site. *J Am Acad Dermatol* 1992;**27**:406–10.
12 Thestrup-Pedersen K, Ravnborg L, Reymann F. Morbus Bowen: a description of the disease in 617 patients. *Acta Derm Venereol* 1988;**68**:236–9.
13 Holman CD, Armstrong BK, Evans PR, *et al.* Relationship of solar keratosis and history of skin cancer to objective measures of actinic skin damage. *Br J Dermatol* 1984;**110**:129–38.
14 Green A, Beardmore G, Hart V, Leslie D, Marks R, Staines D. Skin cancer in a Queensland population. *J Am Acad Dermatol* 1988;**19**:1045–52.
15 Schwartz RA. Therapeutic perspectives in actinic and other keratoses. *Int J Dermatol* 1996;**35**:533–8.
16 Preston DS, Stern RS. Nonmelanoma cancers of the skin. *N Engl J Med* 1992;**327**:1649–62.
17 Sanchez Yus E, de Diego V, Urrutia S. Large cell acanthoma. A cytologic variant of Bowen's disease? *Am J Dermatopathol* 1988; **10**:197–208.
18 Reizner GT, Chuang TY, Elpern DJ, Stone JL, Farmer ER. Bowen's disease (squamous cell carcinoma in situ) in Kauai, Hawaii. A population-based incidence report. *J Am Acad Dermatol* 1994;**31**:596–600.
19 Fiertz U. Catamnestic investigations of the side effects of therapy of skin diseases with inorganic arsenic. *Dermatologica* 1965;**131**: 41–58.
20 Yeh S, How SW, Lin CS. Arsenical cancer of skin. Histologic study with special reference to Bowen's disease. *Cancer* 1968; **21**:312–39.
21 Yeh S. Skin cancer in chronic arsenism. *Hum Pathol* 1967;**4**:469–85.
22 Shannon RL, Strayer DS. Arsenic-induced skin toxicity. *Hum Toxicol* 1989;**8**:99–104.
23 Cox NH, Eedy DJ, Morton CA. Guidelines for management of Bowen's disease. British Association of Dermatologists. *Br J Dermatol* 1999;**141**:633–41.
24 Kettler AH, Rutledge M, Tschen JA, Buffone G. Detection of human papillomavirus in nongenital Bowen's disease by in situ DNA hybridization. *Arch Dermatol* 1990;**126**:777–81.
25 Collina G, Rossi E, Bettelli S, Cook MG, Cesinaro AM, Trentini GP. Detection of human papillomavirus in extragenital Bowen's disease using in situ hybridization and polymerase chain reaction. *Am J Dermatopathol* 1995;**17**:236–41.

26 Czarnecki D, Staples M, Mar A, Giles G, Meehan C. Metastases from squamous cell carcinoma of the skin in southern Australia. *Dermatology* 1994;**189**:52–4.

27 Boddie AW Jr, Fischer EP, Byers RM. Squamous carcinoma of the lower lip in patients under 40 years of age. *South Med J* 1977;**70**:711–2, 715.

28 Glogau RG. The risk of progression to invasive disease. *J Am Acad Dermatol* 2000;**42**:23–4.

29 Dodson JM, DeSpain J, Hewett JE, Clark DP. Malignant potential of actinic keratoses and the controversy over treatment. A patient-oriented perspective. *Arch Dermatol* 1991;**127**:1029–31.

30 Frost C, Williams G, Green A. High incidence and regression rates of solar keratoses in a Queensland community. *J Invest Dermatol* 2000;**115**:273–7.

31 Kao GF. Carcinoma arising in Bowen's disease. *Arch Dermatol* 1986;**122**:1124–6.

32 Saida T, Okabe Y, Uhara H. Bowen's disease with invasive carcinoma showing sweat gland differentiation. *J Cutan Pathol* 1989;**16**:222–6.

33 Beerman H. Tumors of the skin. *Am J Med Sci* 1946;**211**:480–504.

34 Graham JH, Helwig EB. Bowen's disease and its relationship to systemic cancer. *AMA Arch Derm* 1959;**80**:133–59.

35 Epstein E. Association of Bowen's disease with visceral cancer. *Arch Dermatol* 1960;**82**:349–51.

36 Callen JP, Headington J. Bowen's and non-Bowen's squamous intraepidermal neoplasia of the skin. Relationship to internal malignancy. *Arch Dermatol* 1980;**116**:422–6.

37 Lycka BA. Bowen's disease and internal malignancy. A meta-analysis. *Int J Dermatol* 1989;**28**:531–3.

38 Stevens A, Raftery J. Health care needs assessment. In: Williams HC, ed. *Dermatology*. Oxford: Radcliffe Medical Press, 1997: 261–341.

39 Pierre P, Weil E, Chen S. Cryotherapy versus topical 5-flurouracil therapy of actinic keratoses: a systematic review. *Allergologie* 2001;**24**:204–5.

40 Morton C, Campbell S, Gupta G, *et al.* Intraindividual, right-left comparison of topical methyl aminolaevulinate-photodynamic therapy and cryotherapy in subjects with actinic keratoses: a multicentre, randomized controlled study. *Br J Dermatol* 2006; **155**:1029–36.

41 Freeman M, Vinciullo C, Francis D, *et al.* A comparison of photodynamic therapy using topical methyl aminolevulinate (Metvix) with single cycle cryotherapy in patients with actinic keratosis: a prospective, randomized study. *J Dermatolog Treat* 2003;**14**:99–106.

42 Szeimies RM, Karrer S, Radakovic-Fijan S, *et al.* Photodynamic therapy using topical methyl 5-aminolevulinate compared with cryotherapy for actinic keratosis: a prospective, randomized study. *J Am Acad Dermatol* 2002;**47**:258–62.

43 Jorizzo J, Weiss J, Vamvakias G. One-week treatment with 0.5% fluorouracil cream prior to cryosurgery in patients with actinic keratoses: a double-blind, vehicle-controlled, long-term study. *J Drugs Dermatol* 2006;**5**:133–9.

44 Thai KE, Fergin P, Freeman M, *et al.* A prospective study of the use of cryosurgery for the treatment of actinic keratoses. *Int J Dermatol* 2004;**43**:687–92.

45 Lubritz RR, Smolewski SA. Cryosurgery cure rate of actinic keratoses. *J Am Acad Dermatol* 1982;**7**:631–2.

46 Gold MH, Nestor MS. Current treatments of actinic keratosis. *J Drugs Dermatol* 2006;**5**:17–25.

47 Jeffes EW III, Tang EH. Actinic keratosis. Current treatment options. *Am J Clin Dermatol* 2000;**1**:167–79.

48 Morton CA, Whitehurst C, Moseley H, McColl JH, Moore JV, MacKie RM. Comparison of photodynamic therapy with cryotherapy in the treatment of Bowen's disease. *Br J Dermatol* 1996; **135**:766–71.

49 Morton C, Horn M, Leman J, *et al.* Comparison of topical methyl aminolevulinate photodynamic therapy with cryotherapy or fluorouracil for treatment of squamous cell carcinoma in situ: results of a multicenter randomized trial. *Arch Dermatol* 2006; **142**:729–35.

50 Ahmed I, Berth-Jones J, Charles-Holmes S, O'Callaghan CJ, Ilchyshyn A. Comparison of cryotherapy with curettage in the treatment of Bowen's disease: a prospective study. *Br J Dermatol* 2000;**143**:759–66.

51 Cox NH, Dyson P. Wound healing on the lower leg after radiotherapy or cryotherapy of Bowen's disease and other malignant skin lesions. *Br J Dermatol* 1995;**133**:60–5.

52 Dinehart SM. The treatment of actinic keratoses. *J Am Acad Dermatol* 2000;**42**:25–8.

53 Ostertag JU, Quaedvlieg PJ, van der GS, *et al.* A clinical comparison and long-term follow-up of topical 5-fluorouracil versus laser resurfacing in the treatment of widespread actinic keratoses. *Lasers Surg Med* 2006;**38**:731–9.

54 Wollina U, Konrad H, Karamfilov T. Treatment of common warts and actinic keratoses by Er:YAG laser. *J Cutan Laser Ther* 2001;**3**:63–6.

55 Jiang SB, Levine VJ, Nehal KS, Baldassano M, Kamino H, Ashinoff RA. Er:YAG laser for the treatment of actinic keratoses. *Dermatol Surg* 2000;**26**:437–40.

56 Dmovsek-Olup B, Vedlin B. Use of Er:YAG laser for benign skin disorders. *Lasers Surg Med* 1997;**21**:13–9.

57 Iyer S, Friedli A, Bowes L, Kricorian G, Fitzpatrick RE. Full face laser resurfacing: therapy and prophylaxis for actinic keratoses and non-melanoma skin cancer. *Lasers Surg Med* 2004;**34**:114–9.

58 Ostertag JU, Quaedvlieg PJ, Neumann MH, Krekels GA. Recurrence rates and long-term follow-up after laser resurfacing as a treatment for widespread actinic keratoses on the face and scalp. *Dermatol Surg* 2006;**32**:261–7.

59 Tantikun N. Treatment of Bowen's disease of the digit with carbon dioxide laser. *J Am Acad Dermatol* 2000;**43**:1080–3.

60 Gordon KB, Garden JM, Robinson JK. Bowen's disease of the distal digit. Outcome of treatment with carbon dioxide laser vaporization. *Dermatol Surg* 1996;**22**:723–8.

61 Dave R, Monk B, Mahaffey P. The role of the ultrapulse laser in treatment of Bowen's disease of the legs. *Lasers Surg Med* 2001;**28**:53.

62 Dave R, Monk B, Mahaffey P. Treatment of Bowen's disease with carbon dioxide laser. *Lasers Surg Med* 2003;**32**:335.

63 Barta U, Grafe T, Wollina U. Radiation therapy for extensive actinic keratosis. *J Eur Acad Dermatol Venereol* 2000;**14**:293–5.

64 Stevens DM, Kopf AW, Gladstein A, Bart RS. Treatment of Bowen's disease with grenz rays. *Int J Dermatol* 1977;**16**:329–39.

65 Dupree MT, Kiteley RA, Weismantle K, Panos R, Johnstone PA. Radiation therapy for Bowen's disease: lessons for lesions of the lower extremity. *J Am Acad Dermatol* 2001;**45**:401–4.

66 Caccialanza M, Piccinno R, Beretta M, Sopelana N. Radiotherapy of Bowen's disease. *Skin Cancer* 1993;**8**:115–8.

67 Umebayashi Y, Uyeno K, Tsujii H, Otsuka F. Proton radiotherapy of skin carcinomas. *Br J Dermatol* 1994;**130**:88–91.

68 Chung YL, Lee JD, Bang D, Lee JB, Park KB, Lee MG. Treatment of Bowen's disease with a specially designed radioactive skin patch. *Eur J Nucl Med* 2000;**27**:842–6.

69 Marrero GM, Katz BE. The new fluor-hydroxy pulse peel. A combination of 5-fluorouracil and glycolic acid. *Dermatol Surg* 1998;**24**:973–8.

70 Humphreys TR, Werth V, Dzubow L, Kligman A. Treatment of photodamaged skin with trichloroacetic acid and topical tretinoin. *J Am Acad Dermatol* 1996;**34**:638–44.

71 Lawrence N, Cox SE, Cockerell CJ, Freeman RG, Cruz PD Jr. A comparison of the efficacy and safety of Jessner's solution and 35% trichloroacetic acid vs 5% fluorouracil in the treatment of widespread facial actinic keratoses. *Arch Dermatol* 1995;**131**:176–81.

72 Witheiler DD, Lawrence N, Cox SE, Cruz C, Cockerell CJ, Freemen RG. Long-term efficacy and safety of Jessner's solution and 35% trichloroacetic acid vs 5% fluorouracil in the treatment of widespread facial actinic keratoses. *Dermatol Surg* 1997;**23**:191–6.

73 Spira M, Freeman RF, Arfai P, Gerow FJ, Hardy SB. A comparison of chemical peeling, dermabrasion, and 5-fluourouracil in cancer prophylaxis. *J Surg Oncol* 1971;**3**:367–8.

74 Winton GB, Salasche SJ. Dermabrasion of the scalp as a treatment for actinic damage. *J Am Acad Dermatol* 1986;**14**:661–8.

75 Sturm HM. Bowen's disease and 5-fluorouracil. *J Am Acad Dermatol* 1979;**1**:513–22.

76 Hiruma M, Kawada A. Hyperthermic treatment of Bowen's disease with disposable chemical pocket warmers: a report of 8 cases. *J Am Acad Dermatol* 2000;**43**:1070–5.

77 Misiewicz J, Sendagorta E, Golebiowska A, Lorenc B, Czarnetzki BM, Jablonska S. Topical treatment of multiple actinic keratoses of the face with arotinoid methyl sulfone (Ro 14-9706) cream versus tretinoin cream: a double-blind, comparative study. *J Am Acad Dermatol* 1991;**24**:448–51.

78 Alirezai M, Dupuy P, Amblard P, *et al.* Clinical evaluation of topical isotretinoin in the treatment of actinic keratoses. *J Am Acad Dermatol* 1994;**30**:447–51.

79 Smit JV, Cox S, Blokx WA, van de Kerhof PC, de Jongh GJ, de Jong EM. Actinic keratoses in renal transplant recipients do not improve with calcipotriol cream and all-trans retinoic acid cream as monotherapies or in combination during a 6-week treatment period. *Br J Dermatol* 2002;**147**:816–8.

80 Kang S, Goldfarb MT, Weiss JS, *et al.* Assessment of adapalene gel for the treatment of actinic keratoses and lentigines: a randomized trial. *J Am Acad Dermatol* 2003;**49**:83–90.

81 Gupta AK, Davey V, Mcphail H. Evaluation of the effectiveness of imiquimod and 5-fluorouracil for the treatment of actinic keratosis: critical review and meta-analysis of efficacy studies. *J Cutan Med Surg* 2005;**9**:209–14.

82 Kulp-Shorten C, Konnikov N, Callen JP. Comparative evaluation of the efficacy and safety of masoprocol and 5-fluorouracil cream for the treatment of multiple actinic keratoses of the head and neck. *J Geriatr Dermatol* 1993;**1**:161–8.

83 Loven K, Stein L, Furst K, Levy S. Evaluation of the efficacy and tolerability of 0.5% fluorouracil cream and 5% fluorouracil cream applied to each side of the face in patients with actinic keratosis. *Clin Ther* 2002;**24**:990–1000.

84 Jury CS, Ramraka-Jones VS, Gudi V, Herd RM. A randomized trial of topical 5% 5-fluorouracil (Efudix cream) in the treatment of actinic keratoses comparing daily with weekly treatment. *Br J Dermatol* 2005;**153**:808–10.

85 Smith S, Piacquadio D, Morhenn V, Atkin D, Fitzpatrick R. Short incubation PDT versus 5-FU in treating actinic keratoses. *J Drugs Dermatol* 2003;**2**:629–35.

86 Breza T, Taylor R, Eaglstein WH. Noninflammatory destruction of actinic keratoses by fluorouracil. *Arch Dermatol* 1976;**112**:1256–8.

87 Carter VH, Smith KW, Noojin RO. Xeroderma pigmentosum. Treatment with topically applied fluorouracil. *Arch Dermatol* 1968;**98**:526–7.

88 Simmonds W. Topical management of actinic keratoses with 5-fluorouracil: results of a 6-year follow-up study. *Cutis* 1972;**10**:737–41.

89 Neldner KH. Prevention of skin cancer with topical 5-fluorouracil. *Rocky Mt Med J* 1966;**63**:74–8.

90 Epstein E. Treatment of lip keratoses (actinic cheilitis) with topical fluorouracil. *Arch Dermatol* 1977;**113**:906–8.

91 Klein E, Stoll HL Jr, Milgrom H, Helm F, Walker MJ. Tumors of the skin. XII. Topical 5-Fluorouracil for epidermal neoplasms. *J Surg Oncol* 1971;**3**:331–49.

92 Schultz E, Falkson G. Benign and malignant skin diseases response to topical 5-fluorouracil. *Med Proc* 1970;**Feb**:41–6.

93 Dogliotti M. Actinic keratoses in Bantu albinos. Clinical experiences with the topical use of 5-fluoro-uracil. *S Afr Med J* 1973;**47**:2169–72.

94 Dillaha CJ, Jansen GT, Honeycutt WM, Holt GA. Further studies with topical 5-fluorouracil. *Arch Dermatol* 1965;**92**:410–7.

95 Ott F, Storck H, Eichenberger-De Beer H. The local treatment of precancerous skin conditions with 5-fluorouracil ointment. *Dermatologica* 1970;**140**(Suppl 1):109.

96 Robinson TA, Kligman AM. Treatment of solar keratoses of the extremities with retinoic acid and 5-fluorouracil. *Br J Dermatol* 1975;**92**:703–6.

97 Bercovitch L. Topical chemotherapy of actinic keratoses of the upper extremity with tretinoin and 5-fluorouracil: a double-blind controlled study. *Br J Dermatol* 1987;**116**:549–52.

98 Goncalves JC. Treatment of solar keratoses with a 5-fluorouracil and salicylic acid varnish. *Br J Dermatol* 1975;**92**:85–8.

99 Jorizzo J, Stewart D, Bucko A, *et al.* Randomized trial evaluating a new 0.5% fluorouracil formulation demonstrates efficacy after 1-, 2-, or 4-week treatment in patients with actinic keratosis. *Cutis* 2002;**70**:335–9.

100 Weiss J, Menter A, Hevia O, *et al.* Effective treatment of actinic keratosis with 0.5% fluorouracil cream for 1, 2, or 4 weeks. *Cutis* 2002;**70**:22–9.

101 Shuttleworth D, Marks R. A comparison of the effects of intralesional interferon alpha-2b and topical 5% 5-fluorouracil cream in the treatment of solar keratoses and Bowen's disease. *J Dermatolog Treat* 1989;**1**:65–8.

102 Dillaha CJ, Jansen GT, Honeycutt WM, Bradford AC. Selective cytotoxic effect of topical 5-fluorouracil. *Arch Dermatol* 1963;**88**:247–56.

103 Salim A, Leman JA, McColl JH, Chapman R, Morton CA. Randomized comparison of photodynamic therapy with topical

5-fluorouracil in Bowen's disease. *Br J Dermatol* 2003;**148**:539–43.

104 Welch ML, Grabski WJ, McCollough ML, *et al*. 5-fluorouracil iontophoretic therapy for Bowen's disease. *J Am Acad Dermatol* 1997;**36**:956–8.

105 Bell HK, Rhodes LE. Bowen's disease: a retrospective review of clinical management. *Clin Exp Dermatol* 1999;**24**:338–9.

106 Stone N, Burge S. Bowen's disease of the leg treated with weekly pulses of 5% fluorouracil cream. *Br J Dermatol* 1999;**140**: 987–8.

107 Bargman H, Hochman J. Topical treatment of Bowen's disease with 5-fluorouracil. *J Cutan Med Surg* 2003;**7**:101–5.

108 Dillaha CJ, Jansen GT, Honeycutt WM. Topical therapy with fluorouracil. *Prog Dermatol* 1966;**1**:1–2.

109 Jansen GT, Dillaha CJ, Honeycutt WM. Bowenoid conditions of the skin: treatment with topical 5-fluorouracil. *South Med J* 1967;**60**:185–8.

110 Unis ME. Short-term intensive 5-fluorouracil treatment of actinic keratoses. *Dermatol Surg* 1995;**21**:162–3.

111 Pearlman DL. Weekly pulse dosing: effective and comfortable topical 5-fluorouracil treatment of multiple facial actinic keratoses. *J Am Acad Dermatol* 1991;**25**:665–7.

112 Epstein E. Does intermittent "pulse" topical 5-fluorouracil therapy allow destruction of actinic keratoses without significant inflammation? *J Am Acad Dermatol* 1998;**38**:77–80.

113 Hadley G, Derry S, Moore RA. Imiquimod for actinic keratosis: systematic review and meta-analysis. *J Invest Dermatol* 2006;**126**: 1251–5.

114 Falagas ME, Angelousi AG, Peppas G. Imiquimod for the treatment of actinic keratosis: a meta-analysis of randomized controlled trials. *J Am Acad Dermatol* 2006;**55**:537–8.

115 Ooi T, Barnetson RS, Zhuang L, *et al*. Imiquimod-induced regression of actinic keratosis is associated with infiltration by T lymphocytes and dendritic cells: a randomized controlled trial. *Br J Dermatol* 2006;**154**:72–8.

116 Korman N, Moy R, Ling M, *et al*. Dosing with 5% imiquimod cream 3 times per week for the treatment of actinic keratosis: results of two phase 3, randomized, double-blind, parallel-group, vehicle-controlled trials. *Arch Dermatol* 2005;**141**:467–73.

117 Lebwohl M, Dinehart S, Whiting D, *et al*. Imiquimod 5% cream for the treatment of actinic keratosis: results from two phase III, randomized, double-blind, parallel group, vehicle-controlled trials. *J Am Acad Dermatol* 2004;**50**:714–21.

118 Chen K, Yap LM, Marks R, Shumack S. Short-course therapy with imiquimod 5% cream for solar keratoses: a randomized controlled trial. *Australas J Dermatol* 2003;**44**:250–5.

119 Szeimies RM, Gerritsen MJ, Gupta G, *et al*. Imiquimod 5% cream for the treatment of actinic keratosis: results from a phase III, randomized, double-blind, vehicle-controlled, clinical trial with histology. *J Am Acad Dermatol* 2004;**51**:547–55.

120 Stockfleth E, Christophers E, Benninghoff B, Sterry W. Low incidence of new actinic keratoses after topical 5% imiquimod cream treatment: a long-term follow-up study. *Arch Dermatol* 2004;**140**:1542.

121 Stockfleth E, Meyer T, Benninghoff B, *et al*. A randomized, double-blind, vehicle-controlled study to assess 5% imiquimod cream for the treatment of multiple actinic keratoses. *Arch Dermatol* 2002;**138**:1498–502.

122 Stockfleth E, Meyer T, Benninghoff B, Christophers E. Successful treatment of actinic keratosis with imiquimod cream 5%: a report of six cases. *Br J Dermatol* 2001;**144**:1050–3.

123 Patel GK, Goodwin R, Chawla M, *et al*. Imiquimod 5% cream monotherapy for cutaneous squamous cell carcinoma in situ (Bowen's disease): a randomized, double-blind, placebo-controlled trial. *J Am Acad Dermatol* 2006;**54**:1025–32.

124 Mackenzie-Wood A, Kossard S, de Launey J, Wilkinson B, Owens ML. Imiquimod 5% cream in the treatment of Bowen's disease. *J Am Acad Dermatol* 2001;**44**:462–70.

125 Smith KJ, Germain M, Skelton H. Bowen's disease (squamous cell carcinoma in situ) in immunosuppressed patients treated with imiquimod 5% cream and a cox inhibitor, sulindac: potential applications for this combination of immunotherapy. *Dermatol Surg* 2001;**27**:143–6.

126 Peris K, Micantonio T, Fargnoli MC, Lozzi GP, Chimenti S. Imiquimod 5% cream in the treatment of Bowen's disease and invasive squamous cell carcinoma. *J Am Acad Dermatol* 2006; **55**:324–7.

127 Pirard D, Vereecken P, Melot C, Heenen M. Three percent diclofenac in 2.5% hyaluronan gel in the treatment of actinic keratoses: a meta-analysis of the recent studies. *Arch Dermatol Res* 2005;**297**:185–9.

128 Wolf JE Jr, Taylor JR, Tschen E, Kang S. Topical 3.0% diclofenac in 2.5% hyaluronan gel in the treatment of actinic keratoses. *Int J Dermatol* 2001;**40**:709–13.

129 Rivers JK, Arlette J, Shear N, Guenther L, Carey W, Poulin Y. Topical treatment of actinic keratoses with 3.0% diclofenac in 2.5% hyaluronan gel. *Br J Dermatol* 2002;**146**:94–100.

130 Gebauer K, Brown P, Varigos G. Topical diclofenac in hyaluronan gel for the treatment of solar keratoses. *Australas J Dermatol* 2003;**44**:40–3.

131 McEwan LE, Smith JG. Topical diclofenac/hyaluronic acid gel in the treatment of solar keratoses. *Australas J Dermatol* 1997;**38**: 187–9.

132 Solaraze. Diclofenac Sodium 3%—package insert. Fairfield, NJ: Doak Dermatologics, 2004.

133 Dawe SA, Salisbury JR, Higgins E. Two cases of Bowen's disease successfully treated topically with 3% diclofenac in 2.5% hyaluronan gel. *Clin Exp Dermatol* 2005;**30**:712–3.

134 Piacquadio DJ, Chen DM, Farber HF, *et al*. Photodynamic therapy with aminolevulinic acid topical solution and visible blue light in the treatment of multiple actinic keratoses of the face and scalp: investigator-blinded, phase 3, multicenter trials. *Arch Dermatol* 2004;**140**:41–6.

135 Jeffes EW, McCullough JL, Weinstein GD, Kaplan R, Glazer SD, Taylor JR. Photodynamic therapy of actinic keratoses with topical aminolevulinic acid hydrochloride and fluorescent blue light. *J Am Acad Dermatol* 2001;**45**:96–104.

136 DUSA. Levulan Kerastick (aminolevulinic acid HCI) for topical solution, 20%—product monograph revision C. Wilmington, MA: DUSA Pharmaceuticals, Inc., 2004.

137 Kurwa HA, Yong-Gee SA, Seed PT, Markey AC, Barlow RJ. A randomized paired comparison of photodynamic therapy and topical 5-fluorouracil in the treatment of actinic keratoses. *J Am Acad Dermatol* 1999;**41**:414–8.

138 Blecha-Thalhammer U, Honigsmann H, Tanew A. Comparison of incoherent versus pulsed monochromatic light for

photodynamic therapy of actinic keratosis. *J Eur Acad Dermatol Venereol* 2003;**17**:143.

139 Radakovic-Fijan S, Blecha-Thalhammer U, Kittler H, Honigsmann H, Tanew A. Efficacy of 3 different light doses in the treatment of actinic keratosis with 5-aminolevulinic acid photodynamic therapy: a randomized, observer-blinded, intrapatient, comparison study. *J Am Acad Dermatol* 2005;**53**:823–7.

140 Ericson MB, Sandberg C, Stenquist B, *et al.* Photodynamic therapy of actinic keratosis at varying fluence rates: assessment of photobleaching, pain and primary clinical outcome. *Br J Dermatol* 2004;**151**:1204–12.

141 Pariser DM, Lowe NJ, Stewart DM, *et al.* Photodynamic therapy with topical methyl aminolevulinate for actinic keratosis: results of a prospective randomized multicenter trial. *J Am Acad Dermatol* 2003;**48**:227–32.

142 Dragieva G, Prinz BM, Hafner J, *et al.* A randomized controlled clinical trial of topical photodynamic therapy with methyl aminolaevulinate in the treatment of actinic keratoses in transplant recipients. *Br J Dermatol* 2004;**151**:196–200.

143 Tarstedt M, Rosdahl I, Berne B, Svanberg K, Wennberg AM. A randomized multicenter study to compare two treatment regimens of topical methyl aminolevulinate (Metvix)-PDT in actinic keratosis of the face and scalp. *Acta Derm Venereol* 2005;**85**:424–8.

144 Morton CA, Whitehurst C, Moore JV, MacKie RM. Comparison of red and green light in the treatment of Bowen's disease by photodynamic therapy. *Br J Dermatol* 2000;**143**:767–72.

145 Jones CM, Mang T, Cooper M, Wilson BD, Stoll HL Jr. Photodynamic therapy in the treatment of Bowen's disease. *J Am Acad Dermatol* 1992;**27**:979–82.

146 Svanberg K, Andersson T, Killander D, *et al.* Photodynamic therapy of non-melanoma malignant tumours of the skin using topical delta-amino levulinic acid sensitization and laser irradiation. *Br J Dermatol* 1994;**130**:743–51.

147 Wong TW, Sheu HM, Lee JY, Fletcher RJ. Photodynamic therapy for Bowen's disease (squamous cell carcinoma in situ) of the digit. *Dermatol Surg* 2001;**27**:452–6.

148 Stables GI, Stringer MR, Robinson DJ, Ash DV. Large patches of Bowen's disease treated by topical aminolaevulinic acid photodynamic therapy. *Br J Dermatol* 1997;**136**:957–60.

149 Fijan S, Honigsmann H, Ortel B. Photodynamic therapy of epithelial skin tumours using delta-aminolaevulinic acid and desferrioxamine. *Br J Dermatol* 1995;**133**:282–8.

150 Olsen EA, Abernethy ML, Kulp-Shorten C, *et al.* A double-blind, vehicle-controlled study evaluating masoprocol cream in the treatment of actinic keratoses on the head and neck. *J Am Acad Dermatol* 1991;**24**:738–43.

151 Epstein E. Warning! Masoprocol is a potent sensitizer. *J Am Acad Dermatol* 1994;**31**:295–7.

152 Burgess GH, Bloch A, Stoll H, Milgrom H, Helm F, Klein E. Effect of topical tubercidin on basal cell carcinomas and actinic keratoses. *Cancer* 1974;**34**:250–3.

153 Cham BE, Daunter B, Evans RA. Topical treatment of malignant and premalignant skin lesions by very low concentrations of a standard mixture (BEC) of solasodine glycosides. *Cancer Lett* 1991;**59**:183–92.

154 Moriarty M, Dunn J, Darragh A, Lambe R, Brick I. Etretinate in treatment of actinic keratosis. A double-blind crossover study. *Lancet* 1982;**i**:364–5.

155 Watson AB. Preventative effect of etretinate therapy on multiple actinic keratoses. *Cancer Detect Prev* 1986;**9**:161–5.

156 Thianprasit M. Chronic cutaneous arsenism treated with aromatic retinoid. *J Med Assoc Thai* 1984;**67**:93–100.

157 Edwards L, Levine N, Weidner M, Piepkorn M, Smiles K. Effect of intralesional alpha 2-interferon on actinic keratoses. *Arch Dermatol* 1986;**122**:779–82.

158 Edwards L, Levine N, Smiles KA. The effect of topical interferon alpha 2b on actinic keratoses. *J Dermatol Surg Oncol* 1990;**16**:446–9.

159 Dyall-Smith D. Intralesional bleomycin. *Australas J Dermatol* 1998;**39**:123–4.

160 Weinstock MA, Bingham SF, Cole GW, *et al.* Reliability of counting actinic keratoses before and after brief consensus discussion: the VA topical tretinoin chemoprevention (VATTC) trial. *Arch Dermatol* 2001;**137**:1055–8.

161 Cox NH, Eedy DJ, Morton CA. Guidelines for management of Bowen's disease: 2006 update. *Br J Dermatol* 2007;**156**:11–21.

162 de Berker D, McGregor JM, Hughes BR. Guidelines for the management of actinic keratoses. *Br J Dermatol* 2007;**156**:222–30.

32 Kaposi's sarcoma

Rosamaria Corona, Margaret F. Spittle, Russell N. Moule, Michael Bigby

Background

Kaposi's sarcoma (KS), described by Moritz Kaposi in 1872, is a mesenchymal tumor involving blood and lymphatic vessels. It is characterized histologically by a proliferation of spindle-shaped tumor cells surrounding abnormal slit-like vascular channels with extravasated erythrocytes. It may present with cutaneous or mucosal lesions (mouth, gastrointestinal, bronchial), visceral lesions, or lymphadenopathy (Figures 32.1 and 32.2). There are four clinical variants of KS, which appear in specific populations but have identical histological features.

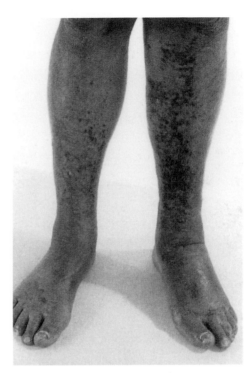

Figure 32.2 Endemic (African) Kaposi's sarcoma.

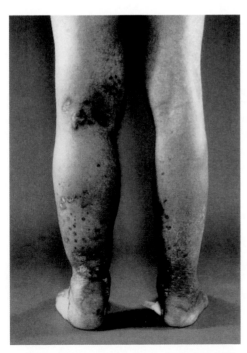

Figure 32.1 Classic Kaposi's sarcoma, with edema of the left leg.

Classical KS
Classical KS (Figure 32.1) typically affects elderly men of Mediterranean or Jewish descent, with a peak incidence after the sixth decade of life. It presents with purple-blue plaques on the lower legs, which progress over a period of years.

AIDS-KS
In 1981, Friedman-Kien *et al.* reported a cluster of young homosexual men with aggressive KS involving skin, lymph nodes, and viscera, in association with a syndrome of opportunistic infections and a defect in cell-mediated immunity,

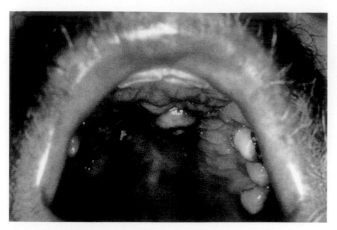

Figure 32.3 Kaposi's sarcoma affecting the hard palate in a patient with AIDS.

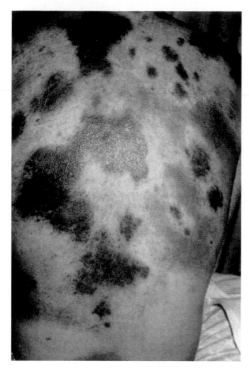

Figure 32.4 Extensive AIDS-related Kaposi's sarcoma.

subsequently named the acquired immune deficiency syndrome (AIDS).[1] This aggressive form of KS (Figures 32.3 and 32.4) was estimated to be 20 000 times more frequent in AIDS patients than in the general population, and 300 times more frequent than in other immunosuppressed patients.[2] It usually presents with multifocal and symmetrical, fast-evolving lesions. KS is an AIDS-defining illness. Before the era of highly active antiretroviral therapy (HAART), oral KS lesions were the first clinical manifestation in about 25% of AIDS patients, whereas today it is infrequently seen

in patients infected with human immunodeficiency virus (HIV).

Endemic (or African) KS

Endemic (or African) KS (Figure 32.2) is common in sub-Saharan Africa. It presents in one of four clinically distinct patterns:
1 Benign nodular cutaneous disease, mimicking classic KS, predominantly in young adults
2 Aggressive localized cutaneous disease, invading soft tissue and bones, with a fatal course of 5–7 years
3 Florid mucocutaneous and visceral disease
4 Fulminant lymphadenopathic disease, without cutaneous involvement, occurring in young children (mean age 3 years)

Iatrogenic/immunosuppression-related KS

Transplant recipients and patients receiving immunosuppressive therapy are another group in which KS occurs. The same ethnic groups in which classical KS is seen are at higher risk. The disease can be chronic or rapidly progressive, but spontaneous regression after discontinuation of the immunosuppressive treatment is the rule.[3]

Incidence/prevalence

Classical KS is rare. It is much more common in men than in women, with a ratio of up to 15 : 1. The peak age of onset is 50–70 years. With the AIDS epidemic, KS has become the most frequently occurring tumor in central Africa, in both men and women, accounting for up to 50% in some countries.[4] Since the introduction of HAART, the proportion of patients with AIDS-related KS is decreasing, but KS remains the most common AIDS-associated malignancy, affecting 20–40% of homosexual men who are HIV-positive.[4] The EuroSIDA study, a pan-European multicenter cohort study of 9803 HIV patients, reported an estimated annual reduction in KS incidence of 39% for patients receiving HAART between 1994 and 2003. The overall incidence of KS among patients with HIV is currently less than 10% of the incidence reported in 1994, while the proportion of AIDS diagnoses made on the basis of KS remains around 6%.[5] Endemic KS is a common tumor in equatorial Africa, and in 1971, in the pre-AIDS era, comprised up to 9% of all cancers seen in Uganda.[6] Its incidence in Africa has since greatly increased, with a narrowing of the gender ratio from 19 : 1 in 1960–1971 to 1.7 : 1 in 1991–1997. The current incidence estimates, as reported in CancerMondial (Globocan 2002)—an extensive database on the occurrence of cancer worldwide held by the Descriptive Epidemiology Group (DEP) of the International Agency for Research on Cancer (IARC)—are the sum of the sex- and age-specific rates (ASR) of endemic and epidemic KS. The ASR per 100 000 per year ranged between 0.3 in northern Africa and 30 in central Africa in males, and between 0.3 in northern Africa and 9.5 in eastern

Table 32.1 AIDS Clinical Trials Group (ACTG) staging classification

	Good risk (0): all of the following		Poor risk (1): any of the following
Tumor (T)	Confined to skin and/or lymph nodes and/or minimal oral disease*		Tumor-associated edema or ulceration Extensive oral KS Gastrointestinal KS KS in other nonnodal viscera
Immune system (I)	CD4 count ≥ 200 × 10⁶/L		CD4 count < 200 × 10⁶/L
Systemic illness (S)	No history of opportunistic infections or thrush No "B" symptoms† Performance status ≥ 70% (Karnofsky)		History of opportunistic infections and/or thrush "B" symptoms present Performance status < 70% Other HIV-related illness (e.g., neurological disease, lymphoma)

* Minimal oral disease is nonnodular Kaposi's sarcoma confined to the palate.
† "B" symptoms are unexplained fever, night sweats, > 10% involuntary weight loss, or diarrhea persisting for more than 2 weeks.

Africa.[7] The incidence of KS among transplant recipients has been estimated at 8.8 per 100 000 person-years in the USA, with most cases occurring in the first 2 years after transplantation (incidence 12.5 per 100 000 person-years). The KS risk increased steadily with recipient age (P < 0.001).[8]

Etiology

The unusual geographical distribution of KS has long suggested an infective cause. Epidemiological evidence, including the 20 times greater frequency of AIDS-related KS in homosexual men in comparison with hemophiliacs, suggested a sexually transmitted cofactor. In 1994, Chang et al. identified DNA sequences of human herpes virus 8 (HHV8), also known as the Kaposi's sarcoma herpes virus (KSHV).[9] It has been identified in virtually all KS specimens, regardless of subtype, but is absent from uninvolved skin. The KSHV genome encodes proteins that are homologous with human oncoproteins and have the potential to induce cellular proliferation and inhibit apoptosis. The presence of KSHV appears to be necessary for the development of KS, but the role of cofactors such as host immunosuppression, cytokines, and HIV is unclear.

Prognosis

The prognosis is determined by the type of KS, the extent of tumor and the organs involved, the general clinical condition, and the virological, immune, and hematological status. Classical KS typically runs an indolent course over years or decades, with gradual development of new lesions and complications such as lower limb lymphedema and hyperkeratosis. An excess of non-Hodgkin's lymphoma has been reported among patients with classic KS, although the overall risk of developing a second malignancy is not increased. AIDS-KS may be a disseminated and fulminant disease. The extent of the tumor (T), the immune status (I), and the severity of the systemic illness (S) are all prognostic determinants that, in the pre-HAART era, have been used in the TIS staging classification proposed by the AIDS Clinical Trials Group (ACTG) and prospectively validated (Table 32.1).[10] In the HAART era, a redefinition of the prognostic factors used in the ACTG TIS has been proposed, based on the observation that a CD4 count of < 200 cells/μL and tumor extension are no longer discriminants of a worse prognosis, whereas a CD4 count < 100 and associated systemic diseases have a more important role in patients on HAART.[11,12] Endemic (African) KS may run an indolent course similar to that of classical KS, with nodules and plaques in association with lower limb edema. The lymphadenopathic form of African KS in children has an aggressive course and carries a poor prognosis.

Aims of treatment

Effective palliation of symptoms related to lymph-node or visceral involvement (pain, edema, bleeding), and cosmetic improvement of disfiguring lesions are of primary importance for all patients suffering from KS. Patients with classic KS generally respond well to local therapies, although the recurrence rate is high. For patients with AIDS-KS, the introduction of HAART improves the overall survival and is associated with an 80% reduction in the risk of death,[13] prolongs the time to treatment failure,[14] and prolongs the survival of patients with pulmonary KS who also receive chemotherapy.[15] The precise mechanism by which HAART induces the regression of KS lesions is not well understood, but it includes immune reconstitution,[16] a general improvement in the immune status, and perhaps a direct anti-angiogenic effect.[17] It is still unclear, however, whether patients with AIDS-KS on HAART should receive concurrent chemotherapy or wait for a response to HAART alone. New prognostic indexes are being proposed to help identify those patients who have a poor prognosis and might need simultaneous chemotherapy in addition to HAART.[12] Endemic African KS, except for the lymphadenopathic form, responds to systemic therapies. Transplantation-related or immunosuppression-related KS regresses after the reduction or cessation of the immunosuppressive treatment.

Relevant outcomes

The most relevant outcome is the complete disappearance of the disease, although it is not commonly achieved or reported in trials specific for the treatment of Kaposi's sarcoma. Response rates in terms of the number and size of lesions, flattening, and degree of pigmentation, are important end points of systemic and local therapies. One of the problems in comparing studies of systemic therapy in KS is the subjective nature of the assessment of response. Recently, the ACTG criteria for assessment of response (Table 32.2) have been adopted in clinical studies.[18] The overall cosmetic effect is also an important end point, particularly for local therapies such as radiotherapy that have long-term effects on the normal skin surrounding lesions. Palliation of tumor-related symptoms such as edema or pain is another end point for which assessment is highly subjective.

Methods of search

We searched Medline and Embase from 1966 to December 2006. We first performed a highly sensitive search using the truncated term "Kaposi*", which generated over 10 000 abstracts. We then performed a more specific Medline search using "sarcoma, Kaposi" (MeSH terms) or "Kaposi's sarcoma" (text word), combined with the following interventions: surgery, laser*, photodynamic therapy, cryotherapy, cryosurgery, intralesional therapy, intralesional vincristine or vinblastine, radiotherapy, interferon, chemotherapy, anthracycline, bleomycin, vinca-alkaloid, vincristine, vinblastine, taxane, paclitaxel, liposomal therapy, gemcitabine, Navelbine, thalidomide, antiangiogenic agent, retinoids, retinoic acid, antiretroviral therapy, zidovudine, ganciclovir, cidofovir, or foscarnet. We also searched the Cochrane Central Register of Controlled Trials and Database of Systematic Reviews using the search terms "Kaposi*" and "Kaposi's sarcoma."

Table 32.2 AIDS Clinical Trials Group (ACTG) response criteria

Complete response (CR)
The absence of any detectable residual disease, including tumor-associated edema, persisting for at least 4 weeks

Clinical complete response (CCR)
In patients in whom pigmented (brown or tan) macular skin lesions persist after apparent CR, biopsy of at least one representative lesion is required to document the absence of malignant cells. In patients known to have had visceral disease, an attempt at restaging with appropriate endoscopic or radiographic procedures should be made. If such procedures are medically contraindicated, the patient may be classified as having CCR

Partial response (PR)
The absence of new cutaneous or oral lesions, new visceral sites of involvement, or the appearance or worsening of tumor-associated edema or effusions, in addition to at least one of the following:
- A 50% or greater decrease in the number of all previously existing skin lesions (skin, oral, measurable or evaluable visceral disease)
- A 50% decrease in the size of lesions (includes a 50% decrease in the sum of the products of the largest perpendicular diameters of bidimensionally measurable marker lesions and/or complete flattening of at least 50% of the lesions (i.e., 50% of previously nodular or plaque-like lesions become macules)
- In those patients with predominantly nodular lesions, flattening to an indurated plaque of 75% or more of the nodules
- Patients with residual tumor-associated edema or effusion who otherwise meet the criteria for CR

Stable disease (SD)
Any response not meeting the criteria for progression or PR

Progressive disease (PD)
An increase of 25% or more in the size of previously existing lesions, and/or the appearance of new lesions or new sites of disease, and/or a change in the character of 25% or more of the skin or oral lesions from macular to plaque-like or nodular. The development of new or increasing tumor-associated edema or effusion is also considered to represent disease progression

Questions

What are the effects of local therapies in Kaposi's sarcoma (surgical excision, cryotherapy, photodynamic therapy, radiotherapy, topical alitretinoin, intralesional interferon and intralesional chemotherapy)?

Radiotherapy

No randomized studies of radiotherapy in classic KS, endemic KS, or immunosuppression-related KS were found. Many retrospective case series of radiotherapy as a local therapy for classic KS indicate that it is a radiosensitive tumor. Patients were treated with local or extended-field radiotherapy, or local electron beam, and high response rates of 80–90% were reported. The criteria for assessment of the response were generally not stated, or varied remarkably across studies. A Cochrane review on the treatment of AIDS-related KS in resource-poor settings[19] included one randomized clinical trial of radiotherapy in patients with AIDS-KS. This randomized study by Stelzer and Griffin compared three different radiotherapy regimens.[20] Fourteen AIDS-KS patients with biopsy-proven KS were included. The trial was not blinded, the randomization criteria were not stated, and the lesions were analyzed on an intention-to-treat (ITT) basis. None of the participants was receiving HAART, but seven were taking zidovudine. A total of 71 lesions were randomized to receive either 8 Gy in one fraction, 20 Gy in 10 fractions, or 40 Gy in 20 fractions, given 5 days a week. At the time of the study, 8 Gy in a single fraction was considered the treatment of choice. Due to the randomization process, the same participant could receive different radiotherapy regimens to separate KS lesions. The trial was confined to the treatment of cutaneous lesions, either for cosmetic reasons or pain relief. The main outcome was complete response to therapy, defined as resolution of palpable tumor within the radiotherapy area, regardless of residual pigmentation. The initial complete response rate of lesions to 40 Gy given in 20 fractions or 20 Gy given in 10 fractions was greater than the one achieved with 8 Gy in a single fraction (83% and 79% vs. 50%), and the median times to recurrence were 43, 26, and 13 weeks, respectively. Adverse events were more common in lesions treated with 20 or 40 Gy than with those treated with 8 Gy.

Drawbacks

In the randomized trial by Stelzer and Griffin, toxicity was graded using the Radiation Therapy Oncology Group scoring system. Grade 1 acute toxicity (skin erythema, dry desquamation, or alopecia) was seen in three of 24 (12%) patients who received 8 Gy, 11 of 24 (46%) patients who received 20 Gy, and 22 of 23 (96%) patients who received 40 Gy. No acute toxicity greater than grade 1 was seen. Late toxicity occurred only in the 40-Gy group (six of 23 patients) but did not exceed grade 1 (slight hyperpigmentation or alopecia).

Comments

Before the AIDS epidemic, radiation therapy was the primary form of local treatment for non-AIDS KS. Radiotherapy, either given as a local or extended field, gives high response rates in the treatment of cutaneous KS and is an effective local palliative therapy, able to control temporarily large or disfiguring patches or plaques. In AIDS patients, it is still widely used to control oral KS lesions. The rates of complete response and duration of lesion control are higher with higher cumulative doses of radiotherapy. However, in

this group of patients, the prognosis is that of the underlying AIDS diagnosis, and in the HAART era it is strongly influenced by the concurrent antiretroviral therapy. Most low-risk patients, as defined by the ACTG staging classification (Table 32.2), show tumor regression with HAART alone, and it is now debated whether and when these patients should receive specific anti-KS treatment.

Implications for clinical practice

Radiotherapy can improve the appearance of cutaneous KS lesions and provide temporary local control. In the population with AIDS-related cutaneous KS, a single 8-Gy fraction of radiotherapy with superficial roentgen rays or electrons gives a high response rate. Higher response rates and a greater duration of local control are seen with fractionated radiotherapy courses to a higher total dose, although more toxic reactions such as cellulitis, blistering, and desquamation are observed.

Topical alitretinoin

Alitretinoin (9-cis-retinoic acid) gel, a retinoid receptor panagonist, has been recently licensed for the treatment of cutaneous KS lesions in AIDS patients. A Cochrane review on the treatment of Kaposi's sarcoma[19] included two trials on topical alitretinoin in patients with AIDS-KS.[21,22] The results could not be combined due to heterogeneity. Bodsworth et al. randomly allocated 134 HIV infected participants with KS to either topical 0.1% alitretinoin gel or placebo vehicle gel.[21] The trial was carried out in centers in Australia, the UK, and the USA. All of the participants had biopsy-proven KS. The participants were treated in a double-blind fashion for 12 weeks and then allowed to continue the treatment on an open-label basis. Both the alitretinoin gel and vehicle gel were applied by the patient to three to eight indicator lesions twice a day for the 12-week period of the study. Application was reduced to once daily if the participant developed grade 3 irritation, and was stopped altogether if this persisted. Seventy-three percent of the treatment group and 81% of the control group were taking HAART. The main outcome measures were the response to treatment as assessed using the ACTG objective criteria for applied topical therapy and toxicity. Adverse events were graded using the National Cancer Institute grading system. The overall response rate (complete and partial) was 37% in the alitretinoin group and 7% in the vehicle group (risk difference 30%, number needed to treat 4). Walmsley et al. randomly allocated 268 HIV-infected KS participants to either topical alitretinoin gel or a placebo vehicle gel.[22] The trial was conducted in Canada and the USA. All of the participants had biopsy-proven KS. The participants were treated in a double-blind fashion for 12 weeks and then allowed to continue the treatment on an open-label basis. Both the alitretinoin gel and the vehicle gel were applied by the participant to six selected indicator lesions three times a day for 2 weeks and then four times a day for the remainder of the study. The median CD4 count was 154 for the treatment group and 144 for the control group; 84% of the participants were receiving HAART. The main outcome measure was the response to treatment, as assessed by ACTG criteria as applied to topical therapy. Toxicity was also assessed and graded. The overall response rate (complete and partial) was 35% in the alitretinoin group and 18% in the vehicle group (risk difference 17%, NNT 6).

Drawbacks
Irritation at the application site was the main adverse effect.

Comments
Alitretinoin gel appears to be effective and safe for use in the treatment of cutaneous AIDS-KS. However, the overall response rates are modest, and the duration of the response could not be determined from the published trials. It is not commonly used in clinical practice.

Intralesional interferon
We found no systematic reviews. In one small controlled clinical trial of non–AIDS-related Kaposi's sarcoma, lesions in 12 patients were treated with intralesional and perilesional human interferon alfa (IFN-α; 50 000 international units twice weekly for 4–6 weeks) and compared with an untreated lesion in the same patient; and lesions in eight patients were treated with IFN-α in combination with interleukin-2 (IL-2) and compared with an untreated lesion in the same patient.[23] All treated lesions were cured in all cases, and the untreated lesions were not cured. Cure was verified histologically. The authors concluded that intralesional IFN-α is an effective treatment for non–AIDS-related Kaposi's sarcoma.

In a small study of 17 patients with AIDS-related KS who were receiving zidovudine (500 mg/day), up to five KS lesions per patient were injected with recombinant IFN-α (1 million units three times weekly for 6 weeks) and compared with one lesion per patient injected with sterile water.[24] Three patients were lost to follow-up and three patients were injected only with IFN-α because they had only one lesion. A complete response (disappearance of all treated lesions) was seen in seven of 14 (50%) of the per-protocol patients, in comparison with three of 11 lesions injected with sterile water (response difference 0.23; 95% CI, 0.60 to −0.14; NNT 5, 95% CI, 2 to −7). The corresponding worst-case scenario ITT response difference was 0.14 (95% CI, 0.49 to −0.21), NNT 8 (95% CI, 2 to −5). A complete response was seen in 41 of 54 (76%) treated lesions, in comparison with three of 11 (27%) lesions injected with sterile water. ITT results were not provided or calculable, since the number of lesions injected in the patients who were lost to

follow-up was not provided. On biopsy, two of 15 (13%) lesions injected with IFN-α and one of two lesions injected with sterile water that had shown clinically complete responses were found to have microfocal KS.

Drawbacks
Injected patients had flu-like symptoms. Local pain was common and inflammation occurred at the injection site. Two to three weekly visits for up to 6 weeks were required.

Comments
Intralesional IFN-α is not commonly used in clinical practice, especially in the HAART era.

Intralesional chemotherapy
A small randomized trial compared intralesional vinblastine (VNB) and 3% sodium tetradecyl sulfate (STS), a sclerosing agent, as a treatment for oral Kaposi's sarcoma.[25] The authors observed the same reduction in the tumor mass for the two agents and concluded that both agents are effective in controlling intraoral AIDS-KS and that the advantages of STS are its low cost and ease of use.

Comment
Intralesional vinblastine (0.1–0.2 mg/mL) has been used in a few series of patients with cutaneous AIDS-KS, with reported response rates ranging from 60% to 92%. Very high response rates were also recorded for patients with intraoral AIDS-KS. We found no systematic reviews or randomized clinical trials of surgical excision, cryotherapy, or photodynamic therapy for KS.

Is interferon alfa an effective systemic treatment for Kaposi's sarcoma?

Classic and African KS
No randomized clinical trials were found. Only case reports and small case series were found in the literature.

Comment
The data are insufficient for firm conclusions to be drawn regarding the effectiveness of systemic interferon alfa in the treatment of classical Kaposi's sarcoma.

AIDS-related Kaposi's sarcoma
We found no systematic reviews of the use of interferon in AIDS-related KS. Phase II trials demonstrated activity of interferon as monotherapy for AIDS-related KS, with higher doses. The drawbacks were the dose-dependent side effects. Gradual dose escalation was shown to reduce the immediate toxicity (flu-like symptoms).[26,27]

On the basis of *in vitro* studies suggesting a synergy between interferon alfa and antiretroviral drugs, multiple subsequent phase II trials have examined the combination of interferon alfa at low or intermediate doses and zidovudine in the treatment of AIDS-related KS. These studies have documented activity for relatively low doses of IFN-α (in comparison with those used as monotherapy) when combined with zidovudine, but have also confirmed a relatively high degree of antitumor activity in patients with CD4 counts below 200/μL, who rarely respond to high doses of IFN alone.[28,29] A phase II trial including 68 patients examined the efficacy of low and intermediate doses of interferon alfa-2b in combination with didanosine. The response rate was 40% in the low-dose group (95% CI, 24 to 58) and 55% in the intermediate-dose group (95% CI, 36 to 72), and the median duration of remission was 110 weeks in both groups.[30]

Comments

The advent of HAART has changed the clinical course of AIDS-related KS. The effectiveness of interferon combined with HAART is unknown. Zidovudine or didanosine alone are no longer standard therapy for HIV infection.

What are the effects of systemic chemotherapy in KS?

Classic and epidemic KS

We found one randomized study comparing oral etoposide with vinblastine in the treatment of classical KS in elderly Mediterranean patients.[31] Sixty-five patients were randomly assigned to receive either oral etoposide (60 mg/m^2 on days 1–3 during the first course; 60 mg/m^2 on days 1–4 during the second course; and 60 mg/m^2 on days 1–5 during the third course; the courses were recycled every 3 weeks) or an intravenous bolus of vinblastine (3 mg/m^2 weekly for 3 weeks, and then 6 mg/m^2 every 3 weeks). The study was not masked due to the differing treatments given. Complete or partial responses were seen in eight of 34 or 17 of 34, and eight of 31 or 10 of 31 patients treated with etoposide or vinblastine, respectively. A response (complete or partial) was observed in 25 of 34 (73.5%) and 18 of 31 (58%) patients treated with etoposide or vinblastine, respectively (response difference 16; 95% CI, –0.08 to 0.38; NNT 7, 95% CI, 3 to –14, $P = 0.3$). There were no statistically significant differences in the duration of response or survival at a median follow-up of 38 months. Side effects of both treatments were limited, although myelotoxicity was more evident in the vinblastine arm.

Comment

Neither etoposide nor vinblastine is commonly used to treat classic KS.

AIDS-KS

A Cochrane systematic review of treatments for AIDS-KS[19] included two studies[32,33] comparing pegylated liposomal doxorubicin (PLD) with standard KS treatment regimens in patients with very advanced disease. These two studies were randomized but not blinded. The randomization method was not described in either study. Patients were analyzed on an intention-to-treat basis. A meta-analysis of these two studies was performed. A total of 499 patients were included in the meta-analysis of PLD versus a standard regimen. The standard regimen was doxorubicin, bleomycin, and vincristine in the first trial, and bleomycin and vincristine in the second trial. None of the participants in either study was receiving HAART. The main outcome measure was the response to treatment as assessed by ACTG criteria. Toxicities were assessed using the standard World Health Organization criteria in the study by Northfelt *et al.*[32] and the National Cancer Institute Common Toxicity Criteria in the study by Stewart *et al.*[33] The relative risk of death was not significantly different between the two treatments (RR 1.26; 95% CI, 0.83 to 1.91). The response to PLD was superior to that of the control regimen (RR 2.16; 95% CI, 1.68 to 2.78). The trials reported adverse events in different ways and so could not be analyzed together, but serious adverse events (number of patients 258) and any adverse event (number of patients 241) did not significantly differ between PLD and the control regimens (RR 0.97; 95% CI, 0.91 to 1.04; and RR 1.01; 95% CI, 0.96 to 1.06, respectively). There were fewer withdrawals from treatment in the PLD group (RR 0.57; 95% CI, 0.48 to 0.68), but more cases of opportunistic infection (RR 1.42; 95% CI, 1.12 to 1.80). The duration of response was measured in one of the studies[33] (number of patients 241) and was not significantly different between the two groups, with a weighted mean difference of 3.70 (95% CI, –1.78 to 9.18). Another phase III trial[34] of pegylated daunorubicin versus a reference regimen of doxorubicin (Adriamycin), bleomycin, and vincristine (ABV) in advanced AIDS-related Kaposi's sarcoma was not included in the meta-analysis because it did not report results on an intention-to-treat basis. The trial was a prospective randomized phase III trial in which 232 patients were randomly assigned to receive pegylated daunorubicin 40 mg/m^2 or a combination regimen of doxorubicin 10 mg/m^2, bleomycin 15 U, and vincristine 1 mg, administered intravenously every 2 weeks. Treatment was continued until complete response (CR), disease progression, or unacceptable toxicity. Of 232 patients randomized, 227 were treated; 116 received pegylated daunorubicin and 111 received ABV. The overall response rate—CR or partial response (PR)—was 25% (three CRs and 26 PRs) for pegylated daunorubicin and 28% (one CR and 30 PRs) for ABV. The difference in the response rates was not statistically significant. The median survival time was 369 days for pegylated daunorubicin patients and 342 days for ABV patients ($P = 0.19$). The median time to treatment failure was 115 days for pegylated daunorubicin and 99 days for ABV ($P = 0.13$).

Comments

Most low-risk patients, as defined by the AIDS Clinical Trials Group, show tumor regression with HAART alone. High-risk patients usually require a combination of HAART and chemotherapy, with discontinuation of the chemotherapy after disappearance of the skin lesion.

Drawbacks

Neutropenia. The incidence of grade 3 neutropenia—absolute neutrophil count (ANC) > 500 and < 1000—in a randomized study comparing liposomal daunorubicin and ABV chemotherapy was similar in both groups (36% versus 35%, respectively). However, grade 4 neutropenia (ANC < 500) was more frequent as an adverse effect of liposomal daunorubicin than of ABV chemotherapy in the same randomized trial (15% versus 5%; $P = 0.021$).[34] The most common adverse event in both arms of an RCT comparing PLD with ABV chemotherapy was leukopenia, affecting 36% of 133 patients who received PLD and 42% of 125 patients in the ABV group.[33] No episodes of febrile neutropenia (neutrophils $< 500 \times 10^6$ cells/L) occurred in the PLD group, but 37% developed opportunistic infections and 6% experienced episodes of sepsis.[33] In a further RCT, 29% of 121 patients who received PLD developed grade 3 leukopenia, in comparison with 12% in the comparative BV chemotherapy arm.[34]

Cardiotoxicity. Of 24 patients who received a cumulative dose of > 500 mg/m^2 of liposomal anthracycline in one randomized study, none were found to have a 20% or greater decline in their left ventricular ejection fraction (LVEF).[34] Liposomal daunorubicin was discontinued in one patient whose LVEF fell from 47% to 33%. An angiogram then showed that this patient had had a complete occlusion of the left anterior descending artery. In one RCT of liposomal doxorubicin versus ABV, pre- and post-treatment estimations of LVEF were available for 47 patients who received PLD. Of these, two patients were found to have had a > 20% fall in LVEF.[32] One death attributable to cardiomyopathy occurred in 133 patients treated with PLD.[32] It appears that, unlike conventional anthracyclines, liposomal anthracyclines are not associated with significant cumulative cardiotoxicity.

Nausea and vomiting. Of the patients receiving liposomal daunorubicin, 51% experienced mild nausea.[34] Grade 3 nausea and vomiting was significantly more frequent with ABV than with PLD (34% versus 15%; $P < 0.001$).[32]

Alopecia. In the randomized trial reported by Gill *et al.*, alopecia occurred more frequently amongst the patients who received ABV chemotherapy than among those receiving liposomal daunorubicin.[34] In the ABV group, 36% experienced grade 1–2 alopecia, in comparison with 8% in

the liposomal daunorubicin group ($P < 0.0001$). In another RCT comparing PLD with ABV chemotherapy, grade 3 alopecia was also more frequent in the ABV group than in those receiving a liposomal anthracycline (19% versus 1%; $P < 0.001$).[32]

Peripheral neuropathy. Peripheral neuropathy was seen in 41% of patients treated with ABV and 13% of those given liposomal daunorubicin ($P < 0.0001$) in the study by Gill *et al.*[34] In another randomized study, peripheral neuropathy was also less common with liposomal doxorubicin than with ABV chemotherapy (6% versus 14%; $P < 0.002$).[32]

Acute infusion reactions. In the only large phase III study of liposomal daunorubicin, the incidence of acute infusion reactions was 2% (two of 116 patients). In an RCT of PLD, six of 133 patients (5%) experienced an acute infusion-related reaction presenting as flushing, chest pain, hypotension, and back pain. Five of the six patients needed premedication for subsequent cycles, but were able to continue on the study.[32] In another study, the frequency of acute infusion reactions with PLD was similar, affecting five of 121 patients (4%), but a severe anaphylactic reaction occurred in one patient.[33]

Mortality. In the RCT by Stewart *et al.*, five of 121 patients in the PLD arm died during the study. The cause of death for four of these patients was progression of AIDS, and the remaining patient died from progression of KS. The investigators attributed none of the deaths to the liposomal drug.[33] In another RCT, 24 of 133 patients who received PLD died, mostly as a result of complications of HIV infection, with one death resulting from cardiomyopathy.[32] There was no significant difference in the death rates in comparison with the ABV arm of the study.[32] In an RCT comparing liposomal daunorubicin with ABV chemotherapy, five of 117 patients who received PLD and five of 115 patients who received ABV chemotherapy died because of complications of HIV infection.[34] The median survival in the two groups did not differ.[34]

Comments

Three large RCTs have provided good evidence, using the ACTG criteria to assess response, that liposomal anthracyclines are at least as effective in AIDS-related cutaneous KS as standard ABV or BV combination chemotherapy.[32–34] The two RCTs that specifically compared pegylated doxorubicin with ABV or BV chemotherapy provide good evidence that PLD is more effective than standard combination chemotherapy.[32,34] The better toxicity profiles found in all three studies, associated with less frequent early termination of therapy because of adverse events, also favor the use of liposomal chemotherapy over standard combination chemotherapy. The addition of bleomycin and vincristine to liposomal doxorubicin is unlikely to be of benefit. Although overall response rates to PLD are higher than for ABV or BV chemotherapy, the median duration of response is similar. In the RCT comparing PLD with ABV chemotherapy, the median durations of response were 90 days and 92 days, respectively.[32] In the RCT comparing PLD with BV chemotherapy, the median durations of response were 142 days and 123 days, respectively, but the difference was not statistically significant.[33] Although we found no RCTs directly comparing the two liposomal drugs, the response rates for patients with advanced AIDS-related KS appear to be higher with liposomal doxorubicin than with daunorubicin. There have been no studies of sequential chemotherapy. Newer single-agent cytotoxic therapies such as paclitaxel, vinorelbine, and gemcitabine should be compared with liposomal anthracyclines in large phase III studies.

Implications for practice
There is good evidence that liposomal doxorubicin is likely to be beneficial for the palliative treatment of advanced AIDS-related KS. In view of its better toxicity profile than conventional chemotherapy, liposomal doxorubicin should be used as first-line systemic therapy for patients with advanced AIDS-related KS who have poor immune function and significant mucocutaneous disease or visceral disease. However, the liposomal anthracyclines are expensive and not readily available in the developing countries, where most HIV-related disease occurs. There have been no recent RCTs of chemotherapy in the other less common types of KS. However, previous uncontrolled studies and case series have suggested that patients with classical KS or African KS are at least as chemosensitive as those with AIDS-related KS, without the underlying immune suppression.

What are the effects of antiretrovirals in the treatment of AIDS-related Kaposi's sarcoma?

We found no systematic reviews or large RCTs of antiretroviral therapy as a systemic treatment for AIDS-related KS. A small prospective cohort study and one larger retrospective cohort study examining the effect of HAART were found.[35,36] A small clinical trial compared a new HAART regimen plus pegylated liposomal doxorubicin (PLD) to the HAART regimen alone.[37] One small RCT of oral zidovudine, intravenous zidovudine, or oral placebo in AIDS-related KS was identified, but zidovudine monotherapy is no longer standard treatment for HIV infection.[38]

Efficacy
Highly active antiretroviral therapy (HAART), which includes two nucleoside reverse transcriptase inhibitors with either a non-nucleoside reverse transcriptase inhibitor or one or two protease inhibitors, has changed the natural history of AIDS-associated Kaposi's sarcoma. Since HAART became widely available, the incidence of KS has declined sharply,[13-15] and the survival and the time to treatment failure increased.[16] Population-based studies worldwide have shown that HAART has decreased the incidence of KS as an AIDS-defining diagnosis.[39-41] In a huge study by the National Cancer Institute, 41 data sets from AIDS and cancer registries in 11 regions of the USA (1980–2002) were used to identify cancers in 375 933 people with AIDS. KS was reported in 25 284 (6.7%). The proportion with KS decreased, beginning in the mid-1980s and continuing through the mid-1990s (declining from 25% to 2–4%), leveling off subsequently at approximately 2%. Risk for KS declined by 83.5% between 1990–1995 and 1996–2002 (standardized incidence ratio 22 100 and 3640, respectively; $P < 0.0001$). The trial that compared HAART therapy to HAART plus PLD[37] was a randomized, open-label trial of patients with moderate to advanced KS (greater than 10 KS lesions, or mucosal or visceral involvement). The methods of randomization and concealment of allocation were not specified. PLD/HAART patients received a median of 11 cycles of intravenous PLD treatment. After 48 weeks of follow-up, the intention-to-treat analysis indicated that nonresponses, partial responses, and complete responses occurred in four, six, and three patients in the HAART/PLD group and in two, one, and 12 patients in the HAART alone group, respectively (chi-squared test 9.5; $P = 0.008$). The significant difference was in the number of partial responders (six versus one). Partial response was not defined. The authors concluded that HAART therapy alone does not provide adequate treatment for some patients with moderate to advanced KS.

A small, prospective cohort study involving 39 patients with KS who were treated with HAART indicated that at 24 months, there were complete and partial response rates of 46% and 28% respectively.[35] In a retrospective analysis of 78 patients, Bower *et al.*[36] observed that the time to relapse of KS was 0.5 years and 1.7 years before and after the initiation of HAART therapy, respectively.

Drawbacks
The side effects of combination HAART depend on the profile of individual drugs used and interactions with other drugs. More frequent side effects include nausea and vomiting, lethargy, diarrhea, peripheral neuropathy, headache, deranged liver function, hypersensitivity reactions, myelosuppression, lactic acidosis and pancreatitis.

Implications for practice
HAART prevents the development of KS in patients with HIV, and has dramatically decreased the incidence of KS as an AIDS-defining diagnosis. HAART may induce the regression of individual KS lesions through different postulated mechanisms (immune reconstitution, inhibition of

HIV replication, anti-angiogenic and anticytokine effects). Patients with high viral loads, low CD4 counts, or with other HIV-related symptoms require antiretroviral therapy for control of HIV infection. HAART alone in these patients is a reasonable initial therapy for KS, which may be combined later with other local or systemic treatments.

Key points

- HAART therapy has had a significant impact in decreasing the prevalence and severity of AIDS-related KS.

Local therapy

- In people with classical and AIDS-related KS, radiotherapy is highly likely to improve the cosmetic outcome of individual cutaneous lesions, with minimal harm. The optimum dose fractionation schedule in these conditions is yet to be determined.
- There is insufficient evidence for any firm recommendations to be made as to the value of surgical excision, cryotherapy, photodynamic therapy, and intralesional chemotherapy.

Systemic therapy

- Interferon alfa is likely to be a beneficial systemic treatment for good-prognosis AIDS-related KS. Interferon can be safely combined with antiretroviral therapy and is most suitable as first-line therapy for patients with CD4 counts > 200 x 10^6 cells/L, no "B" symptoms, and no history of prior opportunistic infection.
- We found good evidence that liposomal doxorubicin is more effective in AIDS-related KS than standard combination chemotherapy containing bleomycin and vincristine, with or without an anthracycline. Unlike conventional anthracyclines, liposomal anthracyclines do not appear to be associated with significant cardiotoxicity.

References

1 Friedman-Kien AE, Laubenstein L, Marmor M, *et al.* Kaposi's sarcoma and *Pneumocystis* pneumonia among homosexual men—New York City and California. *MMWR Morb Mortal Wkly Rep* 1981;**30**:305–8.

2 Beral V, Peterman TA, Berkelman RL, Jaffe HW. Kaposi's sarcoma among persons with AIDS: a sexually transmitted infection? *Lancet* 1990;**335**:123–8.

3 Brooks JJ. Kaposi's sarcoma: a reversible hyperplasia. *Lancet* 1986;**2**:1309–11.

4 Biggar RJ, Rabkin CS. The epidemiology of AIDS-related neoplasms. *Hematol Oncol Clin North Am* 1996;**10**:997–1010.

5 Mocroft A, Kirk O, Clumeck N, *et al.* The changing pattern of Kaposi sarcoma in patients with HIV, 1994–2003: the EuroSIDA Study. *Cancer* 2004;**100**:2644–54.

6 Taylor JF, Templeton AC, Vogel CL, *et al.* Kaposi's sarcoma in Uganda: a clinico-pathological study. *Int J Cancer* 1971;**8**:122–35.

7 CancerMondial, at: http://www-dep.iarc.fr/, last accessed 28 Jan 2007.

8 Mbulaiteye SM, Engels EA. Kaposi's sarcoma risk among transplant recipients in the United States (1993–2003). *Int J Cancer* 2006;**119**:2685–91.

9 Chang Y, Cesarman E, Pessin MS, *et al.* Identification of herpesvirus-like DNA sequences in AIDS-associated Kaposi's sarcoma. *Science* 1994;**266**:1865–9.

10 Krown SE, Testa MA, Huang J, *et al.* for the AIDS Clinical Trials Group Oncology Committee: AIDS-related Kaposi's sarcoma: prospective validation of the AIDS Clinical Trials Group staging classification. *J Clin Oncol* 1997;**15**:3085–92.

11 Nasti G, Talamini R, Antinori A, *et al.* AIDS-related Kaposi's sarcoma: evaluation of potential new prognostic factors and assessment of the AIDS Clinical Trial Group Staging System in the HAART era—the Italian Cooperative Group on AIDS and Tumors and the Italian Cohort of Patients Naive From Antiretrovirals. *J Clin Oncol* 2003;**21**:2876–82.

12 Stebbing J, Sanitt A, Nelson M, Powles T, Gazzard B, Bower M. A prognostic index for AIDS-associated Kaposi's sarcoma in the era of highly active antiretroviral therapy. *Lancet* 2006;**367**:1495–502.

13 Tam HK, Zhang ZF, Jacobson LP, *et al.* Effect of highly active antiretroviral therapy on survival among HIV-infected men with Kaposi sarcoma or non-Hodgkin lymphoma. *Int J Cancer* 2002;**98**:916–22.

14 Bower M, Fox P, Fife K, Gill J, Nelson M, Gazzard B. Highly active anti-retroviral therapy (HAART) prolongs time to treatment failure in Kaposi's sarcoma. *AIDS* 1999;**13**:2105–11.

15 Holkova B, Takeshita K, Cheng DM, *et al.* Effect of highly active antiretroviral therapy on survival in patients with AIDS-associated pulmonary Kaposi's sarcoma treated with chemotherapy. *J Clin Oncol* 2001;**19**:3848–51.

16 Bower M, Nelson M, Young AM, *et al.* Immune reconstitution inflammatory syndrome associated with Kaposi's sarcoma. *J Clin Oncol* 2005;**23**:5224–8.

17 Sgadari C, Barillari G, Toschi E, *et al.* HIV protease inhibitors are potent anti-angiogenic molecules and promote regression of Kaposi sarcoma. *Nat Med* 2002;**8**:225–32.

18 Krown SE, Metroka C, Wernz JC. Kaposi's sarcoma in the acquired immune deficiency syndrome: a proposal for uniform evaluation, response, and staging criteria. *J Clin Oncol* 1989;**7**:1201–7.

19 Dedicoat M, Vaithilingum M, Newton R. Treatment of Kaposi's sarcoma in HIV-1 infected individuals, with emphasis on resource poor settings (Cochrane review). *Cochrane Library* 2006;(**1**). Oxford: Update Software.

20 Stelzer KJ, Griffin TW. A randomized prospective trial of radiation therapy for AIDS-associated Kaposi's sarcoma. *Int J Radiat Oncol Biol Phys* 1993;**27**:1057–61.

21 Bodsworth NJ, Bloch M, Bower M, *et al.* Phase III vehicle-controlled, multi-centred study of topical alitretinoin gel 0.1% in cutaneous AIDS-related Kaposi's sarcoma. *Am J Clin Dermatol* 2001;**2**:77–87.

22 Walmsley S, Northfelt DW, Melosky B, *et al.* Treatment of AIDS-related cutaneous Kaposi's sarcoma with alitretinoin (9-*cis*-retinoic acid) gel. Panretin Gel North American Study Group. *J Acquir Immune Defic Syndr* 1999;**22**:235–46.

23 Ghyka G, Alecu M, Halalau F, Coman G. Intralesional human leukocyte interferon treatment alone or associated with IL-2 in non-AIDS related Kaposi's sarcoma. *J Dermatol* 1992;**19**:35–9.

24 Dupuy J, Price M, Lynch G, Bruce S, Schwartz M. Intralesional interferon-alpha and zidovudine in epidemic Kaposi's sarcoma. *J Am Acad Dermatol* 1993;**28**:966–72.

25 Ramirez-Amador V, Esquivel-Pedraza L, Lozada-Nur F, *et al.* Intralesional vinblastine vs. 3% sodium tetradecyl sulfate for the treatment of oral Kaposi's sarcoma. A double blind, randomized clinical trial. *Oral Oncol* 2002;**38**:460–7.

26 Evans LM, Itri LM, Campion M, *et al.* Interferon-alpha 2a in the treatment of acquired immunodeficiency syndrome-related Kaposi's sarcoma. *J Immunother* 1991;**10**:39–50.

27 Volberding PA, Mitsuyasu RT, Golando JP, Spiegel RJ. Treatment of Kaposi's sarcoma with interferon alfa-2b (Intron A). *Cancer* 1987;**59**(3 Suppl):620–5.

28 Shepherd FA, Beaulieu R, Gelmon K, *et al.* Prospective randomized trial of two dose levels of interferon alfa with zidovudine for the treatment of Kaposi's sarcoma associated with human immunodeficiency virus infection: a Canadian HIV Clinical Trials Network study. *J Clin Oncol* 1998;**16**:1736–42.

29 Fischl MA, Finkelstein DM, He W, Powderly WG, Triozzi PL, Steigbigel RT. A phase II study of recombinant human interferon-alpha 2a and zidovudine in patients with AIDS-related Kaposi's sarcoma. AIDS Clinical Trials Group. *J Acquir Immune Defic Syndr Hum Retrovirol* 1996;**11**:379–84.

30 Krown SE, Li P, Von Roenn JH, Paredes J, Huang J, Testa MA. Efficacy of low-dose interferon with antiretroviral therapy in Kaposi's sarcoma: a randomized phase II AIDS clinical trials group study. *J Interferon Cytokine Res* 2002;**22**:295–303.

31 Brambilla L, Labianca R, Boreschi V, *et al.* Mediterranean Kaposi's sarcoma in the elderly. A randomised study of oral etoposide versus vinblastine. *Cancer* 1994;**74**:2873–8.

32 Northfelt DW, Dezube BJ, Thommes JA, *et al.* Pegylated-liposomal doxorubicin versus doxorubicin, bleomycin and vincristine in the treatment of AIDS-related Kaposi's sarcoma: results of a randomized phase III clinical trial. *J Clin Oncol* 1998;**16**:2445–51.

33 Stewart S, Jablonowski H, Goebel FD, *et al.* Randomized comparative trial of pegylated liposomal doxorubicin versus bleomycin and vincristine in the treatment of AIDS-related Kaposi's sarcoma. *J Clin Oncol* 1998;**16**:683–91.

34 Gill PS, Wernz J, Scadden DT, *et al.* Randomized phase III trial of liposomal daunorubicin versus doxorubicin, bleomycin, and vincristine in AIDS-related Kaposi's sarcoma. *J Clin Oncol* 1996;**14**:2353–64.

35 Dupont C, Vasseur E, Beauchet A, *et al.* Long-term efficacy on Kaposi's sarcoma of highly active antiretroviral therapy in a cohort of HIV-positive patients. CISIH 92. Centre d'Information et de Soins de l'Immunodéficience Humaine. *AIDS* 2000;**14**:987–93.

36 Bower M, Fox P, Fife K, *et al.* Highly active anti-retroviral therapy (HAART) prolongs time to treatment failure in Kaposi's sarcoma. *AIDS* 1999;**13**:2105–11.

37 Martin-Carbonero L, Barrios A, Saballs P, *et al.* Pegylated liposomal doxorubicin plus highly active antiretroviral therapy versus highly active antiretroviral therapy alone in HIV patients with Kaposi's sarcoma. *AIDS* 2004;**18**:1737–40.

38 Lane HC, Falloon J, Walter RE, *et al.* Zidovudine in patients with human immunodeficiency virus (HIV) infection and Kaposi's sarcoma. A phase II randomized placebo-controlled trial. *Ann Intern Med* 1989;**111**:41–50.

39 Grulich AE, Li Y, McDonald AM, *et al.* Decreasing rates of Kaposi's sarcoma and non-Hodgkin's lymphoma in the era of potent combination anti-retroviral therapy. *AIDS* 2001;**15**:629–33.

40 Pezzotti P, Serraino D, Rezza G, *et al.* The spectrum of AIDS-defining diseases: temporal trends in Italy prior to the use of highly active anti-retroviral therapies, 1982–1996. *Int J Epidemiol* 1999;**28**:975–81.

41 Engels EA, Pfeiffer RM, Goedert JJ, *et al.* Trends in cancer risk among people with AIDS in the United States 1980–2002. *AIDS* 2006;**20**:1645–54.

Photoaging

Miny Samuel, Jean-Paul Deslypere, Christopher E.M. Griffiths

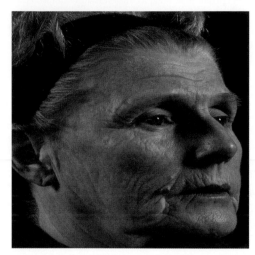

Figure 33.1 Photoaging in a 54-year-old woman.

A 54-year-old woman (Figure 33.1) had been an avid sunbather since her teenage years. She visited the dermatology clinic because she was depressed and conscious that her skin had started to look "old." She had a high-profile job involving frequent interaction with the public; she was concerned about losing confidence and also worried that the condition might lead to skin cancer. From advertisements published in magazines and the media, she was aware of various oral and topical medications that could improve the condition of her skin. Due to convenience and a preference for natural products, she had tried an oral medication containing natural polysaccharides for 6 months, but had not noticed any improvement. The diagnosis was that her skin had mottled hyperpigmentation, fine wrinkles, and roughness associated with "photoaging."

Background

Definition

Photoaging and photodamage (dermatoheliosis) are synonymous terms used to describe the alterations in the structure, function, and appearance of the skin as a result of prolonged or repeated exposure to ultraviolet (UV) radiation from the sun or other sources.

The changes of photoaging are superimposed on the changes caused by chronological aging and are responsible for many of the unwanted "age-associated" features of skin appearance. Sun-protected but aged skin is thin and less elastic, but otherwise largely unblemished and smooth. By contrast, photodamaged skin on sun-exposed parts of the body such as the face, neck, hands, and forearms is characterized by:

- Fine and coarse wrinkles (wrinkles are visible creases or folds in the skin, less than 1 mm in width and depth; coarse wrinkles are more than 1 mm width and depth).
- Mottled hyperpigmentation (uneven discoloration of the skin).
- Roughness.
- Laxity (looseness).
- Sallowness (a yellow discoloration of the skin).
- Telangiectasia (dilated blood vessels).

It is known that the overall loss of collagens in the dermis is linked to aging of the skin, which in turn is influenced both by intrinsic factors (intrinsic aging due to chronologic age, hormonal status, intercurrent diseases) and extrinsic influences (ultraviolet and infrared irradiation and cigarette smoke). Loss of collagen is linked to wrinkle formation. The severity of the skin damage, however, depends on the skin type (Table 33.1), which includes skin color and the capacity to tan.[1]

Table 33.1 Fitzpatrick skin phenotype classification

I	Always burns easily, never tans
II	Always burns easily, tans minimally
III	Burns moderately, tans gradually (light brown)
IV	Burns minimally, always tans well (brown)
V	Rarely burns, tans profusely (dark brown)
VI	Never burns, deeply pigmented (black)

Mottled hyperpigmentation is a heterogeneous condition ranging from freckles to actinic lentigines or "age spots," all of which arise from excessive sun exposure. Invariably, there is an increase in melanin deposition in the epidermis. The condition is harmless, but cosmetically embarrassing for some people.

Incidence/prevalence

Exposure to environmental and artificial UV radiation has increased significantly in recent years due to changes in social behavior, leisure activities, lifestyle, and traveling to equatorial regions.[2] Most studies on the incidence of sun damage have been reported from industrialized countries such as Australia, the USA, and the UK, probably because of the greater awareness of skin cancer and the emphasis on prevention and treatment methods. Photoaging or photodamage (rather than the normal intrinsic aging process) may account for 90% of age-associated cosmetic skin problems in both men and women.[3] In an Australian study[4] of 1539 Queensland residents aged 20–55 years, clinical changes of moderate to severe photoaging were observed in 72% of men and 47% of women under 30 years of age. The severity of photoaging was found to be significantly associated with increasing age, and independently with the presence of keratoses ($P < 0.01$), and skin cancer ($P < 0.05$). It is also increasingly clear that brief incidental sun exposures that occur during activities of daily living add significantly to the average individual's daily UV exposure. A survey performed in Merseyside in north-west England (Caucasians aged 40 years and above) concluded that the sun exposure received during normal daily activity may be sufficient to produce skin malignancies in a significant proportion of the population.[5] The overall prevalence of actinic keratoses in this population was 15.4% in men and 5.9% in women. The prevalence was reported to be strongly related to age in both sexes (34.1% in men and 18.2% in women aged $\geq$ 70 years) and also very strongly related to two objective signs of sun exposure—solar elastosis and the presence of actinic lentigines.

Etiology

The causes of photoaging are multifactorial and depend on age, sex, skin phototype, skin color, and geographic location. In general, the fairer and less pigmented the skin, the greater the risk for photoaging and other sun-induced skin problems, including skin cancer. Photodamage was observed more often in individuals with white skin, especially skin phototypes I and II (people with fair skin who burn easily and tan with difficulty). A study[6] reported that the incidence of photodamage in European and North American populations with Fitzpatrick skin types I–III is approximately 80–90%. In Asian skin, wrinkling is not readily apparent until the age of about 50 years, and even then the severity is not as marked as in white skin of similar age.[7,8] It was observed by Griffiths *et al.* in 1994[8] that Chinese and Japanese people primarily photoage by developing darkly pigmented lesions such as actinic lentigines and flat pigmented seborrheic keratoses, and that wrinkling is less of a problem. Few reports exist for black skin (phototypes V and VI), suggesting that photodamage may be less of a problem for this group.

Excessive exposure to UV radiation—for instance, by sunbathing—contributes to adverse effects such as sunburn and suppression of cellular immunity in the short term and photoaging and skin cancer in the long term. Observational studies show that incidence rates of the main types of skin cancer, basal cell carcinoma (BCC), squamous cell carcinoma (SCC) and melanoma are observed mainly in populations in which ambient sun exposure is high and skin (epidermal) transmission of solar radiation is high, suggesting strong associations between sun exposure and fair skin.[5,9,10] Photodamage in men is associated with outdoor occupations and activities. Unlike intrinsic aging, extrinsic aging may be prevented or partially reversed by sun avoidance. There is also an association between smoking status and pack-years of smoking with facial wrinkling in both men and women.[11,12] In postmenopausal women, estrogen deficiency is thought to be an important contributory factor for the development of wrinkles.[13]

Prognosis

Although photoaging cannot be considered a medical illness requiring intervention, concerns about aging and skin damage that affect quality of life are becoming increasingly common. Such concerns are influenced by geographical differences, culture, and personal values. In some cases, concerns about physical appearance can lead to difficulties with interpersonal relationships, ability to work, and self-esteem.[14] In societies in which the aging population is growing and a high value is placed on the maintenance of a youthful appearance, there is a growing desire for interventions that ameliorate the visible signs of aging. The guidelines developed by the U.S. Preventive Services Task Force suggest that avoiding direct sunlight by staying indoors or in the shade, or by wearing protective clothing, is the most effective measure for reducing exposure to UV light, but there are no randomized trials of sun avoidance to prevent photoaging and skin cancer. One randomized trial[15] of 1621 residents in Australia reported that daily sunscreen use on the hands and face reduced the total incidence of squamous cell cancer (RR 0.61; 95% CI, 0.46 to 0.81), but that sunscreen had no effect on basal cell cancer. Most epidemiological studies describing an association between ultraviolet radiation-induced skin damage and actinic keratoses have been conducted in Australia, the USA, and the UK, but there have been very few studies from other parts of the world.[15–17]

Aims of treatment

It has been estimated that the incidence of both short-term and long-term hazards of UV radiation can be reduced by nearly 80% over a person's lifetime if sunscreens are applied generously to the skin from the age of 6 months until 18 years of age. Other treatments that may help prevent photoaging include sunscreens, retinoids, antioxidants including vitamin C and E and beta-carotene, alpha-hydroxyacids, and estrogen,[18–21] the effects of which are unclear.

Photoaging had been thought to be irreversible. However, during the last decade it has been recognized that some topical compounds and surgical procedures can improve age-related skin damage.[22–25] Nowadays, a variety of topical (applied directly to the skin) and oral prescription and nonprescription agents are widely available, but the effectiveness of these treatments largely remains unclear. Common surgical interventions recommended by dermatologists and cosmetic surgeons include facelifts, dermabrasion, laser resurfacing, botulinum toxin, collagen injection, and chemical peeling. These surgical treatments are believed to produce visible and microscopic improvement in photodamaged skin, but are not without risk and contain no element of prevention.

Relevant outcomes

Clinically relevant outcomes include:
- The physician's and participant's overall evaluation of improvement in facial photoaging.
- The physician's evaluation of improvement in mottled hyperpigmentation, wrinkling, and skin roughness.
- Adverse events.

Methods of search

The Cochrane Skin Group specialized skin register; the Cochrane Library issue 1, 2006; Medline from 1965 to June 2006; and Embase from 1974 to June 2006 were searched for articles reporting trials of treatment for photodamage and photoaging. Medline was searched using OVID and PubMed; Embase was searched using Dialog Datastar. The searches involved the following terms:
- Treatment of skin in subjects with hyperpigmentation and roughness related to photodamage/photoaging/dermatoheliosis.
- Treatment of photodamage with any of the following agents: topical and oral treatments, ascorbic acid, retinoids, alpha hydroxyl acids, natural polysaccharides.

Due to space limitations, the effectiveness of surgical interventions (laser techniques versus other surgical tech-

niques: CO_2 laser, chemical peels, dermabrasion, Er:YAG laser) will be covered in the next update of this chapter.

Questions

Are there effective topical treatments to improve hyperpigmentation, wrinkles, roughness, and overall photoaging of the face?

The following is the evidence extracted from a Cochrane systematic review and other relevant randomized controlled trials (RCTs).

Vitamins

Vitamin C (ascorbic acid) is known to be a powerful antioxidant and a stimulant of collagen production. Researchers have suggested that topical application of ascorbic acid could be beneficial to prevent photoaging of the skin, as oral intake is thought to be incapable of generating an adequate level of response in the skin.[26] However, currently only a small number of studies have dealt with topical application of vitamin C in photodamage. We found one systematic review[27] that reported on one RCT comparing topical L-ascorbic acid 0.5 mL in a vehicle cream versus the vehicle cream alone applied once daily for 12 weeks.[28] The results showed that ascorbic acid, when applied to the face for 12 weeks, improved roughness by 36% ($P = 0.04$), mottled hyperpigmentation by 32%, and overall improvement in photodamage by 84% ($P = 0.002$) according to the assessment by the physician in comparison with placebo. The participant's self-appraisal also showed an improvement of 84% ($P = 0.002$). However, this RCT was limited by its small sample size, the short duration of the study period, and the high rate of loss to follow-up (nine of 28, 32%); in addition, the analysis was not conducted on an intention-to-treat basis. There were also reports of adverse effects such as stinging (55%), erythema (24%), and dry skin (5%). However, the symptoms responded to moisturization and usually resolved within the first 2 months of treatment.

There is no clear evidence to suggest that vitamins are useful, implying a need for well-conducted studies. Studies on ascorbic acid in particular should focus on a good double-blinded RCT with a sufficient sample size and should compare the effectiveness of treatment between patients rather than using a within-patient comparison.

Tretinoin

Tretinoin, the major metabolite of naturally occurring Vitamin A, is one of the few topical agents approved for treating photoaging. Since the first report of the effectiveness of tretinoin for the treatment of photoaging by Kligman et al.[29] 20 years ago, there has been increased interest in its potential as an antiaging agent. There is now considerable evidence that tretinoin can stimulate new collagen synthesis and reduce collagen breakdown in photoaged skin, and that it can inhibit the production of melanin.

We found one systematic review[27] summarizing the evidence from 13 double-blind, vehicle-controlled RCTs (Table 33.1). The RCTs included people with mild to moderate photodamage with Fitzpatrick skin types I–III[30–36] and with moderate to severe photodamage,[22,37,38] as well as two RCTs that did not define clearly the extent of photodamage.[39,40] The RCTs compared tretinoin (0.1%, 0.05%, 0.02%, 0.01%, 0.025%, and 0.001%) once daily, three times weekly, or once weekly versus a vehicle cream for 12–48 weeks. All RCTs that examined creams containing high concentrations (0.1% and 0.05%) of tretinoin reported improved fine wrinkles, coarse wrinkles, and hyperpigmentation compared with vehicle cream. However, significant improvement in roughness was observed only with 0.05% tretinoin. Lower-concentration tretinoin creams (0.01% and 0.001%) in people with mild to moderate photodamage did not improve wrinkles, hyperpigmentation, or roughness. The investigators' assessments also showed that higher concentrations of tretinoin resulted in an overall significant improvement in photodamage. Only a few trials assessed the patients' perception of improvement; the results show that tretinoin concentrations of 0.01%, 0.02%, and 0.05% when applied for 24 weeks resulted in satisfactory improvement. Assessment of improvement in skin texture by participants and investigators was consistent, although the degree of improvement varied (Table 33.2).[27]

The most common adverse effects reported after application of tretinoin were dry skin/peeling, which were most frequent and severe after 12–16 weeks and tended to be persistent; and also itching, burning/stinging, and erythema, which peaked during the first 2 weeks of treatment and decreased with time. The meta-analysis found that erythema occurred in a significantly greater proportion of people using tretinoin 0.05% and 0.1% than in those using lower concentrations. A similar trend was found with scaling/dryness of the skin. Burning/stinging was also reported to be high with higher concentrations. Signs and symptoms of skin irritation (erythema, peeling, dryness, burning, or stinging) tended to peak during the first 4 weeks of the trial period.

Current evidence shows that topical 0.05% tretinoin, when applied once daily for 24 weeks, improves fine wrinkles, coarse wrinkles, mottled hyperpigmentation, and roughness of the skin and also overall photodamage to the face. There is only limited evidence from one study to suggest that topical cream of 0.1% tretinoin for 40 weeks improves fine wrinkles, coarse wrinkles, mottled hyperpigmentation, and roughness. It is also important to caution the users of higher concentrations of tretinoin about potential side effects during the first 2–4 weeks of treatment when it is applied once or twice daily.

Tazarotene

Tazarotene is the first of a new generation of retinoids selective for particular acid receptors. It is approved by the U.S. Food and Drug Administration (FDA) for the treatment of photoaging. Since this is a relatively new drug on the market in comparison with tretinoin, there are only limited data available on the effectiveness and safety of treatment. We found one systematic review[27] that included RCTs. However, only one RCT[41] studied the effects on the face. We found an additional RCT[42] not pooled in the meta-analysis (Table 33.3).[27,42,43]

Fine wrinkles and mottled hyperpigmentation on the face showed a trend towards improvement with increasing concentration of tazarotene. The effect was statistically significant with 0.1% tazarotene only when applied daily for 24 weeks. There were no data on its effectiveness on roughness of the skin. With tazarotene 0.05%, a significant improvement in fine wrinkles resulted. However, the investigators' assessments reported that all concentrations of tazarotene produced significant improvement in overall photodamage. The most beneficial effect was seen with the highest concentration, 0.1%. We found an RCT[42] not included in the meta-analysis (men and women aged 18 years or older with Fitzpatrick skin types I–IV) that compared tazarotene 0.1% versus placebo cream applied once daily for 24 weeks. Once-daily application of tazarotene 0.1% resulted in an improvement in fine wrinkles, coarse wrinkles, hyperpigmentation, and roughness of at least one grade on a 5-point scale at 24 weeks, and an overall integrated assessment was reported. It is difficult to know whether a change of at least one grade can be translated into meaningful clinical improvement.

The most frequent adverse events of topical tazarotene were signs and symptoms of local skin irritation, such as mild to moderate desquamation, burning, erythema, pruritus, and dryness. "Severe" treatment-related adverse events were reported by fewer than 3% of people in the 0.1%, 0.05%, and 0.01% tazarotene groups and by 5% in the tretinoin 0.05% group. In the RCT, adverse events were reported mainly during the first few weeks of treatment,[42] mainly involving desquamation (37.1%), erythema (29.7%), and a burning sensation (29%) in the tazarotene group, and the difference was statistically significant in comparison with the control group ($P < 0.001$).

Tazarotene versus tretinoin. We found one RCT[27] in the systematic review. The study did not observe a statistically significant difference in either overall clinical improvement or fine wrinkles and hyperpigmentation with concentrations of 0.01%, 0.025%, 0.05%, and 0.1% in comparison with tretinoin 0.05%. We found one RCT that was not included in the meta-analysis.[43] The trial included people with Fitzpatrick skin types I–IV and compared tazarotene 0.1% with tretinoin 0.05% applied once daily in the evening for

Table 33.2 Summary of results for tretinoin treatment (Samuel et al.[27])

Tretinoin	Hyperpigmentation	Fine wrinkles	Coarse wrinkles	Roughness	Overall photodamage
0.1%	Improved hyperpigmentation (RR 2.92; 95% CI, 1.58 to 5.38) at 40 weeks	Improved fine wrinkles (RR 20.0; 95% CI, 1.89 to 445.86) at 16 weeks	Improved coarse wrinkles (RR 13.0; 95% CI, 0.80 to 212.02) at 16 weeks	No significant improvement (RR 11.0; 95% CI, 0.66 to 182.87) at 16 weeks	Investigators' assessment showed significant improvement at 16 weeks (RR 29.0; 95% CI, 1.89 to 445.86) and 48 weeks (RR 3.13; 95% CI, 1.67 to 5.85)
0.05%	Improved hyperpigmentation (RR 1.39; 95% CI, 1.21 to 1.60) at 24 weeks	Improved fine wrinkles (RR 1.76; 95% CI, 1.47 to 2.12) at 24 weeks	Improved coarse wrinkles (RR 1.68; 95% CI, 1.17 to 2.42) at 24 weeks	Improved roughness (RR 1.44; 95% CI, 1.19 to 1.76) at 24 weeks	Investigators' assessment reported significant improvement at 24 weeks (RR 1.73; 95% CI, 1.39 to 2.14). Patients' assessment reported significant improvement at 24 weeks (RR 2.04; 95% CI, 1.57 to 2.66)
0.025%	Improved mottled hyperpigmentation (WMD 0.60; 95% CI, 0.07 to 1.13) at 48 weeks	Improved fine wrinkles (WMD 0.75; 95% CI, 0.22 to 1.28) at 48 weeks	NR	NR	Investigators' assessment showed significant improvement at 48 weeks (RR 3.09; 95% CI, 1.65 to 5.77)
0.02%	No significant improvement at 24 weeks (RR 1.66; 95% CI, 0.81 to 3.40)	Improved fine wrinkles (RR 1.60; 95% CI, 1.28 to 2.01) at 24 weeks	Improved coarse wrinkles (RR 1.70; 95% CI, 1.22 to 2.37) at 24 weeks	No significant improvement (RR 1.17; 95% CI, 1.01 to 1.34) at 24 weeks	Investigators' assessment showed significant improvement at 24 weeks (RR 1.60; 95% CI, 1.07 to 2.37). Patients' assessment reported significant improvement at 24 weeks (RR 1.22; 95% CI, 1.07 to 1.38)
0.01%	Improved hyperpigmentation at 24 weeks (RR 1.14; 95% CI, 0.92 to 1.42) but the difference was not statistically significant	Improved fine wrinkles (RR 1.57; 95% CI, 0.91 to 2.71) at 24 weeks but the difference was not statistically significant	Improved coarse wrinkles (RR 7.0; 95% CI, 0.96 to 50.93) at 24 weeks but the difference was not statistically significant	No significant improvement (RR 1.24; 95% CI, 0.83 to 1.84) at 24 weeks	Investigators' assessment: improved at 24 weeks (RR 1.44; 95% CI, 0.90 to 2.31) but the result was not statistically significant. Patients' assessment: improvement at 24 weeks (RR 1.67; 95% CI, 1.26 to 2.23)
0.001%	No improvement at 24 weeks (RR 0.85; 95% CI, 0.59 to 1.23)	No improvement at 24 weeks (RR 0.69; 95% CI, 0.43 to 1.10)	NR	No improvement (RR 1.14, 95% CI, 0.64 to 2.04) but it was not significant	Investigators' assessment: improvement at 24 weeks (RR 0.74; 95% CI, 0.49 to 1.14)

24 weeks. There was an improvement of at least one grade (on a seven-point scale) of fine wrinkles, coarse wrinkles, and hyperpigmentation. Tazarotene 0.1% was superior to tretinoin 0.05% at 12 and 16 weeks, but not at 24 weeks after treatment.

Treatment-related adverse events were of mild to moderate severity and mainly occurred in the first week after starting treatment. There were no significant differences in most of the adverse events between tazarotene and tre-

tinoin, but tazarotene significantly increased the sensation of burning on the skin—18 of 88 (21%) described irritation with tazarotene, compared with 30 of 85 (35%; $P < 0.001$) with tretinoin.

Isotretinoin

Isotretinoin (13-*cis*-retinoic acid) is a metabolite of vitamin A, or retinol, and is a structurally related stereoisomer of *all-trans*-retinoic acid (tretinoin). It is currently available on the

Table 33.3 Summary results for tazarotene treatment

Reference	Tazarotene	Hyperpigmentation	Fine wrinkles	Coarse wrinkles	Roughness	Overall photodamage
Samuel et al.[27]	0.1%	Improved at 24 weeks (RR 1.32; 95% CI, 1.06 to 1.63)	Improved fine wrinkles (RR 2.91; 95% CI, 1.63 to 5.20) at 24 weeks	NR	NR	Investigators' assessment: improvement at 24 weeks (RR 2.64; 95% CI, 1.46 to 4.76)
Phillips et al.[42]	0.1%	Improved by at least 1 grade (on a 5-point scale) at 24 weeks in 62% of subjects given tazarotene compared to 20% in subjects given placebo ($P < 0.001$)	Improved fine wrinkles at least one grade (on a 5-point scale) at 24 weeks in 45% of subjects with tazarotene compared to 18% in subjects given placebo ($P < 0.001$)	Improved coarse wrinkles at least one grade (on a 5-point scale) in 24 weeks in 15% of subjects with tazarotene compared to 8% in subjects given placebo ($P < 0.01$)	Improved by at least 1 grade (on a 5-point scale) in 45% of subjects given tazarotene compared to 35% in placebo ($P < 0.01$)	Investigators' assessment: overall integrated assessment improved by at least 1 grade (on 5-point scale) in 38% of subjects given tazarotene compared to 10% in placebo ($P < 0.001$). Patients' assessment: More than 60% of patients considered their photodamage to be somewhat or much improved by week 4 and more than 80% of patients considered their photodamage to be somewhat or much improved from week 12 onward. The incidence of patients achieving treatment success ($\geq 50\%$ global improvement) was also significantly higher with tazarotene (40%) compared with placebo (15%; $P < 0.001$)
Samuel et al.[27]	0.05%	No significant improvement at 24 weeks (RR 1.21; 95% CI, 0.96 to 1.52)	Improved fine wrinkles (RR 2.55; 95% CI, 1.40 to 4.61) at 24 weeks	NR	NR	Investigators' assessment showed improvement at 24 weeks (RR 2.27; 95% CI, 1.24 to 4.18)
Samuel et al.[27]	0.025%	No significant improvement at 24 weeks (RR 1.03; 95% CI, 0.79 to 1.33)	Improved fine wrinkles (RR 1.82; 95% CI, 0.96 to 3.45) at 24 weeks	NR	NR	Investigators' assessment showed improvement at 24 weeks (RR 1.91; 95% CI, 1.01 to 3.59)
Samuel et al.[27]	0.01%	No significant improvement at 24 weeks (RR 1.11; 95% CI, 0.87 to 1.42)	Improved fine wrinkles (RR 2.41; 95% CI, 1.32 to 4.40) at 24 weeks	NR	NR	Investigators' assessment showed improvement at 24 weeks (RR 2.06; 95% CI, 1.11 to 3.82)
Lowe et al.[43]	0.1% vs. tretinoin 0.05%	At 12 and 16 weeks there was significant improvement: tazarotene 70%, tretinoin 55%, $P < 0.05$; tazarotene 80%, tretinoin 65%, $P < 0.01$). At 24 weeks, the incidence of subjects achieving at least one grade of improvement in mottled hyperpigmentation was not significantly different between the two groups (tazarotene 80%, tretinoin 74%)	Improved fine wrinkles by at least one grade in 80% (70/88) of subjects given tazarotene compared to 62% (53/85) with tretinoin ($P < 0.01$)	Improved coarse wrinkles by at least one grade in 39% (34/88) in subjects given tazarotene compared to 32% (29/85) in tretinoin ($P < 0.05$)	NR	*Overall integrated assessment score*: significant at 16 weeks (tazarotene 45%, tretinoin 25%, $P < 0.05$), but not significantly different at 24 weeks (tazarotene 60%, tretinoin 45%)

Table 33.4 Summary results for treatment with 0.1% isotretinoin (Samuel et al.[27])

Hyperpigmentation	Fine wrinkles	Coarse wrinkles	Roughness	Overall photodamage
At 36 weeks, showed significant improvement (WMD 3.40; 95% CI, 2.29 to 4.51)	Fine wrinkles improved (WMD 4.90; 95% CI, 3.79 to 6.01) at 36 weeks	Improved coarse wrinkles (WMD 3.0; 95% CI, 2.17 to 3.83) at 36 weeks	NR	Investigators' assessment: overall appearance improved (WMD 5.60; 95% CI, 4.49 to 6.71) at 36 weeks. Participants assessed a significant overall improvement in photodamage (RR 1.44; 95% CI, 1.30 to 1.59) at 36 weeks

market only for treatment of acne and not for photodam-aged skin. We found one systematic review[27] of one double-blinded RCT (Table 33.4).[27] In this study,[44] the physician's assessment of improvement was expressed as a change in score from the baseline severity score taken prior to treatment on a 100-mm balanced analog scale divided into marked worsening, mild worsening, mild improvement, and marked improvement. A low score indicated less change from the baseline and a high score a greater change from the baseline. However, it is difficult to interpret the observed change in score in terms of clinical improvement.

Isotretinoin 0.1% cream, applied daily for 36 weeks, produced significant improvement in fine wrinkles, coarse wrinkles, mottled hyperpigmentation, and overall improvement. The participants also assessed a significant overall improvement in photodamage on the face. However, erythema (RR 2.59; 95% CI, 2.13 to 3.15), scaling/dryness (RR 6.47; 95% CI, 4.52 to 9.24), and burning/stinging (RR 4.31; 95% CI, 3.34 to 5.57) were observed to be significantly higher than in the control group. It was reported that overall, 119 of the 800 (14.8%) participants were excluded from the analysis, but the reasons for exclusion were given for only 64 of the participants. Thirty-four participants (25 from the isotretinoin group and nine from the placebo group) withdrew due to adverse events, and another 30 subjects

were lost to follow-up or withdrew due to personal reasons unrelated to treatment.

Although isotretinoin 0.1% appears to be a promising treatment for photoaged skin, there is only limited evidence from one study. The significant increase in adverse events is of concern, and future trials should therefore be vigilant in tracking patients who withdraw or who are lost to follow-up during the trial period. However, there is a clear need for more RCTs on isotretinoin for the treatment of photoaging.

Natural polysaccharides

It was first reported in 1992 that extracts from cartilage derived from marine fish appear to have reparative effects on photoaged skin. Currently, such extracts are widely distributed on the market with their respective trademarks, but it is uncertain whether there is sufficient evidence to support such widespread use. With the increasing preference for the use of natural products by some people, it definitely has great potential if indeed it is shown to be beneficial.

We found one systematic review[27] that included a study by Lassus et al.[45] on topical natural polysaccharides (Vivida cream; Table 33.5).[27] This study was a small within-patient comparison, and insufficient details were provided

Table 33.5 Summary results for treatment with natural polysaccharides (1% Vivida cream; Samuel et al.[27])

Hyperpigmentation	Fine wrinkles	Coarse wrinkles	Roughness
At 9 weeks, mottled hyper-pigmentation improved in 13.3% of subjects compared to 6.7% in placebo group. At 17 weeks, mottled hyperpigmentation improved in 40% of subjects compared to 6.7% in placebo group	At 9 weeks, shallow wrinkles (< 1 mm) improved in 43% of subjects compared to 0% in placebo group. At 9 weeks, moderate wrinkles (1 mm) improved in 10% of subjects compared to 0% in placebo group. At 17 weeks, shallow wrinkles improved in 100% of subjects given Vivida compared to 0% in placebo group. At 17 weeks, moderate wrinkles improved in 90% of subjects given Vivida compared to 0% in placebo group	At 9 weeks, deep wrinkles (> 1 mm) improved in 6.7% of subjects compared to 6.7% in placebo group. At 17 weeks, deep wrinkles (> 1 mm) improved in 16.7% of subjects given Vivida compared to 6.7% in placebo group	NR

for calculate appropriate estimates and standard errors to be calculated. It was reported in the study that the polysaccharide-containing cream was applied twice daily for 17 weeks and that effectiveness was assessed at 12 and 17 weeks. The effect on shallow (< 1 mm) and moderate wrinkles and mottled hyperpigmentation was reported to be significant in comparison with the control group. At 17 weeks, shallow wrinkles improved in all subjects, whereas moderate wrinkles improved in 90% of subjects. Forty percent of the participants had clearance of mottled hyperpigmentation when assessed at 17 weeks, in comparison with 7% in the placebo group. When assessed at 12 weeks however, 87% of the Vivida-treated sides still had mild to severe mottled hyperpigmentation. Dryness was not reported in any of the participants when assessed at 17 weeks, while after 9 weeks, 7% of the Vivida-treated sides were reported to have mild to moderate skin dryness in comparison with the control.

It is still unclear whether topical natural polysaccharides can benefit people with photodamaged skin. Since there is only limited evidence available, it would be worthwhile for researchers to embark on a well-designed RCT with an independent control group rather than a within-patient comparison.

Topical treatments: alpha hydroxy acids

Alpha hydroxy acids (AHAs) have been introduced more recently, and it is still uncertain whether they offer any advantage over existing retinoid-containing creams. Depending on pH and concentration, AHAs can act as "chemical peels"—removing stratum corneum and the upper layers of the epidermis. The methods range from simple scrubs to special creams and intensive peeling treatments using AHA.

We found one systematic review[27] that summarized the evidence from three studies comparing topical glycolic acid/lactic acid versus placebo. Significantly more participants using 8% glycolic acid showed an overall improvement in facial photodamage from the participant's perspective after applying the cream twice daily for 22 weeks in comparison with participants using the vehicle.[46] The data on fine wrinkles, hyperpigmentation, and roughness were reported as the mean grade change from baseline and reported to be significant. A similar trend in improvement was reported with 8% lactic acid of overall photodamage, fine wrinkles, hyperpigmentation, and roughness. One study reported on 5% glycolic acid, but did not show any significant improvement of fine wrinkles in comparison with placebo at 3 months when applied once daily.

It was reported that out of 75 participants, only 69 were included in the analysis. Four out of 39 (10.2%) participants from the glycolic acid group and two of 36 (5.6%) from the

placebo group were excluded because of adverse reactions. Glycolic acid was compared with lactic acid, and the overall improvement in facial photodamage did not show a significant difference; the relative risk of improvement was 1.08 (95% CI, 0.76 to 1.53).

The systematic review[27] found one small trial[47] that studied the effectiveness of 70% glycolic acid in comparison with 10% glycolic acid and a moisturizer. The study showed neither statistical significance nor any conclusive evidence for any of the outcomes assessed (fine wrinkles, coarse wrinkles, hyperpigmentation, roughness, overall improvement), but participants who applied 10% glycolic acid and moisturizer in addition to the 70% glycolic acid peels showed a trend towards improvement with regard to overall improvement in photodamage (participant's assessment), with a nonsignificant relative risk of improvement of 0.80 (95% CI, 0.52 to 1.24). The relative risk for mottled hyperpigmentation was 0.50 (95% CI, 0.06 to 3.91). No significant adverse events or complications were reported in the study (Table 33.6).[27]

The effectiveness of topical hydroxy acids in the treatment of photoaging is unclear, although two small studies of 8% glycolic and lactic acids showed a trend towards effectiveness. This needs to be further evaluated to reaffirm safety and effectiveness.

Are there effective oral treatments to improve wrinkles, hyperpigmentation, roughness, and overall photoaging of the face?

Limited research has been conducted on the effects on wrinkles of oral antioxidant supplements. There are no good RCTs studying the effectiveness of oral vitamin supplements on photodamage. There are also no trials comparing the effectiveness of oral tretinoin or isotretinoin for photodamaged skin, because of the known side effect profile, particularly teratogenicity.

Currently, the evidence shows that only natural polysaccharides have been tested, but there is still a need for adequately designed studies to prove effectiveness.

Natural polysaccharides

There are at present two commercially available oral products containing different amounts of active polysaccharides—Vivida (500 mg) and Imedeen (380 mg).

We found one systematic review,[27] which included two studies. The two RCTs compared Vivida to either placebo[48,49] or Imedeen.[50] For 500 mg Vivida when taken orally for 90 days, there is limited evidence to suggest that it can improve fine wrinkles (RR 21.0; 95% CI, 1.34 to 328.86), but there was no evidence of a difference in improvement in mottled hyperpigmentation between the Vivida and placebo groups (RR 1.50; 95% CI, 0.53 to 4.26). When 500 mg

Table 33.6 Summary results for treatment with hydroxy acids (Samuel et al.[27])

Intervention	Hyperpigmentation	Fine wrinkles	Coarse wrinkles	Roughness	Overall photodamage
5% glycolic acid	NR	At 3 months, there was no significant improvement (WMD −0.42; 95% CI, −1.68 to 0.84)	NR	Roughness improvement was reported as mean change in glycolic acid, −0.86 ($P = 0.0001$); placebo −0.29 ($P = 0.004$)	NR
8% glycolic acid	Hyperpigmentation improved in 14% of subjects compared to 7% in placebo ($P < 0.05$). The mean grade change in glycolic acid was −0.57, placebo −0.32	Fine wrinkles improved in 22% of subjects given glycolic acid compared to 15% in placebo ($P < 0.05$). The mean grade change was glycolic acid −1.14, placebo −0.86	NR	Roughness improved in 44% of subjects given glycolic acid compared to 41% in placebo ($P < 0.05$). The mean grade change in glycolic acid was −1.33, placebo −1.27	Participants' assessment showed a significant improvement in photodamage (RR 1.86, 95% CI 1.07 to 3.25) at 22 weeks. Investigators' assessment showed an improvement in 17% of subjects given glycolic acid compared to 8% in placebo group ($P < 0.05$). The mean grade change was glycolic acid −0.90, placebo −0.45
8% lactic acid	Hyperpigmentation improved in 22% of subjects compared to 7% in placebo ($P < 0.05$). The mean grade change in lactic acid was −0.92, placebo −0.32	Fine wrinkles improved in 22% of subjects given glycolic acid compared to 15% in placebo ($P < 0.05$). The mean grade change was lactic acid −1.04, placebo −0.86	NR	Roughness improved in 42% of subjects compared to 41% in placebo group ($P < 0.05$). The mean grade change in lactic acid was −1.33, placebo −1.27	Participants' assessment showed a trend towards improvement in photodamage (RR 1.73; 95% CI, 0.99 to 3.04)
8% glycolic acid vs. 8% lactic acid	NR	NR	NR	NR	Participants' assessment showed no significant improvement in photodamage (RR 1.08; 95% CI, 0.76 to 1.53)
70% Glycolic acid vs. 10% glycolic acid + moisturizer	No significant improvement (RR 0.50; 95% CI, 0.06 to 3.91)	No significant improvement in fine wrinkles (RR 0.25; 95% CI, 0.04 to 1.52)	NR	No significant difference between the two treatments in roughness (RR 1.33; 95% CI, 0.58 to 3.09)	Participants' assessment showed no significant improvement in photodamage (RR 0.80; 95% CI, 0.52 to 1.24)

Vivida was taken for 90 days, there was significant improvement in fine wrinkles (RR 3.33; 95% CI, 1.14 to 9.75), mottled hyperpigmentation (RR 4.00; 95% CI, 1.01 to 15.81) in comparison with the group taking 380 mg Imedeen. Both studies on natural polysaccharides used intention-to-treat analysis by including all randomized participants in the analysis.

No adverse effects were reported in the Imedeen treatment group. However, in the Vivida treatment group, five women developed transient acneiform lesions during the first month of treatment.

The mechanism of action of natural polysaccharides is still unknown; previously reported data suggest a possible role in promoting synthesis of type III collagen in particular.

Current evidence does not provide any information regarding comparisons between topical applications and oral products or surgical interventions.

Key points

Topical treatment

- *Vitamins.* There is no good evidence to suggest that vitamins, especially topical ascorbic acid–containing creams, are beneficial for wrinkles, hyperpigmentation, and roughness associated with photoaged skin.

- *Tretinoin.* From the current evidence, it seems prudent to suggest that topical cream with 0.05% tretinoin when applied once daily for 24 weeks can improve fine wrinkles, mottled hyperpigmentation, and roughness of the skin, as well as overall facial photodamage. There is only limited evidence from one study to suggest that topical cream with 0.1% tretinoin when applied once daily for 40–48 weeks improves fine wrinkles, mottled hyperpigmentation, and overall photodamage to the face.

- *Tazarotene.* Limited evidence suggests that 0.1% tazarotene applied once daily for 24 weeks improves mottled hyperpigmentation. Limited evidence from two trials shows that the effectiveness of all concentrations of tazarotene was similar to that of tretinoin 0.05% in improving mottled hyperpigmentation.

- *Isotretinoin.* Evidence from just one RCT suggests that isotretinoin when applied once daily for 36 weeks is beneficial in improving mottled hyperpigmentation.

- *Natural polysaccharides.* There is only limited evidence from a small, within-patient study showing a trend towards improvement of shallow (< 1 mm) or moderate wrinkles (1 mm) and mottled hyperpigmentation with treatment using Vivida cream twice daily for 17 weeks. It is therefore unclear whether topical creams containing natural polysaccharides will provide any benefit.

- *Hydroxy acids.* The effectiveness of hydroxy acids is unclear, although two small studies of 8% glycolic and lactic acid showed a trend towards effectiveness.

Oral treatment

- *Natural polysaccharides.* There is only limited evidence, from two small studies, to suggest that oral natural polysaccharides improve wrinkles and mottled hyperpigmentation.

References

1 Nagashima H, Hanada K, Hashimoto I. Correlation of skin photo-type with facial wrinkle formation. *Photodermatol Photoimmunol Photomed* 1999;**15**:2–6.

2 Grether-Beck S, Wlaschek M, Krutmann J, Scharffetter-Kochanek K. Photodamage and photoageing: prevention and treatment. *J Dtsch Dermatol Ges* 2005;**3**:S19–25.

3 Guercio-Hauer C, Macfarlane DF, Deleo VA. Photodamage, photoaging and photoprotection of the skin. *Am Fam Physician* 1994;**50**:327–32.

4 Green AC. Premature ageing of the skin in a Queensland population. *Clin Exp Dermatol* 1991;**155**:473–8.

5 Memon AA, Tomenson JA, Bothwell J, Friedmann PS. Prevalence of solar damage and actinic keratosis in a Merseyside population. *Br J Dermatol* 2000;**142**:1154–9.

6 Maddin S, Lauharanta J, Agache P, Burrows L, Zultak M, Bulger L. Isotretinoin improves the appearance of photodamaged skin: results of a 36-week, multicenter, double-blind, placebo-controlled trial. *J Am Acad Dermatol* 2000;**42**:56–63.

7 Goh SH. The treatment of visible signs of senescence: the Asian experience. *Br J Dermatol* 1990;**122**(Suppl 35):105–9.

8 Griffiths CE, Goldfarb MT, Roulia V, *et al.* Topical tretinoin (retinoic acid) treatment of hyperpigmented lesions associated with photoaging in Chinese and Japanese patients: a vehicle-controlled trial. *J Am Acad Dermatol* 1994;**30**:76–84.

9 Harvey I, Frankel S, Marks R, Shalom D, Nolan-Farrell M. Non-melanoma skin cancer and solar keratoses, 1: methods and descriptive results of the South Wales Skin Cancer Study. *Br J Cancer* 1996;**74**:1302–7.

10 Fritschi L, Green A, Solomon PJ. Sun exposure in Australian adolescents. *J Am Acad Dermatol* 1992;**27**:25–8.

11 Crady D, Ernster V. Does cigarette smoking make you ugly and old? *Am J Dermatol* 1992;**135**:839–42.

12 Freiman A, Bird G, Metelitsa AI, Barankin B, Lauzon GJ. Cutaneous effects on smoking. *J Cutan Med Surg* 2004;**8**:415–23.

13 Affinito P, Palomba S, Sorrentino C, *et al.* Effects of post-menopausal hypoestrogenism on skin collagen. *Maturitas* 1999; **33**:239–47.

14 Gupta MA, Gupta AK. Photodamaged skin and quality of life: reasons for therapy. *J Dermatol Treat* 1996;**7**:261–4.

15 Green A, Williams G, Hart V, *et al.* Daily sunscreen application and betacarotene supplementation in prevention of basal-cell and squamous-cell carcinomas of the skin: a randomised controlled trial. *Lancet* 1999;**354**:723–9.

16 Green A, Battistutta D. Incidence and determinants of skin cancer in a high-risk Australian population. *Int J Cancer* 1990;**46**:356–61.

17 English DR, Armstrong BK, Kricker A, *et al.* Demographic characteristics, pigmentary and cutaneous risk factors for squamous cell carcinoma of the skin: a case–control study. *Int J Cancer* 1998;**76**:628–34.

18 Humphreys TR, Werth V, Dzxubow L, Kligman A. Treatment of photodamaged skin with trichloroacetic acid and topical tretinoin. *J Am Acad Dermatol* 1996;**34**:638–44.

19 Thibault PK, Wlodarczyk J, Wenck A. Double-blind randomized clinical trial on the effectiveness of a daily glycolic acid 5% formulation in the treatment of photoaging. *Dermatol Surg* 1998;**24**:573–8.

20 Darlington S, Williams G, Neale R, Frost C, Green A. A randomised controlled trial to assess sunscreen application and beta carotene supplementation in the prevention of solar keratoses. *Arch Dermatol* 2003;**139**:527–30.

21 Lowe NJ. An overview of ultraviolet radiation, sunscreens, and photo-induced dermatoses. *Dermatol Clin* 2006;**24**:9–17.

22 Griffiths CEM, Kang S, Ellis CN, *et al.* Two concentrations of topical tretinoin (retinoic acid) cause similar improvement of photoaging but different degrees of irritation. *Arch Dermatol* 1995;**131**:1037–44.

23 Roger G, Fuleihan NS. Facelift and adjunctive procedures in the treatment of photodamaged skin. In: Gilchrest BA, ed. *Photo-damage.* Cambridge, MA: Blackwell Science, 1995: 259–85.

24 Pierard GE, Pierard-Franchimont C. Comparative effect of short-term topical tretinoin and glycolic acid on mechanical properties of photodamaged facial skin in HRT-treated menopausal women. *Maturitas* 1996;**23**:273–7.

25 Pierard GE, Nikkels TN, Arrese JE, Pierard FC, Leveque JL. Dermo-epidermal stimulation elicited by a beta-lipohydroxyacid: a comparison with salicylic acid and *all-trans*-retinoic acid. *Dermatology* 1997;**194**:398–401.

26 Darr D, Combs S, Dunston S, Manning T, Pinnell S. Topical vitamin C protects porcine skin from ultraviolet radiation-induced damage. *Br J Dermatol* 1992;**127**:247–53.

27 Samuel M, Brooke RC, Hollis S, Griffiths CE. Interventions for photodamaged skin. *Cochrane Database Syst Rev* 2005;(**1**):CD001782.

28 Traikovich SS. Use of topical ascorbic acid and its effects on photodamaged skin topography. *Arch Otolaryngol Head Neck Surg* 1999;**125**:1091–8.

29 Kligman AM, Grove GL, Hirose R, Leyden JJ. Topical tretinoin for photodamaged skin. *J Am Acad Dermatol* 1986;**15**:836–59.

30 Leyden JJ, Grove GL, Grove MJ, et al. Treatment of photodamaged facial skin with topical tretinoin. *J Am Acad Dermatol* 1989;**21**:638–44.

31 Lever L, Kumar P, Marks R. Topical retinoic acid for treatment of solar damage. *Br J Dermatol* 1990;**122**:91–8.

32 Barel AO, Delune M, Clarys P, et al. Treatment of photodamaged facial skin with topical tretinoin: a blinded, vehicle-controlled half-side study. *Nouv Dermatol* 1995;**14**:585–591.

33 Lowe PM, Woods J, Lewis A, et al. Topical tretinoin improves the appearance of photodamaged skin. *Australas J Dermatol* 1994;**35**:1–9.

34 Weinstein GD, Nigra TP, Pochi PE, et al. Topical tretinoin for treatment of photodamaged skin. *Arch Dermatol* 1991;**127**:659–65.

35 Olsen EA, Katz HI, Levine N, et al. Tretinoin emollient cream: a new therapy for photodamaged skin. *J Am Acad Dermatol* 1992;**26**:215–24.

36 Andreano J, Bergfeld WF, Medendorp SV. Tretinoin emollient cream 0.01% for the treatment of photoaged skin. *Cleve Clin J Med* 1993;**60**:49–55.

37 Nyirady J, Bergfeld W, Ellis C, et al. Tretinoin cream 0.02% for the treatment of photodamaged facial skin: a review of 2 double-blind clinical studies. *Cutis* 2001;**68**:135–43.

38 Nyirady J, Gisslen H, Lehmann P, et al. Safety and efficacy of long-term use of tretinoin cream 0.02% for treatment of photodamage: review of clinical trials. *Cosmet Dermatol* 2003;**3**:49–57.

39 Weiss JS, Ellis CN, Headington JT, Tincoff T, Hamilton TA, Voorhees JJ. Topical tretinoin improves photo-aged skin. A double-blind vehicle-controlled study. *JAMA* 1988;**259**:527–32.

40 Salagnac V, Leonard F, Lacharriere Y, et al. Topical treatment of actinic aging with vitamin A acid at various concentrations. *Rev Fr Gynecol Obstet* 1991;**86**:458–60.

41 Kang S, Leyden JJ, Lowe NJ, et al. Tazarotene cream for the treatment of facial photodamage. *Arch Dermatol* 2001;**137**:1597–604.

42 Phillips TJ, Gottlieb AB, Leyden JJ, et al. Efficacy of 0.1% tazarotene cream for the treatment of photodamage. *Arch Dermatol* 2002;**138**:1486–93.

43 Lowe NJ, Gifford M, Tanghetti E, et al. Tazarotene 0.1% cream versus tretinoin 0.05% emollient cream in the treatment of photodamaged facial skin: a multicenter, double-blind, randomized, parallel-group study. *J Cosmet Laser Ther* 2004;**6**:79–85.

44 Maddin S, Lauharanta J, Agache P, et al. Isotretinoin improves the appearance of photodamaged skin: results of a 36-week, multicenter, double blind, placebo-controlled trial. *J Am Acad Dermatol* 2000;**42**:56–63.

45 Lassus A, Eskelinen A, Santalahti J. The effect of Vivida cream as compared with placebo cream in the treatment of sun-damaged or age-damaged facial skin. *J Int Med Res* 1992;**20**:381–91.

46 Stiller MJ, Bartolone J, Stern R, et al. Topical 8% glycolic acid and 8% L-lactic acid creams for the treatment of photodamaged skin. *Arch Dermatol* 1996;**132**:631–6.

47 Piacquadio D, Dobry M, Hunt S, Andree C, Grove G, Hollenbach KA. Short contact 70% glycolic acid peels as a treatment for photodamaged skin: a pilot study. *Dermatol Surg* 1996;**22**:449–52.

48 Eskelinen A, Santalahti J. Special natural cartilage polysaccharides for the treatment of sun-damaged skin in females. *J Int Med Res* 1992;**20**:99–105.

49 Distante F, Scalise F, Rona C, et al. Oral fish cartilage polysaccharides in the treatment of photoageing: biophysical findings. *Int J Cosmet Sci* 2002;**24**:81–7.

50 Eskelinen A, Santalahti J. Natural cartilage polysaccharides for the treatment of sun-damaged skin in females: a double-blind comparison of Vivida and Imedeen. *J Int Med Res* 1992;**20**:227–33.

34 Melanocytic nevi

Paolo Carli, Camilla Salvini

Background

Definition

Melanocytic nevi are benign proliferations of melanocytes located at different skin levels. Acquired nevi are generally smaller than 1 cm, whereas congenital ones are usually larger. Pigmentation in different shades of brown can range from a brown-yellowish to brown-blackish color; sometimes —as in mature cellular nevi—they can be skin-colored.

Classification

Melanocytic nevi, either congenital or acquired, can be classified relative to the histological location of melanocytes into:

- *Junctional nevus*, if the melanocytes are located at the dermoepidermal junction.
- *Dermal nevus*, if the melanocytes are in the dermis.
- *Compound nevus*, if the melanocytes are at both of the above locations.

A new clinical classification for acquired nevi has recently been proposed, based on dividing them into common and atypical nevi; this approach is particularly useful for stratifying the risk of melanoma. *Common nevi* are neoformations with a maximum diameter of 6 mm, with symmetrical shape and with an homogeneous pigmentation. *Atypical nevi* instead have a larger diameter and at least two of the following parameters: irregular borders (edges) and/or not well defined, asymmetric shape, irregular pigmentation, erythema, and accentuation of the cutaneous design (Figure 34.1).[1] It is also possible to diagnose an atypical nevus when some or all of the "ABCD" criteria for melanoma diagnosis are present (*a*symmetry, irregular *b*orders, heterogeneous *c*olor, *d*iameter larger than 6 mm).[2] Using this definition, it can sometimes be very difficult to distinguish between atypical nevi and early melanoma, even with the adoption of recent noninvasive techniques

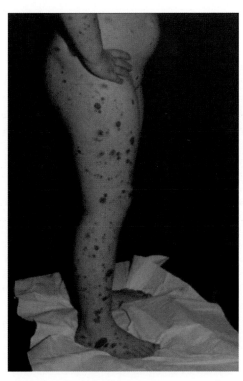

Figure 34.1 The leg of a chid with numerous common and atypical nevi.

such as dermoscopy.[3] In doubtful cases of this type, the lesions should be removed for histological verification.

A congenital nevus is a "melanocytic nevus that has existed since one's birth"; however, a lesion with the same clinical and pathological characteristics as a congenital nevus can also appear within the first 2 years of life. In this case it is called "nevus tardive."[4]

Congenital nevi are normally classified in accordance with diameter into small (< 1.5 cm), medium (1.5–19.9 cm), and large (> 20 cm); the so-called giant nevi are congenital nevi that involve entire anatomic areas (Figure 34.2).[5]

In congenital nevi, melanocytes are typically located on the lowest two-thirds of the dermis. Occasionally, they

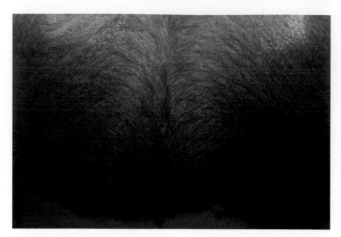

Figure 34.2 A large congenital nevus of the trunk in a girl (13 years old). The lesion is checked every 6 months.

extend into the subcutaneous tissue, with isolated cells or groups of cells within the reticular dermis collagen fibers, with a tendency to be located around cutaneous appendages. However, many congenital nevi do not show these histopathological characteristics, resulting in a picture not dissimilar to that of acquired nevi; this happens most frequently with small congenital nevi.[6]

Incidence/prevalence and etiological factors

In people with the same complexion (i.e., similar skin and eye color and ability to tan), the average nevus density varies in accordance with sun exposure. A study on English twins reported that those who spent at least 410 days by the sea in sunny places had 41 nevi/m² on average, whereas those who did not expose themselves at all only had 24 nevi/m². Larger acquired nevi (≥ 5 mm) were more common in boys than in girls.[7]

A multicenter Italian study on 3127 13–14-year-olds found a higher nevus density in body areas usually exposed to the sun (i.e., face or neck), becoming lower in density in areas of intermittent exposure, and with the lowest density in areas never exposed. A positive correlation was also reported between the number of sunburns and nevus density.[8]

Genetic factors are also an important predictor of nevus development. A recent study based on 221 pairs of teenage twins suggested that genetic factors accounted for about 65% of nevus development, involving factors associated with eye color (7%), hair color (6%), and skin color (1%); the remaining 51% appears to be due to other as yet unidentified genetic factors.[9]

A multivariate analysis reported that the use of sunscreens does not prevent the development of melanocytic nevi; however, a negative correlation between the amount of clothing used and nevi counts has been found.[10] Sunscreens are discussed in more detail in Chapter 26.

It has been estimated that 1% of newborns have a congenital nevus of any size, whereas giant congenital nevi are very rare. One study including over 500 000 newborns has shown that only one baby in 20 000 has a nevus with a diameter larger than 10 cm.[11]

Disease associations

Various disease associations have been reported with congenital nevi, particularly the larger ones. Leptomeningeal melanocytosis (associated with congenital nevi on the head and neck), meningomyelocele, and spina bifida (associated with nevi in the lumbosacral area) are just some of these associations.

There are also reports in the literature of an association between nevi and ocular malformations and glaucoma, auricular malformation, angiomatous lesions, bone atrophy, and neurofibromatosis.[6]

Prognosis

The natural history of melanocytic nevi is still not fully understood. For acquired nevi, an initial development stage is observed within the first two to three decades of life, with an increase in nevus density afterwards, followed by a plateau. Then, in older age, there appears to be a density reduction, probably due to spontaneous regression of some nevi.

Melanocytic nevi can sometimes regress spontaneously during childhood or adolescence. This premature regression is commonly due to immunological mechanisms, as observed when a ring of depigmentation occurs around the nevus (halo or Sutton's nevus).

It is worth mentioning that some varieties of nevi arise at specific ages. For example, the Spitz nevus typically develops in childhood, while Reed's spindle-cell nevus typically occurs in women in their thirties.

Diagnosis

Clinical examination

Most nevi are easy for expert dermatologists to diagnose by clinical examination alone;[12] whenever there are doubtful cases (differential diagnosis with melanoma), dermatoscopy (also known as dermoscopy or epiluminescence microscopy) can be performed in order to increase the diagnostic accuracy. However, dermoscopy is not 100% accurate, and if there is any remaining diagnostic doubt, an excisional biopsy followed by histological examination is recommended. An incisional biopsy is sometimes carried out if the lesions are very large.

Dermoscopic examination

Dermoscopy is a noninvasive technique that enables the observer to examine some morphological characteristics of the lesion that are not visible with the naked eye. In expert hands, dermoscopy improves the diagnostic accuracy for nearly all pigmented skin lesions in comparison with naked-eye examination.[13,14]

Digital dermoscopy also makes it possible to record digital images of specific lesions. This may help in investigating the natural history of a lesion for research purposes, or to follow up a doubtful lesion in order to identify any early malignant behavior. However, the extent to which digital follow-up of a doubtful lesion should be considered an advisable procedure is still a matter of debate.[15] The use of digital follow-up instead of immediate excisional biopsy is associated with a small risk of leaving a melanoma unexcised, with serious consequences. The risk can increase if patients do not comply with regular follow-up surveillance.[16,17]

With regard to the impact of adding dermoscopy to melanoma screening, one controlled randomized trial showed that dermoscopy is associated with a significant reduction in the biopsy rate in comparison with a control group undergoing conventional naked-eye examination only (OR 0.54; 95% CI, 0.30 to 0.88).[15] It is therefore possible that large-scale use of dermoscopy in melanoma screening may be associated with increased specificity in the diagnosis of melanoma, with fewer false-positive cases and consequently fewer surgical excisions for the purpose of diagnostic verification.

Relevant outcomes

There are two main reasons for removing a melanocytic lesion. The first is to prevent a possible melanoma when there is a doubtful lesion, and the second is to relieve discomfort (e.g., a mole rubbing a bra strap) or for cosmetic purposes. Removing clinically banal nevi in order to reduce the incidence of melanoma is disputable practice; the risk of malignant degeneration of a nevus is in fact extremely low.

Methods of search

The databases of the Cochrane Library, Medline, and Embase between 1951 and April 2006 were searched for articles that (a) studied the relationship between nevi and (b) the risk of subsequent melanoma in congenital nevi of various sizes. The search was carried out by combining the following key words: melanocytic nevi, dermoscopy, epiluminescence microscopy, skin self-examination and epidemiology, case–control, meta-analysis.

Questions

What is the risk of a melanocytic nevus developing into a melanoma?

It has been suggested that because the high frequency of melanocytic nevi contrasts with the low incidence rate of nevus-associated melanoma (about 20–30% of all melanomas),[18] the transformation of an acquired nevus into a melanoma should be considered a very rare event, with an estimate of about one nevus out of 200 000 per year for people younger than 40 years of age and one nevus out of 33 000 per year for men over 60 years of age.[19] Little is known about the role of malignant transformation of a preexisting nevus in determining the increased risk of melanoma in people with many nevi. According to a case–control study that compared the risk factor profile of patients with nevus-associated melanoma (cases) with that of patients with melanoma *de novo* (controls), a large number of nevi were associated with a significantly higher risk for melanoma in the former than in the latter group of patients.[20] A history of many sunburns was more strongly associated with nevus-associated melanoma than with melanoma *de novo*. This finding lends support to the role of sunburn in increasing the risk of neoplastic progression of nevus cells. These results are based on a single study and need to be confirmed by further independent studies.

With regard to congenital nevi, their natural history appears to be strongly correlated with the lesion size. A prospective analysis of 80 children affected by large congenital nevi (diameter > 20 cm) who were followed up for 5 years showed a malignant degeneration rate of 3.8%.[21]

Subsequent research on 92 children (maximum age 3 years) with a large congenital nevus who were followed up for 5.4 years reported the occurrence of three melanomas, all of which were located in extracutaneous areas (the central nervous system and retroperitoneal region). This finding is explained by the possible existence of melanocytic hamartomas in noncutaneous areas such as the meninges and retina in some people with giant congenital nevi.

According to these scanty data on giant melanocytic nevi, the risk of developing a melanoma within the first 5 years of life is 4.5% (9.5 CI, 0% to 9.3%), with a standardized incidence ratio over the expected number of the overall population equal to 239.[22]

More controversial than giant nevi is the behavior of nevi with a diameter less than 20 cm. We could not find any reliable evidence assessing the rate of malignant transformation in such lesions. Some authors suggest that malignant transformation of such medium-sized lesions never occurs before adulthood.[21]

Even more controversial is the correlation between the risk of melanoma and small congenital nevi (< 1.5 cm). Only prospective cohort studies, yet to be undertaken, will be able to provide reliable data on the malignant transformation rate of small and intermediate-sized nevi.

How should a patient with an isolated congenital nevus be managed?

There are no widely accepted guidelines on how to deal with congenital nevi[23]—which is not surprising, given the lack of accurate epidemiological evidence regarding their rate of malignant transformation. If strongly required by the patient, the prophylactic removal of a small congenital nevus can be carried out without technical problems.

For medium-sized congenital nevi, the risk of malignant transformation is probably significant, but has not been precisely estimated.[21] However, medium-sized nevi are technically difficult to remove because of their size, and when they are removed they can leave a large and cosmetically unacceptable scar. The logical consequence of this dilemma is that this type of congenital nevus is often managed by regular visits to the doctor, supplemented by instructions being given to parents or to patients to check the lesion frequently.

The management of giant melanocytic nevi poses many difficulties, and the timing of surgery, if contemplated, may be important. Some authors suggest neonatal curettage.[24] The curettage must be carried out during the first month of life, when it is easy to identify the cleavage plane between the nevus and the normal tissue below. However, it is difficult to achieve histological clearance of the nevus, and a risk of malignant transformation can persist. Some authors have suggested that it is easier to identify malignant transformation after curettage than after conventional surgery, because new pigmented lesions are easier to visualize on "normal" skin after curettage.[25]

Unfortunately, while there is an increased risk of melanoma in people with large congenital nevi, there is currently no scientific evidence that traditional surgical intervention reduces the risk of melanoma.[26] The cosmetic effects of extensive surgery and grafting for giant melanocytic nevi in early life can be disappointing and may be complicated by painful scars, through which deeper melanocytic nevi may emerge after many years.

The presence of a larger congenital nevus, often on the upper side of the trunk and the head and associated with leptomeningeal melanocytosis, is a contraindication to surgical removal of the lesion, as the risk of melanoma persists in these areas.[3]

How should a patient with multiple melanocytic nevi be managed?

There is a close correlation between the number of mela-

nocytic nevi and the risk of melanoma; according to one of the numerous case–control studies reported in the literature, the odds ratio (OR) of melanoma associated with more than 45 nevi is 9.7 (95% CI, 5.4 to 17.4).[27] There is therefore an argument that people with approximately 50 nevi should visit a dermatologist at least once a year for surveillance purposes.[27] The presence of atypical nevi, which are often present in people with numerous common nevi and phototype I or II, is another risk factor for melanoma that may require regular surveillance.[28]

One approach is to teach such patients how to carry out self-examination of the skin. Self-examination allows features such as changes in shape and color to be identified at an early stage. One multicenter Italian survey of melanoma cases suggested that this procedure was associated with a reduction in the risk of late diagnosis of melanoma (thickness > 1 mm), even after adjustment for confounding factors such as sex, age, and anatomic area of the lesion (OR 0.70; 95% CI, 0.50 to 0.97).[29] Berwick et al. conducted a case–control study to investigate the relationship between skin self-examination and a reduced risk of fatal melanoma. They found that self-examination is associated with a reduced risk of melanoma incidence (OR 0.66; 95% CI, 0.44 to 0.99) and with a possible reduced risk of advanced disease among melanoma patients (unadjusted risk ratio 0.58; 95% CI, 0.31 to 1.11).[30]

There is no good evidence to suggest that trauma to benign nevi will increase the risk of malignant transformation. Moreover, stratification of nevi on the basis of their risk of transformation is not currently possible. Indeed, there is no good evidence that nevi that have an "atypical" appearance from a clinical point of view should be considered precursors of melanoma. Some clinically atypical nevi can show histological atypia (formerly defined as "dysplastic nevi"). However, even banal nevi can show histological atypia, since the correlation between clinical and histological atypia in nevi is poor.[31]

The approach known as the "mole-mapping technique"—i.e., recording images of all melanocytic lesions on the body and subsequently following them up to identify early possible malignant change—is a controversial procedure.[15,16] It is probably useful for periodic follow-up of people who are at high risk of melanoma. There is no evidence of any benefit of this technique, in comparison with examining the patient without analyzing the baseline characteristics of all the nevi, in other situations.

Skin self-examination (SSE)

How commonly is SSE done and what factors predict regular SSE?

Since skin self-examination may be useful in reducing the rate of late presentation of melanoma,[29] it is possible that promoting SSE in the general population might reduce the overall mortality from melanoma. The American Cancer Society recommends a monthly SSE, a clinical skin examination every 3 years for those over the age of 20, and a clinical examination every year for those over the age of 40.

Little is known about how many people currently perform SSE. In an Australian study, SSE within the previous 12 months was reported by more than 25% of healthy people contacted by means of a telephone interview.[32]

In a study in Connecticut, SSE was noted in 13.2% of melanoma patients and in 17.5% of controls.[30] In an Italian study, 40.5% of people visiting a pigmented-lesion clinic reported that they performed SSE.[33] The higher rates of SSE in the latter study are probably explained by the fact that the participants were examined at a specialized pigmented-lesion clinic aimed at providing melanoma screening and follow-up for those at increased risk of melanoma.

An important point is the frequency of SSE. In a random survey of the adult population in Rhode Island, USA, Weinstock *et al.* found that only 9% of recalled individuals performed a thorough skin examination at least once every few months.[34] Oliveria *et al.* found that 6.0% of men and 7.0% of women performed "rigorous" skin self-examinations.[35]

It is important to identify which factors increase the likelihood of an individual performing skin self-examination, as it may help in refining educational strategies for melanoma prevention. Oliveria *et al.* found that skin awareness was a strong factor associated with skin self-examination for both women and men (OR 4.65 in men; 95% CI, 2.11 to 11.46; OR 2.53 in women; 95% CI, 0.91 to 8.31). For women, variables significantly associated with SSE included previous benign biopsy or the presence of an abnormal mole (OR 4.22; 95% CI, 1.72 to 12.01). In men, a family history of cancer (OR 2.02; 95% CI, 1.02 to 4.13), physician examination (OR 3.44; 95% CI, 1.77 to 6.94), and a change in diet to reduce the cancer risk (OR 2.17; 95% CI, 1.12 to 4.23) increased the likelihood of skin self-examination.[35] The Italian study used a multivariate model that adjusted for eye color, phototype, large numbers of common and atypical melanocytic nevi, sunscreen use, and having had a previous examination and having received a leaflet explaining SSE. The study found that in men, the only variable significantly associated with SSE was a report of having received a leaflet explaining SSE (OR 3.02; 95% CI, 1.24 to 7.38). For women, it was a report of having already had a previous consultation at a pigmented-lesion clinic (OR 4.84; 95% CI, 1.57 to 14.93); the latter may be secondary to the explanations and advice about skin cancer prevention usually provided at a previous visit.[33]

Weinstock *et al.*[36] evaluated the impact of participation in a mole-mapping program on the performance of thorough skin self-examination. They found that 45% of those who were not performing skin self-examination before participation reported performing it after receiving their images. However, 30% had never used the images to assist them in the self-examination. This study has important limitations

—there was a small number of participants and the sample chosen only included a high-risk population.

How accurate is skin self-examination?

In a cohort study of people at high risk of melanoma, Feit *et al.* showed that 32% of the malignancies were diagnosed because patients reported concern about the lesions—suggesting that patients were competent in identifying suspicious lesions using SSE.[37]

Other papers confirm that most melanomas are discovered by the patient: 42–47% of men and 59–69% of women with melanomas reported that their melanomas were self-detected.[38–40]

In a recent population-based study including 3772 Queensland residents with melanoma, McPherson *et al.*[41] found that 44.0% of the patients reported first noticing the melanoma themselves, whereas 25.3% of the melanomas were first noticed by a doctor, 18.6% by partners, and 12.1% by other laypersons (including other relatives, friends, and service people). In comparison with men, a greater proportion of women detected their melanomas themselves (57.1% vs. 33.8%), whereas men had a greater proportion of partner-detected melanomas (26.7% vs. 8.1%). Most commonly, the signs and symptoms reported by patients who are later found to have melanoma are changes in the color, size, or shape of a lesion, or an irritation or itch; they also report that the lesion looked different from other spots.[41]

The sensitivity of SSE for certain risk factors for melanoma was studied by Gruber *et al.*[42] They identified freckles, palpable nevi, and large nevi as potential risk factors for the development of cutaneous malignant melanoma. The sensitivity of self-reporting of the number of freckles on the right forearm was found to be 88%. The sensitivity was 63% for detecting one or more palpable arm nevi and 68% for detecting one nevus larger than 5 mm in diameter on the entire body.

Muhn *et al.*[43] studied the sensitivity of detecting an artificial increase in the size (0, 2, or 4 mm in diameter) of a preexistent nevus on the back using SSE. The patients examined their backs with a mirror before and after the manipulation of the mole. At this point, the patient was asked to determine which mole, if any, had been changed. They found that the sensitivity for detecting a 2-mm change was approximately 58% (95% CI, 49% to 68%). The sensitivity for detecting a 4-mm change was approximately 75% (95% CI, 66% to 83%). The specificity of the test (i.e., the ability to detect no change) was approximately 62% (95% CI, 53% to 72%). These results relate to a difficult area for body examination (on the back) and are thus likely to represent the worst-case scenario for the sensitivity and specificity of SSE for detecting changes in the size of a nevus, although this group of patients were highly selected and motivated. Another limitation of this study is that it only assessed changes in the size of the nevus, whereas it is a combination of changes in shape, thickness, and color, as well as the development of new moles, that allows patients to detect a malignant lesion.

A recent study by Oliveria *et al.*[44] investigated the sensitivity and specificity of SSE for detecting new and changing moles with or without the aid of baseline digital photographs in patients with dysplastic nevi. They found that the sensitivity and specificity of SSE for detecting both new and altered moles without photography were 60.2% and 96.2%, respectively, whereas SSE with photography showed significant improvements in diagnostic accuracy, with a sensitivity and specificity of 72.4% and 98.4%, respectively.

Weinstock *et al.*[45] tested the ability to detect an additional 5-mm pigmented lesion on the back. To improve the accuracy of SSE, they required half of the participants to complete a mole-mapping diagram (intervention group). They found that 33% of the control group and 52% of the intervention group ($P = 0.06$) gave accurate assessments. Participants in the intervention group were better able to identify the added lesion or lesions ($P = 0.01$).

SSE is associated with a reduced incidence of advanced melanoma, but it is prone to error in detecting early melanoma changes. Improving the accuracy of SSE may therefore be important in allowing detection of melanoma at an earlier stage and thereby reducing the mortality.

Key points

- Nevus density is related to sun exposure and genetic factors.
- Dermoscopy improves the diagnostic accuracy for nearly all pigmented skin lesions in comparison with naked-eye examination and may reduce the rate of unnecessary biopsies when used for melanoma screening.
- Nevi may be surgically removed because of discomfort/appearance, or to exclude melanoma or prevent melanoma from occurring.
- There is a link between an increased number of melanocytic nevi and the risk of subsequent malignant melanoma.
- The rate of malignant degeneration of small congenital nevi (< 1.5 cm) is unknown and is difficult to estimate because of their similarity to acquired melanocytic nevi.
- The risk of melanoma developing in medium-sized congenital nevi (1.5–20.0 cm) is only hypothesized on the base of case reports.
- Congenital nevi with a diameter > 20 cm have an approximately 4% risk of melanoma developing.
- The stratification of the risk of neoplastic transformation of acquired melanocytic nevus based on the nevus morphology has not yet been adequately established.
- Clinically atypical nevi are a risk factor for melanoma.
- Removal of giant melanocytic nevi may not be associated with a reduced risk of melanomas, which may appear in noncutaneous sites, and surgical procedures such as grafting are often complicated by scarring and subsequent breakthrough pigmentation.

- Recording images of all the melanocytic lesions on the body for subsequent follow up is a controversial procedure, for which there is at present no evidence that it reduces the risk of late diagnosis of melanoma.
- Self-examination in people with large numbers of moles probably reduces the risk of late diagnosis of melanoma (thickness > 1 mm)
- Skin awareness as a result of a family history of melanoma, previous biopsy of a mole, attendance at a pigmented-lesion clinic, or the provision of written information about melanomas, is associated with an increased frequency of skin self-examination.
- Around 50% of the population probably detect their own melanomas—women more frequently than men.
- Asking patients to self-report the number of freckles or palpable moles on their right forearm has been shown to be a reliable method of assessing the melanoma risk.
- Using baseline photographs and mole-mapping techniques may improve the effectiveness of skin self-examination in picking up melanoma changes.

Editor's note

It is with sadness that we report that Dr Carli passed away in 2007 soon after completing his chapter contribution to this book.

References

1 Carli P, Biggeri A, Giannotti B. Malignant melanoma in Italy: risks associated with common and clinically atypical melanocytic nevi. *J Am Acad Dermatol* 1995;**32**:734–9.
2 Marghoob AA, Kopf AW, Rigel DS, *et al*. Risk of cutaneous malignant melanoma in patients with "classic" atypical-mole syndrome: a case–control study. *Arch Dermatol* 1994;**130**:993–8.
3 Stolz W, Riemann A, Cognetta AB, *et al*. ABCD rule of dermatoscopy: a new practical method for early recognition of melanoma. *Eur J Dermatol* 1994;**4**:521–7.
4 Tannous ZS, Mihm MC, Sober AJ, *et al*. Congenital melanocytic nevi: clinical and histopathologic features, risk of melanoma, and clinical management. *J Am Acad Dermatol* 2005;**52**:197–203.
5 Kopf AW, Bart RS, Hennessey P. Congenital nevocytic nevi and malignant melanomas. *Am Acad Dermatol* 1979;**1**:123–30.
6 Zaal LH, Mooi WJ, Sillevis Smitt JH, van der Horst CMAM. Classification of congenital melanocytic naevi and malignant melanoma transformation: a review of the literature. *Br J Plast Surg* 2004;**57**:707–19.
7 Autier P, Boniol M, Severi G, *et al*. Sex differences in numbers of nevi on the body sites of young European children: implications for the etiology of cutaneous melanoma. *Cancer Epidemiol Biomarkers Prev* 2004;**13**:2203–5.
8 Carli P, Naldi L, Lovati S, *et al*. The density of melanocytic nevi correlates with constitutional variables and history of sunburns: a prevalence study among Italian schoolchildren. *Int J Cancer* 2002;**101**:375–9.

9 Wachsmuth RC, Turner F, Barrett JH, *et al.* The effect of sun exposure in determining nevus density in UK adolescent twins. *J Invest Dermatol* 2005;**124**:56–62.

10 Bauer J, Buttner P, Wiecker TS, *et al.* Effect of sunscreen and clothing on the number of melanocytic nevi in 1812 German children attending day care. *Am J Epidemiol* 2005;**161**:620–7.

11 Castilla EE, da Graca DM, Orioli-Parreiras IM. Epidemiology of congenital pigmented naevi, 1: incidence rates and relative frequencies. *Br J Dermatol* 1981;**104**:307–15.

12 Whited JD, Grichnik JM. Does this patient have a mole or a melanoma? *JAMA* 1998; **279**:696–701.

13 Kittler H, Pehamberger H, Wolff K, Binder M. Diagnostic accuracy of dermoscopy. *Lancet Oncol* 2002;**3**:159–65.

14 Bafounta ML, Beauchet A, Aegerter P, Saiag P. Is dermoscopy (epiluminescence microscopy) useful for the diagnosis of melanoma? *Arch Dermatol* 2001;**137**:1343–50.

15 Carli P, de Giorgi V, Chiarugi A, *et al.* Addition of dermoscopy to conventional naked-eye examination in melanoma screening: a randomized study. *J Am Acad Dermatol* 2004;**50**:683–9.

16 Kittler H, Binder M. Risks and benefits of sequential imaging of melanocytic skin lesions in patients with multiple atypical nevi. *Arch Dermatol* 2001;**137**:1590–5.

17 Schiffner R, Wilde O, Schiffner-Rohe J, Stolz W. Difference between real and perceived power of dermoscopical methods for detection of malignant melanoma. *Eur J Dermatol* 2003;**13**:288–93.

18 Massi D, Carli P, Franchi A, Santucci M. Naevus-associated melanomas: cause or chance? *Melanoma Res* 1999;**9**:85–91.

19 Tsao H, Beona C, Goggins W, Quinn T. The transformation rate of moles (melanocytic nevi) into cutaneous melanoma: a population-based estimate. *Arch Dermatol* 2003;**139**:282–8.

20 Carli P, Massi D, Santucci M, *et al.* Cutaneous melanoma histologically associated with a nevus and melanoma de novo have a different profile of risk: results from a case–control study. *J Am Acad Dermatol* 1999;**40**:549–57.

21 Ruiz-Maldonado R, Tamayo L, Laterza AM, *et al.* Giant pigmented nevi: clinical, histopathologic, and therapeutic considerations. *J Pediatr* 1992;**120**:906–11.

22 Marghoob AA, Schoenbach SP, Kopf AW, *et al.* Large congenital melanocytic nevi and the risk for the development of malignant melanoma: a prospective study. *Arch Dermatol* 1996;**132**:170–5.

23 Kanzler MH. Management of large congenital melanocytic nevi: art versus science. *J Am Acad Dermatol* 2006;**54**:874–6.

24 De Raeve LE, Claes A, Ruiter DJ, van Muijen GN, Roseeuw D, van Kempen LC. Distinct phenotypic changes between the superficial and deep component of giant congenital melanocytic naevi: a rationale for curettage. *Br J Dermatol* 2006;**154**:485–92.

25 De Raeve LE, Roseeuw DI. Curettage of giant congenital melanocytic nevi in neonates: a decade later. *Arch Dermatol* 2002;**138**:943–7.

26 Marghoob AA, Agero AL, Benvenuto-Andrade C, *et al.* Large congenital melanocytic nevi, risk of cutaneous melanoma, and prophylactic surgery. *J Am Acad Dermatol* 2006;**54**:868–70.

27 Naldi L, Imberti GL, Parazzini F, *et al.* Pigmentary traits, modalities of sun reaction, history of sunburns, and melanocytic nevi as risk factors for cutaneous malignant melanoma in the Italian population: results of a collaborative case–control study. *Cancer* 2000;**88**:2703–10.

28 Carli P, Biggeri A, Nardini P, *et al.* Sun exposure and large numbers of common and atypical melanocytic naevi: an analytical study in a southern European population. *Br J Dermatol* 1998;**138**:422–5.

29 Carli P, De Giorgi V, Palli D, *et al.* Dermatologist detection and skin self-examination are associated with thinner melanomas: results from a survey of the Italian Multidisciplinary Group on Melanoma. *Arch Dermatol* 2003;**139**:607–12.

30 Berwick M, Begg CB, Fine JA, Roush GC, Barnhill RL. Screening for cutaneous melanoma by skin self-examination. *J Natl Cancer Inst* 1996;**88**:17–23.

31 Klein LJ, Barr RJ. Histologic atypia in clinically benign nevi: a prospective study. *J Am Acad Dermatol* 1990;**22**:275–82.

32 Aitken JF, Janda M, Lowe JB, Elwood M, Ring IT, Youl PH, Firman DW. Prevalence of whole-body skin self-examination in a population at high risk for skin cancer (Australia). *Cancer Causes Control* 2004;**15**:453–63.

33 Carli P, Nardini P, Chiarugi A, *et al.* Predictors of skin self-examination in subjects attending a pigmented lesion clinic in Italy. *J Eur Acad Dermatol Venereol* 2007;**21**:95–9.

34 Weinstock MA, Martin RA, Risica PM, *et al.* Thorough skin examination for the early detection of melanoma. *Am J Prev Med* 1999;**17**:169–75.

35 Oliveria AS, Christos PJ, Halpern AC, Fine JA, Barnhill RL, Berwick M. Evaluation of factors associated with skin self-examination. *Cancer Epidemiol Biomarkers Prev* 1999;**8**:971–8.

36 Weinstock MA, Nguyen FQ, Martin RA. Enhancing skin self-examination with imaging: evaluation of a mole-mapping program. *J Cutan Med Surg* 2004;**8**:1–5.

37 Feit NE, Dusza SW, Marghoob AA. Melanomas detected with the aid of total cutaneous photography. *Br J Dermatol* 2004;**150**:706–14.

38 Koh HK, Miller DR, Geller AC, *et al.* Who discovers melanoma? Patterns from a population-based survey. *J Am Acad Dermatol* 1992;**26**:914–9.

39 Brady MS, Oliveria SA, Christos PJ, *et al.* Patterns of detection in patients with cutaneous melanoma. *Cancer* 2000;**89**:342–7.

40 Richard MA, Grob JJ, Avril MF, *et al.* Delays in diagnosis and melanoma prognosis, 1: the role of patients. *Int J Cancer* 2000;**89**:271–9.

41 McPherson M, Elwood M, English DR, Baade PD, Youl PH Aitken JF. Presentation and detection of invasive melanoma in a high-risk population *J Am Acad Dermatol* 2006;**54**:783–92.

42 Gruber SB, Roush GC, Barnhill RL. Sensitivity and specificity of self-examination for cutaneous malignant melanoma risk factors. *Am J Prev Med* 1993;**9**:50–4.

43 Muhn CY, From L, Glied M. Detection of artificial changes in mole size by skin self-examination. *J Am Acad Dermatol* 2000;**42**:754–9.

44 Oliveria SA, Chau D, Christos PJ, *et al.* Diagnostic accuracy of patients in performing skin self-examination and the impact of photography. *Arch Dermatol* 2004;**140**:57–62.

45 Chiu V, Won E, Malik M, Weinstock MA. The use of mole-mapping diagrams to increase skin self-examination accuracy. *J Am Acad Dermatol* 2006;**55**:245–50.

IIIc Infective skin diseases and exanthems

Hywel Williams and Thomas Diepgen, Editors

35 Local treatments for cutaneous warts

Sam Gibbs

Background

Definition

Viral warts are extremely common and are benign and usually self-limiting. Infection of epidermal cells with the human papillomavirus (HPV) results in cell proliferation and a thickened, warty papule on the skin. The most common sites involved are the hands and feet, but any area of skin can be infected (Figure 35.1).

Incidence/prevalence

There are few reliable, population-based data on the incidence and prevalence of common warts. The prevalence probably varies widely between different age groups, populations, and periods of time. Two large population-based studies found prevalence rates of 0.84% and 12.9%, respectively.[1,2] The prevalence rates are highest in children and young adults; studies in school populations have shown prevalence rates of 12% in 4–6-year-olds[3] and 24% in 16–18-year-olds.[4]

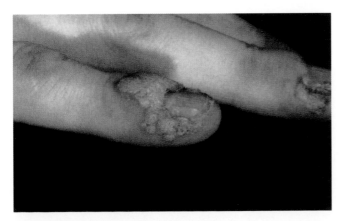

Figure 35.1 Ordinary viral warts on the fingers.

Etiology and risk factors

Warts are caused by HPV, of which there are over 70 different types. Viral warts are most common at sites of trauma such as the hands and feet, and lesions probably result from inoculation of virus into minimally damaged areas of epithelium. Plantar warts are often acquired from common bare-foot areas,[5] and severe hand warts are an occupational risk for butchers and meat handlers.[6] Genital warts are also common and are frequently sexually transmitted; they are not discussed in this chapter.

Prognosis

Extragenital warts in immunocompetent people are harmless and usually resolve spontaneously as a result of natural immunity within months or years. The rate of resolution is highly variable and probably depends on a number of factors, including host immunity, age, HPV type, and site of infection. One frequently cited study of an institutionalized population showed that two-thirds of warts resolved within a 2-year period.[7] Evaluation of control group clearance rates in randomized controlled trials (RCTs) may also give some indication of natural clearance rates, although a nonspecific benefit of vehicle bases may make interpretation difficult. Twenty-three of the RCTs discussed in more depth later in this chapter included a placebo group and used participants rather than warts as the unit of analysis. The average cure rate with placebo preparations in these trials was 18% (range 0–73%) after an average period of 10 weeks (range 4–24 weeks).

Diagnostic tests

Simple warts are nearly always diagnosed clinically. Microscopic examination of warts removed surgically can confirm the diagnosis if there is doubt. HPV typing is used in research laboratories and occasionally in medicolegal cases investigating child abuse.

Aims of treatment

To clear warts completely and permanently.

Relevant outcomes

- Total clearance
- Nonrecurrence
- Adverse reactions, such as pain and blistering

Methods of search

For a systematic review,[8] we searched for all RCTs of local treatments for extragenital warts in immunocompetent people in the Cochrane Central Register of Controlled Trials, Medline, Embase, and a number of other electronic databases using standardized search strategies. The bibliographies of all identified trials and key review articles were searched manually. All relevant pharmaceutical companies were contacted, and a search for unpublished trials was carried out by contacting a number of clinicians and researchers worldwide. The most recent searches were completed in June 2007.

Questions

How effective are the various available local treatments for clearing warts and what are the side effects of these treatments?

Topical treatments containing salicylic acid
Efficacy
The reported cure rates in 13 RCTs ranged from 0% to 84%.[8]

SA versus placebo. Five RCTs[9–13] (including 322 adults and children) compared salicylic acid (SA) with placebo. SA preparations gave higher cure rates—73% versus 48%; risk ratio (RR) 1.60; 95% confidence intervals (CI), 1.16 to 2.23; number needed to treat (NNT) four (95% CI, 3 to 7).

SA versus cryotherapy. Two RCTs[14,15] compared SA with cryotherapy (272 adults and children). The cure rates ranged between 60% and 70% and did not differ significantly between the two treatments (RR 1.04; 95% CI, 0.88 to 1.22).

Other comparisons. Seven other RCTs[14,16–19] compared different products containing SA or compared SA with other topical treatments such as glutaraldehyde and dithranol. The limited evidence provided by these different trials showed no convincing advantage of any particular delivery system for SA, or of the other topical treatments.

Drawbacks
In one RCT that compared a mixture of monochloroacetic acid and 60% SA with placebo,[12] one of the 29 patients in the active treatment group developed cellulitis. Minor skin irritation was noted occasionally in some of the other trials, but generally topical SA was reported to have no significant harmful effects.

Comments
There is some reservation about the validity of pooled data from the different RCTs, because of the generally low quality of trials and the heterogeneity of their design and methodology. For instance, different RCTs used slightly different topical SA products, and while some RCTs included patients with refractory warts, others excluded them. Despite this, we consider that there is good evidence for a modest but definite beneficial clinical effect of SA in treating ordinary warts.

Implications for practice
Topical preparations containing SA are generally effective and safe for treating warts.

Cryotherapy with liquid nitrogen
The reported cure rates in 17 RCTs were highly variable, ranging from 9% to 87%.[8]

Efficacy
Cryotherapy versus placebo or no treatment. Two small RCTs including 69 adults compared cryotherapy with either placebo cream[20] or no treatment.[21] The pooled data did not demonstrate a significant difference in cure rates: 35% vs. 34% (RR 0.88; 95% CI, 0.26 to 2.95). One trial[20] reported a very low cure rate for cryotherapy (one of 11) and the other[21] had a very high cure rate in the placebo group (eight of 20).

Cryotherapy versus SA. Two RCTs[14,15] compared SA with cryotherapy in 320 adults and children. There was no significant difference in the cure rates between the two treatments: 65% vs. 62% (RR 1.04; 95% CI, 0.88 to 1.22).

Length of freeze. Four RCTs[22–25] compared aggressive and gentle cryotherapy in 592 adults and children; however, the definitions of "aggressive" and "gentle" used differed, and some studies included refractory warts, whereas others did not. Overall, cure was achieved in 52% with aggressive cryotherapy and 31% with gentle cryotherapy (RR 1.90; 95% CI, 1.15 to 3.15; NNT 5; 95% CI, 3 to 7).

Interval between freezes. Three RCTs[14,26,27] showed no significant difference in cure rates between 2-week, 3-week, and 4-week intervals. Cure was generally achieved more quickly with shorter treatment intervals.

Optimum number of freezes. Only one RCT[28] examined this question in 115 adults and children not cured after 3 months of 3-weekly cryotherapy and showed no benefit of prolonging cryotherapy for a further 3 months. The cure rates were 43% and 38% in the treated and untreated groups, respectively (no data available for calculating the odds ratio).

Drawbacks

Only two RCTs included precise data on adverse events. Pain or blistering was reported by 64 of 100 participants (64%) treated with an "aggressive" (10-second) regimen, in comparison with 44 of 100 participants (44%) treated with a "gentle" (brief freeze) regimen (RR 1.45; 95% CI, 1.12 to 2.31). Five participants withdrew from the aggressive-regimen group and one from the gentle-regimen group because of pain and blistering.[22] Pain and/or blistering was reported in 29%, 7%, and 0% of those treated at 1-week, 2-week, and 3-week intervals, respectively (no data available for the odds ratio.[26] The rate of reported adverse affects was higher with a shorter interval between treatments, but this is likely to be a reporting artefact, as these participants were seen sooner after each treatment.

Comments

The evidence from the available RCTs for the absolute and relative effectiveness of cryotherapy for warts is both limited and contradictory. Moreover—as with the RCTs on topical SA—the heterogeneity of the study designs and methods and the likely heterogeneity of the populations being studied make it difficult to draw firm conclusions from the pooled data. For instance, some trials included all types of warts on the hands and feet in all age groups, whereas others were more selective and simply looked at hand warts, or excluded certain groups such as those with mosaic plantar warts or refractory warts. Of particular note is the likelihood that the wart clinic "populations" used for these studies may have had very different characteristics at different periods of time. For instance, studies conducted in the 1970s in the UK would have included a higher proportion of participants with incident warts, with a greater chance of cure and/or spontaneous resolution. In the 1980s and 1990s, more people with warts were treated in primary care; thus, hospital wart clinics would have had a more selected population with a higher proportion of refractory warts and correspondingly lower cure rates.

Implications for practice

• The available, rather limited, evidence shows that cryotherapy is probably of equivalent efficacy to topical treatments containing SA and occlusion with duct tape.
• Aggressive cryotherapy (defined by longer freezing times) is more effective than gentle cryotherapy.
• Harmful effects such as pain and blistering are probably more frequent with aggressive cryotherapy.

• There are no significant differences in the cure rates between regimens with intervals of 2 weeks, 3 weeks, or 4 weeks.
• There is no significant benefit of prolonging 3-weekly cryotherapy beyond 3 months.

Occlusive treatment with duct tape
Efficacy

Three RCTs have been published to date, all relatively recently. The reported cure rates range from 16% to 71%.

Duct tape versus cryotherapy. The first of the three trials chronologically compared occlusive treatment with duct tape and cryotherapy in 61 children and young adults.[29] The duct tape was applied for six and a half days every 7 days and cryotherapy was given for 10 seconds every 2–3 weeks up to a maximum of six times. The cure rates in the intention-to-treat population were 22 of 30 (71%) and 15 of 31 (46%), respectively (RR 1.52; 95% CI, 0.99 to 2.31). The trial was relatively small; some would say that 10 seconds of cryotherapy is inadequate; an unspecified number of outcome assessments were carried out over the phone, and it is not entirely clear how long after the treatment period this was done. Despite these weaknesses, this trial added considerable weight to the argument that simpler and safer treatments are likely to be at least as effective as cryotherapy, and possibly more so.

Duct tape versus placebo. Two more recently published trials did not show such good cure rates with duct tape.[30,31] The trial by De Haen *et al.*[30] included 103 primary-school children who were randomly assigned to continuous duct tape or a nonocclusive corn pad applied only once per week to one index wart per child. After 6 weeks, resolution had occurred in eight of 51 (16%) versus three of 52 (6%) of the trial warts, respectively. Curiously, other untreated warts resolved in 21% and 27% of the children, respectively. Wenner *et al.*[31] conducted a trial comparing occlusive duct tape (obscured by a sticky-backed fabric called moleskin) with the moleskin alone as a placebo in 90 adult patients (their trial population had an unusually high mean age of 54 years). After 8 weeks, resolution had occurred in eight of 39 (21%) versus nine of 41 (22%), respectively. Among the cured patients, six of eight and three of nine, respectively, had relapsed again after 6 months.

Drawbacks

Duct tape is simple, safe, and cheap. No significant adverse events were mentioned in any of these trials.

Comments

None of these three trials are particularly strong methodologically and, as with the cryotherapy trials, the results are somewhat contradictory and difficult to summarize meaningfully.

Implications for practice
Duct tape is certainly safe and also relatively cheap, so there is little risk in it being tried. In view of the two more recent trials showing such disappointing cure rates, however, there is little convincing evidence that duct tape has any great advantages over ordinary salicylic acid preparations, which are generally easier to use for patients.

Contact immunotherapy with dinitrochlorobenzene (DNCB)
Efficacy
Two small RCTs[20,32] of DNCB in 80 children and adults achieved a cure rate of 80% (32/40) in comparison with 38% (15/40) in the placebo/no treatment groups (RR 2.12; 95% CI, 1.38 to 3.26; NNT 2; 95% CI, 2 to 4).

Drawbacks
No precise data on adverse effects were reported in either of these trials. Rosado-Cancino et al.[32] commented that six of 20 participants treated with 2% DNCB were sensitized only after the second application. All of them subsequently experienced significant local irritation, with or without blistering, when they were treated with 1% DNCB. None withdrew from the study.

Comments
DNCB, a potent contact allergen, can cause significant local irritation and dermatitis, which probably precludes its use outside specialist centers.

Implications for practice
Contact immunotherapy with DNCB appears to be a promising treatment, but is probably best reserved for highly refractory warts.

Photodynamic therapy (PDT)
Efficacy
Five RCTs[33–37] of different types of PDT reported varying success. Cure rates ranged from 8% (of patients) to 75% (of warts).

PDT versus placebo. One trial[33] including 52 adults and children, using a left–right design (randomizing active and placebo treatments to warts on the left and right side of the body), showed resolution of warts in 40% of the participants. In all those who responded to treatment, the warts on the placebo-treated side also resolved. In another trial in 40 adults,[34] aminolevulinic acid (ALA) PDT achieved a cure rate of 56% of warts compared with 42% of warts in the placebo PDT group. Topical SA was also used for all participants.

A more recently published PDT trial including 67 patients with refractory warts compared ALA-PDT three times with placebo PDT.[37] All of the participants received keratolytic ointment under an occlusive dressing for 7 days prior to PDT. The cure rates were higher in the active treatment group 2 months after the last treatment—48 of 64 warts (75%) versus 13 of 57 warts (23%). Unpublished figures for the cure rates at 22 months were 45 of 64 (71%) versus 13 of 57 (23%), respectively, and—using patients as the unit of analysis—26 of 34 (76%) versus 13 of 33 (42%), respectively.

Local treatments for cutaneous warts
PDT versus SA. One RCT[35] including 120 adults and children compared methylene blue/dimethyl sulfoxide PDT with a mixture of SA and creosote. The cure rates achieved were 8% and 15%, respectively.

PDT versus cryotherapy. One RCT[36] including 28 adults with refractory warts compared four different types of light source for PDT with cryotherapy. PDT was administered three times and cryotherapy four times. The cure rates ranged from 28% to 73% of warts with the different types of PDT; 20% of the warts were cured with cryotherapy. Topical SA was also used for all patients.

Drawbacks
Only three trials provided data on adverse effects.[34,36,37] Burning and itching during treatment and mild discomfort afterwards were reported universally in one trial with ALA PDT.[36] All participants with plantar warts were able to walk after treatment. In another study, severe or unbearable pain during treatment was reported for an average of 17% of warts with active treatment and an average of 4% of warts with placebo PDT.[34] Fabbrocini et al. reported a burning sensation or slight pain at the time of treatment and moderate swelling with mild erythema 24 hours afterwards in patients with ALA-PDT.[37] No treatments were suspended because of pain.

Comments
Methodological heterogeneity makes it difficult to draw conclusions from these different trials. One used a left–right design, three others used warts as the unit of analysis, and each trial used different types of PDT.

Implications for clinical practice
PDT appears to offer no particular advantages in terms of higher cure rates or fewer adverse effects than other simpler and cheaper local treatments available.

Intralesional bleomycin
Efficacy
Conflicting results were reported in five RCTs of intralesional bleomycin. Cure rates ranged from 16% to 94%. Two trials[38,39] reported higher cure rates with bleomycin than with placebo, one[40] showed that placebo was associated

with higher cure rates than bleomycin, and one[41] showed no significant differences between bleomycin and placebo. One other trial found no significant differences in the cure rates between three different concentrations of bleomycin injections.[42]

Bleomycin versus placebo. One RCT[38] using a left–right design in 24 adults showed cure rates of 58% and 10% of warts with 0.1% bleomycin and saline (placebo) injections, respectively. Another RCT[39] including 16 adults and children showed cure rates of 82% and 35% of warts with 0.1% bleomycin and saline injections, respectively. Yet another RCT[40] including 62 adults achieved cure rates of 16% and 44% with 1% bleomycin in oil or saline, and oil or saline placebo injections, respectively. A further RCT[41] in 31 adults and children showed cure rates of 94% and 73% of participants with 0.1% bleomycin and saline injections, respectively.

Different concentrations of bleomycin. One RCT[42] in 26 adults, comparing 0.25, 0.5, and 1.0 units/mL bleomycin showed cure rates of 73%, 88%, and 90% of warts, respectively; the differences were not statistically significant.

Drawbacks

No precise data on adverse effects were provided in any of the RCTs. Munkvad *et al.*[40] reported "adverse events" in 19/62 (31%) participants but the nature of the adverse events and the proportions in the active treatment and placebo groups were not specified. Three of the trials[38,39,42] reported that most participants experienced pain. In two of the five trials, local anesthetic was used routinely[39,41] before the injection of bleomycin. Hayes *et al.*[42] reported pain in most participants, irrespective of dose. In the trial by Bunney *et al.*,[38] of 24 participants who received bleomycin, one withdrew because of the pain of the injections and another because of pain in the period after the injection.

Comments

Again, methodological and statistical heterogeneity (different outcomes, trial periods, units of analysis, numbers of injections, vehicles, and concentrations) make it impossible to synthesize the data from these trials.

Implications for clinical practice

There is no compelling evidence for the efficacy of intralesional bleomycin.

Other local treatments for warts

One trial of the pulsed dye laser[43] including 40 patients showed no significant differences in cure rates between four pulsed dye laser treatments at monthly intervals and "conventional treatment" with either cryotherapy or can-

tharidin. 5-Fluorouracil and intralesional interferons as treatments for warts are more of historical interest. Four[44–47] and six[48–53] trials, respectively, were found for these treatments, most dating from the 1970s and 1980s. Evidence provided by all the trials was severely limited by heterogeneity of methodology and design, and overall did not suggest any striking efficacy for either treatment.

Only two other more recently published trials are worthy of mention, although neither, disappointingly, has significant implications for clinical practice. The first is an RCT of intralesional antigen therapy, a form of local immunotherapy designed to elicit an immune reaction in warts injected with *Candida*, mumps, or *Trichophyton* antigens.[54] Unfortunately, the design of the trial was made more complex by the addition of intralesional interferon (IFN), resulting in four treatment arms (antigen with and without IFN and placebo with and without IFN) rather than two, which would have given much clearer data. Up to five injections were given at 3-weekly intervals into the largest wart in each patient. Blinding involved only the patients and not the investigators, introducing a source of potentially significant bias. The main outcome reported was a reduction of more than 75% in the wart surface area at the end of treatment—an outcome of no relevance to patients (who naturally want their warts cleared). No long-term follow-up appears to have been carried out. A total of 201 patients with refractory warts completed the trial, and 57 of 95 patients (60%) injected with antigen with or without additional interferon experienced the resolution of at least one wart, in comparison with 25 of 106 patients (24%) injected with saline or IFN alone. The number of patients who experienced complete clearance of all warts is a little difficult to ascertain from the paper, but it appears to have been 21 of 95 (22%) in the treatment groups and 11 of 106 (10%) in the "placebo" groups. For an elaborate and presumably fairly painful and expensive treatment, this does not appear to offer any striking advantages.

The other RCT compared topical α-lactalbumin–oleic acid with placebo.[55] This trial employed an unusual hybrid molecule (consisting of a combination of α-lactalbumin from human breast milk and oleic acid), said to be lethal to a wide range of transformed cells but harmless to normal ones. The trial appears to have been properly randomized and double-blinded, but the analysis focuses on the main outcome of a more than 75% reduction in wart volume, rather than the more relevant complete clearance of warts. Unfortunately, the trial defaulted to an open-label design after 3 months, making the long-term follow up data unconvincing. Although 100% of patients in the treatment group were reported to have experienced a reduction in wart volume of more than 75%, only 21% of the lesions in the treatment group resolved completely and only a modest nine of 20 patients (45%) with active treatment experienced the resolution of at least one wart, in comparison with three of 20 (15%) in the placebo group (RR 3.0; 95% CI, 0.95 to 9.48)—an unconvincing difference, given the size of the trial and consequently wide confidence intervals. The number of patients whose warts completely cleared is not clear from the data. The conclusions of this chapter therefore remain much the same as in the previous edition of this book.

No RCTs were identified that studied the efficacy of the following treatments: carbon dioxide laser, surgical excision, curettage and cautery, formaldehyde, podophyllin, and podophyllotoxin.

Key points

- Topical preparations containing SA are generally effective and safe for treating warts.
- The available, rather limited, evidence shows that cryotherapy is probably of equivalent efficacy to topical treatments containing SA.
- Contact immunotherapy with DNCB appears to be a promising treatment, but is probably best reserved for highly refractory warts.
- PDT and pulsed dye laser therapy do not appear to have any particular advantage in terms of higher cure rates or fewer adverse effects than the other simpler and cheaper local treatments available.
- There is no compelling evidence for the efficacy of intralesional bleomycin.

References

1 Johnson M. Skin conditions and related need for medical care among persons 1–74 years. United States, 1971–4. Washington DC. US Department of Health, Education and Welfare/National Centre for Health Statistics, 1978: 1–72 (Vital and Health Statistics, Series 11, No. 212; Department of Health Education and Welfare Publication No. (PHS) 79–1660.)

2 Beliaeva TL. [The population incidence of warts; in Russian.] *Vestn Dermatol Venerol* 1990;**2**:55–8.

3 Williams HC, Pottier A, Strachan D. The descriptive epidemiology of warts in British schoolchildren. *Br J Dermatol* 1993;**128**:504–11.

4 Kilkenny M, Merlin K, Young R, Marks R. The prevalence of common skin conditions in Australian school students: 1. Common, plane and plantar viral warts. *Br J Dermatol* 1998;**138**:840–5.

5 Johnson LW. Communal showers and the risk of plantar warts. *J Fam Pract* 1995;**40**:136–8.

6 Keefe M, al-Ghamdi A, Coggon D, *et al.* Cutaneous warts in butchers. *Br J Dermatol* 1994;**130**:9–14.

7 Massing AM, Epstein WL. Natural history of warts. *Arch Dermatol* 1963;**87**:306–10.

8 Gibbs S, Harvey I, Sterling JC, Stark R. Local treatments for cutaneous warts. *Cochrane Database Syst Rev* 2003;(**3**):CD001781.

9 Bart BJ, Biglow J, Vance JC, Neveaux JL. Salicylic acid in karaya gum patch as a treatment for verruca vulgaris. *J Am Acad Dermatol* 1989;**20**:74–6.

10 Felt BT, Hall H, Olness K, *et al.* Wart regression in children: comparison of relaxation imagery to topical treatment and equal time interventions. *Am J Clin Hypn* 1998;**41**:130–7.

11 Spanos NP, Williams V, Gwynn MI. Effects of hypnotic, placebo, and salicylic acid treatments on wart regression. *Psychosom Med* 1990;**52**:109–14.

12 Steele K, Shirodaria P, O'Hare M, *et al.* Monochloroacetic acid and 60% salicylic acid as a treatment for simple plantar warts: effectiveness and mode of action. *Br J Dermatol* 1988;**118**:537–43.

13 Bunney MH, Hunter JA, Ogilvie MM, Williams DA. The treatment of plantar warts in the home. A critical appraisal of a new preparation. *Practitioner* 1971;**207**:197–204.

14 Bunney MH, Nolan MW, Williams DA. An assessment of methods of treating viral warts by comparative treatment trials based on a standard design. *Br J Dermatol* 1976;**94**:667–79.

15 Steele K, Irwin WG. Liquid nitrogen and salicylic/lactic acid paint in the treatment of cutaneous warts in general practice. *J R Coll Gen Pract* 1988;**38**:256–8.

16 Auken G, Gade M, Pilgaard CE. Treatment of warts of the hands and feet with Verucid. *Ugeskr Laeger* 1975;**137**:3036–8.

17 Flindt-Hansen H, Tikjob G, Brandrup F. Wart treatment with anthralin. *Acta Derm Venereol* 1984;**64**:177–9.

18 Parton AM, Sommerville RG. The treatment of plantar verrucae by triggering cell-mediated immunity. *Br J Pod Med* 1994;**131**:883–6.

19 Veien NK, Madsen SM, Avrach W, Hammershoy O, Lindskov R, Niordson AM. The treatment of plantar warts with a keratolytic agent and occlusion. *J Dermatol Treat* 1991;**2**:59–61.

20 Gibson JR, Harvey SG, Barth J, Darley CR, Reshad H, Burke CA. A comparison of acyclovir cream versus placebo cream versus liquid nitrogen in the treatment of viral plantar warts. *Dermatologica* 1984;**168**:178–81.

21 Wilson P. Immunotherapy v cryotherapy for hand warts; a controlled trial [abstract]. *Scottish Med J* 1983;**28**:191.

22 Connolly M, Basmi K, O'Connell M, Lyons JF, Bourke JF. Efficacy of cryotherapy is related to severity of freeze [abstract]. *Br J Dermatol* 1999;**141**(S55):31.

23 Sonnex TS, Camp RDR. The treatment of recalcitrant viral warts with high dose cryosurgery under local anaesthesia [abstract]. *Br J Dermatol* 1988;**199**(S33):38–9.

24 Berth-Jones J, Bourke J, Eglitis H, *et al.* Value of a second freeze-thaw cycle in cryotherapy of common warts. *Br J Dermatol* 1994;**131**:883–6.

25 Hansen JG, Schmidt H. Plantar warts. Occurrence and cryosurgical treatment. *Ugeskr Laeger* 1986;**148**:173–4.

26 Bourke JF, Berth-Jones J, Hutchinson PE. Cryotherapy of common viral warts at intervals of 1, 2 and 3 weeks. *Br J Dermatol* 1995;**132**:433–6.

27 Larsen PO, Laurberg G. Cryotherapy of viral warts. *J Dermatol Treat* 1996;**7**:29–31.

28 Berth-Jones J, Hutchinson PE. Modern treatment of warts: cure rates at 3 and 6 months. *Br J Dermatol* 1992;**127**:262–5.

29 Focht DR, Spicer C, Fairchok MP. The efficacy of duct tape vs cryotherapy in the treatment of verruca vulgaris. *Arch Paed Adolesc Med* 2002;**156**:971–4.

30 De Haen, Spigt M, van Uden C, van Neer P, Feron F, Knottnerus A. Efficacy of duct tape vs placebo in the treatment of verruca vulgaris (warts) in primary school children. *Arch Paed Adolesc Med* 2006;**160**:1121–5.

31 Wenner R, Askari S, Cham P, Kedrowski R, Liu A, Warshaw E. Duct tape for the treatment of common warts in adults. *Arch Dermatol* 2007;**143**:309–13.

32 Rosado-Cancino MA, Ruiz-Maldonado R, Tamayo L, Laterza AM. Treatment of multiple and stubborn warts in children with 1-chloro-2,4-dinitrobenzene (DNCB) and placebo. *Dermatol Rev Mex* 1989;**33**:245–52.

33 Veien NK, Genner J, Brodthagen H, Wettermark G. Photodynamic inactivation of verrucae vulgares. II. *Acta Derm Venereol* 1977;**57**:445–7.

34 Stender IM, Na R, Fogh H, Gluud C, Wulf HC. Photodynamic therapy with 5-aminolaevulinic acid or placebo for recalcitrant foot and hand warts: randomised double-blind trial. *Lancet* 2000;**355**:963–6.

35 Stahl D, Veien NK, Wulf HC. Photodynamic inactivation of virus warts: a controlled clinical trial. *Clin Exp Dermatol* 1979;**4**:81–5.

36 Stender IM, Lock-Anderson J, Wulf HC. Recalcitrant hand and foot warts successfully treated with photodynamic therapy with topical 5-aminolaevulinic acid: a pilot study. *Clin Exp Dermatol* 1999;**24**:154–9.

37 Fabbrocini G, Di Costanzo MP, Riccardo AM, *et al.* Photodynamic therapy with topical delta-aminolaevulinic acid for the treatment of plantar warts. *J Photochem Photobiol B* 2001;**61**:30–4.

38 Bunney MH, Nolan MW, Buxton PK, Going SM, Prescott RJ. The treatment of resistant warts with intralesional bleomycin: a controlled clinical trial. *Br J Dermatol* 1984;**111**:197–207.

39 Rossi E, Soto JH, Battan J, Villalba L. Intralesional bleomycin in verruca vulgaris. Double-blind study. *Dermatology Review Mexico* 1981;**25**:158–65.

40 Munkvad M, Genner J, Staberg B, Kongsholm H. Locally injected bleomycin in the treatment of warts. *Dermatologica* 1983;**167**(2):86–9.

41 Perez Alfonzo R, Weiss E, Piquero Martin J. Hypertonic saline solution vs intralesional bleomycin in the treatment of common warts. *Dermatology Venezuela* 1992;**30**:176–8.

42 Hayes ME, O'Keefe EJ. Reduced dose of bleomycin in the treatment of recalcitrant warts. *Journal of the American Academy of Dermatology* 1986;**15**(5 Pt 1):1002–6.

43 Robson KJ, Cunningham NM, Kruzan KL, Patel DS, Kreiter CD, O'Donnell MJ, *et al.* Pulsed-dye laser versus conventional therapy for the treatment of warts: a prospective randomized trial. *Journal of the American Academy of Dermatology* 2000;**43**:275–80.

44 Artese O, Cazzato C, Cucchiarelli S, Iezzi D, Palazzi P, Ametetti M. Controlled study: medical therapy (5-fluouracil, salicylic acid) vs physical therapy (DTC) of warts. *Dermatology Clinics* 1994;**14**:55–9.

45 Bunney MH. The treatment of plantar warts with 5-fluorouracil. *British Journal of Dermatology* 1973;**89**:96–7.

46 Hursthouse MW. A controlled trial on the use of topical 5-fluorouracil on viral warts. *British Journal of Dermatology* 1975;**92**(1):93-6.

47 Schmidt H, Jacobsen FK. Double-blind randomized clinical study on treatment of warts with fluouracil-containing topical preparation. *Zeitschrift fur Hautkrankheiten* 1981;**56**:41–3.

48 Berman B, Davis-Reed L, Silverstein L, Jaliman D, France D, Lebwohl M. Treatment of verrucae vulgaris with alpha 2 interferon. *Journal of Infectious Diseases* 1986;**154**(2):328–30.

49 Lee SW, Houh D, Kim HO, Kim CW, Kim TY. Clinical trials of interferon-gamma in treating warts. *Ann Dermatol Venereol* 1990;**2**:77–82.

50 Niimura M. Application of beta-interferon in virus-induced papillomas. *Journal of Investigative Dermatology* 1990;**95**(6 Suppl):149–51S.

51 Pazin GJ, Ho M, Haverkos HW, Armstrong JA, Breinig MC, Wechsler HL, *et al.* Effects of interferon-alpha on human warts. *Journal of Interferon Research* 1982;**2**(2):235–43.

52 Vance JC, Bart BJ, Hansen RC, Reichman RC, McEwen C, Hatch KD, *et al.* Intralesional recombinant alpha-2 interferon for the treatment of patients with condyloma acuminatum or verruca plantaris. *Archives of Dermatology* 1986;**122**(3):272–7.

53 Varnavides CK, Henderson CA, Cunliffe WJ. Intralesional interferon: ineffective in common viral warts. *Journal of Dermatological Treatment* 1997;**8**:169–72.

54 Horn TD, Johnson SM, Helm RM, Roberson PK. Intralesional immunotherapy of warts with mumps, *Candida* and *Trichophyton* skin test antigens: single-blinded, randomized, and controlled trial. *Arch Dermatol* 2005;**141**:589–94.

55 Gustafsson L, Leijonhufvud I, Aronsson A, Mossberg AK, Svanborg C. Treatment of skin papillomas with topical alpha-lactalbumin–oleic acid. *N Engl J Med* 2004;**350**:2663–72.

36 Impetigo

Sander Koning, Lisette W.A. van Suijlekom-Smit,
Johannes C. van der Wouden

Background

Definition

Impetigo (Figure 36.1) is a contagious superficial skin infection, characterized by superficial erosions covered with honey-colored crusts, most often on the face. A distinction is made between bullous and nonbullous impetigo. Impetigo may be primary or secondary to other skin diseases, such as atopic eczema.

Incidence

Impetigo is most frequent in children; the incidence rates peak at 3–6 years of age. Population-based incidence rates are unknown. Impetigo is common in general practice, with incidence rates of around 20 episodes per 1000 children per year seen by the general practitioner.[1–3]

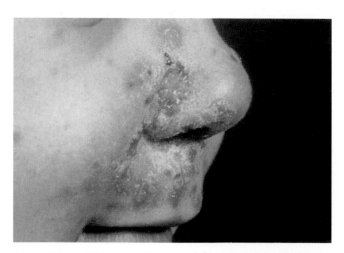

Figure 36.1 A child with impetigo (reproduced with permission from A.P. Oranje).

Etiology

In moderate climates, the primary pathogen in nonbullous impetigo is *Staphylococcus aureus*. However, in warm and humid climates, *Streptococcus pyogenes* or both *S. pyogenes* and *Staphylococcus aureus* are more often isolated. The relative frequency of *S. aureus* infections has also changed with time. It was predominant in the 1940s and 1950s, and then group-A streptococci became more prevalent. Recently, *S. aureus* has become more common again.[4] Bullous impetigo is a staphylococcal disease.

Prognosis

Impetigo is believed to be self-limiting, taking several weeks to cure without intervention. However, no research is available to substantiate this statement. Prompt resolution usually occurs with adequate treatment. The course of the disease is usually mild, but sometimes general symptoms such as fever and lymphadenopathy occur. Streptococcal impetigo can be complicated by nephritis.

Aims of treatment

Impetigo is treated to accelerate cure and to prevent spreading of the infection.

Relevant outcomes

Clinical cure (clearance of crusts, blisters, and redness) is the most relevant outcome. Criteria such as relief of pain, itching, and soreness, and bacteriological cure can be considered as secondary outcomes.

Methods of search

We found three systematic reviews,[5–7] the Cochrane review[7] being an extended update of the first.[5] As the Cochrane review, with 57 included trials, is the most recent and most comprehensive one, it has provided the basis for discussing treatments in this chapter.

The Cochrane review included randomized trials of all interventions for impetigo by using the following search terms in Medline (January 2003): impetigo (Medical Subject Headings, MeSH) or staphylococcal skin infections (MeSH) or impetigo (in title or abstract) or pyoderma (in title or abstract), in combination with the standard search strategy for identifying randomized trials. The authors have also searched for additional randomized controlled trials (RCTs) published since the Cochrane review, up to July 2007. One trial was found that enhanced the evidence base, and this has been incorporated into the text.[8] An update of the Cochrane review is planned for 2008.

Questions

What are the effects of treatments on the clearance of impetiginous lesions after 1 week?

Disinfecting treatments
Efficacy
Versus placebo. We found one randomized controlled trial comparing hexachlorophene with placebo.[9] Scrubbing with hexachlorophene added no notable benefit to placebo treatment.

Versus topical antibiotic treatment. One multicenter RCT compared hydrogen peroxide cream with fusidic acid cream/gel.[10] There was no significant difference in treatment effect, but there was a tendency towards a better effect of fusidic acid cream/gel. There was no significant difference between hexachlorophene and bacitracin ointment in a small and older study.[9]

Versus oral antibiotic treatment. There was no significant difference between hexachlorophene scrubbing and oral treatment with penicillin.[9]

Drawbacks
Eleven percent of the patients using hydrogen peroxide cream reported mild side effects (not specified). No patient was withdrawn from the study because of side effects.[10] No adverse effects of scrubbing with hexachlorophene were recorded.[9]

Comment
Disinfectants, such as povidone iodine and chlorhexidine, advised in some guidelines, have not been compared with a placebo. Hydrogen peroxide cream showed good treatment results in a relatively large trial. However, the procedure for blinding in this trial was considered inappropriate.

Implications for topical disinfectants in clinical practice
There is no good evidence for the value of disinfecting measures in the treatment of impetigo.

Topical antibiotics
Efficacy
Versus placebo. Mupirocin has been studied in two placebo-controlled trials, both of which found a better effect with mupirocin.[11–13] One other RCT showed that fusidic acid was much more effective than placebo (55% of patients cured versus 13%).[14]

Versus each other. Several topical antibiotics have been compared directly. Mupirocin and fusidic acid were compared in four studies,[15–18] none of which showed a significant difference in treatment effect. All other studies comparing topical antibiotics were small and each studied a unique comparison of two antibiotics.

Versus oral antibiotics. When 10 RCTs that compared topical mupirocin with oral erythromycin were pooled,[4,19–27] mupirocin was found to be significantly better than erythromycin.[7] In a small RCT (n = 32), cephalexin and mupirocin were both significantly more effective than bacitracin cream.[28] A recent trial in patients with secondarily infected dermatitis found no difference between oral cephalexin and topical retapamulin ointment.[8]

Drawbacks
RCT reports usually note few, if any, side effects with local antibiotics. The two studies comparing mupirocin with placebo reported none.[11,12] In studies comparing mupirocin with fusidic acid, the greasy nature of mupirocin was reported as a side effect in 7.4% of patients versus 1.0%;[15] minor itching/burning occurred in six of 116 patients (5%) versus two of 50 (4%), respectively.[17] No side effects were reported in Gilbert's study.[16] Studies comparing erythromycin with mupirocin recorded gastrointestinal side effects in 23% versus 8%,[4] none in either group,[26] and an equal distribution between the two groups.[20] Hydrocortisone/potassium hydroxyquinoline caused two cases of mild staining in 65 patients.[29] Miconazole caused "mild burning" in one case.[30] In general, resistance rates against topical antibiotics such as fusidic acid and mupirocin will rise when the antibiotic is used excessively.

Comments
Many RCTs deal with a range of (skin) infections, including impetigo. Only trials that reported separate results for the group of impetigo patients were included here. The follow-up periods and definitions of "cure" and "improvement" differ and are often not clear, making comparison difficult. There is a lack of placebo-controlled studies.

Implications for topical antibiotics in clinical practice

Although they are traditionally considered less effective than oral therapy, there is good evidence that local treatments are equal to or more effective than oral treatment. In general, oral antibiotics have more side effects, especially gastrointestinal side effects. Fusidic acid and mupirocin are equally effective. Most studies date back 10 years or more. Resistance patterns have changed since then. Contemporary and local characteristics and resistance patterns of the causative bacteria should always be taken into account when choosing treatment. When a large area is affected, or when the patient has general symptoms such as fever, oral therapy seems more appropriate.

Systemic antibiotics
Efficacy
Versus placebo. Only one small and inconclusive trial was found, comparing systemic antibiotics to placebo.[9]

Versus topical antibiotics. Discussed under topical antibiotics above.

Versus each other. Two RCTs compared penicillin and erythromycin, both finding erythromycin to be more effective.[31,32] Cloxacillin was significantly superior to penicillin in two studies.[33,34] All other comparisons were each made in only one study, and none of these showed a statistically significant difference between treatments.

Drawbacks
The incidences of side effects were:
- Azithromycin: 16.5%, mainly mild gastrointestinal.[35]
- Cephalexin: 10.9%, mainly mild gastrointestinal,[35] 11% mainly diarrhea,[36] no adverse effects in one study.[31]
- Cefdinir: 16%, mainly diarrhea.[36]

Comments
Many RCTs have been carried out on a range of "soft-tissue" infections, with a subset of impetigo patients. Only trials reporting separate results for the group of impetigo patients were considered in this chapter, although it should be pointed out that most trials in patients with "soft-tissue" infections did not provide results for impetigo separately. There is a lack of placebo-controlled studies. Resistance rates of the bacteria were determined in some studies, and differed from study to study. The follow-up periods differ widely between the studies, making comparison difficult.

Implications for use of systemic antibiotics in clinical practice
There is good evidence that local treatment is equal to or more effective than oral treatment. Macrolide antibiotics provide better treatment results than penicillin. In general,

oral antibiotics have more side effects than topical treatments, especially gastrointestinal side effects. Most studies date back 10 years or more, and resistance patterns have changed since then. Contemporary local characteristics and the resistance patterns of the causative bacteria should always be taken into account when choosing treatment. When a large area is affected, or when the patient has general symptoms such as fever, oral therapy seems preferable.

Key points

- The natural history of impetigo is not known.
- Few placebo-controlled studies have been done.
- Many different antibiotic treatments have been studied against each other, often in small studies showing no significant differences.
- There is no evidence supporting the value of disinfecting treatments.
- Macrolide and cephalosporin antibiotics are more effective than penicillins that are not resistant to beta-lactamase.
- Topical antibiotics such as mupirocin and fusidic acid are equal to or more effective than oral antibiotics such as erythromycin and have fewer side effects.
- For extensive infections accompanied by general symptoms such as fever, oral antibiotics may be preferable.
- Resistance patterns in causative bacteria change over time, and this should be taken into account when choosing a therapy for impetigo.

References

1 Koning S, Mohammedamin RSA, van der Wouden JC, van Suijlekom-Smit LWA, Schellevis FG, Thomas S. Impetigo: incidence and treatment in Dutch general practice in 1987 and 2001—results from two national surveys. *Br J Dermatology* 2006;**154**:239–43.

2 van der Ven-Daane I, Bruijnzeels MA, van der Wouden JC, van Suijlekom-Smit LWA. Occurrence and treatment of impetigo vulgaris in children. *Huisarts Wet* 1993;**36**:291–3.

3 McCormick A, Fleming D, Charlton J. *Morbidity Statistics from General Practice: Fourth National Study 1991–1992*. London: Department of Health, Office of Population Censuses and Royal College of General Practitioners, 1995.

4 Dagan R, Bar-David Y. Double-blind study comparing erythromycin and mupirocin for treatment of impetigo in children: implications of a high prevalence of erythromycin-resistant *Staphylococcus aureus* strains. *Antimicrob Agents Chemother* 1992;**36**:287–90.

5 Van Amstel L, Koning S, van Suijlekom-Smit LWA, Oranje A, van der Wouden JC. The treatment of impetigo contagiosa, a systematic review. *Huisarts Wet* 2000;**43**:247–52.

6 George A, Rubin G. A systematic review and meta-analysis of treatments of impetigo. *Br J Gen Pract* 2003;**53**:480–7.

7 Koning S, Verhagen AP, van Suijlekom-Smit LW, Morris A, Butler CC, van der Wouden JC. Interventions for impetigo. *Cochrane Database Syst Rev* 2004;(2):CD003261.

8 Parish LC, Jorizzo JL, Breton JJ, *et al.* Topical retapamulin ointment (1% wt/wt) twice daily for 5 days versus oral cephalexin twice daily for 10 days in the treatment of secondarily infected dermatitis; results of a randomized controlled trial. *J Am Acad Dermatol* 2006;**55**:1003–13.

9 Ruby RJ, Nelson JD. The influence of hexachlorophene scrubs on the response to placebo or penicillin therapy in impetigo. *Pediatrics* 1973;**52**:854–9.

10 Christensen OB, Anehus S. Hydrogen peroxide cream: an alternative to topical antibiotics in the treatment of impetigo contagiosa. *Acta Derm Venerol* 1994;**74**:460–2.

11 Eells LD, Mertz PM, Piovanetti Y, Pekoe GM, Eaglstein WH. Topical antibiotic treatment of impetigo with mupirocin. *Arch Dermatol* 1986;**122**:1273–6.

12 Gould JC, Smith JH, Moncur H. Mupirocin in general practice: a placebo-controlled trial. *Royal Society of Medicine: International Congress and Symposium Series* 1984;**80**:85–93.

13 Rojas R, Eells LD, Eaglstein W, *et al.* The efficacy of Bactroban ointment and its vehicle in the treatment of impetigo: a double blind comparative study. In: Dobson RL, Leyden JJ, Nobel WC, *et al.*, eds. *Bactroban (Mupirocin): Proceedings of an International Symposium, Nassau, Bahama Islands, 21–22 May 1984.* Amsterdam: Excerpta Medica, 1985: 96–102.

14 Koning S, van Suijlekom-Smit LWA, Nouwen JL *et al.* Fusidic acid cream in the treatment of impetigo in general practice: double blind randomised placebo controlled trial. *BMJ* 2002;**324**:203–6.

15 Morley PAR, Munot LD. A comparison of sodium fusidate ointment and mupirocin ointment in superficial skin sepsis. *Curr Med Res Opin* 1988;**11**:142–8.

16 Gilbert M. Topical 2% mupirocin versus 2% fusidic acid ointment in the treatment of primary and secondary skin infections. *J Am Acad Dermatol* 1989;**20**:1083–7.

17 White DG, Collins PO, Rowsell RB. Topical antibiotics in the treatment of superficial skin infections in general practice—a comparison of mupirocin with sodium fusidate. *J Infect* 1989;**18**:221–9.

18 Sutton JB. Efficacy and acceptability of fusidic acid cream and mupirocin ointment in facial impetigo. *Curr Ther Res* 1992;**51**: 673–8.

19 Barton LL, Friedman AD, Sharkey AM, Schneller DJ, Swierkosz EM. Impetigo contagiosa III. Comparative efficacy of oral erythromycin and topical mupirocin. *Pediatr Dermatol* 1989;**6**:134–8.

20 Britton JW, Fajardo JE, Krafte-Jacobs B. Comparison of mupirocin and erythromycin in the treatment of impetigo. *J Pediatr* 1990;**117**: 827–9.

21 Dux PH, Fields L, Pollock D. 2% topical mupirocin versus systemic erythromycin and cloxacillin in primary and secondary skin infections. *Curr Ther Res* 1986;**40**:933–40.

22 Esterly NB, Markowitz M. The treatment of pyoderma in children. *JAMA* 1970;**212**:667–70.

23 Goldfarb J, Crenshaw D, O'Horo J, Lemon E, Blumer JL. Randomized clinical trial of topical mupirocin versus oral erythromycin for impetigo. *Antimicrob Agents Chemother* 1988;**32**:1780–3.

24 Gratton D. Topical mupirocin versus oral erythromycin in the treatment of primary and secondary skin infections. *Int J Dermatol* 1987;**26**:472–3.

25 McLinn S. Topical mupirocin vs. systemic erythromycin treatment for pyoderma. *Pediatr Infect Dis J* 1988;**7**:785–90.

26 Mertz PM, Marshall DA, Eaglstein WH, Piovanetti Y, Montalvo J. Topical mupirocin treatment of impetigo is equal to oral erythromycin therapy. *Arch Dermatol* 1989;**125**:1069–73.

27 Rice TD, Duggan AK, DeAngelis C. Cost-effectiveness of erythromycin versus mupirocin for the treatment of impetigo in children. *Pediatrics* 1992;**89**:210–4.

28 Bass JW, Chan DS, Creamer KM, *et al.* Comparison of oral cephalexin, topical mupirocin, and topical bacitracin for treatment of impetigo. *Pediatr Inf Dis J* 1997;**16**:708–9.

29 Jaffe GV, Grimshaw JJ. A clinical trial of hydrocortisone/ potassium hydroxyquinoline sulphate (Quinocort) in the treatment of infected eczema and impetigo in general practice. *Pharmatherapeutica* 1986;**4**:628–36.

30 Nolting S, Strauss WB. Treatment of impetigo and ecthyma. A comparison of sulconazole with miconazole. *Int J Derm* 1988; **27**:716–9.

31 Demidovich CW, Wittler RR, Ruff ME, Bass JW, Browning WC. Impetigo: current etiology and comparison of penicillin, erythromycin, and cephalexin therapies. *Am J Dis Child* 1990;**144**: 1313–5.

32 Barton LL, Friedman AD. Impetigo: a reassessment of etiology and therapy. *Pediatr Dermatol* 1987;**4**:185–8.

33 Gonzalez A, Schachner LA, Cleary T, Scott G, Taplin D, Lambert W. Pyoderma in childhood. *Adv Dermatol* 1989;**4**:127–41.

34 Pruksachatkunakorn C, Vaniyapongs T, Pruksakorn S. Impetigo: an assessment of etiology and appropriate therapy in infants and children. *J Med Assoc Thailand* 1993;**76**:222–9.

35 Kiani R. Double-blind, double-dummy comparison of azithromycin and cephalexin in the treatment of skin and skin structure infections. *Eur J Clin Microbiol Infect Dis* 1991;**10**:880–4.

36 Tack KJ, Keyserling CH, McCarty J, Hedrick JA. Study of use of cefdinir versus cephalexin for treatment of skin infections in pediatric patients. *Antimicrob Agents Chemother* 1997;**41**:739–42.

37 Athlete's foot

Fay Crawford

Background

Definition

Athlete's foot, or tinea pedis, is most frequently caused by dermatophyte (ringworm) invasion of the skin of the feet. It usually manifests in one of three ways: interdigital skin appears macerated (white) and soggy; patches of skin on the foot may be affected by recurrent vesicular eruptions, which make the skin itchy and red; and finally, the soles of the feet, including the sides and heels, can appear dry and scaly (Figure 37.1).[1]

Incidence/prevalence

Tinea infections are common. It has been estimated that 15% of the general population have a fungal infection of the feet.[2] Gentles and Evans[3] found the prevalence of athlete's

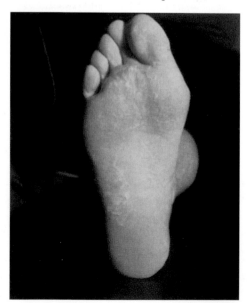

Figure 37.1 Athlete's foot.

foot to be 21.5% in a sample of adult male swimmers, but the prevalence amongst adult females participating in the same survey was only 3.3%.

Etiology

The dermatophytes most frequently reported in clinical trials to be present on patients' skin at trial entry are *Trichophyton rubrum, T. mentagrophytes, Epidermophyton floccosum,* and *T. interdigitale.*[4]

Scaling, fissuring, pruritus, and itching are some of the clinical features of fungal infections of the skin, and it is these irritations that make the patient seek treatment. The natural history of the condition if untreated is a chronic, worsening infection that can lead to fissuring and breaks in the epidermis. Although the condition will not resolve spontaneously, some evidence from cure rates collected from people in the placebo arms of controlled trials suggests that improved foot hygiene alone may cure the infection in a proportion of people.[5,6]

Diagnosis

The use of microscopy and culture laboratory tests to diagnose the presence of dermatophyte infection is very important, because athlete's foot can be mistaken for other skin conditions. For example, interdigital maceration can look exactly like interdigital athlete's foot, and juvenile chronic dermatosis and bacterial infections such as erythrasma can also have a similar appearance to that of fungal infections on the skin of the feet.

Aims of treatment

Treatment aims to reduce the signs and symptoms, such as itching and flaking of the skin, and ultimately to eradicate the infection.

The many creams available for the treatment of athlete's foot differ in cost and availability. The azoles (for example, miconazole and clotrimazole) and allylamines (terbinafine and naftifine) are sold over the counter in pharmacies. Other creams (for example, tolnaftate and undecenoic acid) are available in supermarkets. This last group is the cheapest of the topical preparations and the allylamine creams are the most expensive.

Oral drugs are sometimes used in the management of chronic manifestations of athlete's foot. Griseofulvin is the oldest and cheapest of the oral antifungal drugs, but it must be taken for a long time. Newer azoles—such as itraconazole, ketoconazole, and fluconazole—are effective in a much shorter time. The newest oral antifungal drugs are ally-lamines (terbinafine, naftifine). The allylamines (both topical and oral) are fungicidal, whereas all other antifungal agents are fungistatic.

Relevant outcomes

The effects of treatment on these symptoms are measured in randomized controlled trials (RCTs), but microscopy and culture are usually the primary outcomes. Secondary outcomes are measured using a variety of signs and symptoms (redness, flaking, itching, etc.). A reduction in symptoms may be achieved quite quickly, but the tenacity of tinea infections often means that complete cure takes a long time.

Methods of search

Systematic reviews and RCTs were identified using a search strategy published elsewhere.[7] This was updated to June 2006 with a Medline and Embase search using the same strategy and supplemented by a search of the Cochrane Central Register of Controlled Trials (June 2006).

The inclusion criterion for study selection was the mycological confirmation of the presence of fungi in the trial populations. The search found two systematic reviews, one of topical treatments for skin infections[7] and the other of oral treatments for skin infections.[4] The search also identified three RCTs not included in the reviews, which compared topical allylamines with topical azoles.

Generic drug names are used in the effectiveness analyses below. *Martindale*[8] gives a complete list of brand names of antifungal drugs.

Questions

How effective are allylamine creams in the treatment of athlete's foot?

One systematic review[7] found 12 RCTs comparing ally-lamines (terbinafine 1% cream or naftifine 1% gel) with placebo controls, used for 4 weeks. The two active preparations were similarly effective. A pooled analysis of data from seven trials (n = 683) comparing either naftifine or terbinafine with placebo controls produced a relative risk (RR) of 3.69, with 95% confidence intervals (CI) of 2.41 to 5.66. The allylamine creams, used twice daily for 4 weeks, are highly effective in the management of athlete's foot in comparison with placebo creams.

How effective are azole creams in the treatment of athlete's foot?

One systematic review[7] found 14 RCTs comparing 4–6 weeks treatment with azole creams (1% clotrimazole, 1% tioconazole, 1% bifonazole, 1% econazole, 2% miconazole nitrate) with placebo controls. They were similarly effective.

Treatment with 6 weeks of clotrimazole or tioconazole applied twice daily was evaluated in four trials (n = 434) (RR 1.85; 95% CI, 1.27 to 2.69). Shorter treatment times (4 weeks) with bifonazole, econazole nitrate, or miconazole nitrate gave a RR of 2.25 (95% CI, 1.44 to 3.52; n – 520). All the creams were similarly effective whether used for 4 or 6 weeks. Over-the-counter antifungal creams are very effective in the treatment of athlete's foot in comparison with placebo controls.

How do allylamine creams compare with azole creams in curing athlete's foot?

One systematic review of topical treatments (search date December 1997) indicated slightly better mycological cure rates with the allylamines (terbinafine 1% and butenafine 1% creams) than with azoles (clotrimazole 1% and miconazole 1% creams) used for 4 weeks (RR 1.1; 95% CI, 0.99 to 1.23). This analysis was based on data from 11 RCTs (n = 1554).[7] The analysis showed the allylamines to cure 80% of cases of athlete's foot, compared with a cure rate of 72% achieved with azole creams.

The systematic review[7] included one RCT[9] that compared 1 week of terbinafine 1% cream with 4 weeks of clotrimazole 1% cream. There was no difference in the cure rates (n = 211) after 1 week of treatment, but 6 weeks after the start of treatment, the cure rate for terbinafine was significantly better than that of clotrimazole (RR 1.16; 95% CI, 1.06 to 1.27).

Patel *et al.*[10] found exactly the opposite effect in a smaller but similar trial (n = 104). They compared 1 week of terbinafine cream with 4 weeks of clotrimazole cream in people with interdigital tinea pedis. Terbinafine was found to be more effective after 1 week (RR 1.51; 95% CI, 1.16 to 1.98), but there were no differences in effectiveness for outcomes assessed at later times.

In the smallest of the trials, comparing 1 week of 1% terbinafine with 4 weeks of 2% miconazole (n = 48),[11] no difference in cure rate emerged at any time during the trial (RR at 1 week 0.99; 95% CI, 0.57 to 1.7). At 4 weeks, there were 12/22 cures (54.6%) in the terbinafine group and 15/23 (65.2%) in the miconazole group (RR 0.83; 95% CI, 0.51 to 1.35).

Schopf et al.[12] compared terbinafine cream used for 1 week with clotrimazole cream for 4 weeks in 429 people with interdigital tinea pedis and found no differences in the effectiveness at any time during the trial.

Pooling the data from all three trials (n = 792) comparing 1 week of terbinafine cream with either 2% miconazole or 1% clotrimazole showed no statistical difference between these treatments (RR 1.15; 95% CI, 0.82 to 1.61).

How effectively do creams that can be bought in the supermarket cure athlete's foot?

A systematic review[7] found two three-arm trials comparing undecenoic acid with tolnaftate and placebo, another trial comparing undecenoic acid with placebo and no treatment, a fourth trial comparing undecenoic acid with placebo, and a fifth trial comparing tolnaftate with tea-tree oil and placebo. Pooling the tolnaftate data from the arms of three trials that compared it with placebo indicates that tolnaftate is more effective than placebo against dermatophyte infections (RR 1.56; 95% CI, 1.05 to 2.31). Pooled data from four trials showed undecenoic acid to be more effective than placebo in the management of athlete's foot (RR 2.83; 95% CI, 1.91 to 4.19).

Two trials of ciclopiroxolamine 1% (which is not available in the UK) found it effective in treating athlete's foot. In one placebo-controlled trial (n = 163), the RR was 6.85 (95% CI, 3.10 to 15.15). A second small trial (n = 87) comparing ciclopiroxolamine with clotrimazole found no statistical difference (RR 1.12; 95% CI, 0.90 to 1.38).

A third placebo-controlled RCT (n = 133) of ciclopiroxolamine 0.77% applied twice daily for 28 days found ciclopiroxolamine to be more effective than vehicle in producing a cure (RR 1.39; 95% CI, 1.14 to 1.75). This effect was maintained 2 weeks after treatment.[13]

A fourth RCT comparing ciclopiroxolamine with a vehicle (n = 317) similarly found ciclopiroxolamine to be significantly more effective (RR 0.18; 95% CI, 0.12 to 0.26) 14 days after treatment ended.[14]

Are oral drugs more effective than topical compounds in the treatment of athlete's foot?

Only one small RCT (n = 137) has compared the efficacy of an oral drug with a cream in the management of interdigital athlete's foot.[15] Cure rates were similar in those treated for 1 week with oral terbinafine 250 mg/day and those using clotrimazole 1% cream twice daily for 4 weeks. The relapse rates among those who were cured differed significantly, however: 11 of 39 in the terbinafine group and five of 50 in the clotrimazole group relapsed after 3 months.

What are the most effective oral drugs in the treatment of athlete's foot?

One systematic review[4] found 10 RCTs that compared two antifungal drugs and two RCTs that compared oral antifungal drugs with placebos. The sample sizes in all trials were small (range 14–66).

The review found four trials comparing oral terbinafine 250 mg/day with itraconazole 100 mg/day. One trial (n = 117) compared 2 weeks of terbinafine with 2 weeks of itraconazole and found a significant difference in favor of terbinafine (RR 1.5; 95% CI, 1.23 to 2.02). Three trials (n = 339) comparing 2 weeks of terbinafine with 4 weeks of itraconazole found no statistical differences in cure rates (RR 1.17; 95% CI, 0.94 to 1.46).

The systematic review found two small trials that compared griseofulvin 500 mg/day with terbinafine 250 mg/day for 4 or 6 weeks. The pooled data from the two trials found terbinafine to be significantly more effective (RR 2.20; 95% CI, 1.45 to 3.32).

The systematic review[4] found similar low cure rates for ketoconazole 200 mg (53%) and griseofulvin 1000 mg (57%). The cure rates with fluconazole 50 mg did not differ significantly from those with itraconazole 100 mg or ketoconazole 200 mg, but in both trials the cure rates were high (89–100%). Treatments were taken for 6 weeks in these trials.

Drawbacks

Topical antifungal compounds are well tolerated and are not associated with high rates of adverse events. One systematic review[7] found that few trial reports gave details of adverse events, and the few that were reported were not severe (for example, itching, redness, or burning).

The systematic review of oral treatments for fungal infections of the skin[4] noted that all 12 trials included reported side effects. All drugs produced side effects; the rate was lowest for fluconazole (11%) and highest for terbinafine (18%). Gastrointestinal effects and rashes were reported most frequently.

Comment

The evidence from one small trial[15] shows that oral treatments are no more effective in the management of interdigital athlete's foot than the creams. The same study also found higher relapse rates after oral treatments.

Implications for practice

All antifungal creams, whether over-the-counter drugs or those available in supermarkets, are effective in the treatment of athlete's foot.

There appears to be no therapeutic advantage in using an allylamine cream (terbinafine or naftifine) for 1 week rather than an azole cream for 4 weeks. The hypothesis that higher compliance rates are likely to be associated with shorter treatment times is often quoted, but has not been tested.[16]

If no advantage is gained from treating interdigital athlete's foot with oral antifungals, physicians should be cautious in prescribing oral drugs to manage moccasin-type infection (over the sole of the foot). The belief that recalcitrant cases of athlete's foot are more effectively managed with oral drugs has not been extensively tested.

Key points

- Athlete's foot is common and can be hard to cure.
- Long-standing cases of athlete's foot should be confirmed using microscopy and culture laboratory tests.
- All fungal creams are effective in treating athlete's foot. There is evidence that different antifungal creams are associated with different cure rates; creams containing allylamines are the most effective in producing a cure, followed by the azoles and undecenoic acid, and tolnaftate.
- There is some evidence to suggest that oral drugs (tablets) are no more effective than creams in producing a cure for athlete's foot.

References

1 Springett K, Merriman L. Assessment of the skin and its appendages. In: Merriman L, Tollafield D, eds. *Assessment of the Lower Limb.* Edinburgh: Churchill Livingstone, 1995: 191–225.

2 Gupta AK, Saunder DN, Shear NH. Efficacy of antifungal agent terbinafine in the treatment of superficial dermatophyte infections—an overview. *Today Ther Trends* 1995;**13**:9–20.

3 Gentles JC, Evans EGV. Foot infections in swimming baths. *BMJ* 1973;**3**:260–2.

4 Bell-Syer SEM, Hart R, Crawford F, *et al.* A systematic review of oral treatments for fungal infections of the skin of the feet. *J Dermatol* 2001;**12**:69–74.

5 Smith EB, Graham JL, Ulrich JA. Topical clotrimazole in tinea pedis. *South Med J* 1977;**70**:47–8.

6 Evans EGV, James IGV, Joshipura RC. Two week treatment of tinea pedis with terbinafine a placebo controlled study. *J Dermatol Treat* 1991;**2**:95–7.

7 Crawford F, Hart R, Bell-Syer S, Torgerson D, Young P, Russell I. Topical treatments for fungal infections of the skin and nails of the foot. *Cochrane Database Syst Rev* 2000;(2):CD001434.

8 *Martindale: the Complete Drug Reference*, 32nd ed. London: Pharmaceutical Press, 1999.

9 Evans EGV, Dodman B, Williamson DM. Comparison of terbinafine and clotrimazole in treating tinea pedis. *BMJ* 1993;**307**: 645–7.

10 Patel A, Brookman SD, Bullen MU, *et al.* Topical treatment of interdigital tinea pedis: terbinafine compared with clotrimazole. *Australas J Dermatol* 1999;**40**:197–200.

11 Leenutaphong V, Tangwiwat S, Muanprasat C, Niumpradit N, Spitaveesuawan R. Double-blind study of the efficacy of one week topical terbinafine cream compared to 4 weeks miconazole cream in patients with Tinea pedis. *J Med Assoc Thailand* 1999; **82**:1006–9.

12 Schopf R, Hettler O, Brautigam M, *et al.* Efficacy and tolerability of terbinafine 1% topical solution used for 1 week compared with 4 weeks clotrimazole 1% topical solution in the treatment of interdigital tinea pedis: a randomized, double-blind, multi-centre, 8-week clinical trial. *Mycoses* 1999;**42**:415–20.

13 Aly R, Maibach HI, Bagatell FK, Dittmar W, Hanel H, Falanga V. Ciclopiroxolamine lotion 1% bioequivalence to ciclopiroxolamine cream and clinical efficacy in tinea pedis. *Clin Ther* 1989;**11**:290–302.

14 Aly R, Fisher G, Katz HI, *et al.* Ciclopirox gel in the treatment of patients with interdigital tinea pedis. *Int J Dermatol* 2003; **42**(Suppl 1):29–35.

15 Barnetson RS, Marley J, Bullen M, *et al.* Comparison of one week of oral terbinafine (250 mg/per day) with four weeks of treatment with clotrimazole 1% cream in interdigital tinea pedis. *Br J Dermatol* 1998;**139**:675–8.

16 Williams H. Pragmatic clinical trial is now needed [letter]. *BMJ* 1999;**319**:1070.

38 Onychomycosis

Aditya K. Gupta, Elizabeth A. Cooper

Background

Definition

Onychomycosis is a fungal infection of the nail caused predominantly by anthropophilic dermatophytes, less commonly by yeast (*Candida* spp.), and by nondermatophyte mold infections.[1-3] Onychomycosis may present with hyperkeratosis, subungual debris, thickening, or discoloration of the nail plate (Figure 38.1). Total nail dystrophy may also result with advanced onychomycosis.[3]

Incidence/prevalence

Onychomycosis is the most common nail disorder in adults. It accounts for approximately 50% of all nail diseases[4,5]

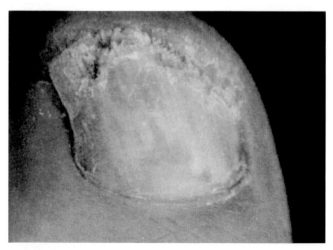

Figure 38.1 Infection of the nail of the left great toe in a 47-year-old nondiabetic male who had no other health problems. He gave a history of a nail abnormality that had persisted for approximately 15 years, possibly related to previous nail trauma. The thickened nail had large areas of yellowish–white discoloration, typical of fungal nail infection. Culture revealed infection with the dermatophyte fungus *Trichophyton rubrum*.

and has increased in individuals over the last 80 years.[3] In North American centers, the prevalence of onychomycosis is between approximately 6.5% and 13.8%.[4,6-8] Onychomycosis predominantly affects toenails in comparison with fingernails; in some reports, the ratio of toenail : fingernail onychomycosis ranges from 4 : 1 to 19 : 1.[4,7,9,10]

Etiology/risk factors

Predisposing factors for onychomycosis include tinea pedis, positive family history, increasing age, male gender, trauma, immunosuppression, diabetes mellitus, poor peripheral circulation, and smoking.[3,4,6,7,11-18] In addition, for fingernails persistent exposure to water, the use of artificial nails, and trauma induced by pushing back the cuticles and aggressive manicuring may also be predisposing factors.

Prognosis

Onychomycosis can be effectively treated with systemic and/or topical antifungal agents. Traditional systemic agents used to treat onychomycosis include griseofulvin and ketoconazole. The newer oral agents used to treat onychomycosis are terbinafine, itraconazole, and fluconazole.[19-26] Recent available data suggest that ravuconazole, a triazole, is effective for this indication.[27] Topical treatments include ciclopirox and amorolfine nail lacquers.[28,29] Only ciclopirox nail lacquer 8% has been approved in the United States for the treatment of onychomycosis.[30]

Relapse of onychomycosis, especially in the toenails, is not uncommon, particularly in predisposed individuals. The reasons why fingernail onychomycosis responds better than toenail disease may be related to the fact that perfusion of the upper extremity is generally better than that of the lower extremity; this may result in improved drug delivery to the fingers in comparison with the toes. Also, fingernails have a faster rate of outgrowth in comparison with toenails

(3 mm/month compared to 1 mm/month),[31] resulting in the infected fingernail growing out faster than its lower-extremity counterpart.

Aims of treatment

Onychomycosis may be a cosmetic problem, especially when fingernails are infected.[32] The treatment objectives are to reduce the fungal burden within the nail, ultimately curing the fungal infection, and to promote healthy regrowth of affected nails. In some instances, when onychomycosis is associated with a degree of morbidity—for example, pain, discomfort, or soft-tissue infection—timely treatment may help eliminate symptoms and prevent complications that could be associated with more severe consequences.[33]

Relevant outcomes

The most commonly reported therapeutic measure of efficacy is mycologic cure, which is defined by most as a negative light-microscopic examination and negative culture. There are several methods by which clinical improvement has been assessed. Some studies have used the parameter of clinical success, which is defined as "cleared" or "markedly improved" (90–100% clear nail).[34] Others have defined clinical success as cure or improvement sufficient to reduce the involved area of the target nail to less than 25% at the end of therapy.[35] Another term that has been used is "clinical effectiveness," which is taken to be mycologic cure and at least 5 mm of new clear toenail growth.[36] Clinical cure refers to the post-therapy nail appearing completely cured to the naked eye. The complete cure rate is the combined result of mycologic and clinical cure.

These outcomes are typically reported in clinical trials in which one toenail is chosen as the target, and "cure" is based on the target toenail alone. While such standards are necessary to provide points of comparison for clinical efficacy, all affected nails would be cured if a regimen was "successful." There is a paucity of clinical data including outcomes for all affected toenails during oral therapy, and there is evidence to suggest that not all toenails can be expected to have equivalent degrees of clinical cure.[37,38] Clinicians should keep in mind that the outcomes measured in clinical studies may not adequately represent all patients being treated for onychomycosis.

The limitations of standard microscopy and culture methods have been recognized for years, particularly in relation to the high rate of false-negative cultures, but until recently no other reliable methods of fungus identification have been available. Reports on the use of molecular-biological methods to identify fungal DNA are increasing.[39–43]

These molecular methods provide faster identification relative to the standard microscopy/culture methods. It remains to be seen what impact such analysis may have on fungal treatment. Greater use of such analyses can be expected in the future, particularly if it can be conclusively demonstrated that such methods can provide an analysis of viable fungus present in nails with higher reliability than standard microscopy/culture methods.

Methods

To identify studies in which oral treatments, itraconazole (continuous and pulse), fluconazole, terbinafine (continuous and pulse), and griseofulvin were used to treat adults with toenail or fingernail onychomycosis caused by dermatophytes, we searched Medline (1966–July 2007) for randomized controlled trials (RCTs). The reference sections of the published reports were also examined for potential studies not listed in the database.

Some of the studies were completely[27,28,44–276] or partially[34,35,277–287] excluded, for various reasons: open trials, studies conducted in special populations (e.g., diabetic patients, Down's syndrome, transplant patients), reports in which we were unable to extract relevant data, double publications, retrospective studies and studies not published in English.

Onychomycosis caused by *Candida* spp. and nondermatophyte molds is less common and will not be considered in this chapter.

The use of the nail lacquers ciclopirox and amorolfine are discussed, as these agents are approved for use in onychomycosis. There are many anecdotal reports of various other topical agents being effective for the management of onychomycosis; however, published reports of the efficacy of topical agents in onychomycosis in the indexed, peer-reviewed literature are far fewer. Other clinical trials have included tioconazole 28% solution, bifonazole with urea, fungoid tincture, miconazole, and tea-tree oil.

The use of other topical agents and cosmetic procedures such as debridement, combined with oral therapy, is not considered here, as most of these studies are single studies and not widely practiced at this time.[145,274–276] However, support for adjunctive therapy, particularly in the more severe cases of onychomycosis, has increased, in an effort to improve cure rates without increasing exposure to oral medications.[288] Further studies of such combinations are anticipated.

This chapter discusses the distal and lateral presentation of onychomycosis, which is the most common type; treatment of the other types of onychomycosis is not considered.[3,289]

Also excluded were studies that used nonstandard treatment dosages or durations for the toenails—e.g., terbinafine therapy < 3 months or > 4 months; itraconazole (continuous) therapy < 3 months or > 4 months or < 200 mg/day; itraconazole (pulse) therapy for less than three pulses or more than four pulses; fluconazole dosage other than 150 mg per week; griseofulvin therapy < 3 months; and for the fingernails—e.g., terbinafine therapy > 6 weeks; itraconazole (continuous) therapy > 6 weeks; itraconazole (pulse) for more than two pulses; fluconazole dosage other than 150 mg per week; or other nonstandard regimens, such as sequential or combination therapy.

We have not considered trials in which ketoconazole was used to treat onychomycosis, given the potential of this agent to cause hepatotoxicity and the availability of alternative agents.

The use of ravuconazole for the management of onychomycosis has not been considered further in this chapter, as only one published report of efficacy is known to the authors currently.[27]

Evidence was graded using the quality-of-evidence scale system employed by Cox *et al.*:[290]

• I: Evidence obtained from at least one properly designed randomized controlled trial.
• II-i: Evidence obtained from well-designed controlled trials without randomization.
• II-ii: Evidence obtained from well-designed cohort or case–control analytic studies, preferably from more than one center or research group.
• II-iii: Evidence obtained from multiple time series with or without the intervention. Dramatic results in uncontrolled experiments could also be included.
• III: Opinions of respected authorities based on clinical experience, descriptive studies, or reports by expert committees.
• IV: Evidence inadequate owing to problems of methodology (e.g., sample size, length or comprehensiveness of follow-up, or conflicts in evidence).

Questions

What is the role of oral antifungal therapy in the management of dermatophyte onychomycosis in adults?

Griseofulvin was the first significant oral antifungal agent available for the management of dermatomycoses. Over the years, the use of griseofulvin in the treatment of onychomycosis has decreased, although it is still widely used for the treatment of tinea capitis.[291] Ketoconazole, an oral imidazole, is no longer recommended for the treatment of onychomycosis, which requires a long duration of therapy, due to the potential for hepatotoxicity.[291] The introduction of the new oral antifungal agents terbinafine, itraconazole, and fluconazole has led to improved efficacy rates, decreased treatment duration, and fewer adverse events.

What are the effects of systemic treatments on fingernail and on toenail onychomycosis?

Griseofulvin

The regimen for treating onychomycosis is continuous therapy using a dosage of 500 mg/day to 1 g/day, typically administered for 6–12 months in fingernail onychomycosis and for 9–18 months in toenail disease.

Fingernails (quality of evidence: I)

One randomized double-blind study compared griseofulvin to terbinafine in the treatment of onychomycosis (Table 38.1).[282]

Fingernails: effectiveness

In a double-blind RCT,[282] griseofulvin was given at a dosage of 500 mg/day for 12 weeks. The mycological cure rate and complete cure rate were 63% and 39%, respectively.

Toenails (quality of evidence: I)

Three double-blind RCTs[281,285,292] and one open RCT[283] compared griseofulvin to terbinafine (continuous) or itraconazole (continuous) in the treatment of onychomycosis (Table 38.2).

Toenails: effectiveness

In the RCTs, 500 mg/day or 1 g/day of griseofulvin was administered to treat onychomycosis. In the double-blind RCTs, the mycological cure rate ranged from 45% to 69%, and complete cure occurred in 2–56% of patients. In the open RCT, 6% of the patients were completely cured.

Drawbacks

The use of griseofulvin may be associated with adverse events such as gastrointestinal upset, nausea, diarrhea, headache, central nervous system symptoms, and urticaria.[293] No drugs are contraindicated with griseofulvin, and few drug interactions are associated with griseofulvin therapy.

Comments

Griseofulvin was the first systemic agent used to treat onychomycosis on a widespread basis. Currently, the newer oral agents (itraconazole, terbinafine, and fluconazole) have been found to be more effective than griseofulvin; the duration of active therapy is also shorter with the more recently introduced antimycotics.[294,295] Moreover, when griseofulvin is used to treat dermatophyte toenail onychomycosis, relapse rates may be higher (40–60%)[137] in comparison with the newer oral antifungal agents.[34,296–299]

Continuous terbinafine

The regimen for fingernail and toenail onychomycosis is 250 mg/day, administered for 6 and 12 weeks, respectively.

Table 38.1 Treatment of dermatophyte fingernail onychomycosis

Year	First author, ref.	Treatment	Study type	Evaluable patients (n)	Regimen	Treatment duration	Follow-up period (after treatment)	Efficacy measure		
								MC*	CR†	CC‡
2001	TER package insert[299]	TERC	DB, R, placebo-controlled	Not stated	250 mg/day	6 wk	24 wk	(79%)	ND	(59%)
1997	Odom[323]	ITRP	DB, R, multicenter placebo-controlled	37	400 mg/day 1 wk/mo	2 mo	Up to 19 wk	16/22 (73%)	17/22 (77%)	15/22 (68%)
1998	Drake[278]	FLUC	DB, R, parallel, multicenter, placebo-controlled	78	150 mg/wk	Up to 9 mo	6 mo	70/78 (90%) ND	69/78 (88%)	61/78 (78%) ND
1995	Haneke[282]	GRIS	DB, R, comparative (TERC)	92	500 mg/day	12 wk, followed by 12 wk placebo	6 mo	45/72 (63%)		(39%)

CC, complete cure; CR, clinical response; DB, double-blind; FLUC, fluconazole; GRIS, griseofulvin; ITRP, itraconazole pulse; MC, mycological cure; mo, months; ND, not defined; R, randomized; TER, terbinafine; TERC, terbinafine continuous; wk, weeks.
* Mycological cure defined as negative microscopy and culture, unless indicated otherwise.
† Clinical response defined as cured or markedly improved, unless indicated otherwise.
‡ Complete cure defined as mycological and clinical cure or improvement, unless indicated otherwise.

Table 38.2 Treatment of dermatophyte toenail onychomycosis using griseofulvin therapy

Year	First author, ref.	Study type	Evaluable patients (n)	Regimen	Treatment duration	Follow-up period (after treatment)	Efficacy measure		
							MC*	CR†	CC‡
1997	Baran[285]	DB, R, parallel, multicenter, comparative (TERC)	58	1 g/day	Up to 12 mo		(69%)		(44%)
1995	Faergemann[292]	DB, R, parallel, comparative (TERC)	41	500 mg/day	13 mo		19/41 (46%) ND		1/41 (2%)§
1995	Hofmann[281]	DB, R, comparative (TERC)	88	1000 mg/day	48 wk	24 wk	42/68 (62%)	ND	49/88 (56%)#
1993	Korting[283]	Open, R, comparative (ITRC)	36 / 36	660 mg/day / 990 mg/day	Up to 18 mo		ND ND	ND ND	2/36 (6%) 2/36 (6%)

CC, complete cure; CR, clinical response; DB, double-blind; ITRC, itraconazole continuous; MC, mycological cure; mo, months; ND, not defined; R, randomized; TERC, terbinafine continuous; wk, weeks.
* Mycological cure defined as negative microscopy and culture, unless indicated otherwise.
† Clinical response defined as cured or markedly improved, unless indicated otherwise.
‡ Complete cure defined as mycological and clinical cure or improvement, unless indicated otherwise.
§ Complete cure defined as clinical cure and negative mycological culture.
# Complete cure defined as mycological cure and continuous growth of unaffected nail.

Fingernails (quality of evidence: I)

Two double-blind RCTs evaluated patients with fingernail onychomycosis only. One study administered terbinafine for 12 weeks and therefore was not included in this analysis.[282]

Fingernails: effectiveness

The double-blind, randomized, placebo-controlled study used terbinafine 250 mg/day for 6 weeks to treat fingernail onychomycosis (Table 38.1).[299] Mycological cure was achieved in 79% of patients and complete cure in 59%.

Toenails (quality of evidence: I)

The majority of studies were double-blind RCTs. Terbinafine was administered at a dose of 250 mg/day terbinafine for 3–4 months (Table 38.3).

Toenails: effectiveness

Six double-blind RCTs compared terbinafine with placebo.[34,286,299–302] Each study reported that terbinafine 250 mg/day was significantly more effective than placebo in treating onychomycosis.

Twelve double-blind, randomized studies compared terbinafine (continuous) with other drug comparators,[36,287,292,303–311] with mycological cure rates ranging from 46% to 95% and the corresponding clinical response rates being 66–97%.

Four open RCTs reported the efficacy of terbinafine (continuous) for 3 or 4 months.[312–315] Mycological cure rates ranged between 75% and 94%. In one study, the clinical response was reported to be 68%.[315] Complete cure ranged between 63% and 79% for reported studies.

Drawbacks

The treatment of onychomycosis with terbinafine (continuous) is associated with a low frequency of adverse events.[294,316] These adverse events are generally mild to moderate in severity, and reversible. The more common adverse events involve the gastrointestinal tract, skin, and central nervous system. Only a small proportion of patients discontinue treatment with terbinafine. Pretreatment serum transaminase tests (alanine transaminase and aspartate transaminase) should be considered in all patients before terbinafine therapy is initiated.[299,317] Terbinafine is an inhibitor of the CYP450 2D6 isozyme, which includes tricyclic antidepressants, selective serotonin reuptake inhibitors, beta-blockers, class 1C antiarrhythmics, and monoamine oxidase inhibitors.[299,318,319] Caution should be used when terbinafine is given to patients using drugs metabolized by CYP 2D6, particularly those drugs with a narrow therapeutic window.[299,317]

Comments

Terbinafine is effective and safe for the treatment of onychomycosis. Terbinafine is an allylamine that inhibits squalene epoxidase, resulting in an accumulation of squalene and a deficiency of ergosterol. The accumulation of squalene may be associated with fungicidal action.[320] In one study, the relapse rate (≥ 90% clear nail at any time and < 90% at last visit) was recorded in 15% of patients when followed up for up to 96 weeks from the start of therapy.[34] There are a substantial number of high-quality studies that demonstrate the effectiveness of terbinafine (continuous) in the treatment of toenail onychomycosis, some of which have stated that this may be the most effective agent available for this indication.[321,322]

Terbinafine (pulse)

Terbinafine (pulse) is administered as 250 mg twice a day for 1 week, followed by 3 weeks off between successive pulses. Typically, two pulses are required to treat fingernail onychomycosis and three or four pulses for toenail disease.

Toenails (quality of evidence: I)

Four studies have reported the use of intermittent terbinafine therapy in the treatment of onychomycosis (Table 38.4). Each of the studies is randomized and against a comparator; two are open, one is single-blind, and one is double-blind. The follow-up periods are approximately 10–18 months.

Toenails: effectiveness

The double-blind, randomized study[311] showed a mycological cure rate of 59% (n = 143) and complete cure rate of 28% (n = 143) after 18 months.

One single-blind, randomized study[277] compared terbinafine pulse to a sequential treatment in which two itraconazole pulses were followed by a terbinafine pulse. The mycological cure rate in the terbinafine group was 49%, and therapy was effective (mycological cure plus at least 5 mm of new nail growth) in 46% of patients, with 32% of patients completely cured (n = 90).

In the two open, randomized comparative studies,[313,314] intermittent terbinafine therapy was associated with complete cure rates of 50% (n = 20)[313] and 74% (n = 23).[314] In the study by Tosti et al.,[313] the mycological cure rate was 80% (n = 20).

Drawbacks

Intermittent terbinafine therapy has been associated with few adverse events. Adverse events are generally mild to moderate, and reversible. The spectrum of adverse effects is similar to that seen with the continuous terbinafine regimen. A terbinafine (pulse) regimen is not indicated for the treatment of onychomycosis, and therefore there are no monitoring guidelines in the United States.

Comments

The preferred regimen for the treatment of onychomycosis using terbinafine is continuous rather than pulse therapy. In comparison with the continuous regimen, which has been well studied, there are relatively few data available on both the efficacy and safety of the pulse regimen.

Pulse itraconazole

Itraconazole pulse therapy is taken to be 200 mg twice a day for 1 week, followed by 3 weeks off between successive pulses. Typically, two pulses are administered for fingernail onychomycosis and three or four pulses for toenail disease. Pulse dosing is the regimen approved by the Food and Drugs Administration (FDA) regimen for

Table 38.3 Treatment of dermatophyte toenail onychomycosis using terbinafine continuous therapy

Year	First author, ref.	Study type	Evaluable patients (n)	Regimen	Treatment duration	Follow-up period (from baseline)	Efficacy measure MC*	CR†	CC‡
2001	TER Package Insert (US)[299]	DB, R, placebo-controlled	Not stated	250 mg/day	12 wk	48 wk	(70%)	ND	(38%)
1999	Billstein[300]	DB, R, parallel, multicenter, placebo-controlled	29 27	250 mg/day	12 wk 16 wk	72 wk	18/21 (86%) 13/16 (81%)	ND ND	ND ND
1997	Drake[34]	DB, R, multicenter, placebo-controlled	142	250 mg/day	12 wk	48 wk	(70%)	58/71 (82%)	ND
1997	Svejgaard[301]	DB, R, multicenter placebo-controlled	48	250 mg/day	3 mo	9 or 12 mo	19/48 (40%)	ND	18/48 (38%)
1995	Watson[302]	DB, R, placebo-controlled	56	250 mg/day	12 wk	24 wk	33/56 (59%)	ND	
1992	Goodfield[286]	DB, R, parallel, multicenter, placebo-controlled	45	250 mg/day	12 wk	48 wk	37/45 (82%)	ND	ND
2006	Sigurgeirsson[287]	DB, DD, R, comparative (TERP)	Trial 1: 390 Trial 2: 405	250 mg/day	12 wk	48 wk	226/390 (58%) 225/405 (56%)	100/390 (26%) 120/405 (30%)	ND ND
2005	Warshaw[311]	DB, DD, R, comparative (TERP)	148	250 mg/day	12 wk (3 mo)	72 weeks (18 mo)	105/148 (71%)	66/148 (45%)§	60/148 (40%)
2002	Heikkila[303]	DB, DD, R, multicenter, comparative (ITRP)	23	250 mg/day	12 wk	72 wk	Negative microscopy: 21/23 (91%) Negative culture: 20/23 (87%)	ND	11/23 (48%) ND
			18		16 wk		Negative microscopy: 18/18 (100%) Negative culture: 17/18 (94%)	ND	9/18 (50%) ND
2002	Sigurgeirsson[304]	DB, DD, R, comparative (ITRP)	74	250 mg/day	12 or 16 wk	Up to 5 years	34/74 (46%)	ND	26/74 (35%)
1999	Evans[36]	DB, DD, R, parallel, multicenter, comparative (ITRP)	110 99	250 mg/day	12 wk 16 wk	72 wk	81/107 (76%) 80/99 (81%)	67/102 (66%)# 67/95 (71%)	49/107 (46%) 54/98 (55%)
1999	Degreef[308]	DB, R, parallel, multicenter, comparative (ITRC)	144	250 mg/day	12 wk	48 mo	(67%)	(87%)	ND
1998	De Backer[306]	DB, R, parallel, multicenter, comparative (ITRC)	186	250 mg/day	12 wk	48 wk	119/163 (73%)	(76%) ND	(38%)

Table 38.3 Cont'd

Year	First author, ref.	Study type	Evaluable patients (n)	Regimen	Treatment duration	Follow-up period (from baseline)	MC*	CR†	CC‡
							Efficacy measure		
1997	Honeyman[307]	DB, DD, R, parallel, multicenter, comparative (ITRC)	64	250 mg/day	4 mo	48 wk	61/64 (95%)¶	62/64 (97%)	61/64 (95%)
1995	Brautigam[309]	DB, R, parallel, multicenter, comparative (ITRC)	86	250 mg/day	12 wk	52 wk	70/86 (81%)	69/86 (80%) / ND	ND
1995	Faergemann[292]	DB, R, parallel, comparative (GRIS)	43	250 mg/day	4 mo		36/43 (84%) ND	ND	18/43 (42%)‡‡
2000	Havu[305]	DB; double-placebo, R, multicenter, comparative (FLUC)	46	250 mg/day	12 wk	60 wk	41/46 (89%)	39/46 (85%)#	ND
1994	De Backer[310]	DB, R, parallel, comparative (TERC)	49 / 51	250 mg/day / 500 mg/day	4 mo	48 wk	41/49 (84%) / 46/51 (90%)	44/49 (90%) / 45/51 (88%)	ND / ND
1997	Tausch[280]	DB, R, multicenter, duration-finding	56	250 mg/day	12 wk	48 wk	46/56 (82%)	33/56 (59%)#	33/56 (59%)
1992	van der Schroeff[284]	DB, R, duration-finding	30 / 34 / 34	250 mg/day	6 wk / 12 wk / 24 wk	48 wk	12/29 (41%) / 24/34 (71%) / 28/34 (82%)	ND / ND / ND	12/30 (40%) / 24/34 (71%) / 27/34 (79%)
2002	Arca[312]	Open, R, comparative (ITRP, FLUC)	16	250 mg/day	3 mo	6 mo	12/16 (75%)	ND	10/16 (63%)
1999	Kejda[315]	Open, R, parallel, comparative (ITRP)	25	250 mg/day	3 mo	12 mo	(76%)	17/25 (68%)	ND
1996	Tosti[313]	Open, R, comparative (ITRP, TERP)	19	250 mg/day	4 mo	10 mo	16/17 (94%)	ND	13/17 (76%)
1996	Alpsoy[314]	Open, R, comparative (TERP)	24	250 mg/day	3 mo	12 mo	ND	ND	19/24 (79%)

CC, complete cure; CR, clinical response; DB, double-blind; DD, double-dummy; FLUC, fluconazole; ITRC, itraconazole continuous; ITRP, itraconazole pulse; MC, mycological cure; mo, months; ND, not defined; R, randomized; TER, terbinafine; TERC, terbinafine continuous; TERP, terbinafine pulse; wk, weeks.

* Mycological cure defined as negative microscopy and culture, unless indicated otherwise.

† Clinical response defined as cured or markedly improved, unless indicated otherwise.

‡ Complete cure defined as mycological and clinical cure or improvement, unless indicated otherwise.

§ Defined as "complete cure—normal appearance with no evidence of onycholysis."

Variable definitions of clinical response used.

¶ Mycological cure defined as negative microscopy.

Table 38.4 Treatment of dermatophyte toenail onychomycosis using terbinafine pulse therapy

Year	First author, ref.	Study type	Evaluable patients (n)	Regimen	Treatment duration	Follow-up period (after treatment)	Efficacy measure		
							MC*	CR†	CC‡
2005	Warshaw[311]	DB, DD, R, comparative (TERC)	143	500 mg/day 1 wk/mo	3 mo	18 mo	84/143 (59%)	42/143 (29%)§	40/143 (28%)
2001	Gupta[277]	SB, R, parallel, comparative (ITRP + TERP)	90	500 mg/day 1 wk/mo	3 mo	18 mo	44/90 (49%)	41/90 (46%)#	29/90 (32%)
1996	Alpsoy[314]	Open, R, comparative (TERC)	23	500 mg/day 1 wk/mo	3 mo	12 mo	ND	ND	17/23 (74%)
1996	Tosti[313]	Open, R, comparative (ITRP, TERC)	20	500 mg/day 1 wk/mo	4 mo	10 mo	16/20 (80%)	ND	10/20 (50%)

CC, complete cure; CR, clinical response; DB, double-blind; DD, double-dummy; ITRP, itraconazole pulse; MC, mycological cure; mo, months; ND, not defined; R, randomized; SB, single-blind; TERC, terbinafine continuous; TERP, terbinafine pulse; wk, weeks.
* Mycological cure defined as negative microscopy and culture, unless indicated otherwise.
† Clinical response defined as cured or markedly improved, unless indicated otherwise.
‡ Complete cure defined as mycological and clinical cure or improvement, unless indicated otherwise.
§ Defined as "complete cure—normal appearance with no evidence of onycholysis."
# Variable definitions of clinical response used.

infections of the fingernails when no toenail involvement has been noted.[298]

Fingernails (quality of evidence: I)
One double-blind, placebo-controlled trial investigated the efficacy of itraconazole (pulse) treatment in fingernail onychomycosis (Table 38.1).[323]

Fingernails: effectiveness
The mycological cure and clinical response rates were 73% and 77%, respectively.[323]

Toenails (quality of evidence: I)
Ten RCTs, four of which were double-blind, evaluated itraconazole pulse in the treatment of toenail onychomycosis (Table 38.5).

Toenails: effectiveness
One double-blind RCT compared three pulses of itraconazole with placebo.[324] A significant difference was observed between the mycological cure rate with itraconazole (62%) and placebo (P < 0.0001). A significant difference also existed between the clinical response rate in the active treatment (65%) in comparison with the placebo group (P < 0.001).

Three double-blind, randomized comparative studies evaluated itraconazole pulse treatment in comparison with continuous terbinafine treatment[36,303] and in comparison with continuous itraconazole treatment.[325] The mycological cure rates for the itraconazole pulse groups ranged

between 38% and 69%. The corresponding range for clinical response rates was 13–81%.

Six open, randomized comparative studies[312,313,315,326–328] reported mycological cure rates of itraconazole that ranged between 61% and 75% and clinical response rates between 77% and 88%.

Drawbacks
Itraconazole (pulse) therapy is approved for fingernail, but not toenail, onychomycosis in the United States. Adverse events occur with a low frequency and are generally mild to moderate in severity, and reversible. These events include gastrointestinal upset, cutaneous eruption, and headache.[329] Studies report a low discontinuation rate due to an adverse event. Itraconazole has the potential for numerous drug interactions, and a thorough review of current medications being used by the patient is required before prescribing.[298,318,319,330] In some cases, the drug interaction may be explained on the basis of an inhibition of cytochrome P450 3A4 by itraconazole. Itraconazole is contraindicated with cisapride, pimozide, quinidine, dofetilide, and levacetylmethadol (levomethadyl).[298,330] Itraconazole is contraindicated in the United States and Canada in patients with evidence of ventricular dysfunction—for example, congestive heart failure or a history of heart failure.[298,331] Liver function monitoring should be done in patients with preexisting hepatic function abnormalities or a history of liver toxicity with a previous medication, and should be considered for all patients using itraconazole.[298,331]

Table 38.5 Treatment of dermatophyte toenail onychomycosis using itraconazole pulse therapy

Year	First author, ref.	Study type	Evaluable patients (n)	Regimen	Treatment duration	Follow-up period (from baseline)	Efficacy measure MC*	CR†	CC‡
2000	Gupta[324]	DB, R, placebo-controlled	78	400 mg/day 1 wk/mo	3 mo	48 wk	48/78 (62%)	51/78 (65%)	ND
2002	Heikkila[303]	DB, DD, R, multicenter, comparative (TERC)	18	400 mg/day 1 wk/mo	12 wk	72 wk	Negative microscopy: 11/18 (61%) Negative culture: 12/18 (67%)	ND	6/18 (33%) ND
			17		16 wk		Negative microscopy: 11/17 (65%) Negative culture: 13/17 (76%)	ND	3/17 (18%) ND
2002	Sigurgeirsson[304]	DB, DD, R, comparative (TERC)	77	400 mg/day 1 wk/mo	12 or 16 wk	Up to 5 y	10/77 (13%)	ND	11/77 (14%)
1999	Evans[36]	DB, DD, R, parallel, multicenter, comparative (TERC)	107	400 mg/day 1 wk/mo	12 wk	72 wk	41/107 (38%)	29/102 (28%)§	25/107 (23%)
			109		16 wk		53/108 (49%)	35/104 (34%)§	28/108 (26%)
1997	Havu[325]	DB, R, parallel, multicenter, comparative (ITRC)	59	400 mg/day 1 wk/mo	3 mo	12 mo	41/59 (69%)	48/59 (81%)	ND
2002	Arca[312]	Open, R, comparative (TERC, FLUC)	18	400 mg/day 1 wk/mo	3 mo	6 mo	11/18 (61%)	ND	11/18 (61%)
1999	Shemer[327]	Open, R, comparative (ITRC)	Minimum of 16 patients in each group	400 mg/day 1 wk/mo	3 mo	48 wk	ND	ND	(50%)
					4 mo		ND	ND	(65%)
1999	Kejda[315]	Open, R, parallel, comparative (TERC)	26	400 mg/day 1 wk/mo	3 mo	12 mo	(75%)	20/26 (77%)	ND
1996	Tosti[313]	Open, R, comparative (TERC, TERP)	21	400 mg/day 1 wk/mo	4 mo	10 mo	15/20 (75%)	ND	8/21 (38%)
1996	De Doncker[228]	Open, R, comparative (ITRP)	25	400 mg/day 1 wk/mo	3 mo	Up to 1 y	16/25 (64%)	22/25 (88%)	ND
			25		4 mo		18/25 (72%)	21/25 (84%)	ND

CC, complete cure; CR, clinical response; DB, double-blind; DD, double-dummy; FLUC, fluconazole; ITRC, itraconazole continuous; ITRP, itraconazole pulse; MC, mycological cure; mo, months; ND, not defined; R, randomized; TERC, terbinafine continuous; TERP, terbinafine pulse; wk, weeks.
* Mycological cure defined as negative microscopy and culture, unless indicated otherwise.
† Clinical response defined as cured or markedly improved, unless indicated otherwise.
‡ Complete cure defined as mycological and clinical cure or improvement, unless indicated otherwise.
§ Variable definitions of clinical response used.

Comments

Itraconazole pulse therapy is effective and safe in onychomycosis. The pulse regimen used to treat toenail onychomycosis decreases the itraconazole required by one-half in comparison with the continuous regimen with this triazole. This may result in cost savings and increased compliance and may reduce the frequency of adverse events.[324,329,332–334] In fact, the pulse regimen is the preferred mode of drug delivery when using itraconazole. No significant difference was found between three-pulse and four-pulse regimens of itraconazole for the primary efficacy parameters in the treatment of toenail onychomycosis.[328] In one report, after the use of three pulses for the treatment of toenail onychomycosis, the relapse rate at follow-up, 12 months after the start of therapy, was 10.4%.[334] Two pulses of itraconazole should be effective and safe in fingernail onychomycosis.

Continuous itraconazole

The regimen for fingernail and toenail onychomycosis is 200 mg/day administered for 6 and 12 weeks, respectively. Continuous itraconazole is used infrequently in current practice, in favor of the pulse itraconazole regimens.

Fingernails (quality of evidence: none)

No studies have been published on the use of continuous itraconazole for fingernail onychomycosis.

Toenails (quality of evidence: I)

The majority of reported studies were double-blind RCTs (Table 38.6).

Toenails: effectiveness

In the four double-blind RCTs that compared itraconazole (continuous) with placebo, significantly more patients receiving the active treatment achieved a mycological cure and clinical response ($P < 0.01$).[298,335–337] The mycological cure rates in the RCTs treating patients with itraconazole continuous ranged from 46% to 84%; the corresponding range for clinical response rates was 58–83%.

Drawbacks

Adverse events associated with the use of continuous itraconazole for the treatment of onychomycosis are not common, and those experienced are generally mild to moderate in severity. Adverse events include gastrointestinal disorders (e.g., nausea, abdominal pain), rashes, and central nervous system effects (e.g., headache).[325,329,332–334] Only a small proportion of patients discontinue treatment with the triazole. There are drugs that are contraindicated with itraconazole (see the section on itraconazole pulse therapy above). In addition, the triazole has several drug interactions (see the section above). Itraconazole is contraindicated in North America in patients with evidence of ventricular dysfunction—for example, congestive heart failure or a history of heart failure. The U.S. package insert suggests that liver function tests should be considered for all patients receiving continuous therapy.[298] Treatment should be stopped immediately and liver function tests should be performed whenever a patient develops signs and symptoms suggestive of liver disease.[298]

Comments

Continuous itraconazole therapy is an effective and well-tolerated treatment for onychomycosis. Historically, the treatment of onychomycosis with itraconazole was with the continuous regimen; later, work done by de Doncker et al.[328,334] resulted in the widespread adaptation of pulse therapy for this indication. The U.S. package insert states that when patients with toenail onychomycosis were treated with itraconazole continuous therapy, 21% of the overall success group had a relapse (worsening of the global score or conversion of KOH or culture from negative to positive).[297]

Fluconazole

The treatment regimen of fluconazole for onychomycosis is 150 mg once weekly, administered until the affected nail has grown out. Typically, the durations of therapy for fingernail and toenail disease have been 4–9 months and 9–15 months, respectively.[338]

Fingernails (quality of evidence: I)

One double-blind RCT assessed the efficacy of fluconazole in the treatment of fingernail onychomycosis (Table 38.1).[278]

Fingernails: effectiveness

The randomized, double-blind study[278] compared various regimens of fluconazole with each other and with placebo in the treatment of fingernail onychomycosis. Fluconazole 150 mg/week administered for up to 9 months resulted in a mycological cure rate of 90% and a clinical response rate of 88%.[278]

Toenails (quality of evidence: I)

Few double-blind RCTs have been reported (Table 38.7).[35,305]

Toenails: effectiveness

In the double-blind RCTs, mycological cure ranged between 49% and 53%. The corresponding clinical response rates were 23–77%. In the open RCT, 31% of patients were mycologically cured.[312]

Drawbacks

Fluconazole is not approved for the treatment of onychomycosis in North America. The more common adverse effects observed with fluconazole affect the gastrointestinal tract, cutaneous system, and central nervous system.[319,338] Adverse events do not commonly occur, and those experienced are usually of mild to moderate severity and reversible. Only

Table 38.6 Treatment of dermatophyte toenail onychomycosis using itraconazole continuous therapy

Year	First author, ref.	Study type	Evaluable patients (n)	Regimen	Treatment duration	Follow-up period (from baseline)	Efficacy measure		
							MC*	CR†	CC‡
2001	ITR package insert[298]	DB, R, placebo-controlled	110	200 mg/day	12 wk		(54%)	ND	(14%)
1996	Jones[336]	DB, R, placebo-controlled	35	200 mg/day	12 wk		24/35 (69%) ND	27/35 (77%) ND	18/35 (51%) ND
1996	Odom[337]	DB, R, placebo-controlled	38	200 mg/day	12 wk	48 wk	18/38 (47%)	26/38 (68%)	14/38 (37%)
1999	Degreef[308]	DB, R, parallel, multicenter, comparative (TERC)	145	200 mg/day	12 wk	48 wk	(61%)	(82%)	ND
1998	Haneke[279]	DB, R, parallel, multicenter, comparative (ITRC + ITRP, MIC)	479	200 mg/day	3 mo	12 mo	354/479 (74%)	395/479 (82%)	ND
1998	De Backer[306]	DB, R, parallel, multicenter, comparative (TERC)	186	200 mg/day	12 wk	48 wk	77/168 (46%)	(58%) ND	(23%) ND
1997	Elewski[335]	DB, R, multicenter, placebo-controlled	109	200 mg/day	12 wk	48 wk	59/109 (54%)	71/109 (65%)	
1997	Havu[325]	DB, R, multicenter, parallel, comparative (ITRP)	62	200 mg/day	3 mo	12 mo	41/62 (66%)	43/62 (69%)	ND
1997	Honeyman[307]	DB, DD, R, parallel, multicenter, comparative (TERC)	70	200 mg/day	4 mo	12 mo	59/70 (84%)§	58/70 (83%)#	53/70 (76%)
1995	Brautigam[309]	DB, R, parallel, multicenter, comparative (TERC)	84	200 mg/day	12 wk	52 wk	53/84 (63%)	63/84 (75%) ND	ND
1999	Shemer[327]	Open, R, comparative (ITRP)	Minimum of 16 patients in each group	200 mg/day	3 mo 4 mo	48 wk	ND ND	ND ND	(68%) (65%)

CC, complete cure; CR, clinical response; DB, double-blind; DD, double-dummy; ITR, itraconazole; ITRC, itraconazole continuous; ITRP, itraconazole pulse; MC, mycological cure; MIC, miconazole; mo, months; ND, not defined; R, randomized; TERC, terbinafine continuous; wk, weeks.

* Mycological cure defined as negative microscopy and culture, unless indicated otherwise.

† Clinical response defined as cured or markedly improved, unless indicated otherwise.

‡ Complete cure defined as mycological and clinical cure or improvement, unless indicated otherwise.

§ Mycological cure defined as negative microscopy.

Variable definitions of clinical response used.

a small proportion of patients discontinue treatment with fluconazole. The drugs contraindicated with fluconazole are cisapride and terfenadine. There are some drug interactions that may occur with the triazole; in certain cases, the drug interactions may be explained by fluconazole inhibiting cytochrome P450 2C9, and at higher doses the triazole may inhibit cytochrome P450 3A4.[318,319]

Comments

Fluconazole is effective and safe in onychomycosis. In comparison with terbinafine and itraconazole, there are relatively few studies that have evaluated the efficacy of fluconazole in the treatment of toenail onychomycosis. The preferred regimen for fluconazole is once-weekly therapy; typically, 150 mg per week administered for several months

Table 38.7 Treatment of dermatophyte toenail onychomycosis using fluconazole therapy

Year	First author, ref.	Study type	Evaluable patients (n)	Regimen	Treatment duration	Follow-up period (from baseline)	Efficacy measure		
							MC*	CR†	CC‡
2000	Havu[305]	DB, double-placebo, R, multicenter, comparative (TERC)	43 41	150 mg/wk	12 wk 24 wk	60 wk	22/43 (51%) 20/41 (49%)	10/43 (23%)§ 18/41 (44%)§	ND ND
1998	Scher[35]	DB, R, parallel, multicenter, placebo-controlled	73	150 mg/wk	Up to 12 mo	6 mo (only patients who were clinically cured or improved)	38/72 (53%)	56/73 (77%)	ND
2002	Arca[312]	Open, R, comparative (ITRP, TERC)	16	150 mg/wk	3 mo	6 mo	5/16 (31%)	ND	5/16 (31%)

CC, complete cure; CR, clinical response; DB, double-blind; ITRP, itraconazole pulse; MC, mycological cure; mo, months; ND, not defined; R, randomized; TERC, terbinafine continuous; wk, weeks.

* Mycological cure defined as negative microscopy and culture, unless indicated otherwise.

† Clinical response defined as cured or markedly improved, unless indicated otherwise.

‡ Complete cure defined as mycological and clinical cure or improvement, unless indicated otherwise.

§ Variable definitions of clinical response used.

until the abnormal-appearing nail plate has grown out. In the study reported by Scher *et al.*,[35] the clinical relapse rate over a 6-month follow-up was 4.4%.[296] Studies evaluating the use of once-weekly fluconazole at higher dosages, such as 300 mg or 450 mg once weekly,[35,278] or continuous fluconazole administration, have not been discussed.

What are the effects of topical nail lacquers on toenail onychomycosis?

Nail lacquers provide a direct application of antifungal medication, with the lacquer formulation providing a stable matrix of concentrated medication that aids drug penetration. Topical medications are associated with fewer and less severe adverse events than oral medications, and with less potential for drug interaction than use of oral antifungals. These make topical lacquers a desirable mode of antifungal treatment.

Amorolfine nail lacquer

Amorolfine 5% nail lacquer can be used once or twice weekly for 6 months for toenail onychomycosis. Amorolfine has not been approved in the United States or Canada for use in onychomycosis.

Quality of evidence: I

One randomized, double-blind study has reported on the efficacy of amorolfine 5% lacquer.[339] Two other studies compared once-weekly dosing with twice-weekly dosing, but the study design details could not be extracted from the

source reporting the trial results.[339] These trials were first reported in 1992,[340–342] and no further clinical trials have reported on monotherapy with amorolfine.

Effectiveness

Follow-up at 3 months post-treatment (month 9 of the study) showed mycological cure rates of 60% and 71%, respectively, for the trials in which sufficient data could be extracted[339] (Table 38.8). The complete cure rates were 38% and 46%, respectively (Table 38.8).

Drawbacks

Amorolfine is not currently approved for onychomycosis therapy in the United States or Canada. The trials reported were relatively small, and required that the patients should have no matrix involvement.[339] No further research has been reported on the use of amorolfine monotherapy.

Comments

Amorolfine has few safety concerns in comparison with oral therapy, with mild topical irritation being the most prevalent event. One patient who inadvertently used amorolfine twice daily rather than twice weekly reported no irritation.[343] Amorolfine may be an effective treatment for patients with milder, nonmatrix onychomycosis.

Amorolfine nail lacquer combined with oral antifungal therapy

Two trials have used amorolfine in combination with oral antifungals—one using continuous terbinafine[344] and the

Table 38.8 Treatment of onychomycosis with nail lacquers as monotherapy or in combination with oral antifungals

Year	First author, ref.	Treatment	Study type	Evaluable patients (n)	Regimen	Treatment duration	Follow-up period (from baseline)	Efficacy measure		
								MC*	CR†	CC‡
1992	Lauharanta[340]	AMOR	DB, R, multicenter, comparative	80	Once weekly	6 mo	9 mo	(60%)		(38%)§
1992	Reinel[341]	AMOR	R, multicenter	Not provided	Once weekly	6 mo	9 mo	(71%)		(46%)§
2000	Gupta[345]	CICL	DB, DD, R, multicenter, placebo-controlled	231	Daily	48 wk	Week 48	63/185 (34%)		16/181 (9%)§

AMOR, amorolfine 5% nail lacquer; CC, complete cure; CICL, ciclopirox 8% nail lacquer; CR, clinical response; DB, double-blind; DD, double-dummy; MC, mycological cure; mo, months; R, randomized; wk, weeks.

* Mycological cure defined as negative microscopy and culture, unless indicated otherwise.
† Clinical response defined as cured or markedly improved, unless indicated otherwise.
‡ Complete cure defined as mycological and clinical cure or improvement, unless indicated otherwise.
§ Mycological cure with a normal nail or a nail with ≤ 10% still affected.

other using continuous itraconazole.[89] Both trials involved onychomycosis with matrix involvement.

Quality of evidence: II
Both trials are randomized, but use an open design rather than blinded design.

Effectiveness
Combined use of amorolfine once weekly for 15 months with continuous terbinafine for 12 weeks led to a global cure (mycologically and clinically clear) in month 15 in 72.3% of cases, in comparison with 37.5% with continuous terbinafine monotherapy for 12 weeks.[344]

Combined use of amorolfine once weekly for 24 weeks, with continuous itraconazole for 12 weeks, showed a global cure rate—negative microscopy and culture, plus disappearance of all visible changes or a 95% reduction in the diseased nail surface area—at week 24 of 93.9%, versus 68.8% for continuous itraconazole alone.[89]

Drawbacks
The open design may produce some bias in assessment. Blinded studies should be done to confirm the results. There was a relatively high drop-out rate in the first study, with many patients leaving due to lack of efficacy. Efficacy definitions are not clearly explained and may not be comparable with other onychomycosis trials.

Comments
The rate and type of adverse events noted with combination therapies were similar to those noted with the respective monotherapies. Combination therapy may increase efficacy, but further blinded trials should be carried out to investigate combination therapy with amorolfine.

Ciclopirox 8% nail lacquer
Ciclopirox 8% nail lacquer is recommended for use once daily for 48 weeks in mild to moderate onychomycosis. This is the first topical therapy to be approved for use in onychomycosis in the United States and Canada.

Quality of evidence: I
The results from two double-blind, double-dummy, randomized multicenter trials have been combined and reported for patients with a 20–65% affected area of nail.[345]

Effectiveness
At the end of therapy (week 48), the mycological cure rate for the combined studies was 34% (63/185) (Table 38.8). Complete cure was observed in 9% of the patients (16/181). Multiple studies performed outside of the United States involving higher degrees of onychomycosis and shorter periods of use of ciclopirox have shown higher rates of efficacy, but the data from these trials have currently not been published individually.[346]

Drawbacks
No further data for 48-week use has been published. The studies outside the United States investigated individuals with a somewhat higher degree of infection than in the 48-week trial, but as different regimens were used, it is difficult to compare the outcomes. Further data on the use of ciclopirox in blinded trials are needed.

Comments
Adverse events were noted rarely with ciclopirox use.[345] Most reactions were localized to the application site, mild in intensity, and transient. No serious adverse events were reported.

Ciclopirox 8% nail lacquer combined with oral antifungal therapy

Quality of evidence: I

One randomized, evaluator-blinded study used a combination of ciclopirox once daily for 48 weeks plus terbinafine 250 mg/day for 12 weeks, compared with terbinafine monotherapy (250 mg/day) for 12 weeks.[347]

A second trial used an open-label design to study the use of ciclopirox once daily for 9 months plus terbinafine 250 mg/day for 16 weeks, in comparison with terbinafine monotherapy (250 mg/day) for 16 weeks.[348]

Effectiveness

The rate of mycological cure at week 48 for the combination of ciclopirox and continuous terbinafine in the blinded trial was 70%, in comparison with 56% for the terbinafine monotherapy.[347] Effective cure rates (mycological cure and a 90% or more reduction in disease area) at week 48 were 33% and 35%, respectively. This study included a third arm, using terbinafine for 4 weeks on, 4 weeks off, and 4 weeks on, combined with ciclopirox nail lacquer for 48 weeks. This arm is not considered here, as it is a nonstandard pulse regimen.

In the open trial, the mycological cure rate for the combination regimen at month 9 was 88%, in comparison with 65% for the terbinafine monotherapy.[348]

Drawbacks

The number of patients in each study is relatively low. Further blinded trials are needed in order to increase the data available on the use of ciclopirox in combination with oral antifungals.

Comments

Most adverse events possibly related to study medication in the blinded trial were minimal and evenly distributed between the treatment groups.[348]

General comments

There have been several pharmacoeconomic analyses of the various oral treatments used in dermatophyte onychomycosis. These studies calculate the cost-effectiveness of each therapy on the basis of the efficacy results of multiple clinical trials. The two most cost-effective regimens for the treatment of onychomycosis are terbinafine (continuous) and itraconazole (pulse).[319,349–353]

In certain nail presentations, the response to therapy may be improved by combining oral antifungal therapy with either an effective topical therapy or mechanical/chemical measures (e.g., mechanical avulsion, debridement, or chemical avulsion). For example, when there is lateral onychomycosis, a dermatophytoma, severe onycholysis, a thickened nail, or severe onychomycosis, it may be advantageous to consider a combination approach.[50,67,76,354–356]

Key points

- The main oral antifungal agents used to treat onychomycosis are terbinafine, itraconazole, and fluconazole. Griseofulvin and ketoconazole are the traditional antifungal agents whose utility for onychomycosis has decreased substantially since the availability of the new oral antifungal agents. In addition, the use of ketoconazole for onychomycosis when long-duration therapy is required has diminished markedly, given the potential for hepatotoxicity.

- The preferred regimens with the new oral antifungal agents are terbinafine (continuous), itraconazole (pulse), and fluconazole (once weekly). The duration of therapy with these agents for fingernail onychomycosis is typically: terbinafine continuous (6 weeks), itraconazole pulse (two pulses), and fluconazole once weekly (6–9 months). The corresponding duration of therapy with these antifungal agents for toenail onychomycosis is 12 or 16 weeks, three or four pulses, and 9–15 months, respectively.

- RCTs have demonstrated that griseofulvin, terbinafine (continuous), itraconazole (pulse and continuous), and fluconazole are effective and safe for the treatment of dermatophyte fingernail onychomycosis.

- RCTs have demonstrated that terbinafine (continuous), itraconazole (pulse and continuous), and fluconazole are effective and safe for treatment of dermatophyte toenail onychomycosis.

- Few RCTs have been conducted for the topical nail lacquer formulations. Although the safety of monotherapy with nail lacquers appears to be good, more rigorous clinical trials need to be done to establish with certainty the efficacy of nail lacquers. Current practice would indicate that the addition of a nail lacquer to an established oral regimen may be a more practical use in clinical settings.

- There are several factors that need to be considered when deciding which agent to prescribe for onychomycosis; these include efficacy, the causative organism, regimen preference (e.g., continuous vs. pulse vs. once weekly, expected duration of therapy), the safety of the antifungal agent, the patient's medical status, the potential for drug interactions, relapse rates, and the cost of therapy.

- None of the newer oral antifungal agents has been approved for the treatment of onychomycosis in children, in whom the disease occurs much less frequently.

References

1 Roberts DT. Onychomycosis: current treatment and future challenges. *Br J Dermatol* 1999;**141**(Suppl 56):1–4.

2 Zaias N. Onychomycosis. *Arch Dermatol* 1972;**105**:263–74.

3 Hay RJ, Baran R, Haneke E. Fungal (onychomycosis) and other infections involving the nail apparatus. In: Baran R, Dawber RPR, eds. *Diseases of the Nails and Their Management*. 2nd ed. Oxford: Blackwell Scientific Publications, 1994:97–134.

4 Gupta AK, Jain HC, Lynde CW, *et al.* Prevalence and epidemiology of onychomycosis in patients visiting physicians' offices: a multicenter Canadian survey of 15,000 patients. *J Am Acad Dermatol* 2000;43:244–8.

5 Gupta AK, Scher RK. Management of onychomycosis: a North American perspective. *Derm Ther* 1997;3:58–65.

6 Ghannoum MA, Hajjeh RA, Scher R, *et al.* A large-scale North American study of fungal isolates from nails: the frequency of onychomycosis, fungal distribution, and antifungal susceptibility patterns. *J Am Acad Dermatol* 2000;43:641–8.

7 Gupta AK, Jain HC, Lynde CW, *et al.* Prevalence and epidemiology of unsuspected onychomycosis in patients visiting dermatologists' offices in Ontario, Canada—a multicenter survey of 2001 patients. *Int J Dermatol* 1997;36:783–7.

8 Elewski BE, Charif MA. Prevalence of onychomycosis in patients attending a dermatology clinic in northeastern Ohio for other conditions. *Arch Dermatol* 1997;133:1172–3.

9 Sais G, Jucgla A, Peyri J. Prevalence of dermatophyte onychomycosis in Spain: a cross-sectional study. *Br J Dermatol* 1995;132:758–61.

10 Williams HC. The epidemiology of onychomycosis in Britain. *Br J Dermatol* 1993;129:101–9.

11 Gupta AK, Gupta MA, Summerbell RC, *et al.* The epidemiology of onychomycosis: possible role of smoking and peripheral arterial disease. *J Eur Acad Dermatol Venereol* 2000;14:466–9.

12 Del Mar M, De Ocariz S, Arenas R, *et al.* Frequency of toenail onychomycosis in patients with cutaneous manifestations of chronic venous insufficiency. *Int J Dermatol* 2001;40:18–25.

13 Gupta AK, Taborda P, Taborda V, *et al.* Epidemiology and prevalence of onychomycosis in HIV-positive individuals. *Int J Dermatol* 2000;39:746–53.

14 Gupta AK, Humke S. The prevalence and management of onychomycosis in diabetic patients. *Eur J Dermatol* 2000;10:379–84.

15 Gupta AK, Konnikov N, MacDonald P, *et al.* Prevalence and epidemiology of toenail onychomycosis in diabetic subjects: a multicentre survey. *Br J Dermatol* 1998;139:665–71.

16 Gupta AK, Lynde CW, Jain HC, *et al.* A higher prevalence of onychomycosis in psoriatics compared with non-psoriatics: a multicentre study. *Br J Dermatol* 1997;136:786–9.

17 Zaias N, Rebell G. Chronic dermatophytosis caused by *Trichophyton rubrum.* *J Am Acad Dermatol* 1996;35:S17–S20.

18 Szepietowski JC, Reich A, Garlowska E, *et al.* Factors influencing coexistence of toenail onychomycosis with tinea pedis and other dermatomycoses: a survey of 2761 patients. *Arch Dermatol* 2006;142:1279–84.

19 Gupta AK. Onychomycosis in the elderly. *Drugs Aging* 2000;16:397–407.

20 Gupta AK, Shear NH. A risk–benefit assessment of the newer oral antifungal agents used to treat onychomycosis. *Drug Saf* 2000;22:33–52.

21 Hart R, Bell-Syer SE, Crawford F, *et al.* Systematic review of topical treatments for fungal infections of the skin and nails of the feet. *BMJ* 1999;319:79–82.

22 Scher RK. Onychomycosis: therapeutic update. *J Am Acad Dermatol* 1999;40:S21–S26.

23 Elewski BE. Onychomycosis: pathogenesis, diagnosis, and management. *Clin Microbiol Rev* 1998;11:415–29.

24 Gupta AK, Scher RK, De Doncker P. Current management of onychomycosis. An overview. *Dermatol Clin* 1997;15:121–35.

25 Hay RJ. Onychomycosis. Agents of choice. *Dermatol Clin* 1993;11:161–9.

26 Haneke E. Fungal infections of the nail. *Semin Dermatol* 1991;10:41–53.

27 Gupta AK, Leonardi C, Stolz R, *et al.* A phase I/II randomized, double-blind, placebo-controlled, dose-ranging study evaluating the efficacy, safety and pharmacokinetics of ravuconazole in the treatment of onychomycosis. *J Eur Acad Dermatol Venereol* 2005;19:437–43.

28 Gupta AK, Fleckman P, Baran R. Ciclopirox nail lacquer topical solution 8% in the treatment of toenail onychomycosis. *J Am Acad Dermatol* 2000;43:S70–S80.

29 Haria M, Bryson HM. Amorolfine. A review of its pharmacological properties and therapeutic potential in the treatment of onychomycosis and other superficial fungal infections. *Drugs* 1995;49:103–20.

30 Dermik Laboratories, Inc. Ciclopirox topical solution 8% nail lacquer. Berwyn, PA: Dermik Laboratories, Inc., 2000.

31 Dawber RPR, De Berker D, Baran R. Science of the nail apparatus. In: Baran R, Dawber RPR, eds. *Diseases of the Nails and their Management.* 2nd ed. Oxford: Blackwell Scientific Publications, 1994: 1–34.

32 Scher RK. Onychomycosis is more than a cosmetic problem. *Br J Dermatol* 1994;130(Suppl 43):15.

33 Drake LA, Patrick DL, Fleckman P, *et al.* The impact of onychomycosis on quality of life: development of an international onychomycosis-specific questionnaire to measure patient quality of life. *J Am Acad Dermatol* 1999;41:189–96.

34 Drake LA, Shear NH, Arlette JP, *et al.* Oral terbinafine in the treatment of toenail onychomycosis: North American multicenter trial. *J Am Acad Dermatol* 1997;37:740–5.

35 Scher RK, Breneman D, Rich P, *et al.* Once-weekly fluconazole (150, 300, or 450 mg) in the treatment of distal subungual onychomycosis of the toenail. *J Am Acad Dermatol* 1998;38:S77–S86.

36 Evans EG, Sigurgeirsson B. Double blind, randomised study of continuous terbinafine compared with intermittent itraconazole in treatment of toenail onychomycosis. The LION Study Group. *BMJ* 1999;318:1031–5.

37 Avner S, Nir N, Henri T. Fifth toenail clinical response to systemic antifungal therapy is not a marker of successful therapy for other toenails with onychomycosis. *J Eur Acad Dermatol Venereol* 2006;20:1194–6.

38 Scher RK, Tavakkol A, Sigurgeirsson B, *et al.* Onychomycosis: diagnosis and definition of cure. *J Am Acad Dermatol* 2007;56:939–44.

39 Binstock JM. Molecular biology techniques for identifying dermatophytes and their possible use in diagnosing onychomycosis in human toenails. *J Am Podiatr Med Assoc* 2007;97:134–44.

40 de Assis Santos D, de Carvalho Araujo RA, Kohler LM, *et al.* Molecular typing and antifungal susceptibility of *Trichophyton rubrum* isolates from patients with onychomycosis pre- and post-treatment. *Int J Antimicrob Agents* 2007;29:563–9.

41 Brillowska-Dabrowska A, Saunte DM, Arendrup MC. Five-hour diagnosis of dermatophyte nail infections with specific detection of *Trichophyton rubrum.* *J Clin Microbiol* 2007;45:1200–4.

42 Savin C, Huck S, Rolland C, *et al.* Multicenter evaluation of a commercial PCR-enzyme-linked immunosorbent assay diagnostic kit (Onychodiag) for diagnosis of dermatophytic onychomycosis. *J Clin Microbiol* 2007;45:1205–10.

43 Gupta AK, Zaman M, Singh J. Fast and sensitive detection of *Trichophyton rubrum* DNA from the nail samples of patients with onychomycosis by a double-round polymerase chain reaction-based assay. *Br J Dermatol* 2007;**157**:698–703.

44 Albanese G, Di Cintio R, Martini C, Nicoletti A. Short therapy for tinea unguium with terbinafine: four different courses of treatment. *Mycoses* 1995;**38**:211–4.

45 Andre J, De Doncker P, Laporte M, *et al.* Onychomycosis caused by *Microsporum canis*: treatment with itraconazole. *J Am Acad Dermatol* 1995;**32**:1052–3.

46 Arenas R, Fernandez G, Dominguez L. Onychomycosis treated with itraconazole or griseofulvin alone with and without a topical antimycotic or keratolytic agent. *Int J Dermatol* 1991;**30**:586–9.

47 Arenas R, Dominguez-Cherit J, Fernandez LM. Open randomized comparison of itraconazole versus terbinafine in onychomycosis. *Int J Dermatol* 1995;**34**:138–43.

48 Assaf RR, Elewski BE. Intermittent fluconazole dosing in patients with onychomycosis: results of a pilot study. *J Am Acad Dermatol* 1996;**35**:216–9.

49 Bahadir S, Inaloz HS, Alpay K, *et al.* Continuous terbinafine or pulse itraconazole: a comparative study on onychomycosis. *J Eur Acad Dermatol Venereol* 2000;**14**:422–3.

50 Baran R, Feuilhade M, Combernale P, *et al.* A randomized trial of amorolfine 5% solution nail lacquer combined with oral terbinafine compared with terbinafine alone in the treatment of dermatophytic toenail onychomycoses affecting the matrix region. *Br J Dermatol* 2000;**142**:1177–83.

51 Baran R, Tosti A, Piraccini BM. Uncommon clinical patterns of Fusarium nail infection: report of three cases. *Br J Dermatol* 1997;**136**:424–7.

52 Baudraz-Rosselet F, Rakosi T, Wili PB, Kenzelmann R. Treatment of onychomycosis with terbinafine. *Br J Dermatol* 1992;**126**(Suppl 39):40–6.

53 Bentley-Phillips B. The treatment of onychomycosis with miconazole tincture. *S Afr Med J* 1982;**62**:57–8.

54 Bohn M, Kraemer KT. Dermatopharmacology of ciclopirox nail lacquer topical solution 8% in the treatment of onychomycosis. *J Am Acad Dermatol* 2000;**43**:S57–S69.

55 Bonifaz A, Carrasco-Gerard E, Saul A. Itraconazole in onychomycosis: intermittent dose schedule. *Int J Dermatol* 1997;**36**:70–2.

56 Brandrup F, Larsen PO. Long-term follow-up of toe-nail onychomycosis treated with terbinafine. *Acta Derm Venereol* 1997;**77**:238.

57 Brautigam M. Terbinafine versus itraconazole: a controlled clinical comparison in onychomycosis of the toenails. *J Am Acad Dermatol* 1998;**38**:S53–S56.

58 Buck DS, Nidorf DM, Addino JG. Comparison of two topical preparations for the treatment of onychomycosis: *Melaleuca alternifolia* (tea tree) oil and clotrimazole. *J Fam Pract* 1994;**38**:601–5.

59 Campbell CK, Johnson EM, Warnock DW. Nail infection caused by *Onychocola canadensis*: report of the first four British cases. *J Med Vet Mycol* 1997;**35**:423–5.

60 Chen J, Liao W, Wen H, *et al.* A comparison among four regimens of itraconazole treatment in onychomycosis. *Mycoses* 1999;**42**:93–6.

61 Coldiron B. Recalcitrant onychomycosis of the toenails successfully treated with fluconazole. *Arch Dermatol* 1992;**128**:909–10.

62 Cribier B, Grosshans E. [Efficacy and tolerance of terbinafine (Lamisil) in a series of 50 cases of dermatophyte onychomycoses; in French.] *Ann Dermatol Venereol* 1994;**121**:15–20.

63 De Backer M, De Keyser P, De Vroey C, Lesaffre E. A 12-week treatment for dermatophyte toe onychomycosis: terbinafine 250 mg/day vs. itraconazole 200 mg/day—a double-blind comparative trial. *Br J Dermatol* 1996;**134**(Suppl 46):16–7.

64 De Cuyper C. Long-term evaluation of terbinafine 250 and 500 mg daily in a 16-week oral treatment for toenail onychomycosis. *Br J Dermatol* 1996;**135**:156–7.

65 De Doncker P, Van Lint J, Dockx P, Roseeuw D. Pulse therapy with one-week itraconazole monthly for three or four months in the treatment of onychomycosis. *Cutis* 1995;**56**:180–3.

66 DiSalvo AF, Fickling AM. A case of nondermatophytic toe onychomycosis caused by *Fusarium oxysporum*. *Arch Dermatol* 1980;**116**:699–700.

67 Dominguez-Cherit J, Teixeira F, Arenas R. Combined surgical and systemic treatment of onychomycosis. *Br J Dermatol* 1999;**140**:778–80.

68 Downs AM, Lear JT, Archer CB. *Scytalidium hyalinum* onychomycosis successfully treated with 5% amorolfine nail lacquer. *Br J Dermatol* 1999;**140**:555.

69 Eastcott DF. Terbinafine and onychomycosis. *N Z Med J* 1991;**104**:17.

70 Effendy I, Kolczak H, Ossowski B, Hohler T. [Topical therapy of onychomycoses with 8% ciclopirox lacquer. An open, non-comparative study; in German.] *Fortschr Med* 1993;**111**:205–8.

71 Elewski BE. Onychomycosis caused by *Scytalidium dimidiatum*. *J Am Acad Dermatol* 1996;**35**:336–8.

72 Galimberti R, Kowalczuk A, Flores V, Squiquera L. Onychomycosis treated with a short course of oral terbinafine. *Int J Dermatol* 1996;**35**:374–5.

73 Galitz J. Successful treatment of onychomycosis with ciclopirox nail lacquer: a case report. *Cutis* 2001;**68**:23–4.

74 Gianni C, Cerri A, Crosti C. Unusual clinical features of fingernail infection by Fusarium oxysporum. *Mycoses* 1997;**40**:455–9.

75 Gianni C, Cerri A, Crosti C. Non-dermatophytic onychomycosis. An underestimated entity? A study of 51 cases. *Mycoses* 2000;**43**:29–33.

76 Goodfield MJ, Evans EG. Combined treatment with surgery and short duration oral antifungal therapy in patients with limited dermatophyte toenail infection. *J Dermatol Treat* 2000;**11**:259–62.

77 Goodfield MJ, Rowell NR, Forster RA, *et al.* Treatment of dermatophyte infection of the finger- and toe-nails with terbinafine (SF 86-327, Lamisil), an orally active fungicidal agent. *Br J Dermatol* 1989;**121**:753–7.

78 Goodfield MJ, Evans EG. Treatment of superficial white onychomycosis with topical terbinafine cream. *Br J Dermatol* 1999;**141**:604–5.

79 Gupta AK, Gregurek-Novak T, Konnikov N, *et al.* Itraconazole and terbinafine treatment of some nondermatophyte molds causing onychomycosis of the toes and a review of the literature. *J Cutan Med Surg* 2001;**5**:206–10.

80 Gupta AK, Horgan-Bell CB, Summerbell RC. Onychomycosis associated with *Onychocola canadensis*: ten case reports and a review of the literature. *J Am Acad Dermatol* 1998;**39**:410–7.

81 Gupta AK, De Doncker P, Haneke E. Itraconazole pulse therapy for the treatment of Candida onychomycosis. *J Eur Acad Dermatol Venereol* 2000;**15**:112–5.

82 Hay RJ, Mackie RM, Clayton YM. Tioconazole nail solution—an open study of its efficacy in onychomycosis. *Clin Exp Dermatol* 1985;**10**:111–5.

83 Hay RJ, Clayton YM, Moore MK. A comparison of tioconazole 28% nail solution versus base as an adjunct to oral griseofulvin in patients with onychomycosis. *Clin Exp Dermatol* 1987;**12**:175–7.

84 Hiruma M, Matsushita A, Kobayashi M, Ogawa H. One week pulse therapy with itraconazole (200 mg day-1) for onychomycosis. Evaluation of treatment results according to patient background. *Mycoses* 2001;**44**:87–93.

85 Kirshbaum BA. Itraconazole therapy for onychomycosis: case reports. *Cutis* 1996;**58**:371–4.

86 Koenig H, Ball C, de Bievre C. First European cases of onychomycosis caused by *Onychocola canadensis*. *J Med Vet Mycol* 1997;**35**:71–2.

87 Lauharanta J. Comparative efficacy and safety of amorolfine nail lacquer 2% versus 5% once weekly. *Clin Exp Dermatol* 1992;**17**(Suppl 1):41–3.

88 Lebwohl MG, Daniel CR, Leyden J, *et al.* Efficacy and safety of terbinafine for nondermatophyte and mixed nondermatophyte and dermatophyte toenail onychomycosis. *Int J Dermatol* 2001;**40**:358–60.

89 Lecha M. Amorolfine and itraconazole combination for severe toenail onychomycosis: results of an open randomized trial in Spain. *Br J Dermatol* 2001;**145**(Suppl 60):21–6.

90 Lee KH, Kim YS, Kim MS, *et al.* Study of the efficacy and tolerability of oral terbinafine in the treatment of onychomycosis in renal transplant patients. *Transplant Proc* 1996;**28**:1488–9.

91 Ling MR, Swinyer LJ, Jarratt MT, *et al.* Once-weekly fluconazole (450 mg) for 4, 6, or 9 months of treatment for distal subungual onychomycosis of the toenail. *J Am Acad Dermatol* 1998;**38**:S95–102.

92 Mahgoub ES. Clinical trial with clotrimazole cream (Bay b 5097) in dermatophytosis and onychomycosis. *Mycopathologia* 1975;**56**:149–52.

93 Mensing H, Polak-Wyss A, Splanemann V. Determination of the subungual antifungal activity of amorolfine after 1 month's treatment in patients with onychomycosis: comparison of two nail lacquer formulations. *Clin Exp Dermatol* 1992;**17**(Suppl 1):29–32.

94 Meyerson MS, Scher RK, Hochman LG, *et al.* Open-label study of the safety and efficacy of Fungoid tincture in patients with distal subungual onychomycosis of the toes. *Cutis* 1992;**49**:359–62.

95 Meyerson MS, Scher RK, Hochman LG, *et al.* Open-label study of the safety and efficacy of naftifine hydrochloride 1 percent gel in patients with distal subungual onychomycosis of the fingers. *Cutis* 1993;**51**:205–7.

96 Molin L, Tarstedt M, Engman C. Oral terbinafine treatment for toenail onychomycosis: follow-up after 5–6 years. *Br J Dermatol* 2000;**143**:682–3.

97 Moncada B, Loredo CE, Isordia E. Treatment of onychomycosis with ketoconazole and nonsurgical avulsion of the affected nail. *Cutis* 1983;**31**:438–40.

98 Montana JB, Scher RK. A double-blind, vehicle-controlled study of the safety and efficacy of fungoid tincture in patients with distal subungual onychomycosis of the toes. *Cutis* 1994;**53**:313–6.

99 Montero-Gei F, Robles-Soto ME, Schlager H. Fluconazole in the treatment of severe onychomycosis. *Int J Dermatol* 1996;**35**:587–8.

100 Nahass GT, Sisto M. Onychomycosis: successful treatment with once-weekly fluconazole. *Dermatology* 1993;**186**:59–61.

101 Ninomiya J, Yamazaki K, Ito Y, *et al.* [Evaluation of the efficacy of small-dose itraconazole pulse therapy (200 mg/day) for tinea unguium; in Japanese.] *Nippon Ishinkin Gakkai Zasshi* 1999;**40**:35–7.

102 Nolting S, Brautigam M, Weidinger G. Terbinafine in onychomycosis with involvement by non-dermatophytic fungi. *Br J Dermatol* 1994;**130**(Suppl 43):16–21.

103 Onsberg P, Stahl D, Veien NK. Onychomycosis caused by Aspergillus terreus. *Sabouraudia* 1978;**16**:39–46.

104 Onsberg P, Stahl D. Scopulariopsis onychomycosis treated with natamycin. *Dermatologica* 1980;**160**:57–61.

105 Piepponen T, Blomqvist K, Brandt H, *et al.* Efficacy and safety of itraconazole in the long-term treatment of onychomycosis. *J Antimicrob Chemother* 1992;**29**:195–205.

106 Piraccini BM, Morelli R, Stinchi C, Tosti A. Proximal subungual onychomycosis due to *Microsporum canis*. *Br J Dermatol* 1996;**134**:175–7.

107 Pittrof F, Gerhards J, Erni W, Klecak G. Loceryl nail lacquer—realization of a new galenical approach to onychomycosis therapy. *Clin Exp Dermatol* 1992;**17**(Suppl 1):26–8.

108 Pollak R, Billstein SA. Efficacy of terbinafine for toenail onychomycosis. A multicenter trial of various treatment durations. *J Am Podiatr Med Assoc* 2001;**91**:127–31.

109 Ramos-e-Silva, Marques SA, Gontijo B, *et al.* Efficacy and safety of itraconazole pulse therapy: Brazilian multicentric study on toenail onychomycosis caused by dermatophytes. *J Eur Acad Dermatol Venereol* 1998;**11**:109–16.

110 Reinel D, Clarke C. Comparative efficacy and safety of amorolfine nail lacquer 5% in onychomycosis, once-weekly versus twice-weekly. *Clin Exp Dermatol* 1992;**17**(Suppl 1):44–9.

111 Reinel D. Topical treatment of onychomycosis with amorolfine 5% nail lacquer: comparative efficacy and tolerability of once and twice weekly use. *Dermatology* 1992;**184**(Suppl 1):21–4.

112 Rollman O. Treatment of onychomycosis by partial nail avulsion and topical miconazole. *Dermatologica* 1982;**165**:54–61.

113 Rollman O, Johansson S. *Hendersonula toruloidea* infection: successful response of onychomycosis to nail avulsion and topical ciclopiroxolamine. *Acta Derm Venereol* 1987;**67**:506–10.

114 Romano C, Miracco C, Difonzo EM. Skin and nail infections due to *Fusarium oxysporum* in Tuscany, Italy. *Mycoses* 1998;**41**:433–7.

115 Romano C, Paccagnini E, Difonzo EM. Onychomycosis caused by *Alternaria* spp. in Tuscany, Italy from 1985 to 1999. *Mycoses* 2001;**44**:73–6.

116 Rosenthal SA, Stritzler R, Vilafane J. Onychomycosis caused by *Aspergillus fumigatus*. Report of a case. *Arch Dermatol* 1968;**97**:685–7.

117 Savin RC, Atton AV. Terbinafine in onychomycosis—a mini study. *Int J Dermatol* 1993;**32**:918–9.

118 Scher RK, Barnett JM. Successful treatment of *Aspergillus flavus* onychomycosis with oral itraconazole. *J Am Acad Dermatol* 1990;**23**:749–50.

119 Seebacher C, Nietsch KH, Ulbricht HM. A multicenter, open-label study of the efficacy and safety of ciclopirox nail lacquer

solution 8% for the treatment of onychomycosis in patients with diabetes. *Cutis* 2001;**68**:17–22.

120 Segal R, Kritzman A, Cividalli L, *et al.* Treatment of *Candida* nail infection with terbinafine. *J Am Acad Dermatol* 1996;**35**:958–61.

121 Shemer A, Bergman R, Cohen A, Friedman-Birnbaum R. [Treatment of onychomycosis using 40% urea with 1% bifonazole; in Hebrew.] *Harefuah* 1992;**122**:159–60.

122 Shuster S, Munro CS. Single dose treatment of fungal nail disease. *Lancet* 1992;**339**:1066.

123 Sigler L, Congly H. Toenail infection caused by *Onychocola canadensis* gen. et sp. nov. *J Med Vet Mycol* 1990;**28**:405–17.

124 Sigler L, Abbott SP, Woodgyer AJ. New records of nail and skin infection due to *Onychocola canadensis* and description of its teleomorph *Arachnomyces nodosetosus* sp. nov. *J Med Vet Mycol* 1994;**32**:275–85.

125 Smith SW, Sealy DP, Schneider E, Lackland D. An evaluation of the safety and efficacy of fluconazole in the treatment of onychomycosis. *South Med J* 1995;**88**:1217–20.

126 Syed TA, Ahmadpour OA, Ahmad SA, Shamsi S. Management of toenail onychomycosis with 2% butenafine and 20% urea cream: a placebo-controlled, double-blind study. *J Dermatol* 1998;**25**:648–52.

127 Syed TA, Qureshi ZA, Ali SM, *et al.* Treatment of toenail onychomycosis with 2% butenafine and 5% *Melaleuca alternifolia* (tea tree) oil in cream. *Trop Med Int Health* 1999;**4**:284–7.

128 Tang WY, Chong LY, Leung CY, *et al.* Intermittent pulse therapy with itraconazole for onychomycosis. Experience in Hong Kong Chinese. *Mycoses* 2000;**43**:35–9.

129 Torok I, Simon G, Dobozy A, *et al.* Long-term post-treatment follow-up of onychomycosis treated with terbinafine: a multicentre trial. *Mycoses* 1998;**41**:63–5.

130 Tosti A, Piraccini BM, Stinchi C, Lorenzi S. Onychomycosis due to *Scopulariopsis brevicaulis*: clinical features and response to systemic antifungals. *Br J Dermatol* 1996;**135**:799–802.

131 Tosti A, Piraccini BM. Proximal subungual onychomycosis due to Aspergillus niger: report of two cases. *Br J Dermatol* 1998;**139**:156–7.

132 Tosti A, Piraccini BM, Lorenzi S. Onychomycosis caused by nondermatophytic molds: clinical features and response to treatment of 59 cases. *J Am Acad Dermatol* 2000;**42**:217–24.

133 Tseng SS, Longley BJ, Scher RK, Treiber RK. *Fusarium* fingernail infection responsive to fluconazole intermittent therapy. *Cutis* 2000;**65**:352–4.

134 Tsuboi R, Unno K, Komatsuzaki H, *et al.* [Topical treatment of onychomycosis by occlusive dressing using bifonazole cream containing 40% urea; in Japanese.] *Nippon Ishinkin Gakkai Zasshi* 1998;**39**:11–6.

135 Tulli A, Ruffilli MP, De Simone C. The treatment of onychomycosis with a new form of tioconazole. *Chemioterapia* 1988;**7**:160–3.

136 Ulbricht H, Worz K. [Therapy with ciclopirox lacquer of onychomycoses caused by molds; in German.] *Mycoses* 1994;**37** (Suppl 1):97–100.

137 Villars VV, Jones TC. Special features of the clinical use of oral terbinafine in the treatment of fungal diseases. *Br J Dermatol* 1992;**126**(Suppl 39):61–9.

138 Walsoe I, Stangerup M, Svejgaard E. Itraconazole in onychomycosis. Open and double-blind studies. *Acta Derm Venereol* 1990;**70**:137–40.

139 Warshaw EM, Carver SM, Zielke GR, Ahmed DD. Intermittent terbinafine for toenail onychomycosis: is it effective? Results of a randomized pilot trial. *Arch Dermatol* 2001;**137**:1253.

140 Wong CK, Cho YL. Very short duration therapy with oral terbinafine for fingernail onychomycosis. *Br J Dermatol* 1995;**133**:329–31.

141 Wu J, Wen H, Liao W. Small-dose itraconazole pulse therapy in the treatment of onychomycosis. *Mycoses* 1997;**40**:397–400.

142 Zaias N, Serrano L. The successful treatment of finger *Trichophyton rubrum* onychomycosis with oral terbinafine. *Clin Exp Dermatol* 1989;**14**:120–3.

143 Zaias N, Rebell G, Zaiac MN, Glick B. Onychomycosis treated until the nail is replaced by normal growth or there is failure. *Arch Dermatol* 2000;**136**:940.

144 Avner S, Nir N, Baruch K, Henri T. Two novel itraconazole pulse therapies for onychomycosis: a 2-year follow-up. *J Dermatolog Treat* 2006;**17**:117–20.

145 Tavakkol A, Fellman S, Kianifard F. Safety and efficacy of oral terbinafine in the treatment of onychomycosis: analysis of the elderly subgroup in Improving Results in ONychomycosis-Concomitant Lamisil and Debridement (IRON-CLAD), an open-label, randomized trial. *Am J Geriatr Pharmacother* 2006;**4**:1–13.

146 Sanchez-Schmidt JM, Gimenez-Jovani S, Peyri-Rey J. [Study on patient satisfaction with the treatment of mycosis on the extremities with terbinafine (SETTA); in Spanish.] *Actas Dermosifiliogr* 2005;**96**:285–90.

147 Sikder AU, Mamun SA, Chowdhury AH, Khan RM, Hoque MM. Study of oral itraconazole and terbinafine pulse therapy in onychomycosis. *Mymensingh Med J* 2006;**15**:71–80.

148 Sigurgeirsson B, Elewski BE, Rich PA, *et al.* Intermittent versus continuous terbinafine in the treatment of toenail onychomycosis: a randomized, double-blind comparison. *J Dermatolog Treat* 2006;**17**:38–44.

149 Mishra M, Panda P, Tripathy S, Sengupta S, Mishra K. An open randomized comparative study of oral itraconazole pulse and terbinafine pulse in the treatment of onychomycosis. *Indian J Dermatol Venereol Leprol* 2005;**71**:262–6.

150 Warshaw EM, St Clair KR. Prevention of onychomycosis reinfection for patients with complete cure of all 10 toenails: results of a double-blind, placebo-controlled, pilot study of prophylactic miconazole powder 2%. *J Am Acad Dermatol* 2005;**53**:717–20.

151 Warshaw EM, Fett DD, Bloomfield HE, *et al.* Pulse versus continuous terbinafine for onychomycosis: a randomized, double-blind, controlled trial. *J Am Acad Dermatol* 2005;**53**:578–84.

152 Warshaw EM, Nelson D, Carver SM, *et al.* A pilot evaluation of pulse itraconazole vs. terbinafine for treatment of *Candida* toenail onychomycosis. *Int J Dermatol* 2005;**44**:785–8.

153 Arnold B, Kianifard F, Tavakkol A. A comparison of KOH and culture results from two mycology laboratories for the diagnosis of onychomycosis during a randomized, multicenter clinical trial: a subset study. *J Am Podiatr Med Assoc* 2005;**95**:421–3.

154 Gupta AK. Ciclopirox topical solution, 8% combined with oral terbinafine to treat onychomycosis: a randomized, evaluator-blinded study. *J Drugs Dermatol* 2005;**4**:481–5.

155 Gupta AK, Leonardi C, Stoltz RR, Pierce PF, Conetta B. A phase I/II randomized, double-blind, placebo-controlled, dose-ranging study evaluating the efficacy, safety and pharmacokinetics of

ravuconazole in the treatment of onychomycosis. *J Eur Acad Dermatol Venereol* 2005;**19**:437–43.

156 Sanmano B, Hiruma M, Mizoguchi M, Ogawa H. Combination therapy consisting of week pulses of oral terbinafine plus topical application of terbinafine cream in the treatment of onychomycosis. *J Dermatolog Treat* 2004;**15**:245–51.

157 Milillo L, Lo ML, Carlino P, Serpico R, Coccia E, Scully C. *Candida*-related denture stomatitis: a pilot study of the efficacy of an amorolfine antifungal varnish. *Int J Prosthodont* 2005;**18**:55–9.

158 Chen X, Hiruma M, Shiraki Y, Ogawa H. Combination therapy of once-weekly fluconazole (100, 150, or 300 mg) with topical application of ketoconazole cream in the treatment of onychomycosis. *Jpn J Infect Dis* 2004;**57**:260–3.

159 Sidou F, Soto P. A randomized comparison of nail surface remanence of three nail lacquers, containing amorolfine 5%, ciclopirox 8% or tioconazole 28%, in healthy volunteers. *Int J Tissue React* 2004;**26**:17–24.

160 Ratajczak-Stefanska V. [Assessment of mycological and clinical factors on the course and results of treatment of mycotic infections in patients with recurrent onychomycosis; in Polish.] *Ann Acad Med Stetin* 2003;**49**:161–71.

161 Watanabe S. [Optimal dosages and cycles of itraconazole pulse therapy for onychomycosis; in Japanese.] *Nippon Ishinkin Gakkai Zasshi* 2004;**45**:143–7.

162 Elewski BE, Haley HR, Robbins CM. The use of 40% urea cream in the treatment of moccasin tinea pedis. *Cutis* 2004;**73**:355–7.

163 Maurer T, Rodrigues LK, Ameli N, *et al.* The effect of highly active antiretroviral therapy on dermatologic disease in a longitudinal study of HIV type 1-infected women. *Clin Infect Dis* 2004;**38**:579–84.

164 Aman S, Akbar TM, Hussain I, Jahangir M, Haroon TS. Itraconazole pulse therapy in the treatment of disto-lateral subungual onychomycosis. *J Coll Physicians Surg Pak* 2003;**13**:618–20.

165 Burzykowski T, Molenberghs G, Abeck D, *et al.* High prevalence of foot diseases in Europe: results of the Achilles Project. *Mycoses* 2003;**46**:496–505.

166 Warshaw EM, Bowman T, Bodman MA, Kim JJ, Silva S, Mathias SD. Satisfaction with onychomycosis treatment. Pulse versus continuous dosing. *J Am Podiatr Med Assoc* 2003;**93**:373–9.

167 Rigopoulos D, Katoulis AC, Ioannides D, *et al.* A randomized trial of amorolfine 5% solution nail lacquer in association with itraconazole pulse therapy compared with itraconazole alone in the treatment of Candida fingernail onychomycosis. *Br J Dermatol* 2003;**149**:151–6.

168 Sommer S, Sheehan-Dare RA, Goodfield MJ, Evans EG. Prediction of outcome in the treatment of onychomycosis. *Clin Exp Dermatol* 2003;**28**:425–8.

169 Larsen GK, Haedersdal M, Svejgaard EL. The prevalence of onychomycosis in patients with psoriasis and other skin diseases. *Acta Derm Venereol* 2003;**83**:206–9.

170 Firooz A, Khamesipour A, Dowlati Y. Itraconazole pulse therapy improves the quality of life of patients with toenail onychomycosis. *J Dermatolog Treat* 2003;**14**:95–8.

171 Jennings MB, Rinaldi MG. Confirmation of dermatophytes in nail specimens using in-office dermatophyte test medium cultures. Insights from a multispecialty survey. *J Am Podiatr Med Assoc* 2003;**93**:195–202.

172 Rich P, Harkless LB, Atillasoy ES. Dermatophyte test medium culture for evaluating toenail infections in patients with diabetes. *Diabetes Care* 2003;**26**:1480–4.

173 Sigurgeirsson B, Paul C, Curran D, Evans EG. Prognostic factors of mycological cure following treatment of onychomycosis with oral antifungal agents. *Br J Dermatol* 2002;**147**:1241–3.

174 Shemer A, Weiss G, Trau H. Oral terbinafine in the treatment of onychomycosis: a comparison of continuous and extended-pause regimens. *J Eur Acad Dermatol Venereol* 2002;**16**:299–301.

175 Tosti A, Piraccini BM, Ghetti E, Colombo MD. Topical steroids versus systemic antifungals in the treatment of chronic paronychia: an open, randomized double-blind and double dummy study. *J Am Acad Dermatol* 2002;**47**:73–6.

176 Salo H, Pekurinen M. Cost effectiveness of oral terbinafine (Lamisil) compared with oral fluconazole (Diflucan) in the treatment of patients with toenail onychomycosis. *Pharmacoeconomics* 2002;**20**:319–24.

177 Pariser D, Opper C. An in-office diagnostic procedure to detect dermatophytes in a nationwide study of onychomycosis patients. *Manag Care* 2002;**11**:43–8, 50.

178 Farkas B, Paul C, Dobozy A, Hunyadi J, Horvath A, Fekete G. Terbinafine (Lamisil) treatment of toenail onychomycosis in patients with insulin-dependent and non-insulin-dependent diabetes mellitus: a multicentre trial. *Br J Dermatol* 2002;**146**:254–60.

179 Elewski BE, El Charif M, Cooper KD, Ghannoum M, Birnbaum JE. Reactivity to trichophytin antigen in patients with onychomycosis: effect of terbinafine. *J Am Acad Dermatol* 2002;**46**:371–5.

180 Maleszka R, Adamski Z, Dworacki G. Evaluation of lymphocytes subpopulations and natural killer cells in peripheral blood of patients treated for dermatophyte onychomycosis. *Mycoses* 2001;**44**:487–92.

181 Baran R. Topical amorolfine for 15 months combined with 12 weeks of oral terbinafine, a cost-effective treatment for onychomycosis. *Br J Dermatol* 2001;**145**(Suppl 60):15–9.

182 Higashi N. [Treatment of tinea unguium with terbinafine: an open study comparing twelve weeks and twenty-four weeks of continuous terbinafine therapy, and determination of terbinafine level in the target nails; in Japanese.] *Nippon Ishinkin Gakkai Zasshi* 2001;**42**:259–65.

183 Fiallo P, Cardo PP. Age as limiting factor of the efficacy of itraconazole for treatment of onychomycosis. *Mycoses* 2001;**44**:191–4.

184 Gupta AK, Gregurek-Novak T. Efficacy of itraconazole, terbinafine, fluconazole, griseofulvin and ketoconazole in the treatment of *Scopulariopsis brevicaulis* causing onychomycosis of the toes. *Dermatology* 2001;**202**:235–8.

185 Tarasenko GN, Patronov IV, Tarasenko I. [Onychomycosis therapy; in Russian.] *Voen Med Zh* 2001;**322**:53–6.

186 Mirmirani P, Hessol NA, Maurer TA, *et al.* Prevalence and predictors of skin disease in the Women's Interagency HIV Study (WIHS). *J Am Acad Dermatol* 2001;**44**:785–8.

187 Gupta AK, Konnikov N, Lynde CW. Single-blind, randomized, prospective study on terbinafine and itraconazole for treatment of dermatophyte toenail onychomycosis in the elderly. *J Am Acad Dermatol* 2001;**44**:479–84.

188 Smith EB, Stein LF, Fivenson DP, Atillasoy ES. Clinical trial: the safety of terbinafine in patients over the age of 60 years: a

multicenter trial in onychomycosis of the feet. *Int J Dermatol* 2000;**39**:861–4.

189 Pierard GE, Pierard-Franchimont C, Arrese JE. The boosted anti-fungal topical treatment (BATT) for onychomycosis. *Med Mycol* 2000;**38**:391–2.

190 Safer LF. Randomized double-blind comparison of short-term itraconazole and terbinafine therapy for toenail onychomycosis. *Acta Derm Venereol* 2000;**80**:317–8.

191 Bonifaz A, Ibarra G. Onychomycosis in children: treatment with bifonazole-urea. *Pediatr Dermatol* 2000;**17**:310–4.

192 Bradley MC, Leidich S, Isham N, Elewski BE, Ghannoum MA. Antifungal susceptibilities and genetic relatedness of serial *Trichophyton rubrum* isolates from patients with onychomycosis of the toenail. *Mycoses* 1999;**42**(Suppl 2):105–10.

193 Huang PH, Paller AS. Itraconazole pulse therapy for derma-tophyte onychomycosis in children. *Arch Pediatr Adolesc Med* 2000;**154**:614–8.

194 Pierard GE, Pierard-Franchimont C, Arrese JE. The boosted oral antifungal treatment for onychomycosis beyond the regular itraconazole pulse dosing regimen. *Dermatology* 2000;**200**:185–7.

195 De Cuyper C, Hindryckx PH. Long-term outcomes in the treat-ment of toenail onychomycosis. *Br J Dermatol* 1999;**141**(Suppl 56): 15–20.

196 Sigurgeirsson B, Billstein S, Rantanen T, *et al.* L.I.ON. Study: efficacy and tolerability of continuous terbinafine (Lamisil) com-pared to intermittent itraconazole in the treatment of toenail onychomycosis. Lamisil vs. itraconazole in onychomycosis. *Br J Dermatol* 1999;**141**(Suppl 56):5–14.

197 Gupta AK, Nolting S, de Prost Y, *et al.* The use of itraconazole to treat cutaneous fungal infections in children. *Dermatology* 1999;**199**:248–52.

198 Warshaw E, Ahmed D. Are mothballs helpful in preventing onychomycosis reinfection? *Arch Dermatol* 1999;**135**:1120–1.

199 Lubeck DP, Gause D, Schein JR, Prebil LE, Potter LP. A health-related quality of life measure for use in patients with ony-chomycosis: a validation study. *Qual Life Res* 1999;**8**:121–9.

200 Wang DL, Wang AP, Li RY, Wang R. Therapeutic efficacy and safety of one-week intermittent therapy with itraconazole for onychomycosis in a Chinese patient population. *Dermatology* 1999;**199**:47–9.

201 Laufen H, Zimmermann T, Yeates RA, Schumacher T, Wildfeuer A. The uptake of fluconazole in finger and toe nails. *Int J Clin Pharmacol Ther* 1999;**37**:352–60.

202 Tarasenko GN, Patronov IV, Tarasenko I. [A clinical trial and the prospects for the Orungal therapy of onychomycoses; in Russian.] *Voen Med Zh* 1999;**320**:37–9.

203 Albreski DA, Gross EG. The safety of itraconazole in the diabetic population. *J Am Podiatr Med Assoc* 1999;**89**:339–45.

204 Matsumoto T, Tanuma H, Nishiyama S. Clinical and pharmaco-kinetic investigations of oral itraconazole in the treatment of onychomycosis. *Mycoses* 1999;**42**:79–91.

205 Havu V, Brandt H, Heikkila H, *et al.* Continuous and inter-mittent itraconazole dosing schedules for the treatment of onychomycosis: a pharmacokinetic comparison. *Br J Dermatol* 1999;**140**:96–101.

206 Haneke E, Abeck D, Ring J. Safety and efficacy of intermittent therapy with itraconazole in finger- and toenail onychomycosis: a multicentre trial. *Mycoses* 1998;**41**:521–7.

207 Brautigam M, Weidinger G, Nolting S. Successful treatment of toenail mycosis with terbinafine and itraconazole gives long term benefits. *BMJ* 1998;**317**:1084.

208 Nolting SK, Sanchez CS, De Boulle K, Lambert JR. Oral treat-ment schedules for onychomycosis: a study of patient preference. *Int J Dermatol* 1998;**37**:454–6.

209 Savin RC, Drake L, Babel D, *et al.* Pharmacokinetics of three once-weekly dosages of fluconazole (150, 300, or 450 mg) in distal subungual onychomycosis of the fingernail. *J Am Acad Dermatol* 1998;**38**:S110–S116.

210 Rich P, Scher RK, Breneman D, *et al.* Pharmacokinetics of three doses of once-weekly fluconazole (150, 300, and 450 mg) in distal subungual onychomycosis of the toenail. *J Am Acad Dermatol* 1998;**38**:S103–S109.

211 Trepanier EF, Nafziger AN, Kearns GL, Kashuba AD, Amsden GW. Absence of effect of terbinafine on the activity of CYP1A2, NAT-2, and xanthine oxidase. *J Clin Pharmacol* 1998;**38**:424–8.

212 Drake LA, Scher RK, Smith EB, *et al.* Effect of onychomycosis on quality of life. *J Am Acad Dermatol* 1998;**38**:702–4.

213 Watson AB, Marley JE, Ellis DH, Williams TG. Long-term follow up of patients with toenail onychomycosis after treatment with terbinafine. *Australas J Dermatol* 1998;**39**:29–30.

214 Pollak R, Billstein SA. Safety of oral terbinafine for toenail ony-chomycosis. *J Am Podiatr Med Assoc* 1997;**87**:565–70.

215 Herranz P, Garcia J, De Lucas R, *et al.* Toenail onychomycosis in patients with acquired immune deficiency syndrome: treatment with terbinafine. *Br J Dermatol* 1997;**137**:577–80.

216 Daniel CR III, Gupta AK, Daniel MP, Daniel CM. Two feet–one hand syndrome: a retrospective multicenter survey. *Int J Dermatol* 1997;**36**:658–60.

217 Elewski BE. Large-scale epidemiological study of the causal agents of onychomycosis: mycological findings from the Multi-center Onychomycosis Study of Terbinafine. *Arch Dermatol* 1997;**133**:1317–8.

218 Hall M, Monka C, Krupp P, O'Sullivan D. Safety of oral terbinafine: results of a postmarketing surveillance study in 25,884 patients. *Arch Dermatol* 1997;**133**:1213–9.

219 Ellis DH, Watson AB, Marley JE, Williams TG. Non-dermatophytes in onychomycosis of the toenails. *Br J Dermatol* 1997;**136**:490–3.

220 Gupta AK, Sibbald RG, Lynde CW, *et al.* Onychomycosis in children: prevalence and treatment strategies. *J Am Acad Der-matol* 1997;**36**:395–402.

221 Ellis DH, Marley JE, Watson AB, Williams TG. Significance of non-dermatophyte moulds and yeasts in onychomycosis. *Dermatology* 1997;**194**(Suppl 1):40–2.

222 Friedman-Birnbaum R, Cohen A, Shemer A, Bitterman O, Bergman R, Stettendorf S. Treatment of onychomycosis: a ran-domized, double-blind comparison study with topical bifonazole-urea ointment alone and in combination with short-duration oral griseofulvin. *Int J Dermatol* 1997;**36**:67–9.

223 Chien RN, Yang LJ, Lin PY, Liaw YF. Hepatic injury during ketoconazole therapy in patients with onychomycosis: a con-trolled cohort study. *Hepatology* 1997;**25**:103–7.

224 Brautigam M, Nolting S, Schopf RE, Weidinger G. German ran-domized double-blind multicentre comparison of terbinafine and itraconazole for the treatment of toenail tinea infection. *Br J Dermatol* 1996;**134** (Suppl 46):18–21.

225 Faergemann J, Laufen H. Levels of fluconazole in normal and diseased nails during and after treatment of onychomycoses in toe-nails with fluconazole 150 mg once weekly. *Acta Derm Venereol* 1996;**76**:219–21.

226 Smith GN. Antifungal pulse therapy for onychomycosis. *J Fam Pract* 1996;**42**:348.

227 Pierard-Franchimont G, De Doncker P, Van de Velde V, Jacqmin P, Arrese JE, Pierard GE. Paradoxical response to itraconazole treatment in a patient with onychomycosis caused by *Microsporum gypseum*. *Ann Soc Belg Med Trop* 1995;**75**:211–7.

228 Schatz F, Brautigam M, Dobrowolski E, *et al*. Nail incorporation kinetics of terbinafine in onychomycosis patients. *Clin Exp Dermatol* 1995;**20**:377–83.

229 Hogan DJ. Short-duration treatment of fingernail dermatophytosis: a randomized, double-blind study with terbinafine and griseofulvin. *J Am Acad Dermatol* 1995;**33**:541–2.

230 Bonifaz A, Guzman A, Garcia C, Sosa J, Saul A. Efficacy and safety of bifonazole urea in the two-phase treatment of onychomycosis. *Int J Dermatol* 1995;**34**:500–3.

231 Korting HC, Ollert M, Abeck D. Results of German multicenter study of antimicrobial susceptibilities of *Trichophyton rubrum* and *Trichophyton mentagrophytes* strains causing tinea unguium. German Collaborative Dermatophyte Drug Susceptibility Study Group. *Antimicrob Agents Chemother* 1995;**39**:1206–8.

232 Matsumoto T, Tanuma H, Kaneko S, Takasu H, Nishiyama S. Clinical and pharmacokinetic investigations of oral terbinafine in patients with tinea unguium. *Mycoses* 1995;**38**:135–44.

233 Takabayashi K, Nawata Y, Sumida T, *et al*. [Effects of fluconazole on onychomycosis in patients with collagen diseases; in Japanese.] *Ryumachi* 1995;**35**:72–6.

234 Nejjam F, Zagula M, Cabiac MD, Guessous N, Humbert H, Lakhdar H. Pilot study of terbinafine in children suffering from tinea capitis: evaluation of efficacy, safety and pharmacokinetics. *Br J Dermatol* 1995;**132**:98–105.

235 Goldstein SM. Advances in the treatment of superficial candida infections. *Semin Dermatol* 1993;**12**:315–30.

236 Blecher P, Korting HC. A new combined diagnostic approach to clinically and microscopically suspected onychomycosis unproven by culture. *Mycoses* 1993;**36**:321–4.

237 Ruping KW, Haas PJ. [Treatment onychomycoses—bifonazole nail set in comparison with urea with ciclopiroxolamine formulation; in German.] *Z Ärztl Fortbild (Jena)* 1993;**87**:425–9.

238 Zaug M, Bergstraesser M. Amorolfine in the treatment of onychomycoses and dermatomycoses (an overview). *Clin Exp Dermatol* 1992;**17**(Suppl 1):61–70.

239 Goodfield MJ, Andrew L, Evans EG. Short term treatment of dermatophyte onychomycosis with terbinafine. *BMJ* 1992;**304**:1151–4.

240 Stevens DA, Greene SI, Lang OS. Thrush can be prevented in patients with acquired immunodeficiency syndrome and the acquired immunodeficiency syndrome-related complex. Randomized, double-blind, placebo-controlled study of 100-mg oral fluconazole daily. *Arch Intern Med* 1991;**151**:2458–64.

241 Wu YC, Chuan MT, Lu YC. Efficacy of ciclopiroxolamine 1% cream in onychomycosis and tinea pedis. *Mycoses* 1991;**34**:93–5.

242 Savin RC. Oral terbinafine versus griseofulvin in the treatment of moccasin-type tinea pedis. *J Am Acad Dermatol* 1990;**23**:807–9.

243 Effendy I, Kolczak H, Friederich HC. [Noncompliance relevant variables in patients with onychomycosis; in German.] *Wien Med Wochenschr* 1989;**139**:356–9.

244 Villars V, Jones TC. Clinical efficacy and tolerability of terbinafine (Lamisil)—a new topical and systemic fungicidal drug for treatment of dermatomycoses. *Clin Exp Dermatol* 1989;**14**:124–7.

245 Hay RJ, Roberts DT, Doherty VR, Richardson MD, Midgley G. The topical treatment of onychomycosis using a new combined urea/imidazole preparation. *Clin Exp Dermatol* 1988;**13**:164–7.

246 Stepanova Z, Smol'iakova LL. [Experience with Nizoral treatment of patients with rubromycosis; in Russian.] *Vestn Dermatol Venerol* 1988;(**1**):66–8.

247 Clissold SP, Heel RC. Tioconazole. A review of its antimicrobial activity and therapeutic use in superficial mycoses. *Drugs* 1986;**31**:29–51.

248 Butareva TA, Kukushkin AM, Unzhakov VP, Nemkaeva RM. [8-Hydroxyquinoline derivatives in the treatment of patients with onychomycoses; in Russian.] *Vestn Dermatol Venerol* 1986;(**12**):50–3.

249 Nilsen A, Hovding G. [Ketoconazole in onychomycosis; in Norwegian.] *Tidsskr Nor Laegeforen* 1985;**105**:141–2.

250 Svejgaard E. Oral ketoconazole as an alternative to griseofulvin in recalcitrant dermatophyte infections and onychomycosis. *Acta Derm Venereol* 1985;**65**:143–9.

251 Zaias N, Drachman D. A method for the determination of drug effectiveness in onychomycosis. Trials with ketoconazole and griseofulvin ultramicrosize. *J Am Acad Dermatol* 1983;**9**:912–9.

252 Ishii M, Hamada T, Asai Y. Treatment of onychomycosis by ODT therapy with 20% urea ointment and 2% tolnaftate ointment. *Dermatologica* 1983;**167**:273–9.

253 Botter AA, Nuijten ST. Further experiences with ketoconazole in the treatment of onychomycosis. *Mykosen* 1981;**24**:156–66.

254 Qadripur SA, Horn G, Hohler T. [On the local efficacy of ciclopiroxolamine in onychomycoses; in German.] *Arzneimittelforschung* 1981;**31**:1369–72.

255 Brugmans J, Scheijgrond H, Van Cutsem J, Van den BH, Baisier A, Horig C. [Oral long-term treatment of onychomycoses with ketoconazole; in German.] *Mykosen* 1980;**23**:405–15.

256 Botter AA, Dethier F, Mertens RL, Morias J, Peremans W. Skin and nail mycoses: treatment with ketoconazole, a new oral antimycotic agent. *Mykosen* 1979;**22**:274–8.

257 Zaias N, Battistini F, Gomez-Urcuyo F, Rojas RF, Ricart R. Treatment of "tinea pedis" with griseofulvin and topical antifungal cream. *Cutis* 1978;**22**:197–9.

258 Bagatell FK. Topical therapy for onychomycosis. *Arch Dermatol* 1977;**113**:378.

259 Emokpare NA. [Clinical evaluation of a new antifungal agent clotrimazole in dermatomycoses; in German.] *Z Ärztl Fortbild (Jena)* 1977;**71**:144–6.

260 Klima J. [A report on the clinical experiences from the comparison of the effectiveness of 0.2% and 0.5% solutions of the antimycotic agent VUFB 9244 (working name Jopargin); in Czech.] *Cesk Dermatol* 1976;**51**:404–6.

261 Schwarz KJ, Much T, Konzelmann M. [Evaluation of econazole in 594 cases of skin mycosis; in German.] *Dtsch Med Wochenschr* 1975;**100**:1497–500.

262 Fredriksson T. Topical treatment of superficial mycoses with clotrimazole. *Postgrad Med J* 1974;**50**(Suppl 1):62–4.

263 Oberste-Lehn H. Ideal properties of a modern antifungal agent—the therapy of mycoses with clotrimazole. *Postgrad Med J* 1974;**50**(Suppl 1):51–3.

264 Grant LV. A further look at the treatment of onychomycosis with topical glutaraldehyde. *J Am Podiatry Assoc* 1974;**64**:158–60.

265 Schubert E. [Clinical experience in the treatment of nail mycoses with the new antibiotic Bay b5097 (clotrimazole); in German.] *Z Hautkr* 1973;**48**:887–91.

266 Kull E. [Local treatment of skin and nail mycoses with Daktarin, a new broad-spectrum antifungal agent. Testing results of a group of dermatologists in practice; in German.] *Schweiz Rundsch Med Prax* 1972;**61**:1308–10.

267 Weuta H. [Clotrimazole cream and solution—clinical assessment in an open trial; in German.] *Arzneimittelforschung* 1972;**22**:1295–9.

268 Botter AA. Topical treatment of nail and skin infections with miconazole, a new broad-spectrum antimycotic. *Mykosen* 1971; **14**:187–91.

269 Dix R, Sloan B. An evaluation of a local and an oral medication in the treatment of onychomycosis. *J Am Podiatry Assoc* 1966;**56**: 450–4.

270 Quintavalle P. Onychomycosis treated with ultrafine griseofulvin. *J Am Podiatry Assoc* 1966;**56**:119–20.

271 El Euch D, Bouassida S, Kourda M, *et al.* [Fluconazole and treatment of onychomycosis. About 86 cases; in French.] *Tunis Med* 2006;**84**:640–3.

272 El Komy MH. Nailfold fluconazole fluid injection for fingernail onychomycosis. *Clin Exp Dermatol* 2006;**31**:465–7.

273 Gupta AK, Gover MD, Lynde CW. Pulse itraconazole vs. continuous terbinafine for the treatment of dermatophyte toenail onychomycosis in patients with diabetes mellitus. *J Eur Acad Dermatol Venereol* 2006;**20**:1188–93.

274 Nakano N, Hiruma M, Shiraki Y, *et al.* Combination of pulse therapy with terbinafine tablets and topical terbinafine cream for the treatment of dermatophyte onychomycosis: a pilot study. *J Dermatol* 2006;**33**:90–105.

275 Jennings MB, Pollak R, Harkless LB, *et al.* Treatment of toenail onychomycosis with oral terbinafine plus aggressive debridement: IRON-CLAD, a large, randomized, open-label, multicenter trial. *J Am Podiatr Med Assoc* 2006;**96**:465–73.

276 Potter LP, Matthias SD, Raut M, *et al.* The impact of aggressive debridement used as an adjunct therapy with terbinafine on perceptions of patients undergoing treatment for toenail onychomycosis. *J Dermatolog Treat* 2007;**18**:46–52.

277 Gupta AK, Lynde CW, Konnikov N. Single-blind, randomized, prospective study of sequential itraconazole and terbinafine pulse compared with terbinafine pulse for the treatment of toenail onychomycosis. *J Am Acad Dermatol* 2001;**44**:485–91.

278 Drake L, Babel D, Stewart DM, *et al.* Once-weekly fluconazole (150, 300, or 450 mg) in the treatment of distal subungual onychomycosis of the fingernail. *J Am Acad Dermatol* 1998;**38**:S87–S94.

279 Haneke E, Tajerbashi M, De Doncker P, Heremans A. Itraconazole in the treatment of onychomycosis: a double-blind comparison with miconazole. *Dermatology* 1998;**196**:323–9.

280 Tausch I, Brautigam M, Weidinger G, Jones TC. Evaluation of 6 weeks treatment of terbinafine in tinea unguium in a double-blind trial comparing 6 and 12 weeks therapy. The Lagos V Study Group. *Br J Dermatol* 1997;**136**:737–42.

281 Hofmann H, Brautigam M, Weidinger G, Zaun H. Treatment of toenail onychomycosis. A randomized, double-blind study with terbinafine and griseofulvin. LAGOS II Study Group. *Arch Dermatol* 1995;**131**:919–22.

282 Haneke E, Tausch I, Brautigam M, *et al.* Short-duration treatment of fingernail dermatophytosis: a randomized, double-blind study with terbinafine and griseofulvin. LAGOS III Study Group. *J Am Acad Dermatol* 1995;**32**:72–7.

283 Korting HC, Schafer-Korting M, Zienicke H, *et al.* Treatment of tinea unguium with medium and high doses of ultramicrosize griseofulvin compared with that with itraconazole. *Antimicrob Agents Chemother* 1993;**37**:2064–8.

284 van der Schroeff JG, Cirkel PK, Crijns MB, *et al.* A randomized treatment duration-finding study of terbinafine in onychomycosis. *Br J Dermatol* 1992;**126**(Suppl 39):36–9.

285 Baran R, Belaich S, Beylot C, *et al.* Comparative multicentre double-blind study of terbinafine (250 mg per day) versus griseofulvin (1 g per day) in the treatment of dermatophyte onychomycosis. *J Dermatol* 1997;**8**:93–7.

286 Goodfield MJ. Short-duration therapy with terbinafine for dermatophyte onychomycosis: a multicentre trial. *Br J Dermatol* 1992;**126**(Suppl 39):33–5.

287 Sigurgeirsson B, Elewski B, Rich PA, *et al.* Intermittent versus continuous terbinafine in the treatment of toenail onychomycosis: a randomized, double-blind comparison. *J Dermatolog Treat* 2006;**17**:38–44.

288 Claveau J, Vender RB, Gupta AK. Multitherapy approach to onychomycosis therapy. *J Cutan Med Surg* 2006;**10**(Suppl 2):S44–S47.

289 Baran R, Hay RJ, Tosti A, Haneke E. A new classification of onychomycosis. *Br J Dermatol* 1998;**139**:567–71.

290 Cox NH, Eedy DJ, Morton CA. Guidelines for management of Bowen's disease. *Br J Dermatol* 1999;**141**:633–41.

291 Gupta AK. Systemic antifungal agents. In: Wolverton SE, ed. *Comprehensive Dermatologic Drug Therapy*. Philadelphia: Saunders, 2001: 55–84.

292 Faergemann J, Anderson C, Hersle K, *et al.* Double-blind, parallel-group comparison of terbinafine and griseofulvin in the treatment of toenail onychomycosis. *J Am Acad Dermatol* 1995;**32**:750–3.

293 Gupta AK, Sauder DN, Shear N. Antifungal agents: an overview. Part I. *J Am Acad Dermatol* 1994;**30**:677–98.

294 Gupta AK, Shear NH. The new oral antifungal agents for onychomycosis of the toenails. *J Eur Acad Dermatol Venereol* 1999;**13**:1–13.

295 Gupta AK, Sauder DN, Shear NH. Antifungal agents: an overview. Part II. *J Am Acad Dermatol* 1994;**30**:911–33.

296 Elewski BE. Once-weekly fluconazole in the treatment of onychomycosis: introduction. *J Am Acad Dermatol* 1998;**38**:S73–S76.

297 De Doncker PR, Scher RK, Baran RL, *et al.* Itraconazole therapy is effective for pedal onychomycosis caused by some nondermatophyte molds and in mixed infection with dermatophytes and molds: a multicenter study with 36 patients. *J Am Acad Dermatol* 1997;**36**:173–7.

298 Janssen Pharmaceutica Products LP. Sporanox® (itraconazole) capsules. Prescribing information. Titusville, NJ: Janssen, 2006.

299 Novartis Pharmaceuticals Corporation. Lamisil® (terbinafine hydrochloride) prescribing information. East Hanover, NJ: Novartis, 2005.

300 Billstein S, Kianifard F, Justice A. Terbinafine vs. placebo for onychomycosis in black patients. *Int J Dermatol* 1999;**38**:377–9.

301 Svejgaard EL, Brandrup F, Kragballe K, *et al.* Oral terbinafine in toenail dermatophytosis. A double-blind, placebo-controlled multicenter study with 12 months' follow-up. *Acta Derm Venereol* 1997;**77**:66–9.

302 Watson A, Marley J, Ellis D, Williams T. Terbinafine in onychomycosis of the toenail: a novel treatment protocol. *J Am Acad Dermatol* 1995;**33**:775–9.

303 Heikkila H, Stubb S. Long-term results in patients with onychomycosis treated with terbinafine or itraconazole. *Br J Dermatol* 2002;**146**:250–3.

304 Sigurgeirsson B, Olafsson JH, Steinsson JB, *et al.* Long-term effectiveness of treatment with terbinafine vs itraconazole in onychomycosis: a 5-year blinded prospective follow-up study. *Arch Dermatol* 2002;**138**:353–7.

305 Havu V, Heikkila H, Kuokkanen K, *et al.* A double-blind, randomized study to compare the efficacy and safety of terbinafine (Lamisil) with fluconazole (Diflucan) in the treatment of onychomycosis. *Br J Dermatol* 2000;**142**:97–102.

306 De Backer M, De Vroey C, Lesaffre E, *et al.* Twelve weeks of continuous oral therapy for toenail onychomycosis caused by dermatophytes: a double-blind comparative trial of terbinafine 250 mg/day versus itraconazole 200 mg/day. *J Am Acad Dermatol* 1998;**38**:S57–S63.

307 Honeyman JF, Talarico FS, Arruda LHF, *et al.* Itraconazole versus terbinafine (Lamisil): which is better for the treatment of onychomycosis? *J Eur Acad Dermatol Venereol* 1997;**9**:215–21.

308 Degreef H, del Palacio A, Mygind S, *et al.* Randomized double-blind comparison of short-term itraconazole and terbinafine therapy for toenail onychomycosis. *Acta Derm Venereol* 1999;**79**:221–3.

309 Brautigam M, Nolting S, Schopf RE, Weidinger G. Randomised double blind comparison of terbinafine and itraconazole for treatment of toenail tinea infection. Seventh Lamisil German Onychomycosis Study Group. *BMJ* 1995;**311**:919–22.

310 De Backer M, De Keyser P, Massart DL, Westelinck KJ. Terbinafine (Lamisil) 250 mg/day and 500 mg/day are equally effective in a 16 week oral treatment of toenail onychomycosis. A double-blind multicentre trial. In: Hay RJ, ed. *International Perspective on Lamisil.* London: CCT Healthcare Communications, 1994: 39–43.

311 Warshaw EM, Fett DB, Bloomfield HE, *et al.* Pulse versus continuous terbinafine for onychomycosis: a randomized, double-blind, controlled trial. *J Am Acad Dermatol* 2005;**53**:578–84.

312 Arca E, Tastan HB, Akar A, *et al.* An open, randomized, comparative study of oral fluconazole, itraconazole and terbinafine therapy in onychomycosis. *J Dermatolog Treat* 2002;**13**:3–9.

313 Tosti A, Piraccini BM, Stinchi C, *et al.* Treatment of dermatophyte nail infections: an open randomized study comparing intermittent terbinafine therapy with continuous terbinafine treatment and intermittent itraconazole therapy. *J Am Acad Dermatol* 1996;**34**:595–600.

314 Alpsoy E, Yilmaz E, Basaran E. Intermittent therapy with terbinafine for dermatophyte toe-onychomycosis: a new approach. *J Dermatol* 1996;**23**:259–62.

315 Kejda J. Itraconazole pulse therapy vs continuous terbinafine dosing for toenail onychomycosis. *Postgrad Med* 1999;Spec No:12–5.

316 Gupta AK, Shear NH. Safety review of the oral antifungal agents used to treat superficial mycoses. *Int J Dermatol* 1999;**38**(Suppl 2):40–52.

317 Novartis Pharmaceuticals Canada. Lamisil® (terbinafine hydrochloride) prescribing information. Dorval, Quebec: Novartis, 2004.

318 Katz HI, Gupta AK. Oral antifungal drug interactions. *Dermatol Clin* 1997;**15**:535–44.

319 Gupta AK, Katz HI, Shear N. Drug interactions with itraconazole, fluconazole and terbinafine and their management. *Int J Dermatol* 1999;**41**:237–49.

320 Ryder NS. Terbinafine: mode of action and properties of the squalene epoxidase inhibition. *Br J Dermatol* 1992;**126**(Suppl 39):2–7.

321 Haugh M, Helou S, Boissel JP, Cribier BJ. Terbinafine in fungal infections of the nails: a meta-analysis of randomized clinical trials. *Br J Dermatol* 2002;**147**:118–21.

322 Crawford F, Young P, Godfrey C, *et al.* Oral treatments for toenail onychomycosis: a systematic review. *Arch Dermatol* 2002;**138**:811–6.

323 Odom RB, Aly R, Scher RK, *et al.* A multicenter, placebo-controlled, double-blind study of intermittent therapy with itraconazole for the treatment of onychomycosis of the fingernail. *J Am Acad Dermatol* 1997;**36**:231–5.

324 Gupta AK, Maddin S, Arlette J, *et al.* Itraconazole pulse therapy is effective in dermatophyte onychomycosis of the toenail: a double-blind placebo-controlled study. *J Dermatolog Treat* 2000;**11**:33–7.

325 Havu V, Brandt H, Heikkila H, *et al.* A double-blind, randomized study comparing itraconazole pulse therapy with continuous dosing for the treatment of toe-nail onychomycosis. *Br J Dermatol* 1997;**136**:230–4.

326 Ginter G, De Doncker P. An intermittent itraconazole 1-week dosing regimen for the treatment of toenail onychomycosis in dermatological practice. *Mycoses* 1998;**41**:235–8.

327 Shemer A, Nathansohn N, Kaplan B, *et al.* Open randomized comparison of different itraconazole regimens for the treatment of onychomycosis. *J Dermatolog Treat* 1999;**10**:245–9.

328 De Doncker P, Decroix J, Pierard GE, *et al.* Antifungal pulse therapy for onychomycosis. A pharmacokinetic and pharmacodynamic investigation of monthly cycles of 1-week pulse therapy with itraconazole. *Arch Dermatol* 1996;**132**:34–41.

329 Gupta AK, De Doncker P, Scher RK, *et al.* Itraconazole for the treatment of onychomycosis. *Int J Dermatol* 1998;**37**:303–8.

330 Gupta AK, Albreski D, Del Rosso JQ, Konnikov N. The use of the new oral antifungal agents, itraconazole, terbinafine, and fluconazole to treat onychomycosis and other dermatomycoses. *Curr Prob Dermatol* 2001;**13**:213–48.

331 Janssen-Ortho Inc. Sporanox® (itraconazole capsules) product monograph. Toronto: Janssen, 2006.

332 De Doncker P, Gupta AK, Del Rosso JQ, *et al.* Safety of itraconazole pulse therapy for onychomycosis. An update. *Postgrad Med* 1999;Spec No:17–25.

333 De Doncker P, Gupta AK. Itraconazole and terbinafine in perspective. From Petri dish to patient. *Postgrad Med* 1999;Spec No:6–11.

334 De Doncker P, Gupta AK, Marynissen G, *et al.* Itraconazole pulse therapy for onychomycosis and dermatomycoses: an overview. *J Am Acad Dermatol* 1997;**37**:969–74.

335 Elewski BE, Scher RK, Aly R, *et al.* Double-blind, randomized comparison of itraconazole capsules vs. placebo in the treatment of toenail onychomycosis. *Cutis* 1997;**59**:217–20.

336 Jones HE, Zaias N. Double-blind, randomized comparison of itraconazole capsules and placebo in onychomycosis of toenail. *Int J Dermatol* 1996;**35**:589–90.

337 Odom R, Daniel CR, Aly R. A double-blind, randomized comparison of itraconazole capsules and placebo in the treatment of onychomycosis of the toenail. *J Am Acad Dermatol* 1996;**35**:110–11.

338 Gupta AK, Scher RK, Rich P. Fluconazole for the treatment of onychomycosis: an update. *Int J Dermatol* 1998;**37**:815–20.

339 Baran R, Kaoukhov A. Topical antifungal drugs for the treatment of onychomycosis: an overview of current strategies for monotherapy and combination therapy. *J Eur Acad Dermatol Venereol* 2005;**19**:21–9.

340 Lauharanta J. Comparative efficacy and safety of Amorolfine nail lacquer 2% versus 5% once weekly. *Clin Exp Dermatol* 1992;**17**(Suppl 1):41–3.

341 Reinel D, Clarke C. Comparative efficacy and safety of amorolfine nail lacquer 5% in onychomycosis, once-weekly versus twice-weekly. *Clin Exp Dermatol* 1992;**17**(Suppl 1):44–9.

342 Zaug M, Bergstrasser M. Amorolfine in the treatment of onychomycoses and dermatomycoses (an overview). *Clin Exp Dermatol* 1992;**17**(Suppl 1):61–70.

343 Downs AM, Lear JT, Archer CB. *Scytalidium hyalinum* onychomycosis successfully treated with 5% amorolfine nail lacquer. *Br J Dermatol* 1999;**140**:555.

344 Baran R, Feuilhade M, Datry A, *et al.* A randomized trial of amorolfine 5% solution nail lacquer combined with oral terbinafine compared with terbinafine alone in the treatment of dermatophytic toenail onychomycoses affecting the matrix region. *Br J Dermatol* 2000;**142**:1177–83.

345 Gupta AK, Joseph WS. Ciclopirox 8% nail lacquer in the treatment of onychomycosis of the toenails in the United States. *J Am Podiatr Med Assoc* 2000;**90**:495–501.

346 Gupta AK, Fleckman P, Baran R. Ciclopirox nail lacquer topical solution 8% in the treatment of toenail onychomycosis. *J Am Acad Dermatol* 2000;**43**:S70–S80.

347 Gupta AK, the Onychomycosis Combination Therapy Study Group. Ciclopirox topical solution, 8% combined with oral terbinafine to treat onychomycosis: a randomized, evaluator-blinded study. *J Drugs Dermatol* 2005;**4**:481–5.

348 Avner S, Nir N, Henri T. Combination of oral terbinafine and topical ciclopirox compared to oral terbinafine for the treatment of onychomycosis. *J Dermatolog Treat* 2005;**16**:327–30.

349 Jansen R, Redekop WK, Rutten FF. Cost effectiveness of continuous terbinafine compared with intermittent itraconazole in the treatment of dermatophyte toenail onychomycosis: an analysis of based on results from the L.I.ON. study. Lamisil versus Itraconazole in Onychomycosis. *Pharmacoeconomics* 2001;**19**:401–10.

350 Gupta AK. Pharmacoeconomic analysis of oral antifungal therapies used to treat dermatophyte onychomycosis of the toenails. A US analysis. *Pharmacoeconomics* 1998;**13**:243–56.

351 Marchetti A, Piech CT, McGhan WF, *et al.* Pharmacoeconomic analysis of oral therapies for onychomycosis: a US model. *Clin Ther* 1996;**18**:757–77.

352 Arikian SR, Einarson TR, Kobelt-Nguyen G, Schubert F. A multinational pharmacoeconomic analysis of oral therapies for onychomycosis. The Onychomycosis Study Group. *Br J Dermatol* 1994;**130**(Suppl 43):35–44.

353 Einarson TR, Arikian SR, Shear NH. Cost-effectiveness analysis for onychomycosis therapy in Canada from a government perspective. *Br J Dermatol* 1994;**130**(Suppl 43):32–4.

354 Gupta AK, Baran R. Ciclopirox nail lacquer solution 8% in the 21st century. *J Am Acad Dermatol* 2000;**43**:S96–102.

355 Roberts DT, Evans EG. Subungual dermatophytoma complicating dermatophyte onychomycosis. *Br J Dermatol* 1998;**138**:189–90.

356 Gupta AK. Are boosters or supplementation of antifungal drugs of any use for treating onychomycosis? *J Drugs Dermatol* 2002;**1**:35–41.

Tinea capitis

Urbà González

Background

Definition

Tinea capitis (scalp ringworm) is an infection of the scalp skin and hair caused by fungi (dermatophytes). mainly of the genera *Trichophyton* and *Microsporum*. The clinical hallmark is single or multiple patches of hair loss, sometimes with a "black dot" pattern (Figure 39.1), which may be accompanied by signs of inflammation such as scaling, pustules and itching.[1,2]

Incidence/prevalence[3,4]

Tinea capitis is uncommon in adults and is seen predominantly in prepubertal children. It has affected mainly disadvantaged communities in both developing and industrialized nations. During the past 30 years, some significant changes have occurred in the reported incidences of tinea capitis. Travel and migration have led to changes in the epidemiology of the species of dermatophyte causing tinea capitis.

Etiology[5,6]

Tinea capitis is contagious. It can be acquired through contact with people, animals, or objects carrying the fungus. The presence of fungi within the scalp may not be sufficient to result in tinea capitis (carrier state). Approximately eight dermatophyte species are characteristically associated with tinea capitis. Infections due to *Trichophyton tonsurans* predominate from Central America to the United States and in parts of western Europe. *Microsporum canis* infections are mainly seen in South America, Southern and Eastern Europe, Africa, and the Middle East.

Prognosis

Tinea capitis is not life-threatening in people with normal immunity. Untreated cases cause persistent symptoms, and in some types of tinea capitis—mainly the inflammatory type or kerion—may lead to scarring alopecia (Figure 39.2).

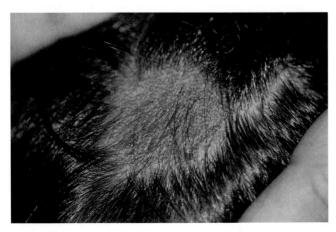

Figure 39.1 Tinea capitis.

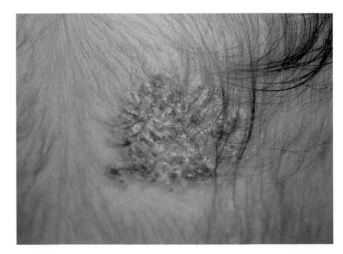

Figure 39.2 Inflammatory tinea capitis.

Diagnostic tests[7–9]

The clinical diagnosis should be confirmed by mycological examination. The main methods of collecting samples for microbiological diagnosis involve either scraping or brushing the scalp. Microscopy provides the most rapid means of diagnosis and allows treatment to commence, but is not always positive. Culture allows accurate identification of the organism involved and may be positive even when microscopy is negative, but may take up to 4 weeks. Wood's light or filtered ultraviolet light can be used to identify infections that fluoresce under this type of light, such as *M. canis* and *M. audouinii*, but not *T. tonsurans*.

Aims of treatment[10–15]

The first aim of treatment is to achieve complete clinical and mycological cure as quickly as possible, with no or minimal adverse effects. Effective short-course therapy is especially desirable in children, because prolonged therapy increases the risk of adverse effects as well as noncompliance. Another goal is prevention of spread to other children from objects, infected animals or children, and from asymptomatic carriers.

Relevant outcomes

Outcomes are based on resolution of the clinical signs (redness, scaling, edema, and hair loss) and symptoms (itch), and negative mycological data, including microscopy and culture. Complete cure (clinical and mycological cure), cure (clinical or mycological cure), improvement (clinical), and failure (ineffective therapy or worsening) are the most widely used outcomes.

Methods of search

The information for this chapter has come from the search strategy used in a Cochrane systematic review (in press) covering the Cochrane Skin Group Specialized Register, the Cochrane Central Register of Controlled Trials (The Cochrane Library), Medline, Embase, *Literatura Latino Americana e do Caribe em Ciências da Saúde* (LILACS), the Cumulative Index to Nursing and Allied Health Literature (CINAHL), the American College of Physicians (ACP) journal club, and HealthStar. Any key randomized clinical trial (RCT) (see web table 39.1) and other relevant information has been included if published by the end of 2006. Because of the limited studies available for some questions, studies with methodological shortcomings were also included.

Systemic antifungal therapy for tinea capitis in children

Griseofulvin has been the most widely used and prescribed treatment for tinea capitis and has served as a standard for the evaluation of any newer agent to be considered for this infection. New drugs being used against other fungal infections in adults, such as ketoconazole, itraconazole, terbinafine, and fluconazole, are being considered more frequently for the treatment of tinea capitis. Sufficient pharmacological and pharmaceutical data exist on these five antifungal drugs to make them suitable for treating tinea capitis in children.[16,17]

Questions

In children with tinea capitis, which oral antifungal drug leads to high rates of cure with the fewest adverse events?

Griseofulvin
There is moderate RCT evidence that griseofulvin at doses of 125–500 mg/day (depending on the patient's weight) for 6–8 weeks is effective and safe for the treatment of tinea capitis caused by *T. tonsurans*, *T. violaceum*, and *M. canis*.

Efficacy
Thirteen RCTs comparing griseofulvin with other oral antifungals in tinea capitis and a further meta-analysis (search date: 1966–2004, six RCTs, 603 patients) involving griseofulvin and terbinafine were identified.

Versus ketoconazole. Four RCTs were identified. In two RCTs[18,19] in which *T. tonsurans* was the most commonly isolated organism, griseofulvin at doses of 10–20 mg/kg/day[18] and 250–500 mg/day[19] was compared with ketoconazole 3.3–6.6 mg/kg/day[18] and 200 mg/day[19] for 12 and 6 weeks, respectively. There were no statistically significant differences between the mycological cure rates of the two drugs. Cure rates in the griseofulvin groups at the end of treatment were 96%[18] and 57.1%.[19] A small RCT[20] including 47 children compared griseofulvin 350 mg/day for 6 weeks with ketoconazole 100 mg/day for 6 weeks in inflammatory tinea capitis (*T. mentagrophytes* and *M. canis*). At the end of treatment, 80% and 100% of the children, respectively, had improved clinically, but no mycological data were reported. An RCT with unknown blinding[21] including 63 children in whom *Trichophyton* spp. predominated compared griseofulvin 15 mg/kg/day with ketoconazole 5 mg/kg/day, each given as a single daily dose, and treatment stopped when there was complete cure or after 6 months. After 8 weeks' therapy, 92% of the patients given griseofulvin had complete cure of their infection, in comparison with only 59% of the ketoconazole-treated patients. After 12 weeks, 96% of the griseofulvin patients were mycologically cured, in comparison with 74% of the ketoconazole-treated group. Hair sample cultures took significantly longer to become sterile in ketoconazole-treated patients (median 8 weeks) than in griseofulvin-treated patients (4 weeks).

Versus itraconazole. One RCT[22] in 34 children (with mainly *M. canis* infections) comparing 6 weeks of ultramicrosized griseofulvin 500 mg/day and itraconazole 100 mg/day showed a complete cure rate of 88% for the two drugs after 14 weeks' follow-up.

Versus terbinafine. Six RCTs were identified and one meta-analysis that included these six RCTs. A double-blind RCT[23] compared 140 children from Pakistan, 87% of whom had *T. violaceum* tinea capitis. They were treated with either terbinafine (by weight) for 4 weeks or with griseofulvin 6–12 mg/kg/day for 8 weeks. After 12 weeks, 93% of the terbinafine group were completely cured, in comparison with 80% of the griseofulvin group; the difference was not significant. A double-blind RCT[24] evaluated 50 children from Peru, 74% of whom had *T. tonsurans* infections. Half were treated with terbinafine according to weight for 4 weeks, plus 4 weeks with placebo; the other half received microsized griseofulvin according to weight for 8 weeks. After 8 weeks of treatment, complete cure was noted in 76% of the griseofulvin group and in 72% of terbinafine group, but 4 weeks later the complete cure rate increased to 76% in the terbinafine group, while in the griseofulvin group it had fallen to 44%—a statistically significant difference. In a large RCT,[25] *T. tonsurans* accounted for 77% of the terbinafine group and 88% of the griseofulvin group; *Microsporum* spp. accounted for 14% of both groups. The RCT compared 8 weeks of griseofulvin suspension 10 mg/kg/day with 4 weeks of terbinafine. The complete cure rates at week 24 were 64% with terbinafine and 67% with griseofulvin— no significant difference. However, there was a trend to better responses in *Microsporum* spp. infections with 8 weeks of griseofulvin than with 4 weeks of terbinafine. In another RCT,[26] the complete cure rate at the final follow-up visit (week 12) was 74% in the group treated for 8 weeks with ultramicrosized griseofulvin, in comparison with 78% in the group treated with terbinafine for 4 weeks, with no significant differences between *M. canis* and *Trichophyton* spp. infections. Another trial[27] compared 50 patients in each treatment group with infections caused by two main organisms (*T. tonsurans* and *T. violaceum*). In this trial, terbinafine for 2–3 weeks was compared with microsized griseofulvin 20 mg/kg for 6 weeks. The complete cure rate was 94% for

the terbinafine group and 92% for the griseofulvin-treated group. Only one RCT[28] assessed medium-term to long-term treatment regimens comparing terbinafine with griseofulvin. In this study, 98.5% of the 165 children included were infected with *M. canis* and the remainder were infected with *M. audouinii*. The patients were treated with terbinafine for 6, 8, 10, or 12 weeks, followed by placebo to complete a 12-week treatment phase in a double-blinded regimen, or griseofulvin for 12 weeks using an unblinded regimen. Medium-term treatment (6 or 8 weeks) resulted in a trend towards an increase in the complete cure rate in the griseofulvin group in comparison with the terbinafine group at 4 weeks after the end of treatment. However, long-term treatment (10 or 12 weeks) resulted in the complete cure rates being significantly higher in the griseofulvin group in comparison with the terbinafine group at 4 weeks after the end of treatment. The meta-analysis[29] of the above six RCTs concluded that a 2–4-week course of terbinafine is at least as effective as a 6–8-week course of griseofulvin for the treatment of *Trichophyton* infections and that griseofulvin is likely to be superior to terbinafine for the less frequent cases of infections by *Microsporum* species.

Versus fluconazole. Three RCTs comparing fluconazole and griseofulvin were found.[27,30,31] The first RCT[27] assessed 100 children who were infected with *T. tonsurans* and/or *T. violaceum* (the exact percentages were not reported). The children were treated either with fluconazole 6 mg/kg/day for 2–3 weeks or with microsized griseofulvin 20 mg/kg/day for 6 weeks, and the complete cure rates were 82% and 92%, respectively. The second RCT[30] compared 40 children: 16 were infected with *T. violaceum*, 16 with *T. verrucosum*, and eight with *M. canis*. The children were treated with 5 mg/kg/day of fluconazole or 15 mg/kg/day griseofulvin for 4 and 6 weeks, respectively. Complete cure was reported for 79% of the fluconazole arm and 76% of the griseofulvin arm. The third study, a three-arm RCT[31] including 880 patients with mainly *T. tonsurans* infection, compared fluconazole 6 mg/kg/day for 3 weeks followed by 3 weeks of placebo, fluconazole 6 mg/kg/day for 6 weeks, and griseofulvin 11 mg/kg/day for 6 weeks. The complete cure rates were 44.5%, 49.6%, and 52.2%, respectively.

Drawbacks

Two patients had nausea and intense stomach ache with severe vomiting at weeks 2 and 4 of treatment and required discontinuation of therapy.[22] One griseofulvin-treated patient showed a twofold increase in serum alanine aminotransferase and aspartate aminotransferase after 3 weeks of treatment, but the values returned to normal at the following weekly clinic visit.[20] The following adverse events have been described as having an uncertain relationship with the study drug: skin infections, skin infestations, rash, urticaria, gastroenteritis, raised hepatic enzymes, raised triglycerides, raised uric acid, anemia, eosinophilia, leukocytosis, and granulocytopenia.[26,27,31] In the largest RCT,[25] a total of 52 adverse events were detected in 27 patients in the griseofulvin group and included abdominal discomfort and vomiting. None of the events was rated as severe, but one patient was withdrawn from the study because of abdominal pain, headaches, and vomiting. In other studies, no adverse effects or no significant adverse effects were reported.[18,19,21,23,24,27,30]

Comments

One study published as an RCT[32] was excluded, as it was still in progress and the codes for concealment of randomization had not yet been broken. Another study described as an RCT[33] was excluded because it did not give separate clinical and mycological data for each group. Two RCTs[34,35] were duplicate publications of other studies.[23,24] All other included studies show that griseofulvin is effective for tinea capitis, although the definition of "cure" varies from study to study and some investigators carefully follow microbiological findings, whereas others place greater emphasis on the clinical response. The high patient drop-out rate in most of the studies may have masked the improvement in the griseofulvin groups, as those who achieve cure may have less incentive to attend follow-up visits. It will also have reduced the power to detect a difference between the groups, indicating that griseofulvin may be even more effective. The duration of follow-up varies from study to study (6–24 weeks) and only RCTs with long-term follow-up can show the relapse rates, which are very important in determining therapeutic efficacy. Five of nine studies were supported by the pharmaceutical industry.[18–20,22,25] The largest RCT[31] showed unusually low cure rates in the group treated with griseofulvin.

Ketoconazole versus griseofulvin

Data from some RCTs[18,21] indicated that ketoconazole may require a longer course of therapy than griseofulvin, and the cure rates with it were no better. However, while ketoconazole is associated with rare but important hepatic and endocrine adverse events, none of these were noted in the pediatric studies described. As oral itraconazole is now available and the safety of long-term use of oral ketoconazole is uncertain, ketoconazole is not considered further as a treatment of choice in children with tinea capitis. Three[18–20] of the four RCTs with ketoconazole were supported by companies producing this drug.

Implications for practice

There is good evidence to support the use of griseofulvin to treat tinea capitis caused by T. tonsurans, M. canis, T. mentagrophytes, and T. violaceum. Overall, griseofulvin is considered to be safe in children. On the basis of the RCTs described, the recommended dosage regimen for children

is continuous therapy with tablets or suspension, adjusted according to the patient's weight (10–20 kg: 125 mg/day; 20–40 kg: 250 mg/day; more than 40 kg: 500 mg/day) for 6–8 weeks, including microsized and ultramicrosized preparations. Other advantages of griseofulvin are that it is inexpensive and that the suspension allows accurate dosage in children. Griseofulvin is licensed for the treatment of tinea capitis in most countries.

Terbinafine

Moderate RCT evidence indicates that terbinafine at doses of 62.5–250 mg/day (depending on body weight) for 2 weeks in T. violaceum infections and for 4 weeks in T. tonsurans infections is effective and safe for the treatment of Trichophyton spp. tinea capitis. A few RCTs (limited evidence) suggest that longer therapeutic regimens of 6 weeks may be necessary to treat Microsporum spp. infections.

Efficacy

One meta-analysis was identified (search date: 1966–2004, six RCTs, 603 patients) involving terbinafine and griseofulvin. Seven RCTs compared terbinafine with other oral antifungals in tinea capitis.

Versus griseofulvin. The meta-analysis[29] concluded that a 2–4-week course of terbinafine is at least as effective as a 6–8 week course of griseofulvin for the treatment of Trichophyton infections and that griseofulvin is likely to be superior to terbinafine for the lest frequent cases of infections by Microsporum species. Six RCTs were identified (the same as those included in the meta-analysis). A double-blind RCT[23] compared 140 children from Pakistan, 87% of whom had T. violaceum infection. They were treated with either terbinafine 62.5–250 mg/day by weight for 4 weeks, or with griseofulvin, 125–500 mg/day depending on the patient's weight, for 8 weeks. Four weeks after the conclusion of the study, 93% of the patients in the terbinafine group were completely cured, in comparison with 80% in the griseofulvin group; the difference was not statistically significant. A double-blind RCT study[24] evaluated 50 children from Lima, Peru, 74% of whom had T. tonsurans infection. Half received terbinafine, 62.5–250 mg/day for 4 weeks, the other half griseofulvin, 125–500 mg/day for 8 weeks; dosage was according to body weight. At the end of week 8, 76% of the terbinafine group and 80% of the griseofulvin group showed complete cure. However, 4 weeks later, the 76% cure rate in the terbinafine group was sustained, whereas in the griseofulvin group the cure rate had decreased to 44%. An RCT[26] compared ultramicrosized griseofulvin for 8 weeks with terbinafine for 4 weeks, both dosed according to body weight. At the final follow-up visit at week 12, 88% of the patients in the terbinafine-treated group were mycologically cured, in comparison with 91% in the griseofulvin-treated group; complete cure was reported in 78% and 74% of patients, respectively. *Trichophyton* spp. and *M. canis* responded similarly to terbinafine. A large RCT[25] compared griseofulvin suspension 10 mg/kg/day for 8 weeks with terbinafine for 4 weeks. *T. tonsurans* infection accounted for 77% of the terbinafine group and 88% of the griseofulvin group; 14% of each group had *Microsporum* spp. infection. At week 24, 4 weeks of terbinafine (complete cure rate: 64%) was at least as effective as 8 weeks of griseofulvin (complete cure rate: 67%). However, the *Microsporum* spp. infections tended to do better with 8 weeks of griseofulvin than with 4 weeks of terbinafine. Another trial[27] compared 50 patients in each treatment group with infections caused by two main organisms (*T. tonsurans* and *T. violaceum*). In this trial, terbinafine for 2–3 weeks was compared with microsized griseofulvin 20 mg/kg for 6 weeks. The complete cure rate was 94% for the terbinafine group and 92% for the griseofulvin-treated group. Only one RCT[28] assessed medium-term to long-term treatment regimens comparing terbinafine with griseofulvin. In this study, 98.5% of the 165 children included were infected with *M. canis* and the remainder infected with *M. audouinii*. Patients were treated with terbinafine for 6, 8, 10, or 12 weeks, followed by placebo to complete a 12-week treatment phase in a double-blinded regimen, or griseofulvin for 12 weeks using an unblinded regimen. Medium-term treatment (6 or 8 weeks) resulted in a trend towards an increase in the complete cure rate in the griseofulvin group in comparison with the terbinafine group at 4 weeks after end treatment. However, long-term treatment (10 or 12 weeks) resulted in the complete cure rates being significantly higher in the griseofulvin group in comparison with the terbinafine group at 4 weeks after the end of treatment.

Versus itraconazole. One RCT[36] compared 2-week courses of terbinafine 62.5–250 mg and itraconazole 50–200 mg (both depending on weight). Twelve weeks after the start of treatment, 78% and 86% of the patients were completely cured in the terbinafine and itraconazole groups, respectively. *T. violaceum* was the major pathogen in both groups, and there were no *Microsporum* spp. infections. With regard to *Trichophyton* species, in another RCT[27] comparing itraconazole and terbinafine in a 2–3-week course of therapy, the complete cure rates at 12 weeks were 94% for the terbinafine group and 82% for the itraconazole group.

Versus fluconazole. The same RCT[27] analyzed the efficacy of fluconazole for 2–3 weeks in comparison with terbinafine, dosed according to weight for 2–3 weeks. The complete cure rates were 82% in the fluconazole arm and 94% in the terbinafine arm, similar to the results for griseofulvin.

Different terbinafine regimens compared. Four RCTs were found. One RCT[37] compared 1, 2, and 4 weeks of terbinafine therapy, 62.5–250 mg depending on weight. The cure rates

were 49% after 1 week of therapy, 61% after 2 weeks, and 67% after 4 weeks. However, this study did not include a griseofulvin control group; 71% of the patients had *T. violaceum* infections. A second RCT[38] compared 1, 2, and 4 weeks of terbinafine, 62.5–250 mg depending on weight, in 79 children and three adults with *T. tonsurans* and *M. ferrugineum* tinea capitis. At week 12, the complete cure rates were 44% in the 1-week therapy group, 57% in the 2-week therapy group, and 78% in the 4-week group. An RCT[39] published in two additional abstracts[40,41] compared 1 week and 2 weeks of terbinafine, 62.5–250 mg depending on weight. At week 12 of follow-up, in *Trichophyton* spp. infections the complete cure rate was 44.4% with 1 week of therapy and 64% with 2 weeks, but acceptable cure rates in *M. canis* infection were achieved only after an additional 4 weeks of treatment. An RCT[42] including 107 children with mainly *M. canis* tinea capitis compared 1, 2, and 4 weeks of terbinafine, 125–250 mg/day depending on weight. At week 12, the mycological cure rate was 46% with only 1 week of therapy, 53% with 2 weeks, and 69% with 4 weeks. In another RCT[43] that compared different regimens of terbinafine at dosages of 3–6 mg/kg/day for 1, 2, or 4 weeks, the complete cure rates were 38%, 46%, and 48% for the 1-week, 2-week, and 4-week arms, respectively. A recently performed study[44] assessed the efficacy of the standard dose of terbinafine in comparison with double doses of terbinafine, both given in a pulsed protocol (1 week on, 3 weeks off) in the treatment of *Microsporum* spp. tinea capitis. There were no statistical differences in the cure rates between standard and double-dose pulsed therapy at week 20; the standard-dose group achieved a complete cure rate of 60.8%, while the double-pulse group reached 68.4%.

Drawbacks
In the RCT comparing itraconazole with terbinafine,[36] fever, body aches, and vertigo occurred in one patient in the terbinafine group, but none of the patients showed any significant hematological or biochemical changes. In some RCTs, tolerability was reported as good, or with no or few adverse events of uncertain relationship or unrelated to the drug.[23,24,40] Cases of tonsillitis, cutaneous infestations, raised hepatic enzymes, raised triglycerides and eosinophilia,[23] and mild elevated triglycerides with an uncertain relationship with the drug[26] have been reported. Fifty-seven adverse events (pruritus, urticaria, skin scaling) were reported by 36 patients, and four patients were withdrawn from a study because of adverse events (vomiting, dizziness, urticaria, and weight loss).[25] The following adverse events were reported in an RCT comparing different regimens of terbinafine:[23] headache, raised hepatic enzymes, raised triglycerides, eosinophilia, and leukocytosis in the 1-week terbinafine group; raised hepatic enzymes and eosinophilia in the 2-week terbinafine group; and

raised hepatic enzymes, raised triglycerides, eosinophilia and leukocytosis in the 4-week terbinafine group. The following adverse events were reported in another RCT comparing different regimens of terbinafine:[42] mild pruritus and mild constipation in the 1-week terbinafine group; mild headache and nausea in the 2-week terbinafine group; mild urticaria, labial edema, mild constipation; and moderate loss of appetite, mild diarrhea, mild nausea, and moderate/partial loss of taste (recovered within 8 weeks) in the 4-week terbinafine group. Other RCTs comparing different regimens of terbinafine reported[39–41] abdominal pain (mild to moderate), epistaxis (mild to moderate), lack of appetite, headache and facial edema (severe), and coughing and fever (mild to moderate) in the 1-week terbinafine group; and abdominal pain, fatigue, nausea, dyspepsia, headache, and fever in the 2-week terbinafine group. One additional patient reported a lack of appetite and gastroenteritis only during the additional 4-week treatment period. A large RCT[28] reported mostly mild to moderate adverse effects, including somnolence, gastrointestinal symptoms, urticaria, and neutropenia.

Comments

A study that was still in progress was excluded.[32] Another[33] was excluded because it did not provide separate clinical and mycological data for each study group. This study was reported as an RCT of a group of New Zealand patients with mainly *M. canis* infections. The authors concluded that 4 weeks of terbinafine was as efficacious as 8 weeks of griseofulvin treatment, using topical econazole cream and ketoconazole shampoo as adjunct therapy. However, complete clinical and mycological data for the end of the study and follow-up time points were not provided. One RCT[34] was presented as a duplicate publication.[23] The manufacturer of terbinafine has been involved in most of the RCTs. Some uncontrolled studies have found oral terbinafine at higher doses or over 6–8 weeks to be effective in the treatment of *M. canis* tinea capitis, and well tolerated.[13] The definition of cure varies from study to study; some investigators follow microbiological findings, while others place greater emphasis on clinical response. High drop-out rates in some studies may artificially decrease the response rate, as those who are cured may be lost to follow-up.

Implications for practice

There is good evidence to support the use of terbinafine for treating *T. tonsurans* tinea capitis in children, and fair evidence to support its use in *M. canis* tinea capitis. Terbinafine has an advantage over griseofulvin in that it produces good results in a shorter time, making patient compliance less of a problem. An important disadvantage is that it is available only in tablet form—there is no suspension. It is also much more expensive in comparison with griseofulvin. According to the RCTs, the recommended regimen in children with tinea capitis is continuous therapy once daily for 4 weeks, with dosage according to body weight: 62.5 mg/day for children weighing 10–20 kg; 125 mg/day for those weighing 20–40 kg; 250 mg/day for those weighing over 40 kg. Analysis of the respective studies showed that a treatment duration of 4 weeks is clearly better than 1 week and 2 weeks. *M. canis* infections may require treatment for 6–8 weeks. Terbinafine is not licensed for this indication in children in some countries.

Itraconazole

Limited RCT evidence shows that oral itraconazole at dosages depending on the patient's weight (< 20 kg: 50 mg/day; > 20 kg: 100 mg/day) for 2–6 weeks is effective and safe for tinea capitis caused by *T. violaceum* (2 weeks of treatment) and *M. canis* (6 weeks of treatment). Only observational data suggest that itraconazole may be effective against *T. tonsurans* infections.

Efficacy

Two RCTs have compared itraconazole with other oral antifungals.

Versus griseofulvin. A double-blind RCT of 34 patients, mostly infected with *M. canis*, compared 6 weeks of itraconazole 100 mg/day with 6 weeks of griseofulvin 500 mg/day.[22] At the 14-week follow-up, the two groups had the same complete cure rate—88%.

Versus terbinafine. A double-blind RCT of 60 patients with predominantly *T. violaceum* tinea capitis compared 2 weeks' treatment with itraconazole with 2 weeks' treatment with terbinafine.[36] After 2 weeks, the complete cure rates in the two groups differed little: 86% in the itraconazole group versus 78% in the terbinafine group. With regard to *Trichophyton* species, in another RCT[27] comparing itraconazole and terbinafine in a 2–3-week course of therapy, the complete cure rates at 12 weeks were 94% in the terbinafine group and 82% in the itraconazole group.

Versus fluconazole. When fluconazole treatment was compared with itraconazole[27] in patients with *Trichophyton* infections, at a dosage of 5 mg/kg/day daily for 2–3 weeks, the complete cure rates were 82% in both groups.

Nine uncontrolled studies including more than 10 patients, using different therapeutic regimens of itraconazole, were identified.[45–54] Some studies used continuous treatment (50–100 mg/day or 5 mg/kg/day for 3–11 weeks) with capsules[46,48,52–54] or oral solution[47] and others used pulse therapy (3–5 mg/kg/day for 1 week per month, with a maximum of 3–5 pulses) with capsules[49,51] or oral solution.[50] Complete cure rates ranged from 81% to 100%; causative fungi were *T. tonsurans* and *M. canis*. One study[52] found a complete cure rate of only 40% in children infected with

T. tonsurans. An unrandomized trial[45] compared 15 children (nine with *M. canis* and six with *T. violaceum* infections) treated with 50 mg itraconazole versus 56 children (38 with *M. canis*, 18 with other *Trichophyton* and *Microsporum* spp. infections) treated with 100 mg itraconazole orally, as capsules, once daily for a minimum of 4 and a maximum of 8 weeks. Two months after the final dose, the mycological cure rates were 60% in the 50-mg group and 89% in the 100-mg group.

Drawbacks

Transient gastrointestinal side effects are the most frequently reported, and rarely a reversible increase in serum aminotransferase. In the RCT comparing itraconazole with griseofulvin,[22] two patients receiving griseofulvin stopped therapy prematurely because of nausea and intense stomach ache with severe vomiting that occurred in weeks 2 and 4 of treatment and subsided after the withdrawal of griseofulvin. In the RCT comparing itraconazole with terbinafine,[36] two patients in the itraconazole group reported urticaria. Other studies have noted a papular skin eruption not clearly related to treatment with itraconazole,[45] minor gastrointestinal disturbances,[46,50,52,53] headache,[52] epistaxis and seizure (not drug-related),[52] and "tired legs."[54]

Comments

The methods of randomization and blinding were not clearly described in either RCT.[22,32] No intention-to-treat analysis was done in these studies, but the drop-out rates were three of 35[22] and five of 60.[36] One of the RCTs[22] was funded by the manufacturer of itraconazole. In one uncontrolled study[52] that reported a complete cure rate of 40%, the high drop-out rate of 54% may have artificially decreased the response rate, as those who are cured may be less likely to return for follow-up. More but less reliable information is available from uncontrolled studies, but additional RCTs comparing itraconazole with other antifungals are clearly needed.

Implications for practice

There is fair evidence to support the use of itraconazole for the treatment of tinea capitis caused by *M. canis*, *T. violaceum* and *T. tonsurans* in children. On the basis of the available evidence, the recommended dosage for itraconazole for tinea capitis in children is 100 mg/day or dose adjusted to body weight, for 6 weeks in *M. canis* and for 2 weeks in *T. violaceum* infections. Uncontrolled studies suggest that shorter or pulse regimens may also be useful.

Fluconazole

Limited evidence suggests that fluconazole continuously at 6–8 mg/kg/day for 3 weeks or intermittently at 6–8 mg/kg/week for 4–8 weeks is effective and safe for treating *T. tonsurans* and *M. canis* tinea capitis in children.

Efficacy

Three RCTs compared fluconazole with other systemic antifungals for tinea capitis.

Versus griseofulvin. Three RCTs[27,30,31] compared fluconazole with griseofulvin. The first[27] assessed 100 children who were infected with *T. tonsurans* and/or *T. violaceum* (the exact percentages were not reported). The children were treated either with fluconazole 6 mg/kg/day for 2–3 weeks or with microsized griseofulvin 20 mg/kg/day for 6 weeks, and the complete cure rates were 82% and 92%, respectively. The second RCT[30] compared 40 children: 16 were infected with *T. violaceum*, 16 with *T. verrucosum*, and eight with *M. canis*. The children were treated with 5 mg/kg/day of fluconazole or 15 mg/kg/day griseofulvin for 4 and 6 weeks, respectively. Complete cure was reported for 79% of those in the fluconazole arm and 76% of those in the griseofulvin arm. The third was a three-arm RCT[31] including 880 patients, comparing fluconazole 6 mg/kg/day for 3 weeks followed by 3 weeks of placebo, fluconazole 6 mg/kg/day for 6 weeks and griseofulvin 11 mg/kg/day for 6 weeks. The complete cure rates were 44.5%, 49.6%, and 52.2%, respectively.

Versus terbinafine. The first RCT[27] analyzed the efficacy of fluconazole for 2–3 weeks in comparison with terbinafine, dosed according to weight for 2–3 weeks. The complete cure rates were 82% in the fluconazole arm and 94% in the terbinafine arm—similar to the results for griseofulvin.

Versus itraconazole. In the same RCT of patients with *Trichophyton* infections,[27] fluconazole treatment was compared with itraconazole at doses of 5 mg/kg/day daily for 2–3 weeks. The complete cure rates were 82% in both groups.

Different fluconazole regimens compared. A small RCT[55] comparing various doses of fluconazole (1.5, 3.0, and 6 mg/kg/day) for 20 days in the treatment of *T. tonsurans* tinea capitis showed a complete cure rate of 25% in the 1.5-mg group, 60% in the 3-mg group, and 89% in the 6-mg group. Three uncontrolled studies of fluconazole in at least 20 patients were identified;[56-58] *M. canis* and *T. tonsurans* were the main causative fungi. The mycological cure rates ranged from 88% to 100%. These studies used intermittent therapy: 6 mg/kg/day for 2 weeks followed after 4 weeks and if indicated by an extra week of treatment at the same dose;[56] 6–8 mg/kg/week for 4–8 weeks;[58] and 8 mg/kg/week for 8–12 weeks.[57]

Drawbacks

Only mild reversible gastrointestinal complaints and asymptomatic and reversible elevated liver function tests were noted.[57] No adverse effects were reported in these trials.[27,30]

Comments

Studies are needed in order to compare fluconazole with other antifungals and to determine the proper dosing and duration of therapy. Only one very small RCT was found.[55] Two studies were supported in part by the manufacturer.[56,57]

Implications for practice

There is some evidence to recommend a dosage regimen with fluconazole for tinea capitis in children. Observational studies suggest that continuous 6 mg/kg/day for 3 weeks or intermittent 6–8 mg/kg/week for 4–8 weeks may be effective. Fluconazole is not licensed for this indication in children in some countries.

What are the effects of topical treatment of tinea capitis in adults and children?

Adjunctive topical therapy has been used together with oral antifungal treatment to eradicate the fungi from the infected site, decrease spread to other people, and speed the cure. Various topical agents are available for adjunctive therapy.[59]

Shampoos

There is moderate RCT evidence that the addition of biweekly shampooing with selenium sulfide substantially reduces the period of active shedding. However, some evidence indicates that topical treatment is not useful for tinea capitis.

Efficacy

An RCT[60] reported that 75% of griseofulvin-treated patients with uncomplicated *T. tonsurans* tinea capitis had sterile hair sample cultures 4 weeks after initiation of griseofulvin. By contrast, 94% of patients who received griseofulvin together with biweekly selenium sulfide shampoos had sterile hair cultures at 4 weeks. Another RCT[61] of 54 patients receiving griseofulvin 15 mg/kg/day for *T. tonsurans* tinea capitis compared selenium sulfide 2.5% lotion or 1% shampoo with a bland, unmedicated shampoo. Patients were observed every 2 weeks until they were clinically and mycologically cured. The selenium sulfide products were statistically superior to the unmedicated shampoo with regard to the time required to eliminate shedding and viable fungi. However, no difference was noted between the two selenium products.

One RCT[62] was conducted in a region of Africa in which griseofulvin is not generally available. It compared 6 weeks of miconazole cream with 6 weeks of Whitfield's ointment (6% benzoic acid plus 3% salicylic acid) in *T. violaceum* and *M. audouinii* tinea capitis and found no significant cure rates. A small open study[63] of children with *T. tonsurans* tinea capitis treated solely with 2% ketoconazole shampoo

daily for 8 weeks reported a clinical cure in 93%, but at the 6-month follow-up only 33% showed a mycological cure and remained cured during the 1-year follow-up.

Drawbacks

No adverse events were reported.

Comments

RCTs of adjunctive therapy were described as randomized, but did not adequately describe the method and were not blinded.[60,61] One of the studies was supported by Janssen, the manufacturer of the ketoconazole shampoo.[63]

Implications for practice

There is some evidence to support the use of adjunctive topical therapy for tinea capitis with antifungal shampoos (for example, 1% selenium sulfide shampoo) to reduce the time of cure and to decrease the spread of infectious fungi to other persons. There is also some evidence not supporting the exclusive use of topical agents to treat tinea capitis.

In children with inflammatory tinea capitis (kerion), does an oral antifungal plus a corticosteroid lead to faster cure and complete hair regrowth than an oral antifungal alone?

Corticosteroids

Moderate RCT evidence indicates that the use of oral or intralesional corticosteroids as adjunctive therapy with griseofulvin for inflammatory tinea capitis (kerion) does not lead to additional or faster improvement.

Efficacy

Three RCTs showed no evidence that the use of oral[64,65] or intralesional[66] corticosteroids as adjunctive therapy with oral griseofulvin in inflammatory tinea capitis (kerion) results in additional or faster improvement of kerion. One RCT[66] of 30 children with *T. tonsurans* tinea capitis showed that intralesional injection of corticosteroid combined with oral griseofulvin is no better than griseofulvin alone for treatment of kerion, and found no significant differences in the time to negative culture, time of onset of new hair growth, complete regrowth of hair, or time to scalp clearing. In this study, all patients were instructed to shampoo their hair with 1% selenium sulfide twice weekly for 3 weeks. Two small RCTs[64,65] using oral corticosteroids showed no additional benefit in terms of improvement, reduction in the severity of clinical signs, or pathogen eradication.

Drawbacks

No adverse events were noted. In particular, none of the patients had post-therapy alopecia, permanent scarring, or biochemical evidence of hepatic dysfunction.[66]

Comments

One RCT[66] described the method of randomization using a table of random numbers, but was not blinded. Triamcinolone acetonide 2.5 mg was used in this study, but whether larger doses of steroid might be effective remains unknown. The other two RCTs[64,65] were described as randomized, but only one[65] was double-blind. In the latter RCT, scaling and pruritus were eliminated more quickly in the group that used erythromycin and prednisone in addition to griseofulvin, but the authors considered that this may have been due to the smaller volume of the kerions in this group rather than the effects of therapy, so that the patients became symptom-free sooner.

Implications for practice

The addition of corticosteroids to oral antifungals is unlikely to be useful. There is some limited evidence questioning the use of oral or intralesional corticosteroids as adjunctive therapy for inflammatory tinea capitis (kerion).

What strategies are best for reducing spread and reinfection in tinea capitis in adults and children?

Carrier state is found in individuals with no signs or symptoms of tinea capitis, but from whom positive cultures from the scalp can be isolated.[1] Strategies for management of the carrier state include: preventive treatments such as fungicidal shampoos, decontamination of objects that come into contact with the scalp, education programs for children to avoid sharing of objects that can spread tinea capitis to others (such as caps, combs, and toys), and shaving of hair.

There is no RCT evidence regarding the optimal management of symptom-free carriers.

Efficacy

No systematic reviews and no RCTs were found concerning the impact of strategies for management of the asymptomatic carrier state. An unrandomized study[67] compared different shampoos in carriers and found that povidone iodine shampoo produced a cure rate of 94%, in comparison with 47% with econazole shampoo, 50% with selenium sulfide 2.5% shampoo, and 50% with a control shampoo.

Drawbacks

None were reported.

Implications for practice

The effectiveness is unknown. Although it is agreed that decontamination of objects that come into contact with the scalp, education programs for children, and avoidance of sharing of objects can reduce the spread of fungal infections,[1] there is no good evidence to support such decontam-

ination procedures. Limited evidence supports the regular use of antifungal shampoos in controlling the carrier state of populations at risk. Povidone iodine shampoo may be the most suitable for prophylaxis.

Key points

Systemic antifungal therapy for tinea capitis in children
- RCT evidence suggests that griseofulvin for 6–8 weeks is effective and safe for tinea capitis.
- The best evidence available also suggests that terbinafine, itraconazole, and fluconazole can cure most patients with tinea capitis with a shorter course of therapy. All these drugs have good safety profiles in children.
- RCT evidence indicates that terbinafine for 4 weeks is effective and safe for treating *Trichophyton* spp. tinea capitis. Some evidence suggests that longer terbinafine therapeutic regimens of 6 weeks are necessary to treat *Microsporum* spp. infections. Terbinafine for 4 weeks and griseofulvin for 8 weeks showed similar efficacy in 3 studies of *Trichophyton* infections involving 382 participants. There was no significant difference in cure between terbinafine and griseofulvin in children with *Microsporum* infections in one small study of 29 children.
- Some RCT evidence suggests that oral itraconazole for 2–6 weeks is effective and safe for treating tinea capitis in children. In *Trichophyton* infections, cure rates following treatment with itraconazole and griseofulvin for 6 weeks were similar in 1 study of 35 children. Another study of 100 children did not show any significant difference in cure between itraconazole for 2 weeks compared with griseofulvin for 6 weeks. There was no difference between itraconazole and terbinafine for treatment periods lasting two to 3 weeks in two studies involving 160 children.
- Some RCT evidence suggests that fluconazole for 3–6 weeks is effective and safe for treating tinea capitis in children. In *Trichophyton* infections, three studies that included 1020 children found similar cure rates between 3–6 weeks of fluconazole and 6 weeks of griseofulvin.
- Regional as well as dermatophyte species variation may play an important role in the response rate, and may determine what dosage regimens are recommended. Resistance to antifungals could be a major concern in some areas.

Adjunctive therapy for tinea capitis in adults and children
- Some RCT evidence suggests that antifungal shampoos can reduce the period of active shedding in patients treated with oral antifungals.
- There is not enough evidence to say whether the addition of oral steroids to antifungal agents improves the resolution of inflammatory tinea capitis.

Strategies to reduce spreading and reinfection in tinea capitis
- No RCT evidence exists regarding the optimal management of symptom-free carriers.
- There is insufficient evidence suggesting that antiseptic shampoos can reduce spread from carriers.

References

1 Eleweski BE. Tinea capitis: a current perspective. *J Am Acad Dermatol* 2000;**42**:1–24.

2 Ceburkovas O, Schwartz RA, Janniger CK. Tinea capitis: current concepts. *J Dermatol* 2000;**27**:144–8.

3 Aly R. Ecology, epidemiology and diagnosis of tinea capitis. *Pediatr Infect Dis J* 1999;**18**:180–5.

4 Figueroa JI, Hay RJ. Skin infections, II: Fungi. In: Williams HC, Strachan DP, eds. *The Challenge of Dermato-epidemiology*. Boca Raton, FL: CRC Press, 1997: 257–9.

5 Al Sogair S. Fungal infections in children: tinea capitis. *Clin Dermatol* 2000;**18**:679–85.

6 Hay RJ, Moore M. Mycology. In: Champion RH, Burton JL, Burns DA, *et al.*, eds. *Textbook of Dermatology, 6th ed.* Oxford: Blackwell Science, 1998: 1303–6.

7 Friedlander SF, Pickering B, Cunningham B, *et al.* Use of the cotton swap method in diagnosing tinea capitis. *Am Acad Pediatrics* 199;**104**:276–9.

8 Hubbard TW, Triquet JM. Brush-culture method for diagnosing tinea capitis. *Pediatrics* 1992;**90**:416–8.

9 Drake LA, Dinehart CSM, Farmer ER, *et al.* Guidelines of care for superficial mycotic infections of the skin: tinea capitis and tinea barbae. *J Am Acad Dermatol* 1996;**34**:290–4.

10 Temple ME, Nahata MC, Koranyi KI. Pharmacotherapy of tinea capitis. *J Am Board Fam Pract* 1999;**12**:236–42.

11 Eleweski BE. Treatment of tinea capitis: beyond griseofulvin. *J Am Acad Dermatol* 1999;**40**:S27–30.

12 Higgins EM, Fuller LC, Smith CH. Guidelines for the management of tinea capitis. *Br J Dermatol* 2000;**143**:53–8.

13 Gupta AK, Hofstader SLR, Adam P, *et al.* Tinea capitis: an overview with emphasis on management. *Pediatr Dermatol* 1999;**16**:171–89.

14 McMichael AJ. Effective management of tinea capitis in the pediatric population. *Today Ther Trends* 2001; **19**:93–104.

15 Nesbitt LT Jr. Treatment of tinea capitis. *Int J Dermatol* 2000; **39**:261–2.

16 Blumer JL. Pharmacologic basis for the treatment of tinea capitis. *Pediatr Infect Dis J* 1999;**18**:191–9.

17 Friedlander SF. The evolving role of itraconazole, fluconazole and terbinafine in the treatment of tinea capitis. *Pediatr Infect Dis J* 1999;**18**:205–10.

18 Tanz RR, Hebert AA, Esterly BN. Treating tinea capitis: should ketoconazole replace griseofulvin? *J Pediatr* 1988;**112**:987–91.

19 Tanz RR, Stagl S, Esterly BN. Comparison of ketoconazole and griseofulvin for treatment of tinea capitis in childhood: a preliminary study. *Pediatr Emerg Care* 1985;**1**:16–8.

20 Martínez-Roig A, Torres-Rodriguez JM, Bartlett-Coma A. Double blind study of ketoconazole and griseofulvin in dermatophytoses. *Pediatr Infect Dis J* 1988;**7**:37–40.

21 Gan VN, Petruska M, Ginsburg CM. Epidemiology and treatment of tinea capitis: ketoconazole *v.* griseofulvin. *Pediatr Infect Dis J* 1987;**6**:46–9.

22 López-Gómez S, Del Palacio A, Cutsem JV, *et al.* Itraconazole versus griseofulvin in the treatment of tinea capitis: a double-blind randomized study in children. *Int J Dermatol* 1994,**33**:743–7.

23 Alvi KH, Iqbal N, Khan KA, *et al.* A randomized, double-blind trial of the efficacy and tolerability of terbinafine once daily compared to griseofulvin once daily in the treatment of tinea capitis.

In: Shuster S, Jafary MH, eds. *Terbinafine in the Treatment of Superficial Fungal Infections*. London: Royal Society of Medicine Services, 1993: 35–40 (Royal Society of Medicine Services International Congress and Symposium Series No. 205).

24 Cáceres-Rios H, Rueda M, Ballona R, *et al.* Comparison of terbinafine and griseofulvin in the treatment of tinea capitis. *J Am Acad Dermatol* 2000;**42**:80–4.

25 Fuller LC, Smith CH, Cerio R, *et al.* A randomized comparison of 4 weeks of terbinafine *v.* 8 weeks of griseofulvin for the treatment of tinea capitis. *Br J Dermatol* 2001;**144**:321–7.

26 Memisoglu HR, Erboz S, Akkaya S, *et al.* Comparative study of the efficacy and tolerability of 4 weeks of terbinafine therapy with 8 weeks of griseofulvin therapy in children with tinea capitis. *J Dermatol Treat* 1999;**10**:189–93.

27 Gupta KA, Adam P, Dlova N, *et al.* Therapeutic options for the treatment of tinea capitis caused by trichophyton species: griseofulvin versus the new oral antifungal agents, terbinafine, itraconazole, and fluconazole. *Pediatr Dermatol* 2001;**18**:433–8.

28 Lipozencic J, Skerlev M, Orofino-Costa R, *et al.* A randomized, double-blind, parallel-group, duration-finding study of oral terbinafine and open-label, high-dose griseofulvin in children with tinea capitis due to *Microsporum* species. *Br J Dermatol* 2002;**146**:816–23.

29 Fleece D, Guaghan JP, Stephen C, Aronoff C. Griseofulvin versus terbinafine in the treatment of tinea capitis: a meta-analysis of randomized, clinical trials. *Pediatrics* 2004;**114**:1312–5.

30 Dastghaib L, Azizzadeh M, Jafari P. Therapeutic options for the treatment of tinea capitis: griseofulvin versus fluconazole. *J Dermatol Treat* 2005;**16**:43–6.

31 Foster KW, Friedlander SF, Panzer H, Ghannoum MA, Elewski BE. A randomized controlled trial assessing the efficacy of fluconazole in the treatment of pediatric tinea capitis. *J Am Acad Dermatol* 2005;**53**:798–809.

32 Haroon TS, Hussain I, Aman S, *et al.* A randomized, double-blind, comparative study of terbinafine *v.* griseofulvin in tinea capitis. *J Dermatol Treat* 1992;**3**(Suppl 1):25–7.

33 Rademaker M, Havill S. Griseofulvin and terbinafine in the treatment of tinea capitis in children. *N Z Med J* 1998;**111**:55–7.

34 Haroon TS, Hussain I, Aman S, *et al.* A randomized double-blind comparative study of terbinafine and griseofulvin in tinea capitis. *J Dermatol Treat* 1995;**6**:167–9.

35 Cáceres H, Rueda M, Ballona R, *et al.* Comparison of terbinafine and griseofulvin in the treatment of tinea capitis. *Ann Dermatol Venereol* 1998;**125**(Suppl 1):1S21.

36 Jahangir M, Hussain M, Hassan M, *et al.* A double-blind, randomized, comparative trial of itraconazole versus terbinafine for 2 weeks in tinea capitis. *Br J Dermatol* 1998;**139**:672–4.

37 Haroon TS, Hussain I, Aman S, *et al.* A randomized double-blind comparative study of terbinafine for 1, 2 and 4 weeks in tinea capitis. *Br J Dermatol* 1996;**135**:86–8.

38 Kullavanijaya P, Reangchainam S, Ungpakorn R. Randomized single-blind study of efficacy and tolerability of terbinafine in the treatment of tinea capitis. *J Am Acad Dermatol* 1997;**37**:272–3.

39 Hamm H, Schwinn A, Bräutigam M, *et al.* Short duration treatment with terbinafine for tinea capitis caused by *Trichophyton* or *Microsporum* species. *Br J Dermatol* 1999;**140**:480–2.

40 Schwinn A, Hamm H, Bräutigam M, *et al.* What is the best approach to tinea capitis with terbinafine? [abstract P199]. *J Eur Acad Dermatol Venereol* 1998;**11**(Suppl 2):S232.

41 Schwinn A, Hamm H, Bräutigam M, *et al.* What is the best approach to tinea capitis with terbinafine? [abstract P147]. *Ann Dermatol Venereol* 1998;**125**(Suppl 1):1S133–4.

42 Talarico Filho S, Cucé LC, Foss NT, *et al.* Efficacy, safety and tolerability of terbinafine for tinea capitis in children: Brazilian multicentric study with daily oral tablets for 1, 2 and 4 weeks. *J Eur Acad Dermatol Venereol* 1998;**11**: 141–6.

43 Friedlander SF, Aly R, Krafchik B, *et al.* Terbinafine in the treatment of trichophyton tinea capitis: a randomized, double-blind, parallel-group, duration-finding study. *Pediatrics* 2002;**109**:602–7.

44 Ungpakorn R, Ayutyanont T, Reangchainam S, Supanya S. Treatment of *Microsporum* spp. tinea capitis with pulsed oral terbinafine. *Clin Exp Dermatol* 2004;**29**:300–3.

45 Degreef H. Itraconazole in the treatment of tinea capitis. *Cutis* 1996;**58**:90–3.

46 Greer DL. Treatment of tinea capitis with itraconazole. *J Am Acad Dermatol* 1996;**35**:637–8.

47 Ginter G. *Microsporum canis* infections in children: results of a new oral antifungal therapy. *Mycoses* 1996;**39**:265–9.

48 Elewski BE. Treatment of tinea capitis with itraconazole. *Int J Dermatol* 1997;**36**:539–41.

49 Gupta AK, Alexis ME, Raboobee N, *et al.* Itraconazole pulse therapy is effective in the treatment of tinea capitis in children: an open multicentre study. *Br J Dermatol* 1997;**137**:251–4.

50 Gupta AK, Solomon R, Adam P. Itraconazole oral solution for the treatment of tinea capitis. *Br J Dermatol* 1998;**139**:104–6.

51 Gupta AK, Hofstader SL, Summerbell RC, *et al.* Treatment of tinea capitis with itraconazole capsule pulse therapy. *J Am Acad Dermatol* 1998;**39**:216–9.

52 Abdel-Rahmen SM, Powell DA, Nahata MC. Efficacy of itraconazole with *Trichophyton tonsurans* tinea capitis. *J Am Acad Dermatol* 1998;**38**:443–6.

53 Möhrenschlager M, Schnopp C, Fesq H, *et al.* Optimizing the therapeutic approach in tinea capitis of childhood with itraconazole. *Br J Dermatol* 2000;**143**:1011–5.

54 Legendre R, Escola-Macre J. Itraconazole in the treatment of tinea capitis. *J Am Acad Dermatol* 1990;**23**:559–60.

55 Solomon BA, Collins R, Sharma R, *et al.* Fluconazole for the treatment of tinea capitis in children. *J Am Acad Dermatol* 1997;**37**:274–5.

56 Gupta AK, Adam P, Hofstader SLR, *et al.* Intermittent short duration therapy with fluconazole is effective for tinea capitis. *Br J Dermatol* 1999;**141**:304–6.

57 Gupta AK, Dlova N, Taborda P, *et al.* Once weekly fluconazole is effective in children in the treatment of tinea capitis: a prospective, multicentre study. *Br J Dermatol* 2000;**142**:965–8.

58 Montero-Gei F. Fluconazole in the treatment of tinea capitis. *Int J Dermatol* 1998;**37**:870–3.

59 Bettoli V, Tosti A. Antifungals. In: Katsambas AD, Lotti TM, eds. *European Handbook of Dermatological Treatments.* Heidelberg: Springer, 2000: 748–55.

60 Allen HB, Honig PJ, Leyden JJ, *et al.* Selenium sulfide: adjunctive therapy for tinea capitis. *Pediatrics* 1982;**69**:81–3.

61 Givens TG, Murray MM, Baker RC. Comparison of 1% and 2.5% selenium sulfide in the treatment of tinea capitis. *Arch Pediatr Adolesc Med* 1995;**149**:808–11.

62 Wright S, Robertson VJ. An institutional survey of tinea capitis in Harare, Zimbabwe and a trial of miconazole cream versus Whitfield's ointment in its treatment. *Clin Exp Dermatol* 1986; **11**:371–7.

63 Greer DL. Successful treatment of tinea capitis with 2% ketoconazole shampoo. *Int J Dermatol* 2000;**39**:302–4.

64 Hussain I, Muzaffar F, Rashid T, *et al.* A randomized, comparative trial of treatment of kerion celsi with griseofulvin plus oral prednisolone *v.* griseofulvin alone. *Med Mycol* 1999;**37**:97–9.

65 Honig PJ, Caputo GL, Leyden JJ, *et al.* Treatment of kerions. *Pediatr Dermatol* 1994;**11**:169–71.

66 Ginsburg CM, Gan VN, Petruska M. Randomized controlled trial of intralesional corticosteroid and griseofulvin *v.* griseofulvin alone for treatment of kerion. *Pediatr Infect Dis J* 1987;**6**:1084–7.

67 Neil G, Hanslo D. Control of the carrier state of scalp dermatophytes. *Pediatr Infect Dis J* 1990;**9**:57–8.

40 Deep fungal infections

Roderick J. Hay

Introduction

Deep fungal infections or mycoses comprise a group of diseases that spread within the subcutaneous tissues (subcutaneous mycoses) or predominantly involve deeper structures including blood and bone marrow, along with other organs such as the lung and the liver (systemic mycoses). They include a number of different diseases (Table 40.1).

Involvement of the skin in subcutaneous mycoses is usually secondary to direct spread from adjacent sites of infection—as in mycetoma, where sinuses from deep abscesses reach the skin surface. The skin is usually breached during the process of infection, and the organisms are often found in the environment with which the patient has contact.

In the case of the systemic mycoses, skin involvement is much less common, but may occur through bloodstream spread, in which the skin lesions are a consequence of dissemination and the formation of active infective foci in the dermis. The lung is usually the portal of entry in infections such as histoplasmosis, known as the endemic respiratory mycoses. Rarely, the skin is the portal of entry in systemic

Table 40.1 The deep mycoses

Disease	Pathogens
Subcutaneous mycoses	*Madurella mycetomatis, M. grisea* (fungi)
Mycetoma	*Nocardia* spp, *Streptomyces somaliensis* (actinomycetes) and others
Chromoblastomycosis (chromomycosis)	*Fonsecaea pedrosoi, Cladophialophora carrionii*, and others
Sporotrichosis	*Sporothrix schenckii*
Lobomycosis	*Lacazia loboi* (previously called *Loboa loboi*)
Subcutaneous zygomycosis	*Basidiobolus* or *Conidiobolus* spp.
Systemic mycoses	
Endemic respiratory infections	
Histoplasmosis	*Histoplasma capsulatum* var. *capsulatum*
African histoplasmosis	*H. capsulatum* var. *duboisii*
Blastomycosis	*Blastomyces dermatitidis*
Coccidioidomycosis	*Coccidioides immitis*
Paracoccidioidomycosis	*Paracoccidioides brasiliensis*
Infections due to Penicillium marneffei	*Penicillium marneffei*
Opportunistic infections	
Systemic candidosis	*Candida albicans, C. tropicalis, C. glabrata*
Aspergillosis	*Aspergillus fumigatus, A. flavus, A. niger*
Cryptococcosis	*Cryptococcus neoformans*
Mucormycosis (invasive zygomycosis)	Species of *Absidia, Rhizopus,* and *Rhizomucor*
Others	Infections due to *Fusarium, Trichosporon*

fungal infections, and the clinical course in such cases may be more benign, sometimes responding to minimal therapy. This pattern of infection, in which there is local inoculation followed by local lesions and regional lymphadenopathy, is referred to as the cutaneous chancriform syndrome. By contrast, fully developed and widely disseminated disease spreading via fungemia to affect the skin is often fatal. Infections with certain fungi such as *Penicillium marneffei* are more likely to result in skin lesions; in the latter infection, over 70% of cases associated with acquired immune deficiency syndrome (AIDS) present with skin lesions. An important subset of systemic mycoses is referred to as the opportunistic mycoses, because there is always an underlying abnormality such as neutropenia or AIDS. Systemic candidosis and aspergillosis belong to this group. Skin involvement is rare and is usually the result of bloodstream spread.

This section is largely concerned with the subcutaneous mycoses. The systemic mycoses are, by definition, severe internal infections, and a discussion of their management is beyond the scope of a dermatological work. In addition, there are no clinical studies directly relevant to the cutaneous manifestations of the systemic diseases, with the exception of a debate about the relevance of direct cutaneous invasion in their pathogenesis.

Subcutaneous infections are rare and are generally confined to developing countries. There are few well-organized clinical studies in these infections, and randomized double-blind controlled trials are exceedingly rare.

The evidence search for this chapter is based on the Cochrane Central Register of Controlled Trials (version 3, 2007) and my own collection of studies and personal contacts in the field. Most drugs used for these infections have been developed to treat other mycotic infections, and their application to deep mycoses is based on individual cases or case clusters. Each of the subcutaneous mycoses is dealt with separately.

Mycetoma

Definition

Mycetoma is a subcutaneous infection caused by either fungi (eumycetoma) or actinomycetes (actinomycetoma) (Figure 40.1). The focus of infection is the subcutaneous tissue, including subcutaneous fat. The hallmark of the infection is that the microorganisms involved form into clusters of filaments called grains, which are surrounded by a dense neutrophil response, forming an abscess. These abscesses subsequently discharge onto the skin surface via draining sinuses, but may affect underlying bone, resulting in osteomyelitis. Infective organisms are implanted into the skin, usually following a thorn injury.[1]

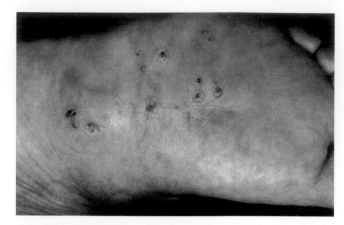

Figure 40.1 Lymphangitic sporotrichosis.

Incidence/prevalence

Mycetoma is an uncommon infection and there are no community-based data on its prevalence. Information on the worldwide incidence is based on an old study conducted by postal questionnaire in which interested departments (133) submitted data on numbers of cases occurring between 1940 and 1960. The results were published in 1963,[2] and indicate that certain countries such as Sudan and Mexico had the highest numbers of cases. However, some countries such as India, in which the disease is endemic, did not participate, so that the data are incomplete.

Etiology and risk factors

Infections follow traumatic implantation of contaminated material from the environment. Because there are no known animal models, the method of infection is unknown. There are also no known risk factors apart from rural occupation. One report suggested that there was a higher incidence of diabetes mellitus in those with the disease, but it did not include appropriate controls and the observation has not been substantiated elsewhere.[3]

Prognosis

There are no studies indicating the prognosis of this infection. Most patients have been found to have some morbidity, usually resulting from limb deformity, but death has been known to occur in cases in which the infection affects the scalp or chest wall.

Treatment aims

The primary aim in the treatment of mycetoma is to eradicate the infection and thereby halt the progression of deformity. This is possible in the case of actinomycetomas; however, there is insufficient evidence to support a particular regimen of treatment for eumycetomas, although individual responses have been recorded for ketoconazole, itraconazole and terbinafine, and amphotericin B.[4] Generally, the response rates amongst eumycetoma infections to chemotherapy are low and unpredictable. Therefore, in eumycetoma a secondary objective is to slow the course of the disease, thus delaying the time when amputation becomes necessary. Amputation provides a radical cure.

Outcomes

Outcomes range from recovery to slowing of the disease progress. Mycetoma is rarely fatal, and the main problems even in extensive disease are deformity and disability. In a few cases in which the disease affects areas close to vital structures, such as the chest wall or cranium, the outcome is fatal.

The main approaches to management are therefore chemotherapy, combined in some cases of eumycetoma with surgery. Surgery itself may cause problems, particularly if this involves removing tissue from weight-bearing areas in which the lack of support may result in pain and further disability.

Can mycetoma be treated successfully?

Efficacy

The usual treatments are chemotherapy for actinomycetomas and surgery and/or chemotherapy for eumycetomas. I have been unable to find any systematic reviews of treatment, and there are no controlled clinical trials. Good responses to drugs such as sulfonamides and sulfones, as well as co-trimoxazole, have been reported in the management of actinomycetomas,[5] and the addition of amikacin has been evaluated in an open study.[6] Treatment of eumycetoma with chemotherapy produces unpredictable results[4] and recovery is unusual. Radical surgery, including limb amputation, is curative in most cases.

Drawbacks

There are also no studies reporting side effects of therapy in the specific case of mycetoma. The adverse events related to azoles such as ketoconazole and itraconazole are symptomatic hepatitis (rare with itraconazole), urticaria, and drug interactions with some common medications such as terfenadine, astemizole, ciclosporin, tacrolimus, digoxin, and statins, interaction with the latter resulting in rhabdomyolysis.

Comments

Mycetoma is a rare disease caused by more than ten different microorganisms distributed throughout much of the developing world. A new generation of clinical trials to provide the foundation for an evidence-based review of treatment remains unlikely and could only be achieved with a coordinated multinational approach.

Implications for clinical practice

Treatment is likely to continue to be based on anecdotal evidence of the efficacy of different regimens.

Key points: mycetoma

- Treatment of actinomycetoma usually depends on two drugs, such as co-trimoxazole plus rifampicin. The latter is given for up to 6 months, while the other medication is continued until clinical recovery.
- Sulfonamides or sulfones can be used instead of co-trimoxazole, and streptomycin instead of rifampicin.[4,6]
- Another proposed two-step regimen based on a small case series involves an intensive phase of therapy with penicillin, gentamicin, and co-trimoxazole for 5–7 weeks, followed by maintenance therapy with amoxicillin and co-trimoxazole.[7]
- A successful outcome of treatment is less likely for eumycetomas. Therapy is therefore based on the premise of control of the infection by suppression of the disease, using fluconazole,[8] itraconazole[9,10] or terbinafine,[11] voriconazole[12] plus amphotericin B.[4] Patients are followed over years.
- Where necessary, surgery is used to supplement the medical approach for slowing eumycetomas. Indications for amputation are advancing disease threatening the whole limb (for example, involvement of the femur) and severe pain.
- Arterial perfusion with amphotericin B has also been tried for eumycetoma, with variable success rates.[13]

Sporotrichosis

Definition

Sporotrichosis (Figure 40.2) is a subcutaneous and systemic infection caused by a single fungus species, *Sporothrix*

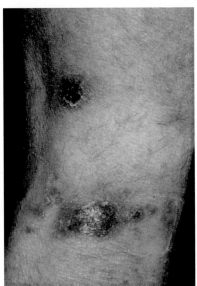

Figure 40.2 Chromoblastomycosis on the site of a traumatic injury.

schenckii, a dimorphic fungal pathogen found in leaf and plant debris. The subcutaneous variety described here presents with solitary or lymphangitic nodules or ulcers on exposed cutaneous sites.

Incidence and prevalence

This is an uncommon infection and there are few data on its prevalence. A problem in estimating the exposure is that the frequency of subclinical infection is unknown. Using the crude antigen sporotrichin, it appears that many of the local unaffected population in endemic areas have positive reactions to the skin test (for example 22%),[14] but it is not clear if this is the result of exposure to *S. schenckii* or to cross-reactive fungal species.

By plotting the spread of cases, it appears that sporotrichosis is mainly seen in the tropics and subtropics and in parts of the United States. Before the 1940s, it was regularly seen in Europe, where it is now uncommon.

It is clear that cutaneous sporotrichosis may occur in the form of isolated cases or in case clusters associated with exposure to a common source of infection, such as straw used in packing.[15] A major and continued outbreak was associated with contaminated pit props used in mines in South Africa. In addition, it appears that there are areas termed hyperendemic in parts of the world—for example, Guatemala, Mexico, and Peru. In the Peruvian focus, for instance, there has been an abnormally high frequency of cases in the vicinity of a single valley in the Andean foothills.[16] A key feature, however, is the absence of any obvious association between the infection and any local or geographical feature.

Etiology and risk factors

Infections follow traumatic implantation of infected material from the environment, although it is not clear whether this is always followed by clinical disease. Risk factors include occupation—for example, miners, flower workers, those using plant material for packing, and armadillo hunters have all been described as being at risk from exposure.

Prognosis

There are no studies to show whether there is spontaneous resolution, but this seems possible. There is clearly a wider spread of cutaneous lesions in patients with AIDS, and there is a risk of internal dissemination from skin lesions in such cases. Rare cases of systemic sporotrichosis usually appear to have arisen independently of skin injury and are thought to have followed inhalation and subsequent dissemination from the lung.

Treatment aims

The aim of treatment is cure of the disease. Generally, full recovery is achievable.

What is the best treatment for sporotrichosis?

Efficacy

The classic treatment of sporotrichosis is a saturated solution of potassium iodide. It is started at a dosage of 1 mL three times daily, and the dose is increased dropwise until 4–6 mL is being administered three times daily.[17,18] The solution is often associated with side effects such as nausea, vomiting, and swelling of the salivary glands. However, terbinafine, itraconazole, and fluconazole have recently been used with some success in this infection.[18,19–21]

Saturated potassium iodide is still widely used because it is cheap. One unblinded randomized comparative study of 57 people with culture-confirmed sporotrichosis showed that there was no advantage in splitting the dose of potassium iodide into three and that a single daily dose was as effective and no more toxic, with cure rates of around 89% in both groups after 45 days of follow up.[22] The alternative therapies are itraconazole 200–600 mg daily and terbinafine 250 mg daily. Itraconazole given for up to 36 months is recommended in a guideline for cutaneous sporotrichosis by the American Infectious Disease Society.[23] The efficacy of itraconazole is mainly supported by open studies[19,20] and there are fewer studies of terbinafine.[11] However, a recent trial comparing terbinafine in two dose forms, 1000 mg versus 500 mg daily, has demonstrated better results (87% vs. 52% clinical cure) and fewer relapses up to 24 weeks after the end of treatment.[24] One study of fluconazole 200–800 mg daily[21] produced a cure in 10 of 14 patients (71%) with lymphocutaneous sporotrichosis.

Other proposed methods of treatment include liquid nitrogen as cryotherapy.[25] I have been unable to find any systematic reviews of treatment, and there are no controlled clinical studies of oral antifungal agents.

Drawbacks

There are no studies reporting side effects of therapy specific for sporotrichosis, and readers are referred to references to itraconazole and terbinafine. Potassium iodide causes other specific side effects, such as sickness, vomiting, hypersalivation, and salivary gland swelling. These side effects are common (affecting around half of the trial participants in the one comparative study described above[22]) and usually mild.

Comments

There are opportunities for controlled studies of therapy in sporotrichosis, even though the disease is uncommon in many areas.

Implications for clinical practice

Given the absence of randomized studies that evaluate different treatment approaches for sporotrichosis, the current recommendations are based mainly on anecdotal experience. One study has suggested that there seems to be little advantage in terms of cure rates in giving potassium iodide three times as opposed to once daily.

Key points: sporotrichosis

- The main treatments in use are saturated potassium iodide solution and itraconazole.
- The disadvantage of potassium iodide is the high frequency of side effects, but the preparation is cheap.
- Fluconazole and terbinafine are alternatives, both of which show promise.
- Itraconazole appears to be effective, but is used for similar long treatment periods to those used with potassium iodide. Comparative studies with terbinafine and fluconazole are needed.

Chromoblastomycosis

Definition

Chromoblastomycosis (Figure 40.3) is a subcutaneous infection caused by a number of different fungi, such as *Clado-phialophora carrionii* and *Fonsecaea pedrosoi*; a less common cause is *Phialophora dermatitidis*. The infection starts in the subcutaneous tissue or dermis, and this is followed by progressive enlargement of cutaneous plaques, which are usually either verrucose or plaque-like, with central scarring. The organisms can be found in skin scrapings or biopsies as small pigmented cells, often divided by a cross-wall.

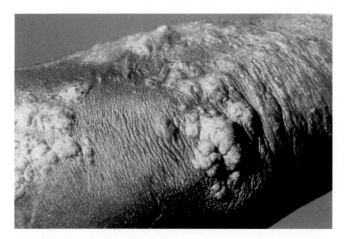

Figure 40.3 A eumycetoma infection.

Incidence and prevalence

This is an uncommon infection and there are no data on its prevalence. The disease is therefore known by clinical anecdote and reported cases. The endemic zone includes the tropics, particularly the humid zones; countries such as Costa Rica, Brazil, and Madagascar probably have the largest number of cases.[26]

Etiology and risk factors

Infection follows traumatic implantation of material from the environment. Fungi such as *Fonsecaea* species can be isolated from leaves and plant material. Although agricultural workers appear to be most at risk, there are no multicenter studies evaluating this issue.[26]

Prognosis

There are no studies indicating the prognosis of this infection. However, a small proportion of patients (5%) may progress to squamous carcinoma of the skin in the affected area.

Treatment aims

The primary aim of treatment is complete recovery.[26] This is not always achievable in advanced disease. A secondary aim is prevention of complications such as squamous cell carcinoma.

Outcomes

As stated above, full recovery is not always achievable, although in early cases full recovery can be expected.

What is the best treatment for chromoblastomycosis?

Efficacy

The treatment of chromoblastomycosis is complex. I have not found any controlled clinical studies of therapy. It is not clear, however, whether a single drug can cure extensive disease. Most of the treatment failures appear to occur when the infection covers a wide area.

The main treatments currently in use are itraconazole and terbinafine. Itraconazole has been used in doses of 100–200 mg daily with good results, particularly in early cases.[27] Terbinafine has been used in doses of 250 mg daily, also with good responses.[28,29] There is less experience with fluconazole, although it has been cited as an effective therapy.[30] There is no clear evidence that there are different responses to the two agents. In unresponsive cases, alternatives include combination therapy with amphotericin B and flucytosine,[31] or itraconazole and flucytosine.[32] Physical methods such as heat therapy and cryotherapy have also been used. Heat therapy involves application of heat-retaining materials to the lesions, repeated daily or less frequently over a number of weeks.[33] Prolonged treatment with repeated episodes of cryotherapy has been shown to lead to the resolution of lesions without relapse during a 3-year follow-up period in 41% of patients.[34] Itraconazole has also been used in a pulsed format[35] and in combination with other agents such as shaving, cryotherapy, and 5-flucytosine.[36] One comparative trial of 12 patients with histologically confirmed chromoblastomycosis evaluated the benefit of cryotherapy in addition to itraconazole.[37] The authors suggested that itraconazole can be used initially to reduce the size of lesions, with cryotherapy being given to the residual lesion. Topically applied ajoene under occlusion has been compared with topical fluorouracil (5-FU) in the management of chromoblastomycosis due to *C. carrionii*. Both were reported to be effective, with over 74% cure rates. There was a higher risk of post-treatment scarring in patients receiving the 5-FU.[38]

Drawbacks

The potential risks of treatment with terbinafine and itraconazole are discussed elsewhere in this volume. Flucytosine is an oral/intravenous drug. Potential side effects include nausea, diarrhea, and headache, and dose-dependent bone-marrow suppression. The latter occurs when plasma flucytosine levels exceed 100 mg/mL. The dose of flucytosine should be reduced in patients with renal impairment (there is a useful guide in the packet insert). Full blood and platelet counts should be followed during therapy; electrolyte and urea levels are also indicative of impending renal impairment. It is possible to monitor serum levels of flucytosine, reducing the dose if necessary. The optimum level is 40–60 mg/mL.

Comments and implications for clinical practice

The best approach to treatment in most cases is to give terbinafine or itraconazole. When the disease is extensive, combination therapy with flucytosine plus itraconazole is of potential use.

Other subcutaneous mycoses

The other subcutaneous mycoses are even rarer and occur in remote areas. It is not possible to provide an evidence base for their diagnosis and treatment. They include the subcutaneous zygomycete infections due to *Conidiobolus* and *Basidiobolus* species, which cause woody swellings infiltrated by the strap-like fungi that cause the infections, fibroblasts, and eosinophils.

Systemic mycoses

The systemic mycoses occasionally exhibit direct skin invasion following infiltration of organisms, or indirect skin manifestations such as erythema nodosum or multiforme, which are thought to develop following immune complex deposition. These are discussed briefly below.

Key points: chromoblastomycosis

- Chromoblastomycosis is caused by a number of different environmental fungi that are implanted through the skin.
- On the basis of several case series, most infections probably respond to terbinafine or itraconazole.
- Physical therapies such as cryotherapy and heat treatment have also been used and may confer additional benefit to drug therapy.
- Flucytosine plus itraconazole may be of value in people who have extensive disease.

The endemic mycoses

Skin involvement is seen as a consequence of one of three different mechanisms: direct penetration, bloodstream spread from a deep focus, and as an immunological reaction to primary, often respiratory, infection. In the latter instance, the skin lesions most commonly seen are erythema nodosum or multiforme.

In the endemic mycoses, the usual portal of entry is the lung. Direct entry via inoculation has been proposed in the case of some mycoses, such as paracoccidioidomycosis caused by *Paracoccidioides brasiliensis*, in which mucocutaneous lesions are common (for example, around the nose or mouth). The incidence of pulmonary disease in *P. brasiliensis* infection, even in the presence of skin lesions, is much higher in the endemic areas, suggesting that widespread subclinical exposure is most likely acquired through the airborne route. The demonstration of dissemination to mucocutaneous areas following fungemia in animal models and the existence of subclinical pulmonary forms of disease support the view that skin lesions of paracoccidioidomycosis result from dissemination to skin from the lung. This is likely to be true of most cases of systemic endemic mycosis.

Opportunistic mycoses

The opportunistic mycoses include infections due to *Candida*, *Aspergillus*, and zygomycete fungi of the genera *Rhizopus*, *Rhizomucor*, and *Absidia*, amongst others. Infection affecting the skin is uncommon, and these infections seldom present to a dermatologist; any skin involvement has to be set against the background of widespread and life-threatening disease. These infections often occur in patients with severe defects of either neutrophil numbers or function, such as recipients of stem cell transplants and cancer patients. *Candida* also affects seriously ill patients in intensive care or after abdominal surgery, neonates, and after prolonged intravenous feeding. Isolated cases of cutaneous aspergillosis and zygomycosis have been recognized following abrasion at a specific site. Disseminated candidosis rarely affects the skin either in neutropenic individuals or in intravenous drug abusers. Systemic *Cryptococcus* infection has been extensively evaluated in at least 16 randomized controlled trials in people with AIDS.

Patients with deep systemic mycoses rarely present directly to the dermatologist. However, there is an extensive literature on the treatment of disseminated fungal infection, and through the involvement of organizations such as the Mycosis Study Group (USA) and the European Organization for the Research and Treatment of Cancer (EORTC), a number of ground-breaking controlled clinical trials have been undertaken independently of, but with full cooperation from, the pharmaceutical industry. These have focused on various forms of treatment, from prevention to specific therapy or empirical therapy.

One form of systemic mycosis that a dermatologist may be called to see is primary cutaneous cryptococcosis. Proving the existence of genuine isolated cutaneous forms of disseminated fungal disease following local trauma and possible direct inoculation, in comparison with localized lesions following bloodstream spread, has been difficult, but the concept is important as it has implications for treatment (for example, the use of smaller doses that might be effective in localized forms of infection). The problem is well encapsulated by consideration of primary cutaneous cryptococcosis.

Cases of primary cutaneous cryptococcosis are rarely reported, and the evidence for direct entry through the skin is often poorly substantiated and generally anecdotal. There are no clinical signs that are likely to provide an accurate indicator that the infection has developed as a result of cutaneous inoculation.[39] The evidence for its occurrence therefore can be summarized as follows:

• The first sign of infection is the development of an isolated skin lesion.

• There are no other signs or symptoms of disease, apart from regional lymphadenopathy.

• There is no circulating cryptococcal antigen or antigen in the cerebrospinal fluid, measured by conventional tests such as the cryptococcal latex antigen test or enzyme-linked immunoabsorbent assay.

• Oral antifungal therapy with fluconazole or itraconazole is effective.

An alternative interpretation for the development of cryptococcal skin lesions was described some time ago by Noble and Fajardo[40] and was based on the subsequent iden-

tification of another focus of infection (for example, lung, prostate) and evidence of positive serology in blood or cerebrospinal fluid.[41,42] This suggests that many cases of cutaneous cryptococcosis are not primary skin lesions at all, but result from fungemia.[43,44] In some cases, this process produces only a single skin lesion.

Examination of the literature shows that there are some patients who meet the criteria for primary cutaneous cryptococcosis.[39] These are generally elderly individuals who do not have any underlying condition known to predispose to cryptococcosis (AIDS, sarcoidosis, T cell lymphoma, or chronic oral steroid therapy). Often, they give a history of local skin injury, sometimes even associated with a peck by a bird that might be carrying *Cryptococcus*. Often, strains isolated from such lesions belong to *C. neoformans* serotype D.[45] In AIDS patients, cutaneous cryptococcal infections may also be superimposed on some other process such as Kaposi's sarcoma[46] and are really part of a disseminated infection.

It is important to emphasize that these are observed criteria and have not, by virtue of the rarity of cutaneous cryptococcosis, been subjected to analysis of sufficient scientific rigor. However, the implications for therapy are sufficiently important that it is recommended that patients who meet the broad criteria for cutaneous cryptococcosis receive treatment with an oral azole antifungal agent, such as fluconazole (at least 200 mg daily) or itraconazole (at least 200 mg daily) until the lesions have resolved, treatment being extended for at least 1 month thereafter. Serology should be monitored again before the end of treatment and for 6 months after the end of treatment. This approach is provided as a guideline based on anecdotal experience and has not been the subject of a clinical trial.

Key points: systemic mycoses

• Systemic mycoses are not usually treated primarily by dermatologists.

• Most opportunistic mycoses are seen in immunocompromised patients.

• Skin lesions in most endemic mycoses, such as paracoccidioidomycosis, probably result from lung dissemination.

• They occasionally exhibit direct skin invasion following infiltration of organisms, or indirect skin manifestations such as erythema nodosum or multiforme, probably from immune complex deposition.

• Although many patients with cutaneous cryptococcal infection probably develop skin involvement as a result of internal spread, some cases of primary cutaneous cryptococcus do exist.

• Anecdotal evidence suggests that itraconazole or fluconazole might be effective in such cases.

• A number of controlled clinical trials on the treatment of systemic mycoses are currently being conducted by the U.S. Mycosis Study Group and the EORTC.

References

1 Mahgoub ES, Murray IG. *Mycetoma*. London: Heinemann, 1973.

2 Mariat F. Sur la distribution géographique et la répartition des agents des mycétomes. *Bull Soc Path Exot* 1963;**56**:35–45.

3 Hay RJ, Mackenzie DWR. Mycetoma (Madura foot) in the United Kingdom—a survey of 44 cases. *Clin Exp Dermatol* 1983;**8**:553–62.

4 Hay RJ, Mahgoub ES, Leon G, *et al.* Mycetoma. *J Med Vet Mycol* 1992;**30**(Suppl 1):41–9.

5 Boiron P, Locci R, Goodfellow M, *et al.* Nocardia, nocardiosis and mycetoma. *Med Mycol* 1998;**36**(Suppl 1):26–37.

6 Welsh O, Sauceda E, Gonzalez J, *et al.* Amikacin alone and in combination with trimethoprim-sulfamethoxazole in the treatment of actinomycotic mycetoma. *J Am Acad Dermatol* 1987;**17**:443–8.

7 Ramam M, Garg T, D'Souza P, *et al.* A two-step schedule for the treatment of actinomycotic mycetomas. *Acta Derm Venereol* 2000;**80**:378–80.

8 Gugnani HC, Ezeanolue BC, Khalil M, *et al.* Fluconazole in the therapy of tropical deep mycoses. *Mycoses* 1995;**38**:485–8.

9 Paugam A, Tourte-Schaefer C, Keita A, *et al.* Clinical cure of fungal Madura foot with oral itraconazole. *Cutis* 1997;**60**:191–3.

10 Lee MW, Kim JC, Choi JS, Kim KH, Greer DL. Mycetoma caused by *Acremonium falciforme*: successful treatment with itraconazole. *J Am Acad Dermatol* 1995;**32**:897–900.

11 Hay RJ. Therapeutic potential of terbinafine in subcutaneous and systemic mycoses. *Br J Dermatol* 1999;**141**(Suppl 56):36–40.

12 Lacroix C. de Kerviler E. Morel P, *et al. Madurella mycetomatis* mycetoma treated successfully with oral voriconazole. *Br J Dermatol* 2005;**152**:1067–8.

13 Subrahmanyam M. Intra-arterial chemotherapy for mycetoma of the foot. *Br J Surg* 1995;**82**:643.

14 Ghosh A, Chakrabarti A, Sharma VK, Singh K, Singh A. Sporotrichosis in Himachal Pradesh (north India). *Trans R Soc Trop Med Hyg* 1999;**93**:41–5.

15 Conias S, Wilson P. Epidemic cutaneous sporotrichosis: report of 16 cases in Queensland due to mouldy hay. *Aust J Dermatol* 1998;**39**:34–7.

16 Pappas PG, Tellez I, Deep AE, *et al.* Sporotrichosis in Peru: description of an area of hyperendemicity. *Clin Infect. Dis* 2000;**30**:65–70.

17 Tobin EH, Jih WW. Sporotrichoid lymphocutaneous infections: etiology, diagnosis and therapy. *Am Fam Phys* 2001;**63**:326–32.

18 Bustamante B, Campos PE. Sporotrichosis: a forgotten disease in the drug research agenda. *Exp Rev Antiinfect Ther* 2004;**2**:85–94.

19 Noguchi H, Hiruma M, Kawada A. Case report. Sporotrichosis successfully treated with itraconazole in Japan. *Mycoses* 1999;**42**:571–6.

20 Karakayali G, Lenk N, Alli N, Gungor E, Artuz F. Itraconazole therapy in lymphocutaneous sporotrichosis: a case report and review of the literature. *Cutis* 1998;**61**:106–7.

21 Kauffman CA, Pappas PG, McKinsey DS, *et al.* Treatment of lymphocutaneous and visceral sporotrichosis with fluconazole. *Clin Infect Dis* 1996;**22**:46–50.

22 Cabezas C, Bustamante B, Holgado W, Begue RE. Treatment of cutaneous sporotrichosis with one daily dose of potassium iodide. *Pediatr Infect Dis J* 1996;**15**:352–4.

23 Kauffman CA, Hajjeh R, Chapman SW. Practice guidelines for the management of patients with sporotrichosis. For the Mycoses Study Group. Infectious Diseases Society of America. *Clin Infect Dis* 2000;**30**:684–7.

24 Chapman SW, Pappas P, Kauffmann C, *et al.* Comparative evaluation of the efficacy and safety of two doses of terbinafine (500 and 1000 mg day^{-1}) in the treatment of cutaneous or lymphocutaneous sporotrichosis. *Mycoses* 2004;**47**:62–8.

25 Bargman H. Successful treatment of cutaneous sporotrichosis with liquid nitrogen: report of three cases. *Int J Dermatol* 1995;**38**:285–7.

26 Minotto R, Bernardi CD, Mallmann LF, *et al.* Chromoblastomycosis: a review of 100 cases in the state of Rio Grande do Sul, Brazil. *J Am Acad Dermatol* 2001;**44**:585–92.

27 Bonifaz A, Carrasco-Gerard E, Saul A. Chromoblastomycosis: clinical and mycologic experience of 51 cases. *Mycoses* 2001;**44**:1–7.

28 Esterre P, Inzan CK, Ramarcel ER, *et al.* Treatment of chromomycosis with terbinafine: preliminary results of an open pilot study. *Br J Dermatol* 1996;**134**(Suppl 46):33–6.

29 Bonifaz A, Saul A, Paredes-Solis V, *et al.* Treatment of chromoblastomycosis with terbinafine: experience with four cases. *J Dermatol Treat* 2005;**16**:47–51.

30 Guerriero C, De Simone C, Tulli A. A case of chromoblastomycosis due to *Phialophora verrucosa* responding to treatment with fluconazole. *Eur J Dermatol* 1998;**8**:167–8.

31 Kombila M, Gomez de Diaz M, Richard-Lenoble D, *et al.* Chromoblastomycosis in Gabon. Study of 64 cases. *Sante* 1995;**5**:235–44.

32 Kullavanijaya P, Rojanavanich V. Successful treatment of chromoblastomycosis due to *Fonsecaea pedrosoi* by the combination of itraconazole and cryotherapy. *Int J Dermatol* 1995;**34**:804–7.

33 Hiruma M, Kawada A, Yoshida M, Kouya M. Hyperthermic treatment of chromomycosis with disposable chemical pocket warmers. Report of a successfully treated case, with a review of the literature. *Mycopathologia* 1993;**122**:107–14.

34 Castro LG, Pimentel ER, Lacaz CS. Treatment of chromomycosis by cryosurgery with liquid nitrogen: 15 years' experience. *Int J Dermatol* 2003;**42**:408–12.

35 Kumarasinghe SP, Kumarasinghe MP. Itraconazole pulse therapy in chromoblastomycosis. *Eur J Dermatol* 2000;**10**:220–2.

36 Poirriez J, Breuillard F, François N, *et al.* A case of chromomycosis treated by a combination of cryotherapy, shaving, oral 5-fluorocytosine, and oral amphotericin B. *Am J Trop Med Hyg* 2000;**63**:61–3.

37 Bonifaz A, Martinez-Soto E, Carrasco-Gerrard E, Peniche J. Treatment of chromoblastomycosis with itraconazole, cryosurgery and a combination of both. *Int J Dermatol* 1997;**36**:542–7.

38 Perez-Blanco M, Valles RH, Zeppefeldt G, *et al.* Ajoene and 5-fluorouracil in the topical treatment of *Cladophialophora carrionii* chromoblastomycosis in humans: a comparative open study. *Med Mycol* 2003;**41**:517–20.

39 Patel P, Ramanathan J, Kayser M, Baran J Jr. Primary cutaneous cryptococcosis of the nose in an immunocompetent woman. *J Am Acad Dermatol* 2000;**43**:344–5.

40 Noble RC, Fajardo LF. Primary cutaneous cryptococcosis: review and morphologic study. *Am J Clin Pathol* 1972;**57**:13–22.

41 Antony SA, Antony SJ. Primary cutaneous cryptococcus in non-immunocompromised patients. *Cutis* 1995;**56**:96–8.

42 Hamann ID, Gillespie RJ, Ferguson JK. Primary cryptococcal cellulitis caused by *Cryptococcus neoformans* var. *gattii* in an immunocompetent host. *Aust J Dermatol* 1997;**38**:29–32.

43 Sanchez P, Bosch RJ, de Galvez MV, *et al.* Cutaneous cryptococcosis in two patients with acquired immune deficiency syndrome. *Int J STD AIDS* 2000;**11**:477–80.

44 Coker LR, Swain R, Morris R, McCall CO. Disseminated cryptococcosis presenting as pseudofolliculitis in an AIDS patient. *Cutis* 2000;**66**:207–10.

45 Naka W, Masuda M, Konohana A, *et al.* Primary cutaneous cryptococcosis and *Cryptococcus neoformans* serotype D. *Clin Exp Dermatol* 1995;**20**:221–5.

46 Glassman SJ, Hale MJ. Cutaneous cryptococcosis and Kaposi's sarcoma occurring in the same lesions in a patient with the acquired immunodeficiency syndrome. *Clin Exp Dermatol* 1995;**20**:480–6.

Streptococcal cellulitis/erysipelas of the lower leg

Neil H. Cox

Background

Definitions and etiology

Cellulitis is inflammation, usually due to infection, of deeper dermis and skin tissues, causing warmth, erythema, induration, and pain. Erysipelas is a spreading infection of the superficial dermis. In practice, these may coexist. Use of the term "erysipelas" to describe spreading mid-facial streptococcal infection is universal, but the same infection in the lower leg may be termed cellulitis (in the UK) or erysipelas (in Europe).

Cellulitis occurs in many situations and due to many organisms. In most studies from dermatology departments, the lower leg is the main site of involvement (75% to over 90%), and most cases are streptococcal. Even amongst unselected or emergency department patients, the lower leg usually accounts for about two-thirds of cases. Proving streptococcal etiology is difficult; staphylococcal infection is the most important differential diagnosis at this site. Several useful reviews discuss aspects of streptococcal infection, the wider spectrum of other sites and organisms involved in cellulitis, differential diagnosis and management.[1-9]

This chapter focuses on presumed streptococcal cellulitis of the lower leg (Figure 41.1), and on clinically important questions for which there is reasonable evidence. These and other issues are also the topic of several guidelines and systematic reviews, published or in progress[10-18] (it should be noted that one of these is aimed mainly at nurses[14]).

Clinical features

Typically, streptococcal cellulitis is initially manifest as swelling of the forefoot, accompanied or preceded by general malaise and/or fever. It progresses as proximally spreading, confluent, tender erythematosus swelling accompanied by malaise, fever, and often rigors. Swelling and pain may be

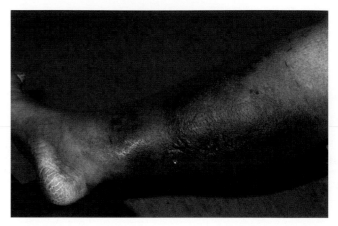

Figure 41.1 Streptococcal cellulitis of the leg: marked erythema, edema and early blistering.

severe; blistering, lymphangitis, and/or lymphadenopathy may occur. Although it is often used as a diagnostic criterion, significant pyrexia may be absent in more than half of patients admitted to hospital;[19,20] this may reflect initial treatment in primary care, or inclusion of milder or localized cellulitis.

Incidence/prevalence

No accurate data are available. The incidence is overestimated if other infections are classified as cellulitis, or underestimated if cellulitis treated in the community is not included. Abscesses or localized wound infections, and/or cellulitis at other body sites, are often included in incidence/prevalence data.

Cellulitis and abscesses accounted for 158 consultations per 100 000 person-years at risk in the UK in 1991, and skin and subcutaneous infections resulted in 29 820 hospital admissions,[21] but these data are not specific to cellulitis of a pattern relevant to this chapter. In a UK district general hospital, about 3% of admissions were for cellulitis.[11]

Importance and prognosis

In those with severe symptoms, or in whom systemic features resolve with antibiotics but redness and swelling persist, hospital admission is usually recommended. In those who do require admission, numerous studies or reviews,[5,20,22] as well as UK National Health Service data (cited in Pearse et al.[21]) document a mean duration of stay of 9–10 days, representing significant health-care costs. Uncommonly, cellulitis may progress to necrotizing fasciitis or streptococcal toxic shock syndrome, each of which has significant mortality.

In addition, long-term sequelae such as persistent edema, leg ulceration, or further episodes are all common (see the section on long-term complications below). Morbidity is therefore significant.

Diagnostic tests

Diagnosis is largely clinical. Streptococci may be identifiable by culture of swabs from macerated toe webs, blister fluid, or ulceration (but leg ulcers, if preceding cellulitis, may be colonized with numerous bacterial species). Aspiration or skin biopsy may yield positive cultures; streptococcal antigen identification by direct immunofluorescence of skin biopsies or using latex agglutination increase the diagnostic rate, but are not routine.

Analysis of the results of cultures in six studies (including 284 patients) documented a causative organism in 29% of cases.[3] One study (229 patients, 79% with leg cellulitis) using cultures and antistreptolysin-O titers (ASOT), isolated group A streptococci from a relevant skin site in 19%; ASOT was elevated acutely in 30%, but more commonly (61%) in convalescent sera.[23] Combining diagnostic methods allows a microbiological/serological diagnosis in 25–95%; a review suggested that even with two diagnostic methods, the etiology remained unknown in 20% of cases.[24] If a relevant organism is identified in the ascending lower leg pattern of cellulitis, streptococci of group A (less frequently group G) account for about 80% of isolates.

Aims of treatment

- To resolve symptoms, reduce the duration of hospital admission, and avoid or reduce sequelae such as edema.
- To prevent subsequent episodes.

Outcome measures

- Resolution of fever/malaise, erythema, edema (or halting progression of erythema; see the discussion below). The "Prodigy" guidelines[13] cite cure at 14 days as a suitable outcome measure.

- Elimination of risk factors, especially tinea pedis if relevant as a portal of entry.

Methods of search

A search was carried out using "cellulitis" or "erysipelas" in the Cochrane Database of Systematic Reviews, Medline, and Embase databases up to May 2007.

Key case series and interventional studies were identified from references obtained and from the author's files. No completed systematic reviews or meta-analyses were identified, apart from one systematic review on the use of blood cultures. A Cochrane review on this subject is in progress at the time of writing.

Questions

The following are currently pertinent questions. Space does not permit discussion of the uncertainty regarding the use of corticosteroids or nonsteroidal anti-inflammatory drugs in cellulitis, suggested on the basis that inflammation appears to persist well beyond presumed microbiological killing; these issues are discussed in several papers.[1,4,25] Similarly, physical therapies to reduce short-term or chronic edema (such as leg elevation, bandaging, compression devices, cycloidal vibration, compression hosiery, etc.) cannot be discussed in detail here, but are discussed elsewhere.[3,13,26]

What are the factors that predispose to lower leg cellulitis?

Evidence summary
Prospective studies
Patients with lower leg cellulitis (n = 167) were compared with controls (n = 294; matched for age, sex and hospital). Risk factors were lymphedema, the strongest risk factor, with an odds ratio (OR) of 71.2 (95% CI, 5.6 to 908), portal of entry (toe web intertrigo, ulcer, wound, dermatosis) (OR 23.8; 95% CI, 10.7 to 52.5), venous insufficiency (OR 2.9; 95% CI, 1.0 to 8.7), leg edema (OR 2.5; 95% CI, 1.2 to 5.1), and being overweight (OR 2.0; 95% CI, 11 to 3.7).[27] Diabetes (identified as a risk factor in some smaller studies) showed no association with the occurrence of cellulitis. Toe web disease was present in 66%, leg edema in 38%, and lymphedema in 18%.

A total of 100 patients were compared with 200 age-matched and sex-matched control individuals, with an emphasis on toe web disease, and using both questionnaires and clinical examinations. Risk factors for cellulitis were previous cellulitis (OR 31.04; 95% CI, 4.15 to 232.2), staphylococci or streptococci in the toe webs (OR 28.97; 95% CI, 5.47 to 153.48), leg erosions or ulceration (OR 11.80; 95%

CI, 2.47 to 56.33), and prior saphenectomy (OR 8.49; 95% CI, 1.62 to 44.52). Toe web tinea infection was only associated when toe web bacterial infection was excluded from analysis (OR 3.86; 95% CI, 1.32 to 11.27).[28]

Retrospective studies

Patients with recurrent cellulitis were compared with a group with single episodes (total n = 574, 81% of which involved the leg, with a retrospective single-institution analysis). Risk factors for recurrence (all statistically significant) were being overweight, venous insufficiency, lymphedema, tinea pedis, and previous regional surgery or trauma.[29]

In a case-note review with questionnaire follow-up at up to 3 years after admission, it was found that of 171 patients, 47% had a history of recurrent episodes and 46% had chronic edema. These two sequelae were strongly associated ($P = 0.0002$).[30] Chronic edema specific to, or greater in, the post-cellulitis lower leg was identified by 37%. Thirteen percent of the patients had leg ulceration attributed to cellulitis.

In a study of 243 patients and 467 control individuals (matched for age ± 5 y, sex, hospital, and timing of admission), mycologically proven foot dermatomycoses of various types were found to be the major risk factor for bacterial cellulitis (overall OR 2.4; interdigital tinea OR 3.2). Other associations with cellulitis were other portals of entry, a history of previous cellulitis, chronic venous insufficiency, and leg edema.[31]

In 647 patients with cellulitis/erysipelas (91.2% in the leg), general or local risk factors were found in 26% (interestingly, only 3.3% had leg edema). Seventy-seven percent of the patients had portals of entry, 50% of which were (predominantly toe web) fungal infections.[11]

In 365 patients with cellulitis (76% in the leg), 24% had fungal infections, described as "mostly tinea pedis." Accurate figures cannot be extracted from the data, but this represents approximately one-third of those with leg cellulitis having tinea pedis.[32]

About a quarter of patients with lymphedema will have at least one episode of cellulitis or related skin infection in the affected limb(s), potentially with recurrences every few weeks, and probably with a higher frequency in those in whom the cause is not related to cancer treatment; although cited in a Cochrane review, this is based on unpublished original data. It is not clear that all such inflammatory episodes are truly infective.[33]

Comments

The publications documenting risk factors for lower leg cellulitis probably represent the strongest evidence in this chapter, with consistent results implicating chronic edema (venous or lymphedema), toe web bacterial and/or fungal infection, and obesity as major risk factors. The importance of distinguishing lymphatic from venous edema may be artificial; the two are typically combined once chronic,[34]

leading to the use of the term "lymphovenous edema." As a risk factor for cellulitis, it is not clear whether it is the chronicity or severity of edema, or both, that is important. It is important to be aware that cellulitis is not only a consequence of edema, but that it also causes chronic edema, so that there is a vicious cycle leading to further episodes.[30,35] The effect of therapy to address these risk factors needs to be assessed.

Other predisposing factors for cellulitis include intravenous drug abuse and conditions in which blood vascular anomalies are associated with lymphatic abnormality (e.g., Klippel–Trénaunay syndrome).

What is the best antibiotic treatment regimen?

Evidence summary

Previous and recent evidence-based reviews have found no satisfactory randomized studies of antibiotics versus placebo or of intravenous antibiotics versus the same agent given by other routes,[4,11] although one such study exists for pediatric orbital cellulitis. There are some published summaries of head-to-head comparisons; most show no difference between the active agents compared.[5,36] The following studies have been chosen as they address specific pertinent issues. Antibiotics used in home treatment programs are discussed later.

Prospective studies

One randomized controlled trial (RCT) of 81 patients with lower leg cellulitis compared flucloxacillin alone versus flucloxacillin and benzylpenicillin. This showed no difference between the two regimens with regard to the number of doses required (mean number of doses 8.71 for flucloxacillin alone and 8.47 for the dual regimen; mean difference −0.24 doses, 95% CI for the difference, −2.38 to −2.01; $P = 0.83$), next-day temperature (mean difference −0.07 °C; 95% CI, −0.76 to −0.62; $P = 0.84$) or area of erythema decrease (mean difference −34 mm; 95% CI, −99 to −31; $P = 0.30$). Pain scores and patients' subjective improvement scores were also similar in the two groups. In conclusion, this study does not support the addition of benzylpenicillin to flucloxacillin.[37]

Another RCT investigating intravenous (IV) benzylpenicillin 4 MU six times daily (n = 55) in comparison with intramuscular (IM) penicillins (a mixture of benzyl penicillin and procaine penicillin) 2 MU b.i.d. (n = 57) found no difference in the cure rate (failure rate 14% IM, 20% IV; $P = 0.40$) or local complications (9.1% IV, 7% IM; $P = 0.477$), but 26% had venous inflammation in the IV group;[38] the intravenous and intramuscular routes were thus equally effective, but there was less treatment-related morbidity with intramuscular penicillin.

A third RCT screened 169 patients, 48 of whom were excluded (neutropenia, abscess, deep infection, incorrect diagnosis, confined to area of a bite, diabetic foot infections, others). All 121 participants received 5 days of levofloxacin 500 mg/day and were then assessed; 87 were randomly assigned to either a further 5 days of treatment (n = 43) or 5 days of placebo (n = 44). Participants were excluded from day 5 randomization if they had worsening cellulitis, no improvement, positive blood culture, ulceration, an alternative diagnosis (e.g., bursitis), abscess, or another nidus of infection. Both groups achieved 98% success (clearance by 14 days, no relapse within 28 days).[39]

A parallel-group open trial of 289 patients with erysipelas (cellulitis) compared oral pristinamycin versus intravenous and then oral penicillin; 102 patients in each limb were able to be assessed for the primary end point (cure rate at 24–25 days). Exclusions were mainly for protocol violations (additional therapy, missed therapy, missing data). Both drugs have a high level of antistreptococcal activity. The cure rates (per protocol and intention to treat) were 81% and 65% for pristinamycin in comparison with 67% and 53% for penicillin, both statistically significant differences.[40] Adverse effects included a higher frequency of (usually nonlimiting) gastrointestinal symptoms with pristinamycin.

Retrospective studies

In 365 patients (76% lower leg site), penicillin alone was used in 45%. Other antibiotics were significantly more frequently used in those with predisposing conditions or in those who were hospitalized. (Patients with bullous cellulitis or with streptococcal toxic shock syndrome were excluded.) The authors documented a median hospital stay of 5 days in the "penicillin alone" and the "other antibiotics" groups, but a longer maximum stay in the "other antibiotic" group (28 vs. 20 days) and an overall statistically different mean duration of stay.[32] The "other antibiotic" group also had a higher rate of predisposing conditions. The authors concluded that there is no advantage with the use of antibiotics other than penicillin (see comments below).

Reviews and other antibiotic-related studies

It is not practical in this chapter to discuss all new antibiotics that may prove to be relevant for cellulitis. However, there are several guidelines, and specific studies of antibiotics for cellulitis, that may prove useful,[3,12,13,41–43] in addition to those discussed in more detail above. Recently suggested antibiotics include intravenous cefazolin twice daily[44–46] or once daily with probenecid,[46] intravenous ceftriaxone once daily,[47] and linezolid.[41,48] Drugs such as cefdinir, linezolid, daptomycin and pristinamycin derivatives are discussed in more general reviews of skin and soft-tissue infections.[41,42,49]

Comments

Benzylpenicillin or phenoxymethylpenicillin have a very low minimal inhibitory concentration (MIC) against strep-

tococci, excellent response rates in most streptococcal disease, and a very low and unchanging (over many decades) risk of streptococcal resistance.[50–52] The main reservations about the use of penicillin alone are nonstreptococcal infections, a large focus of streptococcal infection (in which event clindamycin has benefits[1]), allergy, inconvenience, and uncertainty about the contributory roles of infection and immune-mediated inflammation in ongoing cellulitis symptoms.

Dermatologists usually (in about 80% of cases) use intravenous benzylpenicillin, aminopenicillins, antistaphylococcal penicillins, or cephalosporins as first-line therapy. Intravenous penicillin G is effective in over 80% of cases and is comparable in success rates to second-generation or third-generation cephalosporins or to quinolones.[27]

The argument against using benzylpenicillin or phenoxymethylpenicillin in initial treatment is that flucloxacillin also has perfectly satisfactory antistreptococcal activity with low MICs, and thus that the use of penicillin is unnecessary if flucloxacillin is used and that it does not improve the clinical response.[37] Consequently, unless there are contraindications, flucloxacillin alone has been recommended as first-line therapy for cellulitis by guidelines such as those of the Clinical Resource Efficiency Support Team (CREST),[10] the *British Medical Journal*[11] and Prodigy.[13] The Infectious Diseases Society of America recommends penicillin for erysipelas (well-demarcated tender plaque) and a penicillinase-resistant penicillin or first-generation cephalosporin for cellulitis, although they also state that most cellulitis is streptococcal (staphylococcal infection being rare unless associated with an underlying abscess or penetrating trauma).[12] In France, benzylpenicillin is the gold standard.[16] By contrast, the British Lymphology Society recommend amoxicillin as first-line therapy, on the basis that cellulitis (as opposed to folliculitis or crusted dermatitis) in patients with lymphedema will be due to streptococcal infection.[15]

However, there are some arguments that would still favor the use of penicillin in initial therapy. The study documenting that it does not improve the response obtained with flucloxacillin was not a comparison of the two drugs in isolation (i.e., neither was proven to be superior). In addition, if a longer duration of oral treatment is required for prophylaxis and if streptococcal infection is proven directly or by ASOT, then there is no rationale for using flucloxacillin rather than phenoxymethylpenicillin. Although there is a lack of strong evidence for prophylaxis (see below), when this is required for streptococcal cellulitis, with or without lymphedema, phenoxymethylpenicillin or depot penicillins are viewed as the antibiotic of choice.[10,15,16]

In practice, especially in early streptococcal cellulitis, it may be difficult to distinguish staphylococcal infection—in which case methicillin-resistant *Staphylococcus aureus* (MRSA) should also be considered—or other infections in some cases (especially when there has been overt trauma, human or other bites, or a possibility of waterborne infections). Indeed, the increasing frequency of MRSA, especially as a cause of abscesses, has led to the statement that the evidence used in creating current guidelines for the treatment of skin and skin structure infections has significant limitations, especially as many studies have used comparative noninferiority protocols.[43] There are arguments for wider use of cephalosporins, or empirical use of ciprofloxacin or even linezolid, amongst others.[1,3,41–49] Thus, the study concluding that there is no advantage in the use of antibiotics other than penicillin[32] cannot be supported. Not only were staphylococci and other organisms not sensitive to penicillin identified in some cases (clearly indicating a need for other antibiotics), but the antibiotic choice was clearly biased by the perceived severity, and the analysis was univariate. Equally, the study suggesting that 5 days' therapy is adequate[39] was not strongly supported by the data presented, as there were many exclusion criteria and also numerous patient withdrawals at the 5-day assessment (nearly half of all screened patients were eventually excluded). The 28-day follow-up period in this study was too short for recurrent episodes to be evaluated. In practice, numerous other agents are used in patients perceived as having severe cases or as having cases that are slow to respond, or in patients with penicillin or other relevant drug allergies.

Where should patients be treated?

Most studies of cellulitis have been conducted in secondary care. The number of patients previously treated in primary care is unclear, but the possibility of making a definitive choice for treatment at home has been assessed recently.

Evidence summary
Prospective studies
One RCT was undertaken in patients perceived to have cellulitis requiring intravenous antibiotics and with no contraindication to home therapy (home, n = 98; hospital, n = 96).[45] There were no significant differences in the time to the primary end point, which was cessation of advancement of erythema (mean 1.50 days with home treatment and 1.49 days in the hospital group; mean difference −0.01 days; 95% CI for the difference, −0.3 to −0.28), or in the days on intravenous antibiotics (cephazolin at home; various others also used in hospital), days on oral antibiotics, overall days of treatment, complications, pain, or function; home treatment was preferred. However, there were several exclusion criteria, including previous cellulitis at the same site within 1 month, neutropenia or neutrophilia, signs of sepsis, comorbidities ("severe" diabetes, obesity, peripheral vascular disease, alcoholism, immunosuppression),

directly cellulitis-associated factors (such as blistering, tissue necrosis, severe lymphangitis, or a large area of cellulitis), or refusal to enter the trial. In order to randomly assign 200 patients (into groups of 101 and 99, with 10 rediagnosed after randomization), 658 patients fulfilling the entry criteria had to be screened (thus, only 30% of the potential patients actually entered the trial).

Retrospective studies
A total of 266 episodes of cellulitis treated in a hospital-initiated "hospital-in-the-home" program were reviewed. After accounting for some miscoding (six episodes of ongoing cellulitis, 18 cases of pilonidal sinus), the length of stay was similar in the home and hospital groups (mean 7.3 days at home, 7.1 in hospital).[53]

In a review of 124 patients with cellulitis who were considered suitable for home intravenous therapy in accordance with local "hospital-in-the-home" guidelines,[46] the exclusion criteria included children, bites, deep involvement or surgical review necessary, signs of severe systemic illness, leukopenia, or white cell count $> 20 \times 10^9$/L. Two-thirds of the patients had cellulitis of the leg; over 99% were treated with cephazolin 2 g b.i.d. Eighty-five percent were treated successfully with a mean intravenous antibiotic duration of 6.24 days. The published details are insufficient for separate analysis of the lower-leg subset.

A study compared 112 patients with "uncomplicated cellulitis" and 230 retrospective control individuals to determine the benefits of a protocol for baseline suitability for treatment at home, with recording of symptoms and signs by nurses and criteria for medical review.[54] Most home treatment was initially once-daily intravenous ceftriaxone, then 7 days of oral clindamycin or flucloxacillin. Using a protocol led to a reduction in the median duration of intravenous antibiotic therapy (3 days, versus 4 days in the pre-protocol controls), and reduced physician review (19% versus 100%), but the outcomes, complications, and readmissions were similar. Exclusions, which were also applied to the control group by examination of case records, included severe localized pain, rapid evolution, blistering, hypotension or other features of sepsis, drug or alcohol misuse, some patients with wounds or trauma, and social factors that would make home treatment difficult. The number of exclusions was not stated, but of those entering the home treatment program, 36% had had an immediately preceding hospital admission for their cellulitis (45% in the retrospective controls).

An alternative to home intravenous antibiotic treatment is early discharge once intravenous therapy is no longer considered necessary. In a retrospective study, 17% of 374 patients were discharged on the same day as intravenous antibiotics were stopped, rather than having a further in-patient night for observation.[55] Although only 40 (15%) in this series had cellulitis, none of these had significant pyrexia or local symptom recurrence on the final "observed" or "unobserved" day and none required readmission within 14 days.

Comments

All of these studies suggest that treatment at home is safe and effective, especially if supported by a carefully prepared protocol. However, all need to be interpreted with caution; all of the studies involved decisions about patients' suitability for home treatment and excluded patients with more severe disease or with factors precluding home therapy. None therefore represents an RCT of unselected subjects. In one large retrospective review of 647 patients (91% leg), only 27% were felt to require hospitalization, with a mean duration of stay of 9 days.[22] However, the one prospective study[45] was only able to recruit 30% who fulfilled the criteria for needing intravenous therapy. The number of screened but excluded subjects is not apparent in all of the above studies, but the available data suggest that a minority of patients who would normally require admission can actually be treated at home.

In addition, some of the end points used have uncertain clinical relevance. "Cessation of advancement of erythema" is an end point that appears appropriate, but some hospital admissions are for patients in whom "erythema is not resolving." Indeed, this condition—sometimes (probably incorrectly) termed "chronic cellulitis"—is thought by many to represent an ongoing immunological response to infection,[39] although, particularly if bilateral, it may just represent background lymphedema. The important point is that it is not an end point that automatically excludes subsequent hospital admission.

Early discharge after intravenous antibiotics does not appear to be associated with a greater risk of adverse events,[55] but there was a bias in that patients who were discharged on the day on which intravenous antibiotics were stopped were younger and had less comorbidity.

What factors are associated with or predict short-term morbidity, severe disease, or mortality, and what tests should be done?

Background detail is required here to explain the features that constitute severity.

Short-term complications include severe edema, blistering, leg ulceration, abscess formation, unrecognized infection by rare organisms, necrotizing fasciitis, streptococcal toxic shock syndrome, and death. Severe complications are, however, rare. Clinical features that suggest necrotizing fasciitis are discussed elsewhere;[1,7,9,56] laboratory tests that may be useful in this diagnosis or that of streptococcal toxic shock syndrome (the two are commonly associated) are presented as they are pertinent to the question of "what tests should be done?"

Abbreviated criteria for streptococcal toxic shock syndrome (see Bisno and Stevens[1] for more detailed criteria and a definition of "definite" or "probable" case) include:

I Isolation of group A streptococci
II Signs of severity:
A Hypotension (systolic blood pressure < 90 mmHg)
B Two or more of:
• Renal impairment (creatinine > 177 µmol/L) or > 2 × upper limit of normal for age
• Coagulopathy (platelets < 100 × 10^9/L or evidence of disseminated intravascular coagulation
• Liver involvement—transaminases or bilirubin > 2 × upper limit of normal for age
• Adult respiratory distress syndrome/capillary leak syndrome
• Generalized macular rash
• Soft-tissue necrosis (includes necrotizing fasciitis, myonecrosis, gangrene)

A clinical suspicion of necrotizing fasciitis (especially "crescendo" pain, tender induration, pallor, or cyanosis superimposed on erythema, crepitus, lack of lymphangitis, hypoesthesia, foul exudates, muscle pain or weakness, and increasing systemic disease—e.g., fever, confusion, hypotension) should prompt performance of the above tests. Bullae may occur in either "ordinary" cellulitis or in more severe infection; severe pain often precedes skin signs in necrotizing fasciitis,[56] and bullae, when they appear, are often on a background of vague dusky discoloration rather than of acute erythema.[7] The question regarding laboratory tests is the extent to which they should be routinely performed, or when they should be considered, in patients with cellulitis.

Evidence summary

Systematic review

On the basis of 17 retrospective studies or case series of nonfacial cellulitis,[57] this review showed that blood cultures were usually negative and, if positive, did not alter the empirical therapy already commenced. On the basis of the studies reviewed, the frequency of positive blood cultures in uncomplicated cellulitis is about 2–5%. However, this may increase in more severe infection (see below).

Prospective studies

Using 85 variables in 51 patients, factors associated with prolonged admission (significant on univariate analysis) included various cellulitis severity measures (acuteness of onset, extent of erythema, tachycardia, neutrophilia), factors suggesting edema, lymphedema, or venous disease (chronic edema, leg ulcer, use of diuretics), social issues (living alone, poor mobility) and other medical factors (anemia, raised creatinine). Chronic edema/diuretic use and neutrophilia were independently associated with duration of admission.[58]

Magnetic resonance imaging (MRI) was used in nine patients to assess differentiation between necrotizing and nonnecrotizing fascutis of the leg. All had fascial inflammation (low intensity on T1-weighted images and high intensity on T2-weighted images). An absence of gadolinium enhancement on T1-weighted images was reliable in detecting the presence of necrosis and extent of fasciitis, and was more accurate in detecting necrosis or pyomyositis than elevation of serum creatine kinase or lactate dehydrogenase.[59]

MRI in 69 patients with acute swelling of the limbs included 45 with skin and soft-tissue infections. MRI was sensitive in detecting subtle fascial and muscle signal changes, and was useful in determining the depth of soft-tissue changes, thereby aiding clinical management.[60]

A higher white blood cell count was documented in 18 confirmed cases of necrotizing fasciitis in comparison with 18 suspected cases in which the patients actually had cellulitis or an abscess.[61]

Retrospective studies

In one study,[32] there were no deaths amongst 365 patients, although those with bullous cellulitis were excluded, as were an unspecified number with streptococcal toxic shock syndrome (a condition with a mortality rate of 50%).

In a single-institution analysis of risk factors for poor outcome in 332 adults with cellulitis,[62] the body sites were not stated, but localized cellulitis of the orbit and infections related to surgical wounds, diabetic foot ulcers, or intravenous drug use were excluded. Death occurred in 16 (5%) within 1 month (including eight, 2%, within 72 hours), and was statistically associated with male sex, congestive cardiac failure, morbid obesity, any two comorbid conditions, shock, hypoalbuminemia, elevated creatinine (> 150 μmol/L), and *Pseudomonas* infection (which accounted for five of the 16 deaths).

In the same study,[62] complications in 103 patients (31%) included a need for surgical debridement or other surgery (29%), shock (4.5%), or other systemic complications (11.5%). Although not significantly associated with death, an absence of necrosis at presentation was significantly linked with early discharge without complications. (The C-reactive protein level and white cell count were not analyzed.)

In a review of 647 cases, 91% affecting the leg, only one patient developed necrotizing fasciitis (although only 176 of the patients in this series were felt to have sufficient severity of disease that admission was necessary).[22]

In a series of 229 patients (79% with a leg site), 14% had local skin necrosis or abscess, but none developed streptococcal toxic shock syndrome.[23]

In 200 patients with soft-tissue infection (66% affecting the leg), the mean C-reactive protein (CRP) and erythrocyte sedimentation rate (ESR) at admission were significantly higher in the group requiring more than 10 days' admission in comparison with those discharged earlier.[63]

In a retrospective study of 43 cases of necrotizing fasciitis,[64] streptococcal necrotizing fasciitis was more likely to affect previously healthy individuals, was only initially suspected in 12%, and had a higher mortality than non-streptococcal causes. Mean serum creatine phosphokinase (CPK) levels were much higher in patients with necrotizing fasciitis than in those with cellulitis, presumably reflecting the deeper involvement of musculature, and may be a useful clinical indicator of severity.

The details of 89 patients with necrotizing fasciitis and 225 control individuals (with severe cellulitis or abscess) were used to develop a laboratory risk indicator for necrotizing fasciitis (LRINEC) score, which was then validated on a cohort of 140 patients.[65] Predictive laboratory tests proved to be elevated C-reactive protein (> 150 mg/L), leukocytosis (especially > 25 × 10⁹/L), low hemoglobin (especially < 11 g/dL), hyponatremia < 135 mmol/L, creatinine > 141 μmol/L, and glucose > 10 mmol/L; a scoring system of 0–13 was derived, which has positive and negative predictive values of 92% and 96%, respectively, at a cut-off score of 6.

Comments

Deaths and severe complications are rare. Causes of death are mainly septic shock, multiorgan failure, or related to underlying disease.

There are several factors that contribute to the duration of admission, but this and the duration of antibiotic therapy are often used as end points of cellulitis treatment. They probably reflect costs, but are not necessarily an accurate surrogate for severity (social issues may contribute to prolonged admissions).

There is a case for reducing unnecessary tests. However, very few acutely admitted patients will fail to have a full blood count and basic electrolytes tested. Test results such as elevated creatine phosphokinase (CPK), rising creatinine, rising liver transaminases, or neutrophilia, may all be associated with severity or with development of streptococcal toxic shock syndrome and/or necrotizing fasciitis. Thus, if measurement of CPK or liver enzymes is not felt to be necessary at baseline, it is at least prudent to retain the sample for comparison in the event of clinical deterioration or development of increasing pain.

Bacteremia is uncommon in uncomplicated cellulitis, but occurs in about half of patients with necrotizing fasciitis. It appears reasonable to reserve this test for those with recognized local or systemic severity factors. If standard bacteriology cultures are negative, the streptococcal *speB* gene may be detectable in tissue samples using polymerase chain reaction techniques.

In severe cases, clindamycin has often been recommended as the treatment of choice. However, vancomycin, and more recently linezolid, may have superior effects.

MRI is the most accurate test for diagnosing fasciitis

(reviewed in more detail by Seal[7]). Irrespective of the utility of MRI, which may demonstrate fasciitis before skin changes develop, its sensitivity exceeds its specificity, and cellulitis cannot always be distinguished from fasciitis—thus, it is universally stated that surgical intervention should not be delayed in order to obtain such scans if there is reasonable suspicion of a deep necrotizing infection.

What are the long-term complications?

Evidence summary
Retrospective studies
Recurrent episodes were observed in 48 (21%) of 229 patients (79% of cases affected the leg);[23] 27 of the 229 (12%) had a history of one previous episode, 36 (16%) had had more than one previous episode, and half of those with subsequent episodes had more than one recurrence (most commonly, although not statistically significantly, in those with an underlying cause).

Recurrent episodes were observed in 29% of 143 patients;[66] 13% had two or more further episodes. Risk factors were documented in 26% of those with single episodes, in comparison with 76% of those with recurrent episodes, although only venous insufficiency was statistically significant.

In 70 patients (all with lower-leg sites), morbidity included persistent edema (9%), leg ulceration (3%), and previous or further episodes (28%).[20]

Of 167 admissions (all with lower-leg sites), 77% were for a first-ever episode and 23% for a recurrent episode.[27]

Among 459 patients with leg cellulitis (81% of a series of 574 patients), fewer than 30% were admitted due to a first episode of cellulitis; most (about 37% of leg cellulitis admissions during the study period) were for a second episode at the same site, and one-third were due to a recurrent episode at a different site (not stated, but probably the other leg, as the main risk factors in this study affected the legs).[29]

Among 171 patients (retrospective review with questionnaire follow-up at up to 3 years after admission), 47% had a history of recurrent episodes and 46% had chronic edema. There was a strong association between these two factors (*P* = 0.0002).[30] Chronic edema specific to, or greater in, the previously affected leg was identified by 37%, and 13% had leg ulceration attributed to cellulitis. Both of these complications were less frequent in patients treated with longer courses (> 28 days) of penicillin, the difference but did not reach statistical significance. Half of the recurrent episodes of cellulitis had not required hospital admission.

A UK Dermatology Clinical Trials Network (UKDCTN) pilot study to evaluate possible recruitment into trials of cellulitis showed a similar potential for underestimation of recurrent episodes—40% of patients with cellulitis described previous episodes (multiple in 54% of these), but only 55% had been admitted to hospital during their most recent previous episode.[67]

In 209 episodes of leg cellulitis, 35 patients (16.7%) had recurrences within 2 years;[68] possible predictive factors for recurrence were evaluated, and tibial area involvement, prior malignancy, and dermatitis of the ipsilateral limb were all independent risk factors for recurrence on multivariate analysis, with hazard ratios (HRs) of 5.02, 3.87, and 2.9, respectively. If all three were present, the estimated probability of recurrence was 92.8% (95% CI, 51.9% to 98.9%). Additional factors that had univariate significance included lower leg edema or venous insufficiency (HR 3.52 and 3.88, respectively). Interesting factors that did not have even univariate significance included tinea pedis (HR 1.31) and ipsilateral deep venous thrombosis (HR1.66).

A review of 237 patients with lymphedema and recurrent cellulitis demonstrated a direct correlation between the severity of lymphedema and the frequency of recurrence (only available as an abstract).[35]

In a review of 26 patients with lymphatic disorders, decreased lymphatic flow was found to be related to the time since a venous thrombosis, the occurrence and number of episodes of cellulitis/lymphangitis, and use of the saphenous vein for arterial surgery.[69]

Comments
The main long-term complications are persistent edema, a high risk of further episodes, and a less prominent increase in risk of leg ulceration. In addition, there appears to be a significant link between edema and recurrent cellulitis, which is not unreasonable, as edema is a well-documented risk factor. A vicious cycle of infection and lymphatic damage may thus be encountered.[28,30,69,70]

Thus, any cause of chronic edema, or ongoing portal of entry for streptococci, will predispose to recurrence. It is uncertain why previous malignancy should do so,[68] although this has been suggested previously in the context of lymphedema.[33] It is also uncertain why involvement of the tibial area is linked with a risk of recurrence,[68] although this may have been a surrogate for severity, as the reference comparator was involvement of the foot.

Does prophylaxis work, and in which patients?

Antibiotics
Prospective studies
An RCT of patients with venous or lymphatic edema who had suffered two or more episodes of cellulitis in the preceding 3 years documented two recurrences in an interventional group of 20 patients treated with prophylactic penicillin (n = 15) or erythromycin (n = 5) in comparison with eight recurrences in 20 control individuals (*P* = 0.06).[71]

An RCT of patients with two or more episodes of cellulitis (mainly in the leg) found no recurrences in 16 patients treated with erythromycin, in comparison with 16 control individuals, in whom there were nine recurrences in eight (50%) patients (40 patients entered).[72]

An RCT in patients with recurrent leg cellulitis used intramuscular benzathine penicillin in 24 patients (18 evaluable) in comparison with 34 control individuals (26 evaluable). The active group had no recurrences within a mean of 11.6 months, compared with nine (35%) of the controls.[73]

A controlled, but not randomized, study of intramuscular penicillin G 1 MU monthly for 1 year did not significantly reduce overall recurrences (recurrences were observed in 12.9% of 31 treated patients, in comparison with 19% of 84 control individuals), although the recurrence rate in patients without risk factors was zero, in comparison with 20% in those with risk factors.[74] However, the "controls" in this study were those who declined follow-up or who received incomplete prophylaxis, so there should be some reservations about the conclusions.

In an open study including 15 patients with three or more episodes of cellulitis over 2 years, treated with 10 mega-IU penicillin daily over 10 days every third month for 1 year, together with lymphatic drainage by pneumatic compression, with further follow-up for 1 year, only one patient had a recurrence.[75]

Tinea pedis and toe web intertrigo

Tinea pedis or toe web maceration are well reported risk factors as a portal of entry for infection causing cellulitis[27,31] and have thus been suggested as possible targets for prophylaxis, with some support from individual cases or small groups of cases. However, some larger studies cast some doubt on whether this is likely to work in the long term.

In a study primarily investigating the link between edema and recurrent episodes, toe web disease was not well documented by admitting physicians and was only recognized by 15% of patients in a postal follow-up survey.[30] This compares with a prevalence of 66% in 167 patients with cellulitis who were examined by dermatologists.[27]

Tinea pedis did not have significance as a risk factor for recurrence in a predictive model based on 209 episodes with 35 recurrences.[68]

In a study of antibiotic prophylaxis discussed above,[72] the 50% recurrence rate in the control group occurred despite treatments for tinea pedis.

Control of lymphedema

Although it is logical, and clearly advised by many clinicians (e.g., always used by 18 of 59, and in lymphedema by 32 of 59 dermatologists surveyed in the UK; UKDCTN, unpublished), there are no studies that have specifically quantified the benefit of controlling lymphedema for either primary or secondary prevention. Lymphedema treatment combined with penicillin is discussed above;[75] it is impossible to know which component worked.

Comments

The small studies of oral antibiotic prophylaxis suggest that this is beneficial. In a retrospective study of 143 patients in which 19 (13%) had multiple episodes over the following 3 years, prophylaxis was viewed as possibly cost-effective in those with predisposing factors and severe attacks.[66]

Despite limited evidence, prophylaxis is used relatively widely. Pavlotsky *et al.* discussed the use of long-term (usually permanent) penicillin in their patients with either recurrent or high-risk primary episodes, and mentioned that 8% of their patients with a recurrence had this whilst on prophylaxis.[29] However, they did not put this into the context of numbers of patients receiving prophylaxis or recurrences after stopping prophylaxis. Among 68 dermatologists who had an interest in research into prophylaxis for cellulitis, 31 used long-term (> 1 year) low-dose penicillin for patients with recurrent episodes, and 22 did so if there was a significant risk factor such as lymphedema (UKDCTN, unpublished). The lack of streptococcal resistance to penicillin over many decades,[50–52] and its safe use in postsplenectomy patients, suggest that this approach is safe for prophylaxis. The British Society for Lymphology guidelines suggest that any patient having two or more episodes of cellulitis annually should receive prophylactic phenoxymethylpenicillin.[15] The CREST guideline suggests that prophylaxis "may be worth trying" in patients who have had two or more episodes of cellulitis at the same site;[10] however, there are reservations about the strength of evidence, which antibiotic and route of administration is best, whether patient-initiated treatment may be more effective than long-term prophylaxis, and whether a prolonged course of treatment after an episode may prevent recurrences.

As documented above, the evidence for prophylaxis of tinea pedis or edema is lacking albeit logical.

A wider discussion of prophylaxis is provided by Becq-Giraudon.[76]

Key points

- In a normal immunocompetent person, without skin breaks, wounds, or abscess formation, only a few pathogens (usually streptococci or staphylococci) cause cellulitis or other skin or subcutaneous infection,[2,12] and initial therapy should concentrate on these two organisms.
- Risk factors for lower leg streptococcal cellulitis have been evaluated in large studies; combining studies suggests the following order of importance: lymphedema, other chronic edema, potential breaks in skin integrity (tinea pedis, dermatitis, wounds), venous insufficiency, and (variably) obesity, as significant risk factors in most studies.
- Adequate-dose flucloxacillin is a suitable initial treatment for presumed streptococcal infection, which accounts for most cases, and covers staphylococci as well; selected cephalosporins

are more commonly used for intravenous home treatment, as they can be administered once daily; phenoxymethylpenicillin is the treatment of choice for prophylaxis. Other treatments may be required in patients who respond poorly or on the basis of bacteriology cultures. Choices of antibiotic for different situations are summarized in several papers.[2,3,6,10–17]

- Home treatment has financial advantages, but most protocols exclude about two-thirds of cases; use of once-daily intravenous antibiotics such as cefazolin or ceftriaxone, or of oral agents such as pristinamycin, is simpler for such situations.

- Risk factors for cellulitis are well documented, but proof to support secondary prophylaxis is only moderate, and for primary prophylaxis is minimal. Factors to predict or identify complications are well established, but most have greater sensitivity than specificity.

- Many hospitals have local guidelines for treating cellulitis. National guidelines based on consensus or on surveys of standard practice have been developed in many countries.[10–17] However, the range of potential organisms, altering bacterial resistance, introduction of new antibiotics, the differences between body sites in terms of risk factors and likely organism, different clinical scenarios (e.g., presence of lymphedema, wounds, etc.), the limited evidence for several scenarios, and the noninferiority methodology of many studies, limit the interpretation of the evidence base in this disorder.

- Further studies are required on the role of physical treatments, compression bandaging and hosiery, both for acute management and for prophylaxis.

References

1 Bisno AL, Stevens DL. Streptococcus pyogenes (including streptococcal toxic shock syndrome and necrotizing fasciitis). In: Mandell GL, Bennett JE, Dolin R, eds. *Principles and Practice of Infectious Diseases*. Edinburgh: Churchill Livingstone, 2000: 2101–17.

2 Stevens DL. Cellulitis, pyoderma, abscesses and other skin and subcutaneous infections. In: Armstrong D, Cohen J. *Infectious Diseases*. London: Mosby, 1999: 2.1–2.10.

3 Schwartz MN. Cellulitis. *N Engl J Med* 2004;**350**:904–12.

4 Anonymous. Dilemmas when managing cellulitis. *Drug Ther Bull* 2003;**41**:43–6.

5 Bonnetblanc JM, Bédane C. Erysipelas. Recognition and management. *Am J Clin Dermatol* 2003;**4**:157–63.

6 Tsao H, Johnson RA. Bacterial cellulitis. *Curr Opin Dermatol* 1997;**4**:33–41.

7 Seal DV. Necrotizing fasciitis. *Curr Opin Infect Dis* 2001;**14**:127–32.

8 Cox NH. Management of lower leg cellulitis. *Clin Med* 2002;**2**:23–7.

9 Société Française de Dermatologie. Consensus conference. Erysipelas and necrotizing fasciitis: management. *Ann Dermatol Venereol* 2001;**128**:307–482.

10 Clinical Resource Efficiency Support Team. Guidelines on the management of cellulitis in adults. 2005. http://www.crestni.org.uk/publications/cellulitis/cellulitis-guide.pdf.

11 Morris A. Cellulitis and erysipelas. http://www.clinicalevidence.com/ceweb/conditions/skd/1708/1708.jsp (accessed April 24th, 2006).

12 Stevens DL, Bisno AL, Chambers HF, *et al*. Practice guidelines for the diagnosis and management of skin and soft–tissue infections. *Clin Infect Dis* 2005;**41**:1373–1406.

13 Clinical Knowledge Summaries. Prodigy Guidance, 2006. Cellulitis. http://www.cks.library.nhs.uk/cellulitis (last accessed July 19th, 2007).

14 Beldon P, Burton F. Management guidelines for lower limb cellulitis. *Wounds UK* 2005;**1**(3):16–25.

15 Mortimer PS, Cefai C, Keeley V, *et al*. Consensus document on the management of Cellulitis in Lymphoedema. British Lymphology Society, 2006. www.thebls.com/concensus.php (last accessed July 19th, 2007).

16 Société Française de Dermatologie. Erysipèle et fasciite nécrosante: prise en charge. *Ann Dermatol Venereol* 2001;**128**:463–82.

17 Brenneke S, Hartmann M, Schöfer H, *et al*. Therapie des Erysipels in Deutschland und Österreich—Ergebnisse einer Umfrage an deutschen und österreichischen Hautkliniken. *J Dtsch Dermatol Ges* 2005;**3**:263–70.

18 Kilburn S, Featherstone P, Higgins B, Brindle R, Severs M. Interventions for cellulitis and erysipelas [protocol]. *Cochrane Database Syst Rev* 2003;(**1**):CD004299.

19 Hook EW III, Hooton TM, Horton CA, *et al*. Microbiologic evaluation of cutaneous cellulitis in adults. *Arch Intern Med* 1986;**146**:295–7.

20 Cox NH, Colver GB, Paterson WD. Management and morbidity of lower-leg cellulitis. *J R Soc Med* 1998;**91**:634–7.

21 Pearse RM, Mitra AV, Heymann TD. What the SHO really does. *J R Coll Phys London* 1999;**33**:553–6.

22 Zaraa I, Zeglaoui F, Bechir Z, *et al*. Erysipelas. Retrospective study of 647 patients. *Tunis Med* 2004;**82**:990–5.

23 Eriksson B, Jorup-Ronström C, Karkkonen K, *et al*. Erysipelas: clinical and bacteriologic spectrum and serological aspects. *Clin Infect Dis* 1996;**23**:1091–8.

24 Denis F, Martin C, Ploy MC. Erysipelas: microbiological and pathogenic data. *Ann Dermatol Venereol* 2001;**128**:317–25.

25 Jaussaud R, Kaeppler, Strady C, *et al*. Should NSAID/corticoids be considered when treating erysipelas? *Ann Dermatol Venereol* 2001;**128**:348–51.

26 Johnson S, Leak K, Singh S, *et al*. Can cycloidal vibration plus standard treatment reduce lower limb cellulitis treatment times? *J Wound Care* 2007;**16**:166–9.

27 Dupuy A, Benchikhi H, Roujeau JC, *et al*. Risk factors for erysipelas of the leg (cellulitis): case–control study. *BMJ* 1999;**318**:1591–4.

28 Björnsdóttir S, Gottfredsson M, Thórisdóttir AS, *et al*. Risk factors for acute cellulitis of the lower limb: a prospective case-control study. *Clin Infect Dis* 2005;**41**:1416–22.

29 Pavlotsky F, Amrani S, Trau H. Recurrent erysipelas: risk factors. *J Dtsch Dermatol Ges* 2004;**2**:89–95.

30 Cox NH. Oedema as a risk factor for multiple episodes of cellulitis/erysipelas of the lower leg: a series with community follow-up. *Br J Dermatol* 2006;**155**:947–50.

31 Roujeau JC, Sigurgeirsson B, Korting HC, *et al*. Chronic dermatomycoses of the foot as risk factors for bacterial cellulitis of the leg: a case–control study. *Dermatology* 2004;**209**:301–7.

32 Bishara J, Golan-Cohen A, Robenshtok E, *et al.* Antibiotic use in patients with erysipelas: a retrospective study. *Isr Med Assoc J* 2001;3:722–4.

33 Badger C, Preston N, Seers K, Mortimer P. Antibiotics/anti-inflammatories for reducing acute inflammatory episodes in lymphoedema of the limbs. *Cochrane Database Syst Rev* 2004;(2): CD003143.

34 Mortimer PS, Levick JR. Chronic peripheral oedema: the critical role of the lymphatic system. *Clin Med* 2004;4:448–53.

35 Kosenkov AN, Narenkov VM, Abramov IuA. [Erysipelas as the cause of lymphedema; in Russian.] *Khirurgiia Mosk* 2005;11:51–3.

36 Bedane C. Dermo-hypodermites bactériennes aigües de l'adulte. *Ann Dermatol Venereol* 1977;124:57–60.

37 Leman P, Mukherjee D. Flucloxacillin alone or combined with benzylpenicillin to treat lower leg cellulitis: a randomised controlled trial. *Emerg Med J* 2005;22:342–6.

38 Zeglaui F, Dziri C, Mokhtar I, *et al.* Intramuscular bipenicillin vs. intravenous penicillin in the treatment of erysipelas in adults: randomized controlled study. *J Eur Acad Dermatol Venereol* 2004; 18:426–8.

39 Hepburn MJ, Dooley DP, Skidmore PJ, *et al.* Comparison of short-course (5 days) and standard (10 days) treatment for uncomplicated cellulitis. *Arch Intern Med* 2004;164:1669–74.

40 Bernard P, Chosidow O, Vaillant L, *et al.* Open pristinamycin versus standard penicillin regimen to treat erysipelas in adults: randomised, non-inferiority, open trial. *BMJ* 2002;325:864–6.

41 Rosen T. Update on treating uncomplicated skin and skin structure infections. *J Drugs Dermatol* 2005;4(6 Suppl):S9–14.

42 Guay DRP. Treatment of bacterial skin and skin structure infections. *Expert Opin Pharmacother* 2003;4:1259–75.

43 Jacobs MR, Jones RN, Giordano PA. Oral beta-lactams applied to uncomplicated infections of skin and skin structures. *Diagn Microbiol Infect Dis* 2007;57 (3 Suppl): S55–65.

44 Leder K, Turnidge JD, Grayson ML. Home-based treatment of cellulitis with twice-daily cefazolin. *Med J Aust* 1998;169:519–22.

45 Corwin P, Toop L, McGeoch G, *et al.* Randomised controlled trial of intravenous antibiotic treatment for cellulitis at home compared with hospital. *BMJ* 2005;330:129–132.

46 Donald M, Marlow M, Swinburn E, Wu M. Emergency department management of home intravenous antibiotic therapy for cellulitis. *Emerg Med J* 2005;22:715–7.

47 Grayson ML, McDonald M, Gibson K, *et al.* Once-daily intravenous cefazolin plus oral probenecid is equivalent to once-daily intravenous ceftriaxone plus oral placebo for the treatment of moderate-to-severe cellulitis in adults. *Clin Infect Dis* 2002;34: 1440–8.

48 Vinken AG, Li JZ, Balan DA, *et al.* Comparison of linezolid with oxacillin or vancomycin in the empiric treatment of cellulitis in US hospitals. *Am J Ther* 2003;10:264–74.

49 Schweiger ES, Weinberg JM. Novel antibacterial agents for skin and skin structure infections. *J Am Acad Dermatol* 1994;50:331–4.

50 Kaplan EL, Johnson DR, Del Rosario MC, Horn DL. Susceptibility of group A beta-hemolytic streptococci to thirteen antibiotics: examination of 301 strains isolated in the United States between 1994 and 1997. *Pediatr Infect Dis J* 1999;18:1069–72.

51 Horn DL, Zabriskie JB, Austrian R, *et al.* Why have group A streptococci remained susceptible to penicillin? Report on a symposium. *Clin Infect Dis* 1998;26:1341–5.

52 Macris MH, Hartman N, Murray B, *et al.* Studies of the continuing susceptibility of group A streptococcal strains to penicillin during eight decades. *Pediatr Infect Dis J* 1998;17:377–81.

53 Ioannides DLL, Addicott R, Santamaria NM, *et al.* Differences in length of stay for Hospital in the Home patients: comparing simple coding with medical record review. *Intern Med J* 2001;31: 142–5.

54 Seaton RA, Bell E, Gourlay Y, Semple L. Nurse-led management of uncomplicated cellulitis in the community: evaluation of a protocol incorporating intravenous ceftriaxone. *J Antimicrob Chemother* 2005;55:764–7.

55 Dunn AS, Peterson KL, Schechter CB, *et al.* The utility of an in-hospital observation period after discontinuing intravenous antibiotics. *Am J Med* 1999;106:6–10.

56 Stevens DL. Necrotizing fasciitis, gas gangrene, myositis and myonecrosis. In: Armstrong D, Cohen J, eds. *Infectious Diseases.* London: Mosby, 1999: 3.1–3.9.

57 Stevenson A, Hider P, Than M. The utility of blood cultures in management of non-facial cellulitis appears to be low. *N Z Med J* 2005;118: U1351 (epub).

58 Morpeth SC, Chambers ST, Gallagher K, *et al.* Lower limb cellulitis: features associated with length of hospital stay. *J Infect* 2006;52: 23–9.

59 Brothers TE, Tagge DU, Stutley JE, *et al.* Magnetic resonance imaging differentiates between necrotizing and non-necrotizing fasciitis of the lower extremity. *J Am Coll Surg* 1998;187:416–21.

60 Révelon G, Rahmouni A, Jazaerli N, *et al.* Acute swelling of the limbs: magnetic resonance pictorial review of fascial and muscle signal changes. *Eur J Radiol* 1999;30:11–21.

61 Rodriguez RM, Abdullah R, Miller R, *et al.* A pilot study of cytokine levels and white blood cell counts in the diagnosis of necrotizing fasciitis. *Am J Emerg Med* 2006;24:58–61.

62 Carratalà J, Rosón B, Fernández-Sabé N, *et al.* Factors associated with complications and mortality in adult patients hospitalised for infectious cellulitis. *Eur J Clin Microbiol Infect Dis* 2003;22:151–7.

63 Lazzarini LO, Conti E, Tositti G, de Lalla F. Erysipelas and cellulitis: clinical and microbiological spectrum in an Italian tertiary care hospital. *J Infect* 2005;51:383–9.

64 Simonart T, Nakafusa J, Narisawa Y. The importance of serum creatine phosphokinase in the early diagnosis and microbiological evaluation of necrotizing fasciitis. *J Eur Acad Dermatol Venereol* 2004;18:687–90.

65 Wong CH, Khin LW, Heng KS, *et al.* The LRINEC (laboratory indicator for necrotizing fasciitis) score: a tool for distinguishing necrotizing fasciitis from other soft tissue infections. *Crit Care Med* 2004;32:1535–41.

66 Jorup-Ronström C, Britton S. Recurrent erysipelas: predisposing factors and costs of prophylaxis. *Infection* 1987;15:105–6.

67 Thomas KS, Cox NH, Savelyich BS, *et al.* Feasibility study to inform the design of a UK multi-centre randomised controlled trial of prophylactic antibiotics for the prevention of recurrent cellulitis of the leg. *Trials* 2007;8:3.

68 McNamara DR, Tleyjeh IM, Berbari EF, *et al.* A predictive model of recurrent lower extremity cellulitis in a population-based cohort. *Arch Intern Med* 2007;167:709–15.

69 Collins PS, Villavicencio JL, Abreu SH, *et al.* Abnormalities of lymphatic drainage in lower extremities: a lymphoscintigraphic study. *J Vasc Surg* 1989;9:145–52.

70 Woo PC, Lum PNL, Wong SSY, *et al.* Cellulitis complicating lymphoedema. *Eur J Clin Microbiol Infect Dis* 2000;**19**:294–7.

71 Sjöblom AC, Eriksson B, Jorup-Rönström C, *et al.* Antibiotic prophylaxis in recurrent erysipelas. *Infection* 1993;**21**:390–3.

72 Kremer M, Zuckerman R, Avraham Z, Raz R. Long-term antimicrobial therapy in the prevention of recurrent soft-tissue infections. *J Infect* 1991;**22**:37–40.

73 Chakroun M, Ben-Romdhane F, Battikh R, *et al.* Benzathine penicillin prophylaxis in recurrent erysipelas. *Mal Med Infect* 1994;**24**:894–7.

74 Wang JH, Liu YC, Cheng DL, *et al.* Role of benzathine penicillin G in prophylaxis for recurrent streptococcal cellulitis of the lower legs. *Clin Infect Dis* 1997;**25**:685–9.

75 Allard P, Stücker M, von Kobyletzki G, *et al.* Zyklische intravenöse Antibiose als effizientes Therapiekonzept des chronisch-rezidierenden Erysipels. *Hautarzt* 1999;**50**:34–8.

76 Becq-Giraudon B. L'érysipèle: prévention primaire et secondaire. *Ann Dermatol Venereol* 2001;**128**:368–75.

42 Exanthematic reactions

Sandra R. Knowles, Neil H. Shear

Background

Definitions

Exanthem, originating from the Greek word for efflorescence, derived from *anthos*, flower (*Stedman's Medical Dictionary*), is defined as any eruptive skin rash that may be associated with fever or other constitutional symptoms.[1] This may be the result of an infectious disease, as an adverse drug reaction, or by interaction between viruses and drugs. Viral infections are frequently associated with the development of exanthems, especially in the pediatric population. These virally induced exanthems are generally nonspecific and often lack characteristic morphologic or distributive features. Some viral exanthems may be associated with enanthems (an eruption of the mucous membrane). Exanthems can include erythematous, vesicular, and petechial types, although most viral exanthems are erythematous papules and macules (Table 42.1). Many of these viral exanthems are associated with low-grade fever, myalgias, headache, rhinorrhea, or gastrointestinal symptoms. Due to the large number of viral exanthems, the scope of this chapter will be limited to some of the more common viral exanthems—namely, measles, rubella, hand-foot-and-mouth disease, erythema infectiosum, and roseola infantum.

Drug-induced exanthems are often described as maculopapular, scarlatiniform, or morbilliform eruptions. Because of their nonspecific nature, some nondermatologists frequently use the generic term "drug rash" to depict these cutaneous eruptions. These eruptions manifest as generalized erythematous changes in the skin without evidence of blistering or pustulation. Pruritus is the most frequently associated symptom. In general, these eruptions are observed within the first 10 days of therapy and resolve within 7–14 days. Resolution occurs with a change in color from bright red to a brownish-red, which may be followed by scaling or desquamation. The differential diagnosis in these patients includes a viral exanthem, collagen vascular disease, and bacterial and rickettsial infections. The hypersensitivity syndrome reaction is a complex drug reaction that can affect various organ systems. A triad of fever, skin eruption (usually an exanthematous eruption), and internal organ involvement signals this potentially life-threatening syndrome.

Incidence/prevalence

Infectious agents were identified in 65% of children with acute febrile illness and rash; of these, 72% of cases were caused by viruses and 20% by bacteria.[2] Infection with parvovirus B19 is ubiquitous and occurs worldwide, most commonly in school-aged children.[3,4] The seroprevalence of B19 antibodies increases with direct proportion to age: 2–15% of children 1–5 years of age are immune, 15–60% between 5 and 19 years, and 30–80% of adults.[5] Hand-foot-and-mouth disease is highly contagious, with epidemics occurring every 3 years in the United States. Human herpesvirus 6 (HHV-6) primarily affects children between the ages of 6 months and 2 years, with the peak age of acquisition between 9 and 21 months. Approximately three-quarters of children have been infected with HHV-6 by 2 years of age.[6] Another study concluded that by 12 months, two-thirds of children have been infected with HHV-6, with peak antibody levels reached at 2–3 years.[7] Furthermore, the seroprevalence for HHV-6 among young adults in the United States reaches almost 100%.[8]

Immunization has dramatically reduced the incidence of measles and rubella in developed countries.[9] For example, routine use of the rubella vaccine has reduced the incidence of rubella in the United States by more than 98%. In addition, routine use of the measles vaccine over the last 30–40 years is estimated to have reduced global measles morbidity and mortality by 74% and 85%, respectively. In the United States, the total number of reported cases of measles during 2001–2003 was 216.[10] Yet in Africa and Asia, approximately 30 million cases of measles still contribute to almost 900 000 fatalities annually.[11]

Table 42.1 Distinctive features of some viral exanthems

Disease (synonym)	Causative agent	Season of occurrence	Incubation period	Prodrome	Morphology	Duration of rash	Distribution of rash	Associated symptoms
Rubella (German measles, 3-day measles)	RNA virus of Togaviridae family	Spring	14–21 days	Mild fever and respiratory symptoms	Pink macules or papules	1–2 days	Begins on forehead and spreads to trunk and extremities	Lymphadenopathy, splenomegaly
Measles (rubeola)	Paramyxovirus	Winter/spring	10–14 days	High fever, conjunctivitis, cough	Erythematous, discrete, macular and papular rash	3–5 days	Begins on hair line behind ears and over forehead, spreads to trunk	Koplik spots, photophobia
Erythema infectiosum (fifth disease, slapped cheek disease)	Parvovirus B19	Winter/spring	4–14 days	Fever, malaise, headache, coryza	Bright red macular erythema of cheeks, erythematous macular eruption followed by lacy erythema	1–3 weeks	Face, followed by extremities	Aplastic crisis, papular-purpuric socks syndrome, arthralgia
Roseola infantum (exanthem subitum, sixth disease)	Human herpes virus (HHV)-6 and HHV-7	Spring/fall	9–10 days	High fever for 3–5 days	Rose-pink macules and papules	3–5 days	Trunk, neck, proximal extremities and sometimes face	Mild upper respiratory symptoms, lymphadenopathy, febrile seizures
Hand-foot-and-mouth disease	Enterovirus	Summer/fall	3–6 days	Fever, malaise, abdominal or respiratory symptoms	Vesicular eruption of palms and soles	7–10 days	Hand, foot, mouth	Erosive stomatitis

In the Boston Collaborative Drug Surveillance Program, the prevalence of cutaneous adverse drug reactions (ADRs) in hospitalized patients was 2.2%. Antibiotics were responsible for 7% of detected reactions.[12] Simple exanthematous eruptions are the most common form of drug eruptions, accounting for approximately 95% of skin reactions.[11] The Harvard Medical Practice Study showed that approximately 14% of adverse drug reactions in hospital patients are cutaneous or allergic in nature.[13]

Etiology

The classic childhood exanthems include measles, scarlet fever, rubella, erythema infectiosum, exanthema subitum, and chickenpox.[14] In addition, there have been more than 50 infectious agents (viral, bacterial or rickettsial) identified that cause exanthems in children.[15] One study investigated the causes of morbilliform rash in a highly immunized English population. Among 195 children, laboratory confirmation was obtained in 93 cases (48%): parvovirus B19 in 34 (17%), group A streptococcus in 30 (15%), human

herpesvirus type 6 in 11 (6%), enterovirus in nine (5%), adenovirus in seven, (4%), and group C streptococcus in six (3%).[16]

Measles (rubeola) is a systemic illness caused by a paramyxovirus that is spread by respiratory droplets. Clinical signs and symptoms consist of fever, cough, coryza, conjunctivitis, morbilliform rash, and Koplik spots. Erythematous macules and papules begin at the hairline and behind the ears and spread down the body.

The enteroviruses, a subgroup of the picornavirus family, cause a variety of different illnesses associated with exanthems. Hand-foot-and-mouth disease, a common and well-recognized entity, is characterized by a vesicular eruption of the palms and soles as well as stomatitis; it is most commonly associated with coxsackievirus A16 or enterovirus 71. After an incubation of 3–6 days, low-grade fever, malaise, and abdominal or respiratory symptoms are present. Cutaneous lesions appear as pink to red macules or papules in a characteristic linear arrangement.

Roseola infantum (exanthem subitum, sixth disease) is caused by primary infection with human herpesvirus 6

(HHV-6) and human herpesvirus 7 (HHV-7). High fever in an otherwise well-appearing child and a rash with defervescence are classic findings. The exanthem consists of pink macules and papules that spread from the neck down to the trunk and proximal extremities.[5] One study showed that rash occurred in less than one-third of patients with primary HHV-6 infection.[17]

Erythema infectiosum (fifth disease) is caused by parvovirus B19. After a 3–18-day incubation period, mild symptoms such as fever, malaise and sore throat develop in 20–60% of cases 2 days before the rash. The exanthem has a characteristic "slapped cheek" appearance; erythematous, edematous, confluent plaques appear symmetrically on both cheeks.[3,5] Manifestations significantly associated with acute B19 infection in immunocompetent children were exanthema, anemia, and leukopenia.[18] In healthy adults, parvovirus B19 usually causes a self-limiting febrile illness, accompanied by other features such as polyarthralgia and facial erythema. Clinically significant arthropathy that may persist for weeks to months is found in 50% of adult patients infected with parvovirus B19.[4,19] The skin rash in adults includes the "slapped cheek" appearance and systemic diffuse erythema.[20] Infections in immunocompromised hosts can lead to chronic infection, most often manifested as chronic anemia.[5]

Rubella (German measles), caused by the rubella virus, is usually a mild disease consisting of low-grade fever, generalized erythematous macules and papules which last 3 days, and generalized lymphadenopathy. In adolescents and adults, but not in children, there is a prodromal period with fever, malaise, sore throat, nausea, and anorexia. An enanthem, called Forchheimer spots, consists of petechiae on the hard palate, and may be present in some patients.

Exanthematous eruptions can be caused by many drugs including the penicillins, sulfonamides, nonnucleoside reverse transcriptase inhibitors (e.g., nevirapine), and antiepileptic medications.[12] The incidence of delayed cutaneous eruptions associated with ampicillin or amoxicillin is 9.5%.[21] They can appear 2–3 days after the drug is started, although they usually occur near the end of therapy (i.e., days 8–10). Gemifloxacin, a fluoroquinolone, is associated with a mild to moderate self-limiting maculopapular rash, especially when used beyond 7 days. When used for 5 days for community-acquired respiratory tract infections, the rash rate is typically less than 1.5%, a rate similar to that with other fluoroquinolones.[22] Since most drugs can cause an exanthematous eruption, it is important to obtain a detailed medication history, including over-the-counter preparations and herbal and naturopathic remedies in patients with a history of an ADR. New drugs started within the preceding 6 weeks are potential causative agents for most cutaneous eruptions, as are drugs that have been used intermittently. Approximately 10–20% of all exanthematous eruptions in children are considered to be drug-induced, whereas 50–70% of exanthematous eruptions in adults are triggered by drugs.

The hypersensitivity syndrome reaction has been well described for a number of drugs, including anticonvulsants, sulfonamide antibiotics, dapsone, minocycline, and allopurinol.[23,24] Although this reaction has been estimated to occur in between one in 1000 and one in 10 000 anticonvulsant and sulfonamide antibiotic exposures, its true incidence is unknown because of variable presentation and inaccurate reporting.[25]

Prognosis

Many of the viral exanthems are self-limiting conditions. However, some of the viral illnesses can result in significant morbidity and mortality. For example, in the United States, the mortality rate for measles is 0.3%, but in developing countries it can reach 1–10%. Complications include pneumonia, croup, diarrhea, acute encephalitis, brain damage, and death from respiratory and neurologic complications. The most frequent complication of roseola is febrile seizures. Among 902 children under 3 years of age with primary HHV-6 infection and fever, 149 (16.5%) had a seizure.[26] The most dreaded complication of measles is encephalitis, which occurs in about one in every 800 cases. Approximately 5% of adult patients and 10% of children undergoing chemotherapy for hematological malignancies are persistently infected with the parvovirus B19 virus, resulting in severe and even lethal cytopenias.[19]

Many of the viral illnesses acquired during pregnancy may result in adverse outcomes for the fetus. When rubella occurs during the first trimester of pregnancy, the infection can result in approximately 50% of fetuses with manifestations of congenital rubella syndrome, which includes congenital heart defects, cataracts, microphthalmia, deafness, microcephaly, and hydrocephalus.[27] Similarly, although rare, hand-foot-and-mouth disease acquired during first trimester of pregnancy may result in spontaneous abortion. Erythema infectiosum acquired during fetal development may be complicated by fetal hydrops secondary to infection of erythroid precursors, hemolysis, severe anemia, tissue anoxia, and high-output failure. Fetal loss was 6.5% in a series of 334 cases, with 0.6% with nonfatal hydrops fetalis.[28]

Simple exanthematous eruptions due to medications generally resolve spontaneously without complications or sequelae within 7–14 days. However, hypersensitivity syndrome reactions may, in rare cases, result in significant morbidity and even mortality.

Diagnostic tests

Many viral infections, including hand-foot-and-mouth disease and erythema infectiosum, are straightforward clinical diagnoses. In addition to the clinical presentation of the exanthem and any enanthem, diagnosis is based on the patient's history (e.g., exposure to other infected individuals) and other distinguishing features of the viral infection, such as predilection for certain seasons. However, confirmation of various viral infections can be accomplished via laboratory tests. Viral culture or polymerase chain reaction (PCR)-based tests can be used for diagnosis of enteroviral infection. Rubella can be diagnosed by detection of anti-rubella IgM antibodies, or a fourfold increase in serum IgG levels. Tests for detection of B19 DNA are required in immunocompromised patients who are unable to mount an adequate humoral response. Methods that detect viral particles or viral DNA are amplified by PCR.[5] Detection of serum anti-B19 IgM antibody can also be used when diagnostic confirmation of B19 infection is needed.[19] However, caution is suggested when interpreting serology in immunodeficient individuals and pregnant women, as they may not necessarily be able to mount an antibody response.[19]

In general, skin biopsies are not indicated for diagnosis of viral exanthem, due to the nonspecific findings. In addition, a biopsy of drug-induced exanthematous eruptions is generally not recommended, as nonspecific changes are usually present that consist of a mild perivascular lymphocytic infiltrate and a few necrotic keratinocytes within the epidermis.

Some exanthematous eruptions can be identified through patch or delayed-reading intradermal skin tests. Immediate prick skin testing for drug-induced exanthematous eruptions is not helpful in most cases, as skin testing is usually reserved for the diagnosis of IgE-mediated reactions. However, skin testing has been used in the confirmation of delayed ampicillin and amoxicillin exanthematous eruptions. Patch testing, using the drug in a suitable concentration, can be used to confirm various delayed type IV reactions, including contact dermatitis and delayed exanthematous eruptions.[29] The overall sensitivity of patch testing is estimated to be 30–60%, which suggests that a negative patch test does not exclude a drug-induced reaction.[30] In 165 patients with a cutaneous eruption, patch tests were positive in 33 of 61 patients (54%) with a maculopapular rash.[31] One study concluded that patch testing was found to be a useful screening tool if the reaction was exanthematous and if antimicrobial, cardiovascular, or antiepileptic drugs were suspected. A positive patch test to one or more drug was observed in 89 of 826 patients (10.8%), most often to beta-lactams, clindamycin, and trimethoprim.[32] Another study examined the results of patch testing in individuals who experienced nonimmediate reactions with benzylpenicillin, ampicillin, and amoxicillin. Of the 119 patients with delayed reactions to aminopenicillins, 62 (52%) demonstrated delayed hypersensitivity, as indicated by positive patch or delayed-reading intradermal test responses.[33]

Diagnostic or confirmatory tests are not readily available for patients with the hypersensitivity syndrome reaction. An *in vitro* test employing a mouse hepatic microsomal system is used for research purposes to characterize patients who develop this serious reaction.[25,34] Because of the severity of the reaction, oral rechallenges are not recommended, as reexposure to the offending agent may cause development of symptoms within 1 day.

Differential diagnosis for drug-induced exanthems includes viral exanthems (e.g., enteroviruses, HHV-6, parvovirus B19, Epstein–Barr virus) and other illnesses such as bacterial and rickettsial diseases and Kawasaki's syndrome. It is often difficult to discriminate between a drug-induced morbilliform eruption and a viral exanthem, although the polymorphic nature of the cutaneous eruption favors a drug eruption. Other features that may help distinguish between a drug-induced and a viral eruption include onset of reaction in relationship to drug, history of previous reaction to a medication, exposure to infected individuals with a similar viral infection, and characteristic appearance of the rash (e.g., "slapped cheek" for erythema infectiosum).

Aims of treatment

For most viral and drug-induced exanthems, the aims of treatment are supportive and include reduction of fever, relief of pruritus, and/or management of arthralgias. In immunocompromised patients, the aims of treatment include symptomatic management as well as prevention of complications such as pneumonia, encephalitis, and hepatitis. The aims of treatment in patients with hypersensitivity syndrome reaction include symptomatic management and prevention of serious complications such as hepatitis, nephritis, or pneumonitis.

Relevant outcomes

For viral and drug-induced exanthems:
- Fever
- Extent of exanthem
- Arthralgias and other systemic features such as malaise, nausea/vomiting, diarrhea
- Resolution of symptoms
- Death

For drug-induced exanthems:
- Onset of symptoms, in relationship to initiation of drug therapy
- Internal organ involvement
- Death

Methods

The databases of the Cochrane Library to 2006 and Medline between 1968 and September 2006 were searched for the following terms:

- Measles, rubella, roseola, exanthema subitum, fifth disease, parvovirus B19, human, erythema infectiosum, hand-foot-and-mouth disease
- Exanthema, drug eruptions, drug hypersensitivity, skin diseases viral, viral exanthem, drug exanthems, skin diseases

Subheadings used with the search terms, when appropriate, included "chemically induced," "epidemiology," "drug therapy," "diagnosis," and "treatment." Other search terms used in combination with the above terms included "pregnancy" (e.g., rubella and pregnancy), "skin tests" (e.g., skin tests and drug eruptions), "ampicillin," and "infectious mononucleosis."

Questions

What is the pathogenesis for drug-induced exanthems?

Constitutional factors influencing the risk of cutaneous eruption include pharmacogenetic variation in drug-metabolizing enzymes and human leukocyte antigen (HLA) associations. HLA factors may influence the risk of reactions to nevirapine, abacavir, carbamazepine, and allopurinol.[35–38] Allopurinol-induced adverse reactions, including hypersensitivity syndrome reaction, Stevens–Johnson syndrome (SJS), and toxic epidermal necrolysis (TEN), have been strongly associated with a genetic predisposition among Han Chinese; the HLA-B*5801 allele was found to be an important genetic risk factor.[35] Nevirapine has been associated with hypersensitivity syndrome reaction involving various combinations of fever, hepatitis, or rash. Studies have suggested that HLA-DRB1*0101 and the CD4 status of a patient may determine susceptibility to nevirapine hypersensitivity.[36] Abacavir is also associated with a potentially life-threatening adverse reaction in approximately 8% of patients initiated on this drug. Studies have shown that there is a strong predictive association between abacavir hypersensitivity syndrome reaction and HLA-B*5701.[37]

Many drugs associated with severe idiosyncratic drug reactions are metabolized by the body to form reactive, or toxic, drug products.[39] These reactive products comprise only a small proportion of a drug's metabolites and are usually rapidly detoxified. However, patients with the drug hypersensitivity syndrome, toxic epidermal necrolysis, and Stevens–Johnson syndrome (SJS), resulting from treatment with sulfonamide antibiotics and the aromatic anticonvulsants (e.g., carbamazepine, phenytoin, and phenobarbital) show increased sensitivity in *in vitro* assessments to the oxidative, reactive drug metabolites of these drugs in comparison with control individuals.[25,40]

Acquired factors also alter an individual's risk of drug eruption. Active viral infection and concurrent medications have been shown to alter the frequency of drug-associated eruptions. Drug–drug interactions may also alter the risk of cutaneous eruption. Valproic acid increases the risk of severe cutaneous adverse reactions to lamotrigine, another anticonvulsant.[41] The basis of these interactions and reactions is unknown, but may represent a mixture of factors, including alteration in drug metabolism, drug detoxification, antioxidant defenses, and immune reactivity.

The course and outcome of drug-induced disease are also influenced by host factors. Older age may delay the onset of drug eruptions and has been associated with a higher mortality rate in some severe reactions. A higher mortality rate is also observed in patients with severe reactions with underlying malignancy.[42]

Although the underlying pathogenesis for many drug eruptions remains unknown, certain studies have shown that drug-specific T cells play a major role in exanthematous, bullous, and pustular drug reactions.[43] Immunohistochemical studies have shown that the cell infiltrate in drug-induced maculopapular exanthems is mainly composed of CD3+ T cells (40–70%), with a predominance of CD4+ cells.[44] Cytotoxic T cells (more CD4 cells than CD8 cells) contribute to the characteristic features of interface dermatitis, such as vacuolar alteration and keratinocyte death.[45]

What is the hypersensitivity syndrome reaction?

An exanthematous eruption in conjunction with fever and internal organ involvement (e.g., liver, kidney, central nervous system) signifies a more serious reaction, known as the hypersensitivity syndrome reaction (HSR). The condition is also known as drug rash with eosinophilia and systemic symptoms (DRESS), and as drug-induced hypersensitivity syndrome (DIHS). This syndrome has been well described for a number of drugs, including anticonvulsants, sulfonamide antibiotics, dapsone, minocycline, and allopurinol. Although this reaction has been estimated to occur in between one in 1000 and one in 10 000 anticonvulsant and sulfonamide antibiotic exposures, its true incidence is unknown due to variable presentation and inaccurate reporting.[23] HSR occurs most frequently on first exposure to the drug, with initial symptoms starting 2–6 weeks after exposure to the drug. In patients with a history of HSR, reexposure to the offending agent may cause development of symptoms within 1 day. Hypersensitivity syndrome is not related to dose or serum concentration of the drug.

A mild to high fever ranging from 38 °C to 40 °C and malaise, which can be accompanied by pharyngitis and cervical lymphadenopathy, are the presenting symptoms in most patients. Atypical lymphocytosis with a subsequent prominent eosinophilia may occur during the initial phases of the reaction in many patients.[46] A generalized exanthem occurs in approximately 85% of patients, usually simultaneously with the appearance of the fever or shortly after.

Skin manifestations can range from an exanthematous eruption to more serious eruptions, such as exfoliative dermatitis.[47] Conjunctivitis and angioedema of the face may also be present in some patients, especially patients with anticonvulsant-induced HSR.[47] Liver abnormalities, presenting as elevated transaminases, alkaline phosphatase, prothrombin time, and bilirubin, are present in approximately 50% of patients; in some patients, development of severe hepatitis with jaundice may occur.[24] Other organs, such as the kidney (interstitial nephritis, vasculitis), central nervous system (encephalitis, aseptic meningitis), or lungs (interstitial pneumonitis, respiratory distress syndrome, vasculitis) may less commonly be involved. A small subgroup of patients may become hypothyroid as part of an autoimmune thyroiditis within 2 months of initiation of symptoms.[48] This is characterized by a low thyroxine level, an elevated level of thyroid-stimulating hormone, and thyroid autoantibodies, including antimicrosomal antibodies.

HSR has been associated with the aromatic anticonvulsants—namely, phenytoin, phenobarbital, and carbamazepine.[49] It has been suggested that the formation of toxic metabolites by phenytoin, carbamazepine, and phenobarbital may play a pivotal role in the development of hypersensitivity syndrome.[25] Phenytoin, carbamazepine, and phenobarbital are metabolized by various cytochrome P-450 (CYP) enzymes to chemically reactive metabolites, although the specific metabolite is unknown. This metabolite is thought to be detoxified by epoxide hydroxylases; however, if detoxification is defective, the toxic metabolite may act as a hapten and initiate an immunoresponse, causing cell necrosis directly or indirectly via pathways leading to apoptosis. In one study,[25] 75% of a series of patients with anticonvulsant hypersensitivity syndrome to one aromatic anticonvulsant showed *in vitro* cross-reactivity to the other two. In addition, *in vitro* testing showed that there is a familial occurrence of hypersensitivity to anticonvulsants.[25] Although lamotrigine is not an aromatic anticonvulsant, there have been several reports documenting a hypersensitivity syndrome associated with its use as well.[50]

Sulfonamide antibiotics are also metabolized to toxic metabolites—namely, hydroxylamines and nitroso compounds.[51,52] In most people, detoxification of the metabolite occurs. However, HSRs may occur in patients who are unable to detoxify this metabolite. Because siblings and other first-degree relatives are at increased risk (perhaps as high as one in four) of developing a similar adverse reaction, counseling of family members is essential. Other aromatic amines, such as procainamide, dapsone, and acebutolol, are also metabolized to chemically reactive compounds. We recommend that patients who develop symptoms compatible with a sulfonamide hypersensitivity syndrome reaction avoid these aromatic amines, because the potential exists for cross-reactivity.[53] However, cross-reactivity should not occur between sulfonamides and drugs that are not aromatic amines (e.g., sulfonylureas, thiazide diuretics, furosemide, and acetazolamide).[54]

The differential diagnosis of HSR includes other cutaneous drug reactions, acute viral infections (e.g., Epstein–Barr virus, hepatitis virus, influenza virus, cytomegalovirus), lymphoma, and idiopathic hypereosinophilic syndrome. After HSR has been recognized by the symptom complex of fever, rash, and lymphadenopathy, there are a minimum number of laboratory tests that help to evaluate internal organ involvement, which may be asymptomatic. Liver transaminases, complete blood count, and urinalysis and serum creatinine should be performed at the initial evaluation. In addition, the clinician should be guided by the presence of symptoms, which may suggest specific internal organ involvement (e.g., respiratory symptoms). Thyroid function tests should be measured and repeated after 2–3 months. A skin biopsy may be helpful if the patient has a blistering or a pustular eruption. Unfortunately, readily available diagnostic or confirmatory tests to establish drug causation are not readily available. An *in vitro* test using a mouse hepatic microsomal system is used for research purposes to evaluate patients who develop HSR.[34] Oral rechallenges are not recommended, due to the severity of the HSR reactions.

Although the role of systemic corticosteroid therapy is controversial, most clinicians would elect to start prednisone at a dose of 1–2 mg/kg/day if symptoms are severe. In contrast to the issue of corticosteroids in SJS and TEN, there is no significant barrier function alteration leading to the potential for sepsis in the HSR. There are cases of patients who have been treated with ciclosporin[55] or intravenous immunoglobulin (IVIg).[56] Antihistamines or topical corticosteroids can also be used to alleviate symptoms. Because the risk of HSR is substantially increased in first-degree relatives of patients who have had HSR reactions, counseling of family members is a crucial part of the assessment of this syndrome.[25]

What role do viruses play in the development of drug eruptions?

Various risk factors may contribute to the development of an adverse drug reaction, including genetic predisposition, drug–drug interactions, and viral infections. Viral infections may create biological alterations in the immune system that enhance the risk of adverse drug reactions.

Epstein–Barr virus (EBV) is the cause of most acute infectious mononucleosis syndromes. Patients primarily present with malaise, fever, pharyngitis, and lymphadenopathy. In patients who have infectious mononucleosis, the risk of developing an exanthematous eruption while being treated with an aminopenicillin (e.g., ampicillin) increases from 3–7% to 60–100%.[57] The rash is extensive, maculopapular, pruritic, and usually accompanied by fever. Although the mechanism of the reaction has not been clarified, it does not appear to be IgE-mediated.[58,59] In fact, the patient with infectious mononucleosis who develops a delayed rash while on an aminopenicillin is not at risk from developing the same reaction when reexposed to the aminopenicillin or any penicillin without a concurrent EBV infection.[60]

Approximately 50–60% of patients with human immunodeficiency virus/acquired immune deficiency syndrome (HIV/AIDS) who are exposed to sulfonamide antibiotics for *Pneumocystis carinii* infection develop adverse reactions such as fever, rash, neutropenia, and hepatitis.[61] In addition to the presence of HIV, the increased prevalence of slow acetylation and altered activity of oxidative metabolic pathways in AIDS patients with acute illnesses may partly explain the increased incidence of adverse reactions in these patients.[62–64]

Reactivation of latent viral infection with human herpes virus (HHV)-6 also appears common in the drug hypersensitivity syndrome and may be partly responsible for some of the clinical features and/or course of the disease.[65–67] Viral infections may act as, or generate the production of, danger signals leading to damaging immune responses to drugs, rather than immune tolerance.[68] Allopurinol is associated with the development of serious drug reactions, including hypersensitivity syndrome reaction. In a review of 13 patients with allopurinol adverse reactions, fever and rash were the most common presenting symptoms. Other associated abnormalities included leukocytosis (62%), eosinophilia (54%), renal impairment (54%), and liver dysfunction (69%).[69] In a patient who developed a hypersensitivity syndrome reaction with hepatitis, reactivation of HHV-6 occurred. HHV-6 DNA in blood by PCR analysis was positive. In addition, HHV-6 DNA in the cerebrospinal fluid was detected.[70] Reactivation of HHV-6 may also contribute to the development of hypersensitivity syndrome reaction caused by anticonvulsants.[65,71]

What treatment regimens have been used in patients infected with viral exanthems?

Most viral exanthems are self-limiting conditions that only require symptomatic treatment. This includes the use of antipyretics (e.g., acetaminophen, ibuprofen) and analgesics (i.e., nonsteroidal anti-inflammatory drugs) in cases of arthralgias. For patients with pruritus, relief can be obtained with antihistamines, topical antipruritic lotions (e.g., calamine), or topical corticosteroids.

Parvovirus B19

Intravenous immunoglobulin has been used in the treatment of patients with chronic or persistent infections due to parvovirus B19; this includes children with immunodeficiency syndromes, chemotherapy-induced suppression, transplant patients, and patients with HIV/AIDS.[5] A persistent parvovirus B19 infection responds to a 5-day or 10-day course of immunoglobulin at a dose of 0.4 g/kg of body weight, with a prompt decline in serum viral DNA, accompanied by reticulocytosis and increased hemoglobin levels.[4] IVIg has also been administered at 1 g/kg × 3 days.[18] Intrauterine red-cell transfusions have been used for the treatment of intrauterine infections with fetal hydrops and anemia, although hydrops fetalis may resolve spontaneously.[72]

HHV-6

There are no medications available that are specific for HHV-6. Ganciclovir and foscarnet have been used for serious HHV-6 disease in immunocompromised and transplant patients, but there are no randomized trials. One report described two patients treated early with foscarnet for HHV-6 encephalitis after bone-marrow transplantation. Both patients improved on therapy.[73,74] Antiviral prophylaxis with ganciclovir prevented HHV-6 reactivation in six bone-marrow transplant recipients.[75]

Measles

Vitamin A deficiency is a recognized risk factor for severe measles. The protective effect of vitamin A on measles mortality was shown more than 70 years ago.[76] Measles can decrease serum concentrations of vitamin A in well-nourished children to levels less than those observed in malnourished children without measles. Vitamin A deficiency depresses the immune function and can destroy epithelial tissue; therefore, vitamin A may prevent the complications of measles infection by stimulating the body's impaired immune reaction, by a direct activating effect on helper T cells and by boosting immunoglobulin production.[77]

In 1997, the World Health Organization and United Nations Children's Fund (UNICEF) recommended that 200 000 IU of vitamin A should be given twice to children with measles over the age of 1 year in populations in which vitamin A deficiency may be present. If there is clinical evidence or great risk for vitamin A deficiency, the dose is repeated after 4 weeks.[78] The American Academy of Pediatrics suggests that vitamin A be administered to patients aged 2 years or less who are hospitalized with measles and its complications.[79] It should also be administered to patients who are older than 6 months but have an immunodeficiency, ophthalmological evidence of vitamin A deficiency, impaired intestinal absorption, moderate to severe malnutrition, or recent immigration from areas where a high mortality rate from measles has been observed. There have been several meta-analyses that have evaluated whether vitamin A is beneficial in preventing mortality, pneumonia, and other secondary infections in children with measles.[76,78] In the Cochrane review, eight trials met the inclusion criteria. Overall, there was no significant reduction in the risk of mortality in the vitamin A group when the studies were pooled using the random-effects model (RR 0.70; 95% CI, 0.42 to 1.15). However, two doses of vitamin A 200 000 IU on consecutive days were associated with a reduction in the risk of mortality in children under the age of 2 years (RR 0.18; 95% CI, 0.03 to 0.61) and a reduction in the risk of pneumonia-specific mortality (RR 0.33; 95% CI, 0.08 to 0.92). There was no evidence that vitamin A in a single dose reduced the risk of mortality. There was a decrease in the incidence of croup, but no significant reduction in the incidence of pneumonia or diarrhea with two doses.[76]

In spite of the possible role of oxidative stress in conditions such as viral infections, vitamin E and C have not been shown to provide any benefit in the course of the illness in children with measles and pneumonia.[80] Studies evaluating the efficacy and safety of Chinese medicinal herbs were systematically reviewed in a Cochrane review; unfortunately, none of the trials concealed the allocation or blinding method, and therefore no analyses were performed.[81] There is no specific antiviral therapy for measles, although ribavirin has been used in patients with measles with severe manifestations.[82]

Hand-foot-and-mouth disease

Acyclovir has been studied in the treatment of hand-foot-and-mouth disease in a preliminary report. Symptomatic relief, defervescence, and significant involution of lesions were seen within 12 hours of starting acyclovir (200–300 mg five times daily for 5 days).[82] In another report, an immunocompromised 27-year-old man with a prolonged course of hand-foot-and-mouth disease was started on oral acyclovir 200 mg five times daily, with subsequent resolution of all lesions within 5 days.[84]

Key points

- Most drug-induced exanthems manifest as generalized erythematous changes in the skin without evidence of blistering or pustulation. Pruritus is the most frequently associated symptom. These eruptions generally occur within the first 10 days of therapy and resolve within 7–14 days after discontinuation of the medication.

- Many of the viral illnesses acquired during pregnancy may result in adverse outcomes for the fetus. For example, when rubella occurs during the fist trimester of pregnancy, the infection can result in approximately 50% of fetuses with manifestations of congenital rubella syndrome.

- Diagnosis of viral infections includes the clinical presentation of the exanthem and enanthem, and the patient's history (e.g., exposure to other infected individuals and distinguishing features of the viral infection). Laboratory tests can be done for confirmation, if necessary.

- Diagnosis of drug-induced exanthematous eruptions is based on the clinical history. The use of confirmatory tests, such as patch or delayed reading of intradermal skin tests, has not been well defined.

- The aims of treatment for most viral and drug-induced exanthems are supportive and include reduction of fever, relief of pruritus, and/or management of arthralgias.

- Factors that may influence the risk of a cutaneous eruption include pharmacogenetic variation in drug-metabolizing enzymes and human leukocyte antigen (HLA) associations, acquired factors (e.g., active viral infection and concurrent medications), host factors (e.g., age, underlying malignancy), and drug-specific T cells.

- The hypersensitivity syndrome reaction is a triad of symptoms consisting of a cutaneous eruption (usually exanthematous), fever, and internal organ involvement. This reaction usually occurs on first exposure to the drug, with initial symptoms starting 2–6 weeks after exposure to the drug. This reaction is most commonly associated with the aromatic anticonvulsants (phenytoin, phenobarbital, carbamazepine), sulfonamide antibiotics, allopurinol, dapsone, and minocycline.

References

1 Drago F, Rampini P, Rampini E, Rebora A. Atypical exanthems: morphology and laboratory investigations may lead to an aetiological diagnosis in about 70% of cases. *Br J Dermatol* 2002;**147**: 255–60.

2 Goodyear H, Laidler P, Price E, *et al.* Acute infectious erythemas in children: a clinico-microbiological study. *Br J Dermatol* 1991; **124**:433–8.

3 Vafaie J, Schwartz R. Erythema infectiosum. *J Cutan Med Surg* 2005;**9**:159–61.

4 Young N, Brown K. Parvovirus B19. *N Engl J Med* 2004;**350**: 586–97.

5 Koch W. Fifth (human parvovirus) and sixth (herpesvirus 6) diseases. *Curr Opin Infect Dis* 2001;**14**:343–56.

6 Zerr D, Meier A, Selke S, *et al.* A population-based study of primary human herpesvirus 6 infection. *N Engl J Med* 2005;**352**:768–76.

7 Stoeckle M. The spectrum of human herpesvirus 6 infection: from roseola infantum to adult disease. *Ann Rev Med* 2000;**51**:423–30.

8 Prober C. Sixth disease and the ubiquity of human herpesviruses. *N Engl J Med* 2005;**352**:753–5.

9 Reef S, Cochi S. The evidence for the elimination of rubella and congenital rubella syndrome in the United States: a public health achievement. *Clin Infect Diseases* 2006;**43**:S123–5.

10 Anon. Epidemiology of measles: United States, 2001–2003. MMWR 2004;**53**(31):713–6.

11 Centre for Disease Control. Advances in global measles control and elimination: summary of the 1997 International meeting. *MMWR Recomm Rep* 1998 Jul 24;**47**(RR-11):1–23.

12 Bigby M, Jick S, Jick H, Arndt K. Drug-induced cutaneous reactions: a report from the Boston Collaborative Drug Surveillance Program on 15,438 consecutive inpatients, 1975 to 1982. *JAMA* 1986;**256**:3358–63.

13 Leape L, Brennan T, Laird N, *et al.* The nature of adverse events in hospitalized patients. Results of the Harvard Medical Practice Study II. *N Engl J Med* 1991;**324**:377–84.

14 Bialecki C, Feder H, Grant-Kels J. The six classical exanthems: a review and update. *J Am Acad Dermatol* 1989;**21**:891–903.

15 Gable F, Liu G, Morrell D. Pediatric exanthems. *Primary Care* 2000;**27**:353–69.

16 Ramsay M, Reacher M, O'Flynn C, *et al.* Causes of morbilliform rash in a highly immunised English population. *Arch Dis Child* 2002;**87**:202–6.

17 Hall C, Long C, Schnabel K, *et al.* Human herpesvirus 6 infection in children: prospective evaluation for complications and reactivation. *N Engl J Med* 1994;**331**:432–8.

18 Miron D, Luder A, Horovitz Y, *et al.* Acute human parvovirus B-19 infection in hospitalized children: a serologic and molecular survey. *Ped Infect Dis J* 2006;**25**:898–901.

19 Broliden K, Tolfvenstam T, Norbeck O. Clinical aspects of parvovirus B19 infection. *J Int Med* 2006;**260**:285–304.

20 Hayakawa H, Tara M, Niina K, Osame M. A clinical study of adult human parvovirus B19 infection. *Intern Med* 2002;**41**:295–9.

21 Romano A, Quaratino D, Papa G, Di Fonso M, Venuti A. Aminopenicillin allergy. *Arch Dis Childhood* 1997;**76**:513–7.

22 Iannini P, Mandell L, Patou G, Shear N. Cutaneous adverse events and gemifloxacin: observations from the clinical trial program. *J Chemother* 2006;**18**:3–11.

23 Tennis P, Stern R. Risk of serious cutaneous disorders after initiation of use of phenytoin, carbamazepine, or sodium valproate: a record linkage study. *Neurology* 1997;**49**:542–6.

24 Knowles S, Shapiro L, Shear N. Anticonvulsant hypersensitivity syndrome: incidence, prevention and management. *Drug Saf* 1999;**21**:489–501.

25 Shear N, Spielberg S. Anticonvulsant hypersensitivity syndrome, in vitro assessment of risk. *J Clin Invest* 1988;**82**:1826–32.

26 Millichap J, Millichap J. Role of viral infections in the etiology of febrile seizures. *Pediatr Neurol* 2006;**35**:165–72.

27 DeSantis M, Cavaliere A, Straface G, Caruso A. Rubella infection in pregnancy. *Reprod Toxicol* 2006;**21**:390–8.

28 Levy R, Weissman A, Blomberg G, Hagay Z. Infection by parvovirus B19 during pregnancy: a review. *Obstet Gynecol Surv* 1997;**52**:254–9.

29 Romano A, Blanca M, Torres M, *et al.* Diagnosis of nonimmediate reactions to beta-lactam antibiotics. *Allergy* 2004;**59**:1153–60.

30 Lerch M, Pichler W. The immunological and clinical spectrum of delayed drug-induced exanthems. *Curr Opin Allergy Clin Immunol* 2004;**4**:411–9.

31 Barbaud A. Drug patch testing in systemic cutaneous drug allergy. *Toxicology* 2005;**209**:209–16.

32 Lammintausta K, Kortekangas-Savolainen O. The usefulness of skin tests to prove drug hypersensitivity. *Br J Dermatol* 2005;**152**:968–74.

33 Romano A, Quaratino D, DiFonso M, Papa G, Venuti A, Gasbarrini G. A diagnostic protocol for evaluating nonimmediate reactions to aminopenicillins. *J Aller Clin Immunol* 1999;**103**:1186–90.

34 Neuman M, Malkiewicz I, Shear N. A novel lymphocyte toxicity assay to assess drug hypersensitivity syndromes. *Clin Biochem* 2000;**33**:517–24.

35 Hung S, Chung W, Liou L, Chu C, Lin M, Al E. HLA-B*5801 allele as a genetic marker for severe cutaneous adverse reactions caused by allopurinol. *Proc Natl Acad Sci* 2005;**102**:4134–9.

36 Martin A, Nolan D, James I, Cameron P, Keller J, *et al.* Predisposition to nevirapine hypersensitivity associated with HLA-DRB1*0101 and abrogated by low CD4 T-cell counts. *AIDS* 2005; **19**:97–9.

37 Martin A, Krueger R, Almeida C, *et al.* A sensitive and rapid alternative to HLA typing as a genetic screening test for abacavir hypersensitivity syndrome. *Pharmacogenet Genomics* 2006;**16**:353–7.

38 Hung S, Chung W, Jee S, *et al.* Genetic susceptibility to carbamazepine-induced cutaneous adverse drug reactions. *Pharmacogenet Genomics* 2006;**16**:297–306.

39 Uetrecht J. Is it possible to more accurately predict which drug candidates will cause idiosyncratic drug reactions? *Curr Drug Metab* 2000;**1**:133–41.

40 Shear N, Spielberg S, Grant D, Tang B, Kalow W. Differences in Metabolism of Sulfonamides Predisposing to Idiosyncratic Toxicity. *Annals of Internal Medicine* 1986;**105**:179–184.

41 Sullivan J, Shear N. What are some of the lessons learnt from *in vitro* studies of severe unpredictable drug reactions? *Br J Dermatol* 2000;**142**:205.

42 Bastuji-Garin S, Fouchard N, Bertocchi M, Roujeau JC, Revuz J, Wolkenstein P. SCORTEN: a severity-of-illness score for toxic epidermal necrolysis. *J Invest Dermatol* 2000;**115**:149–53.

43 Pichler W, Yawalkar N, Britschgi M, *et al.* Cellular and molecular pathophysiology of cutaneous drug reactions. *Am J Clin Dermatol* 2002;**3**:229–38.

44 Yawalkar N. Drug-induced exanthems. *Toxicology* 2005;**209**:131–4.

45 Pichler W. Delayed drug hypersensitivity reactions. *Ann Intern Med* 2003;**139**:683–93.

46 Roujeau JC, Stern R. Severe adverse cutaneous reactions to drugs. *N Engl J Med* 1994;**331**:1272–85.

47 Baba M, Karakas M, Aksungur V, Homan S, Acar MA, Memisoglu H. The anticonvulsant hypersensitivity syndrome. *J Eur Acad Dermatol Venereol* 2003;**17**:399–401.

48 Gupta A, Eggo M, Uetrecht J, *et al.* Drug-induced hypothyroidism: the thyroid as a target organ in hypersensitivity reactions to anticonvulsants and sulfonamides. *Clin Pharmacol Ther* 1992;**51**:56–67.

49 Vittorio C, Muglia J. Anticonvulsant hypersensitivity syndrome. *Arch Intern Med* 1995;**155**:2285–90.

50 Schlienger R, Knowles S, Shear N. Lamotrigine-associated anticonvulsant hypersensitivity syndrome. *Neurology* 1998;**51**:1172–5.

51 Ohtani T, Hiroi A, Sakurane M, Furukawa F. Slow acetylator genotypes as a possible risk factor for infectious mononucleosis-like syndrome induced by salazosulfapyridine. *Br J Dermatol* 2003;**148**:1035–9.

52 Cribb A, Spielberg S. Sulfamethoxazole is metabolized to the hydroxylamine in humans. *Clin Pharmacol Ther* 1992;**51**:522–6.

53 Knowles S, Uetrecht J, Shear N. Idiosyncratic drug reactions: the reactive metabolite syndromes. *Lancet* 2000;**356**:1587–91.

54 Knowles S, Shapiro L, Shear N. Should celecoxib be contraindicated in patients who are allergic to sulfonamides? Revisiting the meaning of "sulfa" allergy. *Drug Saf* 2001;**24**:239–47.

55 Harman K, Morris S, Higgins E. Persistent anticonvulsant hypersensitivity syndrome responding to ciclosporin. *Clin Exp Dermatology* 2003;**28**:364–5.

56 Kano Y, Inaoka M, Sakuma K, Shiohara T. Virus reactivation and intravenous immunoglobulin (IVIG) therapy of drug-induced hypersensitivity syndromes. *Toxicology* 2005;**209**:165–7.

57 Kerns D, Shira J, Go S. Ampicillin rash in children. *Am J Dis Child* 1973;**125**:187–90.

58 Haverkos H, Amsel Z, Drotman D. Adverse virus-drug interactions. *Rev Infect Dis* 1991;**13**:697–704.

59 Levy M. The combined effect of viruses and drugs in drug-induced diseases. *Med Hypotheses* 1984;**14**:293–6.

60 Geyman J, Erickson S. The ampicillin rash as a diagnostic and management problem: case reports and literature review. *J Fam Pract* 1978;**7**:493–6.

61 Levy M. Role of viral infections in the induction of adverse drug reactions. *Drug Saf* 1997;**16**:1–8.

62 Koopmans P, van der Ven J, Vree T, *et al*. Pathogenesis of hypersensitivity reactions to drugs in patients with HIV infection: allergic or toxic? *AIDS* 1995;**9**:217–22.

63 Lee B, Wong D, Benowitz N, Sullam P. Altered patterns of drug metabolism in patients with acquired immunodeficiency syndrome. *Clin Pharmacol Ther* 1993;**53**:529–35.

64 Lin D, Tucker M, Rieder M. Increased adverse drug reactions to antimicrobials and anticonvulsants in patients with HIV infection. *Ann Pharmacother* 2006;**40**:1594–601.

65 Descamps V, Valance A, Edlinger C, *et al*. Association of human herpesvirus 6 infection with drug reaction with eosinophilia and systemic symptoms. *Arch Dermatol* 2001;**137**:301–4.

66 Kano Y, Inaoka M, Shiohara T. Association between anticonvulsant hypersensitivity syndrome and human herpesvirus 6 reactivation and hypogammaglobulinemia. *Arch Dermatol* 2004;**140**:183–8.

67 Tohyama M, Yahata Y, Yasukawa M, *et al*. Severe hypersensitivity syndrome due to sulfasalazine associated with human herpesvirus 6. *Arch Dermatol* 1998;**134**:1113–7.

68 Wong G, Shear N. Is a drug alone sufficient to cause the drug hypersensitivity syndrome? *Arch Dermatol* 2004;**140**:226–30.

69 Khoo B, Leow Y. A review of inpatients with adverse drug reactions to allopurinol. *Singapore Med J* 2000;**41**:156–60.

70 Masaki T, Fukunaga A, Tohyama M, *et al*. Human herpes virus 6 encephalitis in allopurinol-induced hypersensitivity syndrome. *Acta Derm Venereol* 2003;**83**:128–31.

71 Fujino Y, Nakajima M, Inoue H, *et al*. Human herpesvirus 6 encephalitis associated with hypersensitivity syndrome. *Ann Neurol* 2002;**51**:771–4.

72 Fairley C, Smoleniec J, Caul O, Miller E. Observational study of effect of intrauterine transfusions on outcome of fetal hydrops after parvovirus B19. *Lancet* 1995;**346**:1335–7.

73 Bethge W, Beck R, Jahn G, *et al*. Successful treatment of human herpesvirus-6 encephalitis after bone marrow transplantation. *Bone Marrow Trans* 1999;**24**:1245–8.

74 Dewhurst S. Human herpesvirus type 6 and human herpesvirus type 7 infections of the central nervous system. *Herpes* 2004;**11**:105A–111A.

75 Rapaport D, Engelhard D, Tagger G, *et al*. Antiviral prophylaxis may prevent human herpesvirus-6 reactivation in bone marrow transplant recipients. *Transpl Infect Dis* 2002;**4**:10–6.

76 Huiming Y, Chaomin W, Meng M. Vitamin A for treating measles in children. *Cochrane Database Syst Rev* 2005;(**4**):CD001479.

77 Ross A. Vitamin A status: relationship to immunity and the antibody response. *Proc Soc Exp Biol Med* 1992;**200**:303–20.

78 D'Souza R, D'Souza R. Vitamin A for the treatment of children with measles: a systematic review. *J Trop Pediatr* 2002;**48**:323–7.

79 American Academy of Pediatrics. *Red Book: Report of the Committee on Infectious Diseases*. 23rd ed. Illinois: American Academy of Pediatrics, 1994.

80 Mahalanabis D, Jana S, Shaikh S, *et al*. Vitamin E and vitamin C supplementation does not improve the clinical course of measles with pneumonia in children: a controlled trial. *J Trop Pediatrics* 2005;**52**:302–3.

81 Gu R, Shi YY, Wu TX, Liu GJ, Zhang MM. Chinese medicinal herbs for measles. *Cochrane Database Syst Rev* 2006;(**2**):CD005531.

82 Chakrabarty A, Beutner K. Therapy of other viral infections: herpes to hepatitis. *Dermatologic Therapy* 2004;**17**:465–90.

83 Shelley W, Hashim M, Shelley E. Acyclovir in the treatment of hand, foot and mouth disease. *Cutis* 1996;**57**:232–4.

84 Faulkner CF, Godbolt AM, DeAmbrosis B, Triscott J. Hand, foot and mouth disease in an immunocompromised adult treated with aciclovir. *Australas J Dermatol* 2005;**44**:203–6.

43 Herpes simplex

Vera Mahler

Background

Definition

Herpes simplex virus (HSV) is a human pathogenic DNA virus that causes a variety of disease manifestations, ranging from localized skin and mucous membrane lesions to severe disseminated infections (such as neonatal herpes simplex, eczema herpeticum, and herpetic meningoencephalitis). In localized manifestations, grouped vesicles are predominantly located at the lips and nostrils, in the mouth and face, and on the genitals. The vesicles may rupture and ulcerate. Lesions are accompanied by pain and/or itching, and in genital lesions also with dysuria and malaise.

Etiology

Herpes simplex virus infections are transmitted by two virus species, HSV-1 and HSV-2, belonging to the group of double-stranded DNA-type viruses (Herpesviridae family, subfamily Alphaherpesvirinae, genus *Simplexvirus*) (Figures 43.1, 43.2). HSV-1 is still most frequently transmitted by saliva and HSV-2 by genital transmission,[1–3] although these findings are no longer reliable in individual cases. Infection is contracted through direct skin contact (not necessarily in the genital area) with an infected person, and less frequently by indirect contact. Transmission can occur not only during an active symptomatic HSV manifestation, but also from virus shedding from the skin in the absence of symptoms.[4,5] The peak viral DNA load has been reported to occur after 48 h, with no virus detected beyond 96 h after the onset of symptoms.[6] In general, symptoms appear 3–6 days after contact with the virus, but may not appear for up to a month or more after infection.

Incidence/prevalence

HSV-1 infection frequently occurs during childhood, and

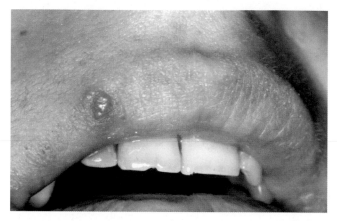

Figure 43.1 Primary herpes simplex infection with HSV-1 may occur at the oral mucocutaneous site. Recalcitrant recurrences of labial herpes may be triggered by a variety of factors.

over 90% of adolescents have specific antibodies in their sera indicating a previous primary (maybe occult) infection. For HSV-2, there is an increasing prevalence of about 20% from the age of puberty onward.[1,3]

Prognosis

Active localized manifestations heal spontaneously within 2–6 weeks without scarring, unless bacterial superinfection has occurred. However, herpes simplex establishes a latent infection in cells of the nervous system by incorporation of dsDNA into the cell nucleus, which can be reactivated by certain trigger factors (e.g., febrile infections, trauma, menstruation, stress, intense ultraviolet exposure). Disseminated systemic disease may be fatal.

Diagnostic tests

In most cases, the diagnosis is based on the characteristic clinical appearance of lesions. In uncertain cases, diagnostic tests and proof of virus can be necessary. HSV can be grown in virus culture from vesicles, swabs from skin and mucous

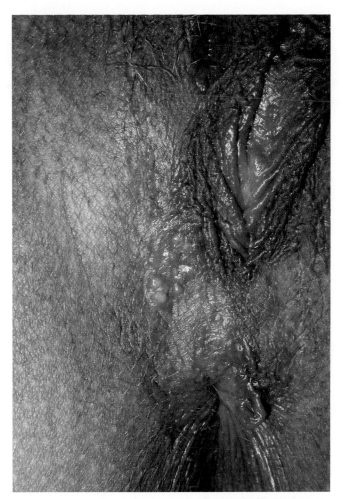

Figure 43.2 Primary herpes simplex infection with HSV-2 may manifest as genital herpes. Recalcitrant recurrences may severely hamper the quality of life for the patients affected.

membranes, tissue biopsies, and cerebrospinal fluid (during the first 2 days of disease manifestation). Whereas these tests take several days to complete, a Tzanck smear from the base of a fresh blister takes only minutes. However, the Tzanck preparation only shows signs of infection (giant cells with multiple nuclei) in 50–79% of patients with a herpes infection, and a negative Tzanck preparation may have to be confirmed by a herpes culture. Detection of HSV antigen (by direct immunofluorescence) or HSV DNA (by polymerase chain reaction) are further diagnostic tests for valid diagnosis of HSV infection. In individuals with a primary HSV infection, specific IgM antibodies can be detected after 10 days (e.g., using a Western blot assay), followed by a subsequent increase in IgG antibodies. Reactivation cannot be adequately confirmed serologically.

Aims of treatment

Episodes of active disease are self-limiting in the immunocompetent adult. However, many patients with primary and recurrent genital and extragenital herpes simplex may seek treatment because of pain associated with the lesions, the duration of the condition, and virus shedding during active disease.

Relevant outcomes

Clinical cure of active lesions is the clinically most relevant outcome. Treatment success is defined as shortening of the duration of pain, active lesions, and virus shedding. Secondary outcomes include time to recurrence and reactivation of latent infection.

Methods of search

The Cochrane Library for Systematic Reviews (third quarter, 2007), the Cochrane Controlled Trials Register (third quarter, 2007) and Medline (1966–August 2007) were searched for randomized controlled trials of all interventions for primary and secondary herpes simplex infections in immunocompetent adults.

If no systematic reviews or randomized controlled trials (RCTs) were found, this is stated and the next best nonrandomized evidence (e.g., large nonrandomized controlled studies, cohort studies, or large case series) are discussed with suitable warnings regarding potential bias.

Questions

Which treatment in primary manifestation of an oral/labial herpes simplex is beneficial with regard to total lesion clearance in the immunocompetent adult?

Efficacy
Neither a systematic review nor RCTs were found on therapeutic interventions with *topical* antiviral agents versus placebo/no treatment at first onset of a primary oral manifestation in immunocompetent adults.

Similarly, no systematic reviews or larger RCTs were found concerning *systemic* interventions for a primary oral manifestation of herpes simplex in immunocompetent adults. A protocol for a systematic review on aciclovir in the treatment of primary herpetic gingivostomatitis in children and young adults (under the age of 25) was recently published.[7]

Data are available from two smaller RCTs conducted in children. The first of these was a double-blind RCT including 20 children with a mean age of 2 years (with a primary manifestation of herpetic stomatitis/gingivitis of less than 4 days' duration), who received oral aciclovir (200 mg five times per day). Active treatment reduced the mean duration of pain (4.3 days with aciclovir versus 5.0 days with placebo; $P = 0.05$).[8] In the second RCT (including 72 children aged 1–6 years with an onset of herpetic gingivostomatitis less than 3 days earlier), oral aciclovir (15 mg/kg five times per day for 7 days) significantly reduced the median time to healing (4 days with aciclovir versus 10 days with placebo; median difference 6 days, 95% confidence interval 4 days to 8 days).[9]

Drawbacks

No significant adverse effects occurred in either group of treated children.[8,9]

Comments

No RCTs on interventions for a primary manifestation of an oral/labial herpes simplex infection in the immunocompetent adult were found. The data are derived from trials conducted in children. Adult patients may not consult physicians until they experience recurrences of oral herpes simplex, making research on the effectiveness of therapeutic interventions in the primary manifestation difficult.

Implications for clinical practice

On the basis of data obtained in affected children, oral antiviral agents (acyclovir) are likely to be beneficial in the first onset of oral/labial herpes simplex. Topical antiviral agents are of unknown effectiveness for primary manifestations of oral/labial herpes simplex in the immunocompetent adult.

Which therapeutic interventions are beneficial for preventing recurrences of labial herpes simplex in immunocompetent adults?

Efficacy

No systematic reviews were found on the prevention of recurrences of labial herpes simplex in immunocompetent adults. Six RCTs were found on the suppression of oral recurrences in immunocompetent adults by prophylactic intake of oral antiviral agents.[10–14] Their results are discordant.

The first RCT observed a reduction in the frequency and duration of labial recurrences in skiers (n = 147) with a history of ultraviolet-precipitated herpes labialis using prophylactic oral aciclovir (400 mg twice daily, beginning 12 h before ultraviolet exposure) in comparison with placebo ($P < 0.05$).[10] Five of 75 aciclovir-treated patients (7%) developed lesions, in comparison with 19 (26%) of 72 persons in the placebo group.

The second, rather small RCT (20 individuals with at least six episodes of herpes labialis/year) found that aciclovir (400 mg twice daily for 4 months) led to 53% fewer clinical recurrences than placebo ($P = 0.05$) and a more than 2.5-fold greater prolongation in the median time to first clinical recurrence (46 to 118 days; $P = 0.05$).[11]

The pooled analysis of two further RCTs[12] (98 adults with at least four episodes of herpes labialis in the previous year) found that oral valaciclovir 500 mg daily significantly increased the interval to recurrence in comparison with placebo (no recurrence within 4 months: 62% with oral valaciclovir versus 40% with placebo; $P = 0.041$; mean time to recurrence 13.1 weeks with oral valaciclovir versus 9.6 weeks with placebo; $P = 0.016$).

In contrast, two RCTs found no effect of prophylactic antiviral treatment. In 239 skiers with a history of recurrent herpes labialis, no significant differences were observed with regard to the occurrence of herpetic lesions between the active treatment group (800 mg aciclovir twice daily, starting on the day before ultraviolet exposure) in comparison with the placebo group—21 of 93 (23%) with aciclovir versus 21 of 102 (21%) with placebo ($P = 0.92$; 95% CI not stated).[13]

In another RCT including 248 adults with a history of sun-induced recurrent herpes labialis, famciclovir was administered in different regimens (125, 250 or 500 mg, respectively, three times a day for 5 days, beginning 48 h *after* artificial ultraviolet exposure) in comparison with placebo.[14] In these conditions, no significant differences were found between the four groups with regard to numbers of lesions (P value not reported). However, a dose–response relationship was found between increasing doses of famciclovir and significantly reduced size and duration of the lesions. The 500-mg dose alone, but not the other doses, significantly reduced the mean time to healing by 2 days (4 vs. 6 days, 33% reduction; $P = 0.01$) and the size of lesions (mean size of lesions; $P = 0.04$; mean time to healing: $P = 0.01$).

Apart from prophylactic treatment with antiviral agents, it has been suggested that L-lysine has antiviral activity due to its antagonism of arginine metabolism, which is required in HSV replication. A double-blind RCT found that L-lysine monohydrochlorine was ineffective administered at daily doses of 624 mg orally, but effective with regard to the recurrence rates of herpes simplex infection in immunocompetent patients when administered at very high oral doses of 1248 mg daily. In the high-dosage lysine group, during the treatment period of 24 weeks, 0.89 recurrences per patient (i.e., 0.037 per patient per week) were seen, in comparison with 1.56 recurrences per patient (i.e., 0.065 recurrences per patient per week) during placebo treatment in the same group. In the low-dose group, 2.27 recurrences per patient and 0.095 recurrences per patient and week were seen during active treatment.[15] The duration of symptoms was not influenced in comparison with placebo.[15]

Drawbacks

Mild to moderate headache and nausea were the most common adverse effects reported. The first RCT found no significant differences between the two treatment groups with regard to adverse effects involving the central nervous system or gastrointestinal tract—seven of 77 (10%) with aciclovir versus three of 76 (4%) with placebo ($P = 0.34$).[10] The second RCT provided no information about adverse effects.[11] The pooled analysis of two RCTs comparing valaciclovir to placebo found slightly fewer adverse events (mostly mild headache) with the active treatment in comparison with placebo (22 events in 33% of those taking valaciclovir versus 29 events in 39% of those taking placebo).[12]

The fourth RCT found no significant differences in frequency of adverse events—58 of 115 (50%) with aciclovir versus 59 of 124 (48%) with placebo ($P = 0.68$).[13] The fifth RCT found no severe adverse events with either dose of famciclovir and no differences (frequencies not reported) in relation to headache or nausea between the different groups.[14]

Comments

The participants in the fourth RCT were allowed to use paracetamol as concomitant medication and were encouraged to use sunscreens.[13] Sunscreens could be a confounder with the effects of aciclovir in this study, since sunscreens *per se* could have a preventive effect on herpetic recurrences. A systematic review on this issue was not found. Two small crossover RCTs are available.[16,17] The first RCT, including 38 individuals with a history of ultraviolet-induced reactivation of herpes labialis, found that sunscreen significantly reduced recurrences at 6 days in comparison with placebo—no recurrences in 35 patients with sunscreen versus 27 of 38 (71%) with placebo ($P < 0.001$).[16] The second RCT (19 individuals exposed to a defined dose of ultraviolet light in artificial conditions) also found that sunscreen significantly reduced recurrences at 6 days in comparison with placebo—one of 19 (5%) with sunscreen versus 11 of 19 (58%) with placebo ($P < 0.01$).[17]

Implications for clinical practice

Oral antiviral agents, as well as the use of sunscreens, are likely to beneficial for prevention of labial recurrences. Prophylactic oral antiviral agents may reduce the frequency and severity of attacks in comparison with placebo.[10-14] However, the optimal timing and duration of treatment is uncertain. Topical antivirals are of unknown effectiveness, since no RCTs are available on the effects of prophylactic use of topical antiviral agents.

Which treatments are effective in treating recurrent oral/labial herpes simplex in the immunocompetent adult?

Efficacy

Topical treatment of recurrences. Several RCTs are available on topical aciclovir/penciclovir versus placebo for treatment in cases of clinical manifestation of recurrent oral/labial herpes simplex in immunocompetent adults.[18-28] Most RCTs found that aciclovir significantly reduced healing time up to 2 days in comparison with placebo (median value to complete healing in placebo: 8 days versus 6 days with aciclovir).[19,20,23-26] In a small RCT (n = 15) with a crossover design, aciclovir in liposomes significantly reduced the time to crusting of lesions in comparison with aciclovir cream (1.8 days vs. 3.5 days; $P = 0.023$).[28] One RCT found no significant difference in healing time between topical aciclovir and placebo.[21]

Four RCTs found no significant differences in the duration of pain between aciclovir and placebo,[18,20,21,23] whereas one large RCT on treatment with penciclovir showed a significantly reduced duration of pain (median 3.5 days with penciclovir versus 4.1 days with placebo; $P < 0.001$),[22] as well as a reduced healing time of up to 2 days.[22,25] A number of the smaller trials found no significant effect of topical antiviral treatment in reactivated labial herpes, possibly due to a lack of statistical power.

In addition to antiviral agents, other topical preparations (e.g., local anesthetics and zinc oxide) have also been suggested in order to reduce the healing time and duration of pain.

One double-blind RCT (n = 72) found that 1.8% tetracaine (amethocaine) cream (applied six times per day) significantly reduced the mean time to loss of crusts (5.1 days with tetracaine versus 7.2 days with placebo; $P = 0.002$) and significantly increased the subjective benefit of treatment.[29]

One double-blind RCT (n = 46) found that zinc oxide/glycine (applied twice per hour during waking hours from the first signs of the herpetic reactivation) significantly reduced time to healing in comparison with placebo (5.0 days with cream versus 6.5 days with placebo; $P = 0.018$).[30]

Systemic treatment of recurrences. Four RCTs were found on systemic antiviral treatment of recurrences in immunocompetent adults.[31-33] The first (including 174 adults with recurrent herpes labialis) found that oral aciclovir (400 mg five times per day for 5 days), taken from the first signs of recurrence (symptoms of labial tingling) significantly reduced the duration of clinical symptoms in comparison with placebo (8.1 days with oral aciclovir versus 12.5 days with placebo; $P = 0.02$).[31] The second RCT (n = 149) compared oral aciclovir (200 mg five times per day for 5 days) started within 12 hours of the recurrence with placebo.[32] No significant differences were found with regard to healing time or duration of pain between oral aciclovir and placebo (mean healing time 7.78 days with aciclovir versus 8.64 days with placebo; P value not reported; mean duration of pain: 1.31 days with aciclovir versus 1.35 days with placebo; P value not reported). Two further RCTs (published in the same paper) compared oral valaciclovir (2 g twice per day administered for 1 day only), oral valaciclovir (2 g twice per day on the first day followed by 1 g twice per day on the second day) and placebo in patients over 12 years of age with a history of recurrent herpes labialis.[33] One of these RCTs (n = 902) found that both regimens significantly reduced the median duration of vesicular and nonvesicular lesions in comparison with placebo (4.0 days with 1-day treatment, $P < 0.001$; 4.5 days with 2-day treatment with valaciclovir, $P = 0.009$ versus 5.0 days with placebo). The other RCT (n = 954) found similar results (5.0 days with 1-day treatment, $P < 0.001$; 5.0 days with 2-day treatment with valaciclovir, $P < 0.001$ versus 5.5 days with placebo). Neither RCT found a significant difference between 1-day treatment and 2-day treatment with valaciclovir (P values not reported).

Drawbacks

Topical treatment. No serious adverse events of topical antiviral agents were reported, and similar rates of minor adverse effects occurred in the active treatment groups and placebo groups.[18–28] No adverse effects were reported as a result of topical treatment with 1.8% tetracaine (amethocaine) cream.[29] Transient mild to moderate sensations of burning, itching, stinging, or tingling were reported in up to 22% (n = 7) of patients treated with zinc oxide, versus 7% (n = 2) with placebo.[30]

Systemic treatment. The first two RCTs on oral antiviral treatment provided no information about adverse events.[31,32] In the large third and fourth RCTs,[33] headache was more common with valaciclovir than with placebo (third RCT: 9% with 1-day treatment; 9% with 2-day treatment with valaciclovir versus 4% with placebo; P values not reported; fourth RCT: 10% with 1-day treatment; 9% with 2-day treatment versus 5% with placebo; P values not reported).[33] The other most common adverse events, nausea and diarrhea, were reported equally in all three treatment groups (1-day treatment with valaciclovir, 2-day treatment with valaciclovir, and placebo).

Comments

Early treatment after onset of the recurrence is apparently feasible, but no RCTs on early versus delayed intervention are available. Firm conclusions about the most feasible timing of systemic antiviral treatment can therefore not be drawn.

Implications for clinical practice

Data from a number of RCTs comparing topical antiviral agents with placebo in the treatment of recurrences of herpes labialis show discordant results with regard to the duration of pain, but provide stronger evidence that topical penciclovir and aciclovir reduce the healing time. One small RCT found limited evidence that topical tetracaine reduced the mean time to scab loss. One small RCT found limited

evidence that zinc oxide cream reduced time to healing, but found a higher proportion of mild skin irritation compared with placebo.

RCTs on the systemic treatment of recurrent episodes of labial herpes provided limited evidence that oral aciclovir and valaciclovir (if taken early at the first symptoms of recurrence) slightly reduced the duration of lesions and pain in comparison with placebo.

Which treatments are beneficial in primary manifestations of genital herpes simplex in the immunocompetent adult?

Efficacy

A systematic review is not yet available. However, a protocol for a Cochrane review does exist (dated 2004).[34] Of three RCTs identified,[35–37] the first (including 119 individuals with primary manifestation of genital herpes) compared aciclovir (200 mg five times per day for 10 days) versus placebo[35] and showed that aciclovir significantly reduced the time to complete healing of lesions (12 days with aciclovir versus 14 days with placebo; $P = 0.005$), reduced the formation of new lesions (18% with aciclovir versus 62% with placebo; $P = 0.001$), reduced the duration of pain (5 days with aciclovir versus 7 days with placebo; $P = 0.05$) and reduced viral shedding in comparison with placebo (2 days with aciclovir versus 9 days with placebo; $P < 0.001$). The second RCT (including 31 individuals with primary manifestation of genital herpes) compared aciclovir (200 mg five times daily for 5 days) with placebo[36] and found similar results with regard to the median time to healing (6 days with aciclovir versus 11 days with placebo; $P = 0.06$), median duration of pain (4 days with aciclovir versus 8 days with placebo; $P < 0.05$) and viral shedding (1 day with aciclovir versus 13 days with placebo; $P < 0.01$). In the third RCT (including 31 women and 17 men), aciclovir (200 mg five times daily for 10 days) or placebo was administered.[37] Aciclovir significantly reduced the time to crusting (mean time to crusting in women: 8.8 days with aciclovir versus 15.0 days with placebo; $P = 0.01$; in men: 5 days with aciclovir versus 15 days with placebo; $P = 0.01$) and viral shedding (in women: 4.9 days with aciclovir versus 17.7 days with placebo; $P = 0.001$; in men: 6 days with aciclovir versus 15 days with placebo; $P = 0.02$).

A systematic review comparing valaciclovir with aciclovir was not found. One large RCT (including 643 individuals with a first episode of genital herpes) compared oral valaciclovir (100 mg twice daily for 10 days) with oral aciclovir (200 mg five times daily for 10 days).[38] It found no significant difference between the treatments with regard to healing time (hazard ratio 1.08; 95% CI, 0.92 to 1.27), duration of symptoms (HR 1.02; 95% CI, 0.85 to 1.22) or duration of viral shedding (HR 1.00; 95% CI, 0.84 to 1.18).

Drawbacks

Adverse effects were rare and similar in the placebo and treatment groups (aciclovir).[36,37] In a large RCT, headache occurred in 11.5% and nausea in 5.9% of patients treated with aciclovir.[38] There were no differences with regard to adverse events between the aciclovir and valaciclovir groups.

Comments

In one of the RCTs,[35] 30 of 180 participants (17%) were excluded before analysis—10 because the study protocol was not completed, 12 due to suspected previous infection, and eight because herpes simplex virus was not isolated.[35] Famciclovir (according to expert guidelines) is also a recommended treatment for the first clinical episode of genital herpes.[39]

Implications for clinical practice

Oral antiviral treatment with aciclovir/valaciclovir in patients with a primary manifestation of genital herpes is effective with regard to the duration of lesions, symptoms, and viral shedding in comparison with placebo. One large RCT found no differences in clinical outcomes between oral aciclovir and valaciclovir.

Which medical interventions are effective in preventing recurrences of genital herpes simplex in immunocompetent adults?

Efficacy

There is a protocol for a Cochrane systematic review on suppressive antiviral therapy for recurrent genital herpes in immunocompetent individuals (dating from 2003).[40] Several oral antiviral agents have been suggested for prophylaxis against the reactivation of genital herpes.

Aciclovir versus placebo. One nonsystematic review based on two RCTs (n = 107)[41] found in the first RCT (n = 32) that aciclovir (800 mg/day) reduced recurrences in comparison with placebo at 2 years—no recurrence at 2 years: five of 18 (28%) with aciclovir versus none of 14 (0%) with placebo; absolute risk reduction (ARR) 28% (95% CI, 1% to 51%).[41] In the second RCT (n = 75), aciclovir (400 mg twice/day) also reduced recurrences in comparison with placebo at 1 year—no recurrence at 1 year: 21 of 48 (44%) with aciclovir versus none of 28 (0%) with placebo (ARR 44%; 95% CI, 26% to 56%).

Four other RCTs[42–45] produced concordant results. A large RCT (n = 1479) found that aciclovir (400 mg twice/day) reduced recurrences in comparison with placebo at 1 year (no recurrence at 1 year: 49% with aciclovir versus 5% with placebo; HR 0.21; 95% CI, 0.16 to 0.27).[42] Another RCT (n = 1146) also found that aciclovir (400 mg twice/day) reduced recurrences in comparison with placebo at 1 year (recurrence rate at 1 year: 1.7% with aciclovir versus 12.5%

with placebo; $P < 0.0001$).[43] During continuous treatment with aciclovir (400 mg twice/day) for 5 years (n = 210) in the same trial, 53–70% of patients were free of recurrence each year.[43] In a small RCT in women with recently acquired genital HSV-2 infection (n = 32), aciclovir (400 mg twice/day for 70 days) reduced viral shedding in comparison with placebo by 95% on days with reported lesions and by 94% on days without lesions.[44]

The fourth RCT (n = 1479)[45] compared the suppressive effects of antiviral agents administered once or twice per day in a six-armed protocol (valaciclovir 1000 mg once/day; valaciclovir 500 mg once/day; valaciclovir 250 mg once/day; valaciclovir 250 mg twice/day; aciclovir 400 mg twice/day; or placebo) with regard to quality of life.[46] Aciclovir significantly improved the health-related quality of life in comparison with placebo after 3 months ($P < 0.05$).[45]

Valaciclovir versus placebo. One systematic review (published in 1999; search date not reported)[47] based on two RCTs (n = 1861)[42,48] compared suppressive treatment with valaciclovir versus placebo for frequently recurring genital herpes. The first RCT included in the review (n = 382) found that valaciclovir (500 mg once/day for 16 weeks) significantly increased the time to recurrence in comparison with placebo (HR 0.10; 95% CI, 0.11 to 0.21).[47] At 16 weeks, 69% of the valaciclovir recipients were recurrence-free, in comparison with 9.5% of placebo recipients.

The second RCT[42] identified by the review (n = 1479 people) compared the suppressive effects of valaciclovir administered once or twice per day in a six-armed protocol (valaciclovir 1000 mg once/day; valaciclovir 500 mg once/day; valaciclovir 250 mg once/day; valaciclovir 250 mg twice/day; aciclovir 400 mg twice/day) versus placebo at 1 year. A dose-dependent effect of valaciclovir was observed in relation to freedom from recurrence in comparison with placebo. Kaplan–Meier estimates of the proportions of patients who were recurrence-free at the end of 1 year were 50% for 250 mg valaciclovir twice daily, 48% for 1 g valaciclovir once daily, 49% for 400 mg aciclovir twice daily, and 40% for 500 mg valaciclovir once daily. The estimated proportions decreased to 22% for 250 mg of valaciclovir once daily and 5% for placebo.[42] Subgroup analysis showed that patients with a history of less than 10 recurrences per year were effectively managed with 500 mg of valaciclovir once daily. One gram of valaciclovir once daily, 250 mg of valaciclovir twice daily, or 400 mg of aciclovir twice daily were more effective in patients with 10 or more recurrences per year.[42] Suppressive treatment with valaciclovir (once or twice daily) significantly improved health-related quality of life in comparison with placebo after 3 months (as measured using a recurrent genital herpes quality-of-life questionnaire; $P < 0.05$).[45,46]

A recent RCT (n = 152; n = 109 receiving 1 g valaciclovir per day versus 43 receiving placebo for 60 days) demonstrated a significantly reduced percentage of days with total (clinical and subclinical) HSV-2 shedding throughout 60 days in comparison with placebo.[49]

In the intention-to-treat population, a 71% reduction in total shedding ($P < 0.001$), a 58% reduction in subclinical shedding ($P < 0.001$), and a 64% reduction in clinical shedding ($P < 0.01$) were observed.[49]

Famciclovir versus placebo. One systematic review (published in 1999, search date not reported)[47] based on two RCTs (n = 830) found that famciclovir significantly increased the median time to first recurrence in comparison with placebo. In the first RCT (n = 455), famciclovir (250 mg twice a day, 125 mg three times per day, or 250 mg three times per day for 1 year) increased the median time to first recurrence significantly in comparison with placebo (11 months with famciclovir 250 mg twice per day, versus 10 months with famciclovir 250 mg three times per day, versus 8 months with famciclovir 125 mg three times per day, versus 1.5 months with placebo). In the second RCT (n = 375), female recipients received famciclovir (125 mg twice a day, 125 mg four times per day, 250 mg twice a day, 250 mg four times per day, or 500 mg four times per day, or placebo for 4 months). Famciclovir 250 mg twice a day was found to be the most effective dosage for reducing recurrences.[47] In comparison with placebo, significant numbers of famciclovir recipients were free of recurrences at 4 months (78% with 250 mg twice a day versus 42% with placebo).

Valaciclovir versus famciclovir. Two RCTs have been reported concerning the comparison of famciclovir (250 mg b.i.d.) and valaciclovir (500 mg/day) administered as daily suppressive therapy for individuals with genital herpes.[50] Study 1 (including 320 participants) compared the clinical effect of the drugs given for 16 weeks; study 2 compared the virological effect of the drugs given for 10 days in 70 HSV-2 seropositive patients. In study 1, the time to first recurrence was similar in the famciclovir and valaciclovir recipients, with a hazard ratio (HR) of 1.17 (95% CI, 0.78 to 1.76), but the time to the first virologically confirmed recurrence was shorter among famciclovir recipients (HR 2.15; 95% CI, 1.00 to 4.60). In study 2, HSV was detected on 3.2% of days among famciclovir recipients and 1.3% of days among valaciclovir recipients (relative risk 2.33; 95% CI, 1.18 to 4.89).[50]

Drawbacks

Daily treatments with aciclovir, famciclovir, and valaciclovir were well tolerated.[42,51] The safety profiles of all of the treatments were comparable.

The aciclovir recipients were followed for up to 7 years, and the famciclovir and valaciclovir recipients for up to 1 year.[51] Nausea and headache were infrequent, and participants rarely discontinued treatment due to adverse effects. No evidence was found that suppressive daily treatment

with aciclovir results in the development of aciclovir resistance during or after stopping treatment in healthy adults.[51]

Comments

Further comparative trials of antiviral drugs for the suppression of genital herpes recurrences should be conducted, as aciclovir and penciclovir appear to have different abilities to abrogate HSV reactivation.

Recurrences of genital herpes often arise during pregnancy and can have serious implications for neonatal herpes if the infections are silent and the child is delivered vaginally. Although prevention and treatment of genital herpes during pregnancy is beyond the scope of this chapter, it should be mentioned that antiviral agents are not approved for the treatment of genital herpes in breast-feeding and pregnant women. A systematic review based on three RCTs dealing with the treatment of genital herpes in pregnant women found no evidence of adverse effects of aciclovir in the women or the newborns.[52] Aciclovir prophylaxis beginning at 36 weeks' gestation was effective in reducing clinical HSV recurrences at the time of delivery (odds ratio 0.25; 95% CI, 0.15 to 0.40), cesarean deliveries for clinical recurrence of genital herpes (OR 0.30; 95% CI, 0.13 to 0.67), total HSV detection at delivery (OR 0.11; 95% CI, 0.04 to 0.31), and asymptomatic HSV shedding at delivery (OR 0.09; 95% CI, 0.02 to 0.39).[53]

A recent RCT in HSV-2 seropositive patients for evaluation of the efficacy of suppressive therapy with oral valaciclovir 500 mg or placebo twice daily from 36 weeks' gestation until delivery did not identify any maternal or neonatal safety concerns.[54] In the 112 women who were included (57 with valaciclovir, 55 with placebo) the number of women with clinical HSV recurrences between the time of randomization and delivery was significantly lower in the valaciclovir versus the placebo group (10.5% versus 27.3%; $P = 0.023$; relative risk 0.4; 95% CI, 0.2 to 0.9). Shedding of HSV within 7 days of delivery was similar in the valaciclovir and placebo groups (10.4% versus 12.0%; $P = 0.804$; RR 0.9; 95% CI, 0.3 to 2.7), as was the number of women with clinical HSV lesions at delivery (5.3% versus 14.6%; $P = 0.121$; RR 0.4; 95% CI, 0.1 to 1.3). No neonates had symptomatic congenital HSV infection before discharge or up to 2 weeks postpartum.[54] In a second RCT (including 350 pregnant women with a history of genital herpes) following the same suppressive treatment approach (170 patients were treated with valaciclovir and 168 received placebo), it was shown that valaciclovir suppression significantly reduces HSV shedding and recurrent genital herpes requiring cesarean delivery. Vaginal delivery was permitted if no clinical recurrence or prodromal symptoms were present. At delivery, 28 women (8%) had recurrent genital herpes requiring cesarean delivery—4% in the valaciclovir group and 13% in the placebo group ($P = 0.009$). Herpes simplex virus was detected by culture in 2% of the valaciclovir group and 9% of the placebo group ($P = 0.02$). No infants were diagnosed with neonatal HSV, and there were no significant differences in neonatal complications.[55]

There is a protocol for a Cochrane systematic review (dated 2004) on third-trimester antiviral therapy to prevent recurrent genital herpes at delivery.[56]

Implications for clinical practice

Oral antiviral maintenance treatment in patients with a history of frequent recurrences is of benefit. Daily maintenance treatment with oral antiviral agents reduces the frequency of recurrences, and improves the quality of life in comparison with placebo.

Valaciclovir appears to be somewhat better than famciclovir for suppressing genital herpes and associated shedding.

What are effective therapeutic interventions for the treatment of recurrent genital herpes simplex in immunocompetent adults?

Efficacy

Aciclovir versus placebo. No systematic reviews were found. In one nonsystematic review (n = 650 people)[41] in comparison with placebo oral aciclovir (200 mg five times/day or 800 mg twice/day, administered early at the first signs of recurrence for 5 days) reduced duration of lesions (5 days with aciclovir vs. 6 days with placebo) and the duration of viral shedding (1 day with aciclovir versus 2 days with placebo).[41]

In another RCT (n = 131 individuals with more than three recurrences during the previous 12 months, followed at least until the next recurrence) aciclovir (800 mg three times/day for 2 days) significantly reduced the duration of episodes (median duration: 4 days with aciclovir versus 6 days with placebo; $P < 0.001$), the duration of lesions (median duration: 4 days with aciclovir versus 6 days with placebo; $P = 0.001$) and viral shedding median duration: 25.0 hours with aciclovir versus 58.5 hours with placebo; $P = 0.04$).[57] The benefit was marked if the treatment was initiated early at the first signs of recurrence.[58]

Valaciclovir versus placebo. One systematic review (based on one RCT, including 987 patients)[47,59] on patient-initiated treatment with oral valaciclovir (500 or 1000 mg twice/day for 5 days) versus placebo found a decreased duration of the lesion and accompanying discomfort (median duration: 4 days with valaciclovir versus 6 days with placebo; HR 1.9; 95% CI, 1.6 to 2.3), a decreased duration of viral shedding (median duration: 2 days with valaciclovir versus 4 days with placebo; HR 2.9; 95% CI, 2.1 to 3.9), and an increased rate of aborted recurrences in comparison with placebo (aborted recurrences: 31% with valaciclovir versus 21% with placebo; RR 1.5; 95% CI, 1.1 to 1.9).[59] No differences in

the outcomes were noted between the two groups who received valaciclovir (500 mg b.i.d. versus 1000 mg b.i.d.) for 5 days. The lower dosage is therefore recommended.

Valaciclovir versus aciclovir/valaciclovir. One systematic review (based on one RCT; n = 739)[60] on valaciclovir versus aciclovir showed that the two regimens (valaciclovir 500 mg b.i.d.) and aciclovir (200 mg five times/day) given for 5 days were equivalent with regard to healing time, symptom duration, and viral shedding.[47]

No differences were observed between a 3-day and 5-day regimen with valaciclovir (500 mg twice/day; n = 531 individuals with more than six recurrences per year) with regard to episode duration (4.7 days with the 3-day treatment versus 4.6 days with the 5-day treatment with valaciclovir; significance not reported) or aborted recurrences (27% with the 3-day treatment versus 21% with the 5-day treatment with valaciclovir (RR 1; 95% CI, 0.92 to 1.65).[61] Initiating treatment within 6 hours of the first symptoms was associated with a greater likelihood of aborted recurrences than initiation later than 6 hours (OR 1.93; 95% CI, 1.28 to 2.9).[61] Another RCT (including 800 individuals with more than four recurrences per year) found concordant results with 3-day and 5-day treatment with valaciclovir (500 mg twice daily) with regard to the healing time of lesions (4.4 days with the 3-day treatment versus 4.7 days with the 5-day treatment with valaciclovir; HR 0.95; 95% CI, 0.81 to 1.13) and aborted lesions (25.4% with the 3-day treatment versus 26.6% with the 5-day treatment with valaciclovir; RR 1.04; 95% CI, 0.83 to 1.32).[62]

Famciclovir versus placebo. One systematic review was found on famciclovir versus placebo (based on one RCT, n = 467).[47,63] It found that patient-initiated oral treatment with famciclovir (125 mg twice/day, 250 mg twice/day, or 500 mg twice/day for 5 days) led to significant reductions in the healing time (median 3.8 days for famciclovir recipients vs. 4.8 days for placebo recipients), the duration of viral shedding (1.7 days with famciclovir vs. 3.3 days with placebo), and the duration of symptoms (3.2 days with famciclovir versus 3.7 days with placebo; P values not reported).[63] Famciclovir (125 mg twice daily) was effective, and higher doses did not confer any additional benefit.

Famciclovir versus aciclovir. No significant differences were found in one RCT (n = 204) between oral famciclovir and aciclovir with regard to the time to healing (mean: 5.1 days with famciclovir versus 5.4 days with aciclovir; mean difference +0.3 days; 95% CI, −0.3 days to +0.8 days).[64]

Drawbacks

Adverse effects (mostly headache and nausea) were rare and occurred at similar frequencies in all of the treatment groups (aciclovir, valaciclovir, famciclovir, placebo).[47]

Comments

Antiviral agents are not approved for the treatment of genital herpes in breastfeeding and pregnant women. One systematic review based on three RCTs dealing with the treatment of genital herpes in pregnant women found no evidence of adverse effects in either the women or the newborn.[52]

Implication for clinical practice

Oral antiviral treatment (aciclovir, famciclovir, or valaciclovir) initiated as soon as the first symptoms of recurrence appear (e.g., within 6 hours)[61] is effective with regard to total lesion clearance in the immunocompetent adult. Oral antiviral agents reduce the duration of lesions and viral shedding and increase the rate of aborted recurrences in comparison with placebo in individuals with recurrent genital herpes. Aciclovir, famciclovir, and valaciclovir are similarly effective in reducing symptom duration, lesion healing time, and viral shedding. The benefit was marked if treatment was initiated early, at the first signs of recurrence.[58,61]

Key points

- For primary manifestations of oral/labial herpes (which may be severe), antiviral agents (such as aciclovir) are likely to be beneficial with regard to the mean time required for healing.

- Recurrences of herpes simplex labialis are common, but their frequency can be significantly reduced with prophylactic oral treatment with antiviral agents. The optimal timing and duration of treatment is uncertain.

- In reactivated herpes labialis, there is some evidence that topical penciclovir and aciclovir reduce the healing time.

- Oral aciclovir and valaciclovir (if taken early at the first symptoms of recurrence of labial herpes) may reduce the duration of lesions and pain.

- Oral antiviral treatment in the primary manifestation of genital herpes reduces the duration of lesions, symptoms, and viral shedding.

- Daily suppressive treatment with oral antiviral agents (aciclovir 400 mg twice/day, famciclovir 250 mg twice/day, or valaciclovir 500 mg once/day) reduces the frequency of recurrences. In patients with 10 or more recurrences per year, 1 g of valaciclovir once daily, 250 mg of valaciclovir twice daily, or 400 mg of aciclovir twice daily were more effective. Valaciclovir appears to be somewhat better than famciclovir in suppressing genital herpes and the associated shedding.

- Suppressive daily treatment with aciclovir in individuals with a history of recurrent herpes with aciclovir does not result in resistant HSV strains during or after the cessation of treatment in immunocompetent adults.

- In a clinically manifest recurrence of genital herpes, aciclovir, famciclovir, and valaciclovir are similarly effective in reducing symptom duration, lesion healing time, and viral shedding.

- No serious adverse events associated with topical antiviral agents (aciclovir, valaciclovir, or famciclovir) have been reported.

- Key research gaps in the field of herpes simplex include trials on interventions in primary oral/labial herpes simplex in the immunocompetent adult; trials to determine the maximal tolerable interval between the onset of disease and the start of treatment; and the optimal timing and duration of treatment to prevent recurrences.

References

1 Fleming DT, McQuillan GM, Johnson RE, *et al.* Herpes simplex virus type 2 in the United States, 1976 to 1994. *N Engl J Med* 1997;**337**:1105–11.
2 Schomogyi M, Wald A, Corey L. Herpes simplex virus-2 infection. An emerging disease? *Infect Dis Clin North Am* 1998;**12**:47–61.
3 Lafferty WE, Downey L, Celum C, Wald A. Herpes simplex virus 1 as a cause of genital herpes: impact on surveillance and prevention. *J Infect Dis* 2000;**181**:1454–7.
4 Gilbert SC. Oral shedding of herpes simplex virus type 1 in immunocompetent persons. *J Oral Pathol Med* 2006;**35**:548–53.
5 Wald A, Zeh J, Selke S, *et al.* Reactivation of genital herpes simplex virus type 2 infection in asymptomatic seropositive persons. *N Engl J Med* 2000;**153**:844–50.
6 Boivin G, Goyette N, Sergerie Y, *et al.* Longitudinal evaluation of herpes simplex virus DNA load during episodes of herpes labialis. *J Clin Virol* 2006;**37**:248–51.
7 Nasser M, Fedorowicz Z, Khoshnevisan MH, *et al.* Aciclovir for treating primary herpetic gingivostomatitis. (protocol). *Cochrane Database Syst Rev* 2007;(**3**):CD006700.
8 Ducoulombier H, Cousin J, DeWilde A, *et al.* Herpetic stomatitis-gingivitis in children: controlled trial of acyclovir versus placebo. *Ann Pediatr* 1988;**35**:212–6.
9 Amir J, Harel L, Smetana Z, *et al.* Treatment of herpes simplex gingivostomatitis with aciclovir in children: a randomised double blind placebo controlled trial. *BMJ* 1997;**314**:1800–3.
10 Spruance SL, Hammil ML, Hoge WS, *et al.* Acyclovir prevents reactivation of herpes labialis in skiers. *JAMA* 1988;**260**:1597–9.
11 Rooney JF, Strauss SE, Mannix ML, *et al.* Oral acyclovir to suppress frequently recurrent herpes labialis: a double-blind, placebo controlled trial. *Ann Intern Med* 1993;**118**:268–72.
12 Baker D, Eisen D. Valacyclovir for prevention of recurrent herpes labialis: 2 double-blind, placebo-controlled studies. *Cutis* 2003;**71**:239–42.
13 Raborn GW, Martel AY, Grace MG, *et al.* Oral acyclovir in prevention of herpes labialis: a randomized, double-blind, placebo controlled trial. *Oral Surg Oral Med Oral Pathol Oral Radiol Endod* 1998;**85**:55–9.
14 Spruance SL, Rowe NH, Raborn GW, *et al.* Peroral famciclovir in the treatment of experimental ultraviolet radiation-induced herpes simplex labialis: a double-blind, dose-ranging, placebo-controlled, multicenter trial. *J Infect Dis* 1999;**179**:303–10.
15 McCune MA, Perry HO, Muller SA, O'Fallon WM. Treatment of recurrent herpes simplex infections with L-lysine monohydrochloride. *Cutis* 1984;**34**:366–73.

16 Rooney JF, Bryson Y, Mannix ML, *et al.* Prevention of ultraviolet-light-induced herpes labialis by sunscreen. *Lancet* 1991;**338**:1419–21.

17 Duteil L, Queille-Roussel C, Loesche C, *et al.* Assessment of the effect of a sunblock stick in the prevention of solar-simulating ultraviolet light-induced herpes labialis. *J Dermatol Treat* 1998;**9**:11–4.

18 Raborn GW, McGraw WT, Grace M, *et al.* Herpes labialis treatment with acyclovir 5% modified aqueous cream: a double-blind randomized trial. *Oral Surg Oral Med Oral Pathol* 1989;**67**:676–9.

19 Fiddian AP, Ivanyi L. Topical acyclovir in the management of recurrent herpes labialis. *Br J Dermatol* 1983;**109**:321–6.

20 Van Vloten WA, Swart RNJ, Pot F. Topical acyclovir therapy in patients with recurrent orofacial herpes simplex infections. *J Antimicrob Chemother* 1983;**12**(Suppl B):89–93.

21 Spruance SL, Schnipper LE, Overall JC, *et al.* Treatment of herpes simplex labialis with topical acyclovir in polyethylene glycol. *J Infect Dis* 1982;**146**:85–90.

22 Spruance SL, Rea TL, Thoming C, *et al.* Penciclovir cream for the treatment of herpes simplex labialis. *JAMA* 1997;**277**:1374–9.

23 Raborn GW, McGraw WT, Grace MG, *et al.* Herpes labialis treatment with acyclovir 5 per cent ointment. *Sci J* 1989;**55**:135–7.

24 Shaw M, King M, Best JM, Banatvala JE, Gibson JR, Klaber MR; Failure of acyclovir cream in treatment of recurrent herpes labialis. *Br Med J (Clin Res Ed)* 1985;**291**:7–9.

25 Boon R, Goodman JJ, Martinez J, *et al.* Penciclovir cream for the treatment of sunlight-induced herpes simplex labialis: a randomized, double-blind, placebo-controlled trial. Penciclovir Cream Herpes Labialis Study Group. *Clin Ther* 2000;**22**:76–90.

26 Evans TG, Bernstein DI, Raborn GW, *et al.* Double-blind, randomized, placebo-controlled study of topical 5% acyclovir 1% hydrocortisone cream (ME-609) for treatment of UV radiation-induced herpes labialis. *Antimicrob Agents Chemother* 2002;**46**:1870–4.

27 Spruance SL, Nett R, Marbury T, *et al.* Acyclovir cream for treatment of herpes simplex labialis: results of two randomized, double-blind, vehicle-controlled, multicenter clinical trials. *Antimicrob Agents Chemother* 2002;**46**:2238–43.

28 Horwitz E, Pisanty S, Czerninski R, *et al.* A clinical evaluation of a novel liposomal carrier for acyclovir in the topical treatment of recurrent herpes labialis. *Oral Surg Oral Med Oral Pathol Oral Radiol Endod* 1999;**87**:700–5.

29 Kaminester LH, Pariser RJ, Pariser DM, *et al.* A double-blind, placebo-controlled study of topical tetracaine in the treatment of herpes labialis. *J Am Acad Dermatol* 1999;**41**:996–1001.

30 Godfrey H, Godfrey N, Godfrey J, *et al.* A randomized clinical trial on the treatment of oral herpes with topical zinc oxide/glycine. *Altern Ther Health Med* 2001;**7**:49–56.

31 Spruance SL, Stewart JC, Rowe NH, *et al.* Treatment of recurrent herpes simplex labialis with oral acyclovir. *J Infect Dis* 1990;**161**:185–90.

32 Raborn GW, McGraw WT, Grace M, *et al.* Oral acyclovir and herpes labialis: a randomized, double-blind, placebo-controlled study. *J Am Dental Assoc* 1987;**115**:38–42.

33 Spruance SL, Jones TM, Blatte MM, *et al.* High-dose, short-duration, early valacyclovir therapy for episodic treatment of cold sores: results of two randomized, placebo-controlled, multicenter studies. *Antimicrob Agents Chemother* 2003;**47**:1072–80.

34 Scoular A, Winston A, Cowan F. Antiviral therapy to reduce the duration and severity of first episode genital herpes in immunocompetent individuals. (protocol) *Cochrane Database Syst Rev* 2004;(**3**):CD004928.

35 Mertz G, Critchlow C, Benedetti J, *et al.* Double-blind placebo-controlled trial of oral acyclovir in the first episode genital herpes simplex virus infection. *JAMA* 1984;**252**:1147–51.

36 Nilsen AE, Aasen T, Halsos AM, *et al.* Efficacy of oral acyclovir in treatment of initial and recurrent genital herpes. *Lancet* 1982;**2**:571–3.

37 Bryson YJ, Dillon M, Lovett M, *et al.* Treatment of first episodes of genital herpes simplex virus infections with oral acyclovir: a randomized double-blind controlled trial in normal subjects. *N Engl J Med* 1983;**308**:916–21.

38 Fife KH, Barbarash RA, Rudolph T, *et al.* Valacyclovir versus acyclovir in the treatment of first-episode genital herpes infection: results of an international, multicenter, double-blind randomized clinical trial. *Sex Transm Dis* 1997;**24**:481–6.

39 Centers for Disease Control and Prevention. Diseases characterized by genital ulcers. Sexually transmitted diseases treatment guidelines 2002. *MMWR Recomm Rep* 2002;**51**:11–25.

40 Evans AL, Pittrof R, Cowan F, *et al.* Suppressive antiviral therapy for recurrent genital herpes in immunocompetent individuals. (protocol). Cochrane Database Syst Rev 2003;(**1**):CD004091.

41 Stone K, Whittington W. Treatment of genital herpes. *Rev Infect Dis* 1990;**12**(Suppl 6):610–9.

42 Reitano M, Tyring S, Lang W, *et al.* Valacyclovir for the suppression of recurrent genital herpes simplex virus infection: a large-scale dose range finding study. *J Infect Dis* 1998;**178**:603–10.

43 Goldberg LH, Kaufman RH, Kurtz TO, *et al.* Continuous five-year treatment of patients with frequently recurring genital herpes simplex virus infection with acyclovir. *J Med Virol* 1993;(Suppl 1):45–50.

44 Wald A, Zeh J, Barnum G, *et al.* Suppression of subclinical shedding of herpes simplex virus type 2 with acyclovir. *Ann Intern Med* 1996;**124**:8–15.

45 Patel R, Tyring S, Strand A, *et al.* Impact of suppressive antiviral therapy on the health related quality of life of patients with recurrent genital herpes infection. *Sex Transm Infect* 1999;**75**:398–402.

46 Doward LC, McKenna SP, Kohlmann T, *et al.* The international development of the RGHQoL: a quality of life measure for recurrent genital herpes. *Qual Life Res* 1998;**7**:143–53.

47 Wald A. New therapies and prevention strategies for genital herpes. *Clin Infect Dis* 1999;**28**:S4–S13.

48 Patel R, Bodsworth NJ, Wooley P, *et al.* Valacyclovir for the suppression of recurrent genital HSV infection: a placebo controlled study of once daily therapy. *Genitourin Med* 1997;**73**:105–9.

49 Fife KH, Warren TJ, Ferrera RD, *et al.* Effect of valacyclovir on viral shedding in immunocompetent patients with recurrent herpes simplex virus 2 genital herpes: a US-based randomized, double-blind, placebo-controlled clinical trial. *Mayo Clin Proc* 2006;**81**:1321–7.

50 Wald A, Selke S, Warren T, *et al.* Comparative efficacy of famciclovir and valacyclovir for suppression of recurrent genital herpes and viral shedding. *Sex Transm Dis* 2006;**33**:529–33.

51 Fife KH, Crumpacker CS, Mertz GJ. Recurrence and resistance patterns of herpes simplex virus following stop of ≥ 6 years of chronic suppression with acyclovir. *J Infect Dis* 1994;**169**:1338–41.

52 Smith J, Cowan FM, Munday P. The management of herpes simplex virus infection in pregnancy. *Br J Obstet Gynaecol* 1998; **105**:255–68.

53 Sheffield JS, Hollier LM, Hill JB, *et al.* Acyclovir prophylaxis to prevent herpes simplex virus recurrence at delivery: a systematic review. *Obstet Gynecol* 2003;**102**:1396–403.

54 Andrews WW, Kimberlin DF, Whitley R, *et al.* Valacyclovir therapy to reduce recurrent genital herpes in pregnant women. *Am J Obstet Gynecol* 2006;**194**:774–81.

55 Sheffield JS, Hill JB, Hollier LM, *et al.* Valacyclovir prophylaxis to prevent recurrent herpes at delivery: a randomized clinical trial. *Obstet Gynecol* 2006;**108**:141–7; erratum in *Obstet Gynecol* 2006;**108**:695.

56 Hollier L, Wendel GL. Third trimester antiviral therapy for preventing recurrent genital herpes at delivery (protocol), *Cochrane Database Syst Rev* 2004;(**4**):CD004946.

57 Wald A, Carrell D, Remington M, *et al.* Two-day regimen of acyclovir for treatment of recurrent genital herpes simplex virus type 2 infection. *Clin Infect Dis* 2002;**34**:944–8.

58 Reichman RC, Badger GJ, Mertz GJ, *et al.* Treatment of recurrent genital herpes simplex infections with oral acyclovir: a controlled trial. *JAMA* 1984;**251**:2103–7.

59 Spruance S, Trying S, Degregorio B, *et al.* A large-scale, placebo-controlled, dose-ranging trial of peroral valacyclovir for episodic treatment of recurrent herpes genitalis. *Arch Intern Med* 1996;**156**:1729–35.

60 Bodsworth NJ, Crooks RJ, Borelli S, *et al.* Valaciclovir versus aciclovir in patient-initiated treatment of recurrent genital herpes: a randomised, double blind clinical trial. International Valaciclovir HSV Study Group. *Genitourin Med* 1997;**73**:110–6.

61 Strand A, Patel R, Wulf H C, *et al.* Aborted genital herpes simplex virus lesions: findings from a randomised controlled trial with valacyclovir. *Sex Transm Infect* 2002;**78**:435–9.

62 Leone PA, Trottier S, Miller JM. Valacyclovir for episodic treatment of genital herpes: a shorter 3-day treatment course compared with 5-day treatment. *Clin Infect Dis* 2002;**34**:958–62.

63 Sacks SL, Aoki FY, Diaz-Mitoma F, *et al.* Patient-initiated, twice-daily oral famciclovir for early recurrent genital herpes: a randomized, double-blind multicenter trial. *JAMA* 1996;**276**:44–9.

64 Chosidow O, Drouault Y, Leconte-Veyriac F, *et al.* Famciclovir versus aciclovir in immunocompetent patients with recurrent genital herpes infections: a parallel-groups, randomized, double-blind clinical trial. *Br J Dermatol* 2001;**144**:818–24.

44 Leprosy

Shamez Ladhani, Weiya Zhang

Background

Clinical scenario

A 32-year-old man presented to the dermatology clinic with a rash. He had developed a single, raised, erythematous patch on his right upper arm 2 months previously, but had ignored it initially. Recently, he had noticed several new lesions developing on his right arm. The lesions were getting bigger and lighter in color, and he was unable to feel any sensation when he pressed on them. There were no other symptoms, and he was otherwise well. He was born in Madagascar and had moved to the United Kingdom 5 years previously. No one in his family had leprosy or tuberculosis. Examination revealed multiple well-demarcated, hypopigmented patches and plaques of different sizes on his right upper arm, with loss of pain and light touch sensation (Figure 44.1). There was no evidence of peripheral nerve thickening or loss of function. Histological examination of a skin smear from one of the lesions showed well-defined granuloma with epithelioid cells and a dense, lymphocytic infiltrate, but no acid-fast bacilli. The clinical and histological findings were consistent with a diagnosis of polar tuberculoid (TT) leprosy. When informed of his diagnosis, the patient mentioned that he had heard that leprosy could now be treated with a single dose of antibiotics. He had also read that some patients with leprosy also took steroids with their antibiotics to protect their nerves from permanent damage, and he wanted to be sure that this would be beneficial because he was concerned about the side effects of long-term steroids.

Definition

Leprosy (from the Greek *lepros,* scaly, scabby, rough) is a chronic infectious granulomatous disease due to *Mycobacterium leprae.*[1] Most people exposed to the organism are able to mount an appropriate immune response and do not

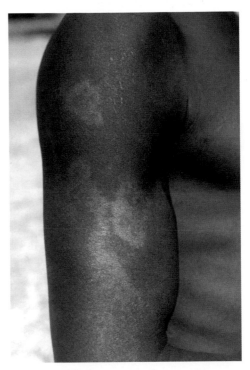

Figure 44.1 Multiple well-demarcated, hypopigmented patches and plaques of different sizes on the right upper arm in a 32-year-old patient.

develop leprosy, and those who do, usually present with single lesions, which often heal without treatment. In a small proportion, however, the lesion may progress to overt disease, the severity of which depends on the host's cell-mediated immune (CMI) response to *M. leprae.* Leprosy is classified according to the degree and type of host immune response as indeterminate (I), tuberculous pole (TT), borderline tuberculoid (BT), borderline (BB), borderline lepromatous (BL), and lepromatous (LL) pole.[2]

For treatment purposes, patients are defined as paucibacillary (PB), with five or fewer skin lesions, or multibacillary (MB), with six or more skin lesions. PB leprosy includes

TT and BT leprosy, while MB leprosy includes BB, BL, and LL patients.[3] Single-lesion leprosy is often defined separately as a subgroup of PB leprosy, as the treatment is different. In 2000, around 39% of leprosy patients worldwide were classified as multibacillary, 52% as paucibacillary (two to five skin lesions) and 9% as having a single lesion.[4]

Indeterminate leprosy (I) is considered to be the early stage of leprosy, which can self-heal and may be underdiagnosed. The lesions are vague, hypopigmented macules without definite anesthesia and/or nerve enlargement. In TT leprosy, however, the lesions may be hypopigmented or erythematous, with loss of pain, touch, hot and cold sensations, and lack of sweating due to sympathetic nerve damage. Skin smears often yield few or no bacilli, and the lesions may heal spontaneously. In borderline leprosy, the skin lesions become more numerous and larger, with less well-defined margins, and nerve damage becomes more prominent. In lepromatous leprosy, the overwhelming bacterial load and the limited host immune response results in generalized multi-system infection which, if left untreated, results in severe multiorgan damage. The skin lesions are larger, less well-defined, symmetrical, more infiltrated, and often develop into plaques and nodules. The patient may present with extensive sensory and motor nerve damage. The nerves commonly affected are the ulnar and median (leading to claw hand), radial (wrist drop), common peroneal (foot drop), posterior tibial (claw toes), the fifth (corneal sensation) and seventh (facial palsy) cranial nerves, cutaneous sensory nerves especially near skin lesions, and auricular nerves. In advanced cases, the patients may present with loss of eyebrows and eyelashes, nasal cartilage damage with collapsed nose, epididymo-orchitis, and iritis, which may progress to blindness. Other forms of leprosy, such as primary neuritic leprosy without skin lesions, are also recognized and can be diagnosed by nerve biopsy.[1]

Reactions in leprosy refer to episodes of acute inflammation of leprosy skin lesions, nerves or other body parts. Type I reactions (T1R), or reversal reactions, occur in borderline leprosies due to spontaneous fluctuations in the host CMI response to *M. leprae*, and can occur before, during, or after treatment, making it difficult to distinguish from relapse.[5,6] Patients present with swelling of the limbs and face and the appearance of new skin lesions, which can ulcerate and scar. Neuritis, particularly involving nerves that are already enlarged, can occur either insidiously and painlessly or as a severe painful episode and may result in permanent nerve damage if not treated promptly. The lesions show infiltration of lymphocytes and monocytes, with elevated levels of interferon gamma. The risk of T1R is associated with facial lesions and more extensive disease.[7] The greatest risk of developing T1R is within the first year of starting treatment and is more severe at the tuberculoid end of the spectrum. With multidrug therapy (MDT), the risk of T1R is estimated at 7–20% in PB and 39–48% in MB patients.[8] It has been proposed that the use of more potent antileprosy drugs increases the risk of T1R by releasing large quantities of *M. leprae* antigens due to more effective killing of the organism, causing an exaggerated host immune response.[9]

Erythema nodosum leprosum (ENL) describes the development of tender red papules and nodules on the skin and sometimes in the nerves and eyes of patients at the lepromatous end of the disease.[5,10] The lesions develop over a few hours and last a few days, and, unlike T1R, usually recur. They can coalesce to form large plaques and may even ulcerate. ENL occurs due to deposition of immune complexes formed by *M. leprae* antigens together with dysfunction of the host CMI response. Increased levels of tumor necrosis factor-α may have a role in the pathogenesis. The severity of ENL varies tremendously from asymptomatic episodes to gross prostration and even death. Systemic symptoms are often present and include fever, malaise, swelling of the hands and feet, and lymphadenitis. The joints, eyes, testes, liver, spleen, and kidneys may also be involved in severe cases. With clofazimine-containing multidrug regimens, ENL accounts for < 1% of all reactions in many large-scale post-surveillance studies.[11]

Incidence/prevalence

The global prevalence of leprosy has declined steadily from its peak of 12 per 100 000 population in 1985 to less than one case per 100 000 by the end of 2000.[4] Trends in new cases detected globally have also been falling since 2001. At the end of 2000, there were around 5.5 million cases registered for treatment globally, with 719 330 new cases detected that year.[4] By 2005, the number of cases registered for treatment had fallen to 286 063, and only 407 791 new cases were detected during 2004.[12] Of the 122 countries in which leprosy was endemic in 1985, only nine had a prevalence rate greater than one per 10 000 population at the beginning of 2005, including six countries in Africa (Angola, Central African Republic, Democratic Republic of Congo, Madagascar, Mozambique, and the United Republic of Tanzania), two in south-east Asia (India and Nepal), and one in South America (Brazil).[12] Together, these nine countries represented 74% of the total registered cases and 84% of new cases detected during 2004. It is estimated that over 14 million leprosy patients globally have been cured through multidrug therapy.

Etiology

Progress in leprosy research has been slow, because it has not been possible to cultivate the organism in artificial media; most research is currently performed on the mouse footpad model.[13] The organism is considered to be of high infectivity but low pathogenicity and is rarely fatal. Humans are the main reservoir of infection, but the organism has been found in several primate species and armadillos. *M. leprae* is a rod-shaped, slightly curved, Gram-positive, obligate intracellular organism. The genome of *M. leprae* was published in 2000 and there are very few differences in genomes from *M. leprae* strains isolated from different geographical regions worldwide.[14] It is found mainly in clumps known as globi inside macrophages, and multiplies very slowly, with a generation time of around 12 days. *M. leprae* has a long and variable incubation period, ranging from 1 to more than 20 years. The optimal temperature for growth is 27–30 °C, which explains its predilection for cooler parts of the human body. The mode of transmission of infection still remains speculative, but it is strongly suspected to involve the respiratory tract, since nasal secretions from infected individuals carry large numbers of the organisms.

Risk factors for leprosy remain poorly understood, but low socio-economic status, overcrowding, nutritional status, and immune response all play an important role. Household contacts have a higher risk of developing leprosy, particularly if the index case has multibacillary leprosy rather than paucibacillary leprosy, and children have a higher risk in comparison with adults.[15] Genetic factors may also influence susceptibility to leprosy and/or progression to overt disease. For example, allelic variants at the human homologue of the mouse natural resistance-associated macrophage protein 1 (Nramp1) gene have been found to be associated with susceptibility to tuberculosis and leprosy in humans.[16] The Nramp1 protein is an integral membrane protein expressed exclusively in the lysosomal compartment of monocytes and macrophages.[17] There is also a strong association between the HLA-DR2 allele and tuberculoid leprosy in ethnically diverse populations and between HLA-DQ1 and lepromatous leprosy.[13,16,18] Other studies have shown an increased risk of leprosy within certain families, high concordance rates among identical twins, and identification of genetic markers on chromosome 10 in linkage studies in south India.[16]

Prognosis and complications

Completion of the antileprosy treatment recommended by the World Health Organization (WHO) leads to cure in almost all cases, with an estimated relapse rate of less than 1% for both PB and MB leprosy.[19] Relapse is defined as reappearance of the disease, gradual worsening of existing lesions, appearance of new skin lesions, thickened, tender nerves, or muscle paralysis after successful completion of the appropriate treatment and can occur many years after treatment completion. Relapse is mainly diagnosed clinically, although some cases may be identified by routine skin smear tests during post-treatment surveillance, and can be difficult to distinguish from late reactions. A delay

in detecting relapse, which often occurs because patients falsely assume they have been cured,[20] can lead to further nerve damage and deformities.

However, the main complication of leprosy is the severe disfigurement and deformity that occurs and progresses even after treatment completion. The International Classification of Impairment, Disease and Handicap emphasizes that deformities, defined as alteration in the form, shape, or appearance of parts of the body, result in impairment and not disability.[21] Disability is defined as any restriction or lack of ability to perform in the manner or within the range considered normal for a human being as a result of impairment. The risk of disability in leprosy is complex and associated with age, sex, occupation, classification, and duration of disease, development of reactions, site of lesions, method of case detection, geographic and socio-economic factors, treatment type, educational attainment, and ethnicity.[22] Deformities in leprosy result from *M. leprae* infection, reactions, and relapse, all of which can cause irreversible nerve damage. The subsequent loss of sensory, motor, and/or autonomic modalities to peripheral limbs often leads to trauma and ulceration of areas supplied by the nerves, eventually leading to gross deformities and even loss of the limb. Psychosocial disabilities are also common and arise from the chronic nature of the disease, the unsightly mutilations that occur, and the stigma associated with leprosy. Thus, loss of confidence, feelings of inadequacy, low self-esteem, anxiety, and frank depression are common among leprosy patients, who are also more likely to be unmarried, divorced, unemployed, and homeless.[20]

In 1969, the WHO redefined its five-point classification of disability to three grades to facilitate its use by field workers worldwide, and simplified it further in 1988 to two grades only (Table 44.1),[22] with the primary aim of collecting data regarding disability for administrative purposes. In 1995, the global prevalence of grade 2 disability among leprosy patients was estimated at 1–2 million, compared to 3.5 million in 1975 and 3.9 million in 1966. By 2000, of almost

Table 44.1 The 1988 World Health Organization grading of disability[22]

Grade	Hands and feet	Eyes
0	No anesthesia, no visible deformity or damage	No eye problems due to leprosy; no evidence of visual loss
1	Anesthesia present, but no visible deformity or damage	Eye problems due to leprosy present, but vision not severely affected as a result (vision 6/60 or better; can count fingers at 6 m)
2	Visible deformity or damage present	Severe visual impairment (vision worse than 6/60; unable to count fingers at 6 m)

700 000 new cases with information on disability status, only 4% had grade 2 disabilities at presentation.[4]

Diagnostic tests

The diagnosis of leprosy is based principally on the clinical features and can be confirmed by skin smears or biopsy. Leprosy should be suspected in any patient presenting with an anesthetized skin lesion, with or without nerve involvement. Sensory loss to pinprick and/or light touch is a typical feature of leprosy.[16] The World Health Organization defines a case of leprosy as involving one or more of the following features in anyone who has not completed antileprosy treatment:

• Hypopigmented or reddish skin lesion(s) with sensory loss

• Involvement of the peripheral nerves, with thickening or loss of sensation in the area supplied by the nerve

• Skin smear positive for acid-fast bacilli[23]

When performed properly, skin smears can help confirm the diagnosis of leprosy, aid correct classification, monitor treatment progress, and diagnose relapse. The bacterial load can be estimated and expressed using the logarithmic Ridley scale or bacterial index (BI; grades 0−6) based on the number of bacilli seen in an average microscopic field using an oil immersion lens.[24] The Morphological Index (MI) can be used to determine the percentage of live organisms—a score of zero means that patient is noninfectious.

A biopsy of the skin lesion may help confirm the diagnosis, improve research, and allow culture of *M. leprae* in mouse footpads. However, the sensitivity is poor, because biopsies can yield negative results despite obvious clinical signs. Leprosy lesions are characterized by the formation of granulomas, which vary from the epithelioid type at the tuberculous end to the "foamy" cell type (macrophages filled with *M. leprae*) at the lepromatous end. Immunohistopathological staining for *M. leprae* antigens, such as phenolic glycolipid-1 (PGL-1), have been shown to be very specific, but are still in the developmental stage.[25]

The Lepromin skin test, which involves injecting inactivated *M. leprae* antigens under the skin, can be used to aid disease classification and predict the type of disease a person is likely to develop, as it measures the host's CMI response against *M. leprae* antigens.[16] The site of injection is examined at 3 days and again at 3−4 weeks after injection for reaction induration. A positive test would suggest the development of leprosy at the tuberculoid end of the spectrum, while a negative test would favor lepromatous leprosy.

Other diagnostic tests have been developed and are currently mainly used for research and epidemiological studies, but many show promise for future use in rapid diagnosis, monitoring therapeutic responses and early diagnosis of relapse. Serological tests include measurement of anti-PGL-1 antibodies in blood or urine. Although these antibodies are often absent at the tuberculoid end of the spectrum, they may play an important role in early detection of relapse in multibacillary patients and in detection of subclinical infection, because they can be present before the onset of clinical symptoms.[13] Detection of *M. leprae* in tissues, using several polymerase chain reaction (PCR) methods and probes targeting stretches of *M. leprae* DNA or ribosomal RNA, has also been developed and is potentially both sensitive and specific, although relatively expensive and impractical for use in the field.[26]

Aims of treatment

Treatment is aimed at:

• Eliminating *M. leprae*

• Reducing reactions and relapse

• Preventing disabilities

Relevant outcomes

• Clinical outcomes
—Percentage of patients with marked clinical improvement
—Percentage of patients completely cured
—Percentage of patients with treatment failure
—Percentage of patients with type I reaction
—Percentage of patients with type II reaction
—Percentage of patients relapsed

• Bactericidal activity
—Bacterial index (BI)
—Morphological Index (MI)
—Mouse footpad test for *M. leprae*

• Histopathological assessment
—Percentage of patients with inactive leprosy

Methods of search

Randomized controlled trials dating back to 1966 were located by searching Medline, Embase, the Scientific Citation Index, and the Cochrane Library. The main search terms were randomized controlled trial(s) or clinical trial(s); leprosy or lepra reactions or erythema nodosum leprosum. A Medical Subject Headings (MeSH) search was conducted if possible, otherwise a keyword search was used. References in original and review articles were reviewed and any randomized controlled trials missed from the electronic search were included. Only English-language trials were assessed.

Questions

Because almost all randomized controlled trials (RCTs) on leprosy have been performed in endemic areas, care must be taken in extrapolating the results to developed countries with a low risk for leprosy.

Is multidrug therapy (MDT) more effective than monotherapy in terms of clinical outcomes and bactericidal activity?

Efficacy

No systematic reviews were found. Five RCTs were identified. Dietrich and colleagues compared two MDT therapy regimens with dapsone monotherapy.[27] A total of 307 patients with lepromatous leprosy and borderline lepromatous leprosy were randomly allocated to dapsone monotherapy, dapsone–rifampin, or dapsone–prothion-amide–isoniazid–rifampin. The patients were treated once daily for 3 years and followed up for 5 years. Clinical improvement, regression of the disease, and bactericidal activity were measured. The results showed that dapsone monotherapy was associated with the same frequency of clinical improvement as both combinations at the end of the 5-year observation period, but with slightly slower regression. The trial did not find any statistical difference in the clearance of bacteria between the monotherapy and either combination. There was no difference in the type or frequency of reactions, but three relapses were observed with dapsone monotherapy. Ji and colleagues compared the efficacy of the combination of ofloxacin 400 mg, dapsone 100 mg, and clofazimine 300 mg daily with ofloxacin (400 mg and 800 mg) daily alone for 56 days.[28] The results showed that all of the treatment regimens were associated with remarkable clinical improvements. Marked improvements were seen in five of eight, six of eight, and six of eight cases for the combination, ofloxacin 400 mg, and ofloxacin 800 mg, respectively. The mouse footpad test showed that all three treatments led to more than 99% *M. leprae* organism clearance. There were no statistically significant differences in clinical improvement and bactericidal activity (BI and MI) between the groups. However, three erythema nodosum leprosum reactions were seen in the combination group.

Four RCTs were undertaken to compare the risk of reaction between MDT and monotherapy. Table 44.2 summarizes the results for relative risk between the two treatments.[9,28–30]

Only one trial showed a significantly lower risk of type I reaction with MDT in paucibacillary leprosy.[9] The relative risk between MDT and the monotherapy was 0.12 (95% CI, 0.04 to 0.35). The number needed to harm was −6 (95% CI, −4 to −16), indicating that one in six patients would be protected from type I reactions when treated with MDT in comparison with the multiple-dose regimen of rifampicin monotherapy. Nevertheless, the single dose of rifampicin monotherapy had no more risk of the reaction than MDT.

Drawbacks

Apart from reaction and relapse, none of the trials reported adverse drug events separately for the various treatment regimens, providing no comparative values for harms with these treatments.

Comment

Except for two studies,[9,27] all of the other trials are under-powered. Although Dietrich and colleagues indicated a rapid regression of the disease with MDT at the early stage of the treatment (6 months), there was no more benefit at the end point of 5 years with this regimen.[27] MDT was superior to multidose monotherapy in reducing type I reactions in paucibacillary leprosy.[9] However, the evidence is sparse, and the benefit of MDT disappears in comparison with single-dose rifampicin. As the trials differ with regard to the treatment regimens used and their duration, pooling is not possible. In addition, there are no RCTs comparing the standard WHO MDT with dapsone monotherapy. Whether MDT is more beneficial than monotherapy has yet to be established.

Implications for clinical practice

MDT may be useful to speed up clinical improvement and reduce type I reactions.

Is single-dose multidrug therapy (MDT)—such as 600 mg rifampicin, 400 mg ofloxacin and 100 mg minocycline (ROM)—as effective as the standard WHO MDT for paucibacillary leprosy in clinical outcomes?

Efficacy

No systematic reviews were identified. Two randomized controlled trials compared single-dose ROM with WHO MDT in the treatment of paucibacillary leprosy, one for a single lesion and another for two or three lesions.[31,32] Both of the trials were double-blinded. The patients were followed up for 18 months. The percentages of patients with marked clinical improvement were slightly in favor of the WHO MDT for single lesion of PB. The rate ratio was 0.90, with a 95% confidence interval of 0.82 to 0.995 ($P < 0.05$) (Table 44.3).[31–33]

The number needed to treat was −18 (95% CI, −9 to −367), indicating that one in 18 patients will obtain marked clinical improvement when treated with WHO MDT in comparison with single-dose ROM. However, this benefit was not seen in multiple lesions of PB (Table 44.3).

Similar results were obtained for the percentage of patients with complete cure (lesion disappearance), with the single-dose ROM regimen showing a lower rate of complete cures than the WHO MDT regimen in patients with single-lesion PB (RR 0.86; 95% CI, 0.77 to 0.95; $P < 0.01$). However, there were no differences in the percentage of

Table 44.2 Randomized controlled trials of MDT versus monotherapy

Trial	MDT	Monotherapy	Follow up	Risk of reaction	MDT Mono	RR (95%CI)
Type I reaction						
Groenen (1986)[9] (PB)	RMP 1500 mg 1x + DDS 100 mg od, 1 y	RMP 40 mg/kg 1x	> 1 y	4/184	5/92	0.40 (0.11, 1.45)
	RMP 900 mg 1/wk, 10 wk			4/184	11/59	0.12 (0.04, 0.35)**
Jamet (1992)[29] (MB)	CLO 50 mg od + CLO 300 mg 1/m, 6 m	CLO 600 mg 1/m, 6 m	6 m	2/16	1/13	1.62 (0.16, 15.99)
	CLO 1200 mg 1/m, 6 m			2/16	7/16	0.29 (0.07, 1.17)
Ji (1994)[28] (MB)	OFL 400 mg od + DDS 100 mg od + CLO 300 mg 1/m + CLO 50 mg od, 2 m	OFL 400 mg od, 2 m	2 m	0/8	0/8	1.00 (0.02, 45.13)
		OFL 800 mg od, 2 m	2 m	0/8	0/8	1.00 (0.02, 45.13)
Ji (1993)[30] (MB)	MIN 100 mg od + CLT 500 mg od, 2 m	MIN 100 mg od, 2 m	2 m	0/12	0/11	0.92 (0.02, 42.98)
		CLT 500 mg od, 2 m		0/12	0/12	1.00 (0.02, 46.71)
Erythema nodosum leprosum						
Ji (1994)[28] (MB)	OFL 400 mg od + DDS 100 mg od + CLO 300 mg 1/m + CLO 50 mg od, 2 m	OFL 400 mg od, 2 m	2 m	3/8	0/8	7.00 (0.42, 116.91)
		OFL 800 mg od, 2 m		3/8	0/8	7.00 (0.42, 116.91)
Ji (1993)[30] (MB)	MIN 100 mg od + CLT 500 mg od, 2 m	MIN 100 mg od, 2 m	2 m	3/12	1/11	2.75 (0.33, 22.69)
		CLT 500 mg od, 2 m		3/12	1/12	3.00 (0.36, 24.92)

* *P* < 0.01.
1/m, once per month; 1/wk, once per week; 1x, single dose; CI, confidence intervals; CLO, clofazimine; CLT, clarithromycin; DDS, dapsone; m, month; MB, multibacillary leprosy; MDT, multidrug therapy; MIN, minocycline; od, once daily; OFL, ofloxacin; PB, paucibacillary leprosy; RMP, rifampicin; RR, relative risk; y, year.

Table 44.3 Randomized controlled trials comparing single-dose rifampicin, ofloxacin, and minocycline (ROM) and World Health Organization multidrug therapy (MDT) in the treatment of paucibacillary leprosy

First author, ref.	Design	Lesions	Follow-up	Marked clinical improvement		
				Single ROM	WHO MDT	RR (95% CI)
Babu (1997)[31]	DB-P	1	18 months	361/697	392/684	0.90 (0.82, 0.995)*
Deenabandhu (2001)[32]	DB-P	2–3	18 months	48/104	55/103	0.86 (0.66, 1.14)

DB-P, double-blind parallel; RR, rate ratio; 95% CI, 95% confidence interval; * *P* < 0.05.

patients with treatment failure (no clinical improvement) between the two regimens in patients with single and multiple lesions. The pooled relative risk was 0.98, with a 95% confidence interval of 0.41 to 2.34 (*P* > 0.05).

Drawbacks

Gastrointestinal and allergic adverse drug events were assessed in both trials. There were no statistically significant differences between the single-dose regimen and the

WHO MDT regimen. The pooled relative risk was 0.48 (95% CI, 0.15 to 1.56).

Reaction and neuritis were also compared, and non-statistical differences were obtained. The relative risks for these between the single-dose treatment and WHO MDT were 2.66 (95% CI, 0.78 to 9.13) and 3.02 (95% CI, 0.31 to 28.97), respectively.

Comment

The two RCTs that compared single-dose ROM with WHO MDT were generally of good quality. The first trial was well powered, with a drop-out rate of only 6%. The results show that clinical improvement (the percentage of patients with marked improvement or complete cure) is slightly in favor of the WHO MDT regimen in a single lesion of PB leprosy, but not with multiple lesions. There are no differences in the other outcomes, such as treatment failure, reaction, and side effects. The studies did not report the relapse rate. Further RCTs with placebo control would be useful.

Implications for clinical practice

The standard WHO MDT regimen is in general superior to the single-dose ROM with regard to clinical improvement in the treatment of PB leprosy. For the patient in the clinical scenario described at the beginning of this chapter, single-dose ROM would not be suitable, as he had more than three lesions at presentation. However, a shorter duration of 3 months' MDT instead of 6 months might have been an option (see the question below), but the results of the relevant RCT will not be available for several years yet.

Are 3 months of MDT for paucibacillary leprosy and 12 months for multibacillary leprosy as effective as 6 and 24 months, respectively?

A multicenter RCT sponsored by WHO is currently being carried out in Myanmar, Guinea, and Senegal to study the efficacy of once-monthly doses of ROM in paucibacillary leprosy patients for 3 or 6 months and multibacillary leprosy patients for 12 or 24 months. The results are due in mid-2007.

Does thalidomide improve clinical outcomes in erythema nodosum leprosum (ENL)?

Efficacy

No systematic reviews were retrieved. Four RCTs were retrieved for this question. Two were considered not relevant, as they were not placebo-controlled (the comparator was acetylsalicylic acid),[34] and thalidomide was used concomitantly with other drugs such as systemic steroids and adrenocorticotropic hormone.[35] Two RCTs comparing the efficacy of thalidomide with a placebo were relevant for the assessment. Sheskin and Convit undertook a double-blind

RCT, comparing thalidomide 100 mg (or 6 mg/kg/day if the patient's weight was less than 50 kg) and placebo four times daily for up to 4 weeks.[36] Each patient was assessed weekly for reaction severity (on a scale of 1 to 3) and clinical improvement (worse, no change, partial, striking, and complete). The complete improvement rate with thalidomide was 51% (43/85), in comparison with 5% (four of 88) with the placebo. The rate ratio was 11.1 (95% CI, 4.2 to 29.7; $P < 0.01$). There were no bacteriological or histopathological differences between the two treatments.

The other RCT was a crossover trial involving 12 patients with long-standing ENL, but not usually requiring steroid treatment.[37] The patients were randomly allocated to thalidomide 100 mg or placebo three times daily for 6 weeks. After 6 weeks, the treatment was switched and continued for another 6 weeks. The response was assessed clinically and by the reduction of the requirement for other anti-ENL treatments (stibophen and/or prednisolone). Thalidomide was shown to be superior to placebo and was also preferred by the patients. However, no statistical tests were conducted and no quantitative data can be re-analyzed.

A recent randomized, double-blind, double-dummy, dose-controlled study of thalidomide showed that a 1-week course of high-dose thalidomide (300 mg/day) followed by slow tapering of the dose over 6 weeks resulted in a lower rate of reemergence of ENL over the 7-week treatment period in comparison with a lower treatment dose of thalidomide (100 mg/day) for one week followed by rapid tapering of the dose over 2 weeks.[38] However, most patients in the study developed new ENL lesions during tapering or soon after stopping treatment—suggesting that a longer duration of treatment with an even slower tapering period may be beneficial, although this needs to be confirmed in future studies.

Drawbacks

Twenty cases of drowsiness, eight cases of dizziness, and seven cases of nausea were seen with thalidomide treatment among 85 patients, whereas none was found with placebo.[36]

Comment

Two trials relevant to the question were undertaken in the late 1960s. The quality of the trials and reports is poor in relation to the Consolidated Standards of Reporting Trials (CONSORT) statement.[39] Although thalidomide shows some benefit for the treatment of ENL, robust, evidence-based and well-conducted RCTs are awaited, particularly in relation to the dose and duration of treatment. However, it must be emphasized that because of its well-known teratogenicity, thalidomide should be given only to males and postmenopausal females. Women of childbearing age should never be given thalidomide. Thalidomide is also known to be associated with irreversible nerve damage. It must therefore be administered under the strictest possible supervision.

Implications for clinical practice
Thalidomide may be useful for improving the clinical symptoms of ENL, but due to its well-known teratogenicity and neurotoxicity, care must be taken when it is being used for ENL.

In patients with leprosy, does steroid prophylaxis prevent nerve impairment?

Efficacy
No systematic reviews were identified, but the use of prophylactic steroids to prevent nerve impairment has been reviewed recently.[40,41] Three clinical trials were identified from the literature.[41–43] A small, unblinded RCT conducted in India in 1985, including 141 histologically-confirmed, Lepromin-positive (grades 2 to 4+), smear-negative TT/BT patients, showed that with 10 mg oral prednisolone once daily for 1 month, given with 100 mg daily dapsone monotherapy for 1 year and followed up for a mean of 15 months, three of 49 patients (6%) receiving steroids developed nerve problems, in comparison with seven of 47 (16%) of those receiving 100 mg daily dapsone alone (the difference between the two proportions was 8.8%; 95% CI, –3.4% to 21.0%; $P = 0.16$).[42] The risk of nerve impairment was therefore not statistically significant. However, there are several problems in interpreting the results of this study; firstly, the primary outcome of the study was not the risk of nerve impairment, but the time taken to reach disease inactivity and the risk of relapse after treatment; secondly, the number of participants was small, so that the study had little power to exclude even large treatment benefits; thirdly, the definition of nerve involvement was vague and included nine cases of nerve abscesses, with only three patients showing evidence of functional deterioration; and fourthly, 32% of the patients were lost to follow-up.[42]

A more recent, uncontrolled trial included 92 new MB patients identified from the large, prospective Bangladesh Acute Nerve Damage Study (BANDS), which has recruited and followed 2664 new leprosy patients since 1995.[41] These 92 patients were given MDT with daily prednisolone 20 mg for 3 months, which was then tapered to zero in the fourth month, and followed up monthly for 12 months. Comparison with a historical control group of 200 patients who received MDT only showed a twofold reduction in the incidence of reactions (14 reaction events during 20 937 days at risk compared to 53 events during 77 316 days at risk; odds ratio 2.01; 95% CI, 1.05 to 3.85). As this was an open series including a relatively small number of patients and with a historical control group, the results were open to confounding bias. A larger, multicenter, double-blind RCT has been undertaken to investigate whether corticosteroids

administered at low doses at the time of diagnosis might reduce the frequency of nerve impairment due to the MDT treatment. A total of 636 newly diagnosed MB leprosy patients in Nepal and Bangladesh were randomly assigned prednisolone 20 mg/day for 3 months, with a tapering dose in month 4, plus MDT, or MDT alone—the TRIPOD study.[44] The results showed that prednisolone alone was associated with a significant reduction in the risk of new reactions and nerve function impairment during the 4 months when the steroid was given (RR 3.9; 95% CI, 2.1 to 7.3), but the effect was not sustained at 1 year (RR 1.3; 95% CI, 0.9 to 1.8).

Drawbacks
The adverse effects of long-term steroid use are well known and include fluid retention, weight gain, redistribution of body fat, osteoporosis, muscle wasting, thinning of skin, and psychological effects including irritability and depression. In addition, the TRIPOD trial identified more minor adverse events, such as fungal skin infection, acne, and epigastric pain in the group receiving prednisolone and MDT in comparison with the group receiving MDT alone ($P < 0.05$).[45]

Comment
The TRIPOD study demonstrates the short-term prophylactic benefit of steroid treatment. However, the effect is not sustained after steroid treatment is stopped, and more adverse effects may occur due to the prophylactic use of steroids. This is the only RCT, and its results are inconsistent with other types of evidence. Further RCTs would be useful to confirm the benefit of using steroids, especially in patients who are at greater risk of nerve damage, who might benefit significantly from prophylactic steroids.

Implications for clinical practice
On the basis of the results of these studies, the patient should be informed that the routine use of prophylactic steroids may only have short-term benefits. It may also cause more adverse effects, such as fungal infection. Studies are needed to confirm the long-term effect of using prophylactic steroids. The benefits of prophylactic steroids should outweigh their potential short-term and long-term adverse effects when this treatment is being considered.

In endemic areas, is chemoprophylaxis effective in preventing leprosy?

Efficacy
One systematic review was retrieved,[46] which identified 14 trials, including six RCTs (four using oral dapsone and two with intramuscular acedapsone), six nonrandomized controlled trials using oral dapsone, and two uncontrolled mass intervention trials (one using oral rifampicin and one

Review: Chemoprophylaxis in leprosy
Comparison: Intervention vs Control
Outcome: Disease Vs No Disease

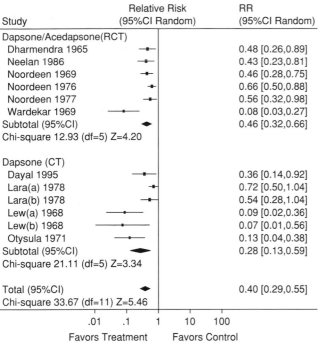

Study	Relative Risk (95%CI Random)	RR (95%CI Random)
Dapsone/Acedapsone(RCT)		
Dharmendra 1965		0.48 [0.26,0.89]
Neelan 1986		0.43 [0.23,0.81]
Noordeen 1969		0.46 [0.28,0.75]
Noordeen 1976		0.66 [0.50,0.88]
Noordeen 1977		0.56 [0.32,0.98]
Wardekar 1969		0.08 [0.03,0.27]
Subtotal (95%CI)		0.46 [0.32,0.66]
Chi-square 12.93 (df=5) Z=4.20		
Dapsone (CT)		
Dayal 1995		0.36 [0.14,0.92]
Lara(a) 1978		0.72 [0.50,1.04]
Lara(b) 1978		0.54 [0.28,1.04]
Lew(a) 1968		0.09 [0.02,0.36]
Lew(b) 1968		0.07 [0.01,0.56]
Otysula 1971		0.13 [0.04,0.38]
Subtotal (95%CI)		0.28 [0.13,0.59]
Chi-square 21.11 (df=5) Z=3.34		
Total (95%CI)		0.40 [0.29,0.55]
Chi-square 33.67 (df=11) Z=5.46		

.01 .1 1 10 100
Favors Treatment   Favors Control

Figure 44.2 Meta-analysis of chemoprophylaxis trials in leprosy. The rectangles represent the point estimates for each study, the size of the rectangle represents the weight allocated to each study, and the horizontal lines represent the 95% confidence intervals. The diamond represents the summary estimate, and the size of the diamond represents the 95% confidence interval. The solid vertical line is the null value. (Reproduced with permission from Smith and Smith, *Journal of Infection* 2000;**41**:137–42).[46]

intramuscular dapsone). All but two involved household contacts of leprosy cases. A meta-analysis of the 12 controlled trials showed a 60% (95% CI, 45% to 71%) protection rate (Figure 44.2).

Drawbacks
The chemoprophylaxis was often continued for several years after the index case was cured; side effects, compliance, and drug resistance would therefore be likely to cause significant long-term problems if such a strategy were to be implemented.

Comment
Almost all of the clinical trials were performed in the 1960s and 1970s using dapsone alone, at a time when dapsone resistance was high. The duration of follow-up was also limited to a few years, and it is possible that chemoprophylaxis may simply delay the onset of leprosy. It is suggested that the single dose of chemoprophylaxis may do more good than harm. One uncontrolled trial has reported that a

single dose of rifampicin 25 mg/kg provided a 35–40% rate of protection against leprosy in the southern Marquesas Islands during 10-year follow-up period.[47] In a recent unblinded study, 4739 individuals living in five Indonesian islands that are highly endemic for leprosy were divided into three groups: a blanket group, including three islands in which chemoprophylaxis was given to all eligible individuals; a contact group on one island, where all eligible household and neighbor contacts of known leprosy patients received chemoprophylaxis; and a control group on one island, who did not receive any chemoprophylaxis.[48] Rifampicin was the chemoprophylactic agent used, and it was given in two doses approximately 3.5 months apart. The annual incidence of leprosy in the control group was 39 in 10 000. After 3 years, the cumulative incidence in the control and contact groups were similar ($P = 0.93$), but there was a significant reduction in the incidence in the blanket group ($P = 0.031$). However, because the follow-up period was only 3 years, it is possible that blanket chemoprophylaxis simply delayed the onset of leprosy rather than eliminating the infection. A longer follow-up period will be needed in order to determine whether blanket prophylaxis prevents leprosy or simply delays onset. In 1996, a chemoprophylaxis study using a single-dose combination of rifampicin, ofloxacin, and minocycline was started in Micronesia, and the results are currently being analyzed. This simpler and more potent combination may have an important role in preventing leprosy in high-risk groups.

Implications for clinical practice
In endemic areas, chemoprophylaxis using oral dapsone or intramuscular acedapsone for household contacts may provide up to 60% protection against leprosy. The results of the recent single-dose combination prophylaxis trial are awaited, because this may have a significant impact on leprosy prevention. There are currently no studies to assess the effectiveness of chemoprophylaxis in developed countries with a low risk for leprosy.

Is BCG effective in the prevention of leprosy?

Efficacy
A systematic review has been recently published with evidence from both clinical trials and observational studies.[49] Seven clinical trials (RCTs or CTs) were included in the meta-analysis. The risk of leprosy in the Bacille Calmette–Guérin (BCG) group was significantly lower than that in the placebo group (pooled RR 0.74; 95% CI, 0.63 to 0.86) (Figure 44.3). The authors also carried out a meta-analysis of 19 observational (cohort and case–control) studies. The results supported the conclusion from the clinical trials, with better statistical power and larger preventive effects (RR 0.39; 95% CI, 0.30 to 0.49).

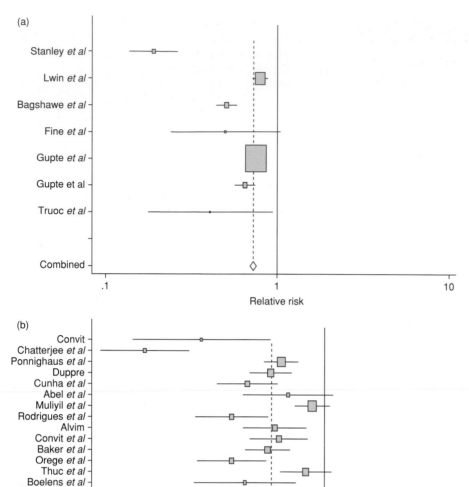

(a)

(b)

Figure 44.3 Meta-analyses of clinical trials (A) and observational studies (B) on the role of BCG in the prevention of leprosy. The rectangles represent the point estimates for each study, the size of the rectangle represents the weight allocated to each study, and the horizontal lines represent the 95% confidence intervals. The diamond and vertical broken line represent the summary estimate and the size of the diamond represents the 95% confidence intervals of the summary estimate. The solid vertical line is the null value. (Reproduced with permission from Setia *et al.*, *Lancet Infectious Diseases* 2006;**6**:162–70).[49]

Drawbacks

BCG vaccine is not free from adverse effects. Fatal disseminated BCG infection has been reported among people with HIV infection.[50] As with other vaccines, the risk of using BCG will need to be assessed against its benefits.

Comment

The BCG vaccine contains a mycobacterium that is closely related to *M. leprae* and is recommended by the WHO's Expanded Programme on Immunization for protection against tuberculosis. It is routinely used to vaccinate children in countries in which leprosy continues to be a public health problem, and it is currently recommended for the household contacts of leprosy patients. It has been well investigated in randomized controlled trials, cohort studies, and case–control studies. The evidence from different studies uniformly supports the use of BCG to prevent leprosy, although the size of the effect in different studies varies, possibly due to differences in the study designs and populations involved.

Implication of clinical practice

Given its protective effects and easy availability, BCG vaccination is warranted in regions in which leprosy continues to be a public health problem and in household contacts who are at greater risk of acquiring the infection.

Key points

- Although chemotherapy is the main treatment for leprosy, there is a lack of robust placebo-controlled trials.

- Multidrug therapy may be useful to speed up clinical improvement, but may offer no greater benefit than single agents in bacterial clearance.

- WHO multidrug therapy (MDT) is superior to the single-dose regimen of 600 mg rifampicin, 400 mg ofloxacin, and 100 mg minocycline (ROM) with regard to clinical improvement, but evidence for other outcomes is awaited.

- The advantages of shortened multidrug therapy (3 months versus 6 months for paucibacillary leprosy and 12 months versus 24 months for multibacillary leprosy) have yet to be established.

- Thalidomide may be useful in controlling reactions, but further robust, randomized controlled trials are needed. It must not be used in women of childbearing age and it has to be monitored carefully because of its neuropathic side effects.

- The evidence for the use of oral steroids to prevent erythema nodosum leprosum reaction is sparse, and the potential harm of such treatment has yet to be assessed.

- Chemotherapy may be useful for preventing leprosy in high-risk populations, but its benefit–risk ratio is unknown. The ongoing trial of single-dose combination prophylaxis may shed further light on this.

- BCG is effective in preventing leprosy. It is recommended to protect people from the infection in endemic areas or among household contacts.

- Care has to be taken when extrapolating the evidence to developed countries, as most of the studies have been carried out in developing countries.

References

1 Hastings RC, ed. *Leprosy.* 2nd ed. Edinburgh: Churchill Livingstone, 1994.

2 Ridley DS, Jopling WH. Classification of leprosy according to immunity. A five-group system. *Int J Lepr Other Mycobact Dis* 1966;**34**:255–73.

3 World Health Organization. *Guide to Eliminate Leprosy as a Public Health Problem.* Geneva: WHO, 2000.

4 World Health Organization. Leprosy. *Wkly Epidemiol Rec* 2002;**77**:1–8.

5 Britton WJ. The management of leprosy reversal reactions. *Lepr Rev* 1998;**69**:225–34.

6 Roche PW, Le Master J, Butlin CR. Risk factors for type 1 reactions in leprosy. *Int J Lepr Other Mycobact Dis* 1997;**65**:450–5.

7 Naafs B. Current views on reactions in leprosy. *Indian J Lepr* 2000;**72**:97–122.

8 Becx-Bleumink M, Berhe D. Occurrence of reactions, their diagnosis and management in leprosy patients treated with multidrug therapy; experience in the leprosy control program of the All Africa Leprosy and Rehabilitation Training Center (ALERT) in Ethiopia. *Int J Lepr Other Mycobact Dis* 1992;**60**:173–84.

9 Groenen G, Janssens L, Kayembe T, Nollet E, Coussens L, Pattyn SR. Prospective study on the relationship between intensive bactericidal therapy and leprosy reactions. *Int J Lepr Other Mycobact Dis* 1986;**54**:236–44.

10 Lockwood DN. The management of erythema nodosum leprosum: current and future options. *Lepr Rev* 1996;**67**:253–9.

11 Ekambaram V, Rao MK. Changing picture of leprosy in North Arcot District, Tamil Nadu after M.D.T. *Indian J Lepr* 1989;**61**:31–43.

12 World Health Organization. Global leprosy situation, 2005. *Wkly Epidemiol Rec* 2005;**80**:289–95.

13 Curtiss R III, Blower S, Cooper K, Russell D, Silverstein S, Young L. Leprosy research in the post-genome era. *Lepr Rev* 2001;**72**:8–22.

14 Brosch R, Gordon SV, Eiglmeier K, Garnier T, Cole ST. Comparative genomics of the leprosy and tubercle bacilli. *Res Microbiol* 2000;**151**:135–42.

15 Smith CM, Smith WC. Current understanding of disability prevention. *Indian J Lepr* 2000;**72**:393–9.

16 Jacobson RR, Krahenbuhl JL. Leprosy. *Lancet* 1999;**353**:655–60.

17 Govoni G, Gros P. Macrophage NRAMP1 and its role in resistance to microbial infections. *Inflamm Res* 1998;**47**:277–84.

18 Fitness J, Tosh K, Hill AV. Genetics of susceptibility to leprosy. *Genes Immun* 2002;**3**:441–53.

19 World Health Organization. *Risk of Relapse in Leprosy.* Geneva: WHO/CTD/LEP/94.1, 1994.

20 Ladhani S. Leprosy disabilities: the impact of multidrug therapy (MDT). *Int J Dermatol* 1997;**36**:561–72.

21 World Health Organization. International classification of impairments, disabilities and handicaps. Geneva: WHO, 1980.

22 World Health Organization Expert Committee on Leprosy. *Sixth Report.* Geneva: WHO, 1988 (WHO Tech Rep Ser 768).

23 World Health Organization Expert Committee on Leprosy. *Seventh Report.* Geneva: WHO, 1998 (WHO Tech Rep Ser 874).

24 Ridley DS. Bacterial indices. In: Cochrane RG, Davey TF, editors. *Leprosy in Theory and Practice.* Bristol: Wright, 1964: 620–2.

25 Weng XM, Chen SY, Ran SP, Zhang CH, Li HY. Immunohistopathology in the diagnosis of early leprosy. *Int J Lepr Other Mycobact Dis* 2000;**68**:426–33.

26 Katoch VM. Advances in the diagnosis and treatment of leprosy. *Expert Rev Mol Med* 2002;**2002**:1–14.

27 Dietrich M, Gaus W, Kern P, Meyers WM. An international randomized study with long-term follow-up of single versus combination chemotherapy of multibacillary leprosy. *Antimicrob Agents Chemother* 1994;**38**:2249–57.

28 Ji B, Perani EG, Petinom C, N'Deli L, Grosset JH. Clinical trial of ofloxacin alone and in combination with dapsone plus clofazimine for treatment of lepromatous leprosy. *Antimicrob Agents Chemother* 1994;**38**:662–7.

29 Jamet P, Traore I, Husser JA, Ji B. Short-term trial of clofazimine in previously untreated lepromatous leprosy. *Int J Lepr Other Mycobact Dis* 1992;**60**:542–8.

30 Ji B, Jamet P, Perani EG, Bobin P, Grosset JH. Powerful bactericidal activities of clarithromycin and minocycline against *Mycobacterium leprae* in lepromatous leprosy. *J Infect Dis* 1993;**168**:188–90.

31 Babu GR, Edward VK, Gupte MD, *et al.* Efficacy of single dose multidrug therapy for the treatment of single-lesion paucibacillary leprosy. Single-lesion Multicentre Trial Group. *Indian J Lepr* 1997;**69**:121–9.

32 Deenabandhu DA, de Britto RL, Emmanuel M, *et al*. A comparative trial of single dose chemotherapy in paucibacillary leprosy patients with two to three skin lesions. *Indian J Lepr* 2001;**73**: 131–43.

33 Babu GR, Edward VK, Gupte MD, *et al*. Efficacy of single-dose multidrug therapy for the treatment of single-lesion paucibacillary leprosy. Single-Lesion Multicentre Trial Group. *Lepr Rev* 1997;**68**:341–9.

34 Iyer CG, Languillon J, Ramanujam K, *et al*. WHO co-ordinated short-term double-blind trial with thalidomide in the treatment of acute lepra reactions in male lepromatous patients. *Bull World Health Org* 1971;**45**:719–32.

35 Waters MF. An internally-controlled double blind trial of thalidomide in severe erythema nodosum leprosum. *Lepr Rev* 1971; **42**:26–42.

36 Sheskin J, Convit J. Results of a double blind study of the influence of thalidomide on the lepra reaction. *Int J Lepr Other Mycobact Dis* 1969;**37**:135–46.

37 Pearson JM, Vedagiri M. Treatment of moderately severe erythema nodosum leprosum with thalidomide—a double-blind controlled trial. *Lepr Rev* 1969;**40**:111–6.

38 Villahermosa LG, Fajardo TT Jr, Abalos RM, *et al*. A randomized, double-blind, double-dummy, controlled dose comparison of thalidomide for treatment of erythema nodosum leprosum. *Am J Trop Med Hyg* 2005;**72**:518–26.

39 Moher D, Schulz KF, Altman D. The CONSORT statement: revised recommendations for improving the quality of reports of parallel-group randomized trials. *JAMA* 2001;**285**:1987–91.

40 Anonymous. Prevention of disabilities and rehabilitation. *Lepr Rev* 2002;**73**:S33–S35.

41 Croft RP, Nicholls P, Anderson AM, Van Brakel WH, Smith WC, Richardus JH. Effect of prophylactic corticosteroids on the incidence of reactions in newly diagnosed multibacillary leprosy patients. *Int J Lepr Other Mycobact Dis* 1999;**67**:75–7.

42 Girdhar BK, Girdhar A, Ramu G, Desikan KV. Short course treatment of paucibacillary (TT/BT) leprosy cases. *Indian J Lepr* 1985;**57**:491–8.

43 Smith WC. Review of current research in the prevention of nerve damage in leprosy. *Lepr Rev* 2000;**71**(Suppl):S138–S144.

44 Smith WC, Anderson AM, Withington SG, *et al*. Steroid prophylaxis for prevention of nerve function impairment in leprosy: randomised placebo controlled trial (TRIPOD 1). *BMJ* 2004;**328**: 1459.

45 Smith WC, Smith CM, Cree IA, *et al*. An approach to understanding the transmission of *Mycobacterium leprae* using molecular and immunological methods: results from the MILEP2 study. *Int J Lepr Other Mycobact Dis* 2004;**72**:269–77.

46 Smith CM, Smith WC. Chemoprophylaxis is effective in the prevention of leprosy in endemic countries: a systematic review and meta-analysis. MILEP2 Study Group. Mucosal Immunology of Leprosy. *J Infect* 2000;**41**:137–42.

47 Nguyen LN, Cartel JL, Grosset JH. Chemoprophylaxis of leprosy in the southern Marquesas with a single 25 mg/kg dose of rifampicin. Results after 10 years. *Lepr Rev* 2000;**71**(Suppl):S33–S35.

48 Bakker MI, Hatta M, Kwenang A, *et al*. Prevention of leprosy using rifampicin as chemoprophylaxis. *Am J Trop Med Hyg* 2005;**72**:443–8.

49 Setia MS, Steinmaus C, Ho CS, Rutherford GW. The role of BCG in prevention of leprosy: a meta-analysis. *Lancet Infect Dis* 2006; **6**:162–70.

50 Grange JM. Complications of bacille Calmette-Guérin (BCG) vaccination and immunotherapy and their management. *Commun Dis Public Health* 1998;**1**:84–8.

45 Cutaneous leishmaniasis

Urbà González, Mayda Delma Villalta Alvarez

Background

Definition[1,2]

Leishmaniasis is a group of diseases caused by infection with protozoan parasites called *Leishmania*, transmitted by bites from sandflies infected with the microorganisms. The parasite may be transmitted from person to person or from a range of animals to humans.

There are several clinical presentation forms, which are associated with a broad range of signs, symptoms, and degrees of severity. Cutaneous leishmaniasis (CL) is the most common form of presentation. After an incubation period of 1–12 weeks, a papule develops at the site of the insect bite. The papule grows and turns into an ulcer (Figures 45.1 and 45.2). Most patients have one or two lesions, usually on exposed parts of the body such as the face, arms, or legs, varying in size from 0.5 to 3 cm in diameter. Most lesions heal spontaneously over months or years, leaving a permanent atrophic scar.

Incidence/prevalence[3]

The World Health Organization considers leishmaniasis to be one of the most serious parasitic diseases, with consequences for socio-economic development in many tropical and subtropical developing countries. The overall prevalence is 12 million, with an estimated 1.5 million new cases of CL per year. Approximately 350 million people are at risk of contracting the disease. CL is endemic in many countries in the Mediterranean area, the Middle East, large parts of the Indian subcontinent, Africa, and Central and South America.

Etiology and prognosis[4]

More than 20 recognized *Leishmania* species are responsible for disease in 88 countries, each one having distinct epidemiological and demographic patterns. The geographical distribution of the species causing CL is: in North Africa, the Mediterranean, the Middle East, north-eastern India, and Central Asia (the Old World), the main species are *L. major*, *L. tropica*, and *L. aethiopica*, and less frequently *L. infantum* and *L. donovani*. In Central and South America, from Mexico to the north of Argentina, there are the *L. mexicana* species complex and subgenus *L. viannia*, most frequently *L. braziliensis*, *L. panamensis*, *L. guyanensis*, and *L. peruviana*. The different presentations of leishmaniasis vary in their prognosis and response to therapy. In general, half of the lesions caused by *L. major* or *L. mexicana* will heal within 3 months, while those caused by *L. tropica* take longer, about 10 months, and those due to *L. braziliensis* persist much longer.

Diagnostic tests[5]

Clinically diagnosed CL cases should be confirmed using

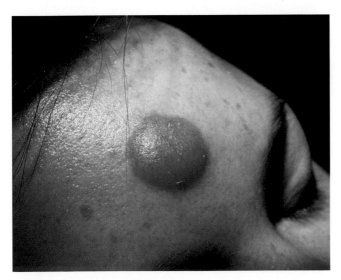

Figure 45.1 Cutaneous leishmaniasis.

451

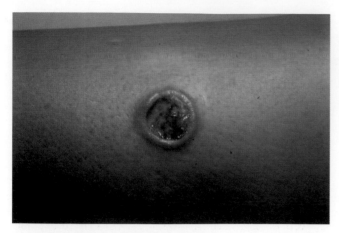

Figure 45.2 Ulcerative cutaneous leishmaniasis.

the traditional diagnostic techniques of smear, culture, and/ or histological analysis of skin biopsies. The polymerase chain reaction test appears to be the most sensitive single diagnostic test for skin samples and aids in identifying the infecting species. Antibodies in circulation are in general low or undetectable. The leishmanin test (Montenegro test) is simple to use and highly specific, but produces negative results in some affected patients and does not distinguish between previous and current infections.

Aims of treatment[6,7]

Many different treatments for CL have been described. The pentavalent antimony derivatives meglumine antimonate (Glucantime) and sodium stibogluconate (Pentostam) remain the mainstay of treatment. Treatments are expensive and require administration over long periods of time. An effective treatment in one area for a given organism may not work in a different geographical area or for a different organism in the same area. In these cases, efficacy also depends on the patient's response. Topical treatments are appropriate for early self-limiting lesions that are not at risk of dissemination, and are attractive options offering reduced systemic toxicity and outpatient treatment. Systemic treatments are indicated when the patient has multiple or complicated lesions or is at risk of mucocutaneous leishmaniasis. The development of drug resistance is a major concern.

Methods of search

We included all randomized controlled trials (RCTs) by searching the Cochrane Library (first issue 2006), Medline (1966–April 2006), and Embase (1988–April 2006). We found no systematic reviews of RCTs. Tables of detailed information for each RCT are available on the web site.

Questions

What is the RCT evidence for local treatments in Old World cutaneous leishmaniasis?

Efficacy

Intralesional meglumine antimonate (Glucantime) or sodium stibogluconate (Pentostam). The mainstay of local treatments for CL has been the intralesional injection of antimony compounds, which have been extensively used as controls in RCTs for several newer treatments.

We found no RCT comparison between the two antimonials. Local versus systemic therapy with meglumine antimonate was compared in an RCT[8] in Saudi Arabia (*L. major*) including 40 patients (70 lesions) treated with an infiltrated solution of meglumine antimonate 0.2–0.8 mL/lesion every other day over a 30-day period, and 40 patients (77 lesions) treated with 12 intramuscular injections of 15 mg/kg/day meglumine antimonate 6 days a week. Follow-up was performed for 1 month after therapy. The results were satisfactory in 84% (57 of 77) of the lesions (46 fully healed and 11 improved) in comparison with 88% (58 of 70) of the lesions (48 fully healed and 10 improved), respectively.

An RCT[9] in Pakistan compared different therapeutic regimens in 49 patients (111 lesions) treated with weekly intralesional meglumine antimonate, and 47 patients (104 lesions) treated with intralesional meglumine antimonate fortnightly, both until complete cure or up to 8 weeks. The patients were followed up for 2 months after therapy. Complete cure was observed in 92% (102 of 111) in comparison with 85.6% (89 of 104) of the lesions, respectively.

Topical paromomycin (aminosidine). We found three RCTs comparing this with placebos. A double-blind RCT[10] from Tunisia (*L. major*) compared 57 patients treated with 15% paromomycin and 10% urea, and 58 patients treated with placebo, twice daily for 14 days. Follow-up was performed for 105 days. The results showed a complete cure in 63% (36 of 57) and 65.5% (38 of 58) of the patients, respectively. A double-blind RCT[11] in Iran (*L. major*) compared 126 patients treated with 15% paromomycin and 10% urea and 125 patients with a placebo, both twice a day for 14 days. The patients were followed up for 105 days. The results showed definitive cure in 68% of patients treated with the drug compared with 68%, with the placebo. Another double-blind RCT[12] in Iran (*L. major*) compared 30 patients treated with 15% paromomycin and 10% urea and 35 with placebo, twice daily for 30 days. The patients were followed-up for 60 days. The results showed definitive cure in 17% of the patients compared with 20%, respectively.

We found two RCTs of different regimens of paromomycin. In a double-blind RCT[13] in Iran (*L. major*), 117 patients were given paromomycin ointment with two applications per day for 4 weeks of treatment, and 116 patients were given 2 weeks of paromomycin followed by 2 weeks of placebo. Follow-up was for 105 days. Complete cure was observed in 53% (62 of 117) compared with 39.6% (46 of 116) of the patients, respectively. A double-blind RCT[14] in Israel (*L. major*) compared 32 patients treated with 15% paromomycin with 12% methylbenzethonium chloride (MBCL) and 11 patients treated with 15% paromomycin with 5% MBCL, both twice a day for 10 days. Follow-up was performed for 10 weeks after treatment. The results were a complete cure in 76% (23 of 32) of the patients, compared with 18% (two of 11), respectively.

We found two RCTs comparing paromomycin with antimonials. An unblinded RCT[15] in Iran (*L. major*) compared 48 patients treated with topical 15% paromomycin and 10% urea, twice per day, and 48 patients treated with intralesional 1.5 g/5 mL meglumine antimonate weekly, for a maximum of 90 days. Follow-up was for 1 year. The results showed cures in 16.6% (eight of 48) compared with 41.7% (20 of 48), respectively. Another open RCT[16] in Iran (*L. major*) compared 30 patients treated with topical 15% paromomycin and 10% urea twice per day, and 30 patients treated with intralesional 1 mL meglumine antimonate every other day, both for 20 days. Follow-up was for 6 weeks. The results showed cures in 69% (20 of 30) compared with 67% (18 of 30), respectively.

We found an open RCT[17] from Turkey (*L. tropica*) comparing 40 patients treated with 15% paromomycin and 12% MBCL twice per day for 15 days and 32 patients treated with 400 mg/day oral ketoconazole for 30 days. At the end of 4 weeks of treatment, 37.5% of patients (15 of 40) showed a complete cure, compared with no complete cure in any of the patients, respectively.

Intralesional zinc sulfate solution. We found three RCTs comparing this with antimonials. An RCT[18] in Iran (*L. major*) compared 36 patients (53 lesions) receiving 2% zinc sulfate solution, and 36 patients (53 lesions) receiving meglumine antimonate, both with six weekly intralesional injections. Follow-up was performed for 1 week. A total of 10.5% of the lesions were cured in comparison with 61.3%, respectively. Another RCT[19] in Iran (*L. major*) compared 31 patients receiving intralesional 2% zinc sulfate and 35 patients treated with intralesional meglumine antimonate. After 6 weeks, the cure rates were 83.8% and 60%, respectively. An RCT[20] in Iraq compared 19 patients (38 lesions) treated with intralesional 2% zinc sulfate and 18 patients (35 lesions) treated with intralesional 100 mg/mL sodium stibogluconate. Follow-up was performed for 6 weeks. A total of 88.5% (31 of 35) of the lesions were cured in comparison with 94.8% (36 of 38), respectively. In this RCT, 17 patients (40 lesions) were also treated with an intralesional hypertonic 7% sodium chloride solution. The results showed complete healing in 85% of the lesions (34 of 40).

Other. We found very limited RCT evidence for the lack of efficacy of treatments such as garlic cream,[21] cream containing interferon beta,[22] topical opium,[23] intralesional interferon gamma,[24] and topical antifungals.[25,26] We found very limited RCT evidence for the use of a topical herbal extract[27] and a topical diminazene solution of cetrimide (Savlon) with chlorhexidine.[28] We found moderate RCT evidence for the benefit of thermotherapy with radiofrequency waves[29] and intralesional metronidazole.[30] An RCT[31] in Iran compared 100 patients treated with cryotherapy and intralesional meglumine antimonate, and 200 patients treated with cryotherapy alone, both every 2 weeks. The groups were followed up for 6 months after treatment. The results showed clinical and parasitological cure in 90% of the lesions compared with 57.3%, respectively.

Drawbacks

Pain at the site of injection is frequently described in intralesional treatments. No other adverse reactions or local reactions were significantly reported. An appreciable number of cases of irritant contact dermatitis have been reported with topical paromomycin. Postinflammatory hypopigmentation and hyperpigmentation have been described with cryotherapy.

Comment

Most of the trials are relatively adequate in size, with short follow-up periods. In comparisons with placebo or no treatment, some trials showed variable rates of self-healing. The results of some of the studies are difficult to interpret due to unusually low cure rates in the group treated with antimonials.

Implications for practice

Local treatment is appropriate for patients with early, not very inflamed, lesions on cosmetically or functionally important sites, but an expectant approach may also be appropriate in Old World endemic areas, due to rapid spontaneous healing and the development of protective immunity.

To limit toxicity, antimony derivatives have been used intralesionally for localized Old World cutaneous leishmaniasis. There are some RCT data on the usefulness of intralesional administration of meglumine antimonate in comparison with other local and systemic treatments. Local pain and time-consuming intralesional treatments have led investigators to seek easier, pain-free treatment modalities such as paromomycin ointment, but on the basis of the best evidence, it is unlikely to be beneficial.

There is limited evidence for the use of intralesional zinc sulfate. Thermotherapy and cryotherapy are simple treatments that require further research. There is no RCT evidence for local excision, curettage, electrodessication, or other physical therapies.

What is the RCT evidence for systemic treatments in Old World cutaneous leishmaniasis?

Efficacy

Intramuscular/intravenous meglumine antimonate or stibogluconate. The mainstay of systemic treatment for Old World CL is the use of pentavalent antimony compounds, which have been extensively used as controls in RCTs for newer treatments. We found no RCTs comparing antimonials with a placebo.

Oral itraconazole. We found six RCTs versus placebo or no treatment. In an RCT[32] from Kuwait (*L. tropica* and *L. major*), 15 patients were given 100 mg (or 3 mg/kg) itraconazole and nine patients were given placebo, both twice per day for 6–8 weeks. Follow-up was 12 weeks after treatment. The results were excellent in 73% of the patients (11 of 15) and good in 20% (three of 15), in comparison with no signs of improvement in the placebo group. A double-blind RCT[33] in Iran (*L. major*) compared 100 patients treated with 200 mg/day itraconazole for 8 weeks with another 100 patients treated with placebo for the same period of time. The follow-up period was 8 weeks. Fifty-nine percent of the patients showed clinical cure and 83% showed parasitological cure, in comparison with 53% and 76%, respectively. In a double-blind RCT[34] in Iran (*L. tropica* and *L. major*), 7 mg/kg/day itraconazole for 3 weeks in 65 patients was compared with placebo in 66 patients. The follow-up was 1 month after treatment. The lesions in 55% of the patients (36 of 65) showed a clinical and biological response, compared with 41% (27 of 66), respectively. A double-blind RCT[35] in India (*L. major* and *L. tropica*) compared 10 patients treated with oral itraconazole 100 mg twice per day for 6 weeks with another 10 treated with placebo. The follow-up period was 3 months. Seven patients were cured, in comparison with only one patient with the placebo. Finally, an RCT[36] in India (*L. major* and *L. tropica*) compared 20 patients treated with 4 mg/kg/day itraconazole for 6 weeks with 20 patients treated with placebo. The follow-up period was 3 months after therapy. Complete healing was observed in 75% of the patients (15 of 20), in comparison with 10% (two of 20) with the placebo. This RCT also compared itraconazole with 20 patients treated with dapsone, in whom complete healing was seen in 90% of the patients (18 of 20). An RCT[37] in India (*L. tropica*) compared 15 patients treated with 4 mg/kg/day itraconazole for 6 weeks with five untreated patients. The follow-up period was 3 months. The results showed that 66.6% of the patients (10 of 15) were cured in comparison with no significant changes, respectively.

Oral ketoconazole. We found two RCTs comparing different doses. In an RCT[38] in India (*L. tropica*), 16 patients were treated with 200 mg ketoconazole twice per day for 10 weeks, and 19 patients were treated with 400 mg ketoconazole, twice per day for 6 weeks. The patients were followed up for 18 weeks. No clinical or parasitological improvement was observed in the patients in the 200-mg group. Four of 19 patients in the 400-mg group showed clinical and parasitological cure. In another RCT[39] in Kuwait, oral 600 mg/day ketoconazole for 28 days was given to 18 patients and oral 800 mg/day ketoconazole for 28 days was given to 15 patients. The patients were followed up for 6 months. Eighty percent of the patients (12 of 18) were cured in comparison with 82% (nine of 15), respectively.

An RCT[40] in Iran (*L. tropica* and *L. major*) compared 64 patients treated with oral 600 mg/day ketoconazole for 30 days and 32 patients treated with intralesional meglumine antimonate, six to eight injections bi-weekly. The follow-up period was 6 months after therapy. The results showed complete cure in 89% (57 of 64) and 72% (23 of 32) of the patients, respectively.

Oral fluconazole. In a double-blind RCT[41] in Saudi Arabia (*L. major*), 106 patients were treated with 200 mg/day fluconazole for 6 weeks and 103 patients were given placebo. At 3 months, complete healing of the lesions was observed in 59% of the patients, (63 of 106) in comparison with 21% (22 of 103).

Oral dapsone. We found three RCTs. A double-blind RCT[42] in India (*L. major* and *L. tropica*) compared 60 patients treated with 100 mg dapsone every 12 hours for 6 weeks, and 60 patients treated with placebo. The patients were followed up for 1 month after therapy. Complete cure was seen in 82% of the patients (49 of 60) compared with 5% (three of 60), respectively. In an RCT[36] in India (*L. major* and *L. tropica*), 20 patients were treated with 4 mg/kg/day dapsone, 20 patients with itraconazole, and 20 patients with placebo, all for 6 weeks. The follow-up period was 3 months after therapy. Complete healing was assessed in 90% of the patients (18 of 20) compared with 75% (15 of 20) and 10% (two of 20), respectively. An RCT[43] in India (*L. tropica*) compared 50 patients treated with 2 mg/kg/day dapsone for 21 days with 15 untreated patients. The follow-up period was 6 months after therapy. The results showed cure in 80% of the patients (40 of 50) and failure in 10% (five of 50), compared with no significant changes, respectively.

Oral allopurinol. We found three RCTs comparing this with systemic antimonials. An RCT[44] in Iran (*L. tropica*) compared 50 patients treated with oral allopurinol 15 mg/kg/day for 3 weeks, 50 patients treated with intramuscular 30 mg/kg/day meglumine antimonate for 2 weeks, and another 50 patients treated with allopurinol plus meglumine antimonate. The follow-up period was 1 month after treatment. The results were excellent in 18% (nine of 50) and good in 6% (three of 50); excellent in 24% (12 of 50) and good in 6% (three of 50); and excellent in 46% (23 of 50) and good in 8% (four of 50) of the patients, respectively. An open RCT[45] in Iran (*L. major*) compared 31 patients treated with 20 mg/kg/day allopurinol plus 30 mg/kg/day meglumine antimonate and 35 patients treated with intramuscular 60 mg/kg/day meglumine antimonate, both for 20 days. Follow-up was for 1 month. The results showed complete cure in 74% (23 of 31) and partial cure in 9.6% (three of 31), compared with complete cure in 60% (21 of 35) and partial cure in 20% (seven of 35) of the patients, respectively. An RCT[46] in Pakistan compared 20 patients treated with 20 mg/kg/day oral allopurinol in three or four doses and 20 patients treated with intravenous 20 mg/kg/day stibogluconate, both for 15 days. Follow-up was performed for 3 months after therapy. The results showed 70% of cure rate compared with 85%, respectively.

Other. We found very limited RCT evidence for the benefit of other treatments such as oral zinc sulfate[47] and rifampicin.[48]

Drawbacks
Parenteral antimonials can produce nausea, vomiting, anorexia, diarrhea, myalgia, body aches, and liver abnormalities. The most common side effects with oral antifungals were gastrointestinal complaints and headache, but the same symptoms were reported in patients from the placebo group and none of the laboratory values were outside normal limits. With oral dapsone, side effects include nausea and anemia. With oral allopurinol, side effects include nausea, macular rash, heartburn, and a mild increase in liver enzymes.

Comment
The results of some of the studies are difficult to interpret because of the small size of the samples, and again unusually low cure rates in the group treated with antimonials, as well as variable rates of self-healing.

Implications for practice
Systemic therapy in Old World CL is appropriate for patients with multiple or more complicated lesions. In these cases, pentavalent antimony compounds have been regarded as the first-line therapy. Their efficacy has been established in RCTs in comparison with other treatments, but not in comparisons between different antimonials or in comparison with a placebo.

When well tolerated and oral agents are needed or preferred, there is moderate RCT evidence to support the use of oral itraconazole, 200 mg/day for 6–8 weeks. There is only limited RCT evidence for the use of oral therapy with fluconazole, ketoconazole, dapsone, and allopurinol.

What is the RCT evidence for systemic treatments in American cutaneous leishmaniasis?

Efficacy
Intravenous/intramuscular meglumine antimonate. The mainstay of systemic treatment for American CL is the use of pentavalent antimony compounds, which have been extensively used in practice and as controls in RCTs for newer treatments. In contrast to Old World CL, we found several RCT comparing different antimonials.

An RCT[49] in Colombia (*L. panamensis*) compared 68 patients treated with 20 mg/kg/day intramuscular meglumine antimonate once a day for 10 days and 68 patients treated with 20 mg/kg/day intramuscular meglumine antimonate for 20 days. The follow-up period was 52 weeks after treatment. The results showed responses in 41% (28 of 68) and 35% (24 of 68), respectively.

In a double-blind RCT[50] in Brazil (*L. braziliensis*), 11 patients were treated with a high dose of intravenous meglumine antimonate (20 mg/kg/day) and 12 patients were treated with a low dose of intravenous meglumine antimonate (5 mg/kg/day), both for 30 days. The results showed complete responses in 81.8% (nine of 11) and 83.3% (10 of 12) of the patients, respectively.

We found three RCTs comparing meglumine antimonate with intramuscular stibogluconate. A single-blind RCT[51] in Brazil (*L. braziliensis*) compared 32 patients treated with 15 mg/kg/day intramuscular meglumine antimonate and 31 patients treated with 15 mg/kg/day intramuscular sodium stibogluconate, both for 20 days. The follow-up period was 3 months. The results showed cure in 81% of the patients (26 of 32) compared with 77% (24 of 31), respectively. In an RCT[52] in Panama (*L. braziliensis panamensis*), 29 patients were treated with 20 mg/kg/day intramuscular meglumine antimonate and 30 patients were treated with 20 mg/kg/day intramuscular stibogluconate, both for 20 days. The follow-up period was 1 year. The results showed complete cure in 72% (21 of 29) and 46% (14 of 30) of the patients, respectively. In a double-blind RCT[53] in Bolivia and Colombia (*L. braziliensis*), 50 patients were treated with 20 mg/kg/day intramuscular meglumine antimonate, 16 patients were treated with 20 mg/kg/day intramuscular stibogluconate (Pentostam) and 48 patients with stibogluconate (generic), all for 20 days. The follow-up period was 6 months. The results showed complete cure in 76% (38 of 50), 75% (12 of 16), and 83% (40 of 48) of patients, respectively.

Intravenous/intramuscular stibogluconate. A double-blind RCT[54] of USA military personnel compared 19 patients treated with 20 mg/kg/day intravenous stibogluconate for 20 days with 19 patients treated with 20 mg/kg/day intravenous stibogluconate for 10 days, followed by placebo for

10 more days. Follow-up was performed for 1 year. The results showed a complete clinical response in six patients and clinical improvement in one patient, compared with a clinical response in five patients and clinical improvement in five patients, respectively. A double-blind RCT[55] in Panama and Central America (*L. braziliensis panamensis*) compared 19 patients treated with 20 mg/kg/day stibogluconate and 21 patients treated with 10 mg/kg/day stibogluconate, both for 20 days. The results, 9 weeks after the start of treatment, showed that 100% versus 76% (16 of 21) of the patients were cured, respectively. An RCT[56] of USA military personnel compared 12 patients treated with 600 mg intravenous stibogluconate once daily for 10 days by rapid infusion; 12 patients treated with 600 mg/day intravenous stibogluconate followed by a continuous infusion of 600 mg stibogluconate for 24 hours every day for 9 days; 12 patients treated with a stibogluconate loading dose of 600 mg followed by 200 mg stibogluconate every 8 hours for 9 days. The patients were followed up for 1 year. The results showed complete cure in 100% (all of 12), 50% (six of 12), and 42% (five of 12) of the patients, respectively.

Intravenous/intramuscular paromomycin. We found three RCTs. In an open RCT[57] in Brazil (*L. braziliensis*) comparing 15 patients treated with 4 mg/kg/day intramuscular pentamidine on alternative days up to a total of eight injections, 15 patients were treated with 20 mg/kg/day intramuscular paromomycin for 20 days and 16 patients were treated with 10 mg/kg/day intramuscular meglumine for 20 days. The patients were followed up for 3 years after the end of treatment. At the end of the follow-up, all of the patients in the paromomycin and pentamidine groups were cured. An open RCT[58] in Belize (*L. braziliensis* and *L. mexicana*) compared 17 patients treated with intravenous paromomycin 14 mg/kg/day and 17 patients treated with intravenous sodium stibogluconate 20 mg/kg/day, both for 20 days. Follow-up was performed for at least 6 months. The results showed clinical cure in 59% (10 of 17) and parasitological cure in 53% (nine of 17) of the patients, compared with 88% (15 of 17) and parasitological cure in 59% (10 of 17), respectively. An RCT[59] in Colombia (*L. panamensis*) compared 30 patients treated with parenteral 12 mg/kg/day paromomycin for 7 days; 29 patients treated with parenteral 12 mg/kg/day paromomycin for 14 days; and 30 patients treated with parenteral paromomycin 18 mg/kg/day for 14 days. The follow-up period was 12 months after treatment. The results showed cures in 10% (three of 30), 45% (13 of 29) and 50% (15 of 30) of patients, respectively.

Oral itraconazole. An RCT[60] in Colombia (*L. panamensis*) compared 20 patients treated with 200 mg oral itraconazole twice a day for 28 days, 23 patients treated with 10 mg/kg intramuscular meglumine antimonate twice a day for 20 days, and 22 untreated patients. The patients were fol-

lowed up for 12 months. Cures were observed in 5% (one of 20), 91% (21 of 23), and 27% (six of 22) of the patients, respectively.

Oral ketoconazole. An RCT[61] in Guatemala compared 38 patients treated with 600 mg/day ketoconazole for 28 days and 40 patients treated with 20 mg/kg/day intravenous stibogluconate for 20 days. The follow-up period was 1 year. The results in patients infected with *L. braziliensis* showed cures in 30% (seven of 23) and 96% (24 of 25), respectively. In the group of patients infected with *L. mexicana*, cures were observed in 89% (eight of nine) and 57% (four of seven), respectively. Another RCT[62] in Panama (*L. braziliensis panamensis*) compared 22 patients treated with oral 600 mg/day ketoconazole for 28 days and 19 patients treated with 20 mg/kg intramuscular stibogluconate for 20 days. The follow-up period was 3 months. The results showed cures in 73% (16 of 22) and 68% (13 of 19) of the patients, respectively.

Oral allopurinol. We found three RCTs comparing this with meglumine antimonate. An open RCT[63] in Colombia (*L. braziliensis panamensis*) compared 33 patients treated with 20 mg/kg/day intramuscular meglumine antimonate for 15 days, 35 patients treated with oral allopurinol plus 20 mg/kg/day intramuscular meglumine antimonate in four divided doses for 15 days, 23 patients treated with 20 mg/kg/day oral allopurinol in four divided doses for 15 days, and 17 untreated patients. The follow-up period was 12 months after treatment. The results showed cures in 36% (12 of 33), 74% (26 of 35), 80% (20 of 23) and 0%, respectively. In an open RCT[64] in Brazil (*L. braziliensis braziliensis*), 16 patients were treated with 10 mg/kg/day intravenous meglumine antimonate once a day and 18 patients were treated with 20 mg/kg oral allopurinol three times a day, both for 20 days. The patients were followed up for 3 months. The results showed healed lesions in 50% (eight of 16) of the patients and no healed lesions (one progressed to mucosal disease), respectively. In a double-blind RCT[65] in Colombia (*L. panamensis*), 56 patients were treated with 20 mg/kg/day intramuscular meglumine antimonate for 20 days, 55 patients were treated with three tablets of allopurinol 100 mg four times daily (20 mg/kg/day) for 28 days, and 46 patients were given placebo. The follow-up period was 12 months. The results showed cures in 92% (52 of 56), 32.7% (18 of 55), and 37% (17 of 46) of the patients, respectively.

We found two RCTs comparing allopurinol with stibogluconate. An open RCT[66] in Colombia (*L. braziliensis panamensis*) compared 49 patients treated with 20 mg/kg/day stibogluconate for 15 days and 51 patients treated with 20 mg/kg/day stibogluconate for 15 days plus oral allopurinol 20 mg/kg/day also for 15 days. The follow-up period was 12 months after therapy. Thirty-nine percent of the patients (19 of 49) were cured, 14% (seven of 49) relapsed, and the treatment failed in 43% (21 of 49), compared with cures in 71% (36 of 51), relapses in 27% (14 of 51), and treatment failure in 12% (six of 51), respectively. In an RCT[67] in Ecuador (*L. panamensis*), 28 patients were treated with 20 mg/kg/day intramuscular stibogluconate for 20 days, 21 patients were treated with oral allopurinol ribonucleoside (1500 mg q.i.d.) plus oral probenecid for 28 days, and 12 patients remained untreated. The follow-up period was 12 months. The results in the stibogluconate group showed cures in 96.4% of the patients (27 of 28). In the allopurinol group, 42.8% of the patients (nine of 21) were cured, and the treatment failed in 10 patients. In the untreated group, 75% of the patients were cured (nine of 12) and the treatment failed in three patients.

Intramuscular pentamidine. In an RCT[60] in Colombia (*L. panamensis*), 23 patients were treated with 10 mg/kg intramuscular meglumine antimonate twice a day for 20 days and 27 patients were treated with 2 mg/kg intramuscular pentamidine every other day, up to a total of seven injections. The patients were followed up for 12 months. Cure was observed in 91% (21 of 23) and 85% (23 of 27) of the patients, respectively. An open RCT[57] in Brazil (*L. braziliensis*) compared 16 patients treated with 10 mg/kg/day intramuscular meglumine for 20 days and 15 patients treated with 4 mg/kg/day intramuscular pentamidine, on alternative days, up to a total of eight injections. The patients were followed up for 3 years. Only one patient in the meglumine group did not achieve a cure, and all of the other patients were cured. In an open RCT[68] in Peru (*L. braziliensis*), 40 patients were treated with 20 mg/kg/day intravenous meglumine antimonate for 20 days and 40 patients were treated with 2 mg/kg intramuscular pentamidine every other day, up to a total of seven injections. The patients were followed up for 6 months. Cures were observed in 78% (31 of 40) and 35% (14 of 40) of the patients, respectively.

Other treatments. We found very limited RCT evidence for the efficacy of other systemic treatments such as immunotherapy with a parasite-derived antigen,[69] oral miltefosine,[70] and adjuvant interferon gamma in intravenous meglumine antimonate therapy.[71] We also found limited RCT evidence of lack of efficacy with oral mefloquine.[72]

Drawbacks

The more frequent side effects of meglumine antimonate are arthralgias, myalgias, asthenia, malaise, nausea, pruritus, headache and fever. There was no evidence of liver, cardiac, bone-marrow, or kidney toxicity. The symptoms reported with stibogluconate include cases of pancreatitis, but no other significant side effects. Intramuscular paromomycin produced myalgia, anorexia, and asthenia. Oral miltefosine showed no side effects different from those of the placebo.

The only severe side effects attributable to allopurinol were headache and epigastric pain. Pentamidine produced cases of hypotension, hypoglycemia, headache, myalgia, anorexia, asthenia, and arthralgia.

Comment

The results of some studies are difficult to interpret, as large numbers of patients were lost to follow-up.

Implications for practice

Systemic therapy with intravenous or intramuscular pentavalent antimony compounds in American CL is regarded as being the first-line therapy, due to the progression to mucocutaneous disease in infections with *L. braziliensis*. There is moderate RCT evidence for the efficacy of these treatments.

There is some limited evidence for the efficacy of intramuscular pentamidine, but its use can be limited by the side effects. There is some RCT evidence for a lack of significant effects with oral itraconazole, oral ketoconazole, and oral allopurinol.

What is the RCT evidence for local treatments in American cutaneous leishmaniasis?

Efficacy

Topical paromomycin/MBCL. A double-blind RCT[73] in Colombia (*L. braziliensis panamensis*) compared 59 patients treated with topical paromomycin/MBCL twice a day for 10 days plus stibogluconate for 7 days; 30 patients treated with topical placebo twice a day for 10 days plus stibogluconate for 7 days; 30 patients treated with topical paromomycin/MBCL twice a day for 10 days plus stibogluconate for 3 days; and 31 patients treated with injectable stibogluconate for 20 days. The follow-up period was 12 months. The percentages of cures were: 58%, 53%, 20% and 84%, respectively. A double-blind RCT[74] in Ecuador (*L. viannia*) compared 40 patients treated with topical 15% paromomycin/12% MBCL twice daily for 30 days; 40 patients treated with topical 15% paromomycin plus 10% urea twice daily for 30 days; and 40 patients treated with 20 mg/kg/day intramuscular meglumine antimonate for 10 days. The percentages of cures were: 57.5% (23 of 40), 52.5% (21 of 40), and 82.5% (33 of 40), respectively, at 12 weeks after the start of treatment.

A double-blind RCT[75] in Guatemala (*L. braziliensis*) compared 35 patients treated with 15% paromomycin and 12% MBCL twice a day for 20 days and 33 patients given placebo. A clinical response was observed after 12 months in 85.7% (31 of 35) and 39.4% (13 of 33), respectively. Another double-blind RCT[76] in Honduras (*L. mexicana* and *L. chagasi*) compared 23 patients treated with 15% paromomycin and 10% urea for 4 weeks and 30 patients receiving a placebo. Complete cure at 15 weeks was seen in two of the 23 patients in the paromomycin group and two of the 30 patients in the placebo group.

Other treatments. We found limited RCT evidence for the efficacy of other treatments such as WR279396 (composed cream)[77] and heat from a radiofrequency generator.[78] Some evidence was found for the utility of adjuvant topical human granulocyte-macrophage colony-stimulating factor[79,80] and for topical 5% imiquimod combined with parenteral antimonials.[81]

Drawbacks
Side effects reported in topical paromomycin therapy included local pruritus, a burning sensation, local pain, and local edema.

Comment
Some adjuvant local therapies are described in one trial that need to be further investigated.

Implications for practice
Local therapy in American cutaneous leishmaniasis is an option only for patients who are not at risk of mucocutaneous disease and with early, not very inflamed, lesions. There is no RCT evidence for local excision, curettage, or electrodessication. However, there is no good RCT evidence to recommend any of the local treatments described. There is some RCT evidence for the lack of efficacy of paromomycin.

Key points

- In our search for the best available evidence on treatments for cutaneous leishmaniasis, we found 25 RCTs of local therapies and 18 RCTs of systemic therapies for Old World cuataneous leishmaniasis. For American cutaneous leishmaniasis, there were 25 RCTs of systemic therapies and nine RCTs of local therapies.
- There is a definite need to identify less expensive, painless, and safer treaments for CL, but definitive recommendations are limited as there have been few rigorously designed randomized clinical trials.
- Varying susceptibility to the different species of *Leishmania* that occur in different geographical regions needs to be taken into account in the response to treatment.
- The development of drug resistance is a major concern when evaluating older trials.

Therapies for Old World cutaneous leishmaniasis
- An expectant approach may be appropriate in Old World endemic areas, in view of rapid spontaneous healing and the development of protective immunity in most cases.
- Pentavalent antimony compounds are considered to be the first-line therapy. Local treatment is used for patients with early, not highly inflamed, lesions on cosmetically or functionally important sites. Systemic therapy may be appropriate for patients with multiple or more complicated lesions.

- The range of affordable and painless treatment modalities includes oral drugs, but on the basis of the best present evidence the latter are unlikely to be beneficial. If well tolerated oral agents are needed or preferred, then there is moderate RCT evidence to support the use of oral itraconazole.

Therapies for American cutaneous leishmaniasis
- Although systemic therapy with pentavalent antimony compounds may be expensive and their administration is associated with severe adverse effects, they are still the first-line drugs for American cutaneous leishmaniasis.

Acknowledgments

Research for this chapter was supported in part by a grant from the International Health Central American Institute Foundation. The authors are grateful for the assistance of Dr. Alireza Firooz in translating some Iranian papers and help from Dr. Mario Tristan in developing this project.

References

1 Herwaldt B. Leishmaniasis. *Lancet* 1999;**354**:1191–9.
2 Salman SM, Rubeiz NG, Kibbi A. Cutaneous leishmaniasis: clinical features and diagnosis. *Clin Dermatol* 1999;**17**:292–6.
3 World Health Organization. Leishmaniasis: background information. http://www.who.int/leishmaniasis/en/ (last accessed 5 April 2006).
4 Hepburn NC. Management of cutaneous leishmaniasis. *Curr Opin Infect Dis* 2001;**14**:151–4.
5 Faber WR, Oskam L, Gool T van, *et al.* Value of diagnostic techniques for cutaneous leishmaniasis. *J Am Acad Dermatol* 2003;**49**:70–4.
6 Moskowitz PF, Kurban AK. Treatment of cutaneous leishmaniasis: retrospectives and advances for the 21st century. *Clin Dermatol* 1999;**17**:305–15.
7 Arana B, Rizzo N, Diaz A. Chemotherapy of cutaneous leishmaniasis: a review. *Med Microbiol Immunol* 2001;**190**:93–5.
8 Alkhawajah AM, Larbi E, Al-Gindan Y, *et al.* Treatment of cutaneous leishmaniasis with antimony: intramuscular versus intralesional administration. *Ann Trop Med Parasitol* 1997;**91**:899–905.
9 Mujtaba G, Khalid M. Weekly vs. fortnightly intralesional meglumine antimoniate in cutaneous leishmaniasis. *Int J Dermatol* 1999;**38**:607–9.
10 Ben Salah A, Zakraoui H, Zaatour A, *et al.* A randomized, placebo-controlled trial in Tunisia treating cutaneous leishmaniasis with paromomycin ointment. *Am J Trop Med Hyg* 1995;**53**:162–6.
11 Asilian A, Jalayer T, Whitworth JAG, *et al.* A randomized, placebo-controlled trial of a two-week regimen of aminosidine (paromomycin) ointment for treatment of cutaneous leishmaniasis in Iran. *Am J Trop Med Hyg* 1995;**53**:648–51.
12 Iraji F, Sadeghinia A. Efficacy of paromomycin ointment in the treatment of cutaneous leishmaniasis: results of a double-blind, randomized trial in Isfahan, Iran. *Ann Trop Med Parasitol* 2005;**99**:3–9.

13 Asilian A, Jalayer T, Nilforooshzadeh M, *et al.* Treatment of cutaneous leishmaniasis with aminosidine (paromomycin) ointment: double-blind, randomized trial in the Islamic Republic of Iran. *Bull World Health Org* 2003,**81**:353–9.

14 El-On J, Halevy S, Grunwald MH, *et al.* Topical treatment of old world cutaneous leishmaniasis caused by Leishmania major: a double-blind control study. *J Am Acad Dermatol* 1992;**27**(Part 1): 227–31.

15 Faghihi G, Tavakoli-kia R. Treatment of cutaneous leishmaniasis with either topical paromomycin or intralesional meglumine antimoniate. *Clin Exp Dermatol* 2003;**28**:13–6.

16 Shazad B, Abbaszadeh B, Khamesipour A. Comparison of topical paromomycin sulfate (twice/day) with intralesional meglumine antimoniate for the treatment of cutaneous leishmaniasis caused by L. major. *Eur J Dermatol* 2005;**15**:85–7.

17 Ozgoztasi O, Baydar I. A randomized clinical trial of topical paromomycin versus oral ketoconazole for treating cutaneous leishmaniasis in Turkey. *Int J Dermatol* 1997;**36**:61–3.

18 Firooz A. Intralesional injection of 2% zinc sulphate solution in the treatment of acute Old World cutaneous leishmaniasis: a randomized, double-blind, controlled trial. *J Drugs Dermatol* 2005; **4**:73–9.

19 Iraji F, Vali A, Asilian A, *et al.* Comparison of intralesionally injected zinc sulfate with meglumine antimoniate in the treatment of acute cutaneous leishmaniasis. *Dermatology* 2004;**209**: 46–9.

20 Sharquie KE, Najim RA, Farjou IB. Comparative controlled trial of intralesionally-administered zinc sulphate, hypertonic sodium chloride and pentavalent antimony compound against acute cutaneous leishmaniasis. *Clin Exp Dermatol* 1997;**22**:169–73.

21 Gholami A, Khamesipour A, Momeni A, *et al.* Treatment of cutaneous leishmaniasis with 5% garlic cream: a randomized, double-blind study. *Iran J Dermatol* 2000;**3**:1.

22 Trau H, Schewach-Millet M, Shoham J, *et al.* Topical application of human fibroblast interferon (IFN) in cutaneous leishmaniasis. *Isr J Med Sci* 1987;**23**:1125–7.

23 Mapar MA, Kavoosi H, Dabbagh MA. Assessment of the effect of topical opium in treatment of cutaneous leishmaniasis. *Iran J Dermatol* 2001;**4**:4.

24 Harms G, Chehade AK, Douba M, *et al.* A randomized trial comparing a pentavalent antimonial drug and recombinant interferon-γ in the local treatment of cutaneous leishmaniasis. *Trans R Soc Trop Med Hyg* 1991;**85**:214–6.

25 Larbi E B, Al-Khawajah, A, Al-Gindan Y. A randomized, double-blind, clinical trial of topical clotrimazole versus miconazole for treatment of cutaneous leishmaniasis in the eastern province of Saudi Arabia. *Am J Trop Med Hyg* 1995;**52**:166–8.

26 Momeni A, Aminjavaheri M, Omid MR. Treatment of cutaneous leishmaniasis with ketoconazole cream. *J Dermatol Treat* 2003; **14**:26–9.

27 Zerehsaz F, Salmanpour R, Handjani F, *et al.* A double-blind randomized clinical trial of a topical herbal extract (Z-HE) vs. systemic meglumine antimoniate for the treatment of cutaneous leishmaniasis in Iran. *Int J Dermatol* 1999;**38**:610–2.

28 Lynen L, Van Damme. Local application of diminazene aceturate: an effective treatment for cutaneous leishmaniasis. *Ann Soc Belge Med Trop* 1992;**72**:13–9.

29 Reithinger R, Mohsen M, Wahid M, *et al.* Efficacy of thermotherapy to treat cutaneous leishmaniasis caused by Leishmania

tropica in Kabul, Afghanistan: a randomized, controlled trial. *Clin Infect Dis* 2005;**40**:1148–54.

30 Al-Waiz MM, Sharquie KE, Al-Assir M. Treatment of cutaneous leishmaniasis by intralesional metronidazole. *Saudi Med J* 2004;**25**: 1512–3.

31 Asilian A, Sadeghinia A, Fghihi G, *et al.* Comparative study of the efficacy of combined cryotherapy and intralesional meglumine antimoniate (Glucantime) vs. cryotherapy and intralesional meglumine antimoniate (Glucantime) alone for the treatment of cutaneous leishmaniasis. *Int J Dermatol* 2004;**43**:281–3.

32 Al-Fouzan AS, Al Saleh QA, Najem NM. Cutaneous Leishmaniasis in Kuwait. *Int J Dermatol* 1991;**30**:519–21.

33 Nassiri-Kashani M, Firooz A, Khamesipour A, *et al.* A randomized, double-blind, placebo-controlled clinical trial of itraconazole in the treatment of cutaneous leishmaniasis. *J Eur Acad Dermatol Venereol* 2005;**19**:80–3.

34 Momeni A, Jalayer T, Emamjomeh M, *et al.* Treatment of cutaneous leishmaniasis with Itraconazole. *Arch Dermatol* 1996;**132**: 784–6.

35 Dogra J, Saxena VN. Itraconazole and leishmaniasis: a randomised double-blind trial in cutaneous disease. *Int J Parasitol* 1996;**26**: 1413–5.

36 Dogra J. Cutaneous Leishmaniasis in India: evaluation of oral drugs (dapsone versus itraconazole). *Eur J Dermatol* 1992;**2**:568– 9.

37 Dogra J, Aneja N, Lal BB, *et al.* Cutaneous Leishmaniasis in India. *Int J Dermatol* 1990;**29**:661–2.

38 Singh S, Singh R, Sundar S. Failure of ketoconazole in oriental sore in India. *J Chemother* 1995;**7**:202–3.

39 Alsaleh QA, Dvorak R, Nanda A. Ketoconazole in the treatment of cutaneous leishmaniasis in Kuwait. *Int J Dermatol* 1995;**34**: 495–7.

40 Salmanpour R, Handjani F, Nouhpisheh MK. Comparative study of the efficacy of oral ketoconazole with intralesional meglumine antimoniate (Glucantime) for the treatment of cutaneous leishmaniasis. *J Dermatolog Treat* 2001;**12**:159–62.

41 Alrajhi A, Ibrahim EA, De Vol EB, *et al.* Fluconazole for the treatment of cutaneous leishmaniasis caused by Leishmania major. *N Engl J Med* 2002;**346**:891–5.

42 Dogra J. A double-blind study on the efficacy of oral dapsone in cutaneous leishmaniasis. *Trans R Soc Trop Med Hyg* 1991;**85**:212–3.

43 Dogra J, Lal BB, Misra SN. Dapsone in the treatment of cutaneous leishmaniasis. *Int J Dermatol* 1986;**25**:398–400.

44 Esfandiarpour I, Alavi A. Evaluating the efficacy of allopurinol and meglumine antimoniate (Glucantime) in the treatment of cutaneous leishmaniasis. *Int J Dermatol* 2002;**41**:521–4.

45 Momeni AZ, Reiszadae MR, Aminjavaheri M. Treatment of cutaneous leishmaniasis with a combination of allopurinol and low-dose meglumine antimoniate. *Int J Dermatol* 2002;**41**:441–3.

46 Mashhood AA, Hussain K. Efficacy of allopurinol compared with pentostam in the treatment of old world cutaneous leishmaniasis. *J Coll Physicians Surg Pak* 2001;**11**:367–70.

47 Sharquie KE, Najim RA, Farjou IB, *et al.* Oral zinc sulphate in the treatment of acute cutaneous leishmaniasis. *Clin Exp Dermatol* 2001;**26**:21–6.

48 Kochar DK, Aseri S, Sharma B, *et al.* The role of rifampicin in the management of cutaneous leishmaniasis. *QJM* 2000;**93**:733–7.

49 Palacios R, Osorio LE, Grajales LF, *et al.* Treatment failure in children in a randomized clinical trial with 10 and 20 days of

meglumine antimonate for cutaneous leishmaniasis due to *Leishmania viannia* species. *Am J Trop Med Hyg* 2001;**64**:187–93.

50 Oliveira-Neto MP, Schubach A, Mattos M, *et al.* Treatment of American cutaneous leishmaniasis: a comparison between low dosage (5 mg/kg/day) and high dosage (20 mg/kg/day) antimony regimens. *Pathol Biol* 1997;**45**:496–9.

51 Deps PD, Viana MC, Falqueto A, Dietze R. [Comparative assessment of the efficacy and toxicity of N-methyl-glucamine and BP88 sodium stibogluconate in the treatment of localized cutaneous leishmaniasis; in Portuguese.] *Rev Soc Bras Med Trop* 2000;**33**: 535–43.

52 Saenz RE, Paz HM, Johnson CM, Narvaez E, de Vasquez AM. [Evaluation of the effectiveness and toxicity of Pentostam and Glucantime in the treatment of cutaneous leishmaniasis; in Spanish.] *Rev Med Panama* 1987;**12**:148–57.

53 Soto J, Valda-Rodriguez L, Toledo J, *et al.* Comparison of generics to branded pentavalent antimony for treatment of new world cutaneous leishmaniasis. *Am J Trop Med Hyg* 2004;**71**:577–81.

54 Wortmann R, Scott Miller R, Oster C, *et al.* A randomized, double-blind study of efficacy of a 10- or 20-day course of sodium stibogluconate for treatment of cutaneous leishmaniasis in United States military personnel. *Clin Infect Dis* 2002;**35**:261–7.

55 Ripley W, McClain, Gordon DM, *et al.* Safety and efficacy of high-dose sodium stibogluconate therapy of American cutaneous leishmaniasis. *Lancet* 1987;**30**:13–6.

56 Oster CN, Chulay JD, Hendricks LD, *et al.* American cutaneous leishmaniasis: a comparison of three sodium stibogluconate treatment schedules. *Am J Trop Med Hyg* 1985;**34**:856–60.

57 Correia D, Macedo VO, Carvalho EM, *et al.* [Comparative study of meglumine antimoniate, pentamidine isethionate and aminosidine sulfate in the treatment of primary skin lesions caused by *Leishmania (viannia) braziliensis*; in Portuguese.] *Rev Soc Bras Med Trop* 1996;**29**:447–53.

58 Hepburn NC, Tidman MJ, Hunter AA. Aminosidine (paromomycin) versus sodium stibogluconate for the treatment of American cutaneous leishmaniasis. *Trans R Soc Trop Med Hyg* 1994;**88**:700–3.

59 Soto J, Grogl M, Berman J, *et al.* Limited efficacy of injectable aminosidine as single-agent therapy for Colombian cutaneous leishmaniasis. *Trans R Soc Trop Med Hyg* 1994;**88**:695–8.

60 Soto-Mancipe J, Grogl M, Berman JD. Evaluation of pentamidine for the treatment of cutaneous leishmaniasis in Colombia. *Clin Infect Dis* 1993;**16**:417–25.

61 Navin TR, Arana BA, Arana FE, *et al.* Placebo-controlled clinical trial of sodium stibogluconate (Pentostam) versus ketoconazole for treating cutaneous leishmaniasis in Guatemala. *J Infect Dis* 1992;**165**:528–34.

62 Saenz RE, Paz H, Berman JD. Efficacy of ketoconazole against *Leishmania braziliensis panamensis* cutaneous leishmaniasis. *Am J Med* 1990;**89**:147–55.

63 Martínez S, Marr J. Allopurinol in the treatment of American cutaneous leishmaniasis. *N Engl J Med* 1992;**326**:741–4.

64 D'Oliveira A, Machado PR, Cravalho E. Evaluating the efficacy of allopurinol for the treatment of cutaneous leishmaniasis. *Int J Dermatol* 1997;**36**:938–40.

65 Velez I, Agudelo S, Hendrickx E, *et al.* Inefficacy of allopurinol as monotherapy for Colombian cutaneous leishmaniasis: a randomized, controlled trial. *Ann Intern Med* 1997;**126**:232–6.

66 Martínez S, González M, Vernaza ME. Treatment of cutaneous leishmaniasis with allopurinol and stibogluconate. *Clin Infect Dis* 1997;**24**:165–9.

67 Guderian RH, Chico ME, Rogers MD, *et al.* Placebo controlled treatment of Ecuadorian cutaneous leishmaniasis. *Am J Trop Med Hyg* 1991;**45**:92–7.

68 Andersen EM, Cruz-Saldarriaga M, Llanos-Cuentas A, *et al.* Comparison of meglumine antimoniate and pentamidine for Peruvian cutaneous leishmaniasis. *Am J Trop Med Hyg* 2005;**72**:133–7.

69 Monjor L, Neogy AB, Vouldoukis J, *et al.* Exploitation of parasite derived antigen in therapeutic success of human cutaneous leishmaniasis in Brazil. *Mem Inst Oswaldo Cruz* 1994;**89**:479–83.

70 Soto J, Arana BA, Toledo J, *et al.* Miltefosine for New World cutaneous leishmaniasis. *Clin Infect Dis* 2004;**38**:1266–72.

71 Arana BA, Navin TR, Arana FE, Berman JD, Rosenkaimer F. Efficacy of a short course (10 days) of high-dose meglumine antimonate with or without interferon-gamma in treating cutaneous leishmaniasis in Guatemala. *Clin Infect Dis* 1994;**18**:381–4.

72 Laguna-Torres VA, Silva CAC, Correia D, *et al.* [Mefloquine in the treatment of cutaneous leishmaniasis in an endemic area of *Leishmania (viannia) braziliensis*; in Portuguese.] *Rev Soc Bras Med Trop* 1999;**32**:529–32.

73 Soto J, Fuya P, Herrera R, Berman J. Topical paromomycin/methylbenzethonium chloride plus parenteral meglumine antimonate as treatment for American cutaneous leishmaniasis: controlled study. *Clin Infect Dis* 1998;**26**:56–8.

74 Armijos RX, Weigel MM, Calvopina M, Mancheno M, Rodriguez R. Comparison of the effectiveness of two topical paromomycin treatments versus meglumine antimoniate for New World cutaneous leishmaniasis. *Acta Trop* 2004;**91**:153–60.

75 Arana BA, Mendoza CE, Rizzo NR, *et al.* Randomized, controlled, double-blind trial of topical treatment of cutaneous leishmaniasis with paromomycin plus methylbenzethonium chloride ointment in Guatemala. *Am J Trop Med Hyg* 2001;**65**:466–70.

76 Neva FA, Ponce C, Ponce E, *et al.* Non-ulcerative cutaneous leishmaniasis in Honduras fails to respond to topical paromomycin. *Trans R Soc Trop Med Hyg* 1997;**91**:473–5.

77 Soto JM, Toledo JT, Gutiérrez P, *et al.* Treatment of cutaneous leishmaniasis with a topical antileishmanial drug WR279396: phase 2 pilot study. *Am J Trop Hyg* 2002;**66**:147–51.

78 Navin TR, Arana BA, Arana FE, de Merida AM, Castillo AL, Pozuelos JL. Placebo-controlled clinical trial of meglumine antimonate (Glucantime) vs. localized controlled heat in the treatment of cutaneous leishmaniasis in Guatemala. *Am J Trop Med Hyg* 1990;**42**:43–50.

79 Santos JB, Ribeiro A, Machado PR, *et al.* Antimony plus recombinant human granulocyte-macrophage colony-stimulating factor applied topically in low doses enhances healing of cutaneous leishmaniasis ulcers: a randomized, double-blind, placebo-controlled study. *J Infect Dis* 2004;**190**:1793–6.

80 Almeida R, D'Oliveira A, Machado P, *et al.* Randomized, double-blind study of stibogluconate plus human granulocyte macrophage colony-stimulating factor versus stibogluconate alone. *J Infect Dis* 1999;**180**:1735–7.

81 Miranda-Verástegui C, Llanos-Cuentas A, Arévalo I, Ward BJ, Matlashewski G. Randomized, double-blind clinical trial of topical imiquimod 5% with parenteral meglumine antimoniate in the treatment of cutaneous leishmaniasis in Peru. *Clin Infect Dis* 2005;**40**:1395–403.

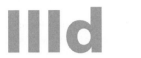

IIId Infestations

Berthold Rzany, Editor

46 Scabies

Ian F. Burgess

Background

Definition

Scabies is an itchy immune hypersensitivity reaction to infestation of the skin by the mite *Sarcoptes scabiei*. Fertilized adult female mites burrow through the skin at the junction of the stratum corneum and the prickle cell layer, where they lay their eggs. Burrows are pushed out progressively towards the skin surface with the stratum corneum. Adult males and juvenile mites (larvae and nymphs) live mostly on the skin surface, but may make temporary burrows for molting from one development stage to another.

Infestation of immune-competent people is most common on the hands, digits and finger webs, and on the wrists. The flexor surfaces of the elbows, the axillae, ankles, buttocks, breasts, and male genitalia may also be infested. In the elderly, infants, and the immunocompromised, the infestation may be more diffuse, including the head and neck, and palms and soles.

Incidence/prevalence

We found no recent published data on the incidence or prevalence from any developed country. Scabies is a common public health problem in developing countries, where the prevalence may exceed 50% in some communities, and the prevalence has been estimated at 300 million cases worldwide.[1] Older studies have shown that the prevalence is highest in teenagers and schoolchildren.[2-4] However, the incidence has increased recently in the institutionalized elderly in nearly all countries. Historical data from Denmark show that epidemic cycles arise at 15–20-year intervals.[2]

Etiology/risk factors

Transmission of scabies mites occurs during relatively prolonged skin–skin contact. The infection is most frequent in communities with long-term conditions of overcrowding, and is believed to increase following social disruption. Reduction of immune competence increases the risk of contracting infestation, with a concomitant risk of high mite numbers. We found no evidence that hygiene influences the risk, although good hygiene may ameliorate symptomatic presentation.[5]

Prognosis

Scabies is not life-threatening, but the severe, persistent itch and secondary infections may be debilitating and disfiguring. Long-term infestations are inherently immunodepressive and in susceptible people may lead to the development of a form of the disease in which large numbers of mites inhabit hyperkeratotic plaques. These shed skin plaques may be a source of reinfection and transmission.[6] In some circumstances, scabies infected with hemolytic streptococci may result in acute glomerulonephritis.[5]

Diagnosis

A diagnosis of active infestation is confirmed only by finding mites, mite ova, or fecal pellets (scybala) (parasitological diagnosis). Mite burrows in the skin, the distribution of papular lesions, and bilateral itch not affecting the head, chest, or back are indicative (clinical diagnosis), as is clustering of cases of nocturnal pruritus associated with a rash in household contacts; but these findings are not confirmation of an active infestation. Nodular lesions around the axillae, navel, or on the penis or scrotum are pathognomonic, but may persist for months after cure.

Aims of treatment

The aim of treatment is to eliminate infestation by killing all mites and their eggs.

Outcomes

There are no established standard criteria for making a

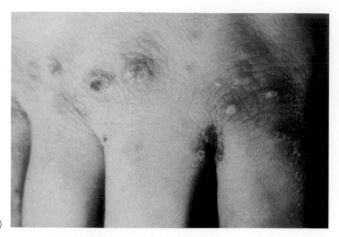 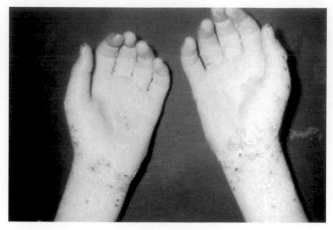

(a)   (b)

Figure 46.1 Papules, pustules and impetiginization in the vicinity of scabies burrows (a) and excoriated rash and papules on the wrists in simple scabies (b).

diagnosis or judging treatment success. Trials have used different methods, and in many cases the method was not stated. Treatment success should be given as the percentage of people completely cleared of scabies mites, ova, or fecal pellets in skin scrapings viewed under magnification. Clinical success includes elimination of papular and vesicular eruptions and pruritus. Ideally, outcomes should be assessed 28 days after the start of treatment, but interim assessments contribute to the clinical and parasitological picture. This allows time for lesions to heal, but assessment after 28 days risks confounding of the result through re-infestation. If treatment fails, eggs hatch within 3 days, and emerging mites become mature 9–10 days later.

Methods of search

• The initial search conducted for a systematic review compiled in 1999[7] used the following primary sources: Cochrane Central Register of Controlled Trials; Medline, 1966 to 1997; Embase, 1974 to 1997; records of military trials from the UK, USA and Russia, and the specialist register of the Cochrane Diseases Group.
• Clinical evidence search, May 2000.
• Medline update search for evidence-based dermatology, March 2006.
• Hand searching of relevant journals.

Questions

How successful are topical treatments for scabies? For example, would a topical treatment be suitable for treating newly diagnosed scabies in a 16-year-old girl? (Figure 46.1)

Insecticide-based pharmaceutical products
Benefits
We found one systematic review (search date 1999) that examined 13 trials (nine compared drug treatments, two compared treatment regimens, one compared the drug vehicle, and one was a community intervention). In each case, a single application of treatment was given, unless stated otherwise.

One study (150 adults and children) compared 5% permethrin cream with 10% crotamiton cream (a noninsecticide) and 1% lindane lotion.[8] It used clinical features as the measure of success. The results showed that at 28 days, permethrin was slightly, but not significantly, more likely to cure patients receiving it (49 of 50; 98%), versus 44 of 50 (88%) with crotamiton. The same study also found that permethrin was significantly more effective than lindane, which cured only 12 of 50 (24%) people (RR 4.08; 95% CI, 2.5 to 6.7).[8] A single randomized controlled trial (RCT) comparing 5% permethrin cream with 10% crotamiton cream evaluated cure by elimination of parasites.[9] It found that permethrin was more effective after 14 and 28 days. After 14 days, 33 of 47 people in the permethrin group (70%) and 41 of 47 in the crotamiton group (87%) still had lesions. At this point, 10 people in the crotamiton group were withdrawn from the study because their infestation was exacerbated. However, after 28 days, 42 of 47 people in the permethrin group (89%) were free from parasites, in comparison with 28 of 47 (60%) in the crotamiton group.[9] This study also recorded patients' subjective reports on the persistence of pruritus, which was found to be closely related to the effectiveness of the treatments.

Three trials compared the effect of 5% permethrin cream with that of 1% lindane lotion. A small study (including 46 patients) found that fewer people improved 14 days after using permethrin (13 of 23; 57%) in comparison with lindane (20 of 23; 87%; $P < 0.02$), but there was a significantly better rate of cure, by parasitological examination, for permethrin at 28 days (21 of 23 versus 15 of 23; $P < 0.025$).[10] A larger trial (including 467 patients) did not identify parasites, but recorded a significant decrease in the number of lesions persisting in both groups after 14 ± 3 days. At 28 ± 7

days, there was no significant difference in the success rates, with 181 of 199 (91%) cured using 5% permethrin cream, compared with 176 of 205 (86%) using 1% lindane lotion.[11] At the final assessment, significantly fewer of the patients in the permethrin group (27 of 194; 14%) had a persistent itch, in comparison with 49 of 197 (25%) in the lindane group ($P = 0.007$).[11]

A medium-sized randomized, double-blind, crossover study (117 patients aged 6–64 years, plus contacts), conducted in Iran, investigated treatment with either 1% lindane cream or 5% permethrin cream.[12] Both treatments were applied for 12 hours and repeated after 7 days. However, there were 11 dropouts from the lindane group and seven from the permethrin group, not adequately explained by the authors. At 2 weeks, 44 of 52 (84.6%) had improved with permethrin and 23 of 47 (48.9%) with lindane. After 14 days, those considered still to be infected, using a mixture of parasitological and clinical criteria, were switched to the other treatment regimen. After 4 weeks one person originally treated with permethrin and then re-treated with lindane still showed severe pruritus. There were two irritation adverse events in the permethrin group and one in the lindane group.

An observational multicenter study conducted in Germany (106 children and adults, aged 3 months–71 years) received a single application of 5% permethrin cream and were assessed after 14 and 28 days.[13] People who were not considered cured by dermatoscopy on day 14 were re-treated, and 95.1% of the participants were diagnosed as being free from infection on day 28.

Two RCTs conducted in Italy evaluated synergized pyrethrins foam (0.16% pyrethrins, 1.65% piperonyl butoxide). In one study (40 adults, 18–75 years) it was compared with 5% permethrin cream.[14] Both treatments were applied three times for 8 hours on days 0, 1, and 14. Efficacy was assessed blindly on day 14 using a mixture of clinical criteria, but an itch index was used as the main criterion of success. A second assessment was made after 4 weeks. The foam was found to produce a significant difference ($P = 0.013$) in reducing the number of lesions and the itch index at day 14 in comparison with permethrin, and the difference increased to $P = 0.0001$ by the 4-week evaluation. The second RCT (including 240 convicted prisoners) compared three applications of synergized pyrethrins foam on consecutive days with five consecutive applications of benzyl benzoate lotion.[15] After 2 weeks, 90 of 120 of the patients in the group treated with pyrethrins (75%) were judged clinically cured, in comparison with 85 of 120 (71%) in the benzyl benzoate group. Those not considered cured were given another course of treatment with the same material, and after 4 weeks the cure rates were 95% and 91%, respectively. Those not considered cured still complained of itching. Burning and irritation due to treatment was significantly ($P = 0.0001$) more common in the benzyl benzoate

group, in which only 41% of participants showed good tolerability, compared with 95% in the pyrethrins group.

The systematic review identified no RCTs comparing 0.5% malathion, in either aqueous or alcohol vehicles, with other treatments. Case series and one quasi-randomized trial suggest that it is effective, with a cure rate of over 80% at 4 weeks.[16–18]

Drawbacks

Only minor adverse effects have been reported for most insecticides. The exception is lindane, for which there are extensive reports of effects related to overdosing and absorption.[19,20] Despite recognized neurotoxicity, lindane is still widely used, partly because alternatives are not readily available in many countries. Lindane passes transdermally during treatment and other exposures, and may be stored in fatty tissues and excreted in breast milk.[21] Acute exposure to lindane during scabies treatment has potentiated seizures in people on medication that reduces the seizure threshold.[22,23] Lindane appears to be contraindicated for those undergoing therapy for human immunodeficiency virus (HIV) infection,[22] attention deficit hyperactivity disorder using amphetamine,[23] and in those who suffer from epileptiform seizures. Concern has been expressed that lindane may be a risk factor for the triggering of seizures in epileptics, as it may alter liver cell function. Lindane does cause oxidative stress, but does not appear to modify liver microsomal function, and in experimental systems these effects were mitigated by prior treatment with phenobarbital.[24,25] Consequently, those being treated with barbiturates may be at lower risk of suffering side effects from lindane. However, it is not clear whether people receiving anticonvulsant drugs in general are at greater risk of having seizures if exposed to lindane.

Various studies have shown that the solvent vehicle plays an important role in the rate of transdermal absorption of lindane.[26,27] In addition, much of the drug can also be absorbed as the treatment is washed off, because a depot of lindane builds up in the stratum corneum.[27–29] In many countries, scabicides are still applied after a hot bath, but the resultant peripheral vasodilation is likely to enhance transdermal absorption. A related increase in the passage of lindane through the dermis has been identified if soap and hot water are used to remove the acaricide at the end of the treatment process. Absorption can be minimized if cool water alone is used to remove residues of lindane products before bathing.[29] An investigation of the absorption of permethrin and lindane through human cadaver skin *in vitro* found that lindane achieved a rate of $2\,\mu g/h/cm^2$ in less than 5 hours, whereas the rate for permethrin was one-tenth of this after 10 hours. However, fresh guinea-pig skin absorbed both at the same rate.[30]

Most RCTs have reported no serious adverse events using these topical insecticide-based products. One RCT reported five serious adverse events, two possibly associated with permethrin (rash and diarrhea) and three possibly associated with lindane use (pruritic rash, papules, and diarrhea).[11] Post-marketing surveillance of permethrin use in the USA from 1990 to 1995 found six adverse events per 100 000 units of product (equivalent to one central nervous system adverse event for each 500 000 units of permethrin used).[31] Case series based on community intervention studies have reported a burning paresthesia as one of the most frequent adverse events following permethrin use, particularly in the immunodeficient.[31,32] A burning sensation was the most frequent adverse event, although not significantly so, in the largest RCT, with 23 events in 233 people following application of 5% permethrin, compared with 12 of 232 after 1% lindane lotion ($P = 0.08$),[11] and one recent case report has suggested that use of even small doses of lindane (60 μg on the body followed by 40 μg on the head 6 days later) may have contributed towards the death of a 91-year-old patient treated for scabies.[33]

Comment

Generally, it is believed that all mites and their eggs are killed soon after treatment. Confirmation of cure is therefore difficult, because mites may not be detectable in post-treatment skin scrapings. It is therefore impossible to determine success until sufficient time has passed to permit the various lesions resulting from the infestation to heal. Many people show considerable improvement after 14 days, but a definitive clinical cure cannot be concluded until about 28 days after treatment, when all lesions present at the time of treatment should either be healed or resolving, without new lesions developing.

Three of the RCTs were conducted in developing countries. The fourth study was divided between the USA and Mexico.[11] It is not known whether scabies mites may be more susceptible to treatment in communities in which treatments are not generally available, but it is likely that prior exposure to acaricidal chemicals may select for reduced sensitivity in mites in developed countries, and some cases of suspected resistance, particularly to lindane, have been recorded.[31,34]

Lindane products are still used against scabies in most Western countries, despite the relative toxicity of the agent. In the UK, the only lindane product was withdrawn on commercial grounds. The former market-leading product in the USA is now no longer produced, for the same reason.

Implications for clinical practice

The evidence indicates that permethrin is more effective than crotamiton, lindane, and malathion, and it has been associated with fewer side effects than lindane. However, the high cost of permethrin may limit its use in some communities. Permethrin is probably more likely to be effective with one application than are other insecticides, but a second treatment may be necessary for all.[35]

Noninsecticide-based acaricides
Benefits

Randomized studies comparing the noninsecticide antiscabies agent crotamiton with insecticide-based treatments were described above.

We found one trial (158 adults and children) comparing 25% benzyl benzoate with sulfur ointment (concentration of sulfur not given) in a community study in India.[36] In this study, patients were first scrubbed in a bath; the treatments were then applied three times in 24 hours (morning, night, and next morning). Assessments were made at approximately 5-day intervals. No significant difference was found between the treatments with regard to improvement of the lesions at 9–10 days—benzyl benzoate 68 of 89 (76%) versus 45 of 69 (65%) with sulfur. If lesions remained at this time, the patients were treated again, so that by 14–15 days there was improvement of symptoms in 81 of 89 patients (91%) in the benzyl benzoate group, in comparison with 67 of 69 (97%) for sulfur, which was also not significantly different. Another RCT conducted in Thailand (100 children aged 6 months–13 years) compared 10% sulfur ointment with 0.3% hexachlorocyclohexane (lindane) gel.[37] After 4 weeks of treatment, there was no significant difference between the treatments whether they were assessed using clinical signs (92% success for sulfur compared with 91% for lindane) or by parasitological findings (83% compared with 84% cure). However, the authors reported a significant difference ($P < 0.05$) in adverse effects due to the foul odor following sulfur treatment.

Noncontrolled studies and case studies have indicated variable effectiveness for both benzyl benzoate (20% emulsion,[38] 25% emulsion,[18] 25% cream[39]) and sulfur ointment (5%,[40] 6%,[41] 10%,[38,41] 2–8%[37]). The activity of these acaricides is related to the concentration of active drug in the vehicle and the number of times they are applied. In general, benzyl benzoate appears to require a minimum of two applications, and sulfur may require several applications over 1 week or longer.[42,43]

We found a single RCT evaluated by the systematic review comparing pork fat containing 1% salicylic acid and cold cream as ointment vehicles for the delivery of sulfur.[44] The numbers in this study were small (51 confirmed cases), and differences in efficacy could have been due to chance effects. Every participant applied the sulfur ointment on three consecutive nights and then again 3 days later. Evaluations were made on the tenth day after the last treatment. This study is more relevant for the side effects observed, described below.

We found that other noninsecticide active materials have only been described in nonrandomized studies and case series. One nonrandomized study comparing 5% sulfur ointment, 1% lindane cream, 25% benzyl benzoate cream, 10% crotamiton lotion, and 0.2% nitrofurazone in a water-soluble ointment, found that nitrofurazone was the least effective, with a 70% cure rate.[39] A case series of 20 patients using the same nitrofurazone ointment produced "complete clinical cure" in 80% of cases.[45]

Monosulfiram (sulfiram) is now little used, either as a liquid (25% before dilution for use) or a soap or in combination with benzyl benzoate (in France). Most studies are of poor quality and more than 50 years old, and more recent case studies show a high incidence of side effects (see below). Thiabendazole has been used as a 5% and a 10% cream applied over several days. In one case series, five of 19 patients (26%) were still infested after 5% cream was used twice daily for 5 days. The remaining patients were cured after a further 5 days of treatment.[46] Another case series, in which 10% cream was used, achieved an 80% success rate after 5 days.[47]

Drawbacks

Generally, studies have reported "only minor adverse reactions" for noninsecticide treatments for scabies. Most of these have been related to skin irritation or dermatitis, often following repeated or multiple applications of the formulation. The RCT comparing vehicles for sulfur ointment[44] did not provide adequate data for a full analysis of effects. Side effects were reported in patients and close contacts within 6 days of first being treated with either cold cream or pork fat with 1% salicylic acid: pruritus (31% versus 60%), xerosis (24% versus 34%), burning sensation (12% versus 17%), erythema (10% versus 2%), and keratosis (2% versus 15%).[44] Where sulfur is used in developed countries, it is normally applied in petroleum jelly, and similar skin reactions have been reported as side effects in case studies and series.[43,48] Similar irritant reactions occur with repeat treatments using benzyl benzoate, particularly if naturally derived rather than synthetic material is used.[43,49] In one RCT, approximately 25% of people reported an increase in pruritus and dermatitis after treatment with two applications of 10% benzyl benzoate.[50]

Monosulfiram has been associated with a systemic adverse event in a number of case reports in which the patients developed dermal edema, flushing, sweating, and tachycardia, especially after ingesting alcohol within 24 hours of treatment.[51-53] This reaction occurs because monosulfiram is chemically related to disulfiram, used in the treatment of alcoholism (Antabuse).

Multiple applications of crotamiton can result in dermatitis, and there is one report of a suspected link with methemoglobinemia.[20,43,54]

Comments

Most studies in this group are not comparable due to differ-

ences in the formulations used, in the concentrations of the active substances, and in the duration or number of applications. Evidence for activity is limited in each case, and it is possible that some of the effectiveness is partially related to a physical effect—for example, sulfur in a heavy greasy base may physically trap and subsequently remove developmental stages of the mite from the skin surface. The mode of action of crotamiton is not understood, and there is doubt about both its acaricidal and antipruritic activities. Similar questions may apply to all of the noninsecticide-based treatments. The fact that these treatments are inexpensive means that they are more likely to be used in developing countries, where source materials may be less well characterized. Most of these compounds have been in use for around 50 years, and there is suspicion that resistance is developing in some areas.[20]

Implications for clinical practice

All of these products are likely to require two to four applications and are not particularly cosmetic. They may therefore suffer from compliance problems—for example, sulfur has a particularly unpleasant odor. However, the low cost and relative safety, apart from skin irritancy, make noninsecticide-based acaricides attractive alternatives to insecticide-based products where mites may have developed resistance or if cost is an issue.

How successful are oral treatments for scabies? Would an oral treatment be suitable for treating an 82-year-old resident in a nursing home?
(Figure 46.2)

Orally administered treatments
Benefits
We found one systematic review examining two small

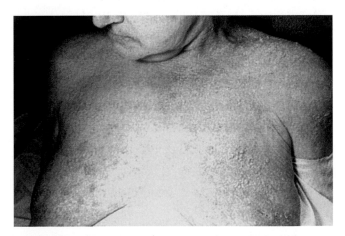

Figure 46.2 Hyperkeratotic crusts may develop in abnormal sites. (Reproduced with permission of the Institute of Dermatology, King's College Hospital, London.)

RCTs, one of which had inadequate follow-up. A placebo-controlled RCT (including 55 adults and children) found that significantly more people (23 of 29; 79%) treated with ivermectin, 200 µg/kg, were free from symptoms at 7 days, in comparison with two of 26 (8%) treated with placebo. The code was then broken and the controls and all patients who had not improved received ivermectin.[55] A comparative RCT (44 people) found no significant difference at 30 days in improvement of lesions between ivermectin 100 µg/kg (16 of 23; 70%) and benzyl benzoate 10%, applied twice over 2 days (10 of 21; 48%).[50]

We also found one RCT (including 85 patients) comparing ivermectin 200 µg/kg with 5% permethrin cream, evaluated at 1, 2, 4, and 8 weeks.[56] In this study, a single dose of ivermectin relieved symptoms in 28 of 40 patients (70%), which was significantly fewer than permethrin (44 of 45; 98%). However, when a second dose of treatment was given after 2 weeks, there was no significant difference in the improvement rate between the ivermectin group (38 of 40; 95%) and the permethrin group, in which everyone was cured. A second small RCT (53 patients, 43 of whom completed the study) found that ivermectin 150–200 µg/kg was statistically equivalent to 1% lindane lotion.[57] After 15 days, 14 of 19 patients (74%) had improved with ivermectin, in comparison with 13 of 24 (46%) treated with lindane. At 29 days, all but one person in each group were cured—18 of 19 (95%) with ivermectin versus 23 of 24 (96%) with lindane. A large RCT conducted in India (including 200 patients) compared ivermectin 200 µg/kg with 1% lindane lotion applied overnight.[58] Assessments were made at 48 hours, 2 weeks, and 4 weeks after treatment. After 4 weeks, 82.6% of the ivermectin group showed marked improvement, based on a clinical assessment, in comparison with 44.4% of those treated with lindane. The only adverse event of note was a severe headache in one person treated using ivermectin. Another RCT (110 children aged 6 months–14 years at the start of the study) conducted in Vanuatu compared a single dose of oral ivermectin 200 µg/kg with one application of 10% benzyl benzoate emulsion.[59] After 3 weeks, an assessment was made using clinical diagnostic criteria, in which 24 of 43 of the ivermectin-treated patients (54%) were considered cured, in comparison with 19 of 37 of those receiving benzyl benzoate (51%). This difference was not significant, but benzyl benzoate was significantly more likely to induce adverse skin reactions ($P = 0.004$; OR 6.4, 95% CI, 1.6 to 25.0). However, this study suffered from a drop-out rate of 27% (30 of 110), which was not adequately explained by the authors.

An observational cohort study (six families, 12 adults and 20 children aged 1–10 years) used a 1% solution of ivermectin in propylene glycol to give a total dose of 400 µg/kg, applied twice with an interval of 1 week.[60] Evaluation was made on the basis of clinical evidence at 2, 4, and 6 weeks. All of the patients were cured without side effects or relapse.

Drawbacks

Most of the RCTs were too small to provide adequate safety data for the use of ivermectin against scabies, particularly in children. What comment there is on adverse experiences is inadequate, as most authors who report adverse events at all generalize comments to stating that adverse experiences "were mild" or treatments were "well tolerated," Such comments are wholly meaningless and no guide to what might be expected in clinical use. Ivermectin has been used extensively in community control programs for onchocerciasis and filariasis, and there have been few reports of serious adverse events.[61,62] There has been one report of a significant increase in the mortality rate in a psychogeriatric unit—15 of 42 (36%; $P = 0.001$) within 6 months of ivermectin use, in comparison with controls in the same care facility over a 3-year period.[63] However, each resident in the unit had previously received several applications of other scabies treatments, including lindane and permethrin. Use of ivermectin in the elderly in other countries has not resulted in any similar increase in mortality.[64]

Comment

Ivermectin has not yet been widely licensed for use against scabies. However, its use on a named-patient basis has become widespread as a component of treatment for hyperkeratotic scabies, in which it is often difficult to kill all the mites due to the limited penetration of the plaques by topical acaricides. In this condition, ivermectin can reach trophic mites by incorporation into the living cell layer on which the mites feed. However, ivermectin is unlikely to have any direct effect on mite eggs, and failures of treatment have been reported unless either dosing is repeated or a topical scabicide is used concurrently.[65–67] So far, no proper dosing studies using ivermectin have been performed, and the relative underdosing using both ivermectin and benzyl benzoate in one study indicates how important a contribution to knowledge this would be.[50]

Implications for practice

A reliable and safe oral treatment is the most attractive option for dosing and compliance with scabies treatment. Ivermectin has not yet been evaluated sufficiently to determine the most appropriate dosing regimen, but it can be a useful adjunct to conventional treatment approaches.

Additional comment

The evidence for the effectiveness of all scabies treatments is still largely rudimentary, and the majority of studies have employed inadequate criteria for diagnosis and evaluation of efficacy. It is almost impossible to compare studies, even when they are sponsored by the same organization, as almost every trial employs a different protocol and set of criteria for making the initial diagnosis, follow-up diagnoses, treatment regimen, and evaluation of success. The majority of studies have been conducted in developing countries, where scabies is not only more highly endemic than in western Europe or North America but is also less likely to have been subjected to any form of therapeutic intervention. As a result, treatments should exhibit exemplary activity against these chemically naive mites. However, the most worrying aspect of reading the study reports is that, even in circumstances in which resistance to treatment cannot be an issue, the treatments of all types exhibit a disturbing lack of efficacy in the absence of re-treatment, and in some cases multiple re-treatments. What evidence exists indicates that none of the topical products is reliable with a single application, and this picture may be further confused by the possibility that resistance to conventional neurotoxic compounds may have developed in some communities. The limited evidence available for oral ivermectin is far from the aspirations expressed by those dealing with problems of long-term infestation, and there are already doubts in some regions as to whether mites are fully sensitive to ivermectin or if they may be developing tolerance already. Consequently, further investigation is required for this and other treatments—firstly, to determine adequate drug regimens and reliable methods of evaluating them, and secondly to confirm the susceptibility of the mites or treatment compounds.

Key points

- Permethrin and lindane are probably effective in scabies treatment, although lindane has been withdrawn from some markets and has a higher potential for toxicity. Malathion and synergized pyrethrins may be effective, but more evidence is required.

- Crotamiton, benzyl benzoate, and sulfur show insufficient evidence of efficacy, as do nitrofurazone, monosulfiram, and thiabendazole.

- There is currently insufficient evidence of the effectiveness of ivermectin. Most studies have been small trials and larger studies have suffered high drop-out rates. Case studies indicate that ivermectin may be effective if used with a topical agent. A proper dose regimen evaluation is required.

References

1 Stein DH. Scabies and pediculosis. *Curr Opin Pediatr* 1991;**3**:660–6.

2 Christopherson J. The epidemiology of scabies in Denmark, 1900 to 1975. *Arch Dermatol* 1978;**114**:747–50.

3 Church RE, Knowlesden J. Scabies in Sheffield: a family infestation. *BMJ* 1978;**i**:761.

4 Palicka P. The incidence and mode of scabies transmission in a district of Czechoslovakia (1961–1979). *Folia Parasitol* 1982;**29**:51–9.

5 Burgess I. *Sarcoptes scabiei* and scabies. *Adv Parasitol* 1994;**33**:235–92.

6 Carslaw RW, Dobson RM, Hood AJK, *et al*. Mites in the environment of cases of Norwegian scabies. *Br J Dermatol* 1975;**92**:333–7.

7 Walker GJ, Johnstone PW. Interventions for treating scabies. *Cochrane Database Syst Rev* 2000;(3):CD000320.

8 Amer M, El-Gharib I. Permethrin versus crotamiton and lindane in the treatment of scabies. *Int J Dermatol* 1992;**31**:357–8.

9 Taplin D, Meinking TL, Chen JA, *et al*. Comparison of crotamiton 10% cream (Eurax) and permethrin 5% cream (Elimite) for the treatment of scabies in children. *Pediatr Dermatol* 1990;**7**:67–73.

10 Taplin D, Meinking TL, Porcelain SL, *et al*. Permethrin 5% dermal cream: a new treatment of scabies. *J Am Acad Dermatol* 1986;**15**:995–1001.

11 Schultz MW, Gomez M, Hansen RC, *et al*. Comparative study of 5% permethrin cream and 1% lindane lotion for the treatment of scabies. *Arch Dermatol* 1990;**126**:167–70.

12 Zargari O, Golchai J, Sobhani A, *et al*. Comparison of the efficacy of topical 1% lindane vs 5% permethrin in scabies: a randomized, double-blind study. *Indian J Dermatol Venereol Leprol* 2006;**72**:33–6.

13 Hamm H, Beiteke U, Hoger PH, *et al*. Treatment of scabies with 5% permethrin cream: results of a German multicenter study. *J Dtsch Dermatol Ges* 2006;**4**:407–13.

14 Amerio P, Capizzi R, Milani M. Efficacy and tolerability of natural synergized pyrethrins in a new thermo labile foam formulation in topical treatment of scabies: a prospective, randomised, investigator-blinded, comparative trial vs permethrin cream. *Eur J Dermatol* 2003;**13**:69–71.

15 Biele M, Campori G, Colombo R, *et al*. Efficacy and tolerability of a new synergized pyrethrins thermofobic foam in comparison with benzyl benzoate in the treatment of scabies in convicts: the ISAC study (Studio Della Scabbia in Ambiente Carcerario). *J Eur Acad Dermatol Venereol* 2006;**20**:717–20.

16 Hanna NF, Clay JC, Harris JRW. *Sarcoptes scabiei* infestation treated with malathion liquid. *Br J Vener Dis* 1978;**54**:354.

17 Thianprasit M, Schuetzenberger R. Prioderm lotion in the treatment of scabies. *Southeast Asian J Trop Med Public Health* 1984;**15**:119–21.

18 Burgess I, Robinson RJ, Robinson J, *et al*. Aqueous malathion 0·5% as a scabicide: clinical trial. *BMJ* 1986;**292**:1172.

19 Schmutz JL, Barbaud A, Trechot P. Intoxication aigue au lindane chez 3 enfants. *Ann Dermatol Venereol* 2001;**128**:799.

20 Elgart ML. A risk–benefit assessment of agents used in the treatment of scabies. *Drug Saf* 1996;**14**:386–93.

21 Schinas V, Leontsinidis M, Alexopoulos A, *et al*. Organochlorine pesticide residues in breast milk from southwest Greece: associations with weekly food consumption patterns of mothers. *Arch Environ Health* 2000;**55**:411–7.

22 Solomon BA, Haut SR, Carr EM, *et al*. Neurotoxic reaction to lindane in an HIV-seropositive patient. An old medication's new problem. *J Fam Pract* 1995;**40**:291–6.

23 Cox R, Krupnick J, Bush N, *et al*. Seizures caused by concomitant use of lindane and dextroamphetamine in a child with attention deficit hyperactivity disorder. *J Miss State Med Assoc* 2000;**41**:690–2.

24 Simon Giavarotti KA, Rodrigues L, Rodrigues T, *et al*. Liver microsomal parameters related to oxidative stress and antioxidant systems in hyperthyroid rats subjected to acute lindane treatment. *Free Radic Res* 1998;**29**:35–42.

25 Videla LA, Arisi AC, Fuzaro AP, *et al*. Prolonged phenobarbital pretreatment abolishes the early oxidative stress component

induced in the liver by acute lindane intoxication. *Toxicol Lett* 2000;**115**:45–51.

26 Dick IP, Blain PG, Williams FM. The percutaneous absorption and skin distribution of lindane in man. I. In vivo studies. *Hum Exp Toxicol* 1997;**16**:645–51.

27 Dick IP, Blain PG, Williams FM. The percutaneous absorption and skin distribution of lindane in man. II. In vitro studies. *Hum Exp Toxicol* 1997;**16**:652–7.

28 Lange M, Nitzsche K, Zesch A. Percutaneous absorption of lindane in healthy volunteers and scabies patients. Dependency of penetration kinetics in serum upon frequency of application, time and mode of washing. *Arch Dermatol Res* 1981;**271**:387–99.

29 Zesch A, Nitsche K, Lange M. Demonstration of the percutaneous resorption of a lipophilic pesticide and its possible storage in the human body. *Arch Dermatol Res* 1982;**273**:43–9.

30 Franz TJ, Lehman PA, Franz SF, *et al.* Comparative percutaneous absorption of lindane and permethrin. *Arch Dermatol* 1996;**132**:901–5.

31 Meinking TL, Taplin D. Safety of permethrin vs lindane for the treatment of scabies. *Arch Dermatol* 1996;**132**:959–62.

32 Carapetis JR, Connors C, Yarmirr D, *et al.* Success of a scabies control program in an Australian Aboriginal community. *Pediatr Infect Dis J* 1996;**15**:1056–7.

33 Katsumata K, Katsumata K. Norwegian scabies in an elderly patient who died after treatment with gammaBHC. *Intern Med* 2003;**42**:367–9.

34 Hernandez-Perez E. Resistance to antiscabietic drugs. *J Am Acad Dermatol* 1983;**8**:121–2.

35 Roberts DT, ed. *Lice & Scabies: a Health Professional's Guide to Epidemiology and Treatment.* London: Public Health Laboratory Service, 2000: 25.

36 Gulati PV, Singh KP. A family based study on the treatment of scabies with benzyl benzoate and sulphur ointment. *Indian J Dermatol Venereol Lepr* 1978;**44**:269–73.

37 Singalavanija S, Limpongsanurak W, Soponsakunkul S. A comparative study between 10 per cent sulfur ointment and 0.3 per cent gamma benzene hexachloride gel in the treatment of scabies in children. *J Med Assoc Thai* 2003;**86**(Suppl 3):S531–6.

38 Srivastava BC, Chandra R, Srivastava VK, *et al.* Epidemiological studies of scabies and community control. *J Commun Dis* 1980;**12**:134–8.

39 Amer M, El-Bayoumi, Rizik MK. Treatment of scabies: preliminary report. *Int J Dermatol* 1981;**20**:289–90.

40 Kenawi MZ, Morsy TA, Abdalla KF, *et al.* Treatment of human scabies by sulfur and permethrin. *J Egypt Soc Parasitol* 1993;**23**:691–6.

41 Henderson C. Community control of scabies. *Lancet* 1991;**337**:1548.

42 Burns DA. The treatment of human ectoparasite infection. *Br J Dermatol* 1991;**125**:89–93.

43 Diaz M, Cazorla D, Acosta M. [Efficacy, safety and acceptability of precipitated sulphur petrolatum for topical treatment of scabies at the city of Coro, Falcon State, Venezuela; in Spanish.] *Rev Invest Clin* 2004;**56**:615–22.

44 Avila-Romay A, Alvarez-Franco M, Ruiz-Maldonado R. Therapeutic efficacy, secondary effects, and patient acceptability of 10% sulfur in either pork fat or cold cream for the treatment of scabies. *Pediatr Dermatol* 1991;**8**:64–6.

45 Chowdhury SPR. Nitrofurazone in scabies. *Lancet* 1977;**i**:152.

46 Biagi F, Delgado Y, Garnica R. First therapeutic trials with thiabendazole cream. *Int J Dermatol* 1974;**13**:102–3.

47 Hernandez-Perez E. topically applied thiabendazole in the treatment of scabies. *Arch Dermatol* 1976;**112**:1400–1.

48 Orkin M, Maibach HI. Treatment of today's scabies. In: Orkin M, Maibach HI, eds. *Cutaneous Infestations and Insect Bites.* New York: Dekker, 1986:103–8.

49 Temesvart E, Soos GY, Podamy B, *et al.* Contact urticaria provoked by balsam of Peru. *Contact Dermatitis* 1978;**4**:65–8.

50 Glaziou P, Cartel JL, Alzieu P, *et al.* Comparison of ivermectin and benzyl benzoate for treatment of scabies. *Trop Med Parasitol* 1993;**44**:331–2.

51 Plouvier B, Lemoine X, de Coninck P, *et al.* Antabuse effect following topical application based on monosulfiram. *Nouvelle Presse Med* 1982;**11**:3209.

52 Blanc D, Deprez P. Unusual adverse reaction to an acaricide. *Lancet* 1990;**335**:1291–2.

53 Burgess I. Adverse reactions to monosulfiram. *Lancet* 1990;**336**:873.

54 Arditti J, Jouglard J. Cutaneous overdose with crotamiton and suspicion of methaemoglobinaemia. *Bull Med Legale Toxicol* 1978;**21**:661–2.

55 Macotela-Ruiz E, Pena-Gonzalez G. Treatment of scabies with oral ivermectin. *Gac Med Mex* 1993;**129**:210–15.

56 Usha V, Gopalakrishnan Nair TV. A comparative study of oral ivermectin and topical permethrin cream in the treatment of scabies. *J Am Acad Dermatol* 2000;**42**:236–40.

57 Chouela EN, Abeldano AM, Pellerano G, *et al.* Equivalent therapeutic efficacy and safety of ivermectin and lindane in the treatment of human scabies. *Arch Dermatol* 1999;**135**:651–5.

58 Madan V, Jaskiran K, Gupta U, Gupta DK. Oral ivermectin in scabies patients: a comparison with 1% topical lindane lotion. *J Dermatol* 2001;**28**:481–4.

59 Brooks PA, Grace RF. Ivermectin is better than benzyl benzoate for childhood scabies in developing countries. *J Paediatr Child Health* 2002;**38**:401–4.

60 Victoria J, Trujillo R. Topical ivermectin: a new successful treatment for scabies. *Pediatr Dermatol* 2001;**18**:63–5.

61 Pacque M, Munoz B, Greene BM, *et al.* Safety of and compliance with community-based ivermectin therapy. *Lancet* 1990;**335**:1377–80.

62 De Sole G, Remme J, Awadzi K, *et al.* Adverse reactions after large-scale treatment of onchocerciasis with ivermectin: combined results from eight community trials. *Bull World Health Organ* 1989;**67**:707–19.

63 Barkwell R, Shields S. Deaths associated with ivermectin treatment of scabies. *Lancet* 1997;**349**:1144–5.

64 Diazgranados JA, Costa JL. Deaths associated with ivermectin treatment of scabies. *Lancet* 1997;**349**:1698.

65 Corbet EL, Crossley I, Holton J, *et al.* Crusted ("Norwegian") scabies in a specialist HIV unit: successful use of ivermectin and failure to prevent nosocomial transmission. *Genitourin Med* 1996;**72**:115–7.

66 Meinking TL, Taplin D, Hermida JL, *et al.* The treatment of scabies with ivermectin. *N Engl J Med* 1995;**333**:26–30.

67 Aubin F, Humbert P. Ivermectin for crusted (Norwegian) scabies. *N Engl J Med* 1995;**332**:612.

47   Head lice

Ian F. Burgess, Ciara S. Casey

Background

Definition

Head lice (*Pediculus capitis*) are blood-feeding insects that are obligate ectoparasites of socially active humans. All stages of the life cycle infest the scalp, where the adult insects attach their eggs to the hair shafts. The juvenile forms (nymphs) are essentially miniature versions of adults, and there is no distinct larval stage.

Incidence/prevalence

We found no data on the incidence and few recent published prevalence data from developed countries. Anecdote suggests that the prevalence has increased in most communities in Europe, the USA, and other developed countries since 1990. One study in Belgium found a prevalence of up to 19.5% in some schools, and in a more recent investigation of 6169 children (2.5–12 years) there was an overall prevalence of 8.9%.[1,2] Low socioeconomic status was a significant risk for the presence of infestation and an inability to treat infestations effectively.[2]

Etiology/risk factors

Observational studies indicate that infestations occur most frequently in schoolchildren, although there is no evidence of a link with school attendance. We found no evidence that either hygiene or hairstyle influence the risk, or that lice prefer clean hair to dirty hair.

Prognosis

This infestation is essentially harmless. However, the stigma associated with head lice and the psychological trauma experienced by some people in their efforts to eliminate the infection greatly outweigh the physical impact of the infestation. Sensitization reactions to louse saliva and feces may cause local irritation and erythema. Secondary infection of scratches may occur. Lice have been identified as primary mechanical vectors of scalp pyoderma caused by streptococci and staphylococci usually found on the skin.[3]

Diagnosis

Only the finding of living lice can confirm a diagnosis of active infestation (Figure 47.1). Eggs glued to hairs, whether hatched (nits) or unhatched, are not proof of active infection, because dead eggs may appear viable for weeks. Itching, resulting from multiple bites, is not diagnostic, but may increase the index of suspicion. Combing is a more effective diagnostic method than visual inspection of the hair.[4–6,46]

Aims of treatment

The aim of treatment is to eliminate infestation by killing or removing all head lice and preventing their eggs from hatching.

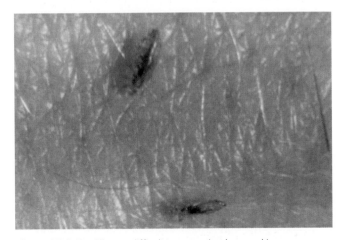

Figure 47.1 Head lice are difficult to see against human skin.

Outcomes

Treatment success is given as the percentage of people completely cleared of head lice. There are no standard criteria for judging treatment success. Trials have used different methods, and in many cases the method was not stated. Few studies are pragmatic.

Method of search

- The Cochrane Infectious Diseases Group at the Liverpool School of Tropical Medicine performed the initial search for a systematic review compiled in July 1998, updated in February 2001 and July 2006; search date March 2006; primary sources: Cochrane Central Register of Controlled Trials, Medline, Embase, Bath Information and Data Services (BIDS SC), BioScience Information Service (BIOSIS), and Toxicology Literature Online (Toxline).
- Dermatological evidence update search November 2006.
- Hand-searching of relevant journals.

Questions

How successful are treatments for head lice?

Case scenario 1

A 10-year-old girl with shoulder-length hair is diagnosed with head louse infestation. How easy would it be to treat her?

Insecticide-based pharmaceutical products
Efficacy

We found two systematic reviews.[7,8] The first (search date March 1995; seven randomized controlled trials, 1808 people), of 11 insecticide products, included lindane, carbaryl, malathion, permethrin, and other pyrethroids in various vehicles.[8] Two randomized controlled trials (RCTs) were identified as showing that only permethrin produced clinically significant differences in the rate of treatment success. Both compared lindane (1% shampoo) with permethrin (1% crème rinse).[9,10] Permethrin was found to be more effective than lindane.

The first Cochrane systematic review (search date May 1998, updated February 2001) set stricter criteria for RCTs and rejected all but four trials.[7] It initially excluded both studies on which the earlier review was based. The most recent update of Cochrane (July 2006), in attempting to address criticisms of the 2001 publication, has evaluated a wider range of studies in greater detail. No clear therapeutic guidelines were obtained from the analyses, as it was impossible to draw up-to-date conclusions from the widely differing results obtained using different formulations of the same materials, different treatment regimens, and different assessment criteria, at different times, especially where resistance to insecticides has had an impact on some of the better-designed trials.

One RCT (193 schoolchildren) compared malathion (0.5% alcoholic lotion) with *d*-phenothrin (0.3% lotion), both applied for 8 h or overnight. One day after treatment, fewer people treated with malathion had lice—eight of 95 (8%) versus 59 of 98 (60%) treated with phenothrin. This difference had increased by day 7—six of 95 (6%) versus 60 of 98 (61%). However, some children not free from lice on day 1 had become louse-free by day 7 in both groups, suggesting that some parental intervention had influenced the results.[11] One RCT (66 people) compared 0.5% malathion (alcoholic lotion applied for 20 min) with 1% permethrin (crème rinse applied for 10 min). One application was used, but a second treatment was given if lice were found after 7 days. At day 7, 33 of 41 people (80%) treated with malathion were louse-free, as were 13 of 22 (59%) treated with permethrin. After the second treatment, the overall cure rate at day 14 was 40 of 41 for malathion (98%) and 15 of 22 (68%) for permethrin.[12]

Drawbacks

Only minor adverse effects have been reported for most insecticides. The exception is lindane, for which there are extensive reports of effects related to overdosing (treatment of scabies), and absorption (treatment of head lice). Lindane passes transdermally during treatment of head lice,[13] but we found no reports of adverse effects in this setting.

We found no confirmed reports of adverse effects from therapeutic exposure to the organophosphorus compound, malathion. A randomized open volunteer study (32 people) examined transdermal absorption of malathion from four head louse treatment products available in the UK.[14] Urinalysis for malathion metabolites found that 0.2–3.2% of the applied dose was eliminated in urine, before decreasing to baseline values by 96 h. Erythrocyte cholinesterase levels were clinically unaffected, irrespective of dose or whether the skin was excoriated.

Pyrethroid insecticides are listed as contraindicated for people with ragweed allergy, but we found only one report of an anaphylactoid reaction to a head louse treatment product.[15]

Comments

Follow-up for less than 7 days is inadequate, because louse eggs normally take 7 days to hatch. A second application of insecticide should be given 7 days after the first treatment. The primary end point of a study is absence of infestation at 14 days after first treatment.

No RCT has yet evaluated the effect of formulation vehicle activity. Studies *in vitro* suggest that excipients of products (for example, terpenoids and solvents) may contribute significantly to pediculicide activity, in some cases more than the insecticide itself.[16]

Resistance to one or more insecticides has now been identified in several countries. There are no data on the prevalence of resistance, and most reports are based on a few cases that may not be representative of the population at large. However, resistance to pyrethroids (permethrin, d-phenothrin, and natural pyrethrum) is widespread in Europe, North America, and Australia, and malathion resistance is present in Europe and Australia.[17–22]

Implications for practice
Evidence for any insecticide-based pediculicide is limited. Early commercial support for permethrin produced a greater body of evidence of its efficacy. However, all insecticides now in use are affected by resistance, which varies considerably both within and between countries. Available data are insufficient to judge this factor other than on a case-by-case basis. In cases of treatment failure, where resistance is indicated by finding all stages of lice immediately after treatment, either an alternative active chemical with a different mode of action should be used, or else an alternative treatment technique—e.g., physical removal, physically disrupting insecticide, or herbal material.

Physically disrupting insecticides
Efficacy
We found one RCT (253 children and adults) comparing 4% dimeticone lotion with 0.5% d-phenothrin aqueous liquid (both products were applied overnight using two applications 7 days apart). At 14 days, no significant difference was found between the numbers of individuals free of lice with phenothrin liquid (94/125, 75%) or with dimeticone lotion (89/127, 70%).[23]

Drawbacks
We found no drawbacks for 4% dimeticone lotion. It was reported as producing fewer irritant reactions (three of 127 patients, 2%) than phenothrin liquid (11 of 125, 9%).[23]

Comment
Dimeticone appears to have a physical mode of action in which it coats the insects and disrupts their ability to manage water. This mode of action circumvents resistance to conventional neurotoxic insecticides and is unlikely to be affected by resistance.

Implications for clinical practice
Because they are less likely to be absorbed transdermally, physically disrupting insecticides offer an alternative method of treatment for people concerned about using insecticides on safety grounds. They also offer a suitable treatment option when resistance to conventional insecticides makes treatment success hard to achieve.

Antimicrobial and other oral treatments
Efficacy
We found one RCT (115 children) in which cotrimoxazole (trimethoprim and sulfamethoxazole), either alone (10 mg/kg/day over 10 days) or in combination with 1% permethrin crème rinse, was compared with 1% permethrin crème rinse alone (one application, with a second after 7 days if lice remained).[24] After 2 weeks, the number of children who were louse-free with cotrimoxazole alone (28/36, 77.8%) did not significantly differ from the number with permethrin alone (28/39, 71.8%) but the combination treatment (37/40, 92.5%) was superior ($P = 0.03$) to permethrin alone. We found one cohort study (114 schoolchildren) in which cotrimoxazole (8 mg/kg daily over 12 days) plus 1% lindane shampoo applied for 10 min was compared with 1% lindane shampoo alone.[25] If lice were found after 2 weeks, a further treatment was given. No significant difference was found between the treatments at either examination. At 2 weeks, the louse-free rate with lindane shampoo was 53 of 69 (76.8%), compared with 39 of 45 (86.7%) for the combination treatment. The cure rate increased following the second treatment to 63 of 69 (91.3%) for lindane shampoo and 44 of 45 (97.8%) with the combined treatment. Other nonrandomized studies have investigated the activity of thiabendazole (20 mg/kg twice daily for 1 day, with repeat treatment after 10 days),[26] levamisole,[27] and ivermectin (200 µg/kg),[28] each of which has shown variable results related to dosing.

Drawbacks
The RCT comparing cotrimoxazole with permethrin reported three cases of scalp irritation with permethrin and nine incidents of intense but transient pruritus following cotrimoxazole alone. Three children treated with cotrimoxazole developed allergic rash and were withdrawn, and three others experienced nausea and/or vomiting. Nausea and mild dizziness also accompanied thiabendazole use.

Comment
Cotrimoxazole is believed to eliminate the symbiotic microorganisms associated with the gut of lice, inhibiting their viability and development. However, its use is inappropriate for this condition, due to the relatively high risk of adverse reactions to the drug. In one RCT, for example, a quarter of children taking cotrimoxazole developed intense pruritus after 3–4 days, even though it disappeared after 1–3 h. Potentially serious, although rare, adverse effects associated with cotrimoxazole include Stevens–Johnson syndrome, erythema multiforme, and blood disorders.

Implications for clinical practice
This is unlikely to be a first choice for treatment despite current problems with resistance, although it may be more acceptable in the USA than Europe. The introduction of

alternatives, such as physically disrupting insecticides and herbal products, is likely to make cotrimoxazole a curious therapeutic anachronism.

Mechanical removal of lice or viable eggs by combing

Efficacy

We found one systematic review that evaluated louse removal by combing compared with insecticide treatment, but none evaluating nit combing to remove eggs. Three studies compared insecticide treatments with "wet combing with conditioner." One study, a community-based pragmatic RCT (72 people) included in the Cochrane review, compared "bug-busting" (wet combing with conditioner) with two applications of 0.5% malathion alcoholic lotion 7 days apart.[29] Seven days after the second treatment (day 14), fewer people using malathion (nine of 40, 23%) had lice in comparison with those using "bug-busting" (20/32, 63%). A second small RCT, in which a trained hairdresser performed the first combing treatment or applied the insecticide product, compared a single application of permethrin (1% crème rinse) with "bug-busting."[4] After 14 days, more people treated with permethrin still had lice (eight of 11, 73% versus eight of 14, 57%). We found one RCT (30 people) that compared 0.2% d-phenothrin lotion (no terpenoids in the vehicle) applied twice at an interval of 7 days, together with some level of combing (not clearly specified) versus "bug-busting."[30] After 14 days, the cure rate with phenothrin lotion (two of 15, 15%) did not significantly differ from that with "bug-busting" (eight of 15, 53%). A more recent RCT (133 young people) compared "bug-busting" with insecticide treatment, divided between 0.5% aqueous malathion liquid and 1% permethrin crème rinse.[31] Nine of 70 individuals treated with insecticide—five of 30 (17%) with malathion and four of 40 (10%) with permethrin—had no lice after 6 days, and 32 of 62 (52%) using "bug-busting" had no lice after 14 days. We found one RCT (95 adults and children) comparing combing with a metal nit/louse comb plus 1% permethrin crème rinse with permethrin alone.[32] Treatments were applied by a health-care professional. If lice were found after 7 days, an additional course of treatment (insecticide or insecticide plus combing) was given. There was no significant difference between the cure rates at 2, 8, and 15 days—louse-free patients at day 2: 49/59 (83%) without combing and 24/33 (73%) with combing; at day 8 before re-treatment: 27/59 (46%) with no combing and 11/33 (33%) with combing; and at day 15: 47/60 (78%) without combing and 24/33 (73%) with combing.

We found one RCT (30 children) comparing nit combs from different manufacturers of insecticide treatments.[33] After using 1% permethrin crème rinse, participants were combed with a different comb on the right and left halves of the head. The combs were not significantly different for

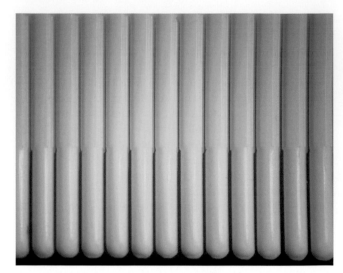

Figure 47.2 A plastic comb with "stepped teeth," which have been found to be more effective for removing nits and eggs.

removing head lice, but one plastic comb with stepped teeth (Figure 47.2) was significantly more effective ($P = 0.0004$) at removing louse eggshells than the other two combs.

Drawbacks

We found no evidence of drawbacks from combing alone, apart from discomfort for both the carer and the person being combed. Potential drawbacks exist for wet combing with conditioner. This requires conditioning crème rinses to be left on the scalp for prolonged periods, but adverse reactions to hair-conditioning agents have occurred after normal limited cosmetic use. Reactions include allergic contact dermatitis, urticaria, urticaria with systemic symptoms, and angioedema.[34–38]

Comment

All four studies comparing insecticide treatments with "bug-busting" were performed in areas in which resistance to the insecticide employed was either recognized before commencing the study or else identified as part of the study. As a result, the potential effectiveness of the insecticides was limited. We found a cohort trial that indicated that a conditioner-like formulation could be an effective pediculicide if allowed to dry on the hair.[39] A similar effect could occur with prolonged combing during "bug-busting." Studies evaluating nit combing as an adjunct to insecticide treatment used combs that differed considerably in material and construction, so it was difficult to attribute efficacy, or lack of it, to either the pediculicide or the comb.

Implications for clinical practice

Although combing may seem an attractive, simple, and safe treatment method, there is no real evidence that it is effective, especially when practiced by carers who may have little skill in the method. What little evidence is available indicates that insecticide-based products are more likely to be effective if applied twice with an interval of 1 week, even in areas in which insecticide resistance has developed. No doubt the success of currently used insecticides will diminish with time, but combing requires better evidence of success before it will replace chemical treatments for the majority of patients.

Herbal treatments and essential oils
Efficacy

We found one RCT (143 children) that compared a spray based on herbal oils (coconut, anise, ylang-ylang; concentrations not given) with an insecticide spray containing a mixture of insecticides (0.5% permethrin, 0.25% malathion, synergized by 2% piperonyl butoxide).[40] Herbal spray was applied three times at 5-day intervals and insecticide twice 10 days apart. There was no significant difference between the cure rate with the herbal spray (60/70, 86%) and that with insecticide (59/73, 81%).

Drawbacks

No clinically detectable adverse effects have been reported for essential oils or herbal extracts, although a potential for toxic effects has been recognized for several essential oils, including anise.[41] Results obtained using one herbal combination are unlikely to translate to other herbal mixes using different active materials at different concentrations.

Comment

Some activity against lice and their eggs has been identified *in vitro*, and in uncontrolled studies, both for essential oils and their constituent terpenoids.[41–44]

Herbal and other alternative therapies have become more popular in this application, despite a lack of evidence for efficacy. Although terpenoids are a major constituent of some registered products, most alternative therapies use these chemicals at low concentrations to reduce the risk of side effects. Such low doses inevitably select for resistant strains of lice, and some resistance to terpenoids has already been observed in the UK (I.F. Burgess, unpublished).

What is the best method for diagnosing louse infection?

Case scenario 2

Head louse infections have been reported on some of the classmates of a 9-year-old girl. A few empty louse eggshells are visible on her hair, and she scratches occasionally. How can this evidence of what may be a past infection be distinguished from an active infestation? Is detection combing or direct observation (Figures 47.3 and 47.4) the most efficient way of finding lice?

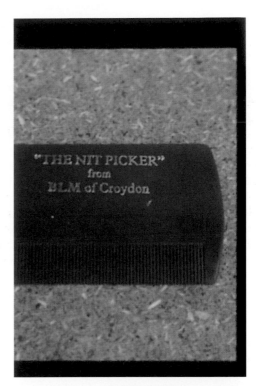

Figure 47.3 Standard detection comb for head lice.

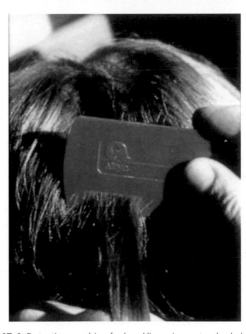

Figure 47.4 Detection combing for head lice using a standard plastic detection comb.

Efficacy

We found no systematic reviews and no RCTs evaluating detection methods. One observational study (224 people) compared traditional scalp inspection with wet combing with conditioner. Wet combing found more cases of louse infection in a school than scalp inspection—49 of 224 (22%)

versus 33 of 224 (15%), respectively. However, visual inspection was claimed to identify a further 13 cases not confirmed either by combing or by follow-up examination 2 weeks later.[45] One RCT of treatments found dry combing with a detection comb to be more effective than visual inspection in identifying positive cases before treatment—all of 25 (100%) versus 12 of 25 (48%).[4] One observational study (268 children) compared the use of a metal louse detection comb with visual inspection of dry or slightly dampened hair.[5] Detection combing was found to be significantly more effective ($P < 0.001$), identifying 68 of 268 (25.4%) children with lice in comparison with 16 of 268 (5.9%) for visual inspection. A second observational study (461 schoolchildren) used a plastic detection comb on dry hair.[46] Detection combing diagnosed lice on 96 of the 461 children (20.8%) in comparison with 30 (6.5%) in whom they were found by visual inspection.[46]

Comment

Accurate diagnosis of an active head louse infestation is fundamental for deciding whether treatment is needed. The presence of apparently viable louse eggs close to the scalp was once considered sufficient evidence of an active infection. Now, only the presence of mobile stages is considered adequate evidence.[7] One cohort study (50 people) confirmed that the presence of eggs close to the scalp is a limited risk factor. Children screened by direct observation of the scalp, and found only to have louse eggs, were evaluated again 14 days later. Those with five eggs or more within 6 mm of the scalp were more likely to develop an active infestation than those with fewer than five eggs (seven of 22 versus two of 28). It was concluded that many children are excluded from school or treated unnecessarily and that repeated examinations to determine whether an infestation develops would be more beneficial.[46]

Unnecessary treatments and school exclusions also arise because caregivers and health professionals misdiagnose items found in the hair. An observational study evaluating 614 samples of presumed head lice found that only 364 (59%) were louse-related, showing that better diagnostic tools are required.[47]

Implications for practice

Accurate diagnosis is essential for developing an appropriate treatment strategy. Treatment should only be given if living lice are found. Too often, children are exposed to insecticides unnecessarily because a parent finds a few empty louse eggshells in the hair. However, if a child has never had head lice before, an infection may run for several weeks before it is discovered by chance, because there is no overt sign of the infestation.[6,16] Prescribers should therefore always ask for evidence of active infestation—e.g., a louse stuck to a piece of paper—before deciding on treatment.

Key points

- Permethrin, malathion, and phenothrin are probably effective against head lice, provided resistance is not present. There is limited evidence for older insecticides such as lindane, which have now been withdrawn in some countries.
- Dimeticone is probably effective against head lice resistant to conventional insecticides and provides an alternative treatment where these have failed.
- There is limited evidence for the effectiveness of oral treatments such as cotrimoxazole, which is supposed to eliminate the symbiotic microorganisms associated with the gut of lice. Potential side effects associated with this material make it of limited applicability to head louse treatment.
- There is insufficient evidence of the effectiveness of combing alone or in combination with insecticide treatment for either removing lice or nit combing.
- There is limited evidence for the effects of herbal treatments and essential oils as alternative treatments for head lice.
- Combing with a plastic detection comb appears to be the most effective method for finding live lice, but diagnostic methods have been little studied.

References

1 Vander Stichele RH, Gyssels L, Bracke C, *et al.* Wet combing for head lice: feasibility in mass screening, treatment preference and outcome. *J R Soc Med* 2002;**95**:348–52.

2 Willens S, Lapeere H, Haedens N, *et al.* The importance of socio-economic status and individual characteristics on the prevalence of head lice in schoolchildren. *Eur J Dermatol* 2005;**15**:387–92.

3 Taplin D, Meinking TL. Infestations. In: Schachner LA, Hansen RC, eds. *Pediatric Dermatology*, vol. 2. New York: Churchill Livingstone, 1988: 1465–93.

4 Bingham P, Kirk S, Hill N, *et al.* The methodology and operation of a pilot randomized control trial of the effectiveness of the Bug Busting method against a single application insecticide product for head louse treatment. *Public Health* 2000;**114**:265–8.

5 Mumcuoglu KY, Friger M, Ioffe-Uspensky I, *et al.* Louse comb versus direct visual examination for the diagnosis of head louse infestations. *Pediatr Dermatol* 2001;**18**:9–12.

6 Williams LK, Reichart A, MacKenzie WR, *et al.* Lice, nits and school policy. *Pediatrics* 2001;**107**:1011–5.

7 Dodd CS. Interventions for treating head lice. Cochrane Database Syst Rev 2001;(**2**):CD001165.

8 Vander Stichele RH, Dezeure EM, Bogaert MG. Systematic review of clinical efficacy of topical treatments for head lice. *BMJ* 1995;**311**:604–8.

9 Brandenburg K, Deinard AS, Di Napoli J, *et al.* 1% permethrin cream rinse *v.* 1% lindane shampoo in treating pediculosis capitis. *Am J Dis Child* 1986;**140**: 894–6.

10 Bowerman JG, Gomez MP, Austin RD, *et al.* Comparative study of permethrin 1% crème rinse and lindane shampoo for the treatment of head lice. *Pediatr Inf Dis J* 1987;**6**:252–5.

11 Chosidow O, Chastang C, Brue C, *et al.* Controlled study of malathion and *d*-phenothrin lotions for *Pediculus humanus* var. *capitis*-infested schoolchildren. *Lancet* 1994;**344**:1724–7.

12 Meinking TL, Vicaria M, Eyerdam DH, *et al.* Efficacy of a reduced application time of Ovide lotion (0.5% malathion) compared to Nix crème rinse (1% permethrin) for the treatment of head lice. *Pediatr Dermatol* 2004;**21**:670–4.

13 Ginsburg CM, Lowry W. Absorption of gamma benzene hexachloride following application of Kwell shampoo. *Pediatr Dermatol* 1983;**1**:74–6.

14 Dennis GA, Lee PN. A phase I volunteer study to establish the degree of absorption and effect on cholinesterase activity of four head lice preparations containing malathion. *Clin Drug Invest* 1999;**18**:105–15.

15 Culver CA, Malina JJ, Talbert RL. Probable anaphylactoid reaction to a pyrethrin pediculocide shampoo. *Clin Pharmacol* 1988;**7**:846–9.

16 Burgess IF. Dermatopharmacology of antiparasitics and insect repellents. In: Gabard B, Elsner P, Surber C, Treffel P, eds. *Dermatopharmacology of Topical Preparations.* Heidelberg: Springer, 1999: 157–78.

17 Rupes V, Moravec J, Chmela J, *et al.* A resistance of head lice (*Pediculus capitis*) to permethrin in Czech Republic. *Cent Eur J Public Health* 1995;**1**:30–2.

18 Mumcuoglu KY, Hemingway J, Miller J, *et al.* Permethrin resistance in the head louse *Pediculus capitis* from Israel. *Med Vet Entomol* 1995;**9**:427–32.

19 Burgess IF, Brown CM, Peock S, *et al.* Head lice resistant to pyrethroid insecticides in Britain [letter]. *BMJ* 1995;**311**:752.

20 Downs AMR, Stafford KA, Harvey I, *et al.* Evidence for double resistance to permethrin and malathion in head lice. *Br J Dermatol* 1999;**141**:508–11.

21 Pollack RJ, Kiszewski A, Armstrong P, *et al.* Differential permethrin susceptibility of head lice sampled in the United States and Borneo. *Arch Pediatr Adolesc Med* 1999;**153**:969–73.

22 Lee SH, Yoon KS, Williamson M, *et al.* Molecular analyses of kdr-like resistance in permethrin-resistant strains of head lice, *Pediculus capitis. Pestic Biochem Physiol* 2000;**66**:130–43.

23 Burgess IF, Brown CM, Lee PN. Treatment of head louse infestation with 4% dimeticone lotion: randomised controlled equivalence trial. *BMJ* 2005;**330**:1423–5.

24 Hipolito RB, Mallorca FG, Zuniga-Macaraig ZO, *et al.* Head lice infestation: single drug versus combination therapy with one percent permethrin and trimethoprim/sulfamethoxazole. *Pediatrics* 2001;**107**:E30.

25 Sim S, Lee IY, Lee KJ, *et al.* A survey of head lice infestation in Korea (2001) and the therapeutic effect of oral trimethoprim/sulfamethoxazole adding to lindane shampoo. *Korean J Parasitol* 2003;**41**:57–61.

26 Namazi MR. Treatment of pediculosis capitis with thiabendazole: a pilot study. *Int J Dermatol* 2003;**42**:973–6.

27 Namazi MR. Levamisole: a safe and economical weapon against pediculosis. *Int J Dermatol* 2001;**40**:292–4 (erratum in: *Int J Dermatol* 2001;**40**:794).

28 Glaziou P, Nguyen LN, Moulia-Pelat JP, *et al.* Efficacy of ivermectin for the treatment of head lice (pediculosis capitis). *Trop Med Parasitol* 1994;**45**:253–4.

29 Roberts RJ, Casey D, Morgan DA, *et al.* Comparison of wet combing with malathion for treatment of head lice in the UK: a pragmatic randomised controlled trial. *Lancet* 2000;**356**:540–4.

30 Plastow L, Luthra M, Powell R, *et al.* Head lice infestation: bug busting vs. traditional treatment. *J Clin Nurs* 2001;**10**:775–83.

31 Hill N, Moor G, Cameron MM, *et al.* Single blind, randomised, comparative study of the Bug Buster kit and over the counter pediculicide treatments against head lice in the United Kingdom. *BMJ* 2005;**331**:384–7.

32 Meinking TL, Clineschmidt CM, Chen C, *et al.* An observer-blinded study of 1% permethrin creme rinse with and without adjunctive combing in patients with head lice. *J Pediatr* 2002;**141**:665–70.

33 De Souza Bueno V, de Oliveira Garcia L, de Oliveira NJ, da Silva Ribeiro DC. [Comparative study on the efficiency of three different fine-tooth combs to remove lice and nits.] *Rev Bras Med* 2001; **58** [www.cibersaude.com.br/revistas.asp?id_materia=1539&fase=imprime].

34 Korting JC, Pursch EM, Enders F, *et al.* Allergic contact dermatitis to cocamidopropyl betaine in shampoo. *J Am Acad Dermatol* 1992;**27**:1013–5.

35 Niinimaki A, Niinimaki M, Makinen-Kiljunen S, *et al.* Contact urticaria from protein hydrolysates in hair conditioners. *Allergy* 1998;**53**:1070–82.

36 Schalock PC, Storrs FJ, Morrison L. Contact urticaria from panthenol in hair conditioner. *Contact Dermatitis* 2000;**43**:223.

37 Pasche-Koo F, Claeys M, Hauser C. Contact urticaria with systemic symptoms caused by bovine collagen in hair conditioner. *Am J Contact Dermatol* 1996;**7**:56–7.

38 Stadtmauer G, Chandler M. Hair conditioner causes angioedema. *Ann Allergy Asthma Immunol* 1997;**78**:602.

39 Pearlman D. A simple treatment for head lice: dry-on, suffocation-based pediculicide. *Pediatrics* 2005;**114**:275–9.

40 Mumcuoglu KY, Miller J, Zamir C, *et al.* The *in vivo* pediculicidal efficacy of a natural remedy. *Isr Med Assoc J* 2002;**4**:790–3.

41 Veal L. The potential effectiveness of essential oils as a treatment for headlice, *Pediculus humanus capitis. Complement Ther Nurs Midwifery* 1996;**2**:97–101.

42 Priestley CM, Burgess IF, Williamson EM. Lethality of essential oil constituents towards the human louse, *Pediculus humanus*, and its eggs. *Fitoterapia* 2006;**77**:303–9.

43 Gauthier R, Agoumi A, Gourai M. Activité d'extraits de *Myrtus communis* contre *Pediculus humanus capitis. Plantes Med Phytother* 1989;**23**:95–108.

44 Schuld M, Jungen C. Control of lice and nits with NeemAzal-FT. In: Kleeberg H, Micheletti V, eds. *Practice Oriented Results on Use and Production of Neem Ingredients and Pheromones. Proceedings of the Fourth Workshop, Bordighera, Italy, Nov. 28th–Dec. 1st 1994.* Lahnau, Germany: Trifolio-M, 1996: 103–4.

45 De Maeseneer J, Blikland I, Willems S *et al.* Wet combing versus traditional scalp inspection to detect head lice in schoolchildren: observational study. *BMJ* 2000;**321**:1187–8.

46 Balcioglu C, Burgess IF, Limoneu ME, *et al.* Plastic detection comb better than visual screening for diagnosis of head louse infestation. *Epidemiol Infect* (in press).

47 Pollack RJ, Kiszewski AE, Spielman A. Overdiagnosis and consequent mismanagement of head louse infestations in North America. *Pediatr Infect Dis J* 2000;**19**:689–93.

Insect bites and stings

Belen Lardizabal Doñtas

Background

Definition

Insects comprise the most diverse group of animals on the earth. The true insects are invertebrate species with six legs and three body segments: head, thorax, and abdomen. Many people would consider spiders, mites, and ticks as insects too, although these are arachnids, having eight legs and two body segments only. A more inclusive term than "insects" would be "arthropods," comprising both insects, arachnids, and other invertebrates with paired jointed legs.[1]

Insect bites and stings are common occurrences. Bites often appear as wheals or extremely pruritic papules. Bee stings produce an immediate burning sensation and pain, followed by localized swelling and redness. Severe reactions such as anaphylactic shock can occur due to venomous stings.[2] Although these bites may seem inconsequential, insect-related diseases constitute a tremendous burden on the world's population.

This chapter focuses on common problems due to mosquito bites and Hymenoptera stings (bees, wasps).

Incidence/prevalence

Insects are found in almost all parts of the world. Mosquitoes are considered the most common nuisance insects and the most important vectors of arthropod-borne diseases.

Blood-feeding insects carry and transmit various pathogens leading to insect-borne diseases such as malaria and dengue. The World Health Organization estimates that there are 300–500 million cases of malaria each year and that approximately 1 million deaths annually are due to malaria.[3] The World Health Organization currently estimates there may be 50 million cases of dengue infection worldwide annually.[4] Systemic allergic reactions to insect stings have been reported to occur in 0.3–4% of individuals.[5] Deaths due to allergic reactions to Hymenoptera stings occur in 0.09–0.45 per million inhabitants.[6]

Nuisance arthropod bites and the diseases they transmit have caused more loss to military troop strength than direct combat itself.[7] About 70% of American army personnel reported experiencing significant problems because of arthropods, especially mosquitoes.[8] Work efficiency is also reduced by the nuisance of painful or pruritic bites, secondary infections, and allergies.[7,9]

Etiology/risk factors

Clinically important insects include mosquitoes, flies, lice, beetles, bedbugs, ants, bees, wasps, butterflies, moths, and fleas, among others.[2]

Most venomous insects bite or sting in defense of their hives or nests. Nonvenomous insects bite in order to feed on human or animal blood. Biting insects such as mosquitoes and sandflies are generally considered a nuisance due to skin reactions to the bites. Substances in the insect's saliva cause allergic or irritant reactions. The bites are rarely harmful, but insects can be vectors of diseases, some of which are potentially fatal.[2]

When bees sting, they leave the sting and venom sac attached. Venom continues to pump in through the stinger until the sack is empty or the sting is removed. Wasps and hornets, however, do not leave their stings behind and can sting repeatedly.[10]

Many factors influence the feeding habits of arthropods, such as season, time of day, or preference for indoor or outdoor feeding.[11] Mosquitoes are attracted to human skin that is moist, warm, and with high levels of natural steroids on the skin surface. Persons who exhale more carbon dioxide (i.e., adults, pregnant women), certain odors, lactic acid, and types of sweat compounds also attract more mosquitoes.[12]

Aims of treatment

The aim of treatment is to reduce the severity and duration

of local and systemic reactions to mosquito bites and Hymenoptera insect stings.

Outcomes

• Risk reductions in the severity and duration of symptoms (itching, pain, swelling, local and systemic reactions such as urticaria, angioedema, hypotension, bronchospasm, anaphylactic shock)
• Adverse effects of treatment

Aims of prevention

• To reduce the risk of mosquito bites or mosquito-borne illnesses

Outcomes

• Number of insect bites or rates of insect catches
• Protective efficacy or risk reductions of insect bites due to protective measure
• Rates of clinical mosquito-borne diseases (e.g., malaria)

Search methods

Search and appraisal (May 2006) of: Medline (1966 to May 2006), Cochrane Library Issue 1, 2006, and the Cochrane Skin Group Specialized Register.

Questions

Case scenario 1

A 19-year-old man developed extremely pruritic, red papules on his arms and legs after an outdoor hike (Figure 48.1).

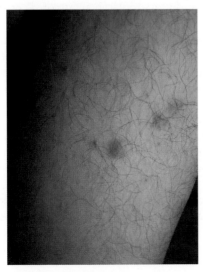

Figure 48.1 Acute insect bite reactions on the leg.

How effective are treatments to reduce mosquito bite allergic reactions?

We found no systematic reviews.

Oral antihistamines versus placebo

We found two randomized, double-blind, placebo-controlled, crossover trials investigating oral antihistamines. Cetirizine 10 mg reduced immediate and delayed cutaneous reactions in 18 mosquito-sensitive patients who were exposed to mosquitoes in the field. After 24 hours, the mean wheal size was reduced by 41% and the mean pruritus score was reduced by 67%.[13]

A study investigated the efficacy of loratadine in 28 children (aged 2–11 years) who were sensitive to mosquito bites. Prophylactically administered loratadine (0.3 mg/kg) significantly decreased the mosquito bite wheal size by 45% and pruritus by 78% and also reduced the size of the bite lesions after 24 hours.[14]

How effective is symptomatic treatment for skin reactions to mosquito bites?

We found no systematic reviews. There were no randomized controlled trials (RCTs) or controlled clinical trials investigating topical corticosteroids.

Topical treatments versus placebo

We found four RCTs that investigated topical remedies for mosquito bite lesions. A double-blind, placebo-controlled RCT conducted in 25 healthy individuals studied the effects of ammonium sulfate solution in relieving immediate cutaneous reactions to controlled mosquito bites. The ammonium solution reduced itching, burning, and pain and gave complete or partial relief in 64% of the treated forearms, in comparison with none in the placebo-treated arms.[15]

Two RCTs studied homeopathic after-bite gels. A placebo-controlled, intraindividual RCT tested 68 healthy volunteers who were each bitten by laboratory-reared mosquitoes on three spots in the volar forearm. There were no statistical differences in pruritus and erythema between the treated, placebo, and untreated bite lesions.[16] A double-blind, intraindividual RCT tested a homeopathic after-bite gel (Prrrikweg gel) in 100 healthy volunteers and found no difference in erythema and pruritus in comparison with the placebo gel.[17]

A double-blind RCT tested a topical antihistamine, dimethindene gel, with regard to relief of pruritus due to insect bites and sunburn. Mosquito bites were most frequently treated. If only the first bite or burn was taken into account, 88% were relieved by dimethindene (n = 49) within 30 minutes of application, in comparison with 64% in the placebo group (n = 52) ($P \leq 0.01$).[18]

Drawbacks

Five patients (18.5%) reported mild sedation after 10 days of taking cetirizine, in comparison with two patients who took placebo after 5 days.[10] The children treated with loratadine had no marked side effects and tolerated the drug well.[14]

No skin irritation or other side effects were reported after the application of topical ammonium or homeopathic gels. Both placebo and dimethindene gel had minor and transient side effects.[15–18]

Comments

There are few RCTs on the treatment of a very common condition—mosquito bites and allergic reactions to these bites. The reduction of symptoms caused by insect bites has been evaluated for just two of the many oral antihistamines available and for only three types of topical treatment, which surprisingly did not include any topical corticosteroids. For such a common inflammatory skin disorder, insect bites and their treatment deserve further RCTs. The pruritus-relieving effects of dimethindene gel were not specifically for mosquito bites alone.

Implications for clinical practice

For mosquito bite–sensitive adults who anticipate exposure to mosquitoes, oral antihistamines such as 10 mg cetirizine may be taken prophylactically to reduce the allergic skin reactions. Loratadine may be given prophylactically to children with allergies to mosquito bites when exposure to these insects are highly possible.

For acute bites by mosquitoes, ammonium sulfate solution may be applied to alleviate the immediate burning, pain, and pruritus. Dimethindene gel may relieve pruritus due to insect bites. The after-bite homeopathic gels tested have not shown significant benefit in persons without mosquito bite allergy. Topical corticosteroids have not been tested for efficacy in treating mosquito bites in controlled clinical trials or RCTs, but are commonly recommended for acute inflammatory skin reactions, including insect bites.

What are effective personal protective measures against mosquito bites for travelers in campsites or wilderness locations?

There were no systematic reviews on this topic.

DEET insect repellent and permethrin-treated clothing

No RCTs were found focusing on travelers, but there was one small RCT on topical insect repellents. An RCT compared the protective effect of N,N-diethyl-m-toluamide (DEET) 75% solution applied on exposed skin and permethrin-treated clothing, used alone or in combination.

Eight male volunteers were exposed to natural populations of mosquitoes for 9-hour daytime periods for 8 days. Unprotected test subjects were also exposed to mosquitoes to determine the overall biting rate. DEET combined with permethrin-treated clothing provided the best biting reduction (94.4%) in comparison with treated clothing alone (89.1%), although the difference was not significant. There was also no significant difference in bite reduction between DEET (68.7%) and unprotected controls (65.9%), due to bites through untreated clothing.[19]

Permethrin-treated tents

One double-blind RCT was conducted among North American campers (n = 545), with campsites being randomly allocated to have permethrin-treated tents or untreated tents. The external surface of canvas tents were sprayed once with 0.4% permethrin. The campers were reminded, by means of handouts and posted signs, to apply DEET insect repellent within 2 hours of dusk. Through daily surveys, mosquito landings and bites (for 5 minutes at dusk) as well as insect repellent use were self-reported by campers. Permethrin treatment of tents significantly reduced the number of mosquito bites at dusk among campers by 44% (relative risk reduction; 95% CI, 2.4 to 3.9; $P < 0.001$). Insect repellent use reduced mosquito landings and bites by 36% (95% CI, 25% to 40%; $P < 0.001$), but no additional benefit was observed among campsites that had permethrin-treated tents. Insect repellent usage only occurred consistently in 15% of subjects.[20]

Herbal insect repellents

There were no RCTs focusing on travelers. We found one RCT that tested a systemic, plant-based repellent against mosquitoes. There were no RCTs that tested the repellency of citronella, oil of eucalyptus, neem oil, soybean oil, IR3535, or picaridin (KBR3023) against mosquitoes.

One intraindividual, placebo-controlled, crossover RCT (n = 51) investigated the mosquito repellence of ingested garlic capsules—two caplets the night before and two caplets at lunch on the day of the study. When volunteers were exposed to laboratory-reared *Aedes aegypti* mosquitoes, no significant mosquito repellence was noted.[21]

Drawbacks

DEET can dissolve plastic and vinyl and damage rayon, spandex, pigmented leather, and acetate. DEET has reportedly caused dermatitis, allergic reactions, and cardiovascular and neurologic toxicities.[12]

Two large case series from poison control centers indicate that the risk of DEET is low. In a 5-year retrospective study conducted in the 1980s, there were five major adverse reactions reported after 9086 exposures to DEET (0.05%). These included hypotension, hypotonic reaction, and syncope, and one death (a suicide ingestion).[22]

In the second report, major adverse reactions to DEET use occurred in 0.1%. These included hypotension, seizures, respiratory distress, and two deaths (0.01%). Among infants and children only, there were 10 major events among 17,252 reported exposures (0.06%), and no deaths. Infants and children accounted for 83.1% of all reported exposures, but the majority of the serious outcomes occurred in adults.[23]

Permethrin-treated clothing or fabric. Although relatively safe and long-lasting when applied to clothing or fabric, permethrin is not recommended as a topical repellent because of safety concerns (e.g., neurotoxicity) upon chronic exposure.[24,25]

Herbal insect repellents. No adverse events were reported after garlic ingestion.

Comments

DEET insect repellent. This RCT had a small sample size and did not have allocation concealment or blinding. RCTs with adequate sample sizes and improved methodology will be able to provide better estimates of the effectiveness and safety of DEET in comparison with no protection or other measures.

Herbal insect repellents and alternatives to DEET. The RCT that investigated garlic may not have detected any effect because only a small dose was ingested. Further clinical trials with increased doses of garlic may be pursued.

There are few RCTs on insect repellents against mosquitoes, but many controlled clinical trials that use DEET as the "gold standard" for testing other chemical and botanical preparations (e.g., IR3535, picaridin, oil of eucalyptus, soy oil, and citronella). RCTs are needed to further validate the effectiveness and safety of these repellents, because some of these are already commercially available, while others may be developed for commercial use and may benefit the countries that possess these indigenous herbs.

Permethrin-treated clothing and tents. The 5-minute counts of mosquito bites and landings were reported by campers themselves, creating variability in the outcome measurement. The large sample size and the "real-world" setting of the trial may have offset this limitation of self-reporting. This RCT did not primarily study the effects of insect repellents or DEET in particular, therefore creating bias in the reported estimate of its efficacy.

Implications for clinical practice

Travelers to mosquito-endemic areas can achieve high levels of sustained protection against bites by using permethrin-treated clothing as well as treated tents. In addition, insect repellents such as DEET may be applied on exposed skin.

Permethrin, like its derivatives, has the advantage of being an insect repellent and an insecticide as well. It is poorly absorbed through the skin and remains active in fabrics even after laundering. It is also quite effective against ticks. DEET has been used worldwide for over 40 years and is found in many commercial insect repellents. It has the added advantage of repelling black flies, chiggers, fleas, and midges as well.[12]

The RCTs identified provide evidence regarding efficacy, but do not delve into the practical use of protective measures. The following are suggestions for use based on non-RCT studies and guidelines.

- Avoidance of the insects' habitats, barrier protection (e.g., clothing, bednets), and insect repellents are general measures to prevent insect bites.[26] The combination of "avoid, cover up, and repel" is recommended.
- Mosquitoes can be avoided by staying indoors in insect-proofed dwellings when mosquitoes actively bite—often from dusk to dawn. When outdoors, clothes covering most body parts would be ideal, and the addition of permethrin or other repellents on the fabric would provide a high degree of protection.
- Users must also be reminded that insect repellents do not repel all insects at all times. The repellents must be applied to all exposed areas of skin, because unprotected skin a few centimeters away from a treated area can be attacked by hungry mosquitoes.[27]
- The following factors may affect the effectiveness of the repellent: the frequency and uniformity of application, the number and species of the insects, the user's inherent attractiveness to blood-sucking arthropods, and the overall activity level of the exposed individual.[28] Topical repellents' effectiveness may be reduced when rubbed off or removed by contact with clothing, evaporation and absorption from the skin surface, wash-off from sweat or rain, higher temperatures, or a windy environment.[27,29]
- On the basis of a controlled clinical trial, increasing the concentration of DEET does not improve protection but does provide a longer duration of protection. Concentrations of 6.65% protect for about 2 hours, while 23.8% DEET can last about 5 hours.[30] The concentrations available for DEET range from 5% to 100%, although the latter is rarely used or indicated. Reapplications are necessary, especially in hot, humid weather, because DEET loses 50% of its effectiveness with every 10° rise in temperature.[26]
- Practice guidelines often recommend only one application of low-dose DEET in children, even though the repellent may provide protection for only a few hours. Since there is a lack of evidence on the toxicity of low-dose DEET, reapplication may be done if the child is outdoors for about 4 hours or more, and especially after swimming or bathing.[31]

- The likelihood of side effects would be minimized if the lowest effective concentration of DEET were used for a given situation. Insect repellents and insecticides may have toxic effects, but with proper adherence to the Environmental Protection Agency guidelines and advisories by disease control agencies, these protective measures can be a safe means of preventing insect bites and vector-borne diseases.

Are insect repellents safe for use among pregnant women?

Safety

One vehicle-controlled RCT was conducted in a refugee camp among pregnant women in their second and third trimester of pregnancy. For an average of 18 weeks, women applied 1.7 g DEET per day with thanaka, a paste derived from *Limonea acidiosima* and used as a carrier of the DEET repellent (n = 449). The control group applied thanaka 3.2 g/ day (n = 448).

The median total DEET dose was 214.2 g per woman (range 0–345.1 g). There were no adverse effects on survival, growth, or development at birth or at 1 year among the patients' infants. DEET was detected in 8% of 50 cord blood samples from babies of randomly selected mothers. DEET was not detected in urine samples, indicating efficient clearing of the chemical from their systems. DEET usage reduced the risk of scabies (RR 0.70; 95% CI, 0.5 to 0.97), but not of fungal infections. There were no significant adverse neurologic or gastrointestinal effects on the women.[32]

Drawbacks

Skin warming was more frequent among DEET users than thanaka users (80% vs. 57.6%; $P < 0.001$). DEET absorption may be enhanced by breaks in the skin—e.g., in the presence of other skin diseases. Liver or kidney impairment may also lead to toxicity.

Comments

In the same cohort of pregnant women, the RCT also investigated the protective effects of DEET against malaria. The relative risk reduction was 28% for falciparum malaria and 9% for vivax malaria. However, these results were not statistically significant.[33]

Implications for clinical practice

Evidence from the single RCT including 897 pregnant women suggests that DEET in 20% solution form is safe for pregnant women in their second and third trimesters and does not result in adverse effects on their infants. There has been no evidence so far that DEET is a health risk to pregnant and lactating women or their infants. Potential toxicity exists in conditions that enhance DEET percutaneous absorption or impair its clearing from the body.

Case scenario 2

A 40-year-old man complained of pain and swelling on his hand after being stung by a bee. He was also experiencing difficulty in breathing.

What symptomatic treatment is effective for skin lesions due to bee or wasp stings?

No systematic reviews were found on this topic. Two RCTs evaluated symptomatic treatment of local reactions after stings by bees, wasps or hornets (Hymenoptera).

Pinching versus scraping off the bee sting left in the skin

We found one RCT with two volunteers who either pinched or scraped off honeybee stings (20 stings in each group). The wheal response was greater for stings removed by pinching than for those removed by scraping (80 mm^2 versus 74 mm^2), but the difference was not statistically significant.[34]

Topical aspirin paste versus ice pack

One RCT studied patients who had just been stung by bees or wasps and who had called a poisons information center for advice. The aspirin group (37 patients) were instructed over the telephone to apply an ice pack followed by topical aspirin paste. The patient was instructed to add a few drops of water to a soluble aspirin tablet and spread this paste over the affected skin. The control group (19 patients) were instructed to apply an ice pack alone to the stings. Swelling at 12 hours had resolved in 57% of the aspirin group and in 74% of the ice-pack group (absolute risk reduction –14%; 95% CI, –39% to –14%). Pain at 12 hours had resolved in 81% of the aspirin group and 95% of the ice-pack group. Redness persisted for a median duration of 6 hours in the aspirin group and only 2 hours in the ice-pack group. In both the intention-to-treat and per-protocol analyses, topical aspirin paste was not significantly better than ice packs in reducing pain, swelling, and pruritus.[35]

Topical corticosteroids

No RCTs or controlled clinical trials were found.

Drawbacks

Topical aspirin paste reportedly increased the duration of redness at the sting sites in comparison with ice-pack application.

Comments

The RCT on methods of removing stingers also determined that the stinger of honeybees should be immediately removed by whatever means possible, because the time during which the stinger remains embedded in the skin determines the degree of envenomization.

The RCT on topical aspirin assessed clinical effects through telephone interviews, not actual physical examination of patients, although care was taken to standardize the quantification of symptoms.

There are very few RCTs on topical or symptomatic treatments for localized reactions to bee or wasp stings, despite the frequency of this condition. Corticosteroids and antihistamines are often mentioned in treatment guidelines, but there are no RCTs focusing on this topic.

Implications for clinical practice
Honeybee stings should be removed immediately either by pinching, scraping, or other means in order to reduce the degree of envenomization. Ice packs or aspirin paste may reduce local swelling, pain, and pruritus, but aspirin may prolong redness due to its inherent irritant properties.

What symptomatic treatment is effective for systemic reactions to accidental bee or wasp stings?

We did not find any systematic reviews or RCTs focusing on this topic.

Implications for clinical practice
Despite the absence of systematic and reliable evidence in the specific context of insect stings, it is important to know that anaphylactic reactions to insect venoms can be treated in the same way as anaphylaxis from any other cause. Sympathomimetics, antihistamines, and corticosteroids are the most effective drugs for dealing with systemic allergic reactions.[36] For severe reactions (e.g., respiratory or cardiovascular symptoms), two RCTs showed that intramuscular epinephrine was superior to subcutaneous injections in terms of the rapid increase in plasma concentration and start of pharmacological effects.[37,38]

An emergency kit for self-medication has been recommended for patients with a known history of systemic reactions. One RCT reported that children (15–30 kg) who self-injected premeasured epinephrine (EpiPen 0.30 mg) had more adverse effects than those using a lower-dose preparation (EpiPen Jr 0.15 mg).[39] One RCT studied the efficacy of subcutaneous versus inhaled epinephrine preparations among healthy individuals and reported that absorption of epinephrine was more rapid with the inhaled epinephrine.[40] Another RCT reported that 19 children with histories of anaphylaxis were unable to inhale sufficient epinephrine, due to the numerous inhalations required and the bad taste.[41]

Is subcutaneous venom immunotherapy (VIT) effective in preventing systemic reactions to Hymenoptera stings?

We found one systematic review on specific immunotherapy

for Hymenoptera venom hypersensitivity that searched the published medical literature from 1966 to 1996. This review involved 453 patients and included studies of different designs (randomized/nonrandomized; placebo-controlled/other control groups; before/after VIT trials). Only VIT by subcutaneous injection of standardized extracts was included. Honeybee and yellow jacket (hornet) venom were the extracts most commonly used in the trials. The reported pooled effect of all eight studies in the meta-analysis was an odds ratio of 2.2 (95% CI, 1.72 to 2.81) indicating a significant protective effect of VIT against systemic reaction after re-stings.[42]

VIT in children
One RCT studied 181 children with a history of non–life-threatening reactions and a positive venom skin-prick test. The difference in occurrence rates of systemic reactions to field insect stings was not significant between the VIT group (6%) and the no-treatment group (17%), indicating a low incidence of severe reactions among insect-allergic children within the 2-year observation period.[43] Another study reported little benefit of VIT in children who had had only local reactions to insect venom.[44]

Long-term effects of VIT in children
A survey was conducted among 512 patients diagnosed with insect sting allergy as children. Within 10–20 years after treatment, VIT in children (mean duration 3.5 years) led to a significantly lower risk of systemic reactions to insect stings (3%) in comparison with those who had not received VIT in childhood (17%). Patients with a history of moderate to severe reactions who did not receive VIT had a significantly higher long-term risk of a systemic allergic reaction to a sting than those who received VIT.[45]

Quality of life with VIT versus self-administered epinephrine
One RCT used a disease-specific instrument to measure health-related quality of life (the Vespid Allergy Quality-of-Life Questionnaire, VQLQ). In an open-label RCT, 36 patients received yellow jacket VIT in a modified semi-rush protocol, while 38 patients had self-administered epinephrine (EpiPen). After 1 year, the mean difference in VQLQ scores between the groups was 1.51 (95% CI, 1.04 to 1.98), favoring VIT. In the VIT group, 72% of the patients fared better overall in comparison with the EpiPen group in terms of quality of life, defined as an increase in VQLQ scores above 0.5.[46]

Tolerance or safety of modified VIT versus standard VIT
One RCT compared the efficacy and tolerability of monomethoxy polyethylene glycol (mPEG)-modified honeybee venom to unmodified honeybee venom (HBV). Occurrences

of local swellings were the same in each group, but systemic reactions to immunotherapy were more frequent in the HBV group. Success rates with mPEG-modified honeybee venom were not significantly lower than with the unmodified honeybee venom.[47]

Another RCT investigated the tolerance of cluster immunotherapy that used aluminum hydroxide–adsorbed honeybee venom extract (depot VIT). Among 55 patients with a history of systemic reactions to honeybee stings, depot VIT administered according to a cluster schedule resulted in only one patient with large, localized swelling and no reported systemic side effects in this regimen ($P < 0.009$ and $P < 0.003$, respectively). Depot VIT was well tolerated in comparison with the aqueous cluster and aqueous rush VIT regimens.[48]

Drawbacks
A prospective multicenter study reported that 20% of 840 patients developed systemic reactions to VIT. Systemic reactions occurred in 1.9% of injections during the dose-increase phase and 0.5% of injections during the maintenance phase. The majority of the reactions were mild. Risk factors for systemic reactions were bee venom extract, female gender, and rapid dose increase (rush regimen), but not the severity of insect sting reactions.[49]

Comments
As Hymenoptera venom hypersensitivity is potentially life-threatening, it appears unethical to perform double-blind, placebo-controlled trials. This may explain why only a few RCTs were found. Some of the evidence has limitations. The only meta-analysis conducted was limited to English publications and needs to be updated.

In one RCT including children, the results of the randomized and nonrandomized patients were not reported separately.[44]

Implications for clinical practice
Subcutaneous VIT showed protective benefit in all studies in terms of reducing the risk of immediate and long-term bee or wasp sting reactions and improving quality of life. Benefit was noted especially for those with prior severe systemic reactions to Hymenoptera venom. In nearly all studies, the effect of VIT was evaluated by measuring the recurrence rates of systemic reactions to re-stings in patients with previous systemic events. Patients with a known history of systemic reactions must be aware that they are at risk of potentially life-threatening reactions to re-stings.

Does pretreatment with antihistamines reduce the risk of adverse effects of VIT?

We found no systematic reviews. Four RCTs have compared oral antihistamines with placebo in rapid dose-increase VIT regimens.

In 140 patients, cetirizine significantly reduced local adverse reactions, but not systemic adverse reactions.[50] In 54 patients, fexofenadine 180 mg given on days 1, 8, 22, and 50 significantly reduced local adverse reactions, but not systemic adverse reactions.[51]

In one RCT (n = 52), terfenadine 120 mg twice daily significantly reduced local adverse reactions, but not respiratory or cardiovascular symptoms.[52]

In the second RCT (n = 121), pretreatment with 120 mg terfenadine or terfenadine plus ranitidine significantly reduced both systemic adverse reactions and local adverse reactions during the first week of rush immunotherapy. Therapeutic benefit was evident during the first 4 weeks of treatment.[53]

Drawbacks
Side effects of the antihistamine pretreatment were reported in only one of the above RCTs: headache in 2% (two of 82) and nausea in 1% (one of 82) of the patients who received terfenadine, and fatigue in 3% (one of 39) of those who received placebo.

Comment
The influence of premedication with terfenadine was assessed after an average of 3 years' follow-up. None of the 20 patients who received terfenadine prior to VIT had reacted to subsequent bee-sting challenges, whereas six of 21 (29%) of the placebo pretreatment group had mild to moderate systemic allergic reactions. These findings indicate that the efficacy of VIT was not adversely affected and may have been enhanced by antihistamine premedication.[54]

Implications for clinical practice
The data suggest that pretreatment with antihistamines such as cetirizine, fexofenadine, and terfenadine may reduce cutaneous adverse reactions to rush or ultra-rush VIT. Terfenadine with or without ranitidine may reduce systemic adverse reactions during the first 4 weeks of rush VIT. The efficacy of VIT is not affected by antihistamine premedication.

Key points

Mosquito bites
- We found fair evidence that 10 mg cetirizine may be taken prophylactically by adults to reduce the allergic skin reactions. Loratadine may be given prophylactically to children with allergies to mosquito bites when exposure to these insects is highly possible.
- We found good evidence that topical ammonium sulfate solution may alleviate immediate burning, pain, and pruritus.
- We found fair evidence that dimethindene gel may relieve pruritus due to insect bites.

- We found good evidence that after-bite homeopathic gels tested have no significant benefit in persons with mosquito-bite allergy.
- We found no controlled clinical trials or RCTs that topical corticosteroids are effective in treating mosquito bites, although corticosteroids are commonly recommended for acute inflammatory skin reactions, including insect bites.
- We found good evidence that travelers to mosquito-endemic areas can achieve high levels of sustained protection against bites by using permethrin-treated clothing as well as treated tents.
- We found fairly reliable evidence that applying DEET only on exposed skin cannot effectively prevent mosquito bites, because bites can penetrate through untreated clothing. The mosquito-repellent efficacy and safety of alternatives to DEET have not been adequately assessed through RCTs.
- The combination of avoidance of the insects' habitats, barrier protection (e.g., clothing, bednets), and insect repellents are general measures for preventing insect bites.
- We found good evidence that DEET in a 20% solution form is reported to be safe for pregnant women in their second and third trimesters and does not result in adverse effects on their infants.

Bee and wasp (Hymenoptera) stings
- We found fair evidence that honeybee stings should be removed immediately either by pinching, scraping, or other means in order to reduce the degree of envenomization.
- We found good evidence that ice packs or aspirin paste may reduce local swelling, pain, and pruritus, but that aspirin may prolong redness.
- We found no reliable evidence on emergency treatment specifically for systemic reactions to Hymenoptera stings. However, anaphylactic reactions to insect venoms can be treated in the same way as anaphylaxis from any other cause. Sympathomimetics, antihistamines, and corticosteroids are the most effective drugs for dealing with systemic allergic reactions.

Subcutaneous venom immunotherapy (VIT) in preventing systemic reactions to Hymenoptera stings
- We found good evidence that subcutaneous VIT has protective benefit among children and adults in terms of reducing the risk of immediate and long-term bee or wasp sting reactions and improving quality of life. Benefit was noted especially for those with prior severe systemic reactions to Hymenoptera venom.
- We found good evidence that modified VIT, such as monomethoxy polyethylene glycol (mPEG)-modified honeybee venom and aluminum hydroxide–adsorbed honeybee venom extract (depot VIT), reduced the risk of systemic side effects compared to standard VIT.

Pretreatment with antihistamines in reducing the risk of adverse effects of VIT
- We found good evidence that pretreatment with antihistamines such as cetirizine, fexofenadine, and terfenadine may reduce cutaneous adverse reactions to rush or ultra-rush VIT.
- Terfenadine with or without ranitidine may reduce systemic adverse reactions during the first 4 weeks of rush VIT.
- The efficacy of VIT is not affected by antihistamine premedication.

Acknowledgment

Michael Kulig and Jacqueline Müller-Nordhorn were contributing authors for this chapter in the first edition of the book.

References

1 Samlaska CP. Arthropod infestations and vectors of disease. In: James WD, ed. *Military Dermatology*. Washington, DC: TMM, 1994 (http://www.bordeninstitute.army.mil/derm/Ch9.pdf. Accessed March 23, 2006).

2 Steen C, Paul C, Robert S. Arthropods in dermatology. *J Am Acad Dermatol* 2004;**50**:819–42.

3 Roll Back Malaria Infosheet. 2006. http://malaria.who.int/cmc. Accessed April 5, 2006.

4 World Health Organization Media Centre. Dengue and dengue hemorrhagic fever fact sheet no. 117. 2006. http://www.who.int/mediacentre/factsheets/fx117/en/. Accessed April 5, 2006.

5 Graft DF. Insect sting allergy. *Med Clin N Am* 2006;**90**:211–32.

6 Müller UR. Epidemiology of insect sting allergy. *Epidemiol Clin Allergy Monogr Allergy* 1993;**31**:131–46.

7 Defense Pest Management Information Analysis Center (DPMIAC), Armed Forces Pest Management Board (AFPMB). *Personal Protective Measures against Insects and Other Arthropods of Military Significance*. Washington, DC: AFPMB, 2002 (Armed Forces Pest Management Board Technical Guide No. 36).

8 Mehr ZA, Rutledge LC, Echano NM, Gupta RK. U.S. Army soldiers' perceptions of arthropod pests and their effects on military missions. *Mil Med* 1997;**162**:804–7.

9 Burgess NRH, Crow IRJ. The incidence and effect of insect bites on servicemen in Belize. *J R Army Med Corps* 1983;**129**:38–42.

10 Scharf MJ, Daly JS. Bites and stings of terrestrial and aquatic life. In: Freedberg IM, Eisen AZ, Wolff K, Austen KF, Goldsmith LA, Katz SI, editors. *Fitzpatrick's Dermatology in General Medicine*, 5th ed. New York: McGraw-Hill, 2003: 2655–76.

11 Rozendaal J. *Vector Control: Methods for Use by Individuals and Communities*. Geneva: World Health Organization, 1997.

12 Brown M, Herbert A. Insect repellents: an overview. *J Am Acad Dermatol* 1997;**36**(Part 1):243–9.

13 Reunala T, Brummer-Korvenkontio H, Karppinen A, Coulie P, Palosuo T. Treatment of mosquito bites with cetirizine. *Clin Exp Allergy* 1993;**23**:72–5.

14 Karppinen A, Kautiainen H, Reunala T, Petman L, Reunala T, Brummer-Korvenkontio H. Loratadine in the treatment of mosquito-bite-sensitive children. *Allergy* 2000;**55**:668–71.

15 Zhai H, Packman EW, Maibach HI. Effectiveness of ammonium solution in relieving type I mosquito bite symptoms: a double-blind, placebo-controlled study. *Acta Derm Venereol* 1998;**78**:297–8.

16 Hill N, Stam C, Tuinder S, van Haselen RA. A placebo controlled clinical trial investigating the efficacy of a homeopathic after-bite gel in reducing mosquito bite induced erythema. *Eur J Clin Pharmacol* 1995;**49**:103–8.

17 Hill N, Stam C, van Haselen RA. The efficacy of Prrrikweg gel in the treatment of insect bites: a double-blind, placebo-controlled clinical trial. *Pharm World Sci* 1996;**18**:35–41.

18 Althaus MA, Berthet P. Dimethindene maleate (Fenistil® gel) in the control of itching due to insect bites and sunburns. *Agents Actions* 1992;**36**:C425–7.

19 Schreck CE, Haile DG, Kline DL. The effectiveness of permethrin and DEET, alone or in combination, for protection against. *Aedes taeniorhynchus. Am J Trop Med* 1984;**33**:725–30.

20 Boulware DR, Beisang AA. Passive prophylaxis with permethrin-treated tents reduces mosquito bites among North American summer campers. *Wilderness Environ Med* 2005;**16**:9–15.

21 Rajan TV, Hein M, Porte P, Wikel S. A double-blinded, placebo-controlled trial of garlic as a mosquito repellant: a preliminary study. *Med Vet Entomol* 2005;**19**:84–9.

22 Veltri JC, Osimitz TG, Bradford DC, Page BC. Retrospective analysis of calls to poison control centers resulting from exposure to the insect repellent N,N-diethyl-m-toluamide (DEET) from 1985–1989. *J Toxicol Clin Toxicol* 1994;**32**:1–16.

23 Bell JW, Veltri JC, Page BC. Human exposures to N,N-diethyl-m-toluamide insect repellents reported to the American Association of Poison Control Centers 1993–1997. *Int J Toxicol* 2002;**21**:341–52.

24 Young GD, Evans S. Safety and efficacy of DEET and permethrin in the prevention of arthropod attack. *Mil Med* 1998;**163**:324–30.

25 Avdel-Rahman A, Dechkovskaia AM, Goldstein LB, *et al.* Neurological deficits induced by malathion, DEET, and permethrin, alone or in combination in adult rats. *J Toxicol Environ Health A* 2004;**67**:331–56.

26 Fradin MS. Mosquitoes and mosquito repellents: a clinician's guide. *Ann Int Med* 1998;**128**:931–40.

27 Maibach HI, Akers WA, Johnson HL, Khan AA, Skinner WA. Insects. Topical insect repellents. *Clin Pharmacol Ther* 1974;**16**(5 Part 2):970–3.

28 Schreck CE. Protection from blood-feeding arthropods. In: Auerbach PS, ed. *Wilderness Medicine: Management of Wilderness and Environmental Emergencies*, 3rd ed. St. Louis: Mosby, 1995: 813–30.

29 Khan AA. Mosquito attractants and repellents. In: Shorey HH, McKelvey JJ, eds. *Chemical Control of Insect Behavior*. New York: J Wiley, 1977: 305–25.

30 Fradin MS, Day JF. Comparative efficacy of insect repellents against mosquito bites. *N Engl J Med* 2002;**347**:13–8.

31 Flake ZA, Hinojosa JR, Brown M. Is DEET safe for children? *J Fam Pract* 2005;**54**:468–9.

32 McGready R, Hamilton KA, Simpson JA, *et al.* Safety of the insect repellent N,N-diethyl-m-toluamide (DEET) in pregnancy. *Am J Trop Med Hyg* 2001;**65**:285–9.

33 McGready R, Simpson JA, Htway M, White NJ, Nosten F, Lindsay SW. A double-blind randomized therapeutic trial of insect repellents for the prevention of malaria in pregnancy. *Trans R Soc Trop Med Hyg* 2001;**95**:137–8.

34 Visscher PK, Vetter RS, Camazine S. Removing bees stings. *Lancet* 1996;**348**:301–2.

35 Balit CR, Isbister GK, Buckley NA. Randomized controlled trial of topical aspirin in the treatment of bee and wasp stings. *J Toxicol Clin Toxicol* 2003;**41**:801–8.

36 Bonifazi F, Jutel M, Bilo M, *et al.* Prevention and treatment of hymenoptera venom allergy: guidelines for clinical practice. *Allergy* 2005;**60**:1459–70.

37 Simons FE, Gu X, Simons KJ. Epinephrine absorption in adults: intramuscular versus subcutaneous injection. *J Allergy Clin Immunol* 2001;**108**:871–3.

38 Simons FE, Roberts JR, Gu X, Simons KJ. Epinephrine absorption in children with a history of anaphylaxis. *J Allergy Clin Immunol* 1998;**101**(1 Pt 1):33–7.

39 Simons FE, Gu X, Silver NA, Simons KJ. EpiPen Jr versus EpiPen in young children weighing 15 to 30 kg at risk for anaphylaxis. *J Allergy Clin Immunol* 2002;**109**:171–5.

40 Heilborn H, Hjemdahl P, Daleskog M, Adamsson U. Comparison of subcutaneous injection and high-dose inhalation of epinephrine—implications for self-treatment to prevent anaphylaxis. *J Allergy Clin Immunol* 1986;**78**:1174–9.

41 Simons FE, Gu X, Johnston LM, Simons KJ. Can epinephrine inhalations be substituted for epinephrine injection in children at risk for systemic anaphylaxis? *Pediatr Rev* 2000;**106**:1040–4.

42 Ross RN, Nelson HS, Finegold I. Effectiveness of specific immunotherapy in the treatment of hymenoptera venom hypersensitivity: a meta-analysis. *Clin Ther* 2000;**22**:351–8.

43 Schuberth KC, Lichtenstein LM, Kagey-Sobotka A, Szklo M, Kwiterovich KA, Valentine MD. Epidemiologic study of insect allergy in children. II. Effect of accidental stings in allergic children. *J Pediatr* 1983;**102**:361–5.

44 Valentine MD, Schuberth KC, Kagey-Sobotka AK, *et al.* The value of immunotherapy with venom in children with allergy to insect stings. *N Engl J Med* 1990;**323**:1601–3.

45 Golden DB, Kagey-Sobotka A, Norma PHS, Hamilton RG, Lichtenstein LM. Outcomes of allergy to insect stings in children, with and without venom immunotherapy. *N Engl J Med* 2004; **351**:668–74.

46 Oude Elberink JN, De Monchy JG, Van Der Heide S, Guyatt GH, Dubois AE. Venom immunotherapy improves health-related quality of life in patients allergic to yellow jacket venom. *J Allergy Clin Immunol* 2002;**110**:174–82.

47 Muller U, Rabson AR, Bischof M, Lomnitzer R, Dreborg S, Lanner AJ. A double-blind study comparing monomethoxy polyethylene glycol-modified honeybee venom and unmodified honeybee venom for immunotherapy. I. Clinical results. *Allergy Clin Immunol* 1987;**80**(3 Pt 1):252–61.

48 Quercia O, Rafanelli S, Puccinelli P, Stefanini GF. The safety of cluster immunotherapy with aluminium hydroxide-adsorbed honey bee venom extract. *J Investig Allergol Clin Immunol* 2001;**11**:27–33.

49 Mosbech H, Müller U. Side-effects of insect venom immunotherapy: results from an EAACI multicenter study. European Academy of Allergology and Clinical Immunology. *Allergy* 2000;**55**:1005–10.

50 Herman D, Melac M. Effect of pretreatment with cetirizine on side effects from rush immunotherapy with honey bee venom. *Allergy* 1996;**51**(Suppl 31):68.

51 Reimers A, Hari Y, Müller U. Reduction of side-effects from ultra-rush immunotherapy with honeybee venom by pretreatment with fexofenadine: a double-blind, placebo-controlled trial. *Allergy* 2000;**55**:483–7.

52 Berchtold E, Maibach R, Müller U. Reduction of side effects from rush-immunotherapy with honey bee venom by pretreatment with terfenadine. *Clin Exp Allergy* 1992;**22**:59–65.

53 Brockow K, Kiehn M, Riethmüller C, Vieluf D, Berger J, Ring J. Efficacy of antihistamine pretreatment in the prevention of adverse reactions to Hymenoptera immunotherapy: a prospective, randomized, placebo-controlled trial. *J Allergy Clin Immunol* 1997;**100**:458–63.

54 Müller U, Hari Y, Berchtold E. Premedication with antihistamines may enhance efficacy of specific-allergen immunotherapy. *J Allergy Clin Immunol* 2001;**107**:81–6.

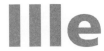

IIIe   Disorders of pigmentation

Berthold Rzany, Editor

49 Vitiligo

Juan Jorge Manriquez

Background

Definition

Vitiligo is an acquired disorder of pigmentation mainly affecting the skin, in which the loss of functioning melanocytes results in white patches. The hair and, rarely, the eyes or other organs and systems may also be affected. The most common form of vitiligo is symmetrical, usually affecting the skin around the orifices, the genitals, sun-exposed areas such as the face and hands, and friction areas such as extensor surfaces of the limbs. The rare segmental type affects only one area of the body.

Incidence/prevalence

Vitiligo is a common skin disorder, affecting about 0.5% of the general population, irrespective of ethnic origin.[1–3] Anyone of any age can develop vitiligo, but generally the disease begins between the ages of 2 and 40. In a Dutch study, 50% of the participants reported the onset of the disease before the age of 20.[4]

Etiology

There appears to be a genetic predisposition to vitiligo, consistent with a polygenic disorder, and up to one-third of patients report a family history of hypopigmentation.[5,6] No definitive precipitating factor responsible for initiating vitiligo has been established, and the basic pathogenesis in general still remains unknown. Current hypotheses range from intrinsic melanocyte dysfunction and/or death to destruction mediated by autoantibodies. Many vitiligo patients also exhibit other autoimmune disorders, and the presence of serum melanocyte-specific autoantibodies appears to correlate with the extent and activity of the disease.[7,8] Köbner phenomenon in response to local trauma may explain the development of vitiligo patches over friction areas.

Prognosis

Although neither lethal nor symptomatic, the effects of vitiligo can be cosmetically and psychologically devastating. The course of the disease is fairly unpredictable, but often progressive (in more than 80% of patients).[9] Periods of slow or rapid enlargement of the lesions, arrest in depigmentation, and spontaneous or partial repigmentation can occur. Spontaneous repigmentation, probably sunlight-induced, is usually also a sign that the patient will respond to medical therapy. On the other hand, as the main reservoir of vital melanocytes is the hair follicle, glabrous skin and hair-bearing skin in which terminal hairs are clearly depigmented might not respond to medical therapies.

Aim of treatment

The aim of treatment is to achieve partial or total repigmentation, at least for body areas that the patients estimate as "most significant," with minimal adverse effects.

Relevant outcomes

- Physician-rated clinical response: success rate in terms of repigmentation (> 75%) or depigmentation (100%), long-term repigmentation rate
- Side effects of treatment

Methods of search

We searched for randomized controlled trials (RCTs) of currently available medical and surgical treatments in the Cochrane Library and Cochrane Central Register of Controlled Trials, Medline, and Embase, using the keyword "vitiligo." The search was completed in June 2007. The references in the key papers were also searched. Where no RCTs were found, information from non-randomized studies or case series was used.

A systematic review without meta-analysis (search date September 2004) on "interventions for vitiligo" is in the Cochrane Database of Systematic Reviews[10] and has been included in this chapter. An older systematic review with meta-analysis (search date December 1997), published in the evidence-based dermatology section of *Archives of Dermatology*, was also included.[11] Finally, a *British Medical Journal* Clinical Evidence systematic review on vitiligo was used as a source of RCTs.[12]

Questions

What are the effects of medical treatment in vitiligo?

Case scenario
A 26-year-old woman reports a 10-year history of depigmented areas. Clinical examination reveals symmetrically distributed depigmented areas affecting the sun-exposed areas, mainly upper arms, face and neck (Figure 49.1).

Phototherapy and photochemotherapy
Efficacy
Photochemotherapy is well established in the treatment of vitiligo, with different modalities essentially related to the

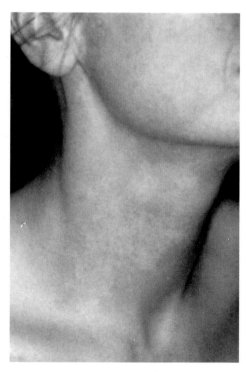

Figure 49.1 Irregularly shaped depigmented areas on the neck in a 26-year-old woman with vitiligo.

equipment available in each geographical area (related to sun exposure). When the photoactive chemical is combined with a light device as a light source it is called psoralen ultraviolet A (PUVA); when a photoactive chemical is used in combination with sunlight as a light source, it is called PUVAsol.

A meta-analysis published in 1998[11] found that the pooled odds ratio (OR) versus placebo (the odds of a patient receiving the active therapy achieving > 75% repigmentation compared with a patient receiving the placebo) was significant for oral methoxsalen plus sunlight as a source of UVA light (one RCT;[13] OR 23.4; 95% confidence intervals, 1.3 to 409.9), oral psoralen plus sunlight (two RCTs;[13,14] OR 19.9; 95% CI, 2.4 to 166.3), and oral trioxsalen plus sunlight (two RCTs;[13,15] OR 3.7; 95% CI, 1.2 to 11.2).

One RCT[13] found that methoxsalen plus trioxsalen plus sunlight was more effective than placebo plus sunlight (RR 19.20; 95% CI, 1.21 to 304.5), but less effective than psoralen plus sunlight (RR 0.51; 95% CI, 0.29 to 0.91). Another RCT[14] found that oral psoralen plus triamcinolone was significantly better than no treatment (RR 33.83; 95% CI, 2.13 to 537.76), oral psoralen alone (RR 6.09; 95% CI, 1.57 to 23.60), and topical psoralen (RR 5.48; 95% CI, 1.42 to 21.07). The same RCT also found no significant differences either between oral and topical psoralens plus sunlight or between topical psoralens plus sunlight and no treatment, in relation to achieving repigmentation (RR 0.90; 95% CI, 0.14 to 5.74 and RR 7.37; 95% CI, 0.37 to 145.06, respectively).

One RCT[16] found that more sessions of broadband ultraviolet B plus oral psoralen were required to produce repigmentation in comparison with ultraviolet A plus oral psoralen, over 30 sessions of treatment. One RCT[17] found that narrowband ultraviolet B was more effective than placebo in increasing the mean repigmentation of affected lesions over 6 months (43% repigmentation with narrowband ultraviolet B in comparison with 3.3% repigmentation with placebo; $P < 0.001$). An additional RCT[18] found that narrowband ultraviolet B (UVB) was equally effective as narrowband UVB plus folic acid and vitamin B_{12} in achieving repigmentation.

Two recent RCTs have demonstrated that narrowband ultraviolet B is more effective than oral PUVA therapy in achieving repigmentation,[19,20] although in the second RCT this difference was only noted after exclusion of traditionally considered therapy-resistant sites.[20] Evidence from a non-randomized controlled trial[21] suggests that narrowband UVB could be more effective than topical PUVA.

Phototherapy or photochemotherapy combined with other treatments
Two RCTs have shown that concurrent topical calcipotriol potentiates the efficacy of PUVAsol (oral psoralen plus sunlight)[22] and PUVA,[23] achieving earlier pigmentation with a lower total UVA dosage.

One non-blinded controlled trial found no significant differences between topical calcipotriol and no treatment in skin repigmentation.[24] One left–right comparison RCT and one parallel RCT found no significant differences between calcipotriol combined with narrowband ultraviolet B and narrowband ultraviolet B alone in achieving repigmentation of lesions.[25,26] In contrast, topical tacalcitol combined with narrowband ultraviolet B was found to be more effective than narrowband ultraviolet B alone in increasing the repigmentation rate in one RCT.[27]

One RCT found that combined treatment with 308-nm monochromatic excimer light and tacalcitol was more effective than monochromatic excimer light alone in attaining repigmentation, with a lower total dosage of light therapy.[28]

One RCT found that a combination of fluticasone propionate and UVA light was more effective than either fluticasone alone or UVA alone in improving repigmentation after 9 months of follow-up.[29]

Finally, one RCT found that a combination of low doses of azathioprine (0.6–0.75 mg/kg) plus oral PUVA was more effective than oral PUVA alone in achieving repigmentation of affected lesions.[30]

No significant differences were found in trials that compared phenylalanine and placebo plus UVA (OR 2.24; 95% CI, 0.35 to 14.28) or oral khellin and placebo plus sunlight (OR 13.16; 95% CI, 0.69 to 249.48).[11,31]

Phototherapy or photochemotherapy in comparison with other treatments

One RCT[32] that compared topical PUVAsol with topical 0.05% clobetasol propionate found that clobetasol was significantly better than PUVAsol at achieving at least 75% repigmentation (RR 4.70; 95% CI, 1.14 to 19.39).

Drawbacks

Photochemotherapy necessitates close monitoring for acute toxicity and cutaneous carcinogenic effects. Oral methoxsalen plus UVA was associated with the highest incidence of side effects. Severe phototoxic reactions (mainly associated with topical psoralen or oral methoxsalen plus UVA) can be avoided by carefully monitoring ultraviolet exposure. Nausea (reported in 29% of the patients treated with methoxsalen) can be reduced by taking food.[11] It seems that wearing UVA-opaque glasses for 24 h after psoralen ingestion makes the risk of cataract development negligible. Liver and renal function tests and ophthalmologic examination should be repeated annually.[33] In the case of phototherapy based on sun exposure, various factors can make it difficult to compare this with phototherapy using artificial ultraviolet devices—not only with regard to the applicability of the findings, but also with regard to the potential side effects, which strongly depend on the patient's compliance, the degree of sun exposure, and the region in which

the treatment is implemented. In patients with psoriasis, long-term PUVA therapy was associated with an increased risk of skin cancer.[34,35] Although the risk appears to be lower in patients with vitiligo (possibly because of lower cumulative dosages and/or darker skin types), guidelines for maximum cumulative PUVA doses should follow those recommended for psoriasis.[36] Both PUVA and UVB therapies should not be continuous, to minimize the carcinogenic potential.

No systemic or local side effects are reported for UVB therapy, except for erythema, pruritus, and xerosis. Long-term side effects and the risk of skin carcinogenesis are unknown.[10,11] Side effects of topical calcipotriol and tacalcitol were negligible in all of the reported trials.[22–28]

Comments/implications for clinical practice

On the basis of the current evidence of efficacy and safety, it appears reasonable to regard narrowband ultraviolet B—alone or plus tacalcitol—as the first-line treatment for moderate to severe generalized vitiligo.

The mean treatment duration of phototherapy and photochemotherapy regimens varied from 6 months to 2 years. Since phototherapy is time-consuming and patients have to remain motivated for long periods, monitoring of compliance is relevant, although seldom reported in trials. Moreover, we found no trials taking quality of life into account as an outcome. These issues need to be better assessed in further studies. In addition, follow-up studies are needed in order to assess the persistence of therapy-induced repigmentation.

Corticosteroids and topical immunomodulators
Efficacy

Topical class 3 corticosteroids have been shown to be effective in localized vitiligo, with a pooled OR[11] of 14.3 (three RCTs;[37–39] 95% CI, 2.4 to 83.7); pooled ORs showed non-significant differences between topical class 4 or intralesional corticosteroids and their respective placebos.[11] The treatment duration in the trials varied from 5 to 8 months, and strongly depended on the response: if no response had occurred by 2–3 months, therapy was stopped. A further RCT[40] showed that a combination of topical calcipotriol and betamethasone dipropionate was more effective than each treatment given alone in hastening the onset of repigmentation, along with reducing side effects.

One left–right RCT[41] that compared 0.1% tacrolimus versus 0.05% clobetasol propionate found them to be equally effective in achieving repigmentation (with average repigmentation rates of 41.3% and 49.3%, respectively; $P = 1.00$). Moreover, a further internally controlled RCT[42] found that tacrolimus plus excimer laser was more effective than excimer laser alone in achieving 75% repigmentation over 10 weeks of treatment. By contrast, one RCT[43] found that the combination of topical tacrolimus and narrowband ultraviolet B was no more effective than narrowband ultraviolet B alone in treating vitiligo lesions. Similarly, one RCT[44] found pimecrolimus to be no more effective than placebo in achieving repigmentation, over 6 months of treatment. No RCTs of imiquimod in vitiligo were found.

The efficacy of oral corticosteroids in generalized vitiligo was low, with fewer than 20% of patients achieving > 75% repigmentation in 4–24 months.[11]

Drawbacks

Atrophy was the most common side effect with local corticosteroids, mainly induced by intralesional and class 4 corticosteroids. Side effects, mainly moon face, weight gain, and acne, were frequent with oral corticosteroids.[11]

The United States Food and Drug Administration has warned of a potential malignancy risk from the use of topical tacrolimus and pimecrolimus, principally based on the theoretical risk of immunomodulator utilization, along with animal and case reports, in a small number of patients. However, a systematic review and a case–control study were not able to confirm such an association in individuals being treated for atopic eczema.[45,46]

Comments/implications for practice

On the basis of the current evidence, it appears reasonable to regard topical corticosteroids as being the first-line treatment for localized vitiligo. The current practice is to prescribe a moderately potent corticosteroid for the face and a more potent corticosteroid for the body. Systemic corticosteroids are not recommended, not only because of the limited evidence of their effectiveness, but also because of the wide range of adverse effects associated with them.

Tacrolimus represents a useful tool, especially for the management of facial skin or eyelid lesions, where the risk of skin atrophy from topical corticosteroids or phototoxicity from phototherapy could be high. More long-term studies are needed in order to establish the safety profile of this drug in the management of vitiligo.

Cognitive–behavioral therapy
Efficacy
We found one controlled trial including 16 patients, showing that cognitive–behavioral therapy is effective in improving the patient's quality of life.[47]

Drawbacks
No drawbacks were reported.

Comments/implications for clinical practice
Studies that take into account the effects of treatments on the patients' quality of life and global health, from the patient's point of view, are needed.

Melagenine, pseudocatalase, levamisole, and systemic antioxidant therapy

One small trial including 20 patients found no clinical differences between melagenine-treated and placebo-treated groups.[48] One trial showed that Dead Sea climatotherapy plus pseudocatalase was more effective than either Dead Sea climatotherapy plus placebo or Dead Sea climatotherapy alone in achieving 50% repigmentation (RR 16.78; 95% CI, 1.11 to 253.02 for each comparison).[49] One RCT found that oral levamisole plus topical mometasone furoate 0.1% was no more effective than topical mometasone furoate 0.1% alone in relation to the development of new lesions in patients with slowly spreading vitiligo over 6 months.[50] One RCT found that oral *Ginkgo biloba* was more effective than placebo in achieving repigmentation in focal, vulgaris, and acrofacial vitiligo (RR 4.40; 95% CI, 1.08 to 17.95).[51] Finally, one recent RCT found that an application of antioxidant and mitochondrial stimulating cream (labeled as VitilVenz AF) and oral administration of antioxidants and phenylalanine could be more effective than placebo in achieving repigmentation over 5 months of treatment.[52]

Drawbacks
Two patients complained of nausea in the *Ginkgo biloba* arm in one RCT.[51] Patients treated with levamisole plus mometasone had an increased rate of nausea and vomiting.[50]

Comments/implications for clinical practice
No clear recommendations on the use of these medications can be made on the basis of the current evidence.

What are the effects of surgical treatment?

In general, autologous transplantation methods are indicated for stable and/or focal lesions that are refractory to medical therapy. Köbner phenomenon should be absent, and the tendency to scar or keloid formation should be ascertained. "Stable" disease is not uniformly defined across the studies.

Even after successful grafting, depigmentation of the grafts may still occur during "reactivation" of the disease.[53]

Autologous noncultured transplantation methods
Efficacy
One RCT found that epidermal noncultured cellular grafting was more effective than placebo in achieving repigmentation of at least 70% of the treated area.[54] One systematic review was found,[55] based on case series only (a total of 39 series, reporting on five different techniques). The highest success rates occurred with split-thickness grafting and suction blister epidermal grafting, with 87% of patients achieving > 75% repigmentation (sample-size weighted averages; 95% CI, 82 to 91 and 83 to 90, respectively). With

minigrafting, 68% of the patients (95% CI, 62 to 64) were successfully grafted. A trial comparing minigrafting and suction blister epidermal grafting[56] confirmed the results of the review, although the outcome measure was the proportion of patches rather than the proportion of patients.

An RCT comparing techniques showed that 25–65% of patients treated with suction blister grafts, in comparison with 90% of those treated with the thin split-thickness graft method, achieved repigmentation 12 weeks after the procedure.[57] One additional RCT found that split-skin grafting was more effective than minipunch grafting in achieving more than 75% repigmentation and in producing excellent cosmetic matching, over larger areas using fewer grafts, especially over the face and extremities.[58] Finally, one RCT that compared the efficacy of two different dilutions of melanocytes in autologous noncultured epidermal suspension found that the minimum number of melanocytes required to produce satisfactory repigmentation was in the range of 210–250/mm^2.[59]

In a placebo-controlled trial including 18 patients, the addition of a melanotropin analogue applied topically on minigrafted patches did not improve the success of the minigrafting.[60] A further RCT[61] found no differences between PUVA therapy and 0.1% fluocinolone acetonide in the repigmentation achieved after punch grafting during a 6-month follow-up period.

Drawbacks

The most frequently reported side effects were scar formation at the donor site (40% of patients) and cobblestone appearance over the recipient area (27%) for minigrafting; scar formation (12% of patients), milia (13%), and partial loss of grafts (11%) for split-thickness grafts; and hyperpigmentation at the donor site (28% of patients) for suction blister epidermal grafts.[55]

Comments/implications for practice

Minigrafting was reported to be the easiest and least expensive method, with the shortest duration for the procedure (45 min for 50 cm^2) and requiring minimal equipment. Suction blister epidermal grafting was the longest procedure, requiring up to 3 h for blister formation and approximately 30 min for the grafting procedure itself.[55]

The data on surgical procedures should be interpreted with caution, as they are derived mainly from small case series and only three comparative trials, with questionable designs and outcome measures.

Autologous cultured transplantation methods

Very little experience has been gained with culturing techniques involving *in vitro* culturing of epidermis containing both melanocytes and keratinocytes (co-culture), or melanocytes alone. One systematic review updated to 1997 includes 10 case series reporting on five different techniques,[55] and two further series have reported on melanocyte grafting.[62,63]

Efficacy

The highest reported percentages of patients with > 75% repigmentation (sample-size weighted averages) were 53% (95% CI, 27–78) for co-cultured melanocyte and keratinocyte grafting (15 patients) and 48% (95% CI, 39–56) for cultured melanocyte grafting (130 patients).[55] However, the results are fairly variable in the different series—reflecting the different techniques, patient selection criteria, and reported outcome measures, in addition to sample variability.

Drawbacks

No adverse effects have been reported. Concern has been raised about the tumorigenic risk of culturing techniques when the culture media are supplemented with tumor promoters.

Comments/implications for practice

Specialized personnel and high-technology laboratory facilities are required.

What are the effects of depigmentation therapy?

Efficacy

Only case series were found, showing efficacy with the monobenzyl ether of hydroquinone (monobenzone), a potent melanocytotoxic agent,[64] methoxyphenol (with 11 of 16 patients achieving total depigmentation) and Q-switched ruby laser (nine of 13 patients).[65]

Drawbacks

When monobenzone is being administered, patients should be warned about possible depigmentation at distant sites and on the skin of others (partners), and should be informed that bleaching is a permanent and irreversible process. Contact dermatitis and corneal and conjunctival melanosis have also been reported.[66]

Repigmentation occurred after total depigmentation was achieved in 36% (95% CI, 11 to 69) of patients treated with methoxyphenol cream and 44% (95% CI, 14 to 79) of patients treated with Q-switched ruby laser.[65]

Comments/implications for clinical practice

Depigmentation therapy may be indicated in patients with extensive vitiligo (> 80% of the body) or disfiguring lesions resistant to repigmentation therapies.[66]

Treatment with monobenzone normally requires 1–3 months in order to initiate a response, and 6 months to 2 years may be required to complete therapy.[64]

Key points

- A meta-analysis of RCTs, one additional systematic review, and several subsequent RCTs showed that narrowband ultraviolet B, psoralen plus UVA light (using sunlight or artificial light sources), and topical class 3 corticosteroids are effective in comparison with placebo in treating generalized and localized vitiligo, respectively.

- There is RCT evidence indicating that narrowband ultraviolet B is more effective than PUVA in achieving repigmentation of treated lesions.

- Two RCTs have reported that concurrent topical calcipotriol potentiates the efficacy of PUVA. Two RCTs have reported that simultaneous use of calcipotriol does not enhance the efficacy ultraviolet B. However, the concurrent use of topical tacalcitol has been shown to increase the efficacy of narrowband ultraviolet B.

- There is some RCT evidence that indicates that tacrolimus is as effective as topical clobetasol propionate in treating vitiligo, although no placebo-controlled trials were found. Evidence from one RCT indicates that topical pimecrolimus is not effective in treating vitiligo. There is concern regarding a theoretical risk of malignancy from the use of topical tacrolimus and pimecrolimus.

- There is scarce RCT evidence on the efficacy of melagenine, pseudocatalase, levamisole, and systemic antioxidant therapy.

- We found limited evidence of the effectiveness of surgical treatments for selected patients and of the effectiveness of depigmentation therapy for widespread vitiligo.

- We found that treatments were evaluated mainly in the short term, with few comparative trials. The maintenance value of therapies and the assessment of patients' preferences, satisfaction, and quality of life have not yet been adequately addressed. Patient compliance is seldom reported in the studies.

Acknowledgment

Cinzia Masini and Damiano Abeni were contributing authors for this chapter in the first edition of the book.

References

1 Jacobson DL, Gange SJ, Rose NR, Graham NM. Epidemiology and estimated population burden of selected autoimmune diseases in the United States. *Clin Immunol Immunopathol* 1997;**84**:223–43.

2 Das SK, Majumder PP, Chakraborty R, Majumdar TK, Haldar B. Studies on vitiligo. I. Epidemiological profile in Calcutta, India. *Genet Epidemiol* 1985;**2**:71–8.

3 Howitz J, Brodthagen H, Schwartz M, Thomsen K. Prevalence of vitiligo. Epidemiological survey on the Isle of Bornholm, Denmark. *Arch Dermatol* 1977;**113**:47–52.

4 Westerhof W, Bolhaar B, Menke HE. Resultaten van een enquete onder vitiligo patienten. *Ned Tjdschr Dermatol Venereol* 1996;**6**:100–5.

5 Bhatia PS, Mohan L, Pandey ON, Singh KK, Arora SK, Mukhija RD. Genetic nature of vitiligo. *J Dermatol Sci* 1992;**4**:180–4.

6 Kim SM, Chung HS, Hann SK. The genetics of vitiligo in Korean patients. *Int J Dermatol* 1998;**37**:908–10.

7 Naughton GK, Reggiardo D, Bystryn JC. Correlation between vitiligo antibodies and extent of depigmentation in vitiligo. *J Am Acad Dermatol* 1986;**15**:978–81.

8 Harning R, Cui J, Bystryn JC. Relation between the incidence and level of pigment cell antibodies and disease activity in vitiligo. *J Invest Dermatol* 1991;**97**:1078–80.

9 Hann SK, Chun WH, Park YK. Clinical characteristics of progressive vitiligo. *Int J Dermatol* 1997;**36**:353–5.

10 Whitton ME, Ashcroft DM, Barrett CW, Gonzalez U. Interventions for vitiligo. *Cochrane Database Syst Rev* 2006;(**1**):CD003263.

11 Njoo MD, Spuls PI, Bos JD, Westerhof W, Bossuyt PM. Nonsurgical repigmentation therapies in vitiligo. Meta-analysis of the literature. *Arch Dermatol* 1998;**134**:1532–40.

12 Martin R. Vitiligo. *Clin Evid* 2007;**15**:1–3.

13 Pathak MA, Mosher DB, Fitzpatrick TB. Safety and therapeutic effectiveness of 8-methoxypsoralen, 4,5,8-trimethylpsoralen, and psoralen in vitiligo. *Natl Cancer Inst Monogr* 1984;**66**:165–73.

14 Farah FS, Kurban AK, Chaglassian HT. The treatment of vitiligo with psoralens and triamcinolone by mouth. *Br J Dermatol* 1967;**79**:89–91.

15 Ruiz Maldonado R, Tamayo Sanchez L. 4-5-8 Trimethylpsoralen in vitiligo: controlled clinical study of its therapeutic and toxic effect in children. *Actas Dermosifiliograficas* 1975;**66**:513–26.

16 Mofty ME, Zaher H, Esmat S, et al. PUVA and PUVB in vitiligo—are they equally effective? *Photodermatol Photoimmunol Photomed* 2001;**17**:159–63.

17 Hamzavi I, Jain H, McLean D, et al. Parametric modeling of narrowband UV-B phototherapy for vitiligo using a novel quantitative tool: the Vitiligo Area Scoring Index. *Arch Dermatol* 2004;**140**:677–83.

18 Tjioe M, Gerritsen MJP, Juhlin L, Van de Kerkhof PCM. Treatment of vitiligo vulgaris with narrowband UVB (311 nm) for one year and the effect of addition of folic acid and vitamin B12. *Acta Derm Venereol* 2002;**82**:369–72.

19 Yones SS, Palmer RA, Garibaldinos TM, Hawk JL. Randomized double-blind trial of treatment of vitiligo: efficacy of psoralen-UV-A therapy vs narrowband UV-B therapy. *Arch Dermatol* 2007;**143**:578–84.

20 Bhatnagar A, Kanwar AJ, Parsad D, De D. Comparison of systemic PUVA and NB-UVB in the treatment of vitiligo: an open prospective study. *J Eur Acad Dermatol Venereol* 2007;**21**:638–42.

21 Westerhof W, Nieuweboer-Krobotova L. Treatment of vitiligo with UV-B radiation vs topical psoralen plus UV-A. *Arch Dermatol* 1997;**133**:1525–8.

22 Parsad D, Saini R, Verma N. Combination of PUVAsol and topical calcipotriol in vitiligo. *Dermatology* 1998;**197**:167–70.

23 Ermis O, Alpsoy E, Cetin L, Yilmaz E. Is the efficacy of psoralen plus ultraviolet A therapy for vitiligo enhanced by concurrent topical calcipotriol? A placebo-controlled double-blind study. *Br J Dermatol* 2001;**145**:472–5.

24 Chiaverini C, Passeron T, Ortonne JP. Treatment of vitiligo by topical calcipotriol. *J Eur Acad Dermatol Venereol* 2002;**16**:137–8.

25 Ada S, Sahin S, Boztepe G, et al. No additional effect of topical calcipotriol on narrow-band UVB phototherapy in patients with

generalized vitiligo. *Photodermatol Photoimmunol Photomed* 2005; **21**:79–83.

26 Arca E, Tastan HB, Erbil AH, Sezer E, Koc E, Kurumlu Z. Narrowband ultraviolet B as monotherapy and in combination with topical calcipotriol in the treatment of vitiligo. *J Dermatol* 2006; **335**:338–43.

27 Leone G, Pacifico A, Iacovelli P, Paro Vidolin A, Picardo M. Tacalcitol and narrow-band phototherapy in patients with vitiligo. *Clin Exp Dermatol* 2006;**31**:200–5.

28 Lu-yan T, Wen-wen F, Lei-hong X, Yi J, Zhi-zhong Z. Topical tacalcitol and 308-nm monochromatic excimer light: a synergistic combination for the treatment of vitiligo. *Photodermatol Photoimmunol Photomed* 2006;**22**:310–4.

29 Westerhof W, Nieuweboer-Krobotova L, Mulder P, Glazenburg EJ. Left–right comparison study of the combination of uticasone propionate and UVA vs either uticasone propionate or UVA alone for the long-term treatment of vitiligo. *Arch Dermatol* 1999;**135**:1061–6.

30 Radmanesh M, Saedi K. The efficacy of combined PUVA and low-dose azathioprine for early and enhanced repigmentation in vitiligo patients. *J Dermatol Treat* 2006;**17**:151–3.

31 Orecchia G, Sangalli ME, Gazzaniga A, Giordano F. Topical photochemotherapy of vitiligo with a new khellin formulation: preliminary clinical results. *J Dermatol Treat* 1998;**9**:65–9.

32 Khalid M, Mujtaba G, Haroon TS. Comparison of 0.05% clobetasol propionate cream and topical PUVAsol in childhood vitiligo. *Int J Dermatol* 1995;**14**:203–5.

33 Drake LA, Ceilley RI, Dorner W. Guidelines of care for phototherapy and photochemotherapy. American Academy of Dermatology Committee on Guidelines of Care. *J Am Acad Dermatol* 1994; **31**:643–8.

34 Stern RS, Laird N. The carcinogenic risk of treatments for severe psoriasis. Photochemotherapy follow-up study. *Cancer* 1994;**73**: 2759–64.

35 Stern RS, Nichols KT, Vakeva LH. Malignant melanoma in patients treated for psoriasis with methoxsalen (psoralen) and ultraviolet A radiation (PUVA). The PUVA Follow-Up Study. *N Engl J Med* 1997;**336**:1041–5.

36 British Photodermatology Group guidelines for PUVA. *Br J Dermatol* 1994;**130**:246–55.

37 Bleehen SS. The treatment of vitiligo with topical corticosteroids. Light and electron-microscopic studies. *Br J Dermatol* 1976;**94** (Suppl 12):43–50.

38 Koopmans-van Dorp B, Goedhart-van Dijjk B, Neering H, *et al.* Treatment of vitiligo by local application of betamethasone 17-valerate in a dimethyl sulfoxide cream base. *Dermatologica* 1973;**146**:310–4.

39 Kandil E. Treatment of vitiligo with 0.1% betamethasone 17-valerate in isopropyl alcohol—a double blind trial. *Br J Dermatol* 1974;**91**:457–60.

40 Kumaran MS, Kaur I, Kumar B. Effect of topical calcipotriol, betamethasone dipropionate and their combination in the treatment of localized vitiligo. *J Eur Acad Dermatol Venereol* 2006; **20**:269–73.

41 Lepe V, Moncada B, Castanedo-Cazares JP, Torres-Alvarez MB, Ortiz CA, Torres-Rubalcava AB. A double-blind randomised trial of 0.1% tacrolimus vs 0.05% clobetasol for the treatment of childhood vitiligo. *Arch Dermatol* 2003;**139**:581–5.

42 Kawalek AZ, Spencer JM, Phelps RG. Combined excimer laser and topical tacrolimus for the treatment of vitiligo: a pilot study. *Dermatol Surg* 2004;**30**(2 Pt 1):130–5.

43 Mehrabi D, Pandya AG. A randomized, placebo-controlled, double-blind trial comparing narrowband UV-B plus 0.1% tacrolimus ointment with narrowband UV-B plus placebo in the treatment of generalized vitiligo. *Arch Dermatol* 2006;**142**:927–9.

44 Dawid M, Veensalu M, Grassberger M, Wolff K. Efficacy and safety of pimecrolimus cream 1% in adult patients with vitiligo: results of a randomized, double-blind, vehicle-controlled study. *J Dtsch Dermatol Ges* 2006;**4**:942–6.

45 Callen J, Chamlin S, Eichenfield LF, *et al.* A systematic review of the safety of topical therapies for atopic dermatitis. *Br J Dermatol* 2007;**156**:203–21.

46 Arellano FM, Wentworth CE, Arana A, Fernandez C, Paul CF. Risk of lymphoma following exposure to calcineurin inhibitors and topical steroids in patients with atopic dermatitis. *J Invest Dermatol* 2007;**127**:808–16.

47 Papadopoulos L, Bor R, Legg C. Coping with the disfiguring effects of vitiligo: a preliminary investigation into the effects of cognitive-behavioural therapy. *Br J Med Psychol* 1999;**72**:385–96.

48 Souto MG, Manhaes AMH, Milhomens CH, Succi ICB. Comparative study of melagenine and placebo for the treatment of vitiligo. *An Bras Dermatol* 1997;**72**:237–9.

49 Schallreuter KU, Moore J, Behrens-Williams S, Panske A. Rapid initiation of repigmentation in vitiligo with Dead Sea climatotherapy in combination with pseudocatalase. *Int J Dermatol* 2002;**41**: 482–7.

50 Agarwal S, Ramam M, Sharma VK, *et al.* A randomized placebo-controlled double-blind study of levamisole in the treatment of limited and slowly spreading vitiligo. *Br J Dermatol* 2005;**153**:163–6.

51 Parsad D, Pandhi R, Juneja A. Effectiveness of oral *Ginkgo biloba* in treating limited, slowly spreading vitiligo. *Clin Exp Dermatol* 2003;**28**:285–7.

52 Rojas-Urdaneta JE, Poleo-Romero AG. [Evaluation of an antioxidant and mitochondria-stimulating cream formula on the skin of patients with stable common vitiligo; in Spanish.] *Invest Clin* 2007;**48**:21–31.

53 Kim HY, Kang KY. Epidermal grafts for treatment of stable and progressive vitiligo. *J Am Acad Dermatol* 1999;**40**:412–7.

54 van Geel N, Ongenae K, De Mil M, Haeghen YV, Vervaet C, Naeyaert JM. Double-blind placebo-controlled study of autologous transplanted epidermal cell suspensions for repigmenting vitiligo. *Arch Dermatol* 2004;**140**:1203–8.

55 Njoo MD, Westerhof W, Bos JD, Bossuyt PM. A systematic review of autologous transplantation methods in vitiligo. *Arch Dermatol* 1998;**134**:1543–9.

56 Gupta S, Jain VK, Saraswat PK. Suction blister epidermal grafting versus punch skin grafting in recalcitrant and stable vitiligo. *Dermatol Surg* 1999;**25**:955–8.

57 Ozdemir M, Cetinkale O, Wolf R, *et al.* Comparison of two surgical approaches for treating vitiligo: a preliminary study. *Int J Dermatol* 2002;**41**:135–8.

58 Khandpur S, Sharma VK, Manchanda Y. Comparison of minipunch grafting versus split-skin grafting in chronic stable vitiligo. *Dermatol Surg* 2005;**31**:436–41.

59 Tegta GR, Parsad D, Majumdar S, Kumar B. Efficacy of autologous transplantation of noncultured epidermal suspension in

two different dilutions in the treatment of vitiligo. *Int J Dermatol* 2006;**45**:106–10.

60 Schwartzmann-Solon AM, Visconti MA, Castrucci AM. Topical application of a melanotropin analogue to vulgar vitiligo dermo-epidermal minigrafts. *Braz J Med Biol Res* 1998;**31**:1557–64.

61 Barman KD, Khaitan BK, Verma KK. A comparative study of punch grafting followed by topical corticosteroid versus punch grafting followed by PUVA therapy in stable vitiligo. *Dermatol Surg* 2004;**30**:49–53.

62 Chen YF, Chang JS, Yang PY, Hung CM, Huang MH, Hu DN. Transplant of cultured autologous pure melanocytes after laser-abrasion for the treatment of segmental vitiligo. *J Dermatol* 2000;**27**:434–9.

63 Guerra L, Capurro S, Melchi F. Treatment of "stable" vitiligo by timed surgery and transplantation of cultured epidermal autografts. *Arch Dermatol* 2000;**136**:1380–9.

64 Mosher DB, Parrish JA, Fitzpatrick TB. Monobenzylether of hydroquinone. A retrospective study of treatment of 18 vitiligo patients and a review of the literature. *Br J Dermatol* 1977;**97**:669–79.

65 Njoo MD, Vodegel RM, Westerhof W. Depigmentation therapy in vitiligo universalis with topical 4-methoxyphenol and the Q-switched ruby laser. *J Am Acad Dermatol* 2000;**42**:760–9.

66 Njoo MD, Westerhof W. Vitiligo. Pathogenesis and treatment. *Am J Clin Dermatol* 2001;**2**:167–81.

50 Melasma

Asad Salim, Mónica Rengifo-Pardo, Sam Vincent,
Luis Gabriel Cuervo-Amore

Background

Definition

Melasma is an acquired increased pigmentation of the skin, characterized by grey–brown symmetrical patches, mostly on the areas of the face exposed to the sun, but occasionally on the neck and forearms.[1] Its clinical and histological presentation does not differ between men and women, apart from differences in the incidence (see below) (Figure 50.1).

Incidence/prevalence

There are few studies showing the prevalence of melasma.

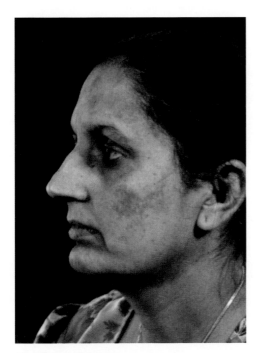

Figure 50.1 Patient with Melasma.

A study conducted in Mexico[2] and another in Peru[3] found that melasma accounted for 4–10% of new dermatology hospital referrals. Melasma was found to be the third most common pigmentary disorder of the skin in a survey of 2000 black people at a private clinic in Washington, DC.[4] Melasma is thought to be more common in people of Hispanic origin who live in areas of high ultraviolet-light exposure, as well as in Asian people.[5] Melasma may also affect men, especially those of Hispanic or Asian origin.

Etiology

Melasma occurs most commonly during pregnancy, and has also been associated with the use of oral contraceptives containing estrogens and/or progestogens, and with certain drugs such as hydantoin.[6–8] Sun exposure appears to be important for the development of melasma,[9] and there also appears to be a familial predisposition.[9] On the basis of a small case series in Puerto Rico, sunlight exposure and family history appear to be the most important determinants for the development of melasma in men.[10] The cause of melasma is unknown; hormonal mechanisms may be involved. Mild ovarian dysfunction has been considered as a cause, after a study found increased levels of luteinizing hormone and low levels of serum estradiol in nine women with melasma.[11] A case–control study of 108 nonpregnant women with melasma found a significant association with increased thyroid antibodies in the blood.[12] Studies measuring levels of immunoreactive β-melanocyte stimulating hormone found normal levels in patients taking oral contraceptives, some of whom had melasma,[13] suggesting that the development of melasma is not related to melanocytic hormone.

Prognosis

Melasma usually persists for several years. It may present as odd streaking on the face, causing cosmetic disfigurement. Pregnancy-related melasma may persist for several months after delivery, and melasma related to hormonal treatments may persist for long periods after oral contraceptives have been stopped. Recurrences are common, particularly after repeat exposure to the sun.[9] The response to treatment can be variable, although dermal-type melasma is less responsive than the epidermal type (see below). The benefits of treatment may not be apparent for many months. Treatment is often unsatisfactory, and has been associated with side effects such as local irritation, scarring, contact dermatitis, and residual patches of lighter color on the skin—known as "confetti pigmentation."

Diagnostic tests

Melasma is a clinical diagnosis. Microscopy studies suggest that there may be two main types of melasma—the epidermal type, characterized by increased melanin pigmentation in the suprabasal layers of the epidermis; and the dermal type, characterized by increased melanin in the dermal macrophages, with associated milder epidermal hyperpigmentation.[9] This distinction may provide a clue to the expected treatment response. The dermal type has been found to be less responsive to conventional therapy.[5] An alternative way of establishing the type of melasma clinically is by using a source of ultraviolet A light, such as a Wood's lamp,[14] in which the dermal type appears much darker than the epidermal type. Ultraviolet-light lamps enhance the lesions in light-colored skins (i.e., skin phototypes I–IV),[12] but may be of little use in dark-skinned people, in whom the enhancement is less prominent.

Aims of treatment

Treatments should aim to prevent the development of melasma, to prevent or reduce the severity of recurrence, to reduce the affected areas, improving the cosmetic defect, and to reduce the time to clearance, with the fewest possible side effects. The time to clearance is important, as current treatments take several months to have any effect.

Relevant outcomes

- Improvement in patient satisfaction measures and quality-of-life assessment measures (Box 50.1)[15] during the time course of the intervention.
- Clearance of lesions as evaluated by objective methods—for example, the Melasma Area and Severity Index (MASI) or the Melasma Area and Melanin Index (MAMI) (Box 50.2),[16,17] or any other objective, semiquantitative measures of disease.
- Lightening of pigmentation (evaluated objectively by a colorimeter or a mexameter, for example).

BOX 50.1 Melasma quality-of-life scale[15]

On a scale of 1 (not bothered at all) to 7 (bothered all the time), patients rate how they feel about:
- The appearance of the skin condition.
- Frustration about the skin condition.
- Embarrassment about the skin condition.
- Feeling depressed about the skin condition
- The effects of the skin condition on interactions with other people (e.g., interactions with family, friends, close relationship).
- The effect of the skin condition on their desire to be with people.
- The skin condition making it hard to show affection.
- Skin discoloration making them feel unattractive to others.
- Skin discoloration making them feel less vital or productive.
- Skin discoloration affecting the sense of freedom.

The melasma quality of life is scored from 7 to 70, with higher scores indicating a poorer melasma-related, health-related quality of life.

BOX 50.2 Melasma scoring indexes

Melasma Area and Melanin Index (MAMI)[16]
This is calculated in the same way as MASI (see below), but darkness and homogeneity are replaced by the single variable of the melanin index. This variable is a measurement of color at involved sites, determined using a reflectance spectrophotometer.

Melasma Area and Severity Index (MASI)[17]
The index evaluates four areas of the face: the forehead (f), the right malar (rm) and left malar (lm) regions, and the chin (c). Each of the first three is weighted with 30% of the score, while the chin is weighted with 10% of the score. The extent of melasma in each *area* (A) is calculated and given a numerical value as follows:

0 No involvement
1 < 10%
2 10–29%
3 30–49%
4 50–69%
5 70–89%
6 < 90–100%.

The *severity* of the melasma is described by a combination of two factors, darkness (D) and homogeneity (H), each evaluated on a scale of 0 to 4, and is calculated as follows:

$$MASI = 0.3(D_f + H_f)A_f + 0.3(D_{rm} + H_{rm})A_{rm} + 0.3(D_{lm} + H_{lm})A_{lm} + 0.1(D_c + H_c)A_c$$

where "f" is forehead, "rm" is right malar, "lm" is left malar, and "c" is chin.

• Adverse effects, such as irregular pigmentation or irritation related to the interventions.

Methods of search

Medline (1966–February 2006), Embase (1980–February 2006) and the Cochrane Library were searched for the terms "melasma," "chloasma," and "mask of pregnancy" as text words and/or key words if present in the database. Randomized controlled trials (RCTs) were searched for first, using a filter; the remaining abstracts from the search were then scanned to see whether any RCTs had been missed using the search filter. References from identified papers were searched. The results of the search were appraised by at least two of the authors.

Categorization of studies: in most studies of melasma, sunscreens are used as a baseline measure with additional interventions. We have therefore not categorized them as combination studies. We have used the term "combination study" when a combined effect of two or more interventions (other than sunscreens) is assessed.

Questions

How effective are preventive interventions in high-risk populations?

Case scenario 1

A Latin-American woman is planning to have children and is concerned about developing melasma. Her three sisters all developed melasma during pregnancy, which lasted for many years.

Efficacy

We found no studies assessing the effects of preventive measures (such as educational interventions to avoid sun exposure or use of prophylactic sunscreens) in high-risk populations.

Comment

Overall, expert opinion supports interventions aimed at reducing exposure to ultraviolet light, which may reduce the risk of developing melasma.

Key messages

We found no good evidence to support preventive interventions in high-risk populations. Current opinion, based on known risk factors, suggests that preventing exposure to ultraviolet light such as sunlight may reduce the risk of developing melasma.

Implications for clinical practice/categorization

Unknown effectiveness.

How effective are therapeutic interventions in childbearing, pregnant, and breastfeeding women?

Case scenario 2

A 30-year-old woman develops melasma in the 20th week of her first pregnancy. She is not on any medication and has not used an oral contraceptive in the past.

Efficacy

We found no studies in pregnant or breastfeeding women. Several studies did not clearly specify whether the women included were pregnant or became pregnant during follow-up. When components used in the study included those that are not recommended in childbearing women (i.e., retinoids), the study was considered to be done in nonpregnant or nursing populations and is discussed under the corresponding question.

Comment

Common expert opinion is that women with a high risk of developing melasma should avoid exposure to the sun or other sources of ultraviolet light. It would seem reasonable to consider the use of broad-spectrum sunscreen with solar protection factors (SPF) > 15 in women who are at high risk of developing melasma.

Key messages

We found no good evidence to support any therapeutic intervention in childbearing, pregnant, or breastfeeding women. Current opinion suggests that such women with melasma may benefit from using broad-spectrum sunscreens and avoiding exposure to ultraviolet light such as sunlight.

Implications for clinical practice/categorization

Unknown effectiveness.

How effective are therapeutic interventions in non-childbearing women?

Case scenario 3

A 35-year-old woman presents with a 3-month history of melasma. She had been taking an oral contraceptive, which she had recently stopped taking after a tubal ligation. She is an outdoor worker.

Sunscreens
Efficacy

We found no systematic reviews. We found one RCT[18] comparing sunscreens with placebo in women receiving hydroquinone. The study included 59 nonpregnant Hispanic women in Puerto Rico. None of the participating women was taking contraceptive hormones and all had had melasma for 2–25 years. All of the women were prescribed a clearing solution of hydroquinone 3% in hydroalcoholic solvent twice daily. The women were randomly assigned to a morning application of broad-spectrum sunscreen or vehicle (placebo) and were then followed for 3 months. Improvement, assessed subjectively by a physician, was seen in 26 of 27 women receiving sunscreen and hydroquinone (96%), in comparison with 21 of 26 women receiving placebo and hydroquinone (81%); relative risk (RR) 1.19, 95% confidence intervals (CI) 0.98 to 1.46. Improvement rates as assessed by participants were high in both groups—27 of 27 (100%) with sunscreen and hydroquinone, in comparison with 25 of 26 (96%) with placebo and hydroquinone; absolute risk reduction (ARR) 4%, 95% CI 1% to 18.9%. Six of the 59 women (10%) withdrew and nine of 53 (17%) women suffered side effects; the report did not mention which group these women were allocated to.

Comment
Sunscreens are commonly prescribed for melasma.

Key messages
We found limited evidence from a single RCT evaluating the effect of therapeutic sunscreens. It showed that during the 3-month follow-up period, the majority of women receiving hydroquinone improved regardless of the addition of sunscreen to their treatment. The study did not describe if women used other strategies to avoid sunlight.

Implications for clinical practice/categorization
Unknown effectiveness.

Topical corticosteroids
Efficacy
We found no systematic reviews. We found one trial of 17 participants (16 consecutive women and one man) followed for 3 months.[19] The trial compared the topical application of a 0.2% betamethasone 17-valerate cream with cream excipient (placebo). Randomization was used to allocate the side of the face to which creams were applied. There was good improvement (subjectively defined by the physician and participants) in eight people, eight of whom considered betamethasone to be better than placebo. Three considered they achieved moderate improvement with either betamethasone or placebo, and four people said they had no improvement at all. One person withdrew from the trial.

Drawbacks
The study reported no significant side effects.[19]

Comment
Although the study reports that betamethasone was effective as a depigmenting agent ($P < 0.05$), the numbers were very small and seven of 16 patients found no therapeutic difference between treatment and placebo.[19] There is con-troversy over the balance between benefits and harms of using topical steroids in the treatment of melasma.

Key messages
We found insufficient evidence to support the use of topical steroids in melasma. There is controversy over the use of topical steroids in melasma.

Implications for clinical practice/categorization
Unknown effectiveness.

Topical retinoids
Efficacy
We found no systematic review. We found three RCTs.

In Caucasian people. The first RCT was done in 50 Caucasian women with facial melasma.[20] The trial compared the daily use of topical 0.1% tretinoin with placebo (vehicle cream for tretinoin) over a period of 40 weeks. The withdrawal rate was 24%. Insufficient baseline data were presented to determine whether the groups were comparable at baseline.

In Asian people. The second RCT[16] included 30 Thai people (26 women and four men) with facial melasma. The RCT compared a titrated daily application of 0.05% isotretinoin gel with a color-matched vehicle used as placebo, for 40 weeks. There were no significant differences in the MASI or MAMI scores in the evaluations done at 2 weeks, 4 weeks, and monthly for up to 40 weeks. The only two participants with dermal melasma were allocated to the isotretinoin group. Participants in both groups improved during the 40-week follow-up.

In black people. One RCT in the United States compared the daily application to the entire face of a cream with 0.1% tretinoin or placebo (vehicle) in 30 Afro-Americans (29 women), followed for 40 weeks.[21] The MASI score was used to assess the severity of melasma. Darkness and homogeneity were also assessed. Colorimetry, photographic, and histology studies were carried out before and after treatment. After 40 weeks, patients receiving tretinoin had higher rates of improvement in their mean ± SD MASI score (the MASI score changed in the tretinoin group from 15.0 ± 1.8 at baseline to 10.2 ± 2, and in the vehicle group from 15.5 ± 2.6 to 13.9 ± 2.7 after 40 weeks of treatment ($P = 0.03$)). Changes were assessed by an independent clinician, who found no significant differences between tretinoin and placebo after 24 weeks—improved or much improved: 11 of 15 (73%) with tretinoin, compared with six of 13 (46%) with placebo (RR 1.6; 95% CI, 0.8 to 3.1).

Drawbacks
In Caucasian people. The first RCT described some causes for withdrawal, such as cutaneous side effects—three of

25 (12%) with tretinoin, in comparison with none of 25 with placebo. Worsening of melasma occurred in a woman in the tretinoin group. Moderate cutaneous reactions were more frequent with tretinoin (22 of 25; 88%) than with placebo (seven of 24; 29%; RR 3.0; 95% CI, 1.6 to 5.7). The number needed to harm was 1.7 (95% CI, 1.3 to 3.1). Severe cutaneous reactions occurred only with tretinoin (four of 25; 16%; NNH 6.3).[20]

In Asian people. The second RCT found similar withdrawals rates in both groups—four of 15 (27%) with isotretinoin, in comparison with three of 15 (20%) with placebo.[16] Mild transient erythema and/or peeling occurred only in the isotretinoin group (four of 15; 27%; NNH 3.8).

In black people. The most frequently found side effects in the third RCT were erythema and/or peeling in the area of application—10 of 15 (67%) with tretinoin, in comparison with one of 15 (7%) with placebo (RR 10, 95% CI, 1.5 to 68.7; NNH 1.7, 95% CI, 1.1 to 2.4).[21]

Comment

The withdrawal rate was high in the first RCT,[20] which compromised the validity of the results. Both RCTs have small samples, making it difficult to draw conclusions with confidence. The RCT in black people[21] may have had insufficient power to rule out an effect, as the confidence intervals for physician-assessed changes were broad. It is impossible to draw reliable conclusions on the effects of retinoids in Caucasian women. The trials done in Asian people[16] and black people[21] were small, so the finding of no differences does not rule out the possibility of a clinically important effect. Side effects, however, were quite common in people receiving retinoids. It is unknown whether the use of sunscreens may have introduced any confounding.

Key messages

We found inconclusive evidence of an effect of retinoids in people with melasma, but side effects were common.

Implications for clinical practice/categorization

Unlikely to be beneficial.

Azelaic acid

Efficacy

We found no systematic reviews. We found three RCTs and one nonrandomized study.

The first RCT done in the USA (52 people: 45 nonpregnant or nonnursing women, seven men; skin phototype IV, V, or VI; clinical diagnosis of facial hyperpigmentation, which could in some cases be caused by melasma) compared azelaic acid with placebo.[22] After 24 weeks, the authors found a statistically significant decrease in the treatment group in pigmentary intensity as measured by chromo-

meter analysis ($P = 0.039$) and the investigators' subjective scale ($P = 0.021$).

The second RCT[23] was a prospective, single-blinded study in 30 Indian patients (25 females, five males) that compared 20% azelaic acid (AZA) versus 20% AZA and 0.05% clobetasol propionate used sequentially. This was a left-to-right comparative study, with 20% AZA used on one side for 24 weeks, in comparison with 8 weeks of topical steroid followed by 16 weeks of 20% AZA. Clinical evaluation, photographic controls, and an assessment for overall response were done at 4, 8, 16, and 24 weeks. Evaluations done at 4-weekly intervals showed improved outcomes at 16 weeks with sequential therapy in comparison with 20% AZA alone ($P > 0.001$). However, at week 24, both groups showed good to excellent responses. Five patients in the AZA group suffered mild irritation, while six patients in the sequential therapy group suffered mild acne form eruptions.

We found one RCT and one left-to-right comparison trial comparing azelaic acid with hydroquinone. The RCT[24] was in 340 patients with nondermal melasma (including 17 men) evenly distributed, and compared twice-daily 20% azelaic acid cream with twice-daily 2% hydroquinone cream for 24 weeks. It found that improvement (defined as a reduction of > 50% in a score including area and pigmentation) was higher with azelaic acid (106 of 154; 69%) than with hydroquinone—88 of 161 (55%), RR 1.26 (95% CI, 1.06 to 1.50), number needed to treat (NNT) 7 (95% CI, 4 to 30). The majority of patients were of skin phototypes III–VI.

A nonrandomized left-to-right comparison trial[25] (60 women with skin phototypes I–IV, centromalar or facial distribution, followed for 24 weeks) included women with epidermal (72%) or mixed melasma (28%), in the age range 18–40 years. Thirty percent of the women were taking oral contraceptives. The trial compared 20% azelaic acid cream with 4% hydroquinone cream. All of the women were given sunscreen (details not provided) and were asked to apply azelaic acid on one side of their face and hydroquinone on the other side twice daily for 24 weeks. No details were provided to explain how the interventions were concealed. Improvement was assessed subjectively by the participants and evaluators. The study was completed by 85% of the participants. The improvement was similar in women receiving azelaic acid (23 of 26; 88%) and hydroquinone (22 of 25; 88%; RR 1.0; 95% CI, 0.8 to 1.3).

Drawbacks

The first study[22] found that people using azelaic acid cream had a higher incidence of burning, particularly at weeks 4 and 12 ($P = 0.046$ and 0.021, respectively; detailed data not provided) and significantly higher stinging symptoms at week 4 ($P = 0.002$; detailed data not provided) than those using placebo. The RCT[23] comparing sequential therapy of azelaic acid and topical steroids showed that although the sequential treatment produced faster improvement at 16 weeks, there was no significant difference between the two groups at 24 weeks.

In the comparison study with hydroquinone, complaints of mild symptoms such as itching and burning were more frequent with azelaic acid (61 of 167; 37%) than with hydroquinone (22 of 173; 12%; RR 3.0, 95% CI, 1.7 to 4.7; NNH 4, 95% CI, 3 to 6). Withdrawals related to intolerance (local irritation) occurred in both groups—four of 167 (2%) with azelaic acid, in comparison with two of 173 (1%) with hydroquinone. Marked irritation was more frequent with azelaic acid (15 of 167; 9%) than with hydroquinone (two of 173; 1%; RR 7.8, 95% CI, 1.8 to 33.5; NNH 12, 95% CI, 7 to 30).[24]

Comment

The results of the nonrandomized clinical trial should be interpreted with caution, as the authors did not describe strategies used to avoid bias, outcomes were assessed subjectively, and no standardized or validated scales were used. The use of topical steroids was associated with faster clearance, but has to be evaluated for side effects in larger studies.

Key messages

Azelaic acid was found to be superior to 2% hydroquinone in achieving improvement in people with melasma. We found no solid evidence in comparison with placebo. Azelaic acid was associated with a higher incidence of side effects. When used sequentially with azelaic acid, topical steroids may result in faster improvement of melasma.

Implications for clinical practice/categorization
Unknown effectiveness.

Hydroquinone
Efficacy
We found no systematic reviews. We found two RCTs. The first RCT was done between autumn and spring in Brazil (48 patients, four men; age range 19–55 years).[26] All participants had a clinical diagnosis of melasma with Wood's lamp evaluation. All participants received an SPF 15 sunscreen. The intervention group received 4% hydroquinone cream applied twice daily, while the control group received a placebo. Outcomes were assessed by subjective clinical evaluation and photography. After 12 weeks, hydroquinone showed higher improvement rates (20 of 21; 95%), in comparison with 16 of 24 (67%) with placebo (RR 1.4, 95% CI, 1.06 to 1.9; NNT 3.5, 95% CI, 1.9 to 12.1). Total clearance of lesions was more frequent in patients receiving hydroquinone (eight of 21; 38%) in comparison with placebo (two of 24, 8%; RR 4.6, 95% CI, 1.1 to 19.2; NNT 3.4, 95% CI, 1.8 to 12.7). We found one RCT comparing hydroquinone with azelaic acid (see above).[24]

A second RCT[27] randomized women's hemifaces to receive 5% ascorbic acid plus sunscreen versus 4% hydroquinone plus sunscreen, in 16 women with melasma in Mexico. Topical application was used once nightly throughout the study period of 16 weeks. The women were evaluated every 4 weeks using digital photography, colorimetry, and subjective assessment—mild (< 25%), moderate (25% to < 50%), good (50 to < 75%) and excellent (> 75%). The women rated clearance better in the hemiface that received hydroquinone, at 93% (good to excellent) versus 62.5% (good to excellent; $P < 0.05$). No significant differences were found between the treatments in the colorimetry evaluation.

Drawbacks
The first RCT[26] found adverse effects in six patients using hydroquinone and five using placebo. Erythema was more frequent with hydroquinone (five patients using hydroquinone, two using placebo). Contact dermatitis occurred in one person receiving hydroquinone. In the placebo group, two patients reported acne, one skin dryness, one solar erythema, and one cutaneous irritation. The RCT comparing azelaic acid with hydroquinone is described above.[24] The second RCT had two withdrawals, one of which was due to skin irritation, while the other was counted as a withdrawal as the patient cleared before completion of the study. Irritation was more frequently seen in the side that received hydroquinone (irritated hemiface: 11 patients with 4% hydroquinone versus one patient with 5% ascorbic acid).[27]

Comment
The trial was small and had exclusion criteria that should be considered when deciding on the applicability of the results. Hydroquinone (4%) plus sunscreen was found to be superior to placebo plus sunscreen in the RCT, while 2% hydroquinone was less effective in comparison with azelaic acid. The second study found that 4% hydroquinone was superior to 5% ascorbic acid by the patients' subjective assessments, but not on objective colorimetry assessment. However, a significant number of patients in both groups (hydroquinone 93%, ascorbic acid 62.5%) found that their melasma improved (with good to excellent results).

Efficacy
Unknown. The second RCT is small and does not explain the differences. Side effects were less frequent with ascorbic acid than with hydroquinone.

Key messages
We found limited evidence from one RCT showing that the use of hydroquinone plus sunscreen was superior to the use of sunscreen and placebo. We found limited evidence of efficacy of 5% ascorbic acid versus 5% hydroquinone.

Implications for clinical practice/categorization
Likely to be beneficial (when used with sunscreen).

Glycolic acid
Efficacy
We found no systematic reviews. We found two RCTs, one nonrandomized study, and one open left- right comparison pilot study.

The first RCT (including 10 nonpregnant and non-nursing Asian women with skin phototypes IV or V, suffering moderate to severe facial melasma) compared the use of peelings with glycolic acid on one side of the face versus no peelings on the other side.[28] All of the women received concomitant twice-daily applications of a cream containing 10% glycolic acid and 2% hydroquinone, as well as SPF 15 sunscreen. An independent evaluator assessed the results using a Munsell color chart and photographs. Participants also assessed the results. Treatments were randomly allocated to a side of the face, and no placebo was used to conceal the intervention. The physician evaluation found improvement on the side using peeling in all cases, and improvement in control sides in eight of 10 cases.

The second RCT was in 40 patients in Pakistan[29] (30 women and 10 men, aged 21–45, with phototypes IV–V, with melasma). They were randomly divided into two groups of 20 each. They all had six fortnightly facial peeling sessions with increasing concentrations of salicylic acid (first two sessions with 20% and subsequently with 30%). Group I was also treated with 4% hydroquinone cream for the subsequent 3 months, but group II had no additional treatment.

Both groups used broad-spectrum sunscreens. Evaluations were made before and after finishing treatment, including a MASI score, photographs, and lesion size. The use of chemical peelings with salicylic acid showed significant improvement in both groups ($P < 0.05$). After an additional 3 months of treatment with 4% hydroquinone cream, 80% of the patients in group I were reported to have continued significant improvement, in comparison with 50% of those in group II ($P \leq 0.05$).

The nonrandoimized study (16 women with skin phototypes II–VI, followed for 6 months), comparing glycolic acid peels against Jessner's solution, found no differences between the two groups.[30] All of the women received nightly 0.05% tretinoin (preparation not specified) for 1–2 weeks and daily applications of sunscreen. They also received three peeling sessions, 1 month apart. Peelings were done using titrated doses of 70% glycolic acid applied to the right side of the face and Jessner's solution applied to the left side. Follow-up was completed by 11 participants (68%), and no differences were found between the groups.

The open-labeled pilot study[31] compared the hemifaces of 10 women in India receiving weekly applications of 1% tretinoin peel on one side of the face and 70% glycolic acid on the other side of the face for 12 weeks. The results were evaluated using the modified MASI scale and with photographs at baseline, 6 weeks, and 12 weeks. Both sides of the face showed a significant decrease in the modified MASI from baseline at 6 weeks, and from 6 weeks to 12 weeks ($P < 0.001$). Nevertheless, no significant differences were observed between the treatments.

Drawbacks
All of the participants in the first RCT[28] experienced stinging and redness during and after each peeling session. One person developed an area of burn after the 20% glycolic acid peeling, resulting in a zone of hyperpigmentation, which disappeared after 2 months. In the second RCT,[29] minor side effects were seen in most of the patients, such as mild burning irritation and stinging. No information is available about three patients who did not finish the treatment.

Glycolic acid peelings were more frequently reported as being more painful than Jessner's solution. One participant developed postinflammatory hyperpigmentation on the side receiving glycolic acid.[30]

The open-label pilot study showed minimal adverse effects in both groups. Compared to 70% glycolic acid peels, 1% tretinoin peel was found to be less irritating and better tolerated[31] (four patients suffered side effects involving erythema, irritation, and vesiculation on the 70% glycolic acid side, in comparison with two patients with such side effects on the 1% tretinoin side).

Comment
The first RCT[28] may have been too small to rule out differences, and concealment may have been difficult to achieve because of the side effects of the peelings.[28] The second RCT[29] has significant methodological flaws. There is no description of inclusion or exclusion criteria, methods of randomization are not described and description of concealment is not provided. The use of chemical peelings with salicylic acid showed significant improvement in both groups ($P < 0.05$) in comparison with the baseline, which can be augmented by subsequent treatments with 4% hydroquinone. Further evaluation in long-term studies with better methodological quality are necessary to evaluate side effects and recurrences.

The open nonrandomized trial[30] has major limitations that compromise the validity of the results. The design of the study is not the most appropriate to answer a clinical question referring to treatment effectiveness. Before–after comparisons do not allow firm conclusions to be drawn, and comparisons with the results of previous reports from different populations may be misleading.[30]

The open-label pilot study suggests that 1% tretinoin peels are as effective as 70% glycolic acid peels, but further RCTs are required to clarify this.

Key messages

We found insufficient evidence to assess the effects of glycolic acid. The above studies suggest some evidence of effectiveness of glycolic acid, salicylic acid, and tretinoin peels in the short-term treatment of melasma, but studies with longer follow-up periods and better methodological qualities will be required. The above three studies found that patients reported more side effects with glycolic acid peels.

Implications for clinical practice/categorization

Unknown effectiveness.

Combined therapies

Efficacy

We found no systematic reviews. We found five RCTs. The first trial was an open RCT (50 Asians, 49 women, with non-dermal melasma and not taking oral contraceptives).[17] It compared the daily use of a cream containing 20% azelaic acid, 0.05% tretinoin, and sunscreen, with a cream containing 20% azelaic acid and sunscreen, for a period of 6 months with monthly evaluations. The number of withdrawals was high and it is therefore difficult to draw conclusions. In addition, some outcome categories overlapped.

A second RCT,[32] including 65 dark-skinned people with skin phototypes > III, with hyperpigmentation, 44 of whom (68%) had melasma—compared a cream containing 20% azelaic acid cream plus 15–20% glycolic acid (first month only) plus sunscreen with 4% hydroquinone plus sunscreen; the participants were followed for 24 weeks. There was no difference between the two groups with regard to overall improvement, and the reductions in lesion area, pigmentary intensity, and disease severity were comparable in the two treatment groups.

A third RCT[33] including 40 Chinese women with pure epidermal melasma, confirmed by Wood's lamp (age range not specified), compared a twice-daily application of a gel containing 2% kojic acid, 2% hydroquinone, and 10% glycolic acid followed by a sunblock with titanium dioxide SPF 15 with a twice-daily application of a control gel containing 2% hydroquinone and 10% glycolic acid, followed by sunblock with titanium dioxide SPF 15. Randomization was used to determine which side of the face would receive each intervention. Data from three women who withdrew were not included in the analysis. The frequency of > 50% clearance of the melasma area was greater when kojic acid was used, although the difference was not significant—24 of 40 (60%) for the combined gel containing kojic acid, versus 19 of 40 (48%) for the combined gel without kojic acid (RR 1.3; 95% CI, 0.8 to 1.9). When the participants assessed improvement, it was found to be better with the gel containing kojic acid.

The fourth RCT[34] included 38 nonchildbearing women with skin phototypes I–IV and melasma (type not specified).

The study randomized affected areas of skin instead of people, and randomization was carried out using a list. The study compared a cream containing 12% alpha hydroxy-acid (particular preparation not specified), 1% polypeptide ascorbate complex, and titanium oxide photoprotector with a preparation containing titanium oxide photoprotector and the vehicle for the cream prepared to the same pH. It found that the patients' global assessment, which was measured using a visual analogue scale for area and pigmentation, improved in more women receiving the active treatment than in those using the placebo preparation. However, the difference did not quite reach significance— 34 of 36 (94%) with the combination treatment versus 17 of 36 (47%) with the placebo (RR 1.51; 95% CI, 0.96 to 2.40). Differences were significant for the melanic index, measured using a mexameter (mean melanic index 15.2 with the active treatment versus 22.1 with placebo; $P < 0.01$ at day 56).

The fifth RCT[35] (39 patients with facial melasma, 5% of whom had dermal melasma under Wood's light; 38 women, followed for 3 months) compared 2% hydroquinone and 5% glycolic acid gel with 2% kojic acid and 5% glycolic acid gel. This study compared interventions applied to the left or right side of the face. Outcomes involved a comparison of facial photographs taken using an ultraviolet filter, clinical evaluation, participants' impressions, and the decrease in the affected area (no formal scales were used). There were no significant differences between the groups (28% reduction with kojic acid and 21% reduction with hydroquinone).

A sixth RCT[36] compared 4% hydroquinone cream plus 10% buffered glycolic acid, plus vitamins C and E plus sunscreen (compound cream, concentrations of vitamins C and E unspecified) versus sunscreen cream alone over a period of 12 weeks in 39 Hispanic women with epidermal melasma, skin types III–V, aged 18–50 years. Changes in pigmentation were measured with a mexameter (Courage & Khazaka Electronic, Cologne, Germany) and MASI, along with global evaluations by the patient and a masked evaluator. Four women were lost to follow-up. Improvement rates were higher with the compound cream—15 of 20 (75%) versus two of 15 (13%) with sunscreen. The MASI score showed a more beneficial effect in the active group in comparison with the group receiving sunscreen alone at week 12 ($P = 0.01$). The mexameter results showed a significant reduction in pigmentation levels with the compound cream ($P < 0.0001$). The physician's global evaluation showed moderate, obvious, or very marked improvement in 14 of 20 women (70%) using the compound cream, versus three of 15 (20%) with sunscreen. However, the patients' global evaluation showed moderate, obvious, or marked improvement in 19 of 20 women (95%) using the compound cream and 13 of 15 (87%) with sunscreen alone.

A seventh multicenter,[37] randomized study included 641 patients, who were randomly assigned to receive either tretinoin 0.05% (RA), hydroquinone 4.0% (HQ), and fluocinolone acetonide 0.01% (FA) (RA+HQ+FA) in a hydrophilic cream base; or (RA+HQ) or (RA+FA) in the same vehicle cream. A baseline photo, an eight-point scale for investigator assessment of global improvement, and a melasma severity rating score (0–4) were used. The patient population consisted predominantly of white women, with skin types 1–4. The patients included had had melasma for at least 3 months and had a melasma severity of at least 2 on the Melasma Severity Score. The end point of the study was the proportion of patients achieving complete clearance at 8 weeks. A secondary end point was the proportion of patients achieving complete or near-complete clearing (severity rating score = 0). At 8 weeks, the authors found that 26.1% of the patients were completely cleared with RA+HQ+FA, in comparison with 9.5% with RA+HQ, 1.9% with RA+FA, and 2.5% for HQ+FA ($P < 0.001$). Complete clearing or near-complete clearing was achieved in 77% of patients in the RA+HQ+FA group, in comparison with 42.2% for HQ+FA, 27.3% for RA+FA, and 46.8% for RA+HQ ($P < 0.001\%$).

Drawbacks

The reasons for withdrawals in the first RCT[17] are not clear. Numbers were similar in the two groups—six of 25 (24%) in the azelaic acid, tretinoin, and sunscreen group versus seven of 25 (28%) in the azelaic acid and sunscreen group (RR 0.9; 95% CI, 0.3 to 2.2).

In the second RCT,[32] the azelaic acid group experienced significantly more burning and peeling. There were two withdrawals in the azelaic acid group and four in the hydroquinone group. However, these were described as not being due to side effects of the preparations.

All participants in the third RCT, comparing a combination of hydroquinone and glycolic acid followed by sunblock with or without 2% kojic acid,[33] complained of redness, stinging, and mild exfoliation on both sides of the face (randomization was done for the side receiving each treatment). Three women withdrew from the study because of adverse effects on both sides of the face, and were replaced by three other women.

In the fourth RCT comparing alpha hydroxyacid, polypeptide ascorbate complex and titanium oxide photoprotector with a preparation containing titanium oxide photoprotector,[34] one woman withdrew after 28 days because of depigmentation. However, no detail is provided on whether this happened on the intervention or control cheek. A second participant was excluded when it became apparent that she did not have melasma. In the active treatment group, a higher frequency of erythema and a burning sensation was reported, and this persisted throughout the follow-up period. However, no further details are provided.

In the fifth RCT,[35] both treatments were described as being well tolerated, although all participants had some degree of

skin irritation. Kojic acid gel was found to be a stronger irritant. No further details are provided.

In the sixth RCT, 17 of 20 women (85%) suffered irritation and mild to moderate erythema at week 12 with the compound cream, and one of them had to stop treatment for 1 week due to excessive irritation. Ten of 15 patients in the sunscreen group (67%) suffered mild erythema at week 12.[36]

In the seventh RCT, a total of 387 of the 642 patients suffered side effects such as erythema, desquamation, burning, dryness, and pruritus, but these were considered to have been related to the study drugs in only 16 of the patients. In the results section, percentages are used instead of numbers of patients, and no description of drop-outs is given. Only one patient receiving HQ+FA suffered from skin atrophy. The authors suggest a protective effect of retinoids as a possible mechanism.

Comments

Methodological limitations compromise the validity of the results in the first RCT comparing azelaic acid, tretinoin, and sunscreen with azelaic acid and sunscreen.[17]

In the second RCT comparing azelaic acid cream, glycolic acid, and sunscreen with hydroquinone and sunscreen, it was not possible to determine if the response varied between people with melasma and people with other hyperpigmentation conditions.[32] It is therefore difficult to draw valid conclusions.

The third RCT—comparing a gel containing kojic acid, hydroquinone, and 10% glycolic acid followed by titanium dioxide sunblock, on the one hand, with a gel containing hydroquinone and glycolic acid followed by titanium dioxide sunblock on the other—had methodological limitations that may compromise its validity, and the sample size may have been insufficient to rule out an effect.[33]

The fourth RCT[34] did not provide details on the melasma type. Melasma type has been associated with treatment response. The study does not give details of the kind of alpha hydroxyacid used and lacks details of demographic data.

The fifth RCT does not allow one to look at variables, but gives percentage improvements and P values. It concludes that the addition of 2% kojic acid gel to glycolic acid is as efficacious as 2% hydroquinone.[35] The addition of 2% kojic acid to a gel containing 10% glycolic acid and 2% hydroquinone further improves melasma. No additional side effects were reported on the kojic acid side.[35]

The sixth RCT[36] found that the patient-assessed results conflicted with other objective measurements. The authors did not give any explanation for these conflicting findings. The added effect of vitamins C and E and glycolic acid is unclear in this study, as the compound cream contained hydroquinone, which is effective in the treatment of melasma.

The seventh RCT[37] has some methodological drawbacks. The publication combines the results of two separate studies, and the authors do not provide any details of these studies. The randomization methods are not clear. The results section only provides percentages, and there is no mention of drop-outs.

We also found one abstract,[38] which did not provide sufficient detail for a critical appraisal of the study methodology to be made.

Key messages

Overall, we found no good evidence of the effects of combined therapies in comparison with placebo or other preparations. These studies had methodological flaws that compromised the validity of the results, including small sample sizes.

Implications for clinical practice/categorization

Unknown effectiveness (all combined preparations).

Laser therapies
Efficacy

We found no systematic reviews. We found one RCT and one nonrandomized study.

The RCT[39] included eight dark-skinned people (skin phototypes IV–VI) with dermal melasma diagnosed using Wood's lamp. The article does not provide any details of the participants' demographic data. All of the participants received a 14-day course of 0.05% tretinoin cream, 4% hydroquinone cream, and 1% hydrocortisone cream, applied twice daily. They were asked to use a sunblock of SPF 15 or higher. The participants had a 1-cm^2 area of the face exposed to one pass of the 950-microsecond pulsed carbon dioxide laser, with a computerized pattern generation set at 300 mJ/cm^2. The intervention group received, in addition to the above, another pass with a Q-switched alexandrite pigmented dye laser at a dose of 6 J/cm^2. The treated area was evaluated after 6 months. Normal skin was found in three participants in the intervention group and one in the control group. However, the sample size is too small for valid conclusions to be drawn, and confounding factors such as the use of different sunblock preparations were not accounted for.

The nonrandomized study[40] was conducted in Taiwanese women with melasma, comparing intense pulsed-light treatment and 4% hydroquinone and sunscreens versus 4% hydroquinone and sunscreens. A total of 33 Taiwanese women with melasma that had been unresponsive to hydroquinone cream for at least 3 months were enrolled. Patients who were pregnant, lactating, taking the contraceptive pill, receiving hormone replacement therapy, or who had major outdoor activities were excluded. This study compared 17 patients in the light group versus 16 in the control group over a period of 36 weeks. Intense pulsed light from a noncoherent source, with a broad spectrum from 500 to 1200 nm, was used. A total of four treatments at 4-weekly intervals were used, and both groups used 4% hydroquinone and broad-spectrum sunscreens throughout the study period. The light group was followed up for 36 weeks, while the control group was evaluated up to 16 weeks. Evaluations were conducted at 4-week intervals using digital photography, reflectance spectrometry, and objective assessment of the improvement rate. The patients also recorded subjective satisfaction rates. After four treatments with intense light, the patients showed a 39.8% improvement in the melanin index (absolute melanin index of melasma/absolute melanin index of normal skin) from the baseline values. This improvement declined to 24.2% at week 36. The patients in the control group showed an 11.6% improvement at 16 weeks, but were not evaluated at 36 weeks. In the intense light group, 23.5% of the patients stated that they were satisfied with their treatment, 53% said they were slightly satisfied, and 23.5% said they were unsatisfied, in comparison with the control group, in which 64% were slightly satisfied and 36% were unsatisfied.

Drawbacks

In the first RCT,[39] two participants in the control group suffered peripheral hyperpigmentation. As mentioned above, the small sample size does not allow firm conclusions to be drawn. In the second nonrandomized study,[40] there were three drop-outs—two in the control group due to poor compliance and one in the intense light group due to relocation. Side effects in the intense light group consisted of erythema, pain, and microcrust formation. Two patients in this group also suffered transient postinflammatory hyperpigmentation.

Comment

The RCT[39] is of particular interest, as it evaluates one of the few interventions currently used for dermal melasma. Properly designed RCTs are needed to determine the effect of laser therapies in dermal melasma. In the nonrandomized study,[40] although the difference between the two groups was statistically significant after 16 weeks ($P < 0.05$), this was not the case after 36 weeks, indicating a requirement for further treatment courses.

Key messages

We found insufficient evidence to evaluate the effect of laser therapies in the treatment of melasma. The second study shows promising short-term results with the use of an intense light source in comparison with the control group. The authors noted repigmentation just 8 weeks after the last course of intense light treatment, despite continuous use of hydroquinone and broad-spectrum sunscreen.

Implications for clinical practice/categorization
Unknown effectiveness.

Key message
We found evidence of short-term improvement in melasma after intense light treatment combined with 4% hydroquinone and broad-spectrum sunscreens.

Oral and topical vitamins
Efficacy
We found no systematic reviews. We found three RCTs.[41–43] The first RCT from Japan included 176 women and two men over a period of 3 months. Melasma was present in 136 of the patients (76%) and pigmented contact dermatitis in 42 (24%). Specific results for melasma were available from the study report. The RCT compared oral vitamin E (50 patients), vitamin C (45 patients) and a combination of vitamins E and C (41 patients). After 12 weeks, the physician-rated color difference and photographic findings were used to assess changes. Using color photographs, an improvement was noticed in 69% of those receiving a combination therapy of vitamins E and C, 60% of those receiving vitamin E, and 50% of those receiving vitamin C. These differences did not reach statistical significance. In the objective clinical improvement evaluation, 72% of the participants in the combined-therapy group showed improvement, in comparison with 63% in the vitamin E group and 44% in the vitamin C group. The difference between the combined-therapy and vitamin C groups reached statistical significance ($P < 0.05$).

The second study[42] was a placebo-controlled, double-blind, within-group comparison conducted in Seoul, South Korea, in 29 women (aged 24–49) with melasma. It compared iontophoresis with a topical compound containing ascorbic acid, magnesium-L-ascorbyl-2-phosphate, against distilled-water iontophoresis. This was a within-group, left–right comparison (with the left and right agents being selected randomly), and the patients were treated twice weekly for 12 weeks, with concomitant use of a sunscreen twice a day on both sides of the face. Interestingly, subjective assessment did not show any differences between the two sides, but measurement of the L value (measured by a colorimeter) showed a significant difference in favor of ascorbic acid (from ΔL 4.60 to 2.78, $P = 0.002$, in comparison with control side from 4.45 to 3.87, $P = 0.142$). The authors considered that the continual use of a sunscreen during the trial might have resulted in some improvement on the placebo side.

A third RCT in Brazil[43] was a double-blind, randomized, prospective study comparing 4% hydroquinone and a skin-whitening complex developed in France. The cream contained: 1, extract of uva ursi, which provokes chemical discoloration of melanin and competes with the tyrosinase enzyme; 2, biofermented *Aspergillus*, which chelates copper ions, which are essential for tyrosinase enzyme activity; 3, grapefruit extract, rich in citric and malic acids, with an exfoliative action; 4, rice extract, rich in oligosaccharides, with a hydrating function. The study was conducted in 30 women aged 38–56, with Fitzpatrick skin types III–V, and with no previous treatments over a period of at least 6 months. The patients were randomly assigned to receive either 4% hydroquinone or skin-whitening complex on one side and a placebo cream on the other side. The treatment was carried out for 3 months, with the addition of a sunblock during the treatment period.

Photographs were taken before and after treatment and clinical evaluation was performed by two independent observers and by the patients themselves. The two groups were evaluated separately. Group 1 (hydroquinone vs. placebo) had an improvement of 76.9% and group 2 (skin-whitening complex vs. placebo) showed an improvement of 66.7%; however, the difference was not statistically significant on Fisher's test ($P = 0.673$).

Additional studies would be necessary to evaluate the long-term effect of the skin-whitening complex.

Drawbacks
There were 10 withdrawals in the Japanese RCT.[41] One participant withdrew because of side effects, while 51 failed to complete the 12-week follow-up. Five people in the group receiving vitamins E and C suffered side effects—two had acne, one had xerosis, one had a mild stomach upset, and one developed metrorrhagia. Eight people in the vitamin E group complained of side effects—four had acne, one had a stomach upset, one had excessive perspiration, and developed two menstrual abnormalities. Side effects were also reported by participants receiving vitamin C: four suffered acne, two hot flushes, one had a stomach upset, and one developed seborrheic dermatitis. The second RCT[42] reported a mild sense of electric shock in 21% patients, itching and erythema in 7%, and burning sensation and dryness in 3%. In the third study,[43] there were no side effects in the skin-whitening complex group, in comparison with the 4% hydroquinone group, in which 25% patients suffered minor side effects.

Comments
The Japanese study did not have a placebo group, and all of the groups improved. Improvement was better in patients receiving preparations containing vitamin E. A placebo-controlled study is needed to determine the effect of these compounds. Thirty-one people suffered side effects, although it is not clear whether this refers to people with chloasma or whether it included people with other pigmentary disorders. In the second RCT, there was improvement in both groups, which may have been due to the use of

sunscreens. The third study did not show any significant improvement in melasma with the use of the skin whitening complex in comparison with hydroquinone 4%.

Key messages
We found limited evidence that a combination of vitamins C and E is better than vitamin C alone. We found no evidence of the effects of these therapies against placebo. We found no evidence in favor of vitamin C iontophoresis versus placebo. We found no evidence in favor of skin whitening complex versus hydroquinone 4%.

Implications for clinical practice/categorization
Unknown effectiveness.

How effective are therapeutic interventions in men?

Case scenario 4
A 40-year-old Latin-American man living in California has had melasma for 3 months. It appeared after a beach holiday. He is not on any regular medication, but has a family history of melasma.

Efficacy
We identified no studies assessing the effects of therapeutic interventions exclusively in men. Although several RCTs included a few men, none of them carried out a subgroup analysis, and none would have had sufficient power to identify any clinically relevant differences.

Comment
On the basis of expert opinion, the same treatments used in nonpregnant women may be considered appropriate in men with melasma.

Key messages
We found no evidence specifically evaluating the effects of treatment in men.

Implications for clinical practice/categorization
Unknown effectiveness.

Implications of the available evidence

For consumers (the public)
Current opinion, based on known risk factors, suggests that measures preventing exposure to sunlight may reduce the risk of the development and recurrence of melasma. From the available trial evidence, therapies likely to be beneficial are azelaic acid and hydroquinone.

For clinical practice (health-care providers)
From the available evidence, a treatment likely to benefit patients with melasma is 2–4% hydroquinone with sunscreens. The use of hydroquinone for melasma has been limited recently, following several case reports of it causing exogenous ochronosis. However, there were no reports of this side effect in any studies with follow-up periods of up to 24 months.

We did not find convincing evidence for the effectiveness of azelaic acid, topical retinoids, topical corticosteroids, glycolic acid, oral vitamins E or C, lasers, or any combined therapies.

For research (research agencies and researchers)
We found inconclusive evidence of the effectiveness of topical azelaic acid, steroids, topical retinoids, glycolic acid, vitamin C, and laser therapy. These are commonly-used therapies for melasma in clinical practice and would require further RCTs to validate their use. Lasers offer a potential advantage over conventional therapies, as the time to clearance can be much reduced. We found only a few studies that looked at patient-based outcomes.

Key points
- No incontrovertible or solid evidence supports preventive interventions in high-risk populations. Current opinion, on the basis of the known risk factors, suggests that preventing exposure to sources of ultraviolet light, such as sunlight, may reduce the risk of developing melasma.
- No incontrovertible evidence supports any therapeutic intervention in pregnant or breastfeeding women. Current opinion suggests that such women with melasma may benefit from using broad-spectrum sunscreens and avoiding exposure to ultraviolet light, such as sunlight.
- Limited evidence from a single RCT evaluating the effect of therapeutic sunscreens shows that during the 3-month study period, the majority of women using hydroquinone had improvement, regardless of the addition of sunscreen to their treatment. The study did not describe whether women used other strategies to avoid sunlight.
- Evidence is insufficient to support the use of topical steroids in melasma. There is controversy over the use of topical steroids in this condition. There is limited evidence from one RCT of a quicker response when topical steroids are used sequentially with azelaic acid.
- An effect of retinoids on melasma has not been shown, but the available studies found that side effects were common.
- In a small trial, azelaic acid was found to be superior to 2% hydroquinone in achieving improvement in people with melasma. We found no solid evidence comparing azelaic acid

with placebo. Azelaic acid was associated with a higher incidence of side effects.

- Limited evidence from one RCT suggests that hydroquinone plus sunscreen was better than sunscreen and placebo.
- The evidence is insufficient to assess the effects of glycolic acid.
- Overall, we found no good evidence of the effects of combined therapies in comparison with a placebo or other preparations. The studies had methodological flaws, including small sample sizes, that compromised the validity of results. There is limited evidence from one RCT suggesting superior results with a combination of retinoids, hydroquinone, and topical steroids.
- We found insufficient evidence to evaluate the effect of laser therapies in the treatment of melasma. One nonrandomized study showed faster improvement with intense pulsed-light therapy.
- We found insufficient evidence that a combination of oral vitamins C and E is better than oral vitamin C alone. We found no evidence of the effects of these therapies in comparison with placebo.
- We found insufficient evidence for the efficacy of a skin-whitening cream containing: extract of uva ursi, biofermented *Aspergillus*, grapefruit extract, and rice extract in comparison with hydroquinone 4%.
- No studies have assessed the effect of treatments specifically in men.

References

1 Newcomer VD. A melanosis of the face ("chloasma"). *Arch Dermatol* 1961;**83**:284–99.

2 Estrada-Castanon R, Torres-Bibiano B, Alarcon-Hernandez H, *et al.* Epidemiología cutánea en dos sectores de atención mèdica en Guerrero, Mexico. *Dermatol Rev Mex* 1992;**36**:29–34.

3 Failmezger C. Incidence of skin disease in Cuzco, Peru. *Int J Dermatol* 1992;**31**:560–1.

4 Halder RN, Grimes PE, McLaurin CI, Kress MA, Kennery JA Jr. Incidence of common dermatoses in a predominantly black dermatologic practice. *Cutis* 1983;**32**:388–90.

5 Pathak MA, Fitzpatrick TB, Kraus EW. Usefulness of retinoic acid in the treatment of melasma. *J Am Acad Dermatol* 1986;**15**:894–9.

6 Bleehem SS. Disorders of skin colour. In: Champion RH, Burton JL, Burns DA, Breathnach SM, eds. *Textbook of Dermatology*, 6th ed. Oxford: Blackwell Science, 1998: 1753–815.

7 Resnick S. Melasma induced by oral contraceptive drugs. *JAMA* 1967;**199**:601–5.

8 Escoda ECJ. Chloasma from progestational oral contraceptives. *Arch Dermatol* 1967;**87**:486.

9 Sanchez NP, Pathak MA, Sato S, Fitzpatrick TB, Sanchez JL, Minhm MC Jr. Melasma: a clinical, light microscopic, ultrastructural and immunofluorescence study. *J Am Acad Dermatol* 1981; **4**:698–710.

10 Vazquez M, Maldonado H, Benaman C, Sanchez JL. Melasma in men: a clinical and histologic study. *Int J Dermatol* 1988;**27**:25–7.

11 Perez M, Samchez JL, Aguilo F. Endocrinologic profile of patients with idiopathic melasma. *J Invest Dermatol* 1983;**81**:543–5.

12 Lufti RJ, Fridmanis M, Misrunas AL. Association of melasma with thyroid autoimmunity and other thyroidal abnormalities and their relationship to the origin of melasma. *J Clin Endocrinol Metab* 1985;**61**:28–31.

13 Smith AG, Shuster S, Thody AJ, Peberdy M. Chloasma, oral contraceptives, and plasma immunoreactive beta-melanocyte-stimulating hormone. *J Invest Dermatol* 1977;**68**:169–70.

14 Gilchrest BA, Fitzpatrick TB, Anderson RR, Parish JA. Localization of melanin pigmentation in the skin with Wood's lamp. *Br J Dermatol* 1977;**96**:245–8.

15 Balkrishnan R, McMichael AJ, Camacho FT, *et al.* Development and validation of a health-related quality of life instrument for women with melasma. *Br J Dermatol* 2003;**149**:572–7.

16 Leenutaphong V, Nettakul A, Rattanasuwon P. Topical isotretinoin for melasma in Thai patients: a vehicle-controlled clinical trial. *J Med Assoc Thai* 1999;**82**:868–75.

17 Graupe K, Verallo RVM, Verallo V, Zaumseil RP. Combined use of 20% azelaic acid cream and 0.05% tretinoin cream in the topical treatment of melasma. *J Dermatol Treat* 1996;**7**:235–7.

18 Vazquez M, Sanchez JL. The efficacy of a broad-spectrum sunscreen in the treatment of melasma. *Cutis* 1983;**32**:92–6.

19 Neering H. Treatment of melasma (chloasma) by local application of a steroid cream. *Dermatologica* 1975;**151**:349–53.

20 Griffiths CE, Finkel LJ, Ditre CM, Hamilton TA, Ellis CN, Voorhees JJ. Topical tretinoin (retinoic acid) improves melasma. A vehicle-controlled, clinical trial. *Br J Dermatol* 1993;**129**:415–21.

21 Krimbrough-Green CK, Griffiths CEM, Finkel LJ, *et al.* Topical retinoic acid (tretinoin) for melasma in black patients. *Arch Dermatol* 1994;**130**:727–33.

22 Lowe NJ, Rizk D, Grimes P, Billips M, Pincus S. Azelaic acid 20% cream in the treatment of facial hyperpigmentation in darker-skinned patients. *Clin Ther* 1998;**20**:945–59.

23 Sarkar R, Bhalla M, Kanwar AJ. A comparative study of 20% azelaic acid cream monotherapy versus a sequential therapy in the treatment of melasma in dark-skinned patients. *Dermatology* 2002;**205**:249–54.

24 Sivayathorn A, Verallo RV, Graupe K. 20% azelaic acid cream in the topical treatment of melasma: a double-blind comparison with 2% hydroquinone. *Eur J Dermatol* 1995;**5**:680–4.

25 Piquero Martin J, Rothe de Arocha J, Beniamini Loker D. [Double-blind clinical study of the treatment of melasma with azelaic acid versus hydroquinone; in Spanish.] *Med Cutan Ibero Lat Am* 1988; **16**:511–4.

26 Ennes SBP, Paschoalick RC, Mota M. A double blind, comparative, placebo-controlled study of the efficacy and tolerability of 4% hydroquinone as a depigmenting agent in melasma. *J Dermatol Treat* 2000;**11**:173–9.

27 Espinal-Perez LE, Moncada B, Castanedo-Cazares JP. A double-blind randomized trial 5% ascorbic acid vs. 4% hydroquinone in melasma. *Int J Dermatol* 2004;**43**:604–7.

28 Lim JT, Tham SN. Glycolic acid peels in the treatment of melasma among Asian women. *Dermatol Surg* 1997;**23**:177–9.

29 Bari AU. Efficacy of facial chemical peeling with salicylic acid and role of 4% hydroquinone as an adjuvant treatment modality in melasma. *J Pak Assoc Dermatol* 2002;**12**:183–9.

30 Lawrence N, Cox SE, Brody HJ. Treatment of melasma with Jessner's solution versus glycolic acid: a comparison of clinical efficacy and evaluation of the predictive ability of Wood's light examination. *J Am Acad Dermatol* 1997;**36**:589–93.

31 Khunger N, Sarkar R, Jain RK, Koppel RA. Tretinoin peels versus glycolic acid peels in the treatment of melasma in dark-skinned patients. *Dermatol Surg* 2004;**30**:756–60.

32 Kakita LS, Lowe NJ. Azelaic acid and glycolic acid combination therapy for facial hyperpigmentation in darker-skinned patients: a clinical comparison with hydroquinone. *Clin Ther* 1998;**20**:960–70.

33 Lim JT. Treatment of melasma using kojic acid in a gel containing hydroquinone and glycolic acid. *Dermatol Surg* 1999;**25**:282–4.

34 Poli F, Lakhdar H, Souissi R, Fiquet E, Chanez JF. Clinical evaluation of a depigmenting cream: Trio-D (R) in melasma of the face. *Nouv Dermatol* 1997;**16**:193–7.

35 Garcia A, Fulton JE Jr. The combination of glycolic acid and hydroquinone or kojic acid for the treatment of melasma and related conditions. *Dermatol Surg* 1996;**22**:443–7.

36 Guevara IL, Pandya AG. Safety and efficacy of 4% hydroquinone combined with 10% glycolic acid, antioxidants, and sunscreen in the treatment of melasma. *Int J Dermatol* 2003;**42**:966–72.

37 Taylor SC, Torok H, Jones T, *et al.* Efficacy and safety of a new triple-combination agent for the treatment of facial melasma. *Cutis* 2003;**72**:67–72.

38 Pathak MA. Treatment of melasma with hydroquinone. *J Invest Dermatol* 1981;**76**:324.

39 Nouri K, Bowes L, Chartier T, Romagosa R, Spencer J. Combination treatment of melasma with pulsed CO_2 laser followed by Q-switched alexandrite laser: a pilot study. *Dermatol Surg* 1999;**25**:494–7.

40 Wang CC, Hui CY, Sue YM, Wong WR. Intense pulsed light for the treatment of refractory melasma in Asian persons. *Dermatol Surg* 2004;**30**:1196–200.

41 Hayakawa R, Ueda H, Nozaki T, *et al.* Effects of combination treatment with vitamins E and C on chloasma and pigmented contact dermatitis: a double blind controlled clinical trial. *Acta Vitaminol Enzymol* 1981;**3**:31–8.

42 Huh CH, Seo KI, Park JY, Lim JG, Eun HC, Park KC. A randomized, double-blind, placebo-controlled trial of vitamin C iontophoresis in melasma. *Dermatology* 2003;**206**:316–20.

43 Haddad AL, Matos LF, Brunstein F, Ferreira LM, Silva A, Costa D. A clinical, prospective, randomized, double-blind trial comparing skin whitening complex with hydroquinone vs. placebo in the treatment of melasma. *Int J Dermatol* 2003;**42**:153–6.

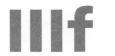

Hair problems

Berthold Rzany, Editor

51 Male and female androgenetic alopecia

Hans Wolff

Background

Definition

The term "androgenetic alopecia" (AGA) describes a genetically determined condition leading to permanent loss of hair in men and women with normal levels of androgens. Synonymous terms are male-pattern and female-pattern hair loss. Most men with AGA show a typical pattern of hair loss, often beginning at the temples and in the vertex area.[1,2] In contrast, most women with AGA have a diffuse thinning in the midline of the scalp.[3] In many, but not all, men and women, the hair loss is accompanied by increased shedding of telogen hair, which is a reflection of shortened anagen growth phases.[4,5]

Prevalence

AGA affects approximately 30% of men under 30 years of age, 50% under 50 years of age, and 70% under 70 years of age.[2,6] In women, the incidence before menopause is 5–10%, rising to 20–30% after the menopause.[7]

Etiology

Microscopically, AGA is characterized by progressive shrinking of scalp hair follicles.[8] In many patients, AGA is accompanied by an acceleration of the hair growth cycle, as reflected by decrease of anagen and increase of telogen hair in the trichogram.[8] However, some patients have a normal anagen/telogen ratio despite slowly progressive AGA. Whether and when a scalp hair follicle miniaturizes is dependent on two factors: genetics and androgens.[9] Several genes responsible for shrinkage of a scalp hair follicle are suspected,[10–12] but are not yet all known. Each scalp hair follicle carries individual genetic information that determines whether and when it will develop a sensitivity towards androgens. Once a scalp hair follicle has become sensitive to androgens, it will progressively shrink during the following years. In men, the most important androgen-driving AGA is dihydrotestosterone (DHT). Within the cells of the hair follicle, DHT is derived from its precursor testosterone by two enzymes: the 5-α-reductase types I and II.[13] DHT appears to be less important in women than in men.[14] In general, androgens can be considered potentially harmful and estrogens potentially beneficial for scalp hair growth in women.

Prognosis

Without treatment, AGA progresses until all hair follicles that have developed a genetically determined sensitivity towards androgens are miniaturized. The extent of AGA depends on the number of hair follicles with genetic sensitivity to androgens. In its maximal expression, all hairs can be lost from the top of the scalp. In both men and women, occipital hair follicles never develop sensitivity to androgens; they are never lost in AGA.

Aims of treatment

Treatment of AGA has two major goals. Firstly, it is important to reliably stop further hair loss. The term "hair loss" does not describe telogen effluvium, but refers to permanent visible thinning of scalp hair density due to miniaturization of hair follicles. Secondly, some men and women benefit so strongly from treatment that they can regrow hair to a certain extent—their hair density can be increased by reenlargement of individual hair follicles.

Relevant outcomes

- Stopping further hair loss: in a clinical study setting, this has to be documented after intervals of at least 1 year by microscopic methods such as hair counts or increase of hair weight in a representative area of hair loss.
- Increase of visible hair density: this has to be documented by standardized scalp hair photography.[15]

A change in the anagen/telogen ratio does not reliably assess the efficacy of treatment against further progression of AGA, because not all men and women with AGA have abnormal anagen/telogen ratios. In addition, some patients with long-standing telogen effluvium never develop AGA.[16] The trichogram therefore cannot reliably measure the efficacy of treatment against AGA.

Methods of literature search

In the PubMed database, different search terms were used for male and female androgenetic alopecia. For male androgenetic alopecia, the search terms were: "((androgenetic and alopecia) or (*male and pattern and baldness)) and (finasteride or minoxidil)." For female androgenetic alopecia, the search terms were "((female and androgenetic and alopecia) or (female and pattern and baldness)) and (minoxidil or antiandrogen* or cyproterone acetate or (cyproterone and acetate) or cyproterone acetate or estrogen* or estrogen* or estradiol)."

Questions

Which topical or systemic treatment can stop further hair loss and increase hair density in men?

Case scenario 1
The patient is a 28-year-old computer specialist with a 3-year history of gradual hair loss starting at the temples and now also involving the top of the scalp (Figure 51.1).

Topical minoxidil for men with AGA
Efficacy
We found no systematic reviews. Several randomized controlled trials (RCTs) show that minoxidil 2% or 5% solution

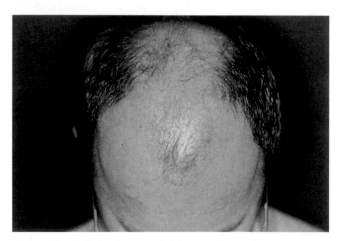

Figure 51.1 Typical male-pattern hair loss in a 28-year-old patient.

applied twice daily can increase test-area hair counts and hair weights in men with AGA.[17–22]

Drawbacks
In approximately 5% of men, minoxidil causes redness and itching of the scalp skin. In most men, this effect appears to be nonspecific irritation by polyethylene glycol or other solvents; in some, however, a specific type IV allergy against minoxidil is possible.[23] Patients sometimes attribute specific systemic effects such as hypotension or an increase in heart rate to minoxidil, but this is implausible, because serum concentrations of minoxidil are very low after twice-daily topical administration. A large 1-year prospective study including more than 10 000 male minoxidil users showed that there are no serious systemic side effects.[24]

Comment
Minoxidil 5% solution applied twice daily is a safe and effective topical treatment for AGA in men. There are no conclusive data on how often minoxidil solution can reliably stop hair loss and increase visible regrowth of hair in men. One of the possible mechanisms is improvement of the microcirculation in the dermal papilla.[25,26]

Implications for clinical practice
Minoxidil 5% solution can stop hair loss in many men, but hair loss resumes when the applications are stopped. There are no systemic side effects.

Systemic finasteride for men with AGA
Efficacy
We found no systematic reviews. Two-year results from the largest RCT were reported by Kaufman *et al.*[27] This international multicenter clinical trial of more than 1500 patients demonstrated a significant increase in hair counts in the finasteride treatment group after 1 year. In the second year, there was stabilization of the increased hair count in the finasteride group. Men on placebo had a progressive loss of hair count in the vertex test area. Men who were switched from finasteride to placebo after 1 year lost the hair gained under finasteride. Therefore, as with other medical treatments for AGA, finasteride needs to be taken permanently to show therapeutic benefit. Visible hair density was also documented by a standardized camera device.[15] After 1 and 2 years, the before and after pictures were judged by an expert panel of dermatologists, who were blinded to the treatment modality. After 1 year, 48% of men in the finasteride treatment group had visibly increased hair density in the vertex area, compared with 7% in the placebo group. After 2 years of treatment, 66% of the men in the finasteride group had visibly increased hair density, compared with only 7% in the placebo group.[27] On the basis of the 5-year data,[28] hair loss can be stopped in 90% of men taking finasteride, compared with 25% in the placebo group. In

addition to stoppage of hair loss, an increase in hair density was seen in 48% of the men in the finasteride group, compared with 6% of men in the placebo group after 5 years of the study.

Other RCTs have demonstrated that finasteride significantly improves the anagen/telogen ratio,[29] increases individual hair weight,[21] also has positive effects on the frontal hair line,[30] is as effective as minoxidil,[22] and also works well in men between 40 and 60 years of age.[31]

Drawbacks

There were no side effects on the liver, kidney, or any other internal organ.[27] Serum hormones were unaffected, with the exception of a desired 70% decline in DHT and a compensatory 10% increase in testosterone. The following sexual side effects were reported the finasteride and placebo groups, respectively: a decrease in libido of 1.9% versus 1.3%; a decrease in potency of 1.4% versus 0.9%; and a decrease in ejaculate volume of 1.0% versus 0.4%. Although the differences between the finasteride and placebo groups were small and statistically not significant,[27] and were not seen in other studies,[32] finasteride must be considered capable of causing such effects in some men. A separate study found sperm function parameters to be unaltered by finasteride 1 mg.[33]

Comment

Finasteride 1 mg is a safe and effective drug for the treatment of AGA in men. Finasteride inhibits the enzyme 5-α-reductase type II, thereby preventing the intracellular conversion of testosterone into its more active metabolite DHT.[34] In men, DHT is essential for the development of AGA, and finasteride decreases DHT by 70%, both in the scalp skin and in serum.[35]

Implications for practice

In 90% of men treated, finasteride 1 mg can stop hair loss (for at least 5 years) while it is being taken. Systemic side effects such as reduction of libido and erectile function are infrequent (1–2%) and often transient.

Which topical or systemic treatment can stop further hair loss and increase hair density in women?

Case scenario 2

The patient is a 35-year-old teacher with a 5-year history of gradual hair loss starting at the midline of her scalp (Figure 51.2). Her mother also had thin hair; her father was bald.

Topical minoxidil for women with AGA

Efficacy

We found no systematic reviews. Several RCTs demonstrate that minoxidil 2% solution applied twice daily can

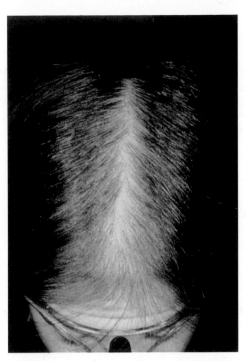

Figure 51.2 Typical female-pattern hair loss in a 35-year-old patient.

increase test-area hair counts and hair weights in women with AGA.[36–38] Most trials were conducted for at least 1 year. When effective, minoxidil solution increased visible hair density within 6 months. After 6 months, no further increase was to be expected. A large American multicenter study included 308 women with AGA; 256 women completed the trial. In the minoxidil group, the increase of nonvellus hairs was significantly larger than in the placebo group. On the investigators' assessment, more minoxidil-treated women had visible regrowth of hair than in the placebo group.[37]

Drawbacks

Patients sometimes attribute specific systemic effects such as hypotension or an increase in heart rate to minoxidil, but the very low serum concentrations of minoxidil after twice-daily topical administration make this implausible. In addition, a large prospective study showed that there are no serious systemic hypotensive side effects in female minoxidil users.[24] Minoxidil causes redness and itching of the scalp skin in approximately 5% of women. In most women, this effect appears to be nonspecific irritation by polyethylene glycol or other solvents; in some, however, a specific type IV allergy against minoxidil is possible.[23] In women with oriental, dark complexion hypertrichosis in the face and other parts of the body can occur as a side effect of minoxidil.[39] Hypertrichosis usually subsides after the drug has been stopped. A study by Lucky *et al.* showed similar efficacy rates of 5% and 2% minoxidil solution for female androgenetic alopecia.[38] However, there was an increased occurrence of pruritus, local irritation, and hypertrichosis in the 5% topical minoxidil group. The manufacturer therefore prefers the use of 2% minoxidil solution in women.

Comment
Minoxidil 2% solution applied twice daily is a safe and effective topical treatment for AGA in some women while it is used. Minoxidil solution can reliably stop hair loss and increase obviously visible regrowth of hair in 10–20% of women.

Implications for clinical practice
Currently, minoxidil 2% solution is the only effective way of treating AGA in women. There are no systemic side effects.

Systemic estrogens and/or antiandrogens for women with AGA
Efficacy
Because estrogens have many antiandrogenic actions, it is thought that they may have a positive influence on hair growth. Antiandrogens such as cyproterone acetate and chlormadinone acetate directly block the androgen receptor. However, most women with AGA have normal estrogen and androgen levels.[40] Positive effects of estrogens and/or antiandrogens on hair growth are therefore questionable. There are no systematic reviews. Recently, one RCT compared the efficacies of the antiandrogen cyproterone acetate, 52 mg daily on days 1–20 of the cycle, with a twice-daily 2% minoxidil application in 66 women with AGA grades Ludwig I (67%), II (31%) and III (2%). The study duration was 1 year, and each treatment group consisted of 33 women. The main outcome was number of strong hairs (> 40 µm in diameter) in a test area as detected by the phototrichogram. After 1 year, hair counts in the 0.32 cm^2 test area were −2.4 ± 6.2 in the cyproterone acetate group and +6.5 ± 9.0 hairs in the minoxidil group.[41] Thus, 2% minoxidil was significantly more effective than cyproterone acetate.

Drawbacks
Systemic 17-β-estrogens are thought to slightly increase the risk of breast cancer and—particularly in women with coagulation disorders—deep venous thrombosis.

Comment
In theory, women using estrogens and/or antiandrogens may benefit from treatment. However, as yet there is little convincing evidence that estrogens and/or antiandrogens can stop or delay AGA.[42]

Implications for practice
There are no convincing data showing that systemic estrogens or antiandrogens are effective in women with AGA.

We are therefore reluctant to treat women with AGA with systemic hormones that increase the risk of deep venous thrombosis and fatal embolism.

Key points

Men with AGA
- Topical minoxidil 2% or 5% solution applied twice daily to the scalp is effective for many men with AGA, but hair loss resumes when the applications cease. The RCTs reported are too small to establish percentages for successful stoppage of hair loss and frequency of visible regrowth of hair.
- Large RCTs show that systemic therapy with finasteride 1 mg per day can stop further hair loss in 90% and increase visible hair density in 48% of treated men. However, hair loss resumes when treatment is stopped.

Women with AGA
- Topical minoxidil 2% solution applied twice daily to the scalp is moderately effective for some women with AGA.
- One RCT using modern methods of hair growth evaluation showed that the systemic antiandrogen cyproterone acetate is less effective than 2% minoxidil solution.

References

1 Norwood OT. Male pattern baldness: classification and incidence. *South Med J* 1975;**68**:1359–65.
2 Hamilton JB. Patterned loss of hair in man: types and incidence. *Ann NY Acad Sci* 1951;**53**:708–28.
3 Ludwig E. Classification of the types of androgenetic alopecia (common baldness) occurring in the female sex. *Br J Dermatol* 1977;**97**:247–54.
4 Sinclair R. Male pattern androgenetic alopecia. *BMJ* 1998;**317**:865–9.
5 Olsen EA. Female pattern hair loss. *J Am Acad Dermatol* 2001;**45**:S70–80.
6 Severi G, Sinclair R, Hopper JL, *et al.* Androgenetic alopecia in men aged 40–69 years: prevalence and risk factors. *Br J Dermatol* 2003;**149**:1207–13.
7 Birch MP, Messenger JF, Messenger AG. Hair density, hair diameter and the prevalence of female pattern hair loss. *Br J Dermatol* 2001;**144**:297–304.
8 Paus R, Cotsarelis G. The biology of hair follicles. *N Engl J Med* 1999;**341**:491–7.
9 Hamilton JB. Male hormone stimulation is a prerequisite and an incitant in common baldness. *Am J Anat* 1942;**71**:451–80.
10 Küster W, Happle R. The inheritance of common baldness: two B or not two B? *J Am Acad Dermatol* 1984;**11**:921–6.
11 Hillmer AM, Kruse R, Macciardi F, *et al.* The hairless gene in androgenetic alopecia: results of a systematic mutation screening and a family-based association approach. *Br J Dermatol* 2002;**146**:601–8.
12 Garton RA, McMichael AJ, Sugarman J, Greer K, Setaluri V. Association of a polymorphism in the ornithine decarboxylase gene with male androgenetic alopecia. *J Am Acad Dermatol* 2005;**52**:535–6.

13 Bayne EK, Flanagan J, Einstein M, *et al.* Immunohistochemical localisation of types 1 and 2 5-alpha reductase in human scalp. *Br J Dermatol* 1999;**141**:481–91.

14 Sawaya ME, Price VH. Different levels of 5alpha-reductase type I and II, aromatase, and androgen receptor in hair follicles of women and men with androgenetic alopecia. *J Invest Dermatol* 1997;**109**:296–300.

15 Canfield D. Photographic documentation of hair growth in androgenetic alopecia. *Dermatol Clin* 1996;14:713–21.

16 Whiting DA. Chronic telogen effluvium: increased scalp hair shedding in middle-aged women. *J Am Acad Dermatol* 1996;**35**: 899–906.

17 Katz HI, Hien NT, Prawer SE, Goldman SJ. Long-term efficacy of topical minoxidil in male pattern baldness. *J Am Acad Dermatol* 1987;**16**:711–8.

18 De Groot A, Nater JP, Herxheimer A. Minoxidil: hope for the bald? *Lancet* 1987;**329**:1019–22.

19 Price VH. Treatment of hair loss. *N Engl J Med* 1999;**341**:964–73.

20 Olsen EA, Dunlap FE, Funicella T, *et al.* A randomized clinical trial of 5% topical minoxidil versus 2% topical minoxidil and placebo in the treatment of androgenetic alopecia in men. *J Am Acad Dermatol* 2002;**47**:377–85.

21 Price VH, Menefee E, Sanchez MR, Ruane P, Kaufman K. Changes in hair weight and hair count in men with androgenetic alopecia after treatment with finasteride, 1 mg, daily. *J Am Acad Dermatol* 2002;**46**:517–23.

22 Saraswat A, Kumar B. Minoxidil vs finasteride in the treatment of men with androgenetic alopecia. *Arch Dermatol* 2003;**139**:1219–21.

23 Friedman ES, Friedman PM, Cohen DE, Washenik K. Allergic contact dermatitis to topical minoxidil solution: etiology and treatment. *J Am Acad Dermatol* 2002;**46**:309–12.

24 Shapiro J. Safety of topical minoxidil solution: a one-year, prospective, observational study. *J Cutan Med Surg* 2003;**7**:322–9.

25 Lachgar S, Charveron M, Gall Y, Bonafe JL. Minoxidil upregulates the expression of vascular endothelial growth factor in human hair dermal papilla cells. *Br J Dermatol* 1998;**138**:407–11.

26 Yano K, Brown LF, Detmar M. Control of hair growth and follicle size by VEGF-mediated angiogenesis. *J Clin Invest* 2001;**107**:409–17.

27 Kaufman KD, Olsen EA, Whiting D, *et al.* Finasteride in the treatment of men with androgenetic alopecia (male pattern hair loss). *J Am Acad Dermatol* 1998;**36**:578–89.

28 The Finasteride Male Pattern Hair Loss Study Group. Long-term (5-year) multinational experience with finasteride 1 mg in the treatment of men with androgenetic alopecia. *Eur J Dermatol* 2002;**12**:38–49.

29 Van Neste D, Fuh V, Sanchez-Pedreno P, *et al.* Finasteride increases anagen hair in men with androgenetic alopecia. *Br J Dermatol* 2000;**143**:804–10.

30 Leyden J, Dunlap F, Miller B, *et al.* Finasteride in the treatment of men with frontal male pattern hair loss. *J Am Acad Dermatol* 1999;**40**:930–7.

31 Kawashima M, Hayashi N, Igarashi A, *et al.* Finasteride in the treatment of Japanese men with male pattern hair loss. *Eur J Dermatol* 2004;**14**:247–54.

32 Tosti A, Pazzaglia M, Soli M, *et al.* Evaluation of sexual function with an international index of erectile function in subjects taking finasteride for androgenetic alopecia. *Arch Dermatol* 2004;**140**: 857–8.

33 Overstreet JW, Fuh VL, Gould J, *et al.* Chronic treatment with finasteride daily does not affect spermatogenesis or semen production in young men. *J Urol* 1999;**162**:1295–300.

34 Rittmaster RS. Finasteride. *N Engl J Med* 1994;**330**:120–5.

35 Drake L, Hordinsky M, Fiedler V, *et al.* The effects of finasteride on scalp skin and serum androgen levels in men with androgenetic alopecia. *J Am Acad Dermatol* 1999;**41**:550–4.

36 Olsen EA. Topical minoxidil in the treatment of androgenetic alopecia in women. *Cutis* 1991;**48**:243–8.

37 DeVillez RL, Jacobs JP, Szpunar CA, Warner ML. Androgenetic alopecia in the female: treatment with 2% topical minoxidil solution. *Arch Dermatol* 1994;**130**:303–7.

38 Lucky AW, Piacquadio DJ, Ditre CM, *et al.* A randomized, placebo-controlled trial of 5% and 2% topical minoxidil solutions in the treatment of female pattern hair loss. *J Am Acad Dermatol* 2004;**50**:541–53.

39 Dawber RP, Rundegren J. Hypertrichosis in females applying minoxidil topical solution and in normal controls. *J Eur Acad Dermatol Venereol* 2003;**17**:271–5.

40 Orme S, Cullen DR, Messenger AG. Diffuse female hair loss: are androgens necessary? *Br J Dermatol* 1999;**141**:521–3.

41 Vexiau P, Chaspoux C, Boudou P, *et al.* Effects of minoxidil 2% vs. cyproterone acetate treatment on female androgenetic alopecia: a controlled, 12-month randomized trial. *Br J Dermatol* 2002;**146**: 992–9.

42 Sinclair R, Wewerinke M, Jolley D. Treatment of female pattern hair loss with oral antiandrogens. *Br J Dermatol* 2005;**152**:466–73.

52 Alopecia areata

Rod Sinclair, Yee Jen Tai

Background

Definition

Alopecia areata is an autoimmune, nonscarring disorder of hair growth affecting genetically predisposed individuals. It is characterized by circular bald areas that contain pathognomonic exclamation-mark hairs and occur on any hair-bearing area of the body.[1] Severe disease may produce total loss of scalp hair (alopecia totalis) or universal loss of body hair (alopecia universalis).

Incidence/prevalence

The true incidence and prevalence of alopecia areata is unknown. It is estimated that 1.7% of the population will experience an episode of alopecia areata during their lifetime.[2] Alopecia areata accounts for 2% of new dermatological outpatient department attendances in the UK and USA.[3] While alopecia areata can develop at any age, 30–40% of cases appear before 21 years of age and 20–30% after 40 years of age.[4] The condition occurs with equal incidence in both sexes. The percentage of patients with alopecia areata who go on to develop alopecia totalis/universalis is not known, but estimates range from 7% to 30%.[5]

Etiology

Alopecia areata is an organ-specific autoimmune disease with genetic predisposition and an environmental trigger.[6] The rate of concordance among monozygotic twins is about 55%, and approximately 20% of patients overall have a positive family history.[5] A large number of potential environmental triggers have been evaluated, including emotional stress, pregnancy, and intercurrent infections. However, no definite associations have been identified.[7]

Prognosis

Regrowth from an initial patch occurs within 6 months in 33% of cases, and within 1 year in 50%; however, 33% never recover from the initial episode.[8] Almost every patient will develop further patches if followed for long enough.[4]

Adverse prognostic factors include age less than 10 years at time of first episode, ophiasis pattern or total alopecia, poor response to previous treatment, and the presence of associated atopy, nail dystrophy, or Down's syndrome.[9] The duration of alopecia areata prior to treatment is also thought to be an independent prognostic factor.[10]

Diagnostic tests

The diagnosis of alopecia areata is a clinical one. Exclamation-mark hairs in circular bald areas are pathognomonic. Rarely, a biopsy is required to exclude other forms of hair loss. The hallmarks of an active lesion are a dense lymphocytic infiltrate around the anagen hair bulbs and uniform miniaturization of terminal hairs into vellus-like hairs.[11] Telogen hairs are not inflamed, and there are decreased numbers of terminal anagen hairs.

Aims of treatment

The aim of treatment is to improve the patient's quality of life either by achieving cosmetically acceptable hair regrowth, or by encouraging the patient to live with the hair loss. Unfortunately, the environmental events that trigger episodes of alopecia areata are unknown, and so relapse can be neither predicted nor prevented. Treatment is often unsatisfactory and centers on the provision of emotional support to distressed patients and their families.

Methods of search

- Clinical evidence search and appraisal (May 2001).

• Supplementary search of Medline from 1966 to 2006.
• Other references obtained from reference lists in all identified review articles and relevant sections of new editions of multiple-author textbooks of dermatology and hair diseases.
• A new literature review was carried out on articles published between 2002 and 2006 for this edition.

Questions

What are the effects of treatment for patchy alopecia areata?

Case scenario 1

Sarah is 22 years old and has two patches of alopecia areata over the frontal and parietal scalp that have been present for 8 months (Figure 52.1). At the age of 10, she developed alopecia totalis, with spontaneous regrowth after 9 months. At the age of 14, she developed a solitary patch of alopecia areata, with regrowth after two intralesional injections of triamcinolone acetonide 6 weeks apart.

She has a history of atopy, her mother has idiopathic hypothyroidism, and a great-aunt became totally bald after receiving a telegram notifying her of her husband's death during the Second World War. Sarah's only recent stress was breaking up with her boyfriend of 4 years; however, that occurred after the hair loss had begun.

Intralesional corticosteroids
Benefits

We found no systematic reviews. One randomized controlled trial (RCT) and one observational comparison study confirm that intradermal injections of triamcinolone acetonide, 5 mg/mL with a needle-less injector produced rapid regrowth of hair in a high proportion of subjects with limited disease, within 4–6 weeks.

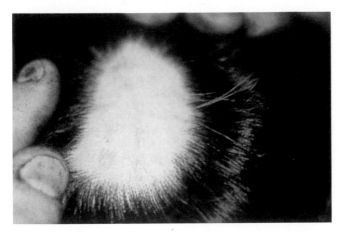

Figure 52.1 Patchy alopecia areata.

Versus placebo

In a report of 84 patients using normal saline controls, 86% of patients treated with triamcinolone responded, in comparison with only 7% of control patients.[12] Injections of triamcinolone acetonide, 0.1 mL of 5 mg/mL, were given at weekly or 2-weekly intervals on three occasions. The number of injections was determined by the size of the area of alopecia, with each injection producing a tuft of hair approximately 0.5 cm². Ninety-two percent of patients with localized disease showed regrowth at 6 weeks, in comparison with 61% of those with alopecia totalis. This decreased to 71% at 12 weeks for alopecia areata and 28% for patients with alopecia totalis, without further treatment. Topical tretinoin was used as an adjunctive treatment to intralesional corticosteroids in one study.[13]

Versus each other

In an observational study comparing triamcinolone acetonide and triamcinolone hexacetonide involving 34 areas of alopecia in 11 patients, 64% of the sites injected with triamcinolone acetonide and 97% of the sites injected with triamcinolone hexacetonide regrew.[14]

Harms

Hemorrhage can occur at the puncture site, but can easily be controlled with pressure.[12] No cases of persistent atrophy of skin were seen. The plasma cortisol level was measured in one patient and showed significant suppression, raising the possibility of a systemic effect.[12]

Comments/implications for clinical practice

Despite the lack of RCTs, intradermal injection of triamcinolone acetonide in concentrations ranging from 2.5 to 10 mg/mL either with a needle or with a needle-less injector is the most widely used first-line treatment for patch alopecia areata. Rapid hair regrowth is achieved in a high proportion of subjects within 4–6 weeks. Dermal atrophy is common, but usually self-limiting. Topical tretinoin is not widely used as an adjunctive treatment, and the reported beneficial effects have not been independently substantiated.

Topical immunotherapy

Three agents have been used for topical immunotherapy: dinitrochlorobenzene, diphencyprone, and squaric acid dibutyl ester (SADBE). All are applied topically at weekly intervals following initial sensitization.

Benefits

We found one systematic review of published case series on the use of topical immunotherapy with diphencyprone, which concluded that 50–60% of patients achieve a worthwhile response. Patients with limited disease have higher response rates than patients with alopecia totalis/universalis.[15]

Versus placebo

We found no RCTs. In the largest series reported to date of diphencyprone in the treatment of alopecia areata, 148 consecutive patients were evaluated for unilateral regrowth following unilateral treatment.[16] At 32 months, cosmetically significant regrowth was obtained in 17.4% of those with alopecia totalis/universalis, in 60.3% of those with 75–99% hair loss, in 88.1% of those with 50–74% hair loss, and in 100% of those with 25–49% hair loss. The only other independent predictor of treatment response was the age of onset of alopecia areata, with an older age of onset portending a better prognosis.[17] Relapse after achievement of cosmetically significant regrowth occurred in 62.6% after a 37-month follow-up period and was not prevented by maintenance therapy.[17]

Versus each other

A controlled trial compared SADBE, diphencyprone, minoxidil, and placebo in patients with patchy alopecia areata involving less than 40% of the scalp.[18] The study included 119 patients and was continued for at least 6 months. No significant differences were found between the different therapies used and placebo.

Harms

Dinitrochlorobenzene is mutagenic on the Ames test.[19] A moderately severe allergic contact dermatitis is necessary for success of the therapy,[20] which if severe may necessitate temporary suspension of treatment. Tender regional lymphadenopathy is common, but usually mild and self-limiting. Generalized dermatitis is uncommon, but may necessitate permanent cessation. Contact urticaria, vitiligo, and erythema multiforme have been reported.[21] Dinitrophenol, a metabolite of dinitrochlorobenzene, has been reported to cause hepatic and renal changes, convulsive seizures, and hyperthermia.[22]

Comments/implications for clinical practice

Diphencyprone is not licensed in the USA. Immunotherapy for alopecia areata is only available in specialist treatment centers. We found no RCTs on the use of topical immunotherapy; however, a number of studies have demonstrated unilateral hair regrowth after unilateral treatment. This protocol conforms to the published investigational guidelines for alopecia areata.[15] In almost all case series, patients with limited disease have higher response rates than patients with alopecia totalis/universalis. In contrast to other studies, Shapiro et al.[23] found that a long duration of disease did not necessarily preclude a positive response to treatment with diphencyprone. Tosti et al. concluded from their work that transferring nonresponder patients with alopecia totalis or universalis to other therapies is generally useless.[24]

Topical corticosteroids

Benefits

We found no systematic reviews. There was one well-conducted RCT with adequate patient numbers to support their use.

Versus placebo

In the RCT, which included 70 patients using 0.2% desoximetasone for 12 weeks, there was a trend to more regrowth in the treatment group, but the complete regrowth rates were higher in the placebo group.[25] In an observational study, 0.2% fluocinolone acetonide was used under night-time occlusion. Of the 47 patients, of whom only 28 were evaluable, 17 (61%) achieved a satisfactory clinical response after 6 months.[26] Another observational study involved the use of clobetasol propionate 0.05% under occlusion in 28 patients with alopecia areata totalis and alopecia universalis.[27] Eight (28.5%) patients achieved successful growth 6–14 weeks after the start of treatment.

Versus each other

A randomized, controlled, investigator-blinded trial compared betamethasone valerate foam and betamethasone dipropionate lotion in patients with mild to moderate patch alopecia areata.[28] Of the 61 patients evaluated, more than 75% regrowth was achieved in 61% of the patients using betamethasone valerate foam, as opposed to 27% of patients using betamethasone dipropionate lotion.

Harms

Side effects of topical therapy include folliculitis, hypertrichosis, acneiform eruption, and the potential for long-lasting local atrophy and telangiectasia.[26]

Comments

Potent topical steroids such as clobetasol propionate and betamethasone valerate foam may be of benefit in alopecia areata—particularly newer formulations and in young children who have relatively thin skin. When used, the treatment should be used continuously for a minimum of 3 months.

Psoralen ultraviolet A (PUVA)

Photochemotherapy involves oral ingestion of psoralen capsules before exposure to ultraviolet A (UVA) radiation. Treatment is performed three times a week, with the dose of UVA being increased gradually.

Benefits

We found no systematic reviews or RCTs. A retrospective audit of 10 years of experience with PUVA showed an effective success rate of 6.3% for disease less severe than the alopecia totalis state.[29]

Topical PUVA has been used in a small study of 22 patients with alopecia areata, of whom 36% achieved a regrowth of at least 75% of the treated scalp.[30]

Harms
Potential risks include sunburn, irritation, accelerated photodamage, and subsequent development of lentigo, nonmelanoma skin cancer, and melanoma.[29]

Implications for clinical practice
PUVA is likely to be beneficial for only a small number of people. The time commitment involved in attending three times a week for up to 6 months, and the potential to induce skin cancer, make this therapy unattractive to most patients. PUVA is contraindicated in children because of the possible increase in the risk of later development of melanoma. Topical PUVA remains an option for this group, but larger-scale studies would need to be done to assess the efficacy of this treatment modality.

Anthralin (dithranol)
Anthralin (dithranol) therapy is thought to act as a contact irritant and possibly also as an immunomodulator. Case series suggest that it needs to be applied on a daily basis in a sufficiently high concentration to produce skin irritation.

Benefits
We found no systematic reviews or RCTs. An uncontrolled, unblinded case series including 68 patients with extensive alopecia areata suggested that up to 25% of patients with patchy alopecia areata may achieve regrowth, compared with 14% with hair loss > 75%. New hair growth was generally seen within 3 months if the treatment was effective, although it may take more than double this time to achieve a cosmetically acceptable response.[31]

Harms
Side effects include irritation, scaling, folliculitis, and regional lymphadenopathy. Patients need to protect treated areas from sun exposure. Reversible staining of the skin occurs, and contact with the eyes must be avoided.[21]

Comments/implications for clinical practice
Anthralin is less effective than contact immunotherapy, but readily available and simple to prescribe.

Topical minoxidil
Benefits
We found no systematic reviews.

Versus placebo
We found 10 RCTs comparing various concentrations of topical minoxidil with placebo. Early reports suggested a significantly increased frequency of regrowth in patchy but not total alopecia areata,[32–38] although subsequent RCTs failed to confirm these results.[39,40]

Versus betamethasone
This incompletely reported study suggested that there was a higher response rate to 5% minoxidil than to 0.005% betamethasone dipropionate. Both were said to be superior to placebo, but strict numbers and statistical analyses were not reported.[41]

Harms
Systemic side effects are rare with topical minoxidil, and are generally only seen when it is combined with penetration enhancers. When used as monotherapy, the very low serum concentrations of minoxidil after twice-daily topical administration produce no serious systemic hypotensive side effects in minoxidil users.[42] Irritant contact dermatitis is seen in fewer than 10%. Allergic contact dermatitis reaction is rare.[32]

Comments
Minoxidil is unlikely to be beneficial. It is a nonspecific hair-growth stimulant with an unknown mechanism of action. Any effect it may have in alopecia areata is not immunologically based.

Cryosurgery
Benefits
We found no systematic reviews and no RCTs. We found a single partially controlled case series of 112 patients with patchy alopecia areata covering < 25% of the scalp. Seventy-two patients with a total of 237 lesions received a 2–3-second application of a cotton swab dipped in liquid nitrogen.[43] Two freeze–thaw cycles were applied once weekly for 4 weeks. New hair growth was seen in over 60% of the involved area in over 97% of patients treated with liquid nitrogen, which was statistically significant compared with the results of the nontreatment group.

Harms
Side effects include skin irritation, vesiculation, and blistering. Temporary hyperpigmentation and permanent hypopigmentation can also occur.

Comments/implications for clinical practice
Cryosurgery is unlikely to be useful. It is not suitable for people with darkly pigmented skin.

Aromatherapy
Benefits
We found one RCT. The use of aromatherapy was compared with carrier oils alone in a randomized, double-blind, controlled trial over 7 months.[44] Treatment with the

essential oils cedarwood, lavender, thyme, and rosemary oils massaged into the scalp every night was seen to be significantly more effective than treatment with carrier oil alone, with an improvement rate of 44%. Although the patients were randomized, treatment groups were small and disease severity was not specified. This result awaits confirmation.

Harms
None were found.

Comments/implications for clinical practice
Aromatherapy is unlikely to be successful.

What are the management options for severe chronic alopecia areata (including alopecia totalis and universalis)?

Case scenario 2
Michael is 15 years old. At the age of 13, he developed a solitary patch of alopecia areata. Two weeks after an intradermal injection of triamcinolone, 5 mg/mL, he developed diffuse generalized hair shedding and within 10 days was totally bald (Figure 52.2). Three months later, he began to lose his eyebrows and eyelashes, and ultimately every hair on his body was lost. Unable to cope with the teasing at school, he had not attended for the previous 8 weeks. A general assumption by his teachers was that he was away from school receiving chemotherapy.

Topical immunotherapy
Benefits
We found one systematic review, no RCTs, but numerous case series.[22,23,45,46] Response rates for patients with severe disease vary from 2% to 50%.

Harms
These are identical to those listed for topical immunotherapy for patchy alopecia areata.

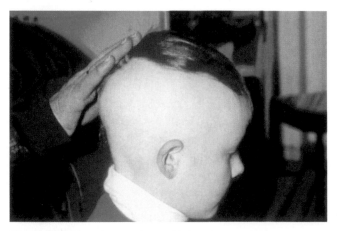

Figure 52.2 Alopecia areata in an ophiasis pattern.

Comments/implications for clinical practice
In all the case series reported, patients with severe alopecia areata and in particular alopecia totalis/universalis responded less frequently to topical immunotherapy. While the response rates are lower when patients have severe alopecia areata, these patients are often highly motivated and prepared to trial the therapy regardless. A minimum trial of 6 months is required. Initial therapy to half the head and only treating the opposite half after demonstrable regrowth is advocated.

Systemic corticosteroids
Oral prednisolone or dexamethasone or intravenous methylprednisolone will stimulate hair regrowth in most, but not all, patients if used at a high enough dosage. It has been suggested that the initial dose threshold for oral prednisolone is 0.8 mg/kg, which is then decreased slowly over 6–8 weeks. Pulse therapy can also be considered in these patients.

Benefits
We found no systematic reviews. A placebo-controlled study evaluated the efficacy of pulse oral prednisolone therapy in severe alopecia areata. The regimen involved 200 mg oral prednisolone once a week for 3 months. Of the 84 patients recruited, 40% experienced significant hair regrowth at the end of 3 months, compared with none in the placebo group. Indicators of poor outcome in this study included atopy, nail involvement, multiple episodes and prolonged duration of disease (more than 2 years). Relapse rates after treatment were not commented on in this study.[47] Numerous case series have been reported as well, but these are not directly comparable because of different patient selection, dose scheduling, and duration of therapy. Winter *et al.*[48] reported a case series of 18 patients with prednisolone on alternate days at doses adjusted according to the clinical response (usually two to four times the daily adrenal replacement dose, and up to 80–120 mg on alternate days in unresponsive patients). A progressively increasing dose of prednisolone was required to maintain cosmetically acceptable hair growth, and most patients experienced rapid hair loss after discontinuation of prednisolone therapy.[48] Oral steroids used in combination with topical and intralesional steroids have shown benefit in nonrandomized trials.[49] The use of topical and intralesional steroids allowed for more rapid lowering of oral doses and thus minimization of side effects. Seven of 15 patients treated with oral steroids showed regrowth of most or all of their hair, with an average remission of 32 months.[49]

Harms
Weight gain and cushingoid facies are the main side effects.[49] Prolonged therapy with oral corticosteroids may retard growth, demineralize bones, and lead to premature

fusion of the bony epiphyses. Nausea and polymenorrhea can occur with pulsed steroid therapy.[50]

Comments/implications for clinical practice

Many patients who are offered systemic corticosteroids decline to take them because of the potential systemic side effects and the high relapse rate. Around 70–80% of patients do regrow hair following a brief course of systemic corticosteroids, but over 50% of those who regrow hair with systemic corticosteroids relapse on dose reduction or within a few months of ceasing therapy. While around 35–40% of patients have sustained remissions following a course of treatment, a similar number will either have to accept the relapse or consider long-term systemic treatment. Some patients can be managed with low-dose systemic corticosteroids (5–10 mg per day) or with a steroid-sparing agent. Long-term high-dose systemic corticosteroids are not desirable and are not recommended for alopecia areata. In view of the limited therapeutic alternatives, systemic corticosteroid use is attractive, but clinicians must contemplate how the dosage will be weaned and relapses managed. Patients who require more than 6 weeks of systemic corticosteroids should receive general measures to prevent bone demineralization.[51]

Ciclosporin
Benefits

We found no systematic reviews or RCTs for oral ciclosporin. In a small case series, six patients received oral ciclosporin, 6 mg/kg/day for 12 weeks.[52] All patients had some regrowth, but cosmetically acceptable regrowth occurred in only two of five patients with alopecia totalis/universalis and in the single patient with patchy alopecia areata. All patients had relapsed within 3 months of stopping therapy. A randomized study of 26 patients with alopecia totalis or universalis compared topical 10% ciclosporin daily with photochemotherapy three times a week and intravenous thymopentin, 50 mg three times a week every 3 months over 9 months.[24] All of the patients had previously been unresponsive to sensitizing therapy for at least 12 months. None of the patients in the study had any cosmetic clinical improvement by the end of the study.

Harms

In the case series of six patients receiving oral ciclosporin, the side effects were mild and transient.[53] Davies *et al.* reported on two patients who had first developed alopecia areata while taking ciclosporin.[53] While the precise mechanism is unknown, alopecia areata can occur in patients who are least partially immunosuppressed.

Comments/implications for clinical practice

The effectiveness of oral ciclosporin for alopecia areata is unknown. A dose of 6 mg/kg/day is a high dose of ciclo-sporin and would require very careful monitoring for renal and other toxicity. The relapse rates on discontinuation of therapy are high, and there is a reluctance to use long-term therapy because of cost and cumulative side effects. Topical ciclosporin is ineffective.

Other therapies
Benefits

Inosine pranobex at a dose of 50 mg/kg/day for 6 months was ineffective in one series[54] and slightly helpful in another.[55]

The combination of SADBE immunotherapy at weekly intervals and interferon alpha 3.0×10^{-6} IU intramuscularly, daily for 15 days, three times a week for 2 weeks, then once a week for 2 months appeared to be better than SADBE alone.[56]

Harms

Flu-like symptoms were observed in patients receiving interferon alpha.[56] No clinically significant side effects attributable to inosine pranobex were reported.[55]

Comments/implications for clinical practice

The low response rate in alopecia totalis should be explained to patients before commencing experimental treatments.

What are the treatment options for alopecia areata in children?

Case scenario 3

Anthony developed 20-nail dystrophy at the age of 30 months. Six months later, he developed a single patch of alopecia areata. Nightly topical application of 0.05% clobetasol dipropionate cream to the patch led to regrowth within 6 weeks, with no obvious cutaneous atrophy. There was some mild associated hypertrichosis of the forehead, which resolved within 6 months of the cream being stopped.

Anthony had no family history of alopecia areata, and no history of atopy. Three years later, he presented again with four patches of alopecia areata, each about 3 cm in diameter.

Topical corticosteroids

Topical corticosteroids are discussed under the section on patchy alopecia areata.

Benefits

In an observational study of 48 patients, children aged 3–10 years had a higher response rate to topical corticosteroids than did adults.[26]

Topical immunotherapy
Benefits

We found no systematic reviews. We found one RCT that

involved small numbers of children. Tosti *et al.*[18] compared SADBE, diphencyprone, minoxidil, and placebo, finding a significant relationship between the age of the patients and the results. Complete hair regrowth was seen in 71.3% of adults, but only 38.9% of children.

We found two case series. Schuttelaar *et al.*[57] treated 26 children with diphencyprone weekly for a period of 3–12 months. Sixteen subjects had alopecia areata totalis, the others having patchy disease only. Eighty-four percent of the children showed hair regrowth, 32% of the total being cosmetically acceptable. Where treatment failed (0–5% hair growth), it was recommended not to continue treatment for longer than 1 year, as hair growth is not promoted by continued treatment. Orecchia and Malagoli[58] treated 28 unresponsive children under the age of 13 years with SADBE for 12 months. Thirty-two per cent of the patients achieved complete or cosmetically acceptable regrowth, and a further 21% achieved significant regrowth.

Harms

Schuttelaar *et al.* noted the problem of psychological dependence on the diphencyprone in certain children and parents, who asked to continue treatment after regrowth had been achieved, fearing a relapse.[57] As with previous studies, itching, erythema, and scaling were noted side effects. Swelling of regional lymph nodes was common and disappeared after discontinuation of treatment.[58]

Comments/implications for clinical practice

Topical immunotherapy has been used in children as young as 4 years by a number of investigators. Taking into consideration that the development of alopecia areata before the age of 10 years is an independent adverse prognostic indicator, side effects and efficacy appear to be similar to those seen in adults. Efficacy is also influenced by the extent of the disease, associated nail changes, and atopy.

Topical minoxidil

Topical minoxidil has not been tested in children. Systemic absorption and systemic side effects may be more likely to occur in children.

---

can be repeated at 4–6-weekly intervals if necessary. We were not able to find data on long-term efficacy.

- One RCT demonstrated that potent topical corticosteroids are marginally more effective than placebo in patchy alopecia areata when used continuously for a minimum of 3 months. In observational case series, children between the ages of 3 and 10 years appear most likely to respond.

- We found one systematic review based on case series on the use of topical immunotherapy. A number of studies have demonstrated unilateral hair regrowth after unilateral treatment. This protocol has been favoured for evaluation of topical immunotherapy because of the inability to blind patients. The systematic review of published case series on the use of topical immunotherapy with diphencyprone concluded that 50–60% of patients achieve a worthwhile response. Patients with limited disease have higher response rates than those with alopecia totalis/universalis.

- We found insufficient evidence on the use of topical minoxidil, topical anthralin therapy, PUVA, aromatherapy, cryosurgery, and ciclosporin A.

Alopecia totalis/universalis

- The prognosis for spontaneous or assisted regrowth is poor.
- In all RCTs, the extent of disease is an adverse prognostic factor for regrowth.
- Systemic corticosteroids can be used, but not for prolonged periods—a tapering schedule and a plan for managing relapses should be thought of from the outset.

Childhood alopecia areata

- In most RCTs, an early age of onset is an adverse prognostic factor for regrowth.
- Topical corticosteroids therapy may be more effective in children than in adults.
- Intralesional injection of corticosteroids is unsuitable for use in children. Most children will not tolerate repeated injections, limiting the usefulness of intralesional corticosteroids.
- Prolonged therapy with oral corticosteroids may retard growth, demineralize bones, and lead to premature fusion of the bony epiphyses.
- PUVA is contraindicated in children because of the possible increase in risk of future development of melanoma.
- Topical PUVA can be tested in this group.

Key points

Patchy alopecia areata

- The spontaneous remission rate in alopecia areata is high, which makes evaluation of treatment in the absence of RCTs very difficult.
- No treatment alters the natural history of alopecia areata.
- We found no good evidence in support of nondrug treatment.
- Small RCTs have shown that intralesional injection of triamcinolone acetonide can effectively stimulate regrowth of patchy alopecia areata. Transient atrophy is common. Treatment

References

1 Safavi K, Muller SA, Suman VJ, Moshell AN, Melton LJ. Incidence of alopecia areata in Olmsted County, Minnesota, 1975 through 1989. *Mayo Clin Proc* 1995;**70**:628–33.

2 Olsen EA. Hair disorders. In: Freedberg IM, Eisen AZ, Wolff K *et al.*, eds. *Fitzpatrick's Dermatology in General Medicine*, 5th ed., vol. 1. New York: McGraw-Hill, 1999: 737–9.

3 Dawber RPR, de Berker D, Wojnarowska F. Disorders of hair. In: Champion RH, Burton JL, Burns DA, Breathnach SM, eds. *Textbook of Dermatology*, 6th ed., vol. 4. Oxford: Blackwell Science, 1998: 2919–27.

4 Messenger AG, Simpson NB. Alopecia areata. In: Dawber RPR, ed. *Diseases of the Hair and Scalp*. Oxford: Blackwell Science, 1997: 338–69.

5 Muller SA, Winkelmann RK. Alopecia areata. *Arch Dermatol* 1963;**88**:290–7.

6 Green J, Sinclair R. Genetics of alopecia areata. *Aus J Dermatol* 2000;**41**:213–8.

7 McDonagh AJG, Messenger AG. Alopecia areata. *Clin Dermatol* 2001;**19**:141–7.

8 Walker SA, Rothman S. Alopecia areata: a statistical study and consideration of endocrine influences. *J Invest Dermatol* 1950;**14**: 403–13.

9 Sinclair RD, Banfield CC, Dawber RPR. *Handbook of Diseases of the Hair and Scalp*. Oxford: Blackwell Science, 1999: 75–84.

10 Van der Steen PHM, van Baar HMJ, Happle R, Boezeman JBM, Perret CM. Prognostic factors in the treatment of alopecia areata with diphenylcyclopropenone. *J Am Acad Dermatol* 1991;**24**:227–30.

11 Weedon D. Diseases of cutaneous appendages. In: Weedon D. *Skin Pathology*. Edinburgh: Churchill Livingstone, 1997: 381–424.

12 Abell E, Munro DD. Intralesional treatment of alopecia areata with triamcinolone acetonide by jet injector. *Br J Dermatol* 1973; **88**:55–9.

13 Kubeyinje EP, C'Mathur M. Topical tretinoin as an adjunctive therapy with intralesional triamcinolone acetonide for alopecia areata. Clinical experience in northern Saudi Arabia. *Int J Dermatol* 1997;**36**:320.

14 Porter D, Burton J. A comparison of intralesional triamcinolone hexacetonide and triamcinolone acetonide in alopecia areata. *Br J Dermatol* 1971;**85**:272–3.

15 Olsen E, Hordinsky M, McDonald-Hull S, *et al*. Alopecia areata investigational assessment guidelines. National Alopecia Areata Foundation. *J Am Acad Dermatol* 1999;**40**:242–6.

16 Rokshar CK, Shupack JL, Vafai JJ, Washenik K. Efficacy of topical sensitizers in the treatment of alopecia areata. *J Am Acad Dermatol* 1998;**39**:751–61.

17 Wiseman MC, Shapiro J, MacDonald N, Lui H. Predictive model for immunotherapy of alopecia areata with diphencyprone. *Arch Dermatol* 2001;**37**:1063–8.

18 Tosti A, De Padova MP, Minghetti G, Veronesi S. Therapies versus placebo in the treatment of patchy alopecia areata. *J Am Acad Dermatol* 1986;**15**:209–10.

19 Swanson NA, Mitchell AJ, Leahy MS, Headington JT, Diaz LA. Topical treatment of alopecia areata. *Arch Dermatol* 1981;**117**: 384–7.

20 Daman LA, Rosenberg EW, Drake L. Treatment of alopecia areata with dinitrochlorobenzene. *Arch Dermatol* 1978;**114**:1036–8.

21 Madani S, Shapiro J. Alopecia areata update. *J Am Acad Dermatol* 2000;**42**:549–66.

22 De Prost Y, Paquez F, Touraine R. Dinitrochlorobenzene treatment of alopecia areata. *Arch Dermatol* 1982;**118**:542–5.

23 Shapiro J, Tan J, Ho V, Abbott F, Tron V. Treatment of chronic severe alopecia areata with topical diphenylcyclopropenone and 5% minoxidil: a clinical and immunopathological evaluation. *J Am Acad Dermatol* 1993;**29**:729–35.

24 Tosti A, Bardazzi F, Guerra L. Alopecia totalis: is treating non-responder patients useful? *J Am Acad Dermatol* 1991;**24**:455–6.

25 Charuwichitratana S, Wattanakrai P, Tanrattanakorn S. Randomized double-blind placebo-controlled trial in the treatment of

alopecia areata with 0.25% desoximetasone cream. *Arch Dermatol* 2000;**136**:1276–7.

26 Pascher F, Kurtin S, Andrade R. Assay of 0.2% fluocinolone acetonide cream for alopecia areata and totalis. *Dermatologica* 1970;**141**:193–202.

27 Tosti A, Piraccini BM, Pazzaglia M, Vincenzi C. Clobetasol propionate 0.05% under occlusion in the treatment of alopecia totalis/universalis. *J Am Acad Dermatol* 2003; **49**:96–8.

28 Mancuso G, Balducci A, Casadio C, *et al*. Efficacy of betamethasone valerate foam formulation in comparison with betamethasone dipropionate lotion in the treatment of mild-to-moderate alopecia areata: a multicenter, prospective, randomized, controlled, investigator-blinded trial. *Int J Dermatol* 2003;**42**:572–5.

29 Taylor CR, Hawk JLM. PUVA treatment of alopecia areata partialis, totalis and universalis: audit of 10 years' experience at St John's Institute of Dermatology. *Br J Dermatol* 1995;**133**:914–8.

30 Mitchell AJ, Douglass MC. Topical photochemotherapy for alopecia areata. *J Am Acad Dermatol* 1985;**12**:644–9.

31 Fiedler-Weiss VC, Buys CM. Evaluation of anthralin in the treatment of alopecia areata. *Arch Dermatol* 1987;**123**:1491–3.

32 Fiedler-Weiss VC, West DP, Fu TS, *et al*. Alopecia areata treated with topical minoxidil. *Arch Dermatol* 1984;**120**:457–63.

33 Vanderveen EE, Ellis CN, Kang S, *et al*. Topical minoxidil for hair regrowth. *J Am Acad Dermatol* 1984;**11**:416–21.

34 Frentz G. Topical minoxidil for extended areata alopecia. *Acta Derm Venereol* 1985;**65**:172–5.

35 Shi YP. Topical minoxidil in the treatment of alopecia areata and male-pattern alopecia. *Arch Dermatol* 1986;**122**:506.

36 Fiedler-Weiss VC. Topical minoxidil solution (1% and 5%) in the treatment of alopecia areata. *J Am Acad Dermatol* 1987;**16**:745–8.

37 Fiedler-Weiss VC, West DP, Buys CM, Rumsfield JA. Topical minoxidil dose–response effect in alopecia areata. *Arch Dermatol* 1986;**122**:180–2.

38 Price V. Double-blind, placebo-controlled evaluation of topical minoxidil in extensive alopecia areata. *J Am Acad Dermatol* 1987; **16**:730–6.

39 White SI, Friedmann PS. Topical minoxidil lacks efficacy in alopecia areata. *Arch Dermatol* 1985;**121**:591.

40 Vestey JP, Savin JA. A trial of 1% minoxidil used topically for severe alopecia areata. *Acta Derm Venereol* 1986;**66**:179–80.

41 Fiedler VC. Alopecia areata: current therapy. *J Invest Dermatol* 1991;**96**(Suppl):69S–70S.

42 Shapiro J. Safety of topical minoxidil solution: a one-year, prospective, observational study. *J Cutan Med Surg* 2003;**7**:322–9.

43 Lei Y, Nie YF, Zhang JM, Liao DY, Li HY. Effect of superficial hypothermic cryotherapy with liquid nitrogen on alopecia areata. *Arch Dermatol* 1991;**127**:1851–2.

44 Hay I, Jamieson M, Ormerod A. Randomized trial of aromatherapy. *Arch Dermatol* 1998;**134**:1349–52.

45 Happle R, Hausen BM, Wiesner-Menzel L. Diphencyprone in the treatment of alopecia areata. *Acta Derm Venereol* 1983;**63**:49–52.

46 Van der Steen PHM, van Baar HMJ, Perret CM, Happle R. Treatment of alopecia areata with diphenylcyclopropenone. *J Am Acad Dermatol* 1991;**24**:253–7.

47 Kar BR, Handa S, Dogra S, Kumar B. Placebo-controlled oral pulse prednisolone therapy in alopecia areata. *J Am Acad Dermatol* 2005;**52**:287–90.

48 Winter RJ, Kern F, Blizzard RM. Prednisolone therapy for alopecia areata. *Arch Dermatol* 1976;**112**:1549–52.

49 Unger WP, Schemmer RJ. Corticosteroids in the treatment of alopecia totalis. *Arch Dermatol* 1978;**114**:1486–90.

50 Sharma VK. Pulsed administration of corticosteroids in the treatment of alopecia areata *Arch Dermatol* 1996;**35**:133–6.

51 Summey BT, Yosipovitch G. Glucocorticoid-induced bone loss in dermatologic patients: an update. *Arch Dermatol* 2006;**142**:82–90.

52 Gupta AK, Ellis CN, Cooper KD *et al*. Oral cyclosporin for the treatment of alopecia areata. *J Am Acad Dermatol* 1990;**22**:242–50.

53 Davies MG, Bowers PW. Alopecia areata arising in patients receiving cyclosporine immunosuppression. *Br J Dermatol* 1995; **132**:827–9.

54 Berth-Jones J, Hutchinson PE. Treatment of alopecia totalis with a combination of inosine pranobex and diphencyprone compared to each treatment alone. *Clin Exp Dermatol* 1991;**16**:172–5.

55 Galbraith GMP, Thiers BH, Jensen J, Hoehler F. A randomized double-blind study of inosiplex (isoprinosine) therapy in patients with alopecia totalis. *J Am Acad Dermatol* 1987;**16**:977–83.

56 Pipoli M, D'Argento V, Coviello C, Dell'Osso A, Mastrolonardo M, Vena GA. Evaluation of topical immunotherapy with squaric acid dibutylester, systemic interferon alpha and the combination of both in the treatment of chronic severe alopecia areata. *J Dermatol Treat* 1995;**6**:95–8.

57 Schuttelaar MLA, Hamstra JJ, Plinck EPB *et al*. Alopecia areata in children: treatment with diphencyprone. *Br J Dermatol* 1996;**135**: 581–5.

58 Orecchia G, Malagoli P. Topical immunotherapy in children with alopecia areata. *J Invest Dermatol* 1995;**104**(Suppl):35S–36S.

53 Evidence-based treatment of hirsutism

Ulrike Blume-Peytavi, Natalie Garcia-Bartels

Background

Definition

Hirsutism is defined as the presence of excess terminal (coarse) hairs in females in a pattern typically seen in adult males.[1,2] Unlike hirsutism, hypertrichosis is independent of androgen influence and is characterized by the superfluous and uniform growth of nonterminal (vellus) hair over the body, particularly in nonsexual areas.[3]

Incidence/prevalence

Approximately 5–10% of women of reproductive age in the general population are hirsute (assessed as having a Ferriman–Gallwey score of 8 or more).[4–6]

Etiology

Hirsutism is usually the result of an underlying adrenal, ovarian, or central endocrine abnormality. Elevated secretion of androgens, increased bioavailability of testosterone, and increased sensitivity of hair follicles to androgens all contribute to the condition.[7,8] The most common cause of androgen excess is polycystic ovary syndrome (PCOS); 70–80% of patients with androgen excess demonstrate hirsutism.[2] Up to 4% of women are affected by PCOS, in whom hirsutism is the most common manifestation of the androgen component.[9] Hirsutism is deemed idiopathic when it develops in the absence of excess androgen levels and in conjunction with normal ovulatory function; these findings account for less than 20% of hirsute women.[10] Other causes of androgen excess, such as nonclassic congenital adrenal hyperplasia (1.5–2.5% of cases)[11,12] and androgen-secreting tumors (0.2% of cases) are less common causes of hyperandrogenism.[13] Cushing's syndrome, hyperprolactinemia, acromegaly, and thyroid dysfunction are other rare but possible causes, and certain prescribed drugs, such as anabolic or androgenic steroids, can also cause hirsutism.[14,15]

Prognosis

If the underlying cause of hirsutism can be well controlled (e.g., ovarian or adrenal dysfunctions), the hirsutism may resolve or at least be well controlled. Since this is not an option with idiopathic hirsutism, its prognosis may be poorer, and resolution will depend on hair removal by physical, chemical, or electrical means. Women presenting with hirsutism due to PCOS may not respond well to epilation treatments unless the specific underlying cause is addressed. The correct evaluation and diagnosis of female hirsutism, coupled with the use of combination therapy, can provide adequate results in many patients, although long-term studies are needed to confirm current findings.

Diagnostic tests

Hirsutism is a clinical diagnosis. A physical examination and medical history are needed to screen for any risk factors for virilizing disorders, PCOS, or hormonal imbalances. It is also important to consider whether any of the patient's current medications could potentially cause or exacerbate the hirsutism. In the case of rapidly progressing hirsutism, or when there is evidence of virilization, it is important to eliminate the presence of an androgen-secreting tumor.[13] The severity of hirsutism can be evaluated using the Ferriman–Gallwey (FG) score,[15] although caution is required, as it is a subjective assessment measure and not as readily applicable in women of Asian origin.[10] A popular adoption of the FG evaluates nine, rather than 11, body sites.[4,16] Each body site is scored from 0 to 4 on the basis of the number of coarse hairs present. A score of 8 or more is consistent with the diagnosis of hirsutism.[16] The FG score is also used in monitoring the patient's individual responses to treatment and is helpful for the clinician in evaluating the patient's degree of hirsutism.

In patients with moderate or severe hirsutism, or in whom other risk factors are present, a screening test for androgen excess is an early-morning.

$$\text{Free androgen index (FAI)} = \frac{\text{Total testosterone} \times 100}{\text{SHB6}}$$

In addition, dehydroepiandrosterone sulphate (DHEAS) should be measured in basic hormonal diagnostic procedures. While normal total testosterone and DHEAS readings in patients with regular menstrual cycles support the diagnosis of idiopathic hirsutism, normal levels do not eliminate peripheral androgen excess. Hair follicles and sebaceous glands can synthesize androgens *de novo* or convert circulating androgens to more potent ones. Furthermore, a monthly curve of basal temperature, in combination with a measurement of 17-OH-progesterone (days 20–24), should help exclude the presence of an asymptomatic anovulatory menstrual cycle or late onset adrenogenital syndrome (AGS). In patients with hirsutism and irregular menstrual cycles, a thorough endocrinological work-up is essential. The following laboratory tests should be undertaken: 17-OH-progesterone, estradiol, sex hormone–binding globulin (SHBG), prolactin, androstene-dione, testosterone (total and free), DHEAS, cortisol, thyroid-stimulating hormone (TSH), and serum glucose. Mildly elevated total testosterone levels or FAI unsatisfactory responses to treatment, or the suspicion of another disorder all warrant an early-morning free plasma testosterone test.[13] Grossly raised total testosterone (> 19 µmol/L) is suggestive of an underlying neoplasm, with elevated levels of DHEAS indicating an adrenal source. Ultrasonography of the adrenal gland and/or pelvic region can also be helpful in the diagnosis of hirsutism. In the case of PCOS in particular, imaging the ovaries and performing hormonal tests (i.e., the luteinizing hormone–follicle-stimulating hormone ratio) can help confirm or refine the diagnosis.

Aims of treatment

The aim of treatment is to rectify any causal hormonal balance and improve the cosmetic appearance of hirsutism, thereby positively affecting the patient's quality of life. The primary goal in the management of hirsutism is to achieve central or peripheral androgen suppression using three groups of drugs: inhibitors of androgen production (oral contraceptives, gonadotropin-releasing hormone analogues), peripheral androgen blockers (cyproterone acetate, flutamide, finasteride, and spironolactone) and insulin-sensitizing agents (rosiglitazone, metformin). A combination of pharmacological, physical and chemical treatment regimens can be used, depending on the particular case, to achieve the optimum result for the patient.

Relevant outcomes

Outcome measures to evaluate the management of hirsutism could include clinical evaluation using the Ferriman–Gallwey score and in addition, hair density, thickness, and length, as well as questionnaires. There is currently a dearth of studies employing objective measurements such as phototrichogram and global photographic evaluation. Further well-designed controlled studies are needed, and clinical trials may in future include trichological measurements to evaluate the hair quantity and quality.

Last but not least, patients' quality of life, based on self-assessment, should also be included.

Methods of search

- Cochrane library
- Medline search
- Embase
- References from reviews on hirsutism and associated clinical conditions
- Use of professional knowledge of publications in the field

Questions

What is the best treatment for idiopathic hirsutism in women?

Case scenario 1 (Figure 53.1)
This case concerns a 25-year-old woman who has suffered from excessive facial hair growth since puberty. There is a family history of the condition, with the patient's mother and sister also suffering. The latter is currently being treated with oral contraceptives. The patient described how she plucks and waxes regularly to remove unwanted facial hair and has also tried electroepilation, although this resulted in some mild scarring. However, she remains unhappy with the frequency with which she has to carry out these hair removal techniques and with the time involved in treating the relatively large skin area affected. Dermatological assessment revealed a modified FG score of about 18, with hypertrichosis mainly on the face and less on the upper legs. No other signs of hyperandrogenemia were noted. Following consultation with a gynecologist, PCOS, non-classic adrenal hyperplasia, androgen-secreting tumors, and prolactinoma were excluded as potential causes of the patient's facial hirsutism.

Antiandrogens
Efficacy
Cyproterone acetate. There is one systematic review of nine randomized controlled trials (RCTs) using cyproterone acetate to treat hirsutism.[17] Cyproterone acetate combined

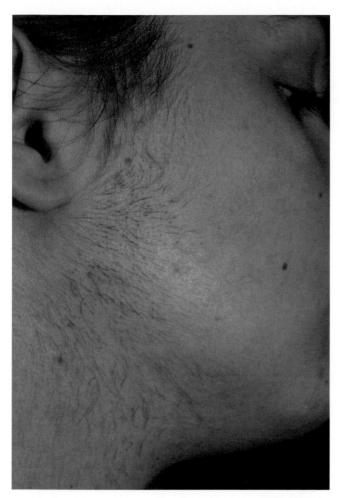

Figure 53.1 A 25 year old woman with excessive facial hair growth in a male pattern distribution 2 weeks after waxing.

with estradiol resulted in a subjective improvement in hirsutism in comparison with placebo. No clinical differences in outcome were found between cyproterone acetate and the other medical therapies (ketoconazole, spironolactone, flutamide, finasteride, and GnRH analogues) included in the review.

A well-designed but small (n = 66) RCT comparing the therapeutic efficacy of different treatments for hirsutism found that cyproterone acetate combined with estradiol resulted in the most rapid reduction of hair growth and the greatest hair growth decrease after 12 months of treatment in comparison with flutamide, finasteride, and ketoconazole.[18]

Chlormadinone acetate. The use of combined oral contraceptives containing chlormadinone acetate or cyproterone acetate plus ethinyl estradiol was shown to produce an improvement of patients' hirsutism in 36% of cases.[19] Chlormadinone acetate-containing combination oral contraceptives have proved similarly effective as cyproterone

acetate/ethinyl estradiol in women with androgen-related skin and hair conditions.[19]

Spironolactone. One systematic review of the use of spironolactone in the treatment of hirsutism and/or acne was found, which included seven small RCTs.[20] The review concluded that 6 months' treatment with spironolactone 100 mg/day was associated with a statistically significant subjective improvement in hair growth and a decrease in the FG score in comparison with placebo.

Spironolactone 100 mg/day has also been shown to be more effective in the treatment of hirsutism than finasteride 5 mg/day and low-dose cyproterone acetate 12.5 mg/day (first 10 days of cycle) up to 12 months after treatment.[21] An open-label trial of 109 women demonstrated that low-dose spironolactone successfully improved hirsutism in 72% of women treated.[22] Another open-label trial comparing the efficacy of spironolactone and metformin in 82 young women with PCOS found that the two drugs were similarly effective in the management of PCOS, although spironolactone was more effective in the treatment of hirsutism.[23]

Flutamide and bicalutamide. Flutamide was found to be more effective than finasteride in the treatment of hirsutism.[24] An RCT comparing low-dose flutamide, finasteride, ketoconazole, and cyproterone acetate–estrogen regimens in the treatment of 66 hirsute women showed that flutamide and cyproterone acetate, combined with estradiol, were the most effective and well-tolerated of the treatments studied.[18] A recent RCT compared the efficacy of flutamide and spironolactone plus Diane 35 (cyproterone), Dianette (2 mg cyproterone acetate and 35 μg ethinyl estradiol) in the treatment of hirsutism.[25] In this study, the FG score decreased significantly and to similar levels in both treatment groups, suggesting that the two therapies are similarly effective in the treatment of hirsutism.

The efficacy of low-dose bicalutamide (25 mg/day) in the treatment of hirsutism was investigated in a small open-label study of 42 women.[26] Clinical improvement in the degree of hirsutism was observed in all patients, with the mean modified FG score decreasing from 22.0 ± 5.1 to 8.6 ± 3.5 after 6 months' treatment ($P < 0.0001$). Hair density was visibly reduced, with a reduction in the FG score of 41.2 ± 11.4% seen at 3 months and of 61.6 ± 11.1% at 6 months.

Drawbacks

Adverse effects that have been reported with the use of antiandrogens include: headache, nausea, weight gain, depression, fatigue, breast symptoms, menstrual irregularity, sexual dysfunction, and elevation of liver enzymes. Spironolactone use was found to be associated with polymenorrhea in 50% of cases.[27]

Comments/implications for clinical practice

Antiandrogens can produce statistically significant improvement in hair growth and decreases in FG scores. However, small study sizes and a lack of standardized assessment and objective measurements of improvements in hirsutism mean that the results should be interpreted with caution. Further studies are required in order to compare efficacy and safety profiles between drug therapies for hirsutism using objective measurements, independently of the opinion of the investigator but providing measurable parameters such as hair density, hair thickness, and hair growth rate. Antiandrogens should always be administered in women of chid bearing age as with an oral controceptive pill.

Enzyme inhibitors: finasteride
Efficacy

The 5α-reductase inhibitor finasteride has been evaluated for the treatment of hirsutism in many randomized and observational trials. The results have shown that finasteride can lower hirsutism scores by 30–60%, in addition to reducing the average hair diameter. In comparative trials, it was found to be as effective as other antiandrogens in the treatment of hirsutism, with its use being associated with fewer adverse effects.[28]

A small randomized, placebo-controlled trial evaluated the clinical and hormonal effects of finasteride in hirsute women with idiopathic hirsutism or PCOS.[29] Twenty-four women received either placebo or finasteride 5 mg/day for 6 months. FG scores were significantly lower during the sixth month of finasteride treatment than at baseline, and all the patients treated with finasteride perceived a reduction in hirsutism at this time.

In an RCT comparing low-dose flutamide, finasteride, ketoconazole, and cyproterone acetate–estrogen regimens in the treatment of 66 hirsute women, finasteride treatment significantly reduced FG scores (−44%), hair diameter (−16%) and daily hair growth rate (−27%).[18] Although finasteride had the slowest onset of action of the drugs studied in the trial, it was still highly effective, with the hair diameter at the end of treatment similar to that in the other therapies studied. Furthermore, finasteride was associated with fewer side effects. In a similar trial of 41 women with idiopathic hirsutism, the short-term results of treatment with cyproterone acetate, finasteride, and spironolactone were similar, but spironolactone demonstrated a higher efficacy over a longer time period.[30]

Drawbacks

Finasteride may cause breast enlargement, breast tenderness, and rash.

Comments/implications for clinical practice

Although finasteride has been shown to be effective in the treatment of hirsutism, it is not licensed for the condition.

It is also contraindicated in women who are potentially pregnant, as it can cause feminization of the male fetus. Women treated with finasteride should therefore also be given appropriate contraception advice.

What is the best topical pharmacologic therapy for treating facial hirsutism?

Enzyme inhibitors: eflornithine
Efficacy

The efficacy of eflornithine in the treatment of facial hirsutism has been evaluated in two multicenter, randomized, double-blind, placebo-controlled trials including 596 patients.[31] Facial hirsutism significantly improved within 8 weeks of treatment with eflornithine. After 24 weeks of treatment, 70% of the patients treated showed some improvements, with 32% of patients said to be clinically improved in comparison with only 8% in the placebo group.

Combination therapy with eflornithine cream plus laser epilation can be effective and results in more rapid hair removal in comparison with laser monotherapy.[32,33] Further long-term prospective trials are needed in this area.

Drawbacks

The most common adverse events associated with eflornithine treatment are mild and skin-related, including burning, tingling, stinging, erythema, and rash at the site of application. All of these are mild and resolve without medical intervention.

Comments/implications for clinical practice

Eflornithine is simple to apply and can therefore be readily incorporated into patients' existing daily skin-care regimens. Treatment with eflornithine can be used alongside medical treatments or mechanical hair removal methods. Treatment with eflornithine is not indicated during pregnancy and lactation. It should be noted that the benefits of treatment start to diminish 8 weeks after therapy is discontinued.

What are the best alternative methods for all types of hypertrichosis in hirsute women?

Electroepilation
Efficacy

No systematic reviews or RCTs were found. Richards et al. reported the results of over 35 000 hours of electroepilation treatment in 281 women over a 4-year period.[34] The study found that electroepilation was beneficial in controlling facial hirsutism, with 93% of patients showing improvement, with no evidence of scarring. The best results were obtained when electroepilation was combined with medical treatment to resolve any androgen excess. Based on observations from 13 years and 140 000 hours of experience, the blend method is reported to be the most effective method for permanent hair removal.[35] In the blend method, heat is created through the modulation of a high-frequency current, and this accelerates the chemical procedure. Although permanent hair removal can be achieved in some cases, the success of the technique ultimately relies on the skill of the operator.

Drawbacks
Electroepilation can cause temporary pain, erythema, and edema. Scarring, keloid formation, and postinflammatory pigment changes are also possible. The technique is not suitable for patients with pacemakers or those with tanned or dark skin tones.[36]

Comments/implications for clinical practice
Electroepilation may take up to 24 months to be effective, and its success is dependent on many factors, such as previous treatments, hair type, and operator skill. There is an increased risk of scarring if probing is inaccurate, if too much current is used, or if hygiene or aftercare are inadequate.

Photoepilation
Efficacy
No systematic reviews were found. In a recent RCT of 88 women with PCOS-related hirsutism, 6 months of photoepilation significantly reduced the severity of facial hair as well as lowering depression scores and anxiety ratings in comparison with controls.[37] In a retrospective study using a solid-state 100 nm pulsed near-infrared diode laser system in 242 patients, retrospective analysis of patient questionnaires revealed that a reduction in pigmented hair was achieved after an average of 1.97 treatments and maintained for a mean period of 8.1 months.[38,39] The habitual hair-plucking interval was also increased from a mean of 3.69 days before treatment to 15.19 days after laser epilation.

In an RCT of single treatment sessions using alexandrite laser, a 40% reduction in hair growth was seen 6 months after treatment,[40] and in a prospective trial using neodymium–yttrium aluminum garnet (Nd:YAG) laser, a single treatment session with the laser and topically applied carbon dye resulted in greater hair reduction in comparison with laser alone.[41] A review of the efficacy of laser hair reduction concluded that hair reduction is less effective with the Nd:YAG laser in comparison with alexandrite, diode, or ruby lasers.[42]

Drawbacks
Photoepilation can cause edema, erythema, pain, hypopigmentation, and hyperpigmentation. Rarely, increased hair growth at the treated site has been reported.[36]

Comments/implications for clinical practice
Further long-term RCTs and comparative studies are

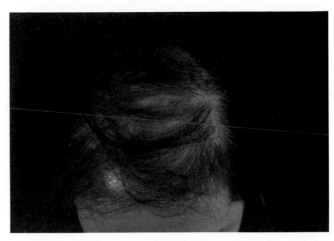

Figure 53.2 Central hair thinning with Ludwig pattern II in a 32-year old woman with PCOS, obesity and hyper insulinemia.

needed to establish the benefits of photoepilation. With the development of lasers to specifically target hair follicles, large areas can be treated rapidly, and long-term hair removal can be achieved, although permanent hair loss is rare.

What is the best way of treating a woman with hyperinsulinemia?

Case scenario 2 (Figure 53.2)
A 32-year-old woman consulted her dermatologist as a result of scalp hair loss. Clinical examination revealed female-pattern hair loss or androgenic alopecia. During consultation with her dermatologist, the patient reported that she felt uncomfortable in public due to her excessive body hair and that recent weight gain had added to her distress. There was no family history of the condition, although the patient's mother had diabetes mellitus. The patient's menstrual cycle was irregular, with cycles ranging from 25 to 38 days, and as a result she was referred to a gynecologist with suspected hyperandrogenemia. She was diagnosed with PCOS, which was found to be the cause of her hirsutism and androgenic alopecia. The patient's body mass index (BMI) was approximately 31, and investigations revealed hyperinsulinemia.

Insulin-sensitizing agents
Efficacy
In a recent RCT, 40 women with PCOS and an impaired glucose tolerance test were randomly assigned to 8 months' treatment with rosiglitazone at either 2 or 4 mg/day.[43] The majority of women in each group achieved improvements in hirsutism, normal glucose tolerance, and ovulatory menses at the end of the study period, with the degree of improvement being superior in the 4-mg rosiglitazone group in comparison with the 2-mg rosiglitazone group.

Another recent RCT compared the effects of metformin and rosiglitazone on hirsutism in 96 patients with PCOS.[44] After 24 weeks of treatment, the patients' FG scores decreased in both treatment groups. However, a significantly greater reduction in scores was reported in the rosiglitazone group. This study found rosiglitazone to be more effective than metformin in the treatment of hirsutism.

An open-label study assessed the effects of rosiglitazone (4 mg/day) versus ethinyl estradiol 35 mg/cyproterone acetate 2 mg, followed by their sequential combinations in 28 overweight women with PCOS.[45] Rosiglitazone reduced insulin levels, but had limited effects on hirsutism. Ethinyl estradiol/cyproterone was not found to modify insulin, but led to an increase in high-density lipoprotein cholesterol and triglycerides and a decrease in androgens and the degree of hirsutism. Similar changes occurred during combined treatments.

A small RCT of metformin was carried out to assess the effects of metformin on hair growth.[46] Sixteen women with PCOS and hirsutism were enrolled into a 14-month double-blind, placebo-controlled crossover study. Throughout the study, the severity of hirsutism was assessed using the FG score, patient self-assessment, and growth velocity. Metformin treatment led to significant improvements in the FG score and patient self-assessment. Growth velocity in millimeters per day at the end of each phase was also improved. The authors concluded that metformin treatment in this patient group led to a clinically and statistically significant improvement in hair growth in comparison with placebo.

An RCT with hirsutism as the primary end point compared the efficacy of metformin with combined ethinyl estradiol and cyproterone acetate.[47] Patients with PCOS (n = 52) received either metformin (500 mg, three times daily) or Diane 35, Dianette (ethinyl estradiol 35 μg and cyproterone acetate 2 mg) for 12 months. Both objective and subjective methods of evaluating hirsutism were used, as well as patients' self-assessment scores. Metformin treatment resulted in greater improvements in the FG score and patient self-assessment scores. Both treatments were moderately effective in reducing the hair diameter at multiple anatomical sites. The data suggest that hirsutism may be effectively treated by reducing hyperinsulinemia.

Other clinical trials have shown that metformin results in a small but significant improvement in hirsutism[48,49] or has no effect.[27]

In an open-label study comparing the efficacy of metformin with spironolactone in 82 women with PCOS, both treatments significantly improved hirsutism scores, but spironolactone was more effective in slowing hair growth.[23]

Drawbacks
Metformin can cause nausea and vomiting, taste disturbances, and loss of appetite. Rosiglitazone can cause anemia, hypercholesterolemia, flatulence, nausea, vomiting, and gastritis.

Comments/implications for clinical practice
The hair-growth cycle is relatively long, and the potential effects of studied drugs should not be evaluated with less than 12 months of treatment. Future trials of longer duration therefore need to be carried out in order to provide adequate data to inform clinical practice. Rosiglitazone may be an appropriate treatment approach for patients with PCOS, particularly those resistant to metformin therapy. However, although these treatments have been found to be effective in some clinical trials, they are not specifically licensed for the treatment of hirsutism.

What is the best treatment for a woman with PCOS and a desire for pregnancy?

Case scenario 3 (Figure 53.3)
A 29-year-old woman and her husband reported that they had been trying for a baby for over a year, but despite a lack of menstruation and some weight gain, her pregnancy

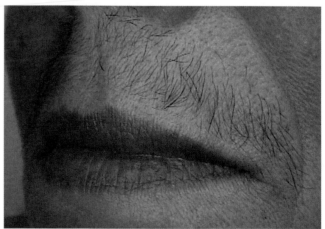
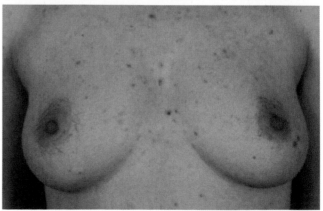

Figure 53.3 (a) Hypertrichosis on the upper lip grade 2 and (b) Papulopustular lesions (acne papulopustulosa) on the chest and perimammilas hypertrichosis in a 29-year-old woman with PCOS.

tests remained negative. During this period, she had noticed an increase of dark-colored hair on her cheeks, upper lip, around her breasts, and on her upper thighs. In addition, she had noticed darkening of the skin in her axillae. The patient was very concerned about these changes in her appearance and consulted her dermatologist to obtain laser hair reduction therapy. The dermatologist suspected that the symptoms might be due to underlying PCOS and recommended further investigation before starting laser therapy. Examination by an endocrinologist confirmed the diagnosis of PCOS, and the patient was referred to a gynecologist.

Due to the patient's desire for a baby, synthetic ovulation induction should be discussed with the gynecologist. If this approach is unsuccessful, treatment with gonadotropin-releasing hormone (GnRH) analogues (leuprolide or nafarelin) may be considered. Alongside the systemic treatment regimen, laser epilation therapy and topical eflornithine treatment can be used to manage the patient's facial hair. However, treatment with eflornithine is not indicated during pregnancy and lactation, and this would therefore need to be discontinued if the patient becomes pregnant.

Gonadotropin-releasing hormone analogues
Efficacy

No systemic reviews were found. One RCT compared the efficacy of finasteride (5 mg) and depot leuprolide (3.75 mg) in 60 women with idiopathic hirsutism.[50] After 6 months of treatment, the mean percentage changes ($\pm$ SD) in hirsutism scores in the GnRH and finasteride groups were 36% $\pm$ 14% and 14% $\pm$ 11% at 6 months, respectively.

In another RCT, 17 hirsute women were treated for 6 months with leuprolide depot (3.75 mg/month) plus conjugated estrogen (0.625 mg/day) and medroxyprogesterone acetate (10 mg, days 1–12; n = 9; leuprolide plus estrogen replacement therapy) or an oral contraceptive pill containing ethynodiol diacetate (1 mg) and ethinyl estradiol (35 µg; n = 8).[51] The patients' FG scores decreased significantly in the group receiving leuprolide plus estrogen replacement therapy (ERT), but not in the group receiving the oral contraceptive. Seventy-eight percent of the patients receiving leuprolide plus ERT and 25% of those receiving an oral contraceptive women noted an improvement in hair growth. Fifty-five percent of the patients receiving leuprolide plus ERT, in comparison with 25% of those receiving an oral contraceptive, noted an improvement in hair texture. Patients treated with leuprolide plus ERT also showed decreases in their hair growth rate. Treatment with leuprolide plus cyclic estrogen/progestin may therefore provide a more rapid and potentially superior improvement in hirsutism in comparison with a standard oral contraceptive pill regimen.

A double-blind RCT evaluated the combined use of a GnRH agonist and an estrogen-containing oral contraceptive in 64 hirsute women.[52] The 24-week trial compared placebo, nafarelin (NAF; 400 µg, intranasal spray, twice daily), norethindrone (1 mg), and ethinyl estradiol (NOR 1/35; 0.035 mg daily for 3 of 4 weeks), or combined use of NAF and NOR 1/35 for 24 weeks. There was a significant decrease in the hair shaft diameter following combination therapy ($P < 0.05$). This was not seen when either drug was used alone. This study showed that combination of GnRH agonist and low-dose oral contraceptive therapy is more effective than monotherapy with either treatment in the management of hirsutism.

In a small, open-label study, six hirsute women were treated with nafarelin (1000 µg/day) for 6 months.[53] The patients showed a good clinical response; hair growth was slower, and new hair was less coarse in texture in comparison with the pretreatment period. Hirsutism scores (determined by FG assessment of the extent and quality of body hair) improved in four of the six patients. Overall, the mean scores decreased significantly from 19.3 $\pm$ 3.3 to 13.2 $\pm$ 2.8 at the end of the treatment period.

Drawbacks

GnRH may cause hot flushes or sudden night sweats, blurred vision, nausea, breast tenderness, a decrease in sexual desire or ability, a decrease in appetite, itching, swelling, and redness at injection site, numbness or tingling in the feet or lower legs, constipation, anxiety, and unstable mood.

Comments/implications for clinical practice

GnRHs should be used as a second-line therapy in women who do not respond to combination hormonal therapy, or who cannot tolerate oral contraceptives. Particular attention should be paid to the possible long-term consequences of GnRH treatment, including atrophic vaginitis, bone demineralization, and hot flushes, and the fact that these treatments are not specifically licensed for the treatment of hirsutism.

Antiestrogens
Efficacy

A review of trials found that clomifene, when used in combination with metformin, increases the incidence of ovulation in women with PCOS and may reduce the effect of abnormal levels of male hormones.[16] Such effects may in turn help to reduce the severity of hirsutism in affected women.

Drawbacks

Clomifene treatment may cause ovarian enlargement, breast tenderness, mild abdominal discomfort, and hot flushes.

Comments/implications for clinical practice

Additional trials are needed to further investigate the effects of antiestrogens on hirsutism, but again it should be noted that such trials would be outside of licensed treatments.

Key points

- The use of combined oral contraceptives containing cyproterone acetate plus ethinyl estradiol or chlormadinone acetate has proved to represent the mainstream in the treatment of idiopathic hirsutism.
- Insulin-sensitizing agents (e.g., rosiglitazone and metformin) have proved to be the first choice in hirsute women with PCOS. Moreover, metformin led to a greater improvement in hirsutism in comparison with a combination of ethinyl estradiol 35 mg plus cyproterone acetate 2 mg or placebo.
- Photoepilation has been shown to reduce hair density effectively in dark hair, with a better result while using alexandrite, diode, or ruby lasers than with the Nd:YAG laser.
- Topical use of the enzyme inhibitor eflornithine has been clinically proven to slow down the rate of hair growth. Combination therapy with eflornithine cream plus laser epilation results in hair removal in comparison with laser monotherapy.

References

1 Deplewski D, Rosenfield RL. Role of hormones in pilosebaceous unit development. *Endocr Rev* 2000;**21**:363–92.
2 Azziz R. The evaluation and management of hirsutism. *Obstet Gynecol* 2003;**101**:995–1007.
3 Ahmed B, Jaspan J. Hirsutism: a brief review. *Am J Med Sci* 1994;**308**:289–94.
4 Hatch R, Rosenfield RL, Kim MH, Tredway D. Hirsutism: implications, etiology, and management. *Am J Obstet Gynecol* 1981;**140**: 815–30.
5 Knochenhauer ES, Key TJ, Kahsar-Miller M. Prevalence of the polycystic ovary syndrome in unselected black and white women of the southeastern United States: a prospective study. *J Clin Endocrinol Metab* 1998;**83**:3078–82.
6 Neithardt AB, Barnes RB. The diagnosis and management of hirsutism. *Semin Reprod Med* 2003;**21**:285–93.
7 Erkkola R, Ruutiainen K. Hirsutism: definitions and etiology. *Ann Med* 1990;**22**:99–103.
8 Rittmaster RS. Hirsutism. *Lancet* 1997;**349**:191–5.
9 Guzick DS. Polycystic ovary syndrome. *Obstet Gynecol* 2004;**103**: 181–93.
10 Azziz R. Idiopathic hirsutism. *Endocr Rev* 2000;**21**:347–62.
11 Azziz R, Sanchez LA, Knochenhauer ES. Androgen excess in women: experience with over 1000 consecutive patients. *J Clin Endocrinol Metab* 2004;**89**:453–62.
12 Ehrmann DA, Rosenfield RL, Barnes RB, Brigell DF, Sheikh Z. Detection of functional ovarian hyperandrogenism in women with androgen excess. *N Engl J Med* 1992;**327**:157–62.
13 Rosenfield RL. Hirsutism. *N Engl J Med* 2005;**353**:2578–88.
14 Leung AK, Robson WL. Hirsutism. *Int J Dermatol* 1993;**32**:773–7.
15 Ferriman D, Gallwey JD. Clinical assessment of body hair growth in women. *J Clin Endocrinol Metab* 1961;21:1440–7.
16 Lord JM, Flight IH, Norman RJ. Insulin-sensitising drugs (metformin, troglitazone, rosiglitazone, pioglitazone, D-chiro-inositol)

for polycystic ovary syndrome. *Cochrane Database Syst Rev* 2003; (3):CD003053.
17 Van der Spuy ZM, le Roux PA. Cyproterone acetate for hirsutism. Cochrane Database Syst Rev 2003;(4)CD001125.
18 Venturoli S, Mareschalchi O, Colombo FM. A prospective randomised trial comparing low dose flutamide, finasteride, ketoconazole and cyproterone acetate-estrogen regimens in the treatment of hirsutism. *J Clin Endocrinol Metab* 1999;**84**:1304–10.
19 Raudrant D, Rabe T. Progestogens with antiandrogenic properties. *Drugs* 2003;**63**:463–92.
20 Farquhar C, Lee O, Toomath R, Jepson R. Spironolactone versus placebo or in combination with steroids for hirsutism and/or acne. *Cochrane Database Syst Rev* 2003;(**4**):CD000194.
21 Lumachi F, Rondinone R. Use of cyproterone acetate, finasteride, and spironolactone to treat idiopathic hirsutism. *Fertil Steril* 2003;**79**:942–6.
22 Crosby PD, Rittmaster RS. Predictors of clinical response in hirsute women treated with spironolactone. *Fertil Steril* 1991;**55**: 1067–81.
23 Ganie MA, Khurana ML, Eunice M, *et al.* Comparison of efficacy of spironolactone with metformin in the management of polycystic ovary syndrome: an open-labeled study. *J Clin Endocrinol Metab* 2004;**89**:2756–62.
24 Falsetti L, Gambera A. Comparison of finasteride versus flutamide in the treatment of hirsutism. *Eur J Endocrinol* 1999;**141**:361–7.
25 Inal MM, Yildirim Y, Taner CE. Comparison of the clinical efficacy of flutamide and spironolactone plus Diane 35 in the treatment of idiopathic hirsutism: a randomized controlled study. *Fertil Steril* 2005;**84**:1693–7.
26 Muderris II, Bayram F, Ozcelik B, Guven M. New alternative treatment in hirsutism: bicalutamide 25 mg/day. *Gynecol Endocrinol* 2002;**16**:63–6.
27 Moghetti P, Tosi F, Tosti A, *et al.* Comparison of spironolactone, flutamide, and finasteride efficacy in the treatment of hirsutism: a randomized, double blind, placebo-controlled trial. *J Clin Endocrinol Metab* 2000;**85**:89–94.
28 Dawber RPR. Guidance for the management of hirsutism. *Curr Med Res Opin* 2005;**21**:1227–33.
29 Lakryc EM, Motta EL, Soares JM, Haidar MA, de Lima GR, Baracat EC. The benefits of finasteride for hirsute women with polycystic ovary syndrome or idiopathic hirsutism. *Gynecol Endocrinol* 2003;**17**:57–63.
30 Beigi A, Sobhi A, Zarrinkoub F. Finasteride versus cyproterone acetate-oestrogen regimens in the treatment of hirsutism. *Int J Gynaecol Obstet* 2004;**87**:29–33.
31 Barman Balfour JA, McClellan K. Topical eflornithine. *Am J Clin Dermatol* 2001;**2**:197–201.
32 Smith SR, Piacquadio DJ, Beger B, Littler C. Eflornithine cream combined with laser therapy in the management of unwanted facial hair growth in women: a randomized trial. *Dermatol Surg* 2006;**32**:1237–43.
33 Hamzavi I, Tan E, Shapiro J, Lui H. A randomized bilateral vehicle-controlled study of eflornithine cream combined with laser treatment versus laser treatment alone for facial hirsutism in women. *J Am Acad Dermatol.* 2007 Jul; **57**(1):54–9.
34 Richards RN, McKenzie MA, Meharg GE. Electroepilation (electrolysis) in hirsutism. 35,000 hours' experience on the face and neck. *J Am Acad Dermatol* 1986;**15**:693–7.

35 Richards RN, Meharg GE. Electrolysis: observations from 13 years and 140 000 hours of experience. *J Am Acad Dermatol* 1995;**33**:662–6.

36 Shenenberger DW, Utecht LM. Removal of unwanted facial hair. *Am Fam Physician* 2002;**66**:1907–11.

37 Clayton WJ, Lipton M, Elford J, Rustin M, Sherr L. A randomized controlled trial of laser treatment among hirsute women with polycystic ovary syndrome. *Br J Dermatol* 2005;**152**:986–92.

38 Kopera D. Hair reduction: 48 months of experience with 800nm diode laser. *J Cosmet Laser Ther* 2003;**5**:146–9.

39 Ash K, Lord J, Newman J, McDaniel DH. Hair removal using a long-pulsed alexandrite laser. *Dermatol Clin* 1999;**17**:387–99.

40 Ash K, Lord J, Newman J, McDaniel DH. Hair removal using a long-pulsed alexandrite laser. *Dermatol Clin* 1999;**17**:387–99.

41 Nanni CA, Alster TS. Optimizing treatment parameters for hair removal using a topical carbon-based solution and 1064nm Q-switched neodymium:YAG laser energy. *Arch Dermatol* 1997;**133**:1546–9.

42 Sanchez LA, Perez M, Azziz R. Laser hair reduction in the hirsute patient: a critical assessment. *Hum Reprod Update* 2002;**8**:169–81.

43 Dereli D, Dereli T, Bayraktar F, Ozgen AG, Yilmaz C. Endocrine and metabolic effects of rosiglitazone in non-obese women with polycystic ovary disease. *Endocr J* 2005;**52**:299–308.

44 Yilmaz M, Karakoc A, Toruner FB, *et al.* The effects of rosiglitazone and metformin on menstrual cyclicity and hirsutism in polycystic ovary syndrome. *Gynecol Endocrinol* 2005;**21**:154–60.

45 Lemay A, Dodin S, Turcot L, Dechene F, Forest JC. Rosiglitazone and ethinyl oestradiol/cyproterone acetate as a single and combined treatment of overweight women with polycystic ovary syndrome and insulin resistance. *Hum Reprod* 2006;**21**:121–8.

46 Kelly CJ, Gordon D. The effect of metformin on hirsutism in polycystic ovary syndrome. *Eur J Endocrinol* 2002;**147**:217–21.

47 Harborne L, Fleming R, Lyall H, Norman J, Sattar N. Descriptive review of the evidence for the use of metformin in polycystic ovary syndrome. *Lancet* 2003;**361**:1894–901.

48 Kolodziejczyk B, Duleba AJ, Spaczynski RZ. Metformin therapy decreases hyperandrogenism and hyperinsulinemia in women with polycystic ovary syndrome. *Fertil Steril* 2000;**73**:1149–54.

49 Pasquali R, Gambineri A, Biscotti D, *et al.* Effect of long-tem treatment with metformin added to hypocaloric diet on body composition, fat distribution, and androgen and insulin levels in abdominally obese women with and without the polycystic ovary syndrome. *J Clin Endocrinol Metab* 2000;**85**:2767–74.

50 Bayhan G, Bahceci M, Demirkol T, Ertem M, Yalinkaya A, Erden AC. A comparative study of a gonadotropin-releasing hormone agonist and finasteride on idiopathic hirsutism. *Clin Exp Obstet Gynecol* 2000;**27**:203–6.

51 Azziz R, Ochoa TM, Bradley EL, Potter HD, Boots LR. Leuprolide and estrogen versus oral contraceptive pills for the treatment of hirsutism: a prospective randomized study. *J Clin Endocrinol Metab* 1995;**80**:3406–11.

52 Heiner JS, Greendale GA, Kawakami AK, *et al.* Comparison of a gonadotropin-releasing hormone agonist and a low dose oral contraceptive given alone or together in the treatment of hirsutism. *J Clin Endocrinol Metab* 1995;**80**:3412–8.

53 Andreyko JL, Monroe SE, Jaffe RB. Treatment of hirsutism with a gonadotropin-releasing hormone agonist (nafarelin). *J Clin Endocrinol Metab* 1986;**63**:854–9.

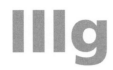

IIIg Leg ulceration

Berthold Rzany, Editor

54 Venous ulcers

Jonathan Kantor, David J. Margolis

Background

Definition

Venous ulcers are wounds that usually occur in a gaiter distribution of the lower leg (Figure 54.1). They are associated with increased pressure in the superficial venous system of the lower legs during ambulation (ambulatory venous hypertension) and are possibly related to failure of the calf muscle pump to return venous flow effectively.[1]

Incidence/prevalence

Venous leg ulcers are common. For example, a recent study showed that the incidence of venous ulcers in people over 65 years of age in the UK is 0.76 (95% confidence interval,

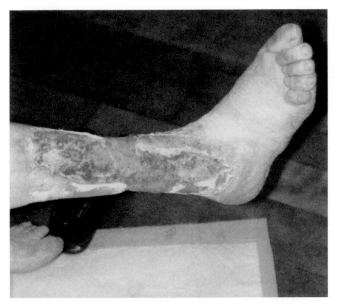

Figure 54.1 Venous ulcer of the lower extremity (case scenario 1).

0.71 to 0.83) per 100 person-years for men and 1.42 (95% CI, 1.35 to 1.48) for women.[2]

Etiology

For a venous leg ulcer to occur, it is hypothesized that the calf muscle pump fails to return blood flow effectively.[1] These wounds are often associated with varicose veins and other clinical signs of venous disease.[3,4] In addition, atherosclerotic vascular disease, diabetes, and many other medical illnesses may also complicate the clinical picture of venous leg ulceration.[5]

Prognosis

Many venous ulcers heal within 24 weeks of care, but the proportion healed after 24 weeks varies widely between studies. Why ambulatory venous hypertension leads to a wound and poor healing is not known. It has been hypothesized that the failure to heal may be associated with senescence of cells in the wound, white blood cell trapping in the microcirculation, fibrin cuffing of the microcirculation, abnormalities of coagulation cascades, and other mechanisms.[1] Unfortunately, none of these hypotheses has been shown to universally explain why a wound occurs and poorly heals. In addition, individuals with venous leg ulcer often have varicose veins and other cutaneous findings consistent with venous disease as well as other medical diseases.[1,3–5]

Aims of treatment

The aims of treatment are to improve the rate of healing and to increase the likelihood that a patient will heal over a given period of time (often 12–24 weeks).

Relevant outcomes

Relevant outcomes include the proportion of wounds healed by the end of the study and the rate of healing.

Methods of search

Medline and the Cochrane Database of Systematic Reviews were searched for the terms "venous ulcer" and "heal" or "treat," as well as bibliographies of relevant articles and systematic reviews.

Questions

What therapies are effective for curing venous leg ulcers?

Case scenario 1

A 56-year-old woman has an ulcer 25 × 6 cm on the medial side of the left ankle (Figure 54.1). The ulcer's red base is covered with yellowish fibrinous debris. On the edges are some signs of reepithelialization. The left lower leg was edematous before use of a limb compression stocking. The limb shows signs of chronic venous insufficiency—pigmentation, enlargement of the cutaneous veins, and fibrosis. What therapies would be effective treatments?

Compression
Benefits

Compression of the lower extremity is one of the oldest and most widely used treatments for venous ulcers. Methods of compression vary and include stockings, single and multi-layer bandages, and pumps.

A Cochrane collaborative review has evaluated the role of compression in the treatment of venous ulcers.[6] This review included 22 trials using a number of different compression methods. Six trials compared compression with no compression, and demonstrated a clear benefit of compression over no compression. Of these, three trials evaluated compression using an Unna boot versus no compression. Two of the three studies demonstrated a benefit of compression. Three additional studies compared compression bandages with noncompressive bandages and demonstrated a benefit of compression bandages. Of note, the results of only four of these six trials were statistically significant, although the preponderance of evidence suggests that compression results in a greater chance of healing than no compression. Three trials compared elastic high-compression bandages with inelastic low-compression bandages. Pooled results from these studies evaluated in the Cochrane review suggest that the relative risk of healing with elastic high-compression bandages over inelastic low-compression bandages was 1.54 (95% CI, 1.19 to 2.00). Four trials compared multilayer high-compression bandages with single-layer (low) compression. A pooled analysis of these studies demonstrated a relative risk of healing of 1.41 (95% CI, 1.11 to 1.80) when using multilayer compression bandages rather than single-layer bandages. Four trials compared multilayer

high-compression bandages with inelastic high-compression bandages. No statistically significant differences were shown between these types of high compression therapy.

These findings have been replicated in other studies. However, in a recent study it was shown that in a sub-group of the hardest-to-heal patients, the four-layered bandage was superior.[7] In addition, studies have shown that the four-layered therapy was less expensive and that individuals who used the four-layered bandage experienced better improvement in their quality of life.[7-9] Finally, it is important to note that in all of these studies, the selection of the bandage directly applied to the wound at a minimum is to maintain it in a moist state. Very few quality randomized studies exist that compare wound bandages, and this topic is beyond the scope of this chapter. In addition, in practice, health-care providers often change their choice of wound bandage during the course of therapy depending on the properties of the bandage and the wound's status.

Complications

Complication rates are not usually noted in trial reports, partly because compression therapy is generally benign. Inexpertly applied high compression could lead to soft-tissue damage, the development of additional wounds, and potentially amputation, although the chance of this occurring is remote.

Comment

Compression has been the mainstay of therapy for venous ulcers, and with good reason. Compression has been shown to have a clear benefit over no compression. Moreover, the evidence suggests that a high level of compression (> 25 mmHg) lends a clear benefit over low-level compression. The method used to apply these bandages is important, and there is some suggestion that the ability to apply compression bandages effectively varies widely. Compression therapy should not be used in patients with an impeded blood supply to the lower extremities.

Implications for clinical practice

Compression represents the cornerstone of the clinical management of patients with venous ulcers. Most studies evaluating novel therapies for venous ulcers use compression as the standard care regimen.

Pentoxifylline
Benefits

Pentoxifylline is a trisubstituted xanthine derivative that has been used to treat a variety of systemic disorders, most notably intermittent claudication. Theoretically, its beneficial effects in vaso-occlusive disease could extend to therapy for venous ulcers. A Cochrane collaborative review has addressed the efficacy of pentoxifylline for the treatment of venous ulcers.[10] Nine trials, including 572 patients, were included in the Cochrane review. Of note, only five of the trials included compression therapy in both the pentoxifylline and placebo groups. Combining the data from the eight trials that compared pentoxifylline (in varying doses) with placebo, pentoxifylline demonstrated a beneficial effect. Most of the studies used the probability of healing by 24 weeks as the end point. The relative risk of healing with pentoxifylline versus placebo was 1.41 (95% CI, 1.19 to 1.66). A separate examination of just the trials that compared pentoxifylline plus compression with placebo plus compression also showed a benefit of pentoxifylline therapy with a relative risk of 1.30 (95% CI, 1.10 to 1.54).

Complications
Pentoxifylline therapy is associated with an increased risk of side effects, mostly gastrointestinal in nature.

Comment
It appears that pentoxifylline is beneficial as an adjuvant treatment for venous ulcers, although all studies included in the meta-analysis did not individually show statistical significance. The dose of pentoxifylline used in the studies varied (800 mg versus 400 mg three times daily), so there is a legitimate question regarding the optimal dosing for the treatment of patients with venous ulcers.[11] Finally, all of the studies described in the meta-analysis did not use limb compression as standard care. Even though a beneficial effect in comparison with placebo was noted when limb compression was not used with pentoxifylline, patients treated with pentoxifylline should be treated with compression therapy as well, because limb compression therapy has been shown to increase the baseline chance of healing.

Implications for clinical practice
Pentoxifylline has been shown to increase the relative risk of healing by 30% over compression therapy alone.[10] Clinicians must ultimately decide whether this potential benefit is worth both the practical and the financial cost of pentoxifylline.

Skin grafting
Benefits
Most venous ulcers respond well to compression therapy. However, some wounds fail to heal with compression therapy alone. One of the options available to the health-care provider is to treat the wound with a skin graft. Grafts can include full-thickness, partial-thickness, allogeneic (cultured), xenografts, and artificial skin (skin equivalent) grafts.

The use of skin grafts for the treatment of venous ulcers is the subject of a Cochrane collaborative review.[12] Overall, seven trials were identified. Two trials evaluated split-thickness autografts, three trials evaluated cultured keratinocyte allografts, one compared artificial skin with a dressing, and one compared artificial skin with a split-thickness skin graft.

The two small studies evaluating split-thickness autografts were pooled by the Cochrane group, but the results did not show a significant benefit of skin grafting. Both studies were small, and used different placebo treatments.

Three studies compared cultured keratinocyte allografts with standard dressings. A pooled analysis of these trials conducted by the Cochrane group did not demonstrate a significant benefit of allografts over control dressings, and the relative risk of healing with the keratinocyte allografts was 1.42 (95% CI, 0.71 to 2.84). These were all small trials and may have been underpowered to demonstrate an effect. A single study compared tissue-engineered skin with a split-thickness allograft, but failed to show any significant benefit of either treatment. Note, however, that this study was small and was conducted before the newest tissue-engineered skin became available. A single study compared tissue engineered skin with a split thickness allograft, but failed to show any significant benefit of one or the other treatment. Of note, this study was small and was also conducted before the newest tissue engineered skin was available.

Graftskin (Apligraf) is a bilayered skin equivalent that includes both dermal and epidermal components. Some health-care providers also call this "artificial skin." It is manufactured by harvesting neonatal foreskins and extracting both keratinocytes and fibroblasts, which are then separately cultured to create the epidermal and dermal components, respectively. Graftskin has been studied for the treatment of venous leg ulcers. In a study that enrolled 240 patients, the percentage of ulcers healed after 24 weeks was significantly higher in those treated with Graftskin plus standard care (compression) than in those treated with compression alone (57% versus 40%).[13] Notably, secondary analyses evaluating the relative efficacy of Graftskin in wounds of more than one year's duration demonstrated that the benefit of Graftskin was most significant for patients with older wounds (47% versus 19%).[13,14] Among patients with wounds of less than one year's duration, there was no statistically significant difference in the percentage healed after 24 weeks between those treated with Graftskin and those treated with placebo (66% versus 73%).[13,14] The Cochrane group analyzed these trial data and concluded that the relative risk of healing with artificial skin versus standard dressings was 1.29 (95% CI, 1.04 to 1.60).[12]

A single multicenter randomized control study also compared the use of porcine extracellular matrix graft (OASIS Wound Material) and a compression bandage with a compression bandage alone.[15] At 12 weeks, significantly more patients in the extracellular matrix group healed (55% vs. 34%; $P = 0.02$).

Complications

A risk of infection, bleeding, and other tissue damage is inherent in any autologous skin grafting procedure. Moreover, there is always an inherent risk that the donor site will prove difficult to heal as well.

Using cultured autologous keratinocytes is likely to delay treatment, because it takes several weeks for the cells to be cultured. Moreover, patients need to undergo a skin biopsy in order to provide the laboratory with the necessary cells.

Artificial skin theoretically could be cultured from samples that are infected with viruses, including human immunodeficiency virus (HIV). Given the aggressive screening associated with this harvesting, however, the chance of infection is remote, although it does remain a possibility that the allogeneic human cells were taken from an HIV-positive but seronegative donor.[13]

Comment

While autologous skin grafts are occasionally used in some centers to aid the closure of recalcitrant wounds, the difficulties associated with harvesting the donor graft, as well as the complexities associated with inducing closure of the grafted site (in addition to the donor site), mean that this procedure cannot be undertaken lightly. Similarly, use of autologous cultured keratinocytes is a time-consuming, expensive, and complex process that demands multiple patient visits and a laboratory capable of culturing the autologous keratinocytes.

Artificial skin for the treatment of venous ulcers is not in widespread use. This may be because of the substantial cost involved. This concern has been addressed in an economics study.[16]

Implications for clinical practice

While most clinicians would not treat all venous ulcers with skin grafts, patients who have wounds recalcitrant to compression therapy could be considered for skin grafts as an adjunct, to improve their likelihood of healing. Of the available skin grafting methods, the use of artificial skin appears to be the most promising, conferring a 29% increase in the likelihood of healing by 24 weeks and an increased rate of healing. These results are based on a randomized controlled trial in patients with recalcitrant venous ulcers.[13,14] However, the short shelf-life of many of these products, the significant costs associated with the therapies, and the theoretical risk of viral infection mean that clinicians need to think carefully before treating patients with artificial skin.

Vitamins and minerals
Benefits

Few practitioners dispute the importance of adequate nutrition for promoting wound healing. However, despite the assumption that vitamin and mineral supplements may aid in healing these wounds, few studies have addressed the potential benefits of supplementation in a rigorous fashion. For example, vitamin C supplements are often prescribed for patients with chronic wounds. Reports evaluating the use of vitamin C as an adjunctive wound-healing agent have failed to demonstrate a clear benefit of vitamin C supplements in patients with chronic wounds of all types.[17,18]

Zinc has been used for more than a century as a topical adjunct for the care of chronic wounds, and Unna incorrectly believed that it was directly responsible for efficacy of his compression bandage. Oral zinc for the treatment of venous ulcers has been addressed in a Cochrane collaborative review evaluating six trials of oral zinc therapy, most of which failed to show a beneficial effect of therapy.[19] Five of these studies included patients with venous ulcers. The doses of zinc varied across studies. One study failed to demonstrate a significant benefit of oral zinc therapy, with a relative risk of healing of 1.5 (95% CI, 0.28 to 7.93). The remaining studies also failed to show any benefit of zinc therapy.

Topical zinc was evaluated in one study, suggesting improved healing in both arterial and venous ulcers. However, a study in porcine skin suggested that the only beneficial action of zinc on the wound bed was that it inhibited bacterial growth.[20]

Several studies have addressed the efficacy of retinoids in decreasing the edema associated with venous insufficiency.[21] Physiologically, it is believed that these agents protect the microcirculation from the increased pressures of ambulatory venous hypertension thereby preventing edema. A meta-analysis of four studies was recently published that evaluated a micronized purified flavonoid fraction (MPFF) of *Rutaceae aurantiae* (Daflon).[21] Basically, 500 mg of MPFF was administered orally twice daily for 2–6 months, which improved the likelihood of a venous leg ulcer healing by about 32%.[21]

Complications

There are few side effects associated with vitamin or mineral therapy for venous ulcers.

Comment

There is a lack of supporting evidence for the supplementary use of vitamin C and zinc. No studies have effectively evaluated the role of daily multivitamins in patients with chronic wounds. Rutosides may be helpful in edema reduction.

Implications for clinical practice

Vitamin supplementation is common and relatively benign. Reasonable evidence exists to support the use of rutosides.

Ultrasound, laser, and electromagnetic therapy
Benefits

Laser therapy using a variety of different lasers, ultrasound, and electromagnetic therapy have been proposed as adjunct treatments for venous leg ulcers. Low-level lasers, ultrasound, and electromagnets have been shown to stimulate cellular function, leading to increased protein synthesis and fibroblast and macrophage proliferation.

Ultrasound, laser therapy, and electromagnetic therapy for venous ulcers are the subject of Cochrane collaborative reviews including seven, four, and three trials, respectively.[22–24] None of the ultrasound studies found a statistically significant treatment effect.[23] The results of the laser studies were pooled in the Cochrane review and failed to demonstrate a significant benefit of laser therapy, with a relative risk of 1.21 (95% CI, 0.73 to 2.03).[24] The results of the electromagnetic therapy also did not demonstrate a statistically significant benefit.[22] However, these are all active areas of research. This is especially true for electromagnetic therapy, where it is also important to note that not all modalities use the same type, dose, or duration of electromagnetic field.

Complications
Complications occur very rarely with these therapies when therapy is administered by well-trained and experienced staff.

Comment
There is some suggestion that laser therapy and electromagnetic therapy may have an effect on end points other than chance of healing, for example pain at the wound site and the amount of granulation tissue. The use and meaningfulness of these end points remains an area in need of further investigation.

Implications for clinical practice
There is currently insufficient evidence to support the use of ultrasound, low-level laser and electromagnetic therapy in treating venous ulcers. Further well-designed trials are needed before these modalities should be widely adopted.

Intermittent pneumatic compression
Benefits
Intermittent pneumatic compression has been used for a number of indications. Since the underlying cause of venous ulceration is postulated to involve deficient blood return in the calf muscle pump, it has been suggested that intermittent pneumatic compression could improve the healing rates of venous ulcers by improving venous return (i.e., acting as a form of lower limb compression).

Intermittent pneumatic compression for the treatment of venous ulcers has been the subject of a Cochrane collaborative review.[25] This review evaluated four randomized controlled trials of intermittent pneumatic compression for the treatment of venous ulcers. One trial of 45 patients compared intermittent pneumatic compression plus standard limb compression with standard limb compression alone,

and found a significant benefit in the intermittent pneumatic compression plus standard compression group, with a relative risk of healing of 11.4 (95% CI, 1.6 to 82). Two other small trials (including 75 people altogether) failed to find a significant benefit of intermittent pneumatic compression plus standard compression over standard compression alone. Notably, the duration of therapy with intermittent pneumatic compression in these trials varied considerably. Moreover, the study end points differed substantially, ranging from 3–6 months. Results of these trials were therefore not pooled by the Cochrane group. One small study compared intermittent pneumatic compression alone (i.e., without standard compression) with standard compression, and failed to show a significant difference between the groups.

Complications
There are few real complications with intermittent pneumatic compression; as long as the equipment is properly set up, patients would not be expected to suffer any injuries.

Comment
Intermittent pneumatic compression may be beneficial as an adjunct to standard limb compression, but this has yet to be conclusively demonstrated. The largest study noted in the Cochrane review did demonstrate a benefit, but the standard compression used was graduated compression stockings—in contrast to the Unna boot used in another study, which failed to show a significant difference in the proportion of ulcers healed after 6 months. Of note, both studies demonstrated an increase in the actual rate of healing, suggesting that the different study end points (3 versus 6 months) may have played a role in the differing results.

The size and method of use of the equipment requires the patient to remain in a single place for the duration of therapy. The equipment is also costly.

Implications for clinical practice
Intermittent pneumatic compression may increase the rate of wound healing for patients already treated with standard compression, but further study is needed for this to be demonstrated conclusively.

What therapies are effective in reducing the risk of recurrence of venous leg ulcers?

Compression
Benefits
Compression therapy has been demonstrated to be an effective therapy for increasing the likelihood that a patient with venous ulcers will heal after 12 to 24 weeks. Since many venous ulcer patients have recurrent ulcers even after they have successfully healed, a pressing question remains as to whether continued compression after wound

healing could reduce the likelihood of recurrent venous ulcer formation.

A Cochrane collaborative review has evaluated compression as a treatment for preventing the recurrence of venous ulcers.[26] The systematic review did not find any studies directly comparing the incidence of recurrent ulcers in patients who did and did not use compression. Two studies were included in the systematic review: one study compared medium-compression and high-compression stockings and did not find a significant difference between the recurrence rates in these two groups. The other study compared two different types of medium-compression stocking and did not find any significant differences between the two groups. The studies did in fact examine differences in recurrence rates between patients who were and were not compliant with compression stockings, and this demonstrated that patients who were noncompliant with compression were more likely to have recurrent ulcerations.[26,27]

Another study conducted after this systematic review also addressed this issue, and found that compression stockings reduced the risk of recurrence of venous ulceration. This study of 153 people found that wearing compression stockings significantly reduced the risk of recurrence of venous ulcers at 6 months, with a relative risk reduction of 54% (95% CI, 24% to 72%).[26]

Complications

Complication rates are not usually noted in trials, partly because compression therapy is generally benign. Inexpertly applied high compression could lead to soft-tissue damage, the development of additional wounds, and potentially amputation, although the chance of this occurring is remote.

Comment

One study has shown that compression reduces the risk of recurrent venous ulceration. Two studies that compared different types of compression found that noncompliant patients had a higher rate of recurrence than those who were compliant with any type of compression regimen.[27] While these data may seem to suggest that ulcers may recur in patients who do not use compression, there are other confounding factors that need to be addressed before this conclusion can be drawn. For example, noncompliant patients may be more or less likely to have serious wounds or to comply with other elements of wound care, including nutrition and avoiding trauma.

The findings of the recent trial—coupled with the implications of the noncompliant patients' increased rate of recurrence from earlier trials and the biological plausibility of this therapy—mean that compression is likely to reduce the risk of recurrence of venous leg ulcers. Finally, compression therapy to prevent recurrence is considered by most wound-care experts to be "standard therapy." It might not be ethically justified to conduct a trial comparing limb compression with no limb compression for prevention of recurrent ulceration.

Implications for clinical practice

Compression appears to reduce the risk of recurrent venous ulceration, and should be recommended for all patients with a history of venous leg ulcers as long as they do not have any other conditions that would make this therapy potentially harmful (for example, arterial disease).

Surgery

Randomized clinical trials that evaluate the effects of surgery are very rare. However, one recent study deserves comment.[28,29] The Effect of Surgery and Compression on Healing and Recurrence (ESCHAR) study was a multicenter randomized controlled study that evaluated compression therapy with superficial venous surgery in comparison with compression therapy alone. While the number of individuals with healing after 24 weeks of therapy was the same in both groups, the individuals in the surgery group had persistence in their hemodynamic improvement and were less likely to have a recurrence on their venous leg ulcer after 12 months of follow-up.[28,29]

Key points

- Limb compression is the mainstay of therapy for venous leg ulcers, and several studies have shown that compression offers a clear benefit over no compression.
- Pentoxifylline and the flavonoid fraction of *Rutaceae aurantiae* as an adjuvant therapy to limb compression has been shown to increase the likelihood of healing.
- Skin equivalents as an adjuvant therapy to limb compression are associated with an increased likelihood of healing.
- The use of long-term limb compression therapy for those with a healed venous leg ulcer is associated with a decreased rate of recurrence, although poor compliance does compromise the effectiveness of this treatment.

References

1 Brem H, Kirsner RS, Falanga V. Protocol for the successful treatment of venous ulcers. *Am J Surg* 2004;**188**:1–8.

2 Margolis DJ, Bilker W, Santanna J, *et al*. Venous leg ulcer: incidence and prevalence in the elderly. *J Am Acad Dermatol* 2002; **46**:381–6.

3 Langer RD, Ho E, Denenberg JO, *et al*. Relationships between symptoms and venous disease: the San Diego population study. *Arch Intern Med* 2005;**165**:1420–4.

4 Criqui MH, Jamosmos M, Fronek A, *et al*. Chronic venous disease in an ethnically diverse population: the San Diego population study. *Am J Epidemiol* 2003;**158**:448–56.

5 Margolis DJ, Knauss J, Bilker W. Medical conditions associated with venous leg ulcers in an outpatient. *Br J Dermatol* 2004;**150**: 267–73.

6 Fletcher A, Cullum F, Sheldon TA. A systematic review of compression treatment for venous leg ulcers. *BMJ* 1997;**315**:576–80.

7 Nelson EA, Iglesias CP, Cullum N, *et al.* Randomized clinical trial of four-layer and short-stretch compression bandages for venous leg ulcers (VenUS I). *Br J Surg* 2004;**91**:1292–9.

8 Iglesias CP, Nelson EA, Cullum N, *et al.* Economic analysis of VenUS I, a randomized trial of two bandages for treating venous leg ulcers. *Br J Surg* 2004;**91**:1300–6.

9 Clarke-Moloney M, O'Brien JF, Grace PA, *et al.* Health-related quality of life during four-layer compression bandaging for venous ulcer disease: a randomised controlled trial. *Ir J Med Sci* 2005;**174**:21–5.

10 Jull A, Arroll B. Pentoxifylline for the treatment of venous leg ulcer: a systemic review. *Lancet* 2002;**359**:1550–4.

11 Falanga V, Fujitani RM, Diaz C, *et al.* Systemic treatment of venous leg ulcers with high doses of pentoxifylline: efficacy in a randomized, placebo-controlled trial. *Wound Repair Regen* 1999; **7**:208–13.

12 Jones JE, Nelson EA. Skin grafting for venous leg ulcers. *Cochrane Database Syst Rev* 2005;(**1**):CD001737.

13 Falanga V, Margolis D, Alvarez O, *et al.* Rapid healing of venous ulcers and lack of clinical rejection with an allogeneic cultured human skin equivalent. Human Skin Equivalent Investigators Group. *Arch Dermatol* 1998;**134**:293–300.

14 Falanga V, Sabolinski M. A bilayered living skin construct (APLIGRAF) accelerates complete closure of hard-to-heal venous ulcers. *Wound Repair Regen* 1999;**7**:201–7.

15 Mostow EN, Haraway GD, Dalsing M, *et al.* Effectiveness of an extracellular matrix graft (OASIS Wound Matrix) in the treatment of chronic leg ulcers: a randomized clinical trial. *J Vasc Surg* 2005;**41**:837–43.

16 Schonfeld WH, Villa KF, Fastenau JM, *et al.* An economic assessment of Apligraf (Graftskin) for the treatment of hard-to-heal venous leg ulcers. *Wound Repair Regen* 2000;**8**:251–7.

17 Margolis DJ, Cohen JH. Management of chronic venous leg ulcers: a literature-guided approach. *Clin Dermatol* 1994;**12**:19–26.

18 Margolis DJ, Lewis VL. A literature assessment of the use of miscellaneous topical agents, growth factors, and skin equivalents for the treatment of pressure ulcers. *Dermatol Surg* 1995;**21**:145–8.

19 Wilkinson EA, Hawke CI. Does oral zinc aid the healing of chronic leg ulcers? A systematic literature review. *Arch Dermatol* 1998;**134**:1556–60.

20 Agren MS. Studies on zinc in wound healing. *Acta Derm Venereol Suppl (Stockh)* 1990;**154**:1–36.

21 Coleridge-Smith P, Lok C, Ramelet AA. Venous leg ulcer: a meta-analysis of adjunctive therapy with micronized purified flavonoid fraction. *Eur J Vasc Endovasc Surg* 2005;**30**:198–208.

22 Flemming K, Cullum N. Electromagnetic therapy for the treatment of venous leg ulcers. *Cochrane Database Syst Rev* 2001;(**1**):CD002933. Update in: *Cochrane Database Syst Rev* 2006;(**2**):CD002933.

23 Flemming K, Cullum N. Therapeutic ultrasound for venous leg ulcers. *Cochrane Database Syst Rev* 2000;(**4**):CD001180.

24 Flemming K, Cullum N. Laser therapy for venous leg ulcers. *Cochrane Database Syst Rev* 2000;(**2**):CD001182.

25 Mani R, Vowden K, Nelson EA. Intermittent pneumatic compression for treating venous leg ulcers. *Cochrane Database Syst Rev* 2001;(**4**):CD001899.

26 Nelson EA, Bell-Syer SE, Cullum NA. Compression for preventing recurrence of venous ulcers. *Cochrane Database Syst Rev* 2000;(**4**):CD002303.

27 Franks PJ, Oldroyd MI, Dickson D, *et al.* Risk factors for leg ulcer recurrence: A randomized trial of two types of compression stockings. *Age Ageing* 1995;**24**:490–4.

28 Gohel MS, Barwell JR, Earnshaw JJ, *et al.* Randomized clinical trial of compression plus surgery versus compression alone in chronic venous ulceration (ESCHAR study): haemodynamic and anatomical changes. *Br J Surg* 2005;**92**:291–7.

29 Gohel MS, Barwell JR, Wakely C, *et al.* The influence of superficial venous surgery and compression on incompetent calf perforators in chronic venous leg ulceration. *Eur J Vasc Endovasc Surg* 2005;**29**:78–82.

IIIh Other important skin disorders

Michael Bigby, Editor

55 Cutaneous lupus erythematosus

Susan Jessop, David Whitelaw

Background

Definition

Systemic lupus erythematosus (SLE) is a multisystem inflammatory disease characterized by the presence of a wide variety of autoantibodies. Skin involvement is common, being present in 55–90% of cases.[1] The characteristic skin lesions can be divided into acute, subacute, and chronic subsets.[2] The acute forms include the malar (butterfly) rash, papular lesions, urticaria, vasculitic lesions, hair loss, and painless mouth ulcers. Subacute cutaneous lupus erythematosus (SCLE) is an uncommon form of cutaneous lupus, described as a clinical subset by Sontheimer in 1979.[3] Chronic discoid lupus erythematosus (DLE) tends to be the most persistent of the skin lesions and may lead to unsightly scarring. It is most frequently seen as an isolated entity, but may also occur in people with the systemic form of lupus (Figure 55.1).

Lupus panniculitis (also known as lupus profundus), neonatal lupus, lupus tumidus, and bullous lupus are less commonly encountered forms of the disease.

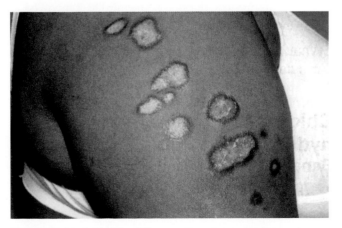

Figure 55.1 Lesions of discoid lupus erythematosus, showing scarring and changes in pigmentation.

What evidence there is for the treatment of cutaneous lupus largely relates to DLE.

Incidence/prevalence

Accurate figures are difficult to obtain, because different methods have been used in the reported studies. Reported prevalence rates vary from 12.5 per 100 000 in England to 50.8 per 100 000 in certain groups in the United States.[4] Many series are hospital-based and probably do not reflect the true incidence. African-American, Chinese, and Malaysian women appear to be the populations with the highest prevalence. Published figures suggest an increasing incidence, but the apparent increase may be due to greater awareness of the condition.

Etiology

Lupus seems to result from an interaction between genetic, hormonal, and environmental factors.[5] SLE is known to be associated with the production of a large range of autoantibodies. In certain specific subsets, such as neonatal lupus, their role in pathogenesis is now clearly established. The greatest risk factor is female sex (the female : male ratio is 9 : 1), and the highest prevalence is in the child-bearing age group. There is now evidence to suggest that estrogens stimulate the immune system, which may be the reason for this observation. The genetic hypothesis is supported by the familial clustering of lupus[6] and the association of certain HLA types with particular subsets of lupus.[7]

Evidence for a viral etiology has not been conclusive.[8]

Prognosis

Mortality is associated with severe systemic disease, and is highest with renal and central nervous system involvement.

Skin involvement, while not associated with mortality *per se*, frequently produces scarring, with considerable morbidity, both physical and psychological.

Diagnostic tests

Diagnosis of cutaneous lupus can generally be made by clinical examination, skin biopsy being used to confirm the diagnosis when the clinician is in doubt. Autoantibody tests (such as antinuclear antibody titer) may be positive in cutaneous lupus, but do not necessarily imply systemic disease. Specific antibodies, notably anti-Ro antibody, are strongly associated with certain subsets, such as SCLE and neonatal lupus.

Aims of treatment

As doctors, we aim to stop inflammation, and prevent further damage. Unfortunately, there may be marked residual pigmentary changes and skin atrophy (most marked in dark-skinned individuals). People with facial DLE may be disappointed by this outcome, as the quality of life remains impaired. Early diagnosis and treatment is important to prevent extensive scarring.

Relevant outcomes

• Improvement in the redness, thickness, or scaling of the lesions
• A reduction in the extent of the lesions
• Total clearing
• No change or worsening of skin lesions
• Development of new lesions

A scoring system, the Cutaneous Lupus Erythematosus Disease Area and Severity Index (CLASI), has been proposed in order to quantify activity and damage in cutaneous lupus.[9] The development of the CLASI is a promising move towards improved consistency in clinical trials, but we would recommend further refinement after testing in larger numbers of people and in different populations.

Methods of search

We searched the Cochrane Library (2006), Medline (1966 to March 2006), Embase (1988 to 2001), Science Direct (2001–March 2006), and the Cochrane Central Register of Controlled Trials. We included all randomized controlled trials (RCTs) and controlled trials. Where no controlled trials were found, we report briefly on observational studies.

Questions

What are the effects of antimalarial treatment in cutaneous lupus?

Chloroquine or hydroxychloroquine
Benefits
We found one systematic review.[10]

We found two RCTs involving antimalarials. Ruzicka et al. studied 39 people with DLE and 19 with SCLE, comparing hydroxychloroquine 400–1200 mg/day with acitretin 50 mg/day over 8 weeks.[11] The groups in the two treatment arms were similar in terms of age, sex, and extent of disease, but SCLE was more strongly represented in the hydroxychloroquine group. Complete clearing or marked improvement occurred in 15 of 30 people on hydroxychloroquine and 13 of 28 on acitretin. The response difference favoring hydroxychloroquine was 4% (95% confidence interval, –23% to 30%; number needed to treat 25, 95% CI, –5 to 4). Four participants dropped out because of treatment side effects (all in the acitretin arm) and three because of total clearing of lesions (all in the hydroxychloroquine arm). In the study by Bezerra et al., 33 people were randomly assigned to receive either 100 mg/day clofazimine (16 participants), or 250 mg chloroquine daily (17 participants). Skin lesions ranged from chronic discoid to acute lupus. There was no significant difference in the response rates at 6 months. The response rate was 14/17 (82%) in the chloroquine group and 12/17 (75%) in the clofazimine group. There were five withdrawals due to flares in the clofazimine group and one in the chloroquine group.[12] We found three RCTs of antimalarials in non–life-threatening SLE. In a Canadian study, people taking hydroxychloroquine for SLE were randomly assigned to continue the drug (n = 25) or to take a placebo (n = 22).[13] At 6 months, 16 of the 22 on placebo and nine of 25 in the active arm had experienced disease flares, a 2.5-fold increase in flares in the untreated participants (risk difference 0.37, 95% CI, 0.10 to 0.63; NNT 3, 95% CI, 2 to 10). Skin lesions were not specifically described. Williams compared hydroxychloroquine 400 mg/day with placebo in 71 people with mild SLE over 48 weeks.[14] Although the study was designed to determine the effect of the trial drug on joint disease, cutaneous, neurological, and cardiopulmonary systems were also evaluated. Placebo and active groups both improved, but overall there was no significant difference in the outcome of skin lesions between the two groups at any stage in the study. The third RCT involved 23 participants, 11 randomly assigned to receive chloroquine and 12 to receive placebo.[15] The chloroquine-treated group showed less skin activity than the placebo group, but the numbers involved were too small to reach significance. Overall, people taking chloroquine experienced fewer flares (two of 11 on chloroquine and 10 of 12 on placebo, relative risk 4.6) and required lower doses of steroids. The nature of the skin lesions was not documented.

We found one double-blind but nonrandomized trial comparing hydroxychloroquine with placebo in DLE.[16] Forty-nine people were treated for 1 year, 24 with hydroxychloroquine and 25 with placebo. Results at both 3 and 12 months indicated that hydroxychloroquine was superior to placebo. Using Wilcoxon's two-sample test, the authors calculated a K^2 value of 0.011 at 1 year, strongly suggesting that hydroxychloroquine was more effective than placebo. We found many observational reports of chloroquine or hydroxychloroquine in cutaneous lupus.[17–22] Christiansen reviewed 13 case series up to 1956 and added his own, giving data on a total of 414 people treated in these studies.[17] He noted that 265 (64%) experienced complete clearing or marked improvement. His series was notable for the duration of treatment (18–53 weeks) and the careful description of outcome, but was flawed by the absence of a parallel control group and the high dose of chloroquine (500–750 mg daily). Open trials of chloroquine in patients with lupus tumidus suggests that it may be useful in this condition.[23,24]

Harms

In the study by Ruzicka *et al.*, adverse events were described in 17 of 30 people taking hydroxychloroquine.[11] Symptoms included dry skin (n = 8), itching (n = 5) and gastrointestinal disturbance (n = 5). The most frequent side effects described by Kraak *et al.* were gastrointestinal (eight in hydroxychloroquine arm versus three in placebo arm), and cutaneous (four in the hydroxychloroquine arm versus three in the placebo arm).[16] However, in addition they identified one person who developed a severe retinopathy while taking hydroxychloroquine. This person had taken chloroquine previously for several years and had taken a high dose of hydroxychloroquine (1200 mg/day) during the trial. A valuable discussion of retinal toxicity is presented by Houpt.[25] A review of the systemic toxicity of chloroquine found little to support regular blood monitoring.[26] A meta-analysis of toxicities places the toxicity of antimalarials in perspective.[27] A small RCT in 20 pregnant women with lupus erythematosus, 10 taking hydroxychloroquine, showed no adverse effects in either mothers or babies.[28]

Comments

We found two randomized controlled trials, each comparing an antimalarial with another agent in cutaneous lupus.[11,12] Neither study demonstrated the superiority of one agent over another. Both studies included more than one type of cutaneous lupus, making interpretation difficult. The older observational studies lacked parallel control groups but included large numbers of participants, who were carefully followed up for long periods. Dosage tended to be unacceptably high by current standards.

We found three RCTs of chloroquine in mild SLE, but skin lesions were not described in detail.

We have not found evidence of a difference between hydroxychloroquine and chloroquine in the treatment of cutaneous lupus, or any information on this disorder regarding dosage in relation to either efficacy or toxicity.

Amodiaquine and quinacrine
Benefits

We found no RCTs or controlled trials. Wallace has

reviewed the literature on quinacrine, finding 20 observational trials.[29] Among 771 people, 209 (27%) showed an excellent response, although cutaneous subsets and outcome measures were not clearly defined. Smaller observational studies of amodiaquine have been published.[30,31]

Harms

Central nervous system, gastrointestinal and cutaneous adverse effects have been reported.

Combinations of antimalarials
Benefits

We found no controlled trials, but three observational trials and a case report of the combination of chloroquine and quinacrine in people with chronic cutaneous lupus.[32–35]

Harms

Yellow skin discoloration, photophobia, insomnia and nausea were noted by some people, but did not usually require withdrawal of treatment.

Intralesional antimalarials
Benefits

We found no controlled trials. We found two observational studies of intralesional chloroquine in a total of 23 people with DLE, with benefit noted in 11.[36,37]

Harms

Local inflammation occurred in one lesion.

What are the effects of systemic steroids in cutaneous lupus?

Oral steroids
Benefits

We found no RCT of oral steroids in cutaneous lupus. We found one observational study, reporting a "very good result" in two of 25 people (8%).[38] There is a case series of 15 people with DLE treated with a combination of antimalarial and oral steroid drugs.[39]

Harms

"Mild cushingoid features" were noted in two people taking oral steroids during the above study.[38] A recent review of side effects of low dose glucocorticoids suggest that the harms associated with these agents may not be as serious as traditionally held.[40]

Comments

There is not sufficient evidence to judge the efficacy of oral steroids in cutaneous lupus.

Intralesional steroids
Benefits

We found no RCTs. We found four case series, including

114 people. There was marked improvement or clearing in 91 participants (80%).[41-44]

Harms

Skin thinning (atrophy) was noted in a small percentage of people in the above studies.[38-42]

What are the effects of other oral agents in cutaneous lupus?

Clofazimine
Benefits

We found one small RCT comparing clofazimine with chloroquine, as reported in the section on antimalarials.[12] The two agents appeared to be comparable. We found four observational studies. A total of 31 of 50 people (62%) with chronic cutaneous lupus showed marked improvement on clofazimine at a dose ranging from 100 mg three times weekly to 100 mg/day.[45-49]

Harms

A pink or red discoloration and darkening of the skin resulting from the deposition of clofazimine has been recorded by several authors. Dry skin and keratosis pilaris were reported by Mackey and Barnes.[47] Jakes[48] reported a transient rise in transaminases. Arbiser and Moschella have reviewed the toxicity of clofazimine.[49]

Comments

A small RCT suggests that clofazimine may be useful in treatment of cutaneous lupus.

Dapsone
Benefits

We found no RCTs or controlled trials of dapsone in lupus erythematosus. Belief in the efficacy of dapsone is based on a number of observational studies. These studies report on a total of 55 people with various forms of cutaneous lupus.[50-52] Marked improvement was noted in 22 people (44%). The use of dapsone has also been reported in several case reports and particularly in people with unusual forms of lupus, such as bullous lupus and urticarial vasculitis.[53-58] Dosage varied from 25 to 150 mg/day.

Harms

Side effects described ranged from nausea, vomiting, headache, and fatigue to hemolysis, methemoglobinemia, and leukopenia. Mok et al. have reviewed the toxicity of dapsone.[59]

Comments

There is inadequate evidence to guide clinical practice.

Long-term remission without maintenance therapy is rare. Dapsone may have a specific role in bullous lupus, but this has not been established in clinical trials.

Methotrexate
Benefits

We found no RCTs, but one controlled trial of methotrexate in systemic lupus. Carneiro and Sato, in their double-blind study, reported that 12 of 20 patients in the active arm and 16 of 21 in the placebo arm had cutaneous lesions, declining to three in the active arm but remaining unchanged in the placebo group.[60] The skin lesions and outcome measures are not described. A retrospective study of cutaneous lupus recorded an improvement in 42 of 43 people.[61] We found small observational studies and case reports describing improvement in a variety of skin lesions of lupus.[62-72]

Harms

Problems encountered with methotrexate in these studies included dyspepsia, mouth ulcers, thrombocytopenia, a rise in transaminases, and an increased rate of infection.[60,63] A thorough discussion of methotrexate toxicity has been published by McKendry.[73]

Comments

The evidence for an improvement of skin lesions is too limited to allow any conclusions to be drawn.

Retinoids
Benefits

We found one RCT including 39 people with DLE and 19 with SCLE, in which hydroxychloroquine, 400–1200 mg/day, was compared with acitretin, 50 mg/day, over 8 weeks,[11] described above in the section on hydroxychloroquine. We found three uncontrolled trials, reporting a 72% improvement and several case reports of oral or topical retinoids in chronic cutaneous lupus.[74-83]

Harms

Retinoids are teratogenic. Side effects were recorded more commonly with acitretin (27 of 28 people) than with chloroquine.[11] Symptoms were predominantly cutaneous, with dry lips, dry skin, itching and hair loss being most common. Raised serum triglycerides were noted in five of 18 people. All improved with dose reduction and resolved when therapy was discontinued. Retinoid toxicity has been reviewed by Lowe and David.[84]

Comments

There is insufficient evidence to assess the value of retinoids in cutaneous lupus. The available evidence suggests that the efficacy is similar to that of hydroxychloroquine, but that side effects appear to be more frequent.

Thalidomide
Benefits

We found no RCTs or controlled trials. The open trials,

in general (but not universally), have included patients resistant to the conventional therapies of antimalarials and topical steroids.

There have been 10 uncontrolled studies and several case series, suggesting benefit in 60–95% of people.[85–95] The number of patients in these trials ranged from seven to 23 and the period of completed treatment varied from weeks to years. Duong *et al.* reported on patients who had been on treatment for 8–9 years. Low-dose maintenance therapy (50–100 mg/day) successfully controlled disease in the majority of cases.[90]

Harms

Thalidomide is teratogenic. Varying incidences of paresthesia and electroneurographic changes have been reported. There is not always a good correlation between clinical findings and conduction studies. Other side effects reported have been drowsiness, dizziness, vertigo, dreams, mood changes, weight gain, and constipation.[96–98] Rarely was it necessary to stop the drug. Calabrese and Fleischer have reviewed the side effects of thalidomide.[97]

Comments

The evidence for efficacy relies on a number of observational studies and a large number of case reports. There is inadequate evidence to guide clinicians in the use of thalidomide in lupus, although published studies do suggest that thalidomide may have a role in the person with disease resistant to other agents.

Implications for clinical practice

Current recommendations for people taking thalidomide include patient education about the risks of pregnancy and the significance of paresthesia, a 3-monthly clinical examination, and electrophysiological studies, if indicated.

Other systemic agents

Short series or case reports describe the use of a range of agents. Some showed benefit, others a lack of benefit, and some were associated with development of cutaneous lupus. Agents include azathioprine,[99–102] ciclosporin,[103–106] gold,[107–111] mycophenolate mofetil,[112,113] phenytoin,[114] and vitamin E,[115–120] but there is no evidence for their effectiveness and we will not discuss these agents further.

While biological agents have been reported to be beneficial in case reports, there are also reports of tumor necrosis factor antagonists inducing lupus-like lesions.[121–125]

What are the effects of topical agents in cutaneous lupus?

Topical steroids

Benefits

We found one RCT of potent topical steroids. In a 12-week crossover study, 0.05% fluocinonide (a potent steroid cream)

was compared with 1% hydrocortisone (a low-potency steroid cream).[126] After 6 weeks, an excellent response was seen in 10 of 37 people (27%) using fluocinonide and in four of 41 people (10%) using hydrocortisone cream (response difference 17%, 95% CI, 0.3% to 34%; NNT 6, 95% CI, 3 to 311). This result suggests that high-potency steroid cream is more effective than low-potency steroid cream.

We found two controlled trials, both flawed by small numbers and short duration. One study compared two potent topical steroids: 0.025% fluocinolone acetonide and 0.1% betamethasone valerate used for 3 weeks. Symmetrical skin lesions were treated, and the participants used the creams on the right or left side of the body. Betamethasone valerate appeared to be superior in 15 of 25 (60%) participants.[127]

Bjornberg and Hellgren used the symmetrical skin lesion design to compare fluocinolone acetonide with ointment base; 17 of 20 people (85%), showed greater improvement with the steroid than with base alone.[128]

We found six observational studies of topical steroids.[129–134] A total of 263 people were treated in these trials, 220 (84%) of whom experienced complete clearing or marked improvement in the treated areas.

Harms

Skin irritation was noted by three people using hydrocortisone, and a burning sensation by one person using fluocinonide.[126] No side effects were reported in the other controlled trials. Toxicity of topical steroids has been reviewed recently by Hengge *et al.*[135]

Comments

All the controlled trials of topical steroid were of short duration, but the evidence does appear to support the use of potent topical steroids in DLE.

The possible impact of skin atrophy with the use of topical steroids in DLE has not been evaluated.

Calcineurin antagonists

Benefits

We found one small, short-term RCT. There were 20 participants with cutaneous LE, randomized to use 0.1% tacrolimus cream on the right or left side of the face, while using 0.05% clobetasol propionate cream on the other side.[136] Clinical outcome, (degree of erythema, desquamation and induration), was recorded weekly for 4 weeks. Only 4 of the participants had DLE and their outcomes were not reported separately. At 4 weeks all treated areas were judged to have improved, with no difference seen between the 2 forms of treatments.

We found case reports and uncontrolled studies on the use of either tacrolimus or pimecrolimus in a total of 47 people, most suggesting some benefit.[137–143]

Harms

RCTs using these agents for other conditions have identified irritation and a sensation of burning as common in the early stages of treatment.[144] Carcinogenesis has been raised as a potential concern.[145]

Comment

Tacrolimus cream may be an effective alternative to topical steroid in people who experience steroid-related adverse effects. However, there is as yet no clear evidence to guide the use of these agents in cutaneous lupus.

What are the effects of non-drug treatments in cutaneous lupus?

Sunscreens
Benefits

We found one double-blind intra-individual trial on the efficacy of sunscreens in the prevention of the skin lesions in SLE. People using three different commercially available sunscreens were tested with ultraviolet light. Protective efficacy varied from 100% to < 30%.[146] We found one further open-label study.[147] Broad-spectrum sunscreen decreased skin disease activity significantly over an 8-week period.

Comments

There is insufficient evidence to guide the clinician in the use of sunscreens.

Surgery
Benefits

We found no RCTs or controlled trials. We found six reports describing 17 people treated with either dermabrasion or excision and grafting.[148–153] The results were favorable in all cases, but with four patients suffering recurrences.

Comments

Insufficient data are available to comment.

Ultraviolet light
Benefits

We found one controlled trial of ultraviolet A1 (UVA1, 350–440 nm) in 11 people with systemic lupus.[154] Although the trial was double blind, the findings cannot be interpreted with confidence because the numbers were small, skin lesions were not clearly described, and the two arms (nine active treatment, two placebo) were disproportionate.

We found several observational studies and case reports.[155–157] We also found case reports describing the use of extracorporeal photopheresis in cutaneous lupus.[158–160]

Harms

No adverse events were reported in the above studies.

Comments

There is currently insufficient evidence to comment on the use of ultraviolet light. There is no evidence to indicate the relative risk of inducing a flare in this light-sensitive disorder.

Laser treatment
Benefits

We found no RCTs or controlled trials. We found two case series and five case reports.[161–167] Clearing or marked improvement was noted in 32 of a total of 54 people with cutaneous lupus, using either pulsed dye or argon laser.

Harms

Transient pigmentation was seen in some people.

Comment

There is insufficient evidence to assess the efficacy of laser treatment in cutaneous lupus.

Key points

- We found limited evidence that potent topical steroids, chloroquine, and acitretin are beneficial in cutaneous lupus.
- We found many observational studies, some involving large numbers of people, followed for several years, including treatment with methotrexate and thalidomide.

References

1 Yell JA, Mbuagbaw J, Burge SM. Cutaneous manifestations of systemic lupus erythematosus. *Br J Dermatol* 1996;**135**:355–62.
2 Gilliam JN, Sontheimer RD. Distinctive cutaneous subsets in the spectrum of lupus erythematosus. *J Am Acad Dermatol* 1981;**4**: 471–5.
3 Sontheimer RD, Thomas JR, Gilliam JN. Subacute cutaneous lupus erythematosus: a cutaneous marker for a distinct lupus erythematosus subset. *Arch Dermatol* 1979;**115**:1409–15.
4 Hochberg MC. The epidemiology of systemic lupus erythematosus. In: Wallace DJ, Hahn BH, eds. *Dubois' Lupus Erythematosus.* Philadelphia: Lea and Febiger, 1993:49–57.
5 Isenberg DA. Systemic lupus erythematosus: immunopathogenesis and the card game analogy. *J Rheumatol* 1997;**24**:62–6.
6 Arnett FC. The genetic basis of lupus erythematosus. In: Wallace DJ, Hahn BH, eds. *Dubois' Lupus Erythematosus.* Philadelphia: Lea and Febiger, 1993:13–36.
7 Millard TP, McGregor JM. Molecular genetics of cutaneous lupus erythematosus. *Clin Exp Dermatol* 2001;**26**:184–91.
8 Vaughan JH. Viruses and autoimmune disease. *J Rheumatol* 1996;**23**:1831–3.
9 Albrecht J, Taylor L, Berlin JA, *et al.* The CLASI (Cutaneous Lupus erythematosus disease Area and Severity Index): an outcome instrument for cutaneous lupus erythematosus. *J Invest Dermatol* 2005;**125**:889–94.
10 Jessop S, Whitelaw D, Jordaan F. Drugs for discoid lupus erythematosus. *Cochrane Database Syst Rev* 2001;(**1**):CD002954.

11 Ruzicka T, Sommerburg C, Goerz G, Kind P, Mensing H. Treatment of cutaneous lupus erythematosus with acitretin and hydroxychloroquine. *Br J Dermatol* 1992;**127**:513–8.

12 Bezerra EL, Vilar MJ, da Trindade Nedo, *et al.* Double blind, randomized, controlled clinical trial of clofazimine compared with chloroquine in patients with systemic lupus erythematosus. *Arthritis Rheum* 2005;**52**:3073–8.

13 Canadian Hydroxychloroquine Study Group. A randomized study of the effect of withdrawing hydroxychloroquine sulphate in systemic lupus erythematosus. *N Engl J Med* 1991;**324**:150–4.

14 Williams HJ, Egger MJ, Singer JZ, *et al.* Comparison of hydroxychloroquine and placebo in the treatment of mild systemic lupus erythematosus. *J Rheumatol* 1994;**21**:1457–62.

15 Meinao IM, Sato EI, Andrade LE, *et al.* Controlled trial with chloroquine diphosphate in systemic lupus erythematosus. *Lupus* 1996;**5**:237–41.

16 Kraak JH, van Ketel WG, Prakken JR. The value of hydroxychloroquine (Plaquenil) for the treatment of chronic discoid lupus erythematosus: a double blind trial. *Dermatologica* 1965;**130**:293–305.

17 Christiansen JV. Treatment of lupus erythematosus with chloroquine. *Br J Dermatol* 1957;**69**:158–68.

18 Brodthagen H. Hydroxychloroquine (Plaquenil) in the treatment of lupus erythematosus. *Acta Derm Venereol* 1959;**39**:233–7.

19 Crissey JT, Murray PF. A comparison of chloroquine and gold in the treatment of lupus erythematosus. *Arch Dermatol* 1956;**74**:69–72.

20 Galla F. L'idrossiclorochina nel trattamento dell'eritematodes cronico. *Minerva Dermatol* 1961;**36**:99–101.

21 Goode P. Plaquenil in the treatment of cutaneous lupus erythematosus. *Br J Dermatol* 1958;**70**:176–8.

22 Tye MJ, Schiff BL, Collins SF, Baler GR, Appel B. Chronic discoid lupus erythematosus. Treatment with Daraprim and chloroquine diphosphate (Aralen). *N Engl J Med* 1954;**251**:52–5.

23 Kuhn A, Richter-Hinz D, Oslislo C, *et al.* Lupus erythematosus tumidus. *Arch Dermatol* 2000;**136**:1033–41.

24 Choonhakarn C, Poonsriaram A, Chaivoremukul J. Lupus erythematosus tumidus. *Int J Dermatol* 2004;**43**:815–8.

25 Houpt JB. A rheumatologist's verdict on the safety of chloroquine versus hydroxychloroquine. *J Rheumatol* 1999:**26**:1864–7.

26 Sontheimer R. Questions answered and a $1 million question raised concerning lupus erythematosus tumidus. *Arch Dermatol* 2000;**136**:1044–9.

27 Felson DT, Anderson JJ, Meenan RF. The comparative efficacy and toxicity of second-line drugs in rheumatoid arthritis. Results of two meta-analyses. *Arthritis Rheum* 1990;**33**:1449–59.

28 Levy RA, Vilela VS, Cataldo MJ, *et al.* Hydroxychloroquine in lupus pregnancy: double-blind and placebo-controlled study. *Lupus* 2001;**10**:401–4.

29 Wallace DJ. The use of quinacrine (Atabrine) in rheumatic diseases: a reexamination. *Semin Arthritis Rheum* 1989;**18**:282–96.

30 Maguire A. Amodiaquine hydrochloride in the treatment of chronic discoid lupus erythematosus. *Lancet* 1962;**31**:665–7.

31 Leeper RW, Allende MF. Antimalarials in the treatment of discoid lupus erythematosus. *Arch Dermatol* 1956;**73**:50–7.

32 Feldmann R, Salomon D, Saurat JH. The association of the two antimalarials chloroquine and quinacrine for treatment-resistant chronic and subacute cutaneous lupus erythematosus. *Dermatology* 1994;**189**:425–7.

33 Lipsker D, Piette JC, Cacoub P, Godeau P, Frances C. Chloroquine–quinacrine association in resistant cutaneous lupus. *Dermatology* 1995;**190**:257–8.

34 Tye MJ, White H, Appel B, Ansell HB. Lupus erythematosus treated with a combination of quinacrine, hydroxychloroquine and chloroquine. *N Engl J Med* 1959;**260**:63–5.

35 Von Schmiedeberg S, Ronnau AC, Schuppe HC, Specker C, Ruzicka T, Lehmann P. [Combination of antimalarial drugs mepacrine and chloroquine in therapy refractory cutaneous lupus erythematosus; in German.] *Hautarzt* 2000;**51**:82–5.

36 Everett MA, Coffey CM. Intradermal administration of chloroquine for discoid lupus erythematosus and lichen sclerosis et atrophicus. *Arch Dermatol* 1961;**83**:977–9.

37 Pelzig A, Witten VH, Sulzberger MB. Chloroquine for chronic discoid lupus erythematosus. *Arch Dermatol* 1961;**83**:146–8.

38 Callen JP. Chronic cutaneous lupus erythematosus. *Arch Dermatol* 1982;**118**:412–6.

39 Alexander S, Cowan MA. The treatment of chronic discoid lupus erythematosus with a combination of antimalarial and corticosteroid drugs. *Br J Dermatol* 1961;**73**:359–61.

40 Da Silva JAP, Jacobs JWG, Kirwan JR, *et al.* Safety of low dose glucocorticoid treatment in rheumatoid arthritis: published evidence and prospective trial data. *Ann Rheum Dis* 2006;**65**:285–93.

41 Smith JF. Intralesional triamcinolone as an adjunct to antimalarial drugs in the treatment of chronic discoid lupus erythematosus. *Br J Dermatol* 1962;**74**:350–3.

42 James APR. Intradermal triamcinolone acetonide in localized lesions. *J Invest Dermatol* 1980;**34**:175–6.

43 Kraak JH. [Local treatment of chronic lupus erythematosus with triamcinolone injections; in Dutch.] *Ned Tijdschr Geneeskd* 1964;**108**:1305–6.

44 Rowell NR. Treatment of chronic discoid lupus erythematosus with intralesional triamcinolone. *Br J Dermatol* 1962;**74**:354–7.

45 Dupré A, Bonafé JL, Lassére J, Albarel N, Christol B. Traitement du lupus érythémateux chronique par le lampréne. *Ann Dermatol Venereol* (Paris) 1978;**105**:423–5.

46 Krivanek J, Paver WKA, Kossard S. (Lamprone) in the treatment of discoid lupus erythematosus. *Dermatol* 1976;**17**:108–10.

47 Mackey JP, Barnes J. Clofazimine in the treatment of discoid lupus erythematosus. *Br J Dermatol* 1974;**91**:93–6.

48 Jakes JT, Dubois EL, Quismorio FP. Antileprosy drugs and lupus erythematosus. *Ann Intern Med* 1982;**97**:788.

49 Arbiser JL, Moschella SL. Clofazimine: review of its medical uses and mechanisms of action. *J Am Acad Dermatol* 1995;**32**:241–7.

50 Coburn PR, Shuster S. Dapsone and discoid lupus erythematosus. *Br J Dermatol* 1982;**106**:105–6.

51 Lindskov R, Reymann F. Dapsone in the treatment of cutaneous lupus erythematosus. *Dermatologica* 1986;**172**:214–7.

52 Ruzicka T, Goerz G. Dapsone in the treatment of lupus erythematosus. *Br J Dermatol* 1981;**104**:53–5.

53 Bohm I, Bruns A, Schupp G, Bauer R. [ANCA-positive lupus erythematodes profundus. Successful therapy with low dosage dapsone; in German.] *Hautarzt* 1998;**49**:403–7.

54 Hall RP, Lawley TJ, Smith HR, Katz SI. Bullous eruption of systemic lupus erythematosus. Dramatic response to dapsone therapy. *Ann Intern Med* 1982;**97**:165–70.

55 Holtman JH, Neustadt DH, Klein J, Callen JP. Dapsone is an effective therapy for the skin lesions of subacute cutaneous

lupus erythematosus and urticarial vasculitis in a patient with C2 deficiency. *J Rheumatol* 1990;**17**:1222–5.

56 McCormack LS, Elgart ML, Turner MLC. Annular subacute cutaneous lupus erythematosus responsive to dapsone. *J Am Acad Dermatol* 1984;**11**:397–401.

57 Neri R, Mosca M, Bernacchi E, Bombardieri S. A case of SLE with acute, subacute and chronic cutaneous lesions successfully treated with dapsone. *Lupus* 1999;**8**:240–3.

58 Tsutsui K, Imai T, Hatta N, *et al.* Widespread pruritic plaques in a patient with subacute cutaneous lupus erythematosus and hypocomplementemia: response to dapsone therapy. *J Am Acad Dermatol* 1996;**35**:313–5.

59 Mok CC, Lau, CS, Wong RW. Toxicities of dapsone in the treatment of cutaneous manifestations of rheumatic diseases. *J Rheumatol* 1998;**25**:1246–7.

60 Carneiro JR, Sato EI. Double blind, randomized, placebo-controlled clinical trial of methotrexate in systemic lupus erythematosus. *J Rheumatol* 1999;**26**:1275–9.

61 Wenzel J, Brahler S, Bauer R, *et al.* Efficacy and safety of methotrexate in recalcitrant cutaneous lupus erythematosus: results of a retrospective study in 43 patients. *Br. J Dermatol* 2005;**153**:157–62.

62 Gansauge S, Breitbart A, Rinaldi N, Schwarz-Eywill M. Methotrexate in patients with moderate systemic lupus erythematosus (exclusion of renal and central nervous system disease). *Ann Rheum Dis* 1997;**56**:382–5.

63 Wilson J, Abeles M. A 2 year, open ended trial of methotrexate in systemic lupus erythematosus. *J Rheumatol* 1994;**21**:1674–7.

64 Arfi S, Numeric P, Grollier L, Panelatti G, Jean-Baptiste G. [Treatment of corticodependent systemic lupus erythematosus with low dose methotrexate; in French.] *Rev Med Interne* 1995;**16**:885–90.

65 Davidson JR, Graziano FM, Rothenberg RJ. Methotrexate therapy for severe systemic lupus erythematosus. *Arthritis Rheum* 1987;**30**:1195–6.

66 Garcia G, Portales G, Nebro F, *et al.* Effectiveness of the treatment of systemic lupus erythematosus with methotrexate. *Med Clin (Barc)* 1993;**101**:361–4.

67 Bohm L, Uerlich M, Bauer R. Rapid improvement of subacute cutaneous lupus erythematosus with low-dose methotrexate. *Dermatology* 1997;**194**:307–8.

68 Rothenberg RJ, Graziano FM, Grandone JT, *et al.* The use of methotrexate in steroid-resistant systemic lupus erythematosus. *Arthritis Rheum* 1988;**31**:612–5.

69 Walz LeBlanc BAE, Dagenais P, Urowitz MB, Gladman DD. Methotrexate in systemic lupus erythematosus. *J Rheum* 1994;**21**:836–8.

70 Bottomley WW, Goodfield M. Methotrexate for the treatment of severe mucocutaneous lupus erythematosus. *Br J Dermatol* 1995;**133**:311–4.

71 Malcangi G, Brandozzi G, Giangiacomi M, *et al.* Bullous SLE: response to methotrexate and relationship with disease activity. *Lupus* 2003;**12**:63–6.

72 Kuhn A, Specker, Ruzicka T. Methotrexate treatment for refractory subacute cutaneous lupus erythematosus. *J Am Acad Dermatol* 2002;**46**:600–3.

73 McKendry RJR. The remarkable spectrum of methotrexate toxicities. *Rheum Dis Clin North Am* 1997;**23**:939–45.

74 Grupper C, Berretti B. Lupus erythematosus and etretinate. In: Cunliffe W, Miller A, eds. *Retinoid Therapy: a Review of Clinical and Laboratory Research.* Lancaster: MTP Press, 1984:73–81.

75 Ruzicka T, Meurer M, Braun-Falco O. Treatment of cutaneous lupus erythematosus with etretinate. *Acta Derm Venereol* 1985;**65**:324–9.

76 Ruzicka T, Meurer M, Bieber T. Efficiency of acitretin in the treatment of cutaneous lupus erythematosus. *Arch Dermatol* 1988;**124**:897–902.

77 Furner BB. Subacute cutaneous lupus erythematosus. Response to isotretinoin. *Int J Dermatol* 1990;**29**:587–90.

78 Green SG, Piette WW. Successful treatment of hypertrophic lupus erythematosus with isotretinoin. *J Am Acad Dermatol* 1987;**17**:364–8.

79 Marks R. Lichen planus and cutaneous lupus erythematosus. In: Lowe N, Marks R, eds. *Retinoids.* London: Dunitz, 1995:143–7.

80 Newton RC, Jorizzo JL, Solomon AR, *et al.* Mechanism-oriented assessment of isotretinoin in chronic or subacute cutaneous lupus erythematosus. *Arch Dermatol* 1986;**122**:170–6.

81 Rubenstein DJ, Huntley AC. Keratotic lupus erythematosus: treatment with isotretinoin. *J Am Acad Dermatol* 1986;**14**:910–4.

82 Shornick JK, Formica N, Parke AL. Isotretinoin for refractory lupus erythematosus. *J Am Acad Dermatol* 1991;**24**:49–52.

83 Seiger E, Roland S, Goldman S. Cutaneous lupus treated with topical tretinoin: a case report. *Cutis* 1991;**47**:351–5.

84 Lowe NJ, David M. Toxicity. In: Lowe N, Marks R, eds. *Retinoids. A Clinician's Guide.* London: Dunitz, 1998:149–65.

85 Knop J, Bonsmann G, Happle R, *et al.* Thalidomide in the treatment of sixty cases of chronic discoid lupus erythematosus. *Br J Derm* 1983;**108**:461–6.

86 Stevens RJ, Andujar C, Edwards CJ, *et al.* Thalidomide in the treatment of the cutaneous manifestations of lupus erythematosus: experience in sixteen consecutive patients. *Br J Rheumatol* 1997;**36**:353–9.

87 Samsoen M, Grosshans E, Basset A. La thalidomide dans le traitement du lupus érythémateux chronique. *Ann Dermatol Venereol* 1980;**107**:515–23.

88 Atra E, Sato EI. Treatment of the cutaneous lesions of systemic lupus erythematosus with thalidomide. *Clin Exp Rheumatol* 1993;**11**:487–93.

89 Ordi-Ros J, Cortes F, Cucurull E, *et al.* Thalidomide in the treatment of cutaneous lupus refractory to conventional therapy. *J Rheumatol* 2000;**27**:1429–33.

90 Duong DJ, Spigel T, Moxley RT, *et al.* American experience with low dose thalidomide therapy for severe cutaneous lupus erythematosus. *Arch Dermatol* 1999;**135**:1079–87.

91 Hasper MF. Chronic cutaneous lupus erythematosus. Thalidomide treatment of 11 patients. *Arch Dermatol* 1983;**119**:812–5.

92 Naafs B, Faber WR. Thalidomide therapy. An open trial. *Int J Dermatol* 1985;**24**:131–4.

93 Coelho A, Souto MI, Cardoso CR, *et al.* Long-term thalidomide use in refractory cutaneous lesions of lupus erythematosus: a 65 series of Brazilian patients. *Lupus* 2005;**14**:434–9.

94 Cuadrado MJ, Karim Y, Sanna G, *et al.* Thalidomide for the treatment of resistant cutaneous lupus: efficacy and safety of different therapeutic regimens. *Am J Med* 2005;**118**:246–50.

95 Gambini D, Carrera C, Passoni E, *et al.* Thalidomide treatment for hypertrophic cutaneous lupus erythematosus. *J Dermatolog Treat* 2004;**15**:365–71.

96 Tseng S, Pak G, Washenik K, *et al.* Rediscovering thalidomide: a review of its mechanism of action, side effects and potential uses. *J Am Acad Dermatol* 1996;**35**:969–79.

97 Calabrese L, Fleischer AB. Thalidomide: current and potential clinical applications. *Am J Med* 2000;**108**:487–95.

98 Briani C, Zara G, Rondinone R, *et al.* Positive and negative effects of thalidomide on refractory cutaneous lupus erythematosus. *Autoimmunity* 2005;**38**:549–55.

99 Callen J, Spencer LV, Burruss JB, Holtman J. Azathioprine. *Arch Dermatol* 1991;**127**:515–22.

100 Ashinoff R, Werth VP, Franks AG. Resistant discoid lupus erythematosus of palms and soles: successful treatment with azathioprine. *J Am Acad Dermatol* 1988;**19**:961–5.

101 Shehade S. Successful treatment of generalised discoid skin lesions with azathioprine. *Arch Dermatol* 1986;**122**:376–7.

102 Tsokos GC, Caughman SW, Klippel JH. Successful treatment of generalised discoid skin lesions with azathioprine. *Arch Dermatol* 1985;**121**:1323–5.

103 Yell JA, Burge SM. Cyclosporin and discoid lupus erythematosus. *Br J Dermatol* 1994;**131**:132–3.

104 Saeki Y, Ohshima S, Kurimoto I, Miura H, Suemura M. Maintaining remission of lupus erythematosus profundus (LEP) with cyclosporin A. *Lupus* 2000;**9**:390–2.

105 Di Lernia V, Biosighini G. Discoid lupus erythematosus during treatment with cyclosporine. *Acta Derm Venereol* 1996;**76**:87–8.

106 Obermoser G, Weber F, Sepp N. Discoid lupus erythematosus in a patient receiving cyclosporin for liver transplantation. *Acta Derm Venereol* 2001;**81**:319.

107 Wright CS. Ten years experience in the treatment of lupus erythematosus with gold compounds. *Arch Dermatol Syph* 1936;**33**:413–29.

108 Rutledge WU. Lupus erythematosus. Treatment with gold preparations. *Arch Dermatol Syph* 1931;**23**:874–83.

109 Strandberg J. Six years' experience of the treatment of lupus erythematosus with gold compounds. *Acta Med Scand* 1931;**75**:296–317.

110 Pascher F. Treatment of lupus erythematosus with calciferol, antibiotics and gold preparations. *Arch Dermatol Syph* 1950;**61**:906–12.

111 Dalziel K, Going G, Cartwright PH, *et al.* Treatment of chronic discoid lupus erythematosus with an oral gold compound (auranofin). *Br J Dermatol* 1986;**115**:211–6.

112 Goyal S, Nousari HC. Treatment of resistant discoid lupus erythematosus of the palms and soles with mycophenolate mofetil. *J Am Acad Dermatol* 2001;**45**:142–4.

113 Pisoni CN, Obermoser G, Cuadrado MJ, *et al.* Skin manifestations of systemic lupus erythematosus refractory to multiple treatment modalities: poor results with mycophenolate mofetil. *Clin Exp Rheumatol* 2005;**23**:393–6.

114 Rodriguez-Castellanos MA, Rubio JB, Gomez JFB, Mendonza AG. Phenytoin in the treatment of discoid lupus erythematosus. *Arch Dermatol* 1995;**131**:620–1.

115 Morgan J. A note on the treatment of lupus erythematosus with vitamin E. *Br J Dermatol* 1951;**63**:224–5.

116 Burgess JF, Pritchard JE. Tocopherols (vitamin E). Treatment of lupus erythematosus: preliminary report. *Arch Dermatol Syph* 1948;**57**:953–64.

117 Pascher F, Sawicky HH, Silverberg MF, *et al.* Tocopherol (vitamin E) for discoid lupus erythematosus and other dermatoses. *J Invest Dermatol* 1951;**17**:261–2.

118 Sawicky HH. Therapy of lupus erythematosus. *Arch Dermatol Syph* 1950;**61**:906–9.

119 Sweet RD. Vitamin E in collagenoses. *Lancet* 1948;**ii**:310–1.

120 Yell JA, Burge S, Wojnarowska F. Vitamin E and discoid lupus erythematosus. *Lupus* 1992;**1**:303–5.

121 Drosou A, Kirsner RS, Welsh E, Sullivan TP, Kerdel FA. Use of infliximab, an anti-tumour necrosis alpha antibody, for inflammatory dermatoses. *J Cutan Med Surg* 2003;**7**:382–6.

122 Norman R, Greenberg RG, Jackson M. Case reports of etanercept in inflammatory dermatoses. *J Am Acad Dermatol* 2006;**54** (3 Suppl 2):S139–42.

123 Scheinfeld N. The medical uses and side effects of etanercept with a focus on cutaneous disease. *J Drugs Dermatol* 2004;**3**:653–9.

124 Stratigos AJ, Antoniou C, Stamathioudaki S, *et al.* Discoid lupus erythematosus-like eruption induced by infliximab. *Clin Exper Dermatol* 2004;**29**:150–3.

125 Prinz JC, Meurer M, Reiter C, *et al.* Treatment of severe cutaneous lupus erythematosus with a chimeric CD4 monoclonal antibody, cM-T412. *J Am Acad Dermatol* 1996;**34**:244–52.

126 Roenigk HH, Martin JS, Eichorn P, Gilliam JN. Discoid lupus erythematosus. Diagnostic features and evaluation of topical corticosteroid therapy. *Cutis* 1980;**25**:281–5.

127 Bjornberg A, Hellgren L. Topical treatment of chronic discoid lupus erythematosus with betamethason-17-valerate and fluocinolone acetonideaa double blind study. *Indian J Dermatol* 1966;**12**:17–8.

128 Bjornberg A, Hellgren L. Treatment of chronic discoid lupus erythematosus with fluocinolone acetonide ointment. *Br J Dermatol* 1963;**75**:156–60.

129 Bjornberg A, Hellgren L. Treatment of chronic discoid lupus erythematosus with betamethasone-17,21 dipropionate. *Curr Ther Res* 1976;**19**:442–3.

130 Haneke E. Long-term treatment with 6 α-methylprednisolone aceponate. *J Eur Acad Dermatol Venereol* 1994;**3**:S19–S22.

131 Jansen GT, Dillaha CJ, Honeycutt WM. Discoid lupus erythematosus. *Arch Dermatol* 1965;**92**:283–5.

132 Marsden CW. Fluocinolone acetonide 0.2% cream—a co-operative clinical trial. *Br J Dermatol* 1968;**80**:614–7.

133 Mitchell AD, Mitchell DM. Fluocinolone acetonide in the treatment of chronic discoid lupus erythematosus. *Lancet* 1962;**ii**:359.

134 Reymann F. Treatment of discoid lupus erythematosus with betamethasone-valerate cream 1%. *Dermatologica* 1974;**149**:65–8.

135 Hengge UR, Ruzicka T, Schwartz RA, Cork MJ. Adverse effects of glucocorticosteroids. *J. Am Acad Dermatol* 2006;**54**:1–15.

136 T-y. Tzung, y-s. Liu, h-w. Chang Tacrolimus vs. clobetasol propionate in the treatment of facial cutaneous lupus erythematosus: a randomized, double-blind, bilateral comparison study. *British Journal of Dermatology* 2007;**156**(1):191–192.

137 Walker SL, Kirby B, Chalmers RJG. Letter. *Eur J Dermatol* 2002;**12**:387–8.

138 Kanekura T, Yoshii N, Terasaki K, Miyoshi H, Kanzaki T. Efficacy of topical tacrolimus for treating the malar rash of systemic lupus erythematosus. *Br J Dermatol* 2003;**148**:353–6.

139 Böhm M, Gaubitz M, Luger TA, Metze D, Bonsmann G. Topical tacrolimus as a therapeutic adjunct in patients with cutaneous lupus erythematosus. A report of three cases. *Dermatology (Basel)* 2003;**207**:381–5.

140 Kreuter A, Gambichler T, Breuckmann F, *et al*. Pimecrolimus 1% cream for cutaneous lupus erythematosus. *J Am Acad Dermatol* 2004;**51**:407–10.

141 Lampropoulos CE, Sangle S, Harrison P, Hughes GRV, D'Cruz DP. Topical tacrolimus therapy of resistant cutaneous lesions in lupus erythematosus: a possible alternative. *Rheumatology (Oxford)* 2004;**43**:1383–5.

142 Heffernan MP, Nelson MM, Smith DI, Chung JH. 1% Tacrolimus ointment in the treatment of discoid lupus erythematosus. *Arch Dermatol* 2005;**141**:1170–1

143 Yoshimasu T, Ohtani T, Oshima A, Sakamoto T, Furukawa F. Topical FK506 (tacrolimus) therapy for facial erythematous lesions of cutaneous lupus erythematosus and dermatomyositis. *Eur J Dermatol* 2002;**12**:50–2.

144 Ashcroft DM, Dimmock P, Garside R, Stein K, Williams HC. Efficacy and tolerability of topical pimecrolimus and tacrolimus in the treatment of atopic dermatitis: meta-analysis of randomised controlled trials. *Br Med J* 2005;**330**:516.

145 Becker JC, Houben R, Vetter CS, Eva B. The carcinogenic potential of tacrolimus ointment suppression; a hypothesis creating case report. *BMC Cancer* 2006;**6**:7–11.

146 Stege H, Budde MA, Grether-Beck S, Krutmann J. Evaluation of the capacity of sunscreens to photoprotect lupus erythematosus patients by employing the photoprovocation test. *Photoderm Photoimmunol Photomed* 2000;**16**:256–9.

147 Callen JP, Roth DE, McGrath C, Dromgoole SH. Safety and efficacy of a broad-spectrum sunscreen in patients with discoid or subacute cutaneous lupus erythematosus. *Cutis* 1991;**47**:130–2.

148 Cornbleet T, Barsky S, Hoit L. Discoid lupus erythematosus scars treated by plastic surgery. *Arch Dermatol* 1957;**74**:219.

149 Neuman Z, Shulman J, Ben-hur N. Successful skin grafting in discoid lupus erythematosus. *Ann Surg* 1961;**154**:142–4.

150 Friederich HC. [Skin moving and skin transplantation in chronic lupus erythematosus integumentalis; in German.] *Hautarzt* 1969; **20**:119–22.

151 Kurwa AR, Evans AJ. Discoid lupus erythematosus treated by dermabrasion. *Br J Dermatol* 1970;**101**:S53.

152 Schiödt M. Local excision in the treatment of oral discoid lupus erythematosus. *Acta Derm Venereol Suppl* 1978;**59**:274–6.

153 Ratner D, Skouge JW. Discoid lupus erythematosus scarring and dermabrasion. a case report and discussion. *J Am Acad Dermatol* 1990;**22**:314–6.

154 Polderman MC, Huizinga, TW, Le-Cessie S, Pavel S. UVA-1 cold light treatment of SLE: a double blind, placebo controlled cross-over trial. *Ann Rheum Dis* 2001;**60**:112–5.

155 McGrath H. Ultraviolet A1 irradiation decreases clinical disease activity and autoantibodies in patients with systemic lupus erythematosus. *Clin Exp Rheumatol* 1994;**12**:129–35.

156 Molina JF, McGrath H. Long-term ultraviolet-A1 irradiation therapy in systemic lupus erythematosus. *J Rheum* 1997;**24**:1072–4.

157 Sonnichsen NH, Meffert V, Kunzelmann V, Audring H. UVA1 therapy of subacute cutaneous lupus erythematosus. *Hautarzt* 1993;**44**:723–5.

158 Richter HI, Krutmann J, Goerz G. Extracorporeal photopheresis in therapy-refractory disseminated discoid lupus erythematosus. *Hautarzt* 1998;**49**:487–91.

159 Wollina U, Looks A. Extracorporeal photochemotherapy in cutaneous lupus erythematosus. *J Eur Acad Dermatol Venereol* 1999;**13**:127–30.

160 Knobler RM, Graninger W, Graninger W, Lindmaier A, Trautinger F, Smolen JS. Extracorporeal photochemotherapy for the treatment of systemic lupus erythematosus. A pilot study. *Arthritis Rheum* 1992;**35**:319–24.

161 Raulin C, Schmidt C, Hellwig S. Cutaneous lupus erythematosus: treatment with pulsed dye laser. *Br J Dermatol* 1999;**141**:1046–50.

162 Gupta G, Roberts DT. Pulsed dye laser treatment of subacute cutaneous lupus erythematosus. *Clin Exp Dermatol* 1999;**24**:498–9.

163 Núñez M, Boixeda P, Miralles ES, de Misa RF, Ledo A. Pulsed dye laser treatment of telangiectatic chronic erythema of cutaneous lupus erythematosus. *Arch Dermatol* 1996;**132**:354–5.

164 Zachariae H, Bjerring P, Cramers M. Argon laser treatment of cutaneous vascular lesions in connective tissue diseases. *Acta Derm Venereol* 1952;**68**:179–82.

165 Nürnberg W, Algermissen B, Hermes B, Henz BM, Kolde G. [Successful treatment of chronic discoid lupus erythematosus with argon laser; in German.] *Hautarzt* 1996;**47**:767–70.

166 Kuhn A, Becker-Wegerich PM, Ruzicka T, Lehmann P. Successful treatment of discoid lupus erythematosus with argon laser. *Dermatology* 2000;**201**:175–7.

167 Baniandres O, Boixeda P, Belmar P, Perez A. Treatment of lupus erythematosus with pulsed dye laser. *Lasers Surg Med* 2003;**32**: 327–30.

56 Dermatomyositis

David F. Fiorentino, Jeffrey P. Callen

Background

Definition

Dermatomyositis (Figure 56.1) is one of the idiopathic inflammatory myopathies.[1,2] In a set of criteria to aid in the diagnosis and classification of dermatomyositis and polymyositis, first proposed in 1975 by Bohan and Peter,[3,4] four of the five criteria are related to the muscle disease:

1 Progressive proximal symmetrical weakness
2 Elevated muscle enzymes
3 Abnormal electromyogram (EMG)
4 Abnormal muscle biopsy
5 Presence of compatible cutaneous disease

Unfortunately, these criteria are not sensitive in identifying the full spectrum of patients with idiopathic inflammatory dermatomyopathy. It has subsequently been recognized that there are many patients with compatible cutaneous disease who never develop any manifestation of muscle disease such as weakness or abnormal changes on muscle biopsy, EMG, or magnetic resonance imaging studies. Sontheimer[5] has used the term "amyopathic dermatomyositis" for those who fulfill these criteria for at least 6 months in the absence of disease-modifying therapies such as corticosteroids and/or immunosuppressive agents.

Incidence/prevalence

Dermatomyositis is a rare disorder. It may be slightly more frequent in women, and all ethnic groups are affected. It has been estimated that dermatomyositis or its related condition polymyositis occur in 5.5 patients per million. However, this figure includes patients with polymyositis and dermatomyositis and most likely does not include patients with amyopathic dermatomyositis.

Etiology

The etiology of dermatomyositis is unknown. Probably the mechanism behind the skin disease differs from that of the muscle disease.

Prognosis

In the patient with amyopathic dermatomyositis, the prognosis is good in the absence of malignancy. For patients with muscle disease, the prognosis depends on the severity of the muscle disease, the presence of lung disease, esophageal dysfunction, and/or malignancy. Children and adolescents with dermatomyositis often develop calcinosis, which can result in disability or discomfort.

Diagnostic tests

The diagnosis of amyopathic dermatomyositis is confirmed by clinical–pathological correlation. The pattern of the skin disease is relatively characteristic, and when an interface dermatitis is demonstrated on skin biopsy, the diagnosis may be relatively firm. However, some subtle cases can be confused with cutaneous lupus, and immunofluorescence studies of skin biopsies can often be helpful in making this distinction.[6,7] For patients with myositis, the diagnosis of dermatomyositis is confirmed by the presence of typical muscle symptoms and findings, together with elevated muscle enzymes, or an abnormal EMG and/or an abnormal muscle biopsy. Magnetic resonance imaging is becoming widely available and abnormalities on this test might be useful in diagnosis.

Aims of treatment

Treatment provides control of the muscle inflammation and allows the patient to return to normal function; the patient might otherwise become disabled from the weakness. The skin disease is often symptomatic and is cosmetically displeasing, and the goal of therapy is therefore to relieve the symptoms and improve the patient's self-image and ability to interact with other people. Some patients

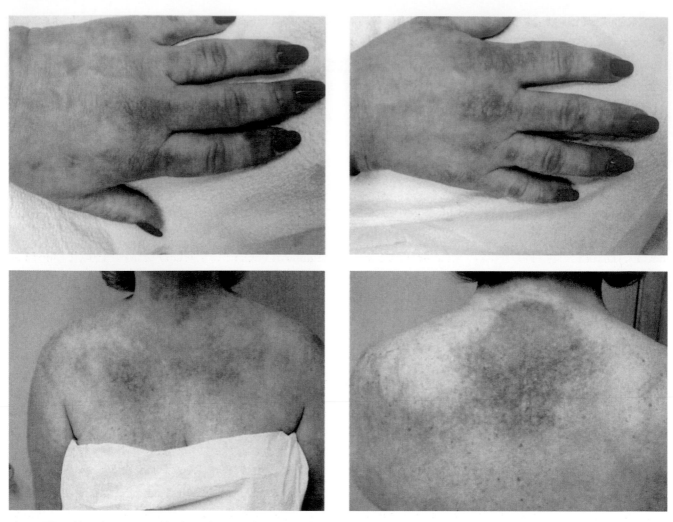

Figure 56.1 This patient presented for the evaluation and treatment of her skin condition, which had been present for the past 6 months. A previous biopsy had revealed an interface dermatitis and her antinuclear antibody was positive. A working diagnosis of lupus erythematosus was made. Treatment with sunscreens and topical corticosteroids were ineffective. Hydroxychloroquine administration resulted in a severe cutaneous drug reaction that required hospitalization.

with dermatomyositis have an associated malignancy, and treatment of the malignancy may in some patients result in a control of the disease process. In children with dermatomyositis, treatment also aims to prevent calcinosis, or to eradicate calcinosis if it does occur. Using partially validated assessment criteria, an international effort has produced consensus statements regarding the definition of "clinically meaningful improvement."[8]

Relevant outcomes

Return of the patient to normal muscle function and improvement in the quality of life for those with skin disease only are important measures of outcome. Improvement in lung function is important in patients with pulmonary disease. In addition, identification and treatment of a potential malignancy is important. Outcome measures of muscular and extramuscular function have been recently defined.[9]

Methods of search

The databases of the Cochrane Skin Group, the *Cochrane Library* to issue 1, 2006, and Medline and Embase between 1968 and February 2006 were searched for articles reporting trials of therapy of skin disease, or dermatomyositis, or the relationship of dermatomyositis to malignancy. Both Embase and Medline were searched using the Ovid search engine at Nottingham University. The searches involved the following terms:

- The relationship of dermatomyositis to cancer (malignancy, neoplasia).
- Treatment of skin disease in patients with dermatomyositis (idiopathic inflammatory myopathy, polymyositis, juvenile dermatomyositis).
- Treatment of dermatomyositis with any of the following agents: antimalarials (hydroxychloroquine, chloroquine), corticosteroids (prednisone, methylprednisolone), dapsone, thalidomide, methotrexate, mycophenolate mofetil, azathioprine, intravenous immunoglobulin (IVIG), rituximab, etanercept, infliximab, adalimumab, efalizumab, abatacept, anakinra, physiotherapy, physical therapy, plasma exchange, plasmapheresis, cyclophosphamide, cyclosporine, tacrolimus, FK506, probenecid, alendronate, diltiazem, Coumadin and sunscreens.

Questions

What is the risk of malignancy in the patient with dermatomyositis or amyopathic dermatomyositis (ADM)?

Population-based studies from Scandinavia clearly demonstrate an increase in the risk of cancer in dermatomyositis, while the modest increase in polymyositis is explained primarily by diagnostic suspicion bias and is not reflected in an increase in mortality (Table 56.1).[10-17] It is also clear that these patients have an increased risk for ovarian cancer.[10-13,18-20] What is not clear is whether these data are applicable to other populations such as south-east Asians, African-Americans, or other ethnic groups.

A recent study from Australia[14] calls into question much of the data that have been based on clinical diagnosis. It does appear that dermatomyositis and polymyositis are not the same disease and that their histopathological abnormalities differ significantly and are recognizable by muscle pathologists. Therefore, there may exist a group of patients who were thought to have polymyositis but who might be classified as having dermatomyositis *sine* dermatitis. This concept is intriguing and might explain why some studies have shown little difference in the prevalence/incidence of malignancy in the two groups. In addition, the existence of this subset might well explain some of the differences that are observed in the studies of therapy (see below).

It is not known whether the increased cancer association is also valid for patients with amyopathic dermatomyositis, because the only published data are individual case reports and small case series.[21] However, a systematic review of the available published cases suggests that these patients

are also at increased risk for cancer, as well as interstitial lung disease.[17] One of the difficulties regarding this issue relates to the manner in which ADM is diagnosed. Because the Sontheimer criteria do not require any testing beyond muscle enzymes, many of the patients defined as having ADM might not actually have amyopathic disease if they were analyzed using all of the available modalities (magnetic resonance imaging, muscle biopsy, etc.).

Another issue that is discussed almost universally in the case–control studies is whether the use of immunosuppressive drugs is associated with an elevated risk of subsequent malignancy. In all of the Scandinavian studies,[10-13] it appears that there is no increase in the prevalence of malignancy in patients who have been treated with an immunosuppressive agent; however, there are many individual case reports of subsequent malignancy in dermatomyositis patients. Several reports[22] have linked the use of methotrexate with lymphoma associated with Epstein–Barr virus. Some, but not all, of these patients can have a spontaneous resolution of their lymphoma when the drug therapy is stopped.

Are there clinical or laboratory findings in dermatomyositis patients that suggest underlying malignancy?

Several studies have suggested that there might be certain clinical or laboratory features that are associated with a greater risk of malignancy (Table 56.2).[11,13,15,23-45] Most studies, including population-based studies from Scandinavia and Scotland, have shown that advanced age is a significant risk factor for malignancy.[11,13,15] Clinical findings of severe vasculopathy (or vasculitis), such as cutaneous necrosis, ulceration, nodules, and/or periungual infarcts have also been associated with malignancy.[31,33,34,40,43,46] Although many studies claim that these findings represent vasculitis, most of them do not present skin biopsy data. Hunger *et al.* provide the only biopsy-based data that cutaneous vasculitis may be a sign of internal malignancy.[32] However, the numbers are too small for firm conclusions to be drawn, and other studies have rejected such an association.[38,39,41] Elevated erythrocyte sedimentation rates have been correlated with malignancy. In contrast, arthralgia/arthritis, Raynaud's, interstitial lung disease, and autoantibodies have been shown to have a "protective" effect against malignancy in many studies. Many of these findings can be found in association with one another (the so-called "antisynthetase syndrome").[45] In general, there have been no consistent associations with regard to muscle disease severity (i.e., strength or enzymes), cutaneous findings (other than the necrosis), or constitutional symptoms that appear to distinguish idiopathic from paraneoplastic dermatomyositis.

Table 56.1 What is the risk of malignancy in patients with dermatomyositis or a myopathic dermatomyositis?

First author (ref.)	Population-based?	Patients with CA in the DM/ADM group	Patients with CA in the PM group	Statistically different?	Comment(s)
Sigurgeirsson[10]	Yes	59/392	37/396	Both groups had elevated rate vs. controls. Cancer mortality raised only in DM	Ovarian cancer increased 17-fold Authors suggest increase in PM due to more extensive evaluation
Airio[11]	Yes	19/71	12/175	SIR DM: 6.5 PM: 1.0	Risk rises with age, slight risk for overlap patients Nonmelanoma skin cancers, myelofibrosis, polycythemia vera, *in situ* cervical cancer and 12 preceding cancers eliminated Overrepresentation of ovarian cancer
Chow[12]	Yes	31/203	26/336	SIR DM: 3.8 PM: 1.7 reduced to 1.0 by 3rd year following diagnosis	Excess lymphoma/leukemia Surveillance for prolonged periods may not be needed
Hill[13]	Yes	115/618	95/914	SIR DM: 3.0 PM: 1.3	Plan for evaluation based on the results of their study suggested data derived from Swedish, Finnish, and Danish studies, but included additional follow-up from Denmark and Finland
Buchbinder[14]	Yes, population-based, retro-spective cohort study based on pathological findings	36/85	57/321	OR All cases: 2.6 DM: 6.2 PM: 2.0 IBM: 2.4 JDM: 29.0 Myositis with CTD: 4.6	Authors feel diagnosis of DM possible without the presence of a rash, based on the changes observed in the muscle biopsy Increased malignancy rate found in all groups, including children
Stockton[15]	Yes	50/286 Women: 30/189 Men: 20/97	40/419 Women: 28/244 Men 12/175	SIR DM: 7.7 PM: 2.1	27 patients with DM and 31 with PM had cancer before DM/PM diagnosed; not known whether any of these patients had metastatic disease at the time of diagnosis. Increase in ovarian, cervical and lung cancer in DM and in Hodgkin's disease in PM found
Zantos[16]	Meta-analysis of 4 CC cohort studies	97/513	56/565	OR	Increased malignancy in the preceding and subsequent 4 years DM: 4.4 PM: 2.1
Gerami[17]	Systematic review of case series/reports	29/197 All cases amyopathic			No control population. Mostly case reports.

ADM, amyopathic dermatomyositis; CA, cancer; CC, case–control; DM, dermatomyositis; CTD, connective tissue disease; IBM, inclusion body myositis; JDM, juvenile dermatomyositis; OR, odds ratio; PM, polymyositis; SIR, standardized incidence ratio.

Table 56.2 Are there clinical or laboratory findings in dermatomyositis patients that suggest underlying malignancy?

First author (ref.)	Population-based?	Patients with CA in DM/ADM group	Risk factor(s)	Effect (CA vs. no CA group)	P/95% CI	Comments
Hill[13]	Yes	115/618	Age > 45	Pos (SIR = 3.1)	CI 2.6–3.7	
Stockton[15]	Yes	50/286	Age 45–74	Pos (SIR = 3.6)	CI 2.0–5.9	
Airio[11]	Yes	63/311 (PM and DM)	Age > 49	Pos (SIR = 8.2)	CI 4.9–13	
Koh[23]	No	17/60 (PM and DM)	Arthralgia	Neg (48 vs. 12%)	ND	Referrals from EMG lab or single hospital. Vasculitis, arthralgia not
			Interstitial lung disease	Neg (29% vs. 12%)	ND	risk factors
			Mean age	Higher in CA group	< 0.001	
Hochberg[24]	No	6/58 (PM and DM)	Mean age	No sign. difference	ND	Statistics not given. Small number of patients. Raynaud's not a risk
			Dysphagia	Pos (67% vs. 40%)		factor
			Arthralgia	Neg (0% vs. 19%)		
			Vasculitis	Pos (33% vs. 10%)		
Bohan[25]	No	13/110 (PM and DM)	Mean age	Higher in CA (62 vs. 47 y)	ND	Statistics not given. Dysphagia not a risk factor. Small number of
			Arthralgia	Neg (0% vs. 23%)		patients
			Raynaud's	Neg (0% vs. 13%)		
Pautas[26]	No (CC)	7/42 (PM and DM)	Age > 65	Pos (OR of CA = 2.97)	0.24	
Marie[27]	No (CC)	16/79 (PM and DM)	Age > 65	Pos (OR of CA = 9.35)	0.0001	
Henriksson[28]	No	7/70 (PM and DM)	Mean age	Higher in CA (57 vs. 52 y)	ND	
Duncan[29]	No	10/39	Mean age	Higher in CA (60 vs. 46 y)	0.02	Dysphagia, ESR not risk factors
Chen[30]	No	18/105 (PM and DM)	Age > 45	Pos (OR of CA = 9.1)	0.004	Multivariate analysis for age, sex, and ILD
			Male sex	Pos (OR of CA = 4.06)	0.04	
			Interstitial lung disease	Neg (OR of CA = 0.04)	< 0.001	
			Elevated CPK	Pos (OR of CA = 5.16)	0.03	
			Arthralgia	Neg (OR of CA = 0.16)	0.08	
Feldman[31]	No	6/76 (PM and DM)	Cutaneous "vasculitis"	Pos (OR = 6.5)	0.09	Statistical trend only. Vasculitis only biopsied in one case
Hunger[32]	No	5/23	Cutaneous vasculitis	Pos (80% vs. 17%)	< 0.05	All cases biopsy-proven vasculitis as incidental finding on biopsy
Basset-Seguin[33]	No	13/32	Cutaneous necrosis	Pos (31% vs. 5%)	0.05	Mean age not a significant risk factor
			Elevated ESR	Pos (54% vs. 26%)	0.02	
Burnouf[34,35]	No (prospective)	8/26	Cutaneous necrosis	Pos (63% vs. 11%)	0.01	Multivariate analysis
Mautner[36]	No	6/11	Cutaneous necrosis	Pos (100% vs. 0%)	ND	Small study. Necrosis vaguely defined. Possible recall bias

Table 56.2 *Cont'd*

First author (ref.)	Population-based?	Patients with CA in DM/ADM group	Risk factor(s)	Effect (CA vs. no CA group)	P/95% CI	Comments
Hidano[37]	No	171/569	Interstitial lung disease	Neg (4.7% vs. 19%)	< 0.01	Large number of cases. All diagnoses by questionnaire
Sparsa[38]	No	16/40 (PM and DM)	Elevated ESR	Pos (48% vs. 25%)	0.008	Mean age, cutaneous necrosis, autoantibodies not risk factors
			Mean CPK	Higher in CA (2840 vs. 1346 U/L)	0.01	
			Raynaud's	Neg (0% vs. 42%)	0.003	
			Constitutional symptoms	Pos (75% vs. 29%)	0.009	
			Rapid-onset disease	Pos (63% vs. 21%)	0.02	
			Interstitial lung disease	Neg (19% vs. 46%)	0.1	
Cox[39]	No	23/53	Mean age	Higher in CA (66 vs. 53 y)	0.001	UK hospital referral base. Vasculitis not a risk factor
Ponyi[40]	No	16/84	Mean age	Higher in CA (56 vs. 46 y)	0.005	Only malignancies < 2 y before or < 5 y after diagnosis of DM were considered. Dysphagia not a risk factor in this study
			Cutaneous ulceration	Pos (44% vs. 13%)	< 0.05	
			Distal weakness	Pos (50% vs. 6%)	0.007	
			Fever	Neg (0% vs. 29%)	< 0.05	
			Arthritis	Neg (25% vs. 51%)	< 0.05	
			Raynaud's	Neg (17% vs. 26%)	0.038	
			Interstitial lung disease	Neg (19% vs. 25%)	0.043	
			Mean CPK	Lower in CA (945 vs. 3612 U/L)	0.039	
			Positive ANA	Neg (19% vs. 39%)	< 0.05	
			Anti-Jo-1 antibody	Neg (0% vs. 16%)	< 0.05	
Amerio[41]	No	14/59	ESR > 35 mm/h	Pos (OR of CA = 197.5)	< 0.05	Multivariate analysis. Age, cutaneous necrosis, ANA, and muscle enzymes not risk factors
Marie[42]	No	28/156 (PM and DM)	Interstitial lung disease	Neg (7% vs. 27%)	0.028	
Dourmishev[43]	No	12/50	Mean age	Higher in CA (59 vs. 49 y)	ND	No statistics available. Hospital-based study
			Poikiloderma	Pos (75% vs. 32%)		
			Cutaneous ulceration	Pos (25% vs. 2.7%)		
			Raynaud's	Neg (0% vs. 17%)		
Nishikai[44]	No	12/36	Positive ANA	Neg (17% vs. 54%)	< 0.03	No data given on malignancies
Love[45]	No	13/92	Raynaud's	Neg (0% vs. 40%)	ND	No statistics available. First study to link these protective effects into the "anti-synthetase syndrome"
			Arthritis	Neg (8% vs. 55%)		
			Dyspnea	Neg (27% vs. 59%)		
			Interstitial lung disease	Neg (0% vs. 37%)		
			Positive ANA	Neg (31% vs. 62%)		
			Anti-Ro/SSA	Neg (0% vs. 11%)		
			Anti-U1RNP	Neg (0% vs. 13%)		
			Anti-synthetase antibody	Neg (0% vs. 33%)		

ADM, amyopathic dermatomyositis; ANA, antinuclear antibody; CA, cancer; CI, confidence intervals; CPK, creatine phosphokinase; DM, dermatomyositis; EMG, electromyography; ESR, erythrocyte sedimentation rate; ILD, interstitial lung disease; ND, no data; Neg, negative; OR, odds ratio; PM, polymyositis; Pos, positive; SIR, standardized incidence ratio.

How should the patient with dermatomyositis/ADM be assessed for possible cancer?

The search for malignancy in patients with dermatomyositis should include a careful history, physical examination, and standard laboratory evaluation (complete blood count, comprehensive metabolic panel, chest radiograph and stool Hematest). Any abnormalities found should be thoroughly investigated. In addition, testing should include tests that would be ordered in a "healthy" person of the same age, sex, and ethnic group as the patient with newly diagnosed dermatomyositis (for example, it is recommended that persons over 50 years of age should have a colonoscopy). Many authors have suggested that "blind" screening tests (beyond those mentioned above) are not fruitful in retrospective studies of patients with dermatomyositis.[39,47–53] One study found that "blind" computed tomography (CT) scans led to a cancer diagnosis in 40 patients with dermatomyositis, but the majority of these appeared to be in patients experiencing cancer recurrence; this observation suggests that CT scans may be justified particularly in patients with a known history of cancer. In women, pelvic CT and mammography are justified.[38] A recent study demonstrated that sustained elevation of CA125 or CA19-9 are very specific findings in patients with cancer-associated dermatomyositis/polymyositis.[54] For patients with polymyositis, a chest radiograph and urinalysis should be performed at the time of diagnosis. Continued surveillance is necessary for patients with dermatomyositis, but perhaps not for those with polymyositis.[13–15] However, what testing should be done beyond age-specific cancer screening is not clear, and the clinician must form a plan in the absence of supporting data. Lastly, nasopharyngeal cancer is much more common among Asian patients in southeast Asia, and a careful ear, nose and throat evaluation is therefore needed. A recent study suggests that dermatomyositis patients residing outside south-east Asia are also at increased risk of developing nasopharyngeal cancer.[55]

Are there effective treatments for dermatomyositis?

The following are some quotes from "major" dermatologic texts that deal with treatment of patients with dermatomyositis:

• "Most forms of polymyositis and dermatomyositis are approached in a similar manner. Corticosteroids are the main pillar of drug therapy . . . However, early use of corticosteroid-sparing drugs should be considered, including combined therapy, from onset. The main drugs for combined therapy are methotrexate, azathioprine and antimalarials."[56]
• "Systemic glucocorticoids remain the traditional first line therapy for classic dermatomyositis."[57]
• "Treatment with corticosteroids is required in almost all cases, the dose depending upon the degree of activity."[58]
• "Prednisone is the therapeutic mainstay."[59]

All of the above authorities recommend corticosteroids as first-line therapy, and relatively high doses are generally suggested. In addition, the early use of a corticosteroid-sparing agent is often proposed, with methotrexate or azathioprine being the most frequently suggested agents. Do we know that these medications are effective, what the proper dosing should be, when a second-line agent should be introduced, which agent should be utilized, and what the likelihood of success is? Unfortunately, as is illustrated in Table 56.3,[25,60–100] the evidence available to answer these questions is poor. It is unclear whether the rate of remission is affected by corticosteroids, whether they are used in high or low doses. In addition, there is little evidence regarding these therapeutic maneuvers for the treatment of cutaneous disease that might accompany dermatomyositis. Well-controlled randomized trials for this disease are lacking, and even the ones that have been conducted often lack power, or have design flaws or potential biases. Many of the studies have included patients with malignancy-associated myositis, a condition that is believed to respond less well than dermatomyositis. In addition, most studies mix dermatomyositis and polymyositis patients in their analyses, and it has become evident that these disorders are probably different in their pathogenesis and most likely have a differential response to therapy.

Current recommendations

It seems that there are no strong data that support the use of corticosteroids in dermatomyositis, whether considering the muscle component, systemic disease such as pulmonary involvement, or the skin disease. Despite this lack of data, most authorities state that corticosteroids are a mainstay of therapy. Therefore, it seems prudent to use corticosteroids for as short a period of time as is possible, substituting a steroid-sparing agent early in the course of treatment. Which of the agents to use is, in our view, dependent on the clinician's comfort level with the specific agent. For muscle disease, no high-quality trials support the use of a particular agent, with the possible exception of IVIG (see below). The addition of azathioprine to a corticosteroid regimen demonstrated a trend towards improvement.[66] Another study suggested that methotrexate and azathioprine do not appear to differ with respect to efficacy, although methotrexate was better tolerated.[67] Observations from individual case reports and small case series suggest that for skin disease, hydroxychloroquine, methotrexate, and mycophenolate mofetil are effective corticosteroid-sparing agents. A retrospective series suggests that patients with dermatomyositis may have an increased risk of hydroxychloroquine reactions.[101] Calcineurin inhibitors (such as ciclosporin and

Table 56.3 Treatments for patients with dermatomyositis

First author (ref.)	Treatments compared/studied	Type of study	Outcome	Comments
Corticosteroids				
Winkelmann[60]	CS therapy	Retrospective review of DM and PM Primary end point: outcome of myositis	High-dose regimen (> 50 mg/d) favored	No statistical analysis Mixture of patients Identified some with an acute, fulminant course
Klein-Gitelman[61]	IVCS vs. OCS	Retrospective comparison of 10	IVCS more costly, but more effective	Small group of patients
Bohan[25]	CS therapy	Retrospective of 124 patients	72% normalized CK levels	Mixture of patients
Nzeusseu[62]	Low-dose vs. high-dose prednisolone (< 0.5 vs. > 0.5 mg/kg/day)	Retrospective review of DM and PM (n = 25)	No difference in functional outcome	Vertebral fractures less common in low-dose group
Dawkins[63]	1 mg/kg/d prednisone with slow taper (over > 2 y)	Prospective DM (14 adult, 7 juvenile)	11/12 adults with normal strength/CPK 4/7 juveniles with normal strength/CPK	Cutaneous disease more difficult to treat
Immunosuppressives				
Mosca[64]	CS alone vs. CS with immunosuppressive	Retrospective analysis	CS first-line therapy	—
Bohan[25]	MTX for CS-resistant DM/PM Initial dose 10–15 mg/wk, raised to 30–60 mg/wk	Retrospective study. 25 patients (PM/DM)	16/25 improved strength	Minor, reversible toxicity
Ramanan[65]	CS alone vs. CS with MTX	Retrospective study of juvenile DM	Addition of MTX resulted in decrease in total dose of CS, more rapid taper of CS. No difference in efficacy	Rapid CS taper only in MTX group, may have been tolerated in CS-only group
Bunch[66]	Prednisone 60 mg/d plus AZA 2 mg/kg/d vs. prednisone plus placebo	3-month DB-PC trial 16 patients with PM	No significant differences	—
Miller[67]	CS + MTX vs. CS + AZA	Double-blind, randomized (n = 28)	Equivalent efficacy on hand grip strength	MTX better tolerated than AZA
Villalba[68]	Oral weekly MTX and daily AZA vs. i.v. MTX with leucovorin rescue	Randomized, open-label cross-over study, 18 PM and 11 DM	ITT analysis showed trend in favor of oral combination	Toxicity slightly more common in i.v. group
Takada[69]	CYA (mean 156 mg/kg/d)	Retrospective analysis of 32 hospitals in Japan. 23 DM patients	Good response in 8/17 acute cases and 3/6 chronic cases	Only ILD measured as outcome. Unclear what parameters were measured
Kameda[70]	CYA (2–4 mg/kg/d) + CYT (10–30 mg/kg/d i.v.) + CS	Prospective study of 10 DM patients with severe ILD	5/10 survived. 5/10 died of respiratory failure	May compare favorably with historical controls (25% survival)
Heckmatt[71]	CYA (2.5–7.5 mg/kg/d)	Retrospective study of 14 patients with juvenile DM	Increased strength	

tacrolimus) also appear to be effective in skin disease, and may have a particular role.

IVIG has been the subject of a randomized controlled trial (RCT) and was found to be effective for both the muscle disease and the skin disease in patients with dermatomyositis refractory to corticosteroids and immunosuppressive agents. However, at least one open-label analysis reported that only seven of 19 patients treated with IVIG improved.

What about the therapy for juvenile dermatomyositis? This condition is complicated in two major ways. First, patients with juvenile dermatomyositis are more prone to calcinosis; and second, they may be permanently disabled by contractures. The results of retrospective case series suggest that the use of early "aggressive" therapy will limit the possibility of calcinosis.[102] Klein-Gitelman et al.[61] believe that high-dose intravenous pulsed methylprednisolone limits the risk and severity of calcinosis. However, adequate RCTs have not yet corroborated this belief. It does appear that whatever the treatment, combination with physical therapy will prevent contractures from developing and that even if contractures occur, the use of physical therapy may improve the long-term disability. Once established, calcinosis may resolve spontaneously after a period of months to years; however, there are multiple individual case reports and some small series suggesting that various therapies—including warfarin, diltiazem, and probenecid—are effective in reversing the calcinosis.

References

1 Callen JP. Dermatomyositis. *Lancet* 2000;**355**:53–7.
2 Plotz PH, Rider LG, Targoff IN, Raben N, O'Hanlon TP, Miller FW. NIH conference. Myositis: immunologic contributions to understanding cause, pathogenesis, and therapy. *Ann Intern Med* 1995;**122**:715–24.
3 Bohan A, Peter JB. Polymyositis and dermatomyositis (first of two parts). *N Engl J Med* 1975;**292**:344–7.
4 Bohan A, Peter JB. Polymyositis and dermatomyositis (second of two parts). *N Engl J Med* 1975;**292**:403–7.
5 Sontheimer RD. Cutaneous features of classic dermatomyositis and amyopathic dermatomyositis. *Curr Opin Rheumatol* 1999;**11**:475–82.
6 Crowson AN, Magro CM. The role of microvascular injury in the pathogenesis of cutaneous lesions of dermatomyositis. *Hum Pathol* 1996;**27**:15–9.
7 Magro CM, Crowson AN. The immunofluorescent profile of dermatomyositis: a comparative study with lupus erythematosus. *J Cutan Pathol* 1997;**24**:543–52.
8 Rider LG, Giannini EH, Brunner HI, *et al.* International consensus on preliminary definitions of improvement in adult and juvenile myositis. *Arthritis Rheum* 2004;**50**:2281–90.
9 Isenberg DA, Allen E, Farewell V, *et al.* International consensus outcome measures for patients with idiopathic inflammatory myopathies. Development and initial validation of myositis activity and damage indices in patients with adult onset disease. *Rheumatology (Oxford)* 2004;**43**:49–54.
10 Sigurgeirsson B, Lindelof B, Edhag O, Allander E. Risk of cancer in patients with dermatomyositis or polymyositis. A population-based study. *N Engl J Med* 1992;**326**:363–7.
11 Airio A, Pukkala E, Isomäki H. Elevated cancer incidence in patients with dermatomyositis: a population based study. *J Rheumatol* 1995;**22**:1300–3.
12 Chow WH, Gridley G, Mellemkjaer L, McLaughlin JK, Olsen JH, Fraumeni JF. Cancer risk following polymyositis and dermatomyositis: a nationwide cohort study in Denmark. *Cancer Causes Control* 1995;**6**:9–13.
13 Hill CL, Zhang Y, Sigurgeirsson B, *et al.* Frequency of specific cancer types in dermatomyositis and polymyositis: a population-based study. *Lancet* 2001;**357**:96–100.
14 Buchbinder R, Forbes A, Hall S, Dennett X, Giles G. Incidence of malignant disease in biopsy-proven inflammatory myopathy. A population-based cohort study. *Ann Intern Med* 2001;**134**:1087–95.
15 Stockton D, Doherty VR, Brewster DH. Risk of cancer in patients with dermatomyositis or polymyositis, and follow-up implications: a Scottish population-based cohort study. *Br J Cancer* 2001;**85**:41–5.
16 Zantos D, Zhang Y, Felson D. The overall and temporal association of cancer with polymyositis and dermatomyositis. *J Rheumatol* 1994;**21**:1855–9.
17 Gerami P, Schope JM, McDonald L, Walling HW, Sontheimer RD. A systematic review of adult-onset clinically amyopathic dermatomyositis (dermatomyositis sine myositis): a missing link within the spectrum of the idiopathic inflammatory myopathies. *J Am Acad Dermatol* 2006;**54**:597–613.
18 Scaling ST, Kaufman RH, Patten BM. Dermatomyositis and female malignancy. *Obstet Gynecol* 1979;**54**:474–7.
19 Cherin P, Piette JC, Herson S, *et al.* Dermatomyositis and ovarian cancer: a report of 7 cases and literature review. *J Rheumatol* 1993;**20**:1897–9.
20 Whitmore SE, Rosenshein NB, Provost TT. Ovarian cancer in patients with dermatomyositis. *Medicine (Baltimore)* 1994;**73**:153–60.
21 Whitmore SE, Watson R, Rosenshein NB, Provost TT. Dermatomyositis sine myositis: association with malignancy. *J Rheumatol* 1996;**23**:101–5.
22 Kamel OW, van de Rijn M, Weiss LM, *et al.* Brief report: reversible lymphomas associated with Epstein–Barr virus occurring during methotrexate therapy for rheumatoid arthritis and dermatomyositis. *N Engl J Med* 1993;**328**:1317–21.
23 Koh ET, Seow A, Ong B, Ratnagopal P, Tjia H, Chng HH. Adult onset polymyositis/dermatomyositis: clinical and laboratory features and treatment response in 75 patients. *Ann Rheum Dis* 1993;**52**:857–61.
24 Hochberg MC, Feldman D, Stevens MB. Adult onset polymyositis/dermatomyositis: an analysis of clinical and laboratory features and survival in 76 patients with a review of the literature. *Semin Arthritis Rheum* 1986;**15**:168–78.
25 Bohan A, Peter JB, Bowman RL, Pearson CM. Computer-assisted analysis of 153 patients with polymyositis and dermatomyositis. *Medicine (Baltimore)* 1977;**56**:255–86.
26 Pautas E, Cherin P, Piette JC, *et al.* Features of polymyositis and dermatomyositis in the elderly: a case–control study. *Clin Exp Rheumatol* 2000;**18**:241–4.

27 Marie I, Hatron PY, Levesque H, *et al.* Influence of age on characteristics of polymyositis and dermatomyositis in adults. *Medicine (Baltimore)* 1999;**78**:139–47.

28 Henriksson KG, Sandstedt P. Polymyositis: treatment and prognosis. A study of 107 patients. *Acta Neurol Scand* 1982;**65**:280–300.

29 Duncan AG, Richardson JB, Klein JB, Targoff IN, Woodcock TM, Callen JP. Clinical, serologic, and immunogenetic studies in patients with dermatomyositis. *Acta Derm Venereol* 1991;**71**:312–6.

30 Chen YJ, Wu CY, Shen JL. Predicting factors of malignancy in dermatomyositis and polymyositis: a case–control study. *Br J Dermatol* 2001;**144**:825–31.

31 Feldman D, Hochberg MC, Zizic TM, Stevens MB. Cutaneous vasculitis in adult polymyositis/dermatomyositis. *J Rheumatol* 1983;**10**:85–9.

32 Hunger RE, Dürr C, Brand CU. Cutaneous leukocytoclastic vasculitis in dermatomyositis suggests malignancy. *Dermatology (Basel)* 2001;**202**:123–6.

33 Basset-Seguin N, Roujeau JC, Gherardi R, Guillaume JC, Revuz J, Touraine R. Prognostic factors and predictive signs of malignancy in adult dermatomyositis. A study of 32 cases. *Arch Dermatol* 1990;**126**:633–7.

34 Burnouf M, Mahe E, Verpillat P, *et al.* [Cutaneous necrosis is predictive of cancer in adult dermatomyositis; in French.] *Ann Dermatol Venereol* 2003;**130**:313–6.

35 Mahe E, Descamps V, Burnouf M, Crickx B. A helpful clinical sign predictive of cancer in adult dermatomyositis: cutaneous necrosis. *Arch Dermatol* 2003;**139**:539.

36 Mautner GH, Grossman ME, Silvers DN, Rabinowitz A, Mowad CM, Johnson BL Jr. Epidermal necrosis as a predictive sign of malignancy in adult dermatomyositis. *Cutis* 1998;**61**:190–4.

37 Hidano A, Kaneko K, Arai Y. [Survey of the association of dermatomyositis and pulmonary fibrosis; in Japanese.] *Arerugi* 1985;**34**:245–51.

38 Sparsa A, Liozon E, Herrmann F, *et al.* Routine vs extensive malignancy search for adult dermatomyositis and polymyositis: a study of 40 patients. *Arch Dermatol* 2002;**138**:885–90.

39 Cox NH, Lawrence CM, Langtry JA, Ive FA. Dermatomyositis. Disease associations and an evaluation of screening investigations for malignancy. *Arch Dermatol* 1990;**126**:61–5.

40 Ponyi A, Constantin T, Garami M, *et al.* Cancer-associated myositis: clinical features and prognostic signs. *Ann N Y Acad Sci* 2005;**1051**:64–71.

41 Amerio P, Girardelli CR, Proietto G, *et al.* Usefulness of erythrocyte sedimentation rate as tumor marker in cancer associated dermatomyositis. *Eur J Dermatol* 2002;**12**:165–9.

42 Marie I, Hachulla E, Cherin P, *et al.* Interstitial lung disease in polymyositis and dermatomyositis. *Arthritis Rheum* 2002;**47**:614–22.

43 Dourmishev LA. Dermatomyositis associated with malignancy. 12 case reports. *Adv Exp Med Biol* 1999;**455**:193–9.

44 Nishikai M, Sato A. Low incidence of antinuclear antibodies in dermatomyositis with malignancy. *Ann Rheum Dis* 1990;**49**:422.

45 Love LA, Leff RL, Fraser DD, *et al.* A new approach to the classification of idiopathic inflammatory myopathy: myositis-specific autoantibodies define useful homogeneous patient groups. *Medicine (Baltimore)* 1991;**70**:360–74.

46 Gallais V, Crickx B, Belaich S. [Cutaneous necrotic lesions in dermatomyositis in adults: a predictive sign of cancer? In French.] *Presse Med* 1995;**24**:1907.

47 Rose C, Hatron PY, Brouillard M, *et al.* [Predictive signs of cancers in dermatomyositis. Study of 29 cases; in French.] *Rev Med Interne* 1994;**15**:19–24.

48 Manchul LA, Jin A, Pritchard KI, *et al.* The frequency of malignant neoplasms in patients with polymyositis-dermatomyositis. A controlled study. *Arch Intern Med* 1985;**145**:1835–9.

49 Moss AA, Hanelin LG. Occult malignant tumors in dermatologic disease. The futility of radiological search. *Radiology* 1977;**123**:69–71.

50 Callen JP. The value of malignancy evaluation in patients with dermatomyositis. *J Am Acad Dermatol* 1982;**6**:253–9.

51 Callen JP, Hyla JF, Bole GG Jr, Kay DR. The relationship of dermatomyositis and polymyositis to internal malignancy. *Arch Dermatol* 1980;**116**:295–8.

52 Bonnetblanc JM, Bernard P, Fayol J. Dermatomyositis and malignancy. A multicenter cooperative study. *Dermatologica* 1990;**180**:212–6.

53 Lakhanpal S, Bunch TW, Ilstrup DM, Melton LJ 3rd. Polymyositis-dermatomyositis and malignant lesions: does an association exist? *Mayo Clin Proc* 1986;**61**:645–53.

54 Amoura Z, Duhaut P, Huong DL, *et al.* Tumor antigen markers for the detection of solid cancers in inflammatory myopathies. *Cancer Epidemiol Biomarkers Prev* 2005;**14**:1279–82.

55 Mebazâa A, Boussen H, Nouira R, *et al.* Dermatomyositis and malignancy in Tunisia: a multicenter national retrospective study of 20 cases. *J Am Acad Dermatol* 2003;**48**:530–4.

56 Catoggio L. Inflammatory muscle disease: management. In: Klippel JH, Dieppe PA, eds. *Rheumatology*. London: Mosby, 1998:7.

57 Sontheimer RD. Dermatomyositis. In: Freedberg IM, Eisen AZ, Wolff K, Goldsmith LA, Katz S, Austen KF, eds. *Fitzpatrick's Dermatology in General Medicine*, 5th ed. New York: McGraw-Hill, 1999: 2018–20.

58 Rowell NR, Goodfield MD. The connective tissue diseases. In: Champion RH, Burton J, Burns T, Breathnach S, eds. *Textbook of Dermatology*. Oxford: Blackwell Science, 1998: 2564–5.

59 Provost TT, Flynn JA. Dermatomyositis. In: Provost TT, Flynn JA, eds. *Cutaneous Medicine*. Toronto: Decker, 2001: 82–103.

60 Winkelmann RK, Mulder DW, Lambert EH, Howard FM Jr, Diessner GR. Course of dermatomyositis-polymyositis: comparison of untreated and cortisone-treated patients. *Mayo Clin Proc* 1968;**43**:545–56.

61 Klein-Gitelman MS, Waters T, Pachman LM. The economic impact of intermittent high-dose intravenous versus oral corticosteroid treatment of juvenile dermatomyositis. *Arthritis Care Res* 2000;**13**:360–8.

62 Nzeusseu A, Brion F, Lefebvre C, Knoops P, Devogelaer JP, Houssiau FA. Functional outcome of myositis patients: can a low-dose glucocorticoid regimen achieve good functional results? *Clin Exp Rheumatol* 1999;**17**:441–6.

63 Dawkins MA, Jorizzo JL, Walker FO, Albertson D, Sinal SH, Hinds A. Dermatomyositis: a dermatology-based case series. *J Am Acad Dermatol* 1998;**38**:397–404.

64 Mosca M, Neri R, Pasero G, Bombardieri S. Treatment of the idiopathic inflammatory myopathies: a retrospective analysis of

63 Caucasian patients longitudinally followed at a single center. *Clin Exp Rheumatol* 2000;**18**:451–6.

65 Ramanan AV, Campbell-Webster N, Ota S, *et al*. The effectiveness of treating juvenile dermatomyositis with methotrexate and aggressively tapered corticosteroids. *Arthritis Rheum* 2005;**52**:3570–8.

66 Bunch TW, Worthington JW, Combs JJ, Ilstrup DM, Engel AG. Azathioprine with prednisone for polymyositis. A controlled, clinical trial. *Ann Intern Med* 1980;**92**:365–9.

67 Miller J. Randomised double blind controlled trial of methotrexate and steroids compared with azathioprine and steroids in the treatment of idiopathic inflammatory myopathy. *J Neurol Sci* 2002;**199**(Suppl 1):S53.

68 Villalba L, Hicks JE, Adams EM, *et al*. Treatment of refractory myositis: a randomized crossover study of two new cytotoxic regimens. *Arthritis Rheum* 1998;**41**:392–9.

69 Takada K, Nagasaka K, Miyasaka N. Polymyositis/dermatomyositis and interstitial lung disease: a new therapeutic approach with T-cell-specific immunosuppressants. *Autoimmunity* 2005;**38**:383–92.

70 Kameda H, Nagasawa H, Ogawa H, *et al*. Combination therapy with corticosteroids, cyclosporin A, and intravenous pulse cyclophosphamide for acute/subacute interstitial pneumonia in patients with dermatomyositis. *J Rheumatol* 2005;**32**:1719–26.

71 Heckmatt J, Hasson N, Saunders C, *et al*. Cyclosporin in juvenile dermatomyositis. *Lancet* 1989;**i**:1063–6.

72 Danko K, Szegedi G. Cyclosporin A treatment of dermatomyositis. *Arthritis Rheum* 1991;**34**:933–4.

73 Maeda K, Kimura R, Komuta K, Igarashi T. Cyclosporine treatment for polymyositis/dermatomyositis: is it possible to rescue the deteriorating cases with interstitial pneumonitis? *Scand J Rheumatol* 1997;**26**:24–9.

74 Grau JM, Herrero C, Casademont J, Fernandez-Sola J, Urbano-Marquez A. Cyclosporine A as first choice therapy for dermatomyositis. *J Rheumatol* 1994;**21**:381–2.

75 Vencovsky J, Jarosova K, Machacek S, *et al*. Cyclosporine A versus methotrexate in the treatment of polymyositis and dermatomyositis. *Scand J Rheumatol* 2000;**29**:95–102.

76 Wilkes MR, Sereika SM, Fertig N, Lucas MR, Oddis CV. Treatment of antisynthetase-associated interstitial lung disease with tacrolimus. *Arthritis Rheum* 2005;**52**:2439–46.

77 Tausche AK, Meurer M. Mycophenolate mofetil for dermatomyositis. *Dermatology* 2001;**202**:341–3.

78 Majithia V, Harisdangkul V. Mycophenolate mofetil (CellCept): an alternative therapy for autoimmune inflammatory myopathy. *Rheumatology (Oxford)* 2005;**44**:386–9.

79 Edge JC, Outland JD, Dempsey JR, Callen JP. Mycophenolate mofetil as an effective corticosteroid-sparing therapy for recalcitrant dermatomyositis. *Arch Dermatol* 2006;**142**:65–9.

80 Rowin J, Amato AA, Deisher N, Cursio J, Meriggioli MN. Mycophenolate mofetil in dermatomyositis: is it safe? *Neurology* 2006;**66**:1245–7.

81 Riley P, Maillard SM, Wedderburn LR, Woo P, Murray KJ, Pilkington CA. Intravenous cyclophosphamide pulse therapy in juvenile dermatomyositis. A review of efficacy and safety. *Rheumatology (Oxford)* 2004;**43**:491–6.

82 Cronin ME, Miller FW, Hicks JE, Dalakas M, Plotz PH. The failure of intravenous cyclophosphamide therapy in refractory idiopathic inflammatory myopathy. *J Rheumatol* 1989;**16**:1225–8.

83 Sinoway PA, Callen JP. Chlorambucil. An effective corticosteroid-sparing agent for patients with recalcitrant dermatomyositis. *Arthritis Rheum* 1993;**36**:319–24.

84 Adams EM, Pucino F, Yarboro C, *et al*. A pilot study: use of fludarabine for refractory dermatomyositis and polymyositis, and examination of endpoint measures. *J Rheumatol* 1999;**26**:352–60.

85 Miller FW, Leitman SF, Cronin ME, *et al*. Controlled trial of plasma exchange and leukapheresis in polymyositis and dermatomyositis. *N Engl J Med* 1992;**326**:1380–4.

86 Cherin P, Auperin I, Bussel A, Pourrat J, Herson S. Plasma exchange in polymyositis and dermatomyositis: a multicenter study of 57 cases. *Clin Exp Rheumatol* 1995;**13**:270–1.

87 Danieli MG, Malcangi G, Palmieri C, *et al*. Cyclosporin A and intravenous immunoglobulin treatment in polymyositis/dermatomyositis. *Ann Rheum Dis* 2002;**61**:37–41.

88 Dalakas MC, Illa I, Dambrosia JM, *et al*. A controlled trial of high-dose intravenous immune globulin infusions as treatment for dermatomyositis. *N Engl J Med* 1993;**329**:1993–2000.

89 Al-Mayouf S, Al-Mazyed A, Bahabri S. Efficacy of early treatment of severe juvenile dermatomyositis with intravenous methylprednisolone and methotrexate. *Clin Rheumatol* 2000;**19**:138–41.

90 Gottfried I, Seeber A, Anegg B, Rieger A, Stingl G, Volc-Platzer B. High dose intravenous immunoglobulin (IVIG) in dermatomyositis: clinical responses and effect on sIL-2R levels. *Eur J Dermatol* 2000;**10**:29–35.

91 Efthimiou P, Schwartzman S, Kagen LJ. Possible role for tumour necrosis factor inhibitors in the treatment of resistant dermatomyositis and polymyositis: a retrospective study of eight patients. *Ann Rheum Dis* 2006;**65**:1233–6.

92 Levine TD. Rituximab in the treatment of dermatomyositis: an open-label pilot study. *Arthritis Rheum* 2005;**52**:601–7.

93 Wiesinger GF, Quittan M, Aringer M, *et al*. Improvement of physical fitness and muscle strength in polymyositis/dermatomyositis patients by a training programme. *Br J Rheumatol* 1998;**37**:196–200.

94 Hollar CB, Jorizzo JL. Topical tacrolimus 0.1% ointment for refractory skin disease in dermatomyositis: a pilot study. *J Dermatolog Treat* 2004;**15**:35–9.

95 García-Doval I, Cruces M. Topical tacrolimus in cutaneous lesions of dermatomyositis: lack of effect in side-by-side comparison in five patients. *Dermatology (Basel)* 2004;**209**:247–8.

96 Woo TY, Callen JP, Voorhees JJ, Bickers DR, Hanno R, Hawkins C. Cutaneous lesions of dermatomyositis are improved by hydroxychloroquine. *J Am Acad Dermatol* 1984;**10**:592–600.

97 Ang GC, Werth VP. Combination antimalarials in the treatment of cutaneous dermatomyositis: a retrospective study. *Arch Dermatol* 2005;**141**:855–9.

98 Zieglschmid-Adams ME, Pandya AG, Cohen SB, Sontheimer RD. Treatment of dermatomyositis with methotrexate. *J Am Acad Dermatol* 1995;**32**(5 Pt 1):754–7.

99 Kasteler JS, Callen JP. Low-dose methotrexate administered weekly is an effective corticosteroid-sparing agent for the treatment of the cutaneous manifestations of dermatomyositis. *J Am Acad Dermatol* 1997;**36**:67–71.

100 Gelber AC, Nousari HC, Wigley FM. Mycophenolate mofetil in the treatment of severe skin manifestations of dermatomyositis: a series of 4 cases. *J Rheumatol* 2000;**27**:1542–5.

101 Pelle MT, Callen JP. Adverse cutaneous reactions to hydroxychloroquine are more common in patients with dermatomyositis than in patients with cutaneous lupus erythematosus. *Arch Dermatol* 2002;**138**:1231–3; discussion 1233.

102 Pachman LM, Abbott K, Sinacore JM, *et al*. Duration of illness is an important variable for untreated children with juvenile dermatomyositis. *J Pediatr* 2006;**148**:247–53.

Acquired subepidermal bullous diseases

Gudula Kirtschig, Nonhlanhla P. Khumalo, Vanessa Venning,
Fenella Wojnarowska

Bullous pemphigoid

Background

Definition

Bullous pemphigoid (BP) is an acquired nonscarring autoimmune subepidermal bullous disease characterized by tense blisters. Circulating immunoglobulin G (IgG) autoantibodies (rarely IgA and IgE) typically bind to BP230 and BP180 antigens, which are components of the hemidesmosome adhesion complex found in the basement membrane zone of the skin. Direct antibody–antigen interaction, local activation of complement, and release of cytokines lead to loss of dermoepidermal adherence and formation of subepidermal blisters.[1] Blistering typically occurs on the flexures, although BP may be generalized or localized to one site, such as the lower legs. Erosions and blisters occur on the mucous membranes, particularly the mouth, in about 50% of cases. Blister formation may be preceded by pruritus, an urticarial or eczematous rash, which may precede the blistering for many months (Figure 57.1).

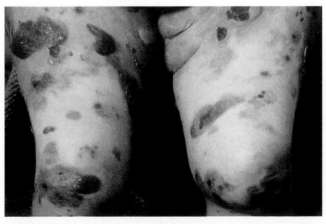

Figure 57.1 Crusted erosions and large hemorrhagic bullae.

Incidence/prevalence

BP is the most common autoimmune blistering disease in the West. The estimated annual incidence varies in different countries between two and 30 cases per million population.[2] It tends to affect the elderly, with a high incidence in men above the age of 85, according to a Scottish study; however, there is no sex preponderance in general.[2]

Etiology

No clear etiological factors have been identified. There are anecdotal reports of BP being preceded by local cutaneous trauma, such as surgery, and exposure to ionizing or ultraviolet radiation. There appears to be a true association between BP and certain neurological diseases.[3,4] BP is possibly triggered by drugs in certain patients.[5] There does not seem to be an increased risk of malignancy in patients with BP in Western countries, in comparison with controls.[2,6]

Prognosis

Both treated and untreated BP show a chronic relapsing course. The majority of patients with BP will have disease remission within 5 years.[7] The mortality rate appears to be highest within the first 2 years of diagnosis;[2,8] according to the Scottish study, 48% of patients died within 2 years (unrelated and related to BP or treatment). Respiratory disease accounted for a higher than expected number of deaths.[2]

Aims of treatment

The aims of treatment are to achieve quick healing of skin and mucous membrane lesions and longer-term disease remission, and to improve the quality of life, with minimal adverse effects of treatment.

Outcomes

• Rate of healing of blisters and suppression of new blister formation
• Effect on quality of life
• Duration of remission while the patient is receiving treatment and after cessation of treatment

- Complications of disease
- Adverse effects of treatment, including mortality

Methods of search

Randomized controlled trials (RCTs) were identified from searches of the Skin Group Specialized Register, the Cochrane Central Register of Controlled Trials, Medline, and Embase up to May 2005. All RCTs on interventions for BP confirmed by immunofluorescence studies were included.

Questions

What are the effects of corticosteroids?

A systematic review of treatments for BP identified only seven RCTs, with a total of 634 patients.[9]

Topical corticosteroids
Benefits

We found one RCT comparing very potent topical steroids (clobetasol propionate) versus prednisone for the treatment of BP.[10] A total of 341 patients with BP were stratified according to disease severity: moderate (≤ 10 new blisters/day, n = 153) or extensive (> 10 new blisters/day, n = 188). Patients were randomly assigned to receive either topical clobetasol propionate cream (40 g per day) or oral prednisone (0.5 mg/kg/day for moderate disease and 1 mg/kg/day for extensive disease). The major outcome in this study was survival. In the extensive disease group, those using topical steroids had a better survival rate at 1 year in comparison with those receiving oral steroids (71/93 vs. 56/95; risk difference 0.17; 95% confidence interval, 0.04 to 0.31; number needed to treat 6; 95% CI, 4 to 24). This difference was consistent with the incidence of severe complications in the two extensive disease groups (29% for topical steroids versus 54% for oral steroids). The disease was controlled in 99% of cases (92/93 vs. 86/95; difference in rate of control 0.08; 95% CI, 0.02 to 0.15; NNT 12; 95% CI, 7 to 47). The difference reaches statistical significance, although this outcome was not assessed blindly and there is therefore a possibility of bias. In the moderate disease group, no significant differences were seen between the topical steroid and 0.5 mg/kg oral steroid groups in terms of overall survival, rate of disease control at 3 weeks, or the incidence of severe complications.

Harms

Skin infection, skin atrophy, and evidence of systemic absorption may be seen.

Comment

The recent RCT suggests the use of topical steroids as the first-line treatment for both localized and mild disease.[10] Relatively few and mild side effects are associated with topical corticosteroid treatment in BP; however, their use in extensive disease may be limited by more side effects and practical factors (e.g., the need for nursing input).

Systemic corticosteroids
Benefits

Two small RCTs looked at the effects of systemic corticosteroids alone.[11,12] Dreno et al. compared biologically equivalent doses of different corticosteroids: methylprednisolone 1.17 mg/kg/day and prednisolone methylsulphobenzoate 1.16 mg/kg/day (at day 10, the overall responders were 22/28 and 18/29, respectively (response difference 0.17; 95% CI, −0.07 to 0.40; NNT 6; 95% CI, 3 to −15). The mean number of blisters was 6.0 for methylprednisolone and 13.0 for prednisolone. The difference between groups was not significant, with a mean difference of seven fewer blisters with methylprednisolone (95% CI, 22 fewer to 8 more).[11] Morel et al. compared different doses of prednisolone: 1.25 mg/kg/day and 0.75 mg/kg/day.[12] This study had only a short follow-up period (51 days). There were 3/22 vs. 2/24 deaths and 12/26 vs. 8/24 responders, respectively (response difference 0.13; 95% CI, −0.14 to 0.40; NNT 8; 95% CI, 3 to −7). Neither trial found any statistical differences in the effectiveness of treatment.

Harms

Higher doses of prednisolone were associated with more side effects, including infection, hepatic and renal impairment, cerebrovascular accidents, hypertension, heart failure, and death.

Comment

Systemic corticosteroids are regarded as being the standard treatment for BP, although a placebo-controlled trial has not been carried out. Higher doses of corticosteroids are associated with increased morbidity and mortality.

Does combination treatment offer any advantage over corticosteroid monotherapy?
Benefits

We found three non-blinded RCTs.[13–15] Burton et al. compared prednisolone 30–80 mg/day alone and in combination with azathioprine 2.5 mg/kg/day. The addition of azathioprine resulted in a 45% reduction in the prednisolone dose over a 3-year period.[13] Roujeau et al. compared prednisolone 0.3 mg/kg/day alone and in combination with plasma exchange. They found that less than half the total prednisolone dose was required in the plasma exchange group.[14] Disease control was achieved within weeks in both groups—in the plasma exchange group with a mean prednisolone dose of 0.52 ± 0.28 mg/kg/day and in the prednisolone-only group with 0.97 ± 0.33 mg/kg/day. Guillaume et al. compared prednisolone 1 mg/kg/day alone or in combination with either azathioprine (100 mg for body weight ≤ 60 kg and 150 mg for body weight > 60 kg) or plasma exchange.[15] This trial failed to confirm any benefit of combination therapy over prednisolone alone.

Harms

The addition of azathioprine and/or plasma exchange did not increase the incidence of side effects; in fact, similar side-effect profiles were seen in the studies by Burton *et al.* and Roujeau *et al.*[13,14] Guillaume *et al.* commented that most side effects were attributable to corticosteroids, but details were not supplied.[15]

Comment

With the evidence currently available, the value of combination treatment remains doubtful.

Are nonantibiotic properties of antimicrobials useful?

Benefits

One small RCT compared tetracycline 2 g/day in four divided doses, plus nicotinamide 1500 mg/day in three divided doses, with prednisolone 40–80 mg/day.[16] There were no deaths in the group of 14 patients treated with tetracyclines and nicotinamide and one death among six patients treated with prednisolone (survival difference 0.17; 95% CI, −0.25 to 0.58; NNT 6; 95%, CI 2 to −4). Five complete responders, five partial responders and one nonresponder and one case of disease progression were described in the tetracycline group, in comparison with one complete and five partial responders in the steroid group; two patients in the tetracycline group were unavailable for follow-up at 8 weeks. The results are not statistically significant for either complete response or complete and/or partial response.

Harms

More serious side effects (including death due to sepsis) were noted in the prednisolone group. One patient with established renal impairment in the tetracycline/ nicotinamide group developed acute tubular necrosis, but concomitant medications included aspirin and ibuprofen.

Comments

This was a small trial of 18 patients, with an unclear method of randomization and a high drop-out rate. To determine if tetracyclines are effective in suppressing BP a RCT comparing prednisolone 0.05 mg/kg/day vs doxycycline 200 mg/ kg/day is in progress.

Mucous membrane pemphigoid

Background

Definition

Mucous membrane pemphigoid (MMP), formerly known as cicatricial pemphigoid, is an acquired autoimmune bullous disease primarily affecting the mucous membranes and to a lesser extent the skin.[17] Autoantibodies are directed against constituents of the hemidesmosomal adhesion complex of the skin and mucous membranes; the main autoantigens are BP180 and laminin 5. Autoantibody–autoantigen interaction leads to blister formation.[17–20] Direct immunofluorescence investigation of patients' skin or mucosa shows linear IgG and C3 deposits at the dermoepidermal junction, and indirect immunofluorescence of patients' serum may reveal circulating autoantibodies. Indirect immunofluorescence using salt-split skin may show binding to the roof (epidermis) in BP180-MMP or to the floor (dermis) in laminin 5-MMP of the artificial blister.[19,20] Scar formation is characteristic, though not usually seen at the oral mucosa, and may result in blindness and respiratory obstruction.

Incidence/prevalence

The incidence of MMP is estimated at 0.87 cases per million population per year in western Europe.[21] There is a slight female preponderance (1.5 : 1) and the elderly are more commonly affected.

Etiology

The etiology is unknown; there are reports of drug-induced MMP.[22]

Prognosis

The course of MMP is variable; usually it is a very chronic disease.[17] The presentation may vary from stable oral involvement to rapidly progressive ocular disease despite immunosuppressive therapy.

Aims of treatment

The aims of treatment are to achieve quick healing of mucosal and skin lesions and longer-term disease remission, and to improve the quality of life with minimal adverse effects.

Key points—bullous pemphigoid

- Few RCTs systematically reviewing treatments for BP were identified.
- The available evidence is inadequate to allow confident recommendation of optimal treatment.
- A less aggressive approach to therapy with low doses of corticosteroids (and topical steroids for localized disease) may be sufficient for disease control and appears to be associated with less morbidity and mortality.
- Tetracyclines and nicotinamide may be effective, but larger trials are needed in order to compare this therapy with low-dose prednisolone.
- The benefits of azathioprine and plasma exchange are difficult to assess.

Relevant outcomes

- Rate of healing of blisters, cessation of blistering and prevention of scarring
- Effect on quality of life
- Duration of remission after cessation of treatment
- Complications of primary disease
- Adverse effects of treatment, including mortality

Methods of search

RCTs of patients with MMP or epidermolysis bullosa acquisita (EBA) were identified from Medline/PubMed and Embase from their inception to April 2005. The Cochrane Skin Group Specialized Register, the Cochrane Central Register of Controlled Trials (Central), www.controlled-trials.com, and www.clinicaltrials.gov were last examined in April 2005. The bibliographies from identified studies were searched. However, because MMP and EBA are rare diseases, we did not expect to find many RCTs and therefore also considered some evidence from nonrandomized studies and case reports with diagnoses confirmed by immunofluorescence studies.

Questions

What are the effects of systemic drug treatments?

There is one systematic review of therapeutic interventions for MMP.[23] It identified two small RCTs for the treatment of ocular MMP, but no placebo-controlled trials.[24]

What are the effects of cyclophosphamide?
Benefits

Cyclophosphamide plus prednisolone versus prednisolone. One double-blind RCT included 24 patients with bilateral ocular, stage III MMP (symblepharon formation). It compared prednisolone (initially 1 mg/kg/day) alone with cyclophosphamide (2 mg/kg/day) plus prednisolone.[24] Cyclophosphamide in combination with prednisolone was found to be more effective in controlling bilateral stage III cicatricial pemphigoid involving the eyes (using chi-squared analysis, $P < 0.005$).

Cyclophosphamide versus dapsone. One double-blind RCT trial included 40 patients with stage III ocular MMP. It compared dapsone (2 mg/kg/day) with cyclophosphamide (2 mg/kg/day) in 40 patients with stage III ocular MMP. It is not clearly stated, but both groups most likely had additional prednisolone, as in the above-mentioned trial.[24] Cyclophosphamide was found to be superior to dapsone in MMP patients with severe (4+) inflammation of the eyes. Dapsone treatment failed in six patients, including four patients with 4+ and two patients with 3+ conjunctival inflammation prior to therapy, all of whom responded to cyclophosphamide after a 3-month trial of dapsone.

Harms

None of the patients withdrew from systemic immunosuppression because of adverse effects. Each of the patients in the prednisone group experienced prednisone-induced complications such as hypertension, diabetes mellitus, osteoporosis, peptic ulcer disease, myopathy, and psychosis. Leukopenia was a routine finding in patients treated with cyclophosphamide, and the dose was adjusted to achieve a white cell count of 2500–4000/μL. Reversible hair loss was a common finding with cyclophosphamide, as was asymptomatic macrocytic anemia. Routine urinalysis detected microcytic hematuria in about 10% of patients taking cyclophosphamide. An alteration in the timing of cyclophosphamide administration and increased fluid intake eliminated this potentially serious side effect (hemorrhagic cystitis). Male sterility may occur, and there is a potential for development of malignancies (DNA damage).

Comments

With careful monitoring, systemic cyclophosphamide may pose fewer risks than long-term corticosteroid therapy.

What are the effects of sulfa drugs?
Benefits

No placebo-controlled trials were identified. Observational studies suggest a beneficial effect of dapsone, sulfapyridine and sulfamethoxypyridazine in most patients with MMP.[25–29]

Sulfa drugs versus other treatments. As mentioned above, one RCT compared dapsone and cyclophosphamide in the treatment of stage III ocular cicatricial pemphigoid.[24] Although cyclophosphamide was superior in the treatment of severe disease, dapsone treatment resulted in disease control in 14 of 20 patients.

Comparisons between sulfa drugs. A small observational study (20 patients) reports that sulfapyridine may be superior to dapsone in moderate ocular MMP.[28] Another study stated that sulfasalazine was effective in maintaining disease control in six of nine patients with ocular MMP who had had previous dapsone-related side effects, although two of the six required additional oral cyclophosphamide.[29]

Harms

Dapsone must not be given to patients with glucose-6-phosphate-dehydrogenase deficiency; some degree of anemia is common in most patients. There are potentially serious adverse effects in treatment with dapsone, but these are very rare. They include severe hemolytic anemia, methemoglobinemia, agranulocytosis, neuropathy, and the dapsone syndrome (rash with fever and eosinophilia), which requires the immediate cessation of dapsone, as it may progress to exfoliative dermatitis and death. In general, most dermatologists will have used dapsone regularly, but most are probably not familiar with the use of cyclophosphamide.

Comments

Cyclophosphamide appears to be more effective in controlling severe ocular disease, but because of the lower side-effect profile, dapsone appears to be a reasonable first choice in patients with little inflammation and disease that is not rapidly progressive.

What are the effects of antibiotics?
Benefits

Small uncontrolled studies (including a total of 25 patients)[30,31] indicate that minocycline (50–100 mg/day) or tetracycline (1 g/day) combined with nicotinamide (2.5–3.0 g/day) may be beneficial in oral disease.

Harms

Hyperpigmentation was a common side effect with minocycline.

Comments

RCTs are required to confirm the benefit of nonantibiotic properties of antimicrobials.

What is the effect of intravenous immunoglobulin therapy?
Benefits

The use of intravenous immunoglobulins has been described in a few reports by the same group of investigators.[32,33] One noncomparative case series of 10 patients with treatment-resistant progressive ocular MMP showed resolution of conjunctivitis after four to 12 cycles of intravenous immunoglobulin treatment (2–3 g/kg body weight per cycle every 2–6 weeks).[32] A nonrandomized comparison between conventional immunosuppressive and intravenous immunoglobulin therapies investigated eight patients in each group.[33] All of the patients had received (various forms of) immunosuppressive treatment initially before treatment with intravenous immunoglobulin was started.

Harms

There were no untoward side effects in these case series.

Comment

Comparative studies are needed. Intravenous immunoglobulin therapy is expensive.[34]

What is the effect of mycophenolate mofetil?
Benefits

Small case series including five and 14 patients have been published.[35,36] One showed nonprogression of ocular MMP in nine of 10 eyes treated with oral mycophenolate mofetil

(MMF) 2 g daily for at least 12 months.[35] MMF helped to control the MMP in 10 of 14 patients in the second series.[36]

Harms

Lack of appetite, nausea, and mild diarrhea were common early side effects. Severe side effects resulting from immunosuppression were not noted in these series.

Comment

Larger comparative studies are needed to assess the treatment efficacy of MMF.

Treatment with topical tacrolimus, topical ciclosporin, tetracycline and nicotinamide, colchicine, thalidomide, leflunomide, plasmapheresis, autologous serum application to ocular epithelial defects and "biologicals" such as tumor necrosis factor-α receptor blocker (etanercept), anti-CD25 (daclizumab), and anti-CD20 (rituximab) has been described in single cases.

Summary

- Cyclophosphamide and dapsone combined with predniso(lo)ne are likely to be beneficial in the treatment of MMP.
- Antibiotics (e.g., tetracyclines), mycophenolate mofetil, and intravenous immunoglobulins are of unknown effectiveness.

Key points—mucous membrane pemphigoid

- The available evidence is inadequate for confident recommendation of optimal treatment.
- Cyclophosphamide combined with systemic corticosteroids appears to suppress inflammation and scarring in ocular MMP.
- Dapsone combined with systemic corticosteroids may be helpful in the management of ocular MMP with modest inflammation.
- More recent studies suggest a beneficial effect of antimicrobials, MMF, and intravenous immunoglobulins, although RCTs are needed to support these observations.

Epidermolysis bullosa acquisita

Background

Definition

Epidermolysis bullosa acquisita (EBA) is an acquired autoimmune bullous disease characterized by tense blisters arising on inflamed or normal appearing skin. Two different presentations of EBA are recognized: a) the blister distribution may resemble bullous pemphigoid with blistering on inflamed skin; and b) the blisters may appear at trauma-exposed sites on often noninflamed skin. Mucous membrane involvement is common and is similar to that found in mucous membrane pemphigoid. Atrophic scar formation is characteristic and may result in blindness and respiratory obstruction. In some patients, EBA is associated with ulcerative colitis.

Autoantibodies are directed against collagen VII, a constituent of the adhesion complex within the basement membrane zone of skin and mucous membranes. Auto-antibody–autoantigen interaction is thought to induce blister formation.[37,38] Direct immunofluorescence shows linear deposition of IgG and C3 at the dermoepidermal junction; indirect immunofluorescence may reveal circulating autoantibodies. Indirect immunofluorescence on salt-split skin shows binding to the floor of the artificial blister.[39]

Incidence/prevalence
EBA is rare, with an estimated annual incidence of 0.22 per million population in western Europe.[40] It tends to affect people over 40 years of age, although children may also be affected.[41] There may be a slight female preponderance.

Etiology
The etiology is unknown.

Prognosis
EBA is a chronic disease with variable severity.[37]

Aims of treatment
The aims of treatment are to achieve quick healing of skin and mucous membrane lesions and longer-term disease remission, and to improve the quality of life with minimal adverse effects.

Relevant outcomes
- Rate of healing of blisters and suppression of new blister formation
- Effect on quality of life
- Duration of remission after stopping treatment
- Complications of primary disease
- Adverse effects of treatment, including mortality

Methods of search
See the methods described for MMP above. All therapeutic interventions for EBA confirmed by immunofluorescence studies were included.

Question

What are the effects of treatment?

There is one systematic review of all treatments for EBA.[42] No RCTs were identified. Ten small observational studies involving two or more patients were identified.[42-51] No

final results were obtained regarding the one prospective uncontrolled trial for EBA.[45]

Various systemic medications have been tested, including corticosteroids, immunosuppressants, dapsone, colchicine, and intravenous immunoglobulins. Various doses of prednisolone or methylprednisolone were used, frequently in combination with other drugs, including dapsone or sulfapyridine and colchicine.

Comments
The uncontrolled studies of EBA suggest that children appear to respond to treatment with a combination of systemic corticosteroids and dapsone. However, in children, EBA appears to remit within a few years, and it is not possible to judge whether this is due to treatment or represents a spontaneous remission.

Summary
No reliable evidence-based recommendations can be given for the treatment of EBA. Glucocorticosteroids, immunosuppressants, dapsone, colchicine, and intravenous immunoglobulins are of unknown effectiveness.

Key points—epidermolysis bullosa acquisita
- It is not possible to draw conclusions regarding the optimum treatment for EBA.
- Children appear to have a better prognosis than adults.

References

1 Sams WM Jr, Gammon WR. Mechanism of lesion production in pemphigus and pemphigoid. *J Am Acad Dermatol* 1982;**6**:431–52.
2 Gudi VS, White MI, Cruickshank N, *et al.* Annual incidence and mortality of bullous pemphigoid in the Grampian region of North-east Scotland. *Br J Dermatol* 2005;**153**:424–7.
3 Seppanen A, Autio-Harmainen H, Alafuzoff I, *et al.* Collagen XVII is expressed in human CNS neurons. *Matrix Biol* 2006;**25**:185–8.
4 Stinco G, Codutti R, Scarbolo M, *et al.* A retrospective epidemiological study on the association of bullous pemphigoid and neurological diseases. *Acta Derm Venereol* 2005;**85**:136–9.
5 Bastuji-Garin S, Joly P, Picard-Dahan C, *et al.* Drugs associated with bullous pemphigoid. A case–control study. *Arch Dermatol* 1996;**132**:272–6.
6 Venning VA, Wojnarowska F. The association of bullous pemphigoid and malignant disease: a case control study. *Br J Dermatol* 1990;**123**:439–45.
7 Venning V, Wojnarowska F. Lack of predictive factors for the course of bullous pemphigoid. *J Am Acad Dermatol* 1992;**26**:585–9.
8 Colbert RL, Allen DM, Eastwood D, Fairley JA. Mortality rate of bullous pemphigoid in a US medical center. *J Invest Dermatol* 2004;**122**:1091–5.

9 Khumalo N, Kirtschig G, Middleton P, Hollis S, Wojnarowska F, Murrell D. Interventions for bullous pemphigoid. *Cochrane Database Syst Rev* 2005;(**3**):CD002292.

10 Joly P, Roujeau J-C, Benichou J, et al. A comparison of oral and topical corticosteroids in patients with bullous pemphigoid. *N Engl J Med* 2002;**346**:321–7.

11 Dreno B, Sassolas B, Lacour P, et al. Methylprednisolone versus prednisolone methylsulphobenzoate in pemphigoid: a comparative multicenter study. *Ann Dermatol Venereol* 1993;**120**:518–21.

12 Morel P, Guillaime JC. Treatment of bullous pemphigoid with prednisolone only: 0.75 mg/kg/day versus 1.25 mg/kg/day. A multicenter randomised study. *Ann Dermatol Venereol* 1984;**111**:925–8.

13 Burton JL, Harman RR, Peachey RD, Warin RP. Azathioprine plus prednisolone in treatment of pemphigoid. *BMJ* 1978;**2**:1190–1.

14 Roujeau JC, Guillaume JC, Morel P, et al. Plasma exchange in bullous pemphigoid. *Lancet* 1984;**2**:486–8.

15 Guillaume JC, Vaillant L, Bernard P, et al. Controlled trial of azathioprine and plasma exchange in addition to prednisolone in the treatment of bullous pemphigoid. *Arch Dermatol* 1993;**129**:49–53.

16 Fivenson D, Breneman D, Rosen G, et al. Nicotinamide and tetracycline therapy of bullous pemphigoid. *Arch Dermatol* 1994;**130**:753–8.

17 Chan LS, Ahmed AR, Anhalt GJ, et al. The first international consensus on mucous membrane pemphigoid: definition, diagnostic criteria, pathogenic factors, medical treatment, and prognostic indicators. *Arch Dermatol* 2002;**138**:370–9.

18 Liu Z, Diaz LA, Troy LJ, et al. A passive transfer model or the organ specific autoimmune disease bullous pemphigoid using antibodies directed against the hemidesmosomal antigen BP120. *J Clin Invest* 1993;**92**:2480–8.

19 Bernard P, Prost C, Durepaire N, et al. The major cicatricial pemphigoid antigen is a 180-kD protein that shows immunologic cross-reactivity with the bullous pemphigoid antigen. *J Invest Dermatol* 1992;**99**:174–9.

20 Domloge-Hultsch N, Gammon WR, Briggaman RA, et al. Epiligrin, the major human keratinocyte integrin ligand, is a target in both an acquired autoimmune and an inherited subepidermal blistering skin disease. *J Clin Invest* 1992;**90**:1628–33.

21 Zillikens D, Wever S, Roth A, et al. Incidence of autoimmune subepidermal blistering dermatoses in a region of Central Germany. *Arch Dermatol* 1995;**131**:957–8.

22 Butt Z, Kaufman D, McNab A, McKelvie P. Drug-induced ocular cicatricial pemphigoid: a series of clinicopathological reports. *Eye* 1998;**12**:285–90.

23 Kirtschig G, Murrell D, Wojnarowska F, Khumalo N. Interventions for mucous membrane pemphigoid and epidermolysis bullosa acquisita. *Cochrane Database Syst Rev* 2003;(**1**):CD004056.

24 Foster CS. Cicatricial pemphigoid. *Trans Am Ophthalmol Soc* 1986;**84**:527–663.

25 Rogers RS, Seehafer JR, Perry HO. Treatment of cicatricial (benign mucous membrane) pemphigoid with dapsone. *J Am Acad Dermatol* 1982;**6**:215–23.

26 Rogers RS, Mehregan DA. Dapsone therapy of cicatricial pemphigoid. *Semin Dermatol* 1988;**7**:201–5.

27 Thornhill M, Pemberton M, Buchanan J, Theaker E. An open clinical trial of sulphamethoxypyridazine in the treatment of mucous membrane pemphigoid. *Br J Dermatol* 2000;**143**:117–26.

28 Elder MJ, Leonard J, Dart JK. Sulphapyridine: new treatment for the treatment of ocular cicatricial pemphigoid. *Br J Ophthalmol* 1996;**80**:549–52.

29 Doan S, Lerouic JF, Robin H, Prost C, et al. Treatment of ocular cicatricial pemphigoid with sulfasalazine. *Ophthalmology* 2001;**108**:1565–86.

30 Poskitt L, Wojnarowska F. Minimizing cicatricial pemphigoid orodynia with minocycline. *Br J Dermatol* 1995;**132**:784–9.

31 Reiche L, Wojnarowska F, Mallon E. Combination therapy with nicotinamide and tetracyclines for cicatricial pemphigoid: further support of its efficacy. *Clin Exp Dermatol* 1998;**23**:254–7.

32 Foster CS, Ahmed AR. Intravenous immunoglobulin therapy for ocular cicatricial pemphigoid: a preliminary study. *Ophthalmology* 1999;**106**:2136–43.

33 Letko E, Miserocchi E, Daoud YJ, et al. A nonrandomized comparison of the clinical outcome of ocular involvement in patients with mucous membrane (cicatricial) pemphigoid between conventional immunosuppressive and intravenous immunoglobulin therapies. *Clin Immunol* 2004;**111**:303–10.

34 Daoud Y, Amin KG, Mohan K, Ahmed AR. Cost of intravenous immunoglobulin therapy versus conventional immunosuppressive therapy in patients with mucous membrane pemphigoid: a preliminary study. *Ann Pharmacother* 2005;**39**:2003–8.

35 Zurdel J, Aboalchamat B, Zierhut M, Stubiger N, Bialasiewicz A, Engelmann K. [Early clinical results with mycophenolate mofetil in immunosuppressive therapy of ocular pemphigoid; in German.] *Klin Monatsbl Augenheilkd* 2001;**218**:222–8.

36 Ingen-Housz-Oro S, Prost-Squarcioni C, Pascal F, et al. Cicatricial pemphigoid: treatment with mycophenolate mofetil. *Ann Dermatol Venereol* 2005;**132**;13–6.

37 Briggaman RA, Gammon WR, Woodley DT. Epidermolysis bullosa acquisita. In: Wojnarowska F, Briggaman RA, eds. *Management of Blistering Disease.* London: Chapman and Hall, 1990:127–38.

38 Borradori L, James B, Caldwell MC, et al. Passive transfer of autoantibodies from a patient with mutilating epidermolysis bullosa acquisita induces specific alterations in the skin of neonatal mice. *Arch Dermatol* 1995;**131**:590–5.

39 Gammon WR, Briggaman RA, Inman AO III, et al. Differentiating anti-lamina lucida and anti-sublamina densa anti-BMZ antibodies by indirect immunofluorescence on 1.0 M sodium chloride-separated skin. *J Invest Dermatol* 1984;**82**:139–44.

40 Zillikens D, Wever S, Roth A, et al. Incidence of autoimmune subepidermal blistering dermatoses in a region of Central Germany. *Arch Dermatol* 1995;**131**:957–8.

41 Kirtschig G, Wojnarowska F, Marsden RA, et al. Acquired bullous disease of childhood: re-evaluation of diagnosis by direct immunofluorescence examination and immunoblotting. *Br J Dermatol* 1994;**130**:610–6.

42 Kirtschig G, Murrell D, Wojnarowska F, Khumalo N. Interventions for mucous membrane pemphigoid and epidermolysis bullosa acquisita. *Cochrane Database Syst Rev* 2003;(**1**):CD004056.

43 Harman KE, Black MM. High-dose intravenous immune globulin for the treatment of autoimmune blistering diseases: an evaluation of its use in 14 cases. *Br J Dermatol* 1999;**140**:865–74.

44 Luke MC, Darling TN, Hsu R et al. Mucosal morbidity in patients with epidermolysis bullosa acquisita. *Arch Dermatol* 1999;**135**:954–9.

45 Gordon KB, Chan LS, Woodley DT. Treatment of refractory epidermolysis bullosa acquisita with extracorporeal photochemotherapy. *Br J Dermatol* 1997;**136**:415–20.

46 Cunningham BB, Kirchmann TT, Woodley D. Colchicine for epidermolysis bullosa acquisita. *J Am Acad Dermatol* 1996;**34**:781–4.

47 Megahed M, Scharffetter-Kochanek K. Epidermolysis bullosa acquisita: successful treatment with colchicine. *Arch Dermatol Res* 1994;**286**:35–46.

48 Rappersberger K, Konrad K, Schenk P, Tappeiner G. [Acquired epidermolysis bullosa. A clinico-pathologic study; in German.] *Hautarzt* 1988;**39**:355–62.

49 Arpey CJ, Elewski BE, Moritz DK, Gammon WR. Childhood epidermolysis bullosa acquisita. *J Am Acad Dermatol* 1991;**24**:706–14.

50 Edwards S, Wakelin SH, Wojnarowska F, *et al.* Bullous pemphigoid and epidermolysis bullosa acquisita: presentation, prognosis and immunopathology in 11 children. *Pediatr Dermatol* 1998;**15**:184–90.

51 Callot-Mellot C, Bodemer C, Caux F, *et al.* Epidermolysis bullosa acquisita in childhood. *Arch Dermatol* 1997;**133**:1122–6.

58 Pemphigus

Brian R. Sperber, Linda K. Martin, Dedee F. Murrell, Victoria P. Werth

Background

Definition

Pemphigus is an intra-epidermal autoimmune blistering disease involving the skin and mucous membranes. Pemphigus is conventionally divided into three distinct subtypes: pemphigus vulgaris, pemphigus foliaceus, and paraneoplastic pemphigus. Pemphigus vulgaris is characterized by blisters affecting both oral and cutaneous surfaces, whereas patients with pemphigus foliaceus have only cutaneous involvement. Patients with paraneoplastic pemphigus invariably have striking mucous membrane disease, as well as a widespread skin eruption that can resemble pemphigus vulgaris, bullous pemphigoid, erythema multiforme, graft-versus-host disease, or lichen planus. In this chapter, we will exclusively address pemphigus vulgaris and foliaceus, except in the discussion of studies that included paraneoplastic pemphigus patients before it was recognized as a distinct clinicopathological entity and was thus not distinguished from other forms of pemphigus (Figure 58.1).

Epidemiology

The incidence of pemphigus has been estimated at approximately one in 1 000 000 to one in 100 000 per year, depending on the population in question.[1] For instance, in regions with many Jewish residents or residents of Mediterranean origin, the incidence of pemphigus is estimated to be much higher than in regions with fewer people from these ethnic groups.

Etiology

As is the case with other autoimmune diseases, the exact pathophysiological mechanism that causes immune dys-

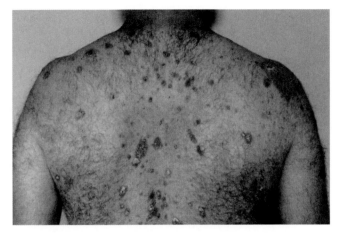

Figure 58.1 A patient with extensive erosions and flaccid bullae due to pemphigus vulgaris.

regulation in pemphigus is unknown. Pemphigus is a T-cell–driven autoantibody-mediated disease, with T cells reacting to specific antigenic adhesion proteins in the skin. The production of autoantibodies to intercellular proteins in the epidermis, along with various inflammatory mediators, is believed to directly elicit acantholysis. The clinical phenotype of pemphigus is defined by the specific profile of autoantibodies. Patients with mucosal-dominant pemphigus vulgaris have only antidesmoglein 3 immunoglobulin G (IgG) autoantibodies. Patients with mucocutaneous pemphigus vulgaris have both antidesmoglein 3 and antidesmoglein 1 autoantibodies. Patients with pemphigus foliaceus, who have only skin lesions, have antidesmoglein 1 antibodies.[1]

Prognosis

The mortality of pemphigus decreased dramatically after corticosteroids were introduced as therapy in the 1950s. Before that time, the mortality was approximately 70%

and usually resulted from sepsis.[2] With corticosteroids and adjuvant therapy, the mortality is now approximately 6%, with most deaths being related to side effects of therapy.[3]

Diagnosis

Diagnosis is based on three measures:
- Clinical features: oral ulcers, flaccid blisters, or erosions with scale.
- Histological features: acantholysis with loss of coherence between epidermal cells; upward growth of papillae lined by a single layer of epidermal cells.
- Direct and indirect immunofluorescence: detection of autoantibodies either in a biopsy specimen (direct) or in the patient's serum (indirect). The enzyme-linked immunosorbent assay (ELISA) is a new diagnostic modality that may prove to be effective for diagnosis, as well as functioning as a prognostic indicator.

Aims of treatment

The main aims of treatment in pemphigus are to suppress new blister formation and promote the healing of old lesions whilst minimizing the side effects of treatment.

Relevant outcomes

Interpretation of evidence is complicated by the lack of uniform outcome measures. Outcomes regarding disease control include prevention of new blister formation, healing of old lesions, and the time required to achieve disease control. In the longer term, the proportion of patients able to discontinue treatment and the proportion of patients who relapse are important. The safety of treatments is especially important, as the major morbidity is derived from complications of treatment. Cumulative steroid dose is often measured as a surrogate for steroid-induced adverse events. Autoantibody titers are reported to correlate with disease activity. Patient-based measures, including quality of life, should also be considered.

Search strategy

Articles were identified from the Cochrane Central Register of Controlled Trials (Central), Medline, and Embase, using the Cochrane Collaboration's highly sensitive search strategy.

Study selection criteria

Only seven randomized controlled trials (RCTs) on interventions for pemphigus were identified. We have restricted our analysis to controlled trials and case series including at least five patients.

Questions

What is the optimal dosing strategy for corticosteroids in newly diagnosed patients?

Corticosteroids are firmly established as the mainstay of treatment for pemphigus. Their introduction in the 1950s was associated with a dramatic decrease in mortality.[4–6] Initially, very high doses were employed, but these doses were associated with significant adverse events, and the rationale for high-dose regimens has been questioned.[7–9]

In the only RCT to address steroid-dosing regimens, Ratnam *et al.* compared the efficacy of different prednisolone doses.[10] Twenty-two previously untreated patients with severe disease (> 50% of the body surface area affected) were randomly assigned to "high-dose" (120–150 mg/day; n = 11) or "low-dose" (30–60 mg/day; n = 11) prednisolone. Patients also received adjuvant therapy with methotrexate or cyclophosphamide when steroids were tapered below 20 mg/day. Patients were followed for 5 years. All patients were seronegative for pemphigus autoantibodies after 3 months of treatment (initial titers ranged from 1 : 40 to 1 : 160). All patients in both groups had resolution of blister formation. There was no difference between the duration of prednisolone therapy required to control disease (average 19 vs. 24 days). There was no difference in the number of relapses between groups, or in the time to relapse. Steroid-related complications occurred in both groups, with a trend towards more complications in the high-dose group. Therefore, this trial suggested that a "high-dose" regimen offered no advantage over a "low-dose" regimen.

Fernandes reported a nonrandomized controlled trial involving 71 patients (41 with pemphigus vulgaris, 30 with pemphigus foliaceus).[11] Patients were allocated to groups receiving 1 mg/kg/day (n = 34) or 2 mg/kg/day (n = 37) prednisone, according to baseline disease severity. No adjuvants were given, and steroids were tapered after 4–6 weeks. Patients were followed for 5 years. Suppression of blister formation was similar in the two groups, with 24 of 34 patients on low-dose treatment and 27 of 37 patients on high-dose treatment responding to therapy. Two patients in the low-dose group and four in the high-dose group died. There was a significant difference in the number of adverse events, in particular infection, with 16 infections reported in the low-dose group and 48 in the high-dose group. Although the lack of randomization in this study detracts from the validity of the results, it suggests that high doses of steroid are no more effective and are associated with higher morbidity.

In summary, the evidence indicates that lower-dose steroid regimens (≤ 1 mg/kg/day) have equivalent efficacy in inducing disease control and that higher-dose regimens are associated with increased morbidity.

Does pulsed corticosteroid therapy increase efficacy or reduce morbidity?

Pulsed therapy is based on the rationale that short-term high-dose steroid may achieve more rapid control of disease and decrease cumulative steroid dose, thus reducing complications resulting from long-term usage. There have been one RCT, one nonrandomized controlled trial, and four case series reporting on the use of pulsed corticosteroid therapy.

Mentink et al. designed a randomized controlled trial in which 20 pemphigus vulgaris patients with new disease or new disease activity were randomly assigned to oral dexamethasone 300 mg pulses 3 days per month (n = 11) or placebo (n = 9).[12] Both treatment groups also received prednisolone 80 mg/day, tapered over 19 weeks, and azathioprine 3 mg/kg/day. Monthly pulses were continued until prednisolone was tapered to zero, and the patients were followed for 1 year. Eight of the 11 patients with pulsed dexamethasone and all nine of the patients on placebo were able to discontinue all steroids. There were no differences in the time to remission, duration of remission, or relapse rate. The mean cumulative steroid dose was higher in the pulsed group. Adverse events occurred more commonly in the pulsed group, and three of nine patients withdrew due to side effects. Adverse events with pulsed therapy included viral hepatitis, muscle weakness, cognitive problems, and weight gain.

Femiano et al. reported an open nonrandomized controlled trial of 20 patients with new-onset pemphigus vulgaris.[13] The patients were treated with a tapering schedule of prednisone 125 mg/day (n = 10) or intravenous betamethasone 20 mg/day for 4 days/month and prednisone 50 mg/day. There was no difference in the time to achieve disease control (30 vs. 25 days). Adverse events were reported less commonly in the pulsed group.

In addition, there have been four retrospective case series reporting on pulsed steroids. Mignogna et al. reported 12 pemphigus vulgaris patients treated with monthly pulses of methylprednisolone 30 mg/kg for 3–5 consecutive days.[14] Disease was controlled in all patients after three or four cycles, but nine of the 12 patients relapsed during the 6-month follow-up. Adverse events were common and included flushing, hyperglycemia, pruritus, headaches, palpitations, mood changes, insomnia, and fatigue. Toth et al. described 14 patients treated with various pulse regimens.[15] Seven of 14 were able to discontinue treatment, and three subsequently relapsed. Adverse events were reported in 60% of the patients and included flushing, sleep disturbance, mood change, hyperglycemia, and cardiovascular accidents. Werth described nine patients with pemphigus vulgaris who had not initially responded to prednisone, who received intravenous methylprednisolone 250–1000 mg/day for 1–5 days in addition to adjunctive

therapy.[16] Six of the nine patients improved during the pulse therapy, and four were able to discontinue treatment for an average of 2 years. A steroid-sparing effect was seen in comparison with a historical control group. One patient died of candidal sepsis during therapy. Chrysomallis et al. reported eight patients with severe or recalcitrant pemphigus vulgaris, treated with six to 10 pulses of intravenous methylprednisolone 8–10 mg/kg on alternate days plus oral prednisone and either azathioprine or cyclophosphamide.[17] All patients achieved disease control, with healing of at least 50% of lesions, following pulsed steroid therapy, but none was able to discontinue medication. Four patients relapsed within 16 months of pulsed therapy. One patient died of cardiac arrest and one developed thrombophlebitis.

Although the early case series of pulsed corticosteroids appeared promising, evidence from controlled trials shows that pulsed corticosteroids confer no additional benefit and may be associated with more severe side effects. However, patients in these controlled trials were predominantly newly diagnosed, and whether pulsed corticosteroid therapy is beneficial for a subset of patients with severe or refractory disease is not clear.

Are immunosuppressive drugs (azathioprine, ciclosporin, cyclophosphamide, methotrexate, mycophenolate) in addition to corticosteroids beneficial in improving efficacy or reducing morbidity?

Immunosuppressive medications are widely used due to their theoretical advantage of improving efficacy while reducing steroid-induced complications. These agents are slow-acting, so their primary role is in maintenance therapy rather than in inducing remission. There have been only two RCTs of immunosuppressants, and the majority of evidence is derived from case series.

Azathioprine

There are no RCTs investigating the use of azathioprine in pemphigus, although it may be the most commonly used adjuvant agent.

Akhtar and Hasan reported a nonrandomized controlled trial in 72 pemphigus vulgaris patients, comparing prednisolone (n = 40), prednisolone plus azathioprine (n = 15), and betamethasone–cyclophosphamide pulse therapy (n = 17).[18] The regimen consisted of prednisolone 30–120 mg/day on a tapering schedule, alone or in combination with azathioprine 100–150 mg/day. Treatment with azathioprine was more effective with regard to the proportion of patients achieving disease control (11/15 vs. 13/40; response difference 0.41, 95% confidence interval, 0.14 to 0.68; number needed to treat 3, 95% CI, 2 to 8). The frequency of relapses and the incidence of complications were lower in the azathioprine group. Eight of the 40 patients in the prednisolone arm died, compared with one of the 15 in the azathioprine arm. The results of the betamethasone–cyclophosphamide arm are reported below in the section in which cyclophosphamide is discussed.

The largest case series was reported by Aberer et al., in a long-term study of 37 patients with pemphigus vulgaris who were treated with steroid plus azathioprine.[19] All patients were treated initially with corticosteroids (80–200 mg daily) plus azathioprine (2–3 mg/kg). In follow-up ranging from 4 to 16 years, 24 of the 37 patients were disease-free; five had improvement, but were not disease-free; the regimen failed in two, who were withdrawn from the study; three died, and three were lost to follow-up. Sixty-six percent of the patients experienced a relapse. Adverse events were common, but mostly steroid-related. There were three deaths, one due to infection and two unrelated to treatment.

Benoit Corven et al. reported a retrospective case series including 22 patients with pemphigus vulgaris.[20] Newly diagnosed patients received what was termed the "low Lever protocol," or prednisone 40 mg on alternate days in addition to azathioprine 100 mg/day; after 1 year, the prednisone is slowly tapered. Eighteen of 22 patients achieved complete healing of lesions after a mean of 4.3 months, and 12 of the 22 were able to stop all treatment after a mean of 2.9 years. Four of the 22 patients did not respond, and three of these died of unrelated conditions. Adverse events included pneumonia, diabetes, hepatitis, and pulmonary embolism.

Mourellou et al. described a retrospective case series including 15 pemphigus vulgaris patients treated with prednisone 40 mg on alternate days and azathioprine 100 mg/day.[21] None of the patients treated with adjuvant azathioprine died, in contrast with 12 of 33 patients in this case series who received prednisone alone. As this was a nonrandomized retrospective series of patients over a 20-year period, there may have been other factors influencing the mortality rate.

Although there are no randomized controlled trials of azathioprine, it appears that adjunctive azathioprine is beneficial. Adjunctive azathioprine may induce remission in the majority of patients, has a lower relapse rate than steroids alone, and reduces steroid-related complications.

Cyclophosphamide

The most substantive evidence is of adjuvant oral cyclophosphamide in combination with corticosteroids. A single small RCT and three case series have reported on the use of oral cyclophosphamide in pemphigus vulgaris.

Chrysomallis et al. conducted a randomized controlled trial of prednisone, cyclophosphamide, and ciclosporin.[22] Twenty-eight patients with newly diagnosed pemphigus vulgaris restricted to the oral cavity were randomized to

prednisone equivalent 40 mg daily (n = 10), alone or in combination with either cyclophosphamide 100 mg/day (n = 10), or ciclosporin 5 mg/kg/day (n = 8). All patients were followed for 5 years. There was no significant difference in the duration of treatment required to achieve disease control (mean 24 vs. 28 days), or in the relapse rate in the three groups. At 5 years, all patients had disease controlled at prednisone doses of 2.5 mg/day or less. Adverse events were mild, although the incidence of complications was higher with combination treatments. There were no deaths.

Cummins et al. described 23 patients (20 with pemphigus vulgaris, three with pemphigus foliaceus) treated with oral cyclophosphamide 2.0–2.5 mg/kg and prednisone 1 mg/kg. Five patients were also treated with concomitant plasmapheresis.[23] Seventeen of the 23 patients were lesion-free when prednisone was tapered below 0.15 mg/kg, although six subsequently relapsed. Adverse events included hematuria in five patients, infection, and one case of transitional cell bladder carcinoma. Piamphongsant described 12 patients treated with prednisone at doses of either 60 or 120 mg/day, depending on disease severity, and cyclophosphamide 100 mg daily, on a tapering schedule.[24] Nine of the 12 patients achieved disease control on prednisone < 15 mg/day plus cyclophosphamide 50 mg on alternate days or once a week, and three of the 12 patients were able to stop treatment. No serious complications of cyclophosphamide therapy were reported. Fellner et al. described five patients with newly diagnosed pemphigus vulgaris who were treated with oral cyclophosphamide 100–200 mg/day plus prednisone 200 mg/day.[25] All of the patients achieved disease control and four were able to discontinue medication.

In summary, adjuvant oral cyclophosphamide has been reported as effective in inducing remission in pemphigus. However, studies have not been carried out to show that the combination of cyclophosphamide and steroids is more effective than steroids alone, and the combination was associated with greater adverse effects.

Methotrexate

No controlled trials have tested the efficacy of methotrexate in pemphigus. Reports of serious side effects associated with methotrexate have largely precluded its use in pemphigus in recent years, but the controversy about methotrexate may be related to the previous use of extremely high doses (up to 150 mg/week).[26] In a series of nine pemphigus vulgaris patients, all of whom had had been treated unsuccessfully with another adjuvant agent, Smith and Bystryn reported the use of methotrexate at doses of 10.0–17.5 mg/week in combination with prednisone.[27] Once the disease was controlled, steroids were rapidly tapered, and six of the nine patients were able to discontinue steroids within 6 months. Adverse events were mild and included nausea and mild elevation of transaminases.

Mashkilleyson and Mashkilleyson reported 53 patients with pemphigus vulgaris who were treated with prednisone 60–200 mg/day and methotrexate 25–50 mg/week.[28] Treatment was reported as "effective" in 42 of the 53 patients and "ineffective" in nine, and two patients withdrew due to adverse events. There were no changes in liver enzymes, and liver biopsies performed after every 1.5 g cumulative methotrexate were unremarkable. A steroid-sparing effect was seen. The most common adverse effect was infection. Twenty-eight of 185 patients in this case series died, but the number of these who were receiving methotrexate was not reported.

There is insufficient evidence to draw conclusions regarding the role of adjuvant methotrexate in pemphigus.

Ciclosporin

Ioannides et al. published the results of an open randomized controlled trial of 33 patients with newly diagnosed pemphigus (29 with pemphigus vulgaris and four with pemphigus foliaceus).[29] The patients were randomly assigned to treatment with prednisolone 1 mg/kg (n = 17) or prednisolone 1 mg/kg plus ciclosporin 5 mg/kg (n = 16). Treatment was tapered and discontinued according to a standardized protocol, and the patients were followed for 4–6 years. There were no differences in any of the variables used to measure the response to treatment (mean 17 days in both groups), the proportion of patients able to taper steroids below 15 mg/day (12/17 and 12/16 at 12 months), the proportion of patients able to stop treatment (five of 17 and four of 16 at 12 months), or the time to achieve remission. Treatment failed in two of the 17 and one of the 16 patients, and complications were more common among patients who received combination therapy—in particular, hypertrichosis, hypertension, and renal function abnormalities. Steroid-related adverse events were similar in both arms; there was no mortality.

Similar results were reported in another RCT of ciclosporin by Chrysomallis, et al. described above in the cyclophosphamide section.[22] There was no benefit from ciclosporin with regard to the time needed to achieve disease control, the proportion of patients responding to treatment, or the relapse rate. The incidence of adverse events, particularly hypertrichosis and renal impairment, was higher in the ciclosporin group.

Lapidoth et al. compared 16 pemphigus vulgaris patients treated with ciclosporin plus prednisone with a historical control group of 15 pemphigus vulgaris patients who had received prednisone alone.[30] The study and control groups did not differ significantly with regard to the time to healing of old lesions. The mean total cumulative prednisone dose was significantly lower in the ciclosporin group, and the duration of hospitalization was also shorter. Overall, more side effects were reported in the ciclosporin treatment group, and two patients treated with ciclosporin

discontinued treatment because of side effects. Mobini et al. described six patients with recalcitrant pemphigus vulgaris who were successfully treated with ciclosporin and prednisone.[31] Clearing of "most lesions" was reported within 16–20 weeks and treatment was discontinued in all patients after 1–2 years, with no relapses. Barthelemy et al. published a case series of nine pemphigus vulgaris patients treated with different regimens of ciclosporin, with or without prednisone.[32] None of the four patients treated with ciclosporin alone demonstrated clinical improvement. In four patients who showed no improvement after being treated for 2 months with prednisone, the addition of ciclosporin induced clearing of lesions within 3 weeks, but three of the four patients relapsed within an unspecified period. One patient treated initially with ciclosporin plus prednisone demonstrated early improvement, but the disease worsened when the dose of prednisone was tapered.

From the available evidence, adjunctive ciclosporin does not appear to be beneficial in pemphigus. Efficacy does not appear to be greater than with steroids alone, and adverse events are more frequent.

Mycophenolate

Mycophenolate mofetil is an immunosuppressive drug reported to be associated with fewer adverse effects than older immunosuppressants. There have been six case series on the treatment of pemphigus with mycophenolate.

The largest series, reported by Mimouni et al., described 42 patients (31 with pemphigus vulgaris and 11 with pemphigus foliaceus).[33] The patients were treated with mycophenolate mofetil 35–45 mg/kg/day in combination with prednisone 1 mg/kg/day for a median of 22 months. The patients included had relapsed or suffered adverse events during treatment with prednisone and azathioprine. Twenty-seven of the 42 patients were in remission with a steroid dose below 0.15 mg/kg/day, and reached remission after a median of 9 months. The treatment was considered to have failed in 10 of the 42 patients. Antibody titers rapidly declined. Adverse events included gastrointestinal problems and neutropenia.

Powell et al. described 17 patients (12 with pemphigus vulgaris, four with pemphigus foliaceus, and one with paraneoplastic pemphigus) who were treated with mycophenolate 2.5 g/day and prednisone at dosages of 15–60 mg/day.[34] The patients included had severe disease refractory to management with multiple adjuvants. Eight of the 17 patients had no clinical lesions within 3 months, four improved with ongoing lesions, the treatment failed in two, and three withdrew. Autoantibody titer returned to normal in five patients. Side effects reported included esthesia, myalgia, herpes, mycobacteria, and lymphopenia. Infections were associated with higher doses of mycophenolate.

Enk and Knop described 12 patients with pemphigus vulgaris who received prednisone 2 mg/kg/day and mycophenolate 2 g/day.[35] The patients had relapsed while being treated with prednisone and azathioprine, although disease severity was not reported. Eleven of the 12 patients achieved clearance within 2 months. In these patients, the prednisone dose was reduced to at least 5 mg/day by the end of the study, and there were no relapses during the 12-month study period. One patient failed to respond, and was withdrawn. Serum titers of pemphigus autoantibodies declined and were undetectable by 2 months. Nearly all of the patients developed lymphopenia. In general, side effects were not serious, and there were no deaths. The rapid clinical and serological improvement described in this study has been questioned by other investigators.[36]

Chams-Davatchi et al. described 10 patients with severe pemphigus vulgaris refractory to azathioprine and multiple other adjuvants.[37] The patients were treated with 2 g/d mycophenolate mofetil for 6 months and a tapering schedule of prednisone. Nine of the 10 patients responded and had clinical resolution of lesions after a mean of 3.4 months. There was a steroid-sparing effect. One patient failed to respond, and two patients relapsed during the trial. Five patients relapsed within 3 weeks of discontinuing mycophenolate, indicating that courses of longer than 6 months are required for sustained remission.

There are two other case series of five patients, in each of whom azathioprine treatment had failed.[36,38] Limited patient history, methods, and data were reported in both series. The patients in both series received prednisone in combination with mycophenolate. All of the patients responded to treatment, with disease controlled at the end of the follow-up period. A steroid-sparing effect was seen. Aside from lymphopenia and diarrhea, no side effects were reported.

In summary, these case series report the use of adjuvant mycophenolate mofetil in patients with refractory disease. The majority of patients achieved clinical resolution and a steroid sparing effect was seen, but treatment failed in a small proportion of patients in these series. Minimal adverse events were reported. Mycophenolate mofetil appears to be a safe treatment that suppresses clinical disease in the majority of patients. However, there are no controlled trials, and these results need to be interpreted with caution. An RCT of adjuvant mycophenolate in pemphigus vulgaris is ongoing at present.

Pulsed cyclophosphamide

Pulsed intravenous cyclophosphamide has been reported in randomized trials to be more effective than oral cyclophosphamide in treating lupus nephritis and autoimmune thrombocytopenic purpura.[39–41] It was therefore anticipated that this mode of therapy might also be effective in pemphigus and might minimize the side effects associated with prolonged daily oral therapy. One randomized controlled trial, one nonrandomized controlled trial, and numerous case series have been reported. There have been no studies comparing oral and pulsed cyclophosphamide in pemphigus.

Rose et al. conducted an open randomized controlled trial comparing intravenous dexamethasone–cyclophosphamide (D/C) and oral methylprednisolone–azathioprine (M/A).[42] Twenty-two patients with newly diagnosed disease (16 with pemphigus vulgaris and six with pemphigus foliaceus) were enrolled. The patients were randomly assigned to methylprednisolone 2 mg/kg plus azathioprine 2.0–2.5 mg/kg (n = 11) or intravenous dexamethasone 100 mg/day for 3 days and cyclophosphamide 500 mg on day one, plus oral cyclophosphamide 50 mg/day (n = 11). The D/C pulse was administered every 2–4 weeks at increasing intervals. At 24 months, five of the 11 patients in the M/A group and one of the 11 in the D/C group had controlled disease on treatment; three of the 11 in each group were in remission and had stopped therapy; and one in the M/A group and six in the D/C group had had progression of disease. Patients who progressed on D/C were subsequently treated with the M/A regimen, and all improved. One patient in the M/A group withdrew due to generalized herpes simplex virus infection. Adverse events were reported more commonly in the M/A group.

Akhtar and Hasan reported a nonrandomized controlled trial comparing prednisolone (n = 40), prednisolone plus azathioprine (n = 15) and betamethasone–cyclophosphamide (B/C) pulse therapy (n = 17) in pemphigus vulgaris.[18] This trial was described in part in the section on azathioprine above. The regimen consisted of pulsed intravenous betamethasone 100 mg/day for 3 days and cyclophosphamide 500 mg on day 1, plus cyclophosphamide 50 mg orally daily. Treatment was considered to have failed in 12 of the 17 patients in the pulsed cyclophosphamide arm, and the patients required additional steroids. An increased susceptibility to infection was seen in the B/C group in comparison with other arms, and four of the 17 patients died.

These controlled trials differ considerably from the numerous case series describing similar protocols of pulsed cyclophosphamide. Sacchidanand et al. reported a case series including 46 patients with extensive pemphigus (44 with pemphigus vulgaris and two with pemphigus foliaceus), and the majority of patients achieved disease control.[43] Pasricha et al. summarized their experience with 300 patients over a 12-year period.[44,45] A total of 190 of the original 300 patients were described as "disease-free" and not receiving any medication. Long-lasting remission was described, with remission continuing over 2 years in 123 patients. Kaur and Kanwar described 50 patients treated with pulsed cyclophosphamide over a course of 2 years.[46] Almost half of the patients improved, but were still receiving monthly pulse treatments. Another five patients had responded well and were receiving only oral cyclophosphamide 50 mg/day. Kanwar *et al.* later reported on the long-term efficacy of this regimen in 36 patients (32 with pemphigus vulgaris and four with pemphigus foliaceus).[47] All of the patients were able to discontinue therapy and remain free of disease over a range of 0.5 to 12 years. Fleischli *et al.* studied the use of pulsed cyclophosphamide without concomitant intravenous corticosteroids in nine patients.[48] Six patients were reported as having an "excellent or good" response, but only two of the nine had remission of skin lesions.

The controlled trials of pulsed cyclophosphamide indicate a high rate of treatment failure. This outcome differs considerably from the predominantly positive outcomes reported in uncontrolled case series. The evidence does not support the use of pulsed cyclophosphamide in pemphigus.

Summary

There are few well-designed trials directly evaluating the efficacy of adjunctive immunosuppressants in comparison with corticosteroids alone. Interpretation of the trials conducted to date is limited by inadequate power, heterogeneous patient characteristics, and limited duration of follow-up. Thus, it is difficult to confidently distinguish the additive benefit of adjunctive immunosuppressants. Most data concerning adjuvant immunosuppressants are derived from retrospective case series, but this type of data is at high risk of bias. Most of the evidence of benefit comes from comparison with historical studies, but improvement in outcomes and the decline in morbidity and mortality associated with the introduction of immunosuppressants may be attributable in part to other advances in care.

When evaluating the efficacy of adjunctive immunosuppressants, it is important to remember the rationale for their use. They are slow-acting agents, and their primary role is as a steroid-sparing agent in the maintenance phase of disease. It is not known whether they have a "disease-modifying" activity in terms of altering the overall remission or relapse rate. Thus, the emphasis in trials should be on long-term efficacy and safety, rather than on short-term and time-to-event outcomes. Moreover, there is a need for improvement in the reporting and weighting of adverse events and overall risk–benefit analyses.

From the limited evidence available, adjunctive immunosuppressants appear to be beneficial. They appear to effectively induce remission in the majority of patients, as well as reducing steroid-related complications. However, they do not appear to influence the duration of treatment required for disease control.

There have been few trials directly comparing different adjunctive immunosuppressive agents. From the trials conducted by Rose *et al.* and Akhtar and Hasan, azathioprine appears to be more efficacious than pulsed cyclophosphamide.[18,42] The studies by Chryssomallis *et al.* and Ioannides *et al.* do not support the use of ciclosporin.[17,29] The most promising data are for azathioprine and mycophenolate, although this needs to be confirmed in randomized controlled trials. At present, it is probably advisable to select an adjuvant immunosuppressive agent after consideration of the adverse effect profile and the patient's comorbidities.

Does immunomodulatory therapy—i.e., plasmapheresis or intravenous immunoglobulin—improve efficacy or reduce morbidity in patients with severe or recalcitrant pemphigus?

Immunomodulatory therapies are appealing, as they target the antibodies, which are directly pathogenic in pemphigus. However, because these agents/modalities are more invasive and involve health-care services other than simple clinic visits, and because they are substantially more costly, these modalities are usually reserved for patients with severe recalcitrant disease.

Plasmapheresis

The use of plasmapheresis is based on the hypothesis that effective therapy can be achieved through removal of pathogenic autoantibodies. Our search revealed one RCT of plasmapheresis and eight case series.

Guillaume *et al.* randomly assigned 40 previously untreated patients with pemphigus vulgaris and foliaceus to prednisolone alone (0.5–2.0 mg/kg/day; n = 18) or prednisolone plus 10 large-volume plasma exchanges (55 mL/kg/exchange) over 4 weeks (n = 22).[49] There were no differences between the two groups with respect to clinical improvement, cumulative steroid dose, or serum autoantibody titers. Eight patients (four in each group) did not achieve disease control. Four patients, all in the plasmapheresis group, died of sepsis or thromboembolism. This study suggests that plasmapheresis in association with steroids is not effective in the treatment of pemphigus. Other authors have argued that concurrent immunosuppressive agents are required to prevent rebound antibody synthesis during plasmapheresis, which may explain the poor efficacy of plasmapheresis in the trial.[50,51] Nevertheless, the high mortality rate in the plasmapheresis arm is concerning.

In a retrospective case series, Tan-Lim and Bystryn described 11 patients treated with plasmapheresis (1–2 L/exchange, five to 12 exchanges over 10–24 days), corticosteroids (70–240 mg/day), and immunosuppressants (azathioprine or cyclophosphamide).[52] The decrease in antibody titer is promising, but no clinical data were presented and long-term follow up was not reported, so these results need to be interpreted with caution.

Turner *et al.* described their experience with plasmapheresis in seven patients with severe pemphigus vulgaris, in all of whom previous treatment with a variety of therapeutic agents had failed.[53] Each patient underwent five plasma exchanges (50 mL/kg/exchange), in combination with pulsed cyclophosphamide or pulsed steroid and azathioprine. Four of the seven patients achieved clinical resolution of lesions, two patients improved and were able to taper steroid dosage, and one patient continued to have active disease. Antibody titers decreased, and there was a steroid-sparing effect. The patients were followed for only 2 months.

Ruocco *et al.* reported the use of plasmapheresis in seven patients with recalcitrant pemphigus. Three different plasmapheresis protocols were used, including weekly small volume (400 mL/exchange), weekly large volume (1200 mL/exchange), and monthly massive volume (4000 mL/exchange) for 6–9 weeks.[54] The patients continued on steroid and immunosuppressant medication, with the dosage being maintained "as low as possible." Clinical improvement was seen in all cases, but healing of lesions was only reported in one case. The large volume did not appear to be more efficacious than the small volume. Antibody titers decreased in four of the seven patients. Adverse events reported included decreased platelet and red cell counts, shivering, nausea, and vomiting.

Blaszczyk *et al.* described a retrospective case series of eight patients treated with plasmapheresis (500–800 mL/exchange) once a week for 6 weeks. The patients continued to receive previous medication, including prednisone 25–100 mg on alternate days and azathioprine 50 mg or cyclophosphamide 100–200 mg on alternate days.[55] After treatment, two of the eight patients were in "remission," four improved, and two had progressed. In the long-term follow-up over 1–6 years, four patients were in remission and four had relapsed.

Roujeau *et al.* described a retrospective case series of 10 patients (eight with pemphigus vulgaris and two with pemphigus foliaceus) who were treated with massive-volume plasmapheresis (3000–5000 mL/exchange).[56] Two patients had new-onset disease, and the remaining eight patients had steroid-resistant or steroid-dependent disease. The patients received concurrent treatment with prednisone 0.1–2.5 mg/kg, and cyclophosphamide, azathioprine, or chlorambucil. Plasmapheresis was administered two or three times per week, with 3–20 sessions per patient over 1–16 weeks. Two of the 10 patients showed no improvement, two patients had transient improvement, and six patients had rapid improvement with no new blisters occurring after four treatment sessions, although three

of the six subsequently relapsed. Adverse events included thrombocytopenia, hypocalcemia, urticaria, fever, and hypotension, and two patients suffered acute hepatitis.

Sondergaard *et al.* described the use of adjunctive plasmapheresis in eight patients (seven with pemphigus vulgaris and one with pemphigus foliaceus) in combination with prednisone 30–120 mg/day and azathioprine, cyclophosphamide, or ciclosporin.[57] Three patients had new-onset disease, two were lesion-free at the start of treatment, and four were resistant to conventional therapy. Massive-volume plasmapheresis (1500–3000 mL/exchange) was performed once or twice per month for 5–73 months, with a total of 5–89 exchanges per patient. All patients achieved clinical remission within 2 months. Six of the eight patients relapsed, and patients remained in remission for 40–100% of the treatment period. A steroid-sparing effect was seen. Adverse events included nausea, dizziness, fever, and leg muscle spasms.

The role of plasmapheresis in pemphigus is unclear. The RCT by Guillaume *et al.* provides the best quality of evidence.[49] The lack of benefit and high mortality rate in this study suggests that plasmapheresis should not be recommended in patients with new-onset disease. However, the role of plasmapheresis in patients with severe recalcitrant disease is unclear. Some case series have shown benefit in patients with severe disease when plasmapheresis is combined with steroids and immunosuppressants, but this has yet to be confirmed in an RCT. The treatment failure rate, relapse rate, and adverse event profile of plasmapheresis demonstrated in these series is concerning.

Immunoadsorption

Immunoadsorption is similar to plasmapheresis, but immunoglobulins are specifically removed from the circulation. There are two case series describing immunoadsorption in pemphigus.

Luftl *et al.* conducted a prospective case series on protein A immunoadsorption, including nine patients (seven with pemphigus vulgaris and two with pemphigus foliaceus).[58] The treatment regimen consisted of two cycles of immunoadsorption separated by 48 hours, given with a pulse of prednisolone. Patients were continued on methylprednisolone 0.5 mg/kg/day and on preexisting adjuvant medication. All of the patients showed clinical improvement, allowing reduction of steroid doses. Antibody titers decreased by 30% after a single treatment, and IgG was preferentially eliminated in comparison with other plasma proteins. One patient had an anaphylactic reaction and immunoadsorption was discontinued.

Schmidt *et al.* described the use of immunoadsorption in five patients (four with pemphigus vulgaris and one with pemphigus foliaceus).[59] The patients were treated with 19 cycles of immunoadsorption over 41 weeks, in addition to 0.5 mg/kg methylprednisolone, which was gradually tapered. Pulsed cyclophosphamide and dexamethasone for administered with the initial cycle of immunoadsorption. Clinical improvement was seen within 2 weeks, and the patients became lesion-free in 3–21 weeks. One patient relapsed, but responded to a second induction cycle. A steroid-sparing effect was seen. Antibody titers decreased by an average of 75% at 1 month. Adverse events reported included deep vein thrombosis, bradycardia and hypertension, symptomatic hypocalcemia, and difficulty with venous access.

Immunoadsorption appears to be an effective treatment in inducing rapid clinical improvement, associated with decreased antibody titers and a steroid-sparing effect. Confirmation of these observations with an RCT would be helpful. Testing in a randomized controlled fashion of immunoadsorption against standard plasmapheresis is also required.

Intravenous immunoglobulin

The proposed mechanisms of intravenous immunoglobulin (IVIG) in autoimmune disorders have been reviewed elsewhere. There have been 10 published case series, but interpretation is complicated, as there has been duplication of data in separate publications. Moreover, when patients have been reported more than once, the outcome has not always been consistent.

In a retrospective case series, Harman and Black described 14 patients with autoimmune blistering disorders, including seven patients with pemphigus vulgaris.[60] The patients had extensive disease refractory to treatment, or side effects of treatment. The treatment regimen consisted of 2 mg/kg IVIG over 5 consecutive days, with one to four cycles per patient given over up to 9 months. IVIG was administered in combination with existing therapy, which consisted of prednisolone 10–120 mg daily, and four patients also received adjunctive immunosuppressants. Rapid clinical improvement was noted in all cases, although the effect was transient and variable. A steroid-sparing effect was seen. Indirect immunofluorescence (IIF) antibody titers decreased in the majority of patients, but this effect also was transient.

Bystryn et al. described six patients with pemphigus vulgaris who were treated with 2 mg/kg over 5 days for one to three cycles, in combination with cyclophosphamide 100–150 mg/day and a tapering schedule of prednisolone.[61] The patients included were unresponsive to prednisone and cyclophosphamide. There was a rapid clinical benefit with cessation of new blister formation, healing of lesions, and reduction of steroid dose within weeks. Similarly, the antibody titer decreased by 72% in 1 week. However, this study had a short follow-up period of only 2–4 months, and evaluation of the long-term benefit is not possible.

Levy et al. described nine patients with pemphigus vulgaris and three patients with pemphigus foliaceus. All of the patients were described as having steroid-dependent or steroid-resistant disease.[62] The treatment regimen consisted of 0.6–2.0 mg/kg/cycle of IVIG over 2–5 days, with a mean of seven cycles per patient, in combination with prednisone (8–100 mg/day). Three patients received adjuvant immunosuppressants. During treatment, eight of the 12 patients had clinical resolution of lesions, two patients improved, and two patients failed to improve. Twelve months after IVIG, five of eight patients had controlled disease and the treatment was considered to have failed in three of five patients. A steroid-sparing effect was seen in the majority of patients.

Enk et al. described the use of IVIG in six patients with pemphigus vulgaris who had initially responded to a regimen of prednisone 1.5–2.0 mg/kg and azathioprine 1.5 mg/kg, but had relapsed when the high-dose steroid was tapered.[63] IVIG was started in combination with the above treatments, at a dose of 2 mg/kg IVIG over 2 days given every 4 weeks, with six to nine cycles per patient. All of the patients experienced resolution of blistering, with no relapses over 1 year. Steroids were able to be tapered, and IIF titers declined.

Ahmed's group have published six case series evaluating IVIG as a monotherapy.[64–69] Systemic steroids and adjuvants were rapidly tapered and discontinued within 2–7 months. In this protocol, patients were treated with 2 mg/kg over 3 days every 4 weeks until lesions healed, typically 3–7 months. Thereafter, the interval between cycles of IVIG was extended to 6, 8, 10, 12, 14, and then 16 weeks, and then discontinued. In the case of relapse, the IVIG was administered more frequently. This regimen was continued from 18 to 40 months. The patients included had severe disease at baseline, or an unsatisfactory response or significant side effects of conventional treatment.

Due to some duplication of publications, it is difficult to evaluate exactly how many patients were treated with Ahmed's regimen, but at least 21 patients with pemphigus vulgaris and 11 patients with pemphigus foliaceus were treated. All of the patients achieved remission, after a mean of 4.5 months in pemphigus vulgaris and 5.3 months in pemphigus foliaceus. All of the patients had relapses during the study period, most of which required an alteration of the treatment regimen. Treatment was stopped after a mean of 29.8 months in pemphigus foliaceus and 22.7 months in pemphigus vulgaris, and patients remained lesion-free after treatment cessation. Overall, the quality of life measured on a five-point scale improved. The autoantibody titer measured with ELISA declined progressively in all patients. The mean cumulative steroid dose after treatment was relatively low, as would be expected, as steroids were rapidly stopped as part of this protocol.

IVIG was generally well tolerated, with minimal adverse events reported in all studies. The adverse events reported include nausea, headache, fatigue, tachycardia, hypertension, myalgia, flushing, urticaria, rigors, and vomiting. These are all documented adverse effects of IVIG and can be treated with premedication and slowing of the infusion rate.

On the basis of the limited evidence provided by these case series, IVIG is portrayed as a safe and effective treatment in recalcitrant pemphigus. IVIG appears to be effective as a monotherapy, but is slow to induce remission and is expensive in comparison with other alternatives. The experience of other groups with IVIG[70,71] does not support the efficacy and safety suggested in the above series, perhaps reflecting the batch-to-batch variation in IVIG. When it has been reported as effective, the onset of action was rapid when IVIG was used as an adjuvant treatment; however, the effect is transient. Better results were achieved when repeated courses were given. All studies demonstrated a steroid-sparing effect. It would appear that the role of IVIG is as an adjuvant in recalcitrant pemphigus, with repeated courses required to sustain the benefit. Further randomized controlled trials to test this hypothesis are required. The current literature probably reflects the fact that treatment failures are less likely to be reported, further emphasizing the need for randomized trials.

Are anti-inflammatory therapies—e.g., gold, dapsone, antibiotics—beneficial in pemphigus?

Anti-inflammatory agents are often prescribed for patients with relatively mild pemphigus, as they have a more favorable safety profile in comparison with immunosuppressants.

Gold

Because gold has a delayed onset of action, it is usually administered as an adjuvant. One controlled study and four retrospective case series were identified.

Auad and Auad described a blinded, placebo-controlled trial of adjuvant gold in 30 patients with pemphigus foliaceus.[72] The patients were initially stabilized on corticosteroids, and gold 3 mg/day or a placebo was then added. Nine of the 30 patients did not complete the trial, and an intention-to-treat analysis was not performed. The results for 10 patients treated with gold and 11 in the placebo arm were reported, with a mean follow-up of 4 years. At 12 months, a steroid-sparing effect was seen, with a mean steroid dose of 37 mg in the placebo group and 5.5 mg/day in the gold arm. Four patients in the gold arm experienced complications, including diarrhea and proteinuria.

Pandya and Dyke described 26 patients treated with gold, either alone or in combination with prednisone.[73]

Patients with severe disease requiring "aggressive" therapy were excluded from the study. Patients were treated with 50-mg intramuscular injections of gold thiomalate until disease control was established, and then monthly for a further 4 months. Twenty-two of the 26 patients (85%) improved and were able to taper steroids below 20 mg/day. Eleven patients were able to discontinue steroids, and four patients discontinued all treatment. The duration of gold therapy required before steroid dosages could be tapered by half was 3 months. Four of the 26 patients did not respond. There was no mortality, but adverse effects were noted in 11 patients, nine of whom discontinued therapy. Adverse events included eosinophilia, "cutaneous reactions," and proteinuria.

Sutej et al. reported a prospective case series of six patients with pemphigus vulgaris, including four patients with new-onset disease.[74] The patients were treated with gold in addition to prednisone. All of the patients improved; four of the six patients tapered steroids below 15 mg/day and two were able to discontinue steroids. The regimen was well tolerated.

Poulin et al. reported their experience in 13 patients with pemphigus vulgaris.[75] The disease severity was not described. Patients were treated with gold and prednisone, and three patients also received either dapsone or sulfapyridine. The treatment regimen consisted of 50 mg intramuscular gold thiomalate or aurothioglucose administered weekly as steroids were gradually tapered, and then decreased to 2–4-week intervals. Seven patients experienced complete resolution of lesions and stopped all treatment after a mean of 18.3 months, although two subsequently relapsed. Four patients did not have any clinical benefit, and one patient died (the cause of death was not reported). Gold therapy was discontinued in five patients because of adverse effects, including proteinuria, eosinophilia, leukopenia, urticaria, and dizziness.

Penneys et al. reported on the long-term follow-up of 18 patients treated with gold.[76] The treatment regimen was the same as that used by Poulin described above. Eight of the 18 patients had clinical resolution of lesions and were able to stop all treatment after a mean of 37.3 months of gold therapy. Remission had been sustained in these eight patients during a follow-up period of 8–34 months. Seven of the 18 patients improved, but required maintenance therapy. Two patients discontinued gold due to adverse events, and one patient was lost to follow-up. Adverse events reported included nephrotic syndrome, proteinuria, dermatitis, erythema nodosum, and agranulocytosis.

Most series have evaluated the use of gold in a population of patients with relatively mild disease. The majority of patients improved, a substantial proportion were able to stop treatment, and a small proportion failed to respond. A steroid-sparing effect was seen. Although side effects related to gold therapy were relatively mild, many patients were unable to tolerate treatment.

Dapsone

The most substantial evidence in favor of dapsone therapy is an RCT reported by Werth et al.[77] Nineteen patients with pemphigus vulgaris who were unable to taper steroid below 15 mg/day after twice following a standardized prednisone-tapering schedule, plus any adjuvant, were randomly assigned to dapsone 125–150 mg/day (n = 9) or placebo (n = 10), in addition to steroid and immunosuppressants. Five of the nine patients receiving dapsone, in comparison with three of the ten receiving the placebo, were able to taper steroids below 7.5 mg/day. There was a trend favoring dapsone, but statistical significance was not reached. Overall side effects included a drug rash, paresthesias, and dyspnea secondary to methemoglobinemia.

Heaphy et al. reported the use of dapsone in a retrospective case series of nine patients with pemphigus vulgaris who where steroid-dependent or had poorly controlled disease.[78] Dapsone was used as a third-line agent, in combination with steroids and immunosuppressive or anti-inflammatory adjuvants, at doses of 125–150 mg/day. Seven of the nine patients were able to successfully taper steroids below 7.5 mg/day, and two patients were able to stop steroids. Two patients who had poorly controlled disease at baseline did not respond. The dapsone dose was adjusted in three of the nine patients in response to decreased hemoglobin.

Basset et al. reported a case series of nine previously untreated patients who received dapsone 200–300 mg/day.[79] Five patients, all with mild to moderate disease, responded with at least a 50% decrease in the extent of their disease within 15 days of starting therapy. Four patients did not respond. Three patients discontinued dapsone due to adverse events, including hemolytic anemia, toxic hepatitis, and methemoglobinemia.

Dapsone appears to be an effective steroid-sparing agent in controlled, but steroid-dependent, disease. Its adverse effect profile is relatively mild.

Tetracyclines

Antibiotics, including tetracycline and minocycline, have been used in pemphigus for their anti-inflammatory properties.

Calebotta et al. conducted a prospective case series with tetracycline.[80] Thirteen pemphigus vulgaris patients received tetracycline 2 g/day and prednisone 0.5–1.0 mg/kg/day. All patients treated with tetracycline and prednisone responded and achieved cessation of new blister formation within a mean of 5.4 days. Prednisone was able to be tapered within a mean of 17 days. Two of the 13 patients discontinued tetracycline due to adverse events, including sepsis and gastrointestinal upset.

In another case series by Alpsoy et al., 15 patients with pemphigus (11 with pemphigus vulgaris and four with pemphigus foliaceus) were treated with tetracycline 2 g/day and nicotinamide 1.5 g/day over 2 months.[81] Five patients were newly diagnosed and 10 had previously been treated with corticosteroids and/or immunosuppressive agents. All of the patients had active disease. At 2 months, two of the 15 patients had complete healing, four had 50% healing of lesions, and nine had no response. Three of the 15 patients had mild gastrointestinal upset. Chaffins et al. described 11 patients (six with pemphigus vulgaris and five with pemphigus foliaceus) who were treated with tetracycline 2 mg/day and nicotinamide 1.5 mg/day.[82] Five of the 11 patients received concurrent prednisone (2.5–30 mg/day). At 2 months, five of the 11 patients had complete healing, four had 50% healing, and two had no response. Adverse events included gastrointestinal upset, headache, and a morbilliform eruption.

Gaspar et al. described 10 patients (seven with pemphigus vulgaris and three with pemphigus foliaceus) who were treated with minocycline 100 mg/day as an adjuvant.[83] Nine of the 10 patients were concurrently treated with prednisone (10–40 mg/day) and five patients also received azathioprine (100–200 mg/day). All of the patients had active disease when minocycline was commenced. Four of the 10 patients had complete clearing of lesions, two improved, and four had no response. A steroid-sparing effect was seen among responders. Minocycline was well tolerated; one patient developed pigmentation and nine developed candidiasis.

The evidence to support the use of antibiotics is inconsistent. Some series report high response rates, while others do not. Anti-inflammatory antibiotics may be of benefit as an adjuvant in the treatment of mild or steroid-dependent patients, but further research, including controlled trials, is required.

Are biologicals effective and safe in pemphigus?

The use of biological agents in pemphigus has generated considerable interest. To date, several case series have been reported.[84] The patients had experienced recurrence of pemphigus on prednisone at doses > 10 mg/day and immunosuppression (azathioprine 2.0–2.5 mg/day or equivalent). The treatment regimen included rituximab 375 mg/week for 4 weeks, in addition to prednisone 10–25 mg and mycophenolate mofetil 2 g/day or methotrexate 20–30 mg/week. Three of the five patients had resolution of clinical disease, and two patients had improvement of disease. All of the patients were able to taper prednisone below 5 mg/day and reduce immunosuppressants. Adverse events were minor and included nausea, vomiting, facial edema, and cough.[85]

Key points

- Low-dose (1 mg/kg) corticosteroids appear to be equally effective as higher-dose regimens for initial disease control.

- Pulsed corticosteroid therapy confers no additional benefit in newly diagnosed patients and is associated with increased morbidity.

- Adjunctive immunosuppressants (azathioprine, cyclophosphamide, methotrexate, ciclosporin, mycophenolate mofetil) have not been shown to provide additional benefit. Adjuvant ciclosporin is thought to increase adverse events. Pulsed cyclophosphamide does not appear to be effective. There is insufficient information to comment on role of azathioprine and mycophenolate.

- Plasmapheresis is not indicated in new-onset disease. Its role in recalcitrant disease has not been established. IVIG appears to be beneficial and relatively safe in recalcitrant disease, but this result has not been confirmed in controlled trials.

- Anti-inflammatory agents may be beneficial in mild or steroid-dependent disease. Dapsone and gold appear to have a steroid-sparing effect.

- Trials evaluating biological agents in pemphigus are in progress.

- There is a need for further randomized controlled trials to clarify the efficacy and safety of interventions in pemphigus. There is a need for improved uniformity of outcome measures to allow comparison of interventions and meta-analysis. There is a need for improved reporting and weighting of adverse events for risk–benefit analyses.

References

1 Stanley JR. Pemphigus. In: Freedberg IM, Eisen AZ, Wolff K, Goldsmith LA, Katz S, Austen KF, eds. *Fitzpatrick's Dermatology in General Medicine*, 5th ed. New York: McGraw-Hill, 1999: 654–66.

2 Bystryn JC. Adjuvant therapy of pemphigus. *Arch Dermatol* 1984;**120**:941–51.

3 Bystryn JC, Steinman NM. The adjuvant therapy of pemphigus. An update. *Arch Dermatol* 1996;**132**:203–12.

4 Lever WF, White H. Treatment of pemphigus with corticosteroids. *Arch Dermatol* 1963;**87**:52–66.

5 Lever WF, Schaumburg-Lever G. Immunosuppressants and prednisone in pemphigus vulgaris: therapeutic results obtained in 63 patients between 1961 and 1975. *Arch Dermatol* 1977;**113**:1236–41.

6 Lever WF, Schaumburg-Lever G. Treatment of pemphigus vulgaris. Results obtained in 84 patients between 1961 and 1982. *Arch Dermatol* 1984;**120**:44–7.

7 Franchin G, Diamond B. Pulse steroids: how much is enough? *Autoimmun Rev* 2006;**5**:111–3.

8 Rosenberg FR, Sanders S, Nelson CT. Pemphigus: a 20-year review of 107 patients treated with corticosteroids. *Arch Dermatol* 1976;**112**:962–70.

9 Ryan JG. Pemphigus. A 20-year survey of experience with 70 cases. *Arch Dermatol* 1971;**104**:14–20.

10 Ratnam KV, Phay KL, Tan CK. Pemphigus therapy with oral prednisolone regimens. A 5-year study. *Int J Dermatol* 1990;**29**:363–7.

11 Fernandes NC, Perez M. Treatment of pemphigus vulgaris and pemphigus foliaceus: experience with 71 patients over a 20 year period. *Rev Inst Med Trop Sao Paulo* 2001;**43**:33–6.

12 Mentink LF, Mackenzie MW, Toth GG, *et al.* Randomized controlled trial of adjuvant dexamethasone pulse therapy in pemphigus vulgaris: PEMPULS trial. *Arch Dermatol* 2006;**142**:570–6.

13 Femiano F, Gombos F, Scully C. Pemphigus vulgaris with oral involvement: evaluation of two different systemic corticosteroid therapeutic protocols. *J Eur Acad Dermatol Venereol* 2002;**16**:353–6.

14 Mignogna MD, Lo Muzio L, Ruoppo E, Fedele S, Lo Russo L, Bucci E. High-dose intravenous "pulse" methylprednisone in the treatment of severe oropharyngeal pemphigus: a pilot study. *J Oral Path Med* 2002;**31**:339–44.

15 Toth GG, van de Meer JB, Jonkman MF. Dexamethasone pulse therapy in pemphigus. *J Eur Acad Dermatol Venereol* 2002;**16**:607–11.

16 Werth VP. Treatment of pemphigus vulgaris with brief, high-dose intravenous glucocorticoids. *Arch Dermatol* 1996;**132**:1435–9.

17 Chryssomallis F, Dimitriades A, Chaidemenos GC, Panagiotides D, Karakatsanis G. Steroid-pulse therapy in pemphigus vulgaris long term follow-up. *Int J Dermatol* 1995;**34**:438–42.

18 Akhtar SJ, Hasan MU. Treatment of pemphigus: a local experience. *J Pak Med Assoc* 1998;**48**:300–4.

19 Aberer W, Wolff-Schreiner EC, Stingl G, Wolff K. Azathioprine in the treatment of pemphigus vulgaris. A long-term follow-up. *J Am Acad Dermatol* 1987;**16**:527–33.

20 Benoit Corven C, Carvalho P, Prost C, *et al.* [Treatment of pemphigus vulgaris by azathioprine and low doses of prednisone (Lever scheme); in French.] *Ann Dermatol Venereol* 2003;**130**:13–5.

21 Mourellou O, Chaidemenos GC, Koussidou T, Kapetis E. The treatment of pemphigus vulgaris. Experience with 48 patients seen over an 11–year period. *Br J Dermatol* 1995;**133**:83–7.

22 Chrysomallis F, Ioannides D, Teknetzis A, Panagiotidou D, Minas A. Treatment of oral pemphigus vulgaris. *Int J Dermatol* 1994;**33**:803–7.

23 Cummins DL, Mimouni D, Anhalt GJ, Nousari CH. Oral cyclophosphamide for treatment of pemphigus vulgaris and foliaceus. *J Am Acad Dermatol* 2003;**49**:276–280.

24 Piamphongsant T. Treatment of pemphigus with corticosteroids and cyclophosphamide. *J Dermatol* 1979;**6**:359–63.

25 Fellner MJ, Katz JM, McCabe JB. Successful use of cyclophosphamide and prednisone for initial treatment of pemphigus vulgaris. *Arch Dermatol* 1978;**114**:889–94.

26 Lever WF, Goldberg HS. Treatment of pemphigus vulgaris with methotrexate. *Arch Dermatol* 1969;**100**:70–8.

27 Smith TJ, Bystryn JC. Methotrexate as an adjuvant treatment for pemphigus vulgaris. *Arch Dermatol* 1999;**135**:1275–6.

28 Mashkilleyson N, Mashkilleyson AL. Mucous membrane manifestations of pemphigus vulgaris. A 25-year survey of 185 patients treated with corticosteroids or with combination of corticosteroids with methotrexate or heparin. *Acta Derm Venereol* 1988;**68**:413–21.

29 Ioannides D, Chrysomallis F, Bystryn JC. Ineffectiveness of cyclosporine as an adjuvant to corticosteroids in the treatment of pemphigus. *Arch Dermatol* 2000;**136**:868–72.

30 Lapidoth M, David M, Ben-Amitai D, Katzenelson V, Lustig S, Sandbank M. The efficacy of combined treatment with prednisone and cyclosporine in patients with pemphigus: preliminary study. *J Am Acad Dermatol* 1994;**30**:752–7.

31 Mobini N, Padilla T Jr, Ahmed AR. Long-term remission in selected patients with pemphigus vulgaris treated with cyclosporine. *J Am Acad Dermatol* 1997;**36**:264–6.

32 Barthelemy H, Frappaz A, Cambazard F, *et al*. Treatment of nine cases of pemphigus vulgaris with cyclosporine. *J Am Acad Dermatol* 1988;**18**:1262–6.

33 Mimouni D, Anhalt GJ, Cummins DL, Kouba DJ, Thorne JE, Nousari HC. Treatment of pemphigus vulgaris and pemphigus foliaceus with mycophenolate mofetil. *Arch Dermatol* 2003;**139**: 739–42.

34 Powell AM, Albert S, Al Fares S, *et al*. An evaluation of the usefulness of mycophenolate mofetil in pemphigus. *Br J Dermatol* 2003;**149**:138–45.

35 Enk AH, Knop J. Mycophenolate is effective in the treatment of pemphigus vulgaris. *Arch Dermatol* 1999;**135**:54–6.

36 Nousari HC, Anhalt GJ. The role of mycophenolate mofetil in the management of pemphigus. *Arch Dermatol* 1999;**135**:853–4.

37 Chams-Davatchi C, Nonahal Azar R, Daneshpazooh M, *et al*. [Open trial of mycophenolate mofetil in the treatment of resistant pemphigus vulgaris; in French.] *Ann Dermatol Venereol* 2002;**129**: 23–5.

38 Enk AH, Knop J. Treatment of pemphigus vulgaris with mycophenolate mofetil. *Lancet* 1997;**350**:494.

39 Austin HA, Klippel JH, Balow JE, *et al*. Therapy of lupus nephritis. Controlled trial of prednisone and cytotoxic drugs. *N Engl J Med* 1986;**314**:614–9.

40 Boumpas DT, Austin HA, Vaughn EM, *et al*. Controlled trial of pulse methylprednisolone versus two regimens of pulse cyclophosphamide in severe lupus nephritis. *Lancet* 1992;**340**:741–5.

41 Reiner A, Gernsheimer T, Slichter SJ. Pulse cyclophosphamide therapy for refractory autoimmune thrombocytopenic purpura. *Blood* 1995;**85**:351–8.

42 Rose E, Wever S, Zilliken D, Linse R, Haustein UF, Brocker EB. Intravenous dexamethasone–cyclophosphamide pulse therapy in comparison with oral methylprednisolone–azathioprine therapy in patients with pemphigus: results of a multicenter prospectively randomized study. *J Dtsch Dermatol Ges* 2005;**3**:200–6.

43 Sacchidanand S, Hiremath NC, Natraj HV, *et al*. Dexamethasone–cyclophosphamide pulse therapy for autoimmune-vesiculobullous disorders at Victoria hospital, Bangalore. *Dermatol Online J* 2003; **9**:2.

44 Pasricha JS, Thanzama J, Khan UK. Intermittent high-dose dexamethasone-cyclophosphamide therapy for pemphigus. *Br J Dermatol* 1988;**119**:73–7.

45 Pasricha JS, Khaitan BK, Raman RS, Chandra M. Dexamethasone-cyclophosphamide pulse therapy for pemphigus. *Int J Dermatol* 1995;**34**:875–82.

46 Kaur S, Kanwar AJ. Dexamethasone–cyclophosphamide pulse therapy in pemphigus. *Int J Dermatol* 1990;**29**:371–4.

47 Kanwar AJ, Kaur S, Thami GP. Long-term efficacy of dexamethasone–cyclophosphamide pulse therapy in pemphigus. *Dermatology* 2002;**204**:228–31.

48 Fleischli ME, Valek RH, Pandya AG. Pulse intravenous cyclophosphamide therapy in pemphigus. *Arch Dermatol* 1999;**135**:57–61.

49 Guillaume JC, Roujeau JC, Morel P, *et al*. Controlled study of plasma exchange in pemphigus. *Arch Dermatol* 1988;**124**:1659–63.

50 Bystryn JC, Graf MW, Uhr JW. Regulation of antibody formation by serum antibody. II. Removal of specific antibody by means of exchange transfusion. *J Exp Med* 1970;**132**:1279–87.

51 Derksen RH, Schuurman HJ, Gmelig Meyling FH, Struyvenberg A, Kater L. Rebound and overshoot after plasma exchange in humans. *J Lab Clin Med* 1984;**104**:35–43.

52 Tan-Lim R, Bystryn JC. Effect of plasmapheresis therapy on circulating levels of pemphigus antibodies. *J Am Acad Dermatol* 1990;**22**:35–40.

53 Turner MS, Sutton D, Sauder DN. The use of plasmapheresis and immunosuppression in the treatment of pemphigus vulgaris. *J Am Acad Dermatol* 2000;**43**:1058–64.

54 Ruocco V, Astarita C, Pisani M. Plasmapheresis as an alternative or adjunctive therapy in problem cases of pemphigus. *Dermatologica* 1984;**168**:219–23.

55 Blaszczyk M, Chorzelski TP, Jablonska S, *et al*. Indications for future studies on the treatment of pemphigus with plasmapheresis. *Arch Dermatol* 1989;**125**:843–4.

56 Roujeau JC, Andre C, Joneau Fabre M, *et al*. Plasma exchange in pemphigus. Uncontrolled study of ten patients. *Arch Dermatol* 1983;**119**:215–21.

57 Søndergaard K, Carstens J, Jørgensen J, Zachariae H. The steroid-sparing effect of long-term plasmapheresis in pemphigus. *Acta Derm Venereol* 1995;**75**:150–2.

58 Lüftl M, Stauber A, Mainka A, Klingel R, Schuler G, Hertl M. Successful removal of pathogenic autoantibodies in pemphigus by immunoadsorption with a tryptophan-linked polyvinylalcohol adsorber. *Br J Dermatol* 2003;**149**:598–605.

59 Schmidt E, Klinker E, Opitz A, *et al*. Protein A immunoadsorption: a novel and effective adjuvant treatment of severe pemphigus. *Br J Dermatol* 2003;**148**:1222–9.

60 Harman KE, Black MM. High-dose intravenous immune globulin for the treatment of autoimmune blistering diseases: an evaluation of its use in 14 cases. *Br J Dermatol* 1999;**140**:865–74.

61 Bystryn JC, Jiao D, Natow S. Treatment of pemphigus with intravenous immunoglobulin. *J Am Acad Dermatol* 2002;**47**:358–63.

62 Levy A, Doutre MS, Lesage FX, *et al*. [Treatment of pemphigus with intravenous immunoglobulin; in French.] *Ann Dermatol Venereol* 2004;**131**:957–61.

63 Enk AH, Knop J. [Adjuvant therapy of pemphigus vulgaris and pemphigus foliaceus with intravenous immunoglobulins; in German.] *Hautarzt* 1998;**49**:774–6.

64 Ahmed AR. Intravenous immunoglobulin therapy in the treatment of patients with pemphigus vulgaris unresponsive to conventional immunosuppressive treatment. *J Am Acad Dermatol* 2001;**45**:679–90.

65 Sami N, Bhol KC, Ahmed RA. Influence of intravenous immunoglobulin therapy on autoantibody titers to desmoglein 3 and desmoglein 1 in pemphigus vulgaris. *Eur J Dermatol* 2003;**13**: 377–81.

66 Sami N, Qureshi A, Ruocco E, Ahmed AR. Corticosteroid-sparing effect of intravenous immunoglobulin therapy in patients with pemphigus vulgaris. *Arch Dermatol* 2002;**138**:1158–62.

67 Ahmed AR, Sami N. Intravenous immunoglobulin therapy for patients with pemphigus foliaceus unresponsive to conventional therapy. *J Am Acad Dermatol* 2002;**46**:42–9.

68 Sami N, Bhol KC, Ahmed AR. Influence of IVIg therapy on autoantibody titers to desmoglein 1 in patients with pemphigus foliaceus. *Clin Immunol* 2002;**105**:192–8.

69 Sami N, Qureshi A, Ahmed AR. Steroid sparing effect of intravenous immunoglobulin therapy in patients with pemphigus foliaceus. *Eur J Dermatol* 2002;**12**:174–8.

70 Wetter DA, Davis MDP, Yiannias JA, *et al*. Effectiveness of intravenous immunoglobulin therapy for skin disease other than toxic epidermal necrolysis: a retrospective review of Mayo Clinic experience. *Mayo Clin Proc* 2005;**30**:41–7.

71 Katz KA, Hivnor CM, Geist DE, Shapiro M, Ming ME, Werth VP. Stroke and deep venous thrombosis complicating intravenous immunoglobulin infusions. *Arch Dermatol* 2003;**139**:991–3.

72 Auad A, Auad T. Terpaeutica coadjuvante no tratamento do penfigo foliaceo sul-americano com auranofina. Estudo duplo-cego. *An Bras Dermatol* 1986;**61**:131–4.

73 Pandya AG, Dyke C. Treatment of pemphigus with gold. *Arch Dermatol* 1998;**134**:1104–7.

74 Sutej PG, Jorizzo JL, White W. Intramuscular gold therapy for young patients with pemphigus vulgaris: a prospective, open, clinical study utilizing a dermatologist/rheumatologist team approach. *J Eur Acad Dermatol Venereol* 2006;**5**:222–8.

75 Poulin Y, Perry HO, Muller SA. Pemphigus vulgaris: results of treatment with gold as a steroid-sparing agent in a series of thirteen patients. *J Am Acad Dermatol* 1984;**11**:851–7.

76 Penneys NS, Eaglstein WH, Frost P. Management of pemphigus with gold compounds: a long-term follow-up report. *Arch Dermatol* 1976;**112**:185–7.

77 Werth VP, Fivenson D, Pandya A, *et al*. Multicenter randomized placebo-controlled clinical trial of dapsone as a Glucocorticoid-sparing agent in maintenance phase Pemphigus Vulgaris. *J Invest Dermatol* 2005;**125**:1088.

78 Heaphy MR, Albrecht J, Werth VP. Dapsone as a glucocorticoid-sparing agent in maintenance-phase pemphigus vulgaris. *Arch Dermatol* 2005;**141**:699–702.

79 Basset N, Guillot B, Michel B, Meynadier J, Guilhou JJ. Dapsone as initial treatment in superficial pemphigus. Report of nine cases. *Arch Dermatol* 1987;**123**:783–5.

80 Calebotta A, Saenz AM, Gonzalez F, Carvalho M, Castillo R. Pemphigus vulgaris: benefits of tetracycline as adjuvant therapy in a series of thirteen patients. *Int J Dermatol* 1999;**38**:217–21.

81 Alpsoy E, Yilmaz E, Basaran E, Yazar S, Cetin L. Is the combination of tetracycline and nicotinamide therapy alone effective in pemphigus? *Arch Dermatol* 1995;**131**:1339–40.

82 Chaffins ML, Collison D, Fivenson DP. Treatment of pemphigus and linear IgA dermatosis with nicotinamide and tetracycline: a review of 13 cases. *J Am Acad Dermatol* 1993;**28**:998–1000.

83 Gaspar ZS, Walkden V, Wojnarowska F. Minocycline is a useful adjuvant therapy for pemphigus. *Australas J Dermatol* 1996;**37**:93–5.

84 Joly P, Mouquet H, Roujeau J-C, *et al*. A single cycle of rituximab for the treatment of severe pemphigus. *N Eng J Med* **337**:545–52.

85 Arin MJ, Hunzelmann N. Anti-B cell-directed immunotherapy (rituximab) in the treatment of refractory pemphigus: an update. *Eur J Dermatol* 2005;**15**:224–30.

59 Cutaneous sarcoidosis

Leonid Izikson, Joseph C. English III

Background

Definition

Sarcoidosis is a systemic, idiopathic disease characterized by the formation of noncaseating epithelioid granulomas that disrupt underlying tissue function. While sarcoidosis can affect virtually any organ system, pulmonary (> 90%), hepatosplenic (50–80%), hematological (40%), musculoskeletal (39%), ocular (30–50%), cutaneous (25%), cardiac (5%), and neurological (5–10%) manifestations are most common.[1]

Cutaneous manifestations of sarcoidosis typically present at disease onset, and—with the exception of erythema nodosum—do not correlate with disease severity. Erythema nodosum tends to be associated with acute, benign, spontaneously resolving sarcoidosis.[2] Skin lesions in sarcoidosis can be divided into specific lesions (i.e., skin biopsy demonstrates noncaseating granulomas) and nonspecific lesions (i.e., reactive states). Specific lesions include papules, nodules, plaques, subcutaneous nodules, infiltrative scars, and lupus pernio. Multiple atypical presentations also exist (i.e., verrucous, ulcerative, and morpheaform). Plaques and papules are the most common cutaneous lesions, while lupus pernio is most specific for sarcoidosis.[3] Lupus pernio tends to affect the face, manifesting as brownish-red, dusky, swollen, and shiny infiltrated plaques with no papulonodular component.[1]

Incidence/prevalence

Sarcoidosis affects all ethnic groups, ages, and both sexes, but incidence peaks in adults under 40 years of age.[4] Sarcoidosis is most common in African-American females, whose disease is typically more acute and severe in comparison with others.[5,6] In the United States, the incidence is 10–14 per 100 000 for whites, and 35.5–64 per 100 000 for African-Americans.[7]

Etiology

The etiology of sarcoidosis remains elusive, with immunologic infectious, genetic, and environmental factors all postulated to play a role. The genetic basis for sarcoidosis has been demonstrated in some family clusters of disease, and serological studies have found increased susceptibility in patients with certain class I and II HLA serotypes.[8–10] Mycobacteria have been investigated as a possible etiological agent because of the granulomatous nature of this disease, but no definitive proof has emerged thus far.[1]

Prognosis

Sarcoidosis has a variable course, with both limited/spontaneously resolving and chronic/progressive forms of disease. Most patients with sarcoidosis do well. The disease resolves spontaneously in up to 60% of patients, and only about 5% of sarcoidosis patients will eventually die of their disease.[11,12] In the United States, patients are most likely to die of pulmonary complications such as pneumonia, pulmonary fibrosis progressing to cor pulmonale, and chronic obstructive pulmonary disease.[13]

Diagnostic tests

Because no specific diagnostic test exists, sarcoidosis remains a diagnosis of exclusion. Diagnostic evaluation of a patient with suspected sarcoidosis may include:[1,12]
- *Detailed history and physical examination:* with emphasis on lungs, skin, eyes, nervous system, and heart.
- *Chest radiography.* The stages are not chronological:
  —Stage 1: bilateral hilar, with or without paratracheal adenopathy
  —Stage 2: adenopathy with pulmonary infiltrate
  —Stage 3: pulmonary infiltrates only
  —Stage 4: pulmonary fibrosis
- *Pulmonary function tests:* restrictive pattern with decreased diffusing capacity (DLCO).

- *Biopsy of affected tissue:* noncaseating granulomas.
- *Serum chemistries:* elevated alkaline phosphatase and/or hypercalcemia, which are not specific for sarcoidosis.
- *Angiotensin-converting enzyme (ACE) levels:* generally, not a useful guide for diagnosis or monitoring of therapeutic response.

Aims of treatment

Disfiguring skin lesions represent an indication for treatment of cutaneous sarcoidosis. Multiple available treatment modalities include topical and intralesional steroids, oral steroids, antimalarials, various immunosuppressive agents, and other medical and physical interventions. Since cutaneous sarcoidosis may spontaneously regress, and since many available therapeutic modalities carry a risk for substantial toxicity, it is important to weigh the risks and benefits carefully. Nonetheless, patients often seek treatment because of poor cosmesis produced by cutaneous sarcoidosis, especially when disease leads to disfiguring or nondisfiguring lesions on the face. Accordingly, dermatologists should become familiarized with the evidence-based treatment options available for cutaneous sarcoidosis.

Relevant outcomes

Outcome measures in cutaneous sarcoidosis are limited to subjective evaluation of whether therapy decreases or resolves active skin lesions. To date, no scoring method, such as an index of severity and/or extent of involvement, is available for this disease. The definition of disfiguring lesions is not well-established among different investigators, and there is a lack of uniformity in measuring clinical end points in response to therapy due to polymorphic cutaneous manifestations.

Methods of search

We searched the Cochrane Library for "sarcoidosis or sarcoid." We searched Medline from 1966 to 2006 using the terms "cutaneous sarcoidosis," or "sarcoidosis," or "lupus pernio" and "therapeutics," or "treatment," or "prednisone," or "steroids," or "glucocorticoids," or "allopurinol," or "chloroquine," or "hydroxychloroquine," or "antimalarial," or "methotrexate," or "thalidomide," or "pentoxifylline," or "tretinoin," or "isotretinoin," or "tetracyclines," or "minocycline" or "allopurinol," or "tacrolimus," or "infliximab," or "adalimumab," or "etanercept," or "ultraviolet," or "photodynamic therapy," or "surgery," or "intralesional," or "pulse dye laser," or "laser" as subject headings or titles or key words.

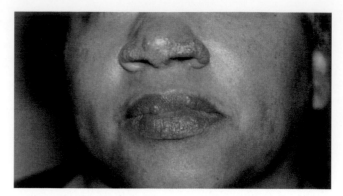

Figure 59.1 Cutaneous sarcoidosis.

Questions

Case scenario

The patient is a 44-year-old African-American woman with a 14-year history of sarcoidosis. The patient has asymptomatic pulmonary involvement that does not require treatment. However, she is requesting treatment for noticeable facial lesions (Figure 59.1).

What are the effects of systemic therapeutic interventions in patients with cutaneous sarcoidosis?

Oral steroids
Benefits
Oral glucocorticoids are used in systemic sarcoidosis because of their anti-inflammatory and immunosuppressive actions, and are often offered as first-line treatment for cutaneous sarcoidosis[14,15] despite scant, and largely anecdotal, evidence to support their use for this indication.[16–27]

Harms
The multiple complications of steroid therapy are well known, and their likelihood and severity correlate with the length of administration. Complications may include glucose intolerance, increased susceptibility to infection, osteoporosis, avascular bone necrosis, cataracts, and neuropsychiatric changes.[28]

Comments/implications for clinical practice
There are no randomized controlled trials (RCTs) or systematic reviews to support the use of oral steroids for cutaneous sarcoidosis. In the articles reviewed above, 17 of 56 patients treated with oral steroids as monotherapy had positive results. This is insufficient evidence to

conclude that oral steroids are effective in cutaneous sarcoidosis. Hence, large RCTs are needed to establish clear benefit.

Despite the lack of definitive studies showing the effectiveness of oral steroids in cutaneous sarcoidosis, many dermatologists still use them as first-line therapy, since steroids reverse the manifestations of pulmonary and other extrapulmonary manifestations of disease.[4,28–30]

Antimalarials

Antimalarials, such as chloroquine and hydroxychloroquine, are 4-aminoquinolones, and represent an effective therapy for connective-tissue diseases. Their immunomodulatory properties form the rationale for their use in cutaneous sarcoidosis.

Benefits

While there are no RCTs to support the effectiveness of antimalarials in cutaneous sarcoidosis, their benefit has been reported in a number of open nonrandomized, noncontrolled, prospective studies. In a 1991 comprehensive literature review of antimalarials in cutaneous sarcoidosis, Zic et al. concluded that chloroquine should be strongly considered in patients for whom the main indication for treatment is disfiguring cutaneous lesions, while corticosteroids should remain first-line treatment for patients with extracutaneous sarcoidosis.[29] The authors recommended an initial 14-day course of chloroquine, 500 mg/day, followed by long-term therapy with 250 mg/day, on the basis of published data.[31–36]

Harms

Long-term administration of either chloroquine or hydroxychloroquine may lead to various ocular complications, the most serious of which are irreversible retinopathy and blindness.[29] Hydroxychloroquine has a lower risk of ocular toxicity, but also less effectiveness in sarcoidosis.[12,29] Thus, periodic ophthalmological examinations should be carried out in any patient on long-term therapy.[37,38] Other common side effects include nausea and vomiting, gastrointestinal upset, central nervous system toxicity (irritability, nervousness, depression), neuromuscular reactions (skeletal muscle palsies, myopathy or neuromyopathy), and cutaneous pigmentation. Millard et al. reported drug-induced bullous pemphigoid in a male patient treated with 3 months of chloroquine for sarcoidosis.[39]

Comments/implications for clinical practice

The articles summarized above describe experience with a total of 103 patients treated with antimalarials, 82 of whom had a positive result. While none of these articles represents a large RCT, these studies as a whole suggest that chloroquine and hydroxychloroquine represent a reasonable treatment option for patients with cutaneous sarcoidosis without substantial systemic disease.

Methotrexate

Methotrexate is a dihydrofolate reductase inhibitor widely used in the treatment of neoplastic diseases due to its antiproliferative actions, and in chronic inflammatory conditions as a nonsteroidal immunosuppressant.

Benefits

There are no RCTs or systematic reviews of methotrexate in cutaneous sarcoidosis,[40,41] and the evidence for its effectiveness is based on open nonrandomized noncontrolled studies. In the first study of methotrexate for cutaneous sarcoidosis, Veien and Brodthagen reported clearance of skin lesions in 12 of 16 patients treated with 25 mg/week. Two patients discontinued treatment because of nausea.[41] Lower and Baughman reported improvement of cutaneous disease in 16 of 17 patients treated with methotrexate as a steroid-sparing agent for over 2 years (the average dose in the 55 study patients was 28 mg/day).[42] Kaye et al. reported complete regression of severe recalcitrant cutaneous sarcoidosis in one patient, and significant improvement in three patients, treated with methotrexate, 10 mg/week, for 30 months.[43] Gedalia et al. reported resolution of cutaneous sarcoidosis in two of three pediatric patients treated with 10–15 mg/week of methotrexate, with significant reduction of oral steroid doses while on methotrexate.[44] Lacher reported improvement of steroid-resistant cutaneous sarcoidosis in one patient after the initial combination of prednisone 75 mg three times weekly and methotrexate 40 mg twice weekly, followed by methotrexate 7.5 mg twice weekly and eventual tapering of the steroid.[45] Webster et al. reported improvement of severe steroid-resistant cutaneous sarcoidosis in three patients after methotrexate 15.0–22.5 mg/week.[46] Henderson et al. reported improvement of cutaneous sarcoidosis in a male patient with steroid-resistant laryngeal and cutaneous disease after 10 mg/week of methotrexate.[47] Gary et al. reported complete remission of recalcitrant cutaneous sarcoidosis in three of four patients after treatment with methotrexate at doses ranging from 12.5 mg to 30 mg/week after a mean treatment duration of 29 months. Side effects of methotrexate were observed in one patient (elevated liver enzymes), leading to discontinuation of methotrexate.[48]

Harms

Complications of methotrexate therapy include bone-marrow suppression, nausea and vomiting, hepatotoxicity, and hypersensitivity pneumonitis.[28] Albertini et al. described a patient with severe systemic and ulcerative sarcoidosis who was started on methotrexate 25 mg/week.[49] Although her ulcerative lesions initially regressed, she soon developed anemia, leukopenia, and an elevated aspartate transaminase level, necessitating the withdrawal of methotrexate. The patient subsequently died of her disease. Major toxic effects noted by Lower and Baughman were hepatotoxicity, leukopenia, and cough.[42]

Comments/implications for clinical practice

The articles published to date describe experience with a total of 50 patients with cutaneous sarcoidosis treated with methotrexate, of whom 42 had positive results. While none of these articles represents a large RCT, and there is little consistency across the trials with regard to the patient population, dosage, or clinical end points, the aggregate evidence from these studies suggests that methotrexate might be useful as a steroid-sparing agent in patients who require an additional or alternative therapeutic option.

Thalidomide

Thalidomide was originally marketed as a sedative, but was withdrawn in 1962 because of its teratogenic effects.[50] Thalidomide at low doses is effective in the treatment of erythema nodosum leprosum and lupus erythematous.[51] Thalidomide inhibits tumor necrosis factor-α (TNF-α), interferon gamma, and interleukin-12 (IL-12), and increases IL-2. TNF-α and interferon gamma are the major cytokines that drive granulomatous inflammation in sarcoidosis, while IL-2 counteracts the effects of interferon gamma and TNF-α.[52] Based on its mechanism of action, thalidomide may be effective in the treatment of cutaneous sarcoidosis.

Benefits

There are no RCTs or systematic reviews of thalidomide in cutaneous sarcoidosis. Estines et al. reported complete regression of severe and disfiguring recalcitrant cutaneous sarcoidosis in three patients and incomplete regression in four among 10 patients treated with thalidomide 1.84 mg/kg. The dose was gradually reduced for five of the seven responders; three of the five relapsed, but improved after re-starting at the same dose.[53] Baughmann et al. reported an open-label, dose-escalation trial of thalidomide in 14 patients with lupus pernio unresponsive to prior therapy who completed 4 months of thalidomide. All patients experienced some subjective improvement of skin lesions, and 10 of 12 evaluable patients showed objective improvement using photograph scoring. Five patients improved after 1 month (treated with 50 mg/day of thalidomide), seven more patients improved after 2 months (treated with 100 mg/day of thalidomide in the second month), and two patients required an additional month of 200 mg/day of thalidomide to achieve a response.[54]

A retrospective evaluation of thalidomide 100–200 mg/day in 12 patients with cutaneous sarcoidosis, by Nguyen et al., found that lesions regressed in 10 of 12 treated patients within 1–5 months of therapy, with an average time of 2–3 months. Four of the patients achieved complete responses, six had partial responses, and two showed no response.[55] In an open study by Oliver et al., five of eight patients with chronic cutaneous sarcoidosis had flattening of skin lesions, while one developed enlarging and ulcerating skin lesions, after 16 weeks of thalidomide. Treatment was started at an initial dose of 50 mg/day, and doubled monthly to a maximum dose of 200 mg/day. All lesions became hyperpigmented during the study period, which the authors characterized as an improvement, and all follow-up biopsies showed decreased granuloma size and decreased epidermal thickness. After discontinuing thalidomide, all of the treated patients relapsed.[56]

Carlesimo et al. reported clinical improvement of steroid-resistant cutaneous sarcoidosis in a 56-year-old woman after 2 weeks of thalidomide 200 mg/day, followed by 100 mg/day for 11 weeks.[50] Rousseau et al. reported clinical improvement of recalcitrant cutaneous sarcoidosis in a 30-year-old woman after thalidomide 100 mg/day for 2 months, gradually tapered to a maintenance dose of 50 mg/day.[51] Lee et al. reported clinical improvement of cutaneous sarcoidosis in a 59-year-old patient after thalidomide 200 mg/day for 2 months and 300 mg/day for 4 months.[57] Hoch et al. reported almost complete resolution of generalized or disseminated cutaneous sarcoidosis in two patients after 8–12 months of treatment with thalidomide, initially with 200 mg/day and later with 100 mg/day.[58] Walter et al. reported rapid improvement of therapy-resistant long-standing cutaneous sarcoidosis in a 36-year-old man after thalidomide 50 mg/day, without major adverse effects.[59]

Harms

Thalidomide therapy may be complicated by neurosensory, gastrointestinal, and teratogenic effects.[50,57] In their analysis of thalidomide for cutaneous sarcoidosis, Baughmann and Lower reported that the most serious adverse effect is peripheral neuropathy, which often resolves by reducing the dose or discontinuing the medication.[60] Baughmann et al. noted neuropathy in seven of 14 patients, somnolence in nine patients, dizziness in two patients, constipation in six patients, rash in one patient, and increasing shortness of breath in one patient.[54] Nguyen et al. also noted nasopharyngeal, pulmonary, hepatic, and neurologic side effects in their retrospective analysis, and reported one patient who developed deep vein thrombosis while on thalidomide.[55]

Comments/implications for clinical practice

The articles published to date describe experience with 50 patients treated with thalidomide, 38 of whom had positive results. While none of these articles represents a large RCT, and there is inconsistency across the trials with regard to patient population, dosage, and clinical end points, the aggregate evidence from these studies suggests that thalidomide may represent a reasonable alternative or additional therapeutic option in cutaneous sarcoidosis. A large RCT will thus be necessary in order to obtain definitive proof.

Tetracyclines
Tetracyclines are antibiotics that inhibit T-cell proliferation and granuloma formation *in vitro*,[61] which forms the rationale for their use in cutaneous sarcoidosis.

Benefits
There are no RCTs or systematic reviews of tetracyclines in cutaneous sarcoidosis. In one nonrandomized, noncontrolled, open prospective study, eight of 12 patients with recalcitrant cutaneous sarcoidosis had complete regression, two had partial regression, and two had treatment failure (one progressed and one remained stable) after 12 months of minocycline 200 mg/day. After withdrawal of therapy, three of the 10 responders relapsed.[61] Antonovich and Callen reported complete clearance of lesions in a patient with cutaneous sarcoidosis induced by cosmetic tattoo after a 4-month course of doxycycline 100 mg twice a day combined with a mid-potency topical steroid.[62]

Harms
General side effects of tetracyclines include photosensitivity, gastrointestinal symptoms, and pseudotumor cerebri. Side effects of minocycline include nausea and vomiting, hypersensitivity reactions, blue skin pigmentation, and vertigo.[61] Hypersensitivity was noted in one patient in this study.[61]

Comments/implications for clinical practice
The articles published to date describe experience with a total of 13 patients treated with tetracyclines, 11 of whom had positive results. While this is insufficient evidence to conclude that tetracyclines are beneficial for the treatment of cutaneous sarcoidosis and a large RCT will be necessary for definitive proof, tetracyclines may represent an easy alternative to oral steroids or other medications with a more serious side-effect profile.

Allopurinol
Allopurinol is a xanthine oxidase inhibitor used in the treatment of gout and other inflammatory diseases. Its anti-inflammatory properties form the basis for its use in cutaneous sarcoidosis.

Benefits
There are no RCTs or systematic reviews of allopurinol in cutaneous sarcoidosis. In one nonrandomized, uncontrolled, open prospective study, four of six patients with cutaneous sarcoidosis had improvement of skin lesions after treatment with allopurinol, starting at 100 mg/day and increased to 600 mg/day by 100 mg every 2–4 weeks.[63] Bregnhoej and Jemec reported a positive response in four of seven patients with cutaneous sarcoidosis who were treated with low-dose allopurinol.[64]

Pfau *et al.* reported complete resolution of scar sarcoidosis in two patients and partial resolution of nodular sarcoidosis in two patients after treatment with allopurinol 300 mg/day over a 3–7-month period.[65] Rosof reported remission of cutaneous sarcoidosis in two patients treated with allopurinol.[66] Pollock *et al.* reported marked improvement of cutaneous sarcoidosis lesions in two patients after treatment with allopurinol, either 100 mg/day or 300 mg/day.[67] Brechtel *et al.* reported improvement of recalcitrant disseminated cutaneous sarcoidosis in one patient after allopurinol 300 mg/day.[68] Antony *et al.* reported improvement of recalcitrant cutaneous acral sarcoidosis after allopurinol 300 mg/day.[69] Voelter-Mahlknecht *et al.* reported one patient whose cutaneous sarcoidosis progressed while on allopurinol.[70]

Harms
Allopurinol therapy may be complicated by a drug rash (including a severe reaction, such as toxic epidermal necrosis), as well as nausea and vomiting, hepatotoxicity, and bone-marrow suppression.[68]

Comments/implications for clinical practice
The articles published to date describe experience with a total of 25 patients treated with allopurinol, 19 of whom had a positive result. This is insufficient evidence to conclude that allopurinol is beneficial for treatment of cutaneous sarcoidosis, particularly because cutaneous sarcoidosis often resolves spontaneously. Large RCTs will be necessary for definitive proof.

Isotretinoin
Isotretinoin, a retinoid that inhibits sebaceous gland function and keratinization, is useful in the treatment of many dermatological conditions. The immunomodulatory effects of isotretinoin form the basis for its use in cutaneous sarcoidosis.[71]

Benefits
There are no RCTs or systematic reviews of isotretinoin in cutaneous sarcoidosis. Georgiou *et al.* described complete resolution of recalcitrant, long-standing cutaneous sarcoidosis in a 31-year-old woman after 8 months of isotretinoin 1 mg/kg/day.[71] Waldinger *et al.* reported resolution or improvement of many long-standing severe disfiguring and recalcitrant lesions in a woman after 30 weeks of isotretinoin (initially 40 mg/day for 6 weeks, increased to 80 mg/day for 16 weeks, and decreased back to 40 mg/day for the last 8 weeks because of side effects).[72]

Spiteri and Taylor reported negligible resolution of chronic cutaneous sarcoid nodules in a woman treated with iso-tretinoin, 75 mg/day (decreased to 50 mg/day because of cheilitis), whose exfoliative dermatitis prompted drug withdrawal after 7 weeks.[73] Vaillant et al. reported improvement of recalcitrant cutaneous sarcoidosis in a woman after 6 months of isotretinoin 0.4–1.0 mg/kg/day.[74] Mosam and Morar reported clearance of multitherapy-resistant cutaneous sarcoidosis in one patient after 6 months of isotretinoin therapy at 25 mg/day.[75]

Harms

Isotretinoin is a teratogenic drug and must not be used by women who are pregnant or who become pregnant during treatment. Other side effects include visual impairment, hepatic dysfunction, and pancreatitis. Side effects noted by study participants included myalgia, xerosis, dryness of nasal mucosa, cheilitis, and exfoliative dermatitis.[71,72,74]

Comments/implications for clinical practice

The articles published to date describe experience with five patients treated with isotretinoin, four of whom had a positive result. This is insufficient evidence to conclude that isotretinoin is beneficial for the treatment of cutaneous sarcoidosis, particularly because cutaneous sarcoidosis often resolves spontaneously. Large RCTs will be necessary for definitive proof.

Fumaric acid esters

Fumaric acid esters (FAEs) represent a form of immunomodulatory therapy that has been used successfully in Europe for the treatment of psoriasis. FAEs inhibit the pathogenetic mechanisms of granuloma formation, namely the downstream effects of TNF-α, maintenance of a Th1 environment, and proliferation of lymphocytes.[76,77] FAEs may therefore have efficacy in treatment of cutaneous sarcoidosis.

Benefits

There are no RCTs or systematic reviews of FAEs in cutaneous sarcoidosis. Breuer et al. treated 11 patients with recalcitrant cutaneous sarcoidosis with FAE. Three of the patients treated with five or six tablets per day for 12–23 months had significant improvement of disease, while three of the patients treated with four to six tablets for 4–7 months had slight to moderate improvement of disease. Treatment was discontinued in five of the patients due to a lack of effect, and four of the patients had side effects that prompted discontinuation of therapy, including leukopenia, nausea, proteinuria, and flushing.[77] Gutzmer et al. reported a 61-year old woman with cutaneous sarcoidosis whose lesions markedly improved after 12 months of therapy with FAEs. A recurrence of cutaneous disease 18 months after discontinuation was treated successfully with a 2-month

course of FAEs.[78] Nowack et al. reported on three women with recalcitrant cutaneous sarcoidosis whose disease completely cleared after 4–12-month courses of FAEs dosed in accordance with the standard therapy regimen for psoriasis. Side effects included flushing, minor gastrointestinal complaints, and lymphopenia.[79] In addition, Dummler et al. described two patients with cutaneous sarcoidosis, one of whom who had a significant improvement after 4 months of treatment with FAE; the second patient showed a slight therapeutic response after 2 months of therapy.[80]

Harms

FAEs have been associated with several types of side effect in most treated patients with granulomatous skin diseases. The most frequent side effects of FAEs are flushing and diarrhea. Others include abdominal discomfort, nausea, flatulence, lack of appetite, and fatigue.[75] FAEs may produce leukopenia, relative lymphopenia, eosinophilia, and elevation of liver function tests, all of which resolve spontaneously after dose reduction or discontinuation of the treatment.[76]

Hoefnagel et al. have evaluated the long-term safety of FAEs in 66 patients with severe psoriasis, 41 of whom received FAEs for at least 1 year and 12 of whom had received FAEs for 10–14 years. Seventy-three percent of the patients reported adverse events, which were usually mild and mainly consisted of flushing (55%), diarrhea (42%), nausea (14%), fatigue (14%), and abdominal complaints (12%). Seventy-six percent of the patients had relative lymphocytopenia during therapy with FAEs, and 14% and 25% of the patients had transient eosinophilia and moderate liver enzyme elevations, respectively. The authors concluded that FAEs are a safe long-term treatment in patients with severe psoriasis.[81]

Comments/implications for clinical practice

The articles published to date describe positive results in 12 of 17 patients, in whom FAE therapy led to improvement or resolution of disease. Patients had only mild or moderate side effects. This is insufficient evidence to conclude that FAEs are beneficial for the treatment of cutaneous sarcoidosis, particularly because cutaneous sarcoidosis often resolves spontaneously. RTCs will therefore be necessary to evaluate fully the efficacy and long-term safety of FAEs in patients with cutaneous sarcoidosis.

Biologic anti-TNF-α agents

Monoclonal anti-TNF-α antibodies (infliximab, adalimumab) as well as the soluble anti-TNF-α receptor (etanercept) neutralize soluble and cell-bound TNF-α, and have been widely used in the treatment of psoriasis and inflammatory bowel disease in the past 15 years. The antibodies appear to have increased potency in comparison with the soluble receptor due to their cytolytic effects against immune cells with membrane-resident TNF-α. The use of these agents—infliximab, in particular—has been associated with suppression of TNF-α-mediated granulomatous responses, leading to exacerbation of pulmonary tuberculosis; possible exacerbation of demyelinating central nervous system disease; and immunosuppression, leading to increased risk of serious infection and possibly decreased immunosurveillance against malignancy.[82] Since TNF-α appears to be a key mediator of granuloma development in sarcoidosis,[82,83] these biologic treatments have been employed to treat isolated cases of cutaneous sarcoidosis. There are no RCTs or systematic reviews of the role of biologic anti-TNF-α agents in the treatment of cutaneous sarcoidosis. Evidence regarding their efficacy has been presented in case series and case reports.

Benefits

Infliximab. Doty *et al.* reported significant improvement of cutaneous sarcoidosis in five patients and resolution in one patient among six patients with recalcitrant cutaneous disease after treatment with infliximab for cutaneous and/or visceral disease using conventional dosing regimens. Some of the patients received concomitant prednisone therapy. Infliximab was generally well tolerated in all patients. Noted adverse events included a drug reaction in one patient after several months of therapy, oral candidiasis in one patient, and angioimmunoblastic lymphoma in one patient.[84] Heffernan and Anadkat reported 90% clearance of severe recalcitrant cutaneous sarcoidosis in a 51-year-old African-American woman treated at weeks 0, 2, and 6 with 5 mg/kg of infliximab. She experienced no adverse events during therapy.[85] Haley *et al.* reported flattening of all cutaneous sarcoidosis lesions in a 39-year-old African-American man with severe and recalcitrant cutaneous sarcoidosis, after treatment at weeks 0, 2, and 6 with 5 mg/kg of infliximab and concomitant oral prednisone. Notably, prednisone alone was ineffective, and the prednisone dose was tapered significantly over the course of therapy with infliximab. The patient did not experience any adverse effects associated with infliximab therapy.[82]

Baughman and Lower reported improvement in two patients with persistent recalcitrant lupus pernio after treatment with infliximab 5 mg/kg at weeks 2, 4, and 12, without any significant adverse events.[86] Mallbris *et al.* reported substantial clinical improvement of severe recalcitrant cutaneous sarcoidosis in a 39-year-old white man after 5 mg/kg treatment with infliximab at weeks 0, 2, 4, 6, and 14, when combined with concomitant methotrexate administration to prevent anti-infliximab antibody production. Notably, methotrexate alone did not produce any clinical effect. The clinical effect of infliximab therapy was noticeable after the first treatment, and became significant after the fourth treatment. The patient experienced no adverse effects.[83] Meyerle and Shorr reported complete resolution of cutaneous sarcoidosis in a female patient after initiation of infliximab.[87] Pritchard and Nadarajah reported rapid resolution of cutaneous sarcoidosis in a 32-year-old white woman with multiorgan involvement. Skin nodules disappeared after 2 days of infliximab therapy. The authors reported no adverse effects, with the exception of infusion-associated complications.[88]

Adalimumab. Philips *et al.* reported resolution of severe ulcerative recalcitrant cutaneous sarcoidosis nodule in a 55-year-old white woman after a 9-week course of adalimumab 40 mg intramuscularly per week. The patient was concomitantly on prednisone, and the dosage was reduced progressively after initiation of adalimumab therapy. The patient experienced no adverse events.[89] Heffernan and Smith reported significant improvement of severe and ulcerating recalcitrant cutaneous sarcoidosis in an African-American woman after 10 weeks of treatment with adalimumab 40 mg weekly, with clinical effects readily apparent after five treatments. She was concomitantly being treated with hydroxychloroquine and pentoxifylline, which by themselves had no clinical effect. The patient experienced no adverse effects.[90]

Etanercept. Khanna *et al.* reported significant improvement of cutaneous sarcoidosis in a 50-year-old African-American woman 2 months after the addition of etanercept 25 mg twice weekly to her regimen of prednisone, hydroxychloroquine, and methotrexate. Etanercept was discontinued transiently during treatment of cellulitis.[91]

Harms

Complications of anti-TNF-α biologic agents include infusion reactions (with intravenously administered infliximab), injection reactions (with subcutaneously or intramuscularly administered adalimumab and etanercept), exacerbation of preexisting tuberculosis, exacerbation of demyelinating neurologic disease, and immunosuppression that may lead to an increased risk of infection and decreased cancer immunosurveillance. Evaluation with a purified protein derivation test (and chest radiography if the test is positive) is therefore necessary before treatment is started, and a thorough history and physical are mandatory to elicit a prior or family history of demyelinating disorders, malignancies, and risk for malignancy.[92]

Comments/implications for clinical practice

The articles published to date describe experience with a total of 13 patients with cutaneous sarcoidosis treated successfully with infliximab, two treated successfully with adalimumab, and one treated successfully with etanercept. While this is insufficient evidence to conclude that anti-TNF-α biologic agents are beneficial for the treatment of cutaneous sarcoidosis, these reports suggest that biological anti-TNF-α agents might be useful as an alternative or additional therapy, particularly in extremely recalcitrant cases. RCTs will therefore be necessary in order to evaluate fully their efficacy and long-term safety in patients with cutaneous sarcoidosis.

Conclusions

A review of the available data on oral and systemic therapy in cutaneous sarcoidosis reveals a dearth of evidence-based medicine, underscoring the need for RCTs. Although oral steroids have been "grandfathered in" as the first-line treatment, on the basis of many clinicians' personal experiences with sarcoidosis, this therapy has not been formally evaluated or proven in appropriate clinical trials.

The reported evidence suggests that chloroquine or hydroxychloroquine, methotrexate, and thalidomide may be the most effective medications for the treatment of cutaneous sarcoidosis. Hence, these agents may represent a reasonable therapeutic option as an alternative or adjunct to oral steroids. Less studied potential alternatives include biological anti-TNF-α agents, tetracyclines, and allopurinol.

Additional drugs reported as successful in isolated cases include tranilast, melatonin, clofazimine, mepacrine, and levamisole.[93–97]

What are the effects of topical and physical therapeutic interventions in patients with cutaneous sarcoidosis?

Topical corticosteroids and intralesional injections

While topical corticosteroids and intralesional injections are often recommended as the first-line treatment for the cutaneous manifestations of sarcoidosis, due to their anti-inflammatory properties,[12,14,15,30] the evidence for their efficacy is scant and has been reported in case series and case reports.[98–100]

Harms

In general, topical or intralesional steroids may lead to hypopigmentation, skin atrophy, tachyphylaxis, or systemic absorption. No major side effects have been reported in any of the above studies. Minimal bleeding from needle puncture and postinflammatory hypopigmentation and hyperpigmentation are additional risks of intralesional hydrocortisone injections.[100,101]

Comments/implications for clinical practice

The articles published to date describe a limited number of patients with cutaneous sarcoidosis treated with intralesional injections or topical steroids. This is insufficient evidence to conclude that this therapy is beneficial for the treatment of cutaneous sarcoidosis. Large RCTs are therefore necessary to evaluate their efficacy and safety. However, many dermatologists still use these modalities as

first-line therapy, due to their general anti-inflammatory properties.

Tacrolimus

Topical tacrolimus, a novel immunosuppressive agent successfully used in atopic dermatitis, inhibits the production of TNF-α by T cells and macrophages, and inhibits hapten-induced production of Th1 cytokines by T cells.[102] Thus, it may suppress the formation of granulomas in cutaneous sarcoidosis.

Benefits

Katoh *et al.* reported on a 62-year-old woman with recalcitrant persistent sarcoidosis of the face that resolved after treatment with topical tacrolimus without any adverse effects.[102] Gutzmer *et al.,* reported on a 56-year-old woman with recalcitrant cutaneous sarcoidosis of the face whose disease almost completely resolved after a 3-month course of topical tacrolimus.[103] Landers *et al.* reported almost complete resolution of persistent cutaneous sarcoidosis in an eyebrow tattoo of a 70-year-old woman after the addition of tacrolimus 0.1% ointment to oral prednisone.[104]

Harms

Topical tacrolimus appears to be a safe and well-tolerated medication, both in the three reported cases of cutaneous sarcoidosis and in more than 1.7 million patients, most with atopic dermatitis. The most common adverse effects are skin burning and pruritus. Topical tacrolimus is not associated with increased rates of infection or malignancy in comparison with topical steroids when used intermittently.[105,106]

Comments/implications for clinical practice

The articles published to date describe three patients who were treated successfully topical tacrolimus. This is insufficient evidence to conclude that this therapy is beneficial for the treatment of cutaneous sarcoidosis. Further RCTs will be necessary in order to evaluate the safety and efficacy of topical tacrolimus in cutaneous sarcoidosis.

Photomedicine
Flashlamp pulsed-dye laser therapy

Flashlamp pulsed-dye laser (fPDL) therapy has been used successfully in the treatment of port-wine stains and telangiectasias, where it selectively ablates the dilated and inflamed vessels.[107] This mechanism forms the rationale for its use in lupus pernio, a disfiguring cutaneous manifestation of sarcoidosis.

Benefits. There are no RCTs or systematic reviews of fPDL therapy in cutaneous sarcoidosis. Goodman and Alpern reported on a woman with a 5-year history of lupus pernio of the nose who responded to fPDL at an energy level of 7–8 J/cm^2. The improvement induced by the laser was temporary; the erythema and papules returned 7 months after the first treatment and 6–15 months after the second treatment, but on both occasions responded again to laser therapy. She received three sessions altogether, without side effects (such as atrophy, scarring, or hypopigmentation).[107] Cliff *et al.* reported on a patient with lupus pernio of the nose, who improved after six treatment sessions at 6-week intervals with fPDL at a setting of 5.6–7.3 J/cm^2. A biopsy of her nose after treatment showed noncaseating sarcoid granulomas, leading the authors to conclude that laser therapy was effective in improving the appearance of the lesions, but not the underlying disease process.[108] Dosik and Ashinoff reported on a woman with a 3-year history of topical and intralesional steroid-resistant lupus pernio who responded successfully to fPDL at an energy of 7.25 J/cm^2. The therapy was given for nine sessions at 1–2-month intervals.[109]

Harms. There were no side effects of laser therapy in the above patients. However, laser treatment has been reported to exacerbate cutaneous sarcoidosis in one patient.[110] The inherent risks of fPDL include erythema, atrophy, scarring, dyspigmentation, and a risk of eye damage when appropriate protection is not provided.

Comments/implications for clinical practice. The articles published to date describe experience with four patients with treatment-resistant chronic lupus pernio who were treated with fPDL, three of whom had a positive result. This is insufficient evidence to conclude that fPDL is beneficial in the treatment of cutaneous sarcoidosis. RCTs will be necessary for definitive proof.

Other laser modalities

Benefits. Nonablative lasers, such as Q-switched ruby laser, that have the capacity to target foreign material in sarcoidal lesions, may be effective in treating cutaneous sarcoidal lesions where foreign material, such as tattoo, may be the nidus of granuloma formation. Additionally, ablative modalities, such as carbon dioxide laser, may effectively remove granulomatous lesions.

Grema *et al.* reported successful resolution of recalcitrant scar sarcoidosis of the elbow and knees in a 50-year-old woman using Q-switched ruby laser. The patient remained recurrence-free for over 3 years. The affected areas also had traumatic tattoos from abrasions, and did not resolve after three previous treatments with pulsed-dye laser.[111] O'Donoghue and Barlow reported on three patients with significant improvement of disfiguring lupus pernio after treatment with CO_2 laser. The sarcoidal granulomas were debulked, and wound healing occurred after 4 weeks. Two of the patients remained disease-free after therapy.[112] Stack *et al.* reported successful resolution of recalcitrant lupus pernio in a 31-year-old African-American man after

excision and fulguration with a CO_2 laser, followed with an intralesional steroid injection in the postoperative period. The site healed well, and the patient had no recurrence. He experienced no adverse effects.[113] Young *et al.* reported on two patients with long-standing recalcitrant lupus pernio who were successfully treated with CO_2 laser resurfacing.[114] Ekback and Molin reported complete healing of long-standing recalcitrant lupus pernio in a 57-year-old white woman after two treatments with a frequency-doubled Nd:YAG laser (532 nm, 50 msec, 12–16 J/cm^2) 7 months apart. Side effects included slight erythema and swelling of the treated skin areas 1 day after treatment. The patient had not experienced a relapse at the 3-month follow-up.[115]

Harms. No significant complications were noted in these reports, but the inherent risks of laser therapy (scarring, dyspigmentation, erythema, as well as exacerbation of sarcoidosis and other photodermatoses) should be considered.

Comments/implications for clinical practice. The articles published to date describe one patient who was successfully treated with Q-switched ruby laser, six patients who were successfully treated with CO_2 laser, and one patient who was treated successfully with a frequency-doubled Nd:YAG laser. This is insufficient evidence to conclude that either therapy is beneficial for the treatment of cutaneous sarcoidosis. Further RCTs will be necessary in order to evaluate the safety and efficacy of laser therapy in cutaneous sarcoidosis.

UVA1 therapy

Ultraviolet A1 (UVA1, 340–440 nm) has many known immunomodulating and immunosuppressive effects that may be responsible for the therapeutic effect in cutaneous inflammatory diseases, such as atopic dermatitis, urticaria pigmentosa, and lichenoid graft-versus-host disease. Long-wave UVA induces apoptosis in T cells. UVA1 irradiation, similar to ultraviolet B, has been shown to induce the expression of immunosuppressive cytokines in human keratinocytes, including TNF-α and IL-10.[116,117] The immunosuppressive properties of UVA1 form the basis for its use in cutaneous sarcoidosis.

Benefits. Mahnke *et al.* reported the disappearance of nearly all lesions of generalized recalcitrant cutaneous sarcoidosis in an 82-year-old white female after 50 sessions of medium-dose UVA1. Treatment was started at four times per week with medium-dose UVA1 at 20 J/cm^2 for the first three treatment sessions and 40 J/cm^2 for the subsequent 12 sessions. The final dose of 60 J/cm^2 was given 35 times. The patient experienced no adverse effects during or after therapy.[116] Graefe *et al.* reported marked improvement of cutaneous sarcoidosis on the forehead in a 63-year-old white woman after 25 sessions of high-dose UVA1, starting with 20 J/cm² for 2 days, 50 J/cm² for 3 days, 90 J/cm² for 5 days, and finishing with the final dose of 130 J/cm² four times weekly. After 25 sessions, a total dose of 2460 J/cm² was administered. The patient had no adverse effects and did not relapse.[117]

Additionally, Patterson and Fitzwater reported significant improvement of hypopigmented sarcoidosis of the face after 8 months of tri-weekly psoralen ultraviolet A (PUVA) therapy.[118]

Harms. The patients experienced no adverse effects during therapy, but the long-term effects of UVA1, such as the carcinogenic effects of therapy, have to be considered.

Comments/implications for clinical practice. To date, only two patients successfully treated for cutaneous sarcoidosis with UVA1, and one patient successfully treated with PUVA, have been reported in the literature. This is insufficient evidence to recommend UVA1 or PUVA therapy for cutaneous sarcoidosis. RCTs are therefore necessary to evaluate the efficacy and safely of UVA1 and PUVA in cutaneous sarcoidosis.

Photodynamic therapy

Photodynamic therapy (PDT) with aminolevulinic acid (ALA) targets rapidly proliferating cells, leading to cytotoxic and immunomodulatory effects. PDT with topical ALA is currently approved for the treatment of actinic keratoses, but has also been used successfully to treat superficial basal cell carcinoma and Bowen's disease, as well as inflammatory conditions such as verrucae, scleroderma, and psoriasis.[119] The anti-inflammatory and immunomodulatory effects of PDT in skin form the rationale for its use in cutaneous sarcoidosis.

Benefits. Karrer *et al.* reported the only use of PDT in cutaneous sarcoidosis.[119] A 3-month course of PDT with topical ALA produced complete resolution of recalcitrant cutaneous lesions that had persisted for 17 years in a 67-year-old white woman. Topical ALA 3% in a gel containing 40% dimethyl sulfoxide was applied, under occlusion with a light-impenetrant paper, to the affected areas for 6 hours. Subsequently, the lesions were irradiated with an incoherent light source emitting wavelengths of 580–740 nm, with a light intensity of 40 mW/cm² and an energy density of 20 J/cm². PDT was performed twice weekly for the first 8 weeks, followed by treatments once a week, for a total of 22 treatments in 3 months. Four weeks after the onset of therapy, the plaques flattened and faded. After 3 months, the skin lesions resolved completely, without the development of new lesions. A biopsy obtained from a former lesional site 4 months after therapy showed histologically normal skin. The patient was free of skin disease and visceral involvement 18 months after PDT.

Harms. The adverse effects included a slight burning sensation during irradiation, followed by erythema and edema of the treated area, lasting for about 2 days. Slight hyperpigmentation of the treated area occurred after 2 weeks of treatment and persisted for about 3 months after the end of PDT.[119]

Comments/implications for clinical practice. To date, only one patient with cutaneous sarcoidosis has been reported with a positive result to PDT with topical ALA. This is insufficient evidence to conclude that this therapy is beneficial for the treatment of cutaneous sarcoidosis. RCTs will therefore be necessary for definitive proof.

Plastic surgery

Benefits. There are no RCTs or systematic reviews of plastic surgery in the treatment of cutaneous sarcoidosis. In 1970, O'Brien described two patients successfully treated with plastic surgery for lupus pernio.[120] In 1984, Shaw *et al.* described a man with a 6-year history of treatment-resistant lupus pernio successfully treated with surgical excision and split skin grafting; the results remained good 2.5 years after surgery.[121] Collison *et al.* described a man with extensive ulcerative nodules of the lower extremities, which were resistant to topical/intralesional steroids, oral steroids, hydroxychloroquine, and methotrexate. He was treated with vigorous operative debridement and partial-thickness skin grafting. While the grafts were well accepted (80%), the patient developed new ulcerating nodules in previously uninvolved skin 2 months after surgery.[122] Streit *et al.* reported on a woman with widespread ulcerative cutaneous sarcoidosis who was treated with Apligraf (graft skin), a bilayered human skin equivalent, with good results.[123]

Harms. No complications were noted in the above studies. However, the inherent risks of general anesthesia and surgery (bleeding, scarring, postoperative infection) should be considered.

Comments/implications for clinical practice. The above articles describe five patients with treatment-resistant chronic lupus pernio who were treated with plastic surgery, all of whom had a positive result. This is insufficient evidence to conclude that this therapy is beneficial in the treatment of cutaneous sarcoidosis.

Conclusions

There is a lack of significant evidence-based data on topical and physical therapies for cutaneous sarcoidosis. There are no RCTs to prove that intralesional or topical steroids are effective in the treatment of cutaneous sarcoidosis. Intralesional and topical steroids, like oral steroids, have been accepted as first-line therapies on the basis of clinicians' experience, with no definitive dosage or duration of therapy identified. Topical tacrolimus has been reported as a successful therapy in three patients. The physical modalities of laser and plastic surgery, as well as UVA1 and PDT, have been reported as successful in isolated treatment-resistant cases, but larger studies are lacking.

Phonophoresis is another beneficial modality, but it has only been described in an isolated case report.[124]

Key points

- There are no randomized, controlled trials of any therapy for the treatment of cutaneous sarcoidosis.

- In a review of the existing literature on nonsteroidal systemic therapies for cutaneous sarcoidosis, only antimalarials, methotrexate, and thalidomide appear to show clinical benefit, and thus may represent a reasonable therapeutic option in patients requiring an additional or alternative therapy. Other medications, such as biologic anti-TNF-α agents, tetracyclines, and allopurinol, need additional study, but could be used in difficult or resistant cases.

- A review of the existing literature on topical and physical therapies for cutaneous sarcoidosis shows that no therapy can be recommended at present.

References

1 English JC, Patel PJ, Greer KE. Sarcoidosis. *J Am Acad Dermatol* 2001;**44**:725–43.

2 Mana J, Salazar A, Manresa F. Clinical factors predicting persistence of activity in sarcoidosis: a multivariate analysis of 193 cases. *Respiration* 1994;**61**:219–25.

3 Mana J, Marcoval J, Graells J, Salazaar A, Pyri J, Pujol R. Cutaneous involvement in sarcoidosis: relationship to systemic disease. *Arch Dermatol* 1997;**133**:882–8.

4 Newman LS, Rose CS, Maier LA. Sarcoidosis. *N Engl J Med* 1997;**336**:1224–34.

5 Edmonstone WM, Wilson AG. Sarcoidosis in Caucasians, blacks and Asians in London. *Br J Dis Chest* 1985;**79**:27–36.

6 Rybicki BA, Major M, Popovich J, Maliarik MJ, Iannuzzi MC. Racial differences in sarcoidosis incidence: a 5-year study in a health maintenance organization. *Am J Epidemiol* 1997;**145**:234–41.

7 Reich JM, Johnson R. Incidence of clinically identified sarcoidosis in a northwest United States population. *Sarcoid Vasc Diffuse Lung Dis* 1996;**13**:173–7.

8 Rybicki BA, Harrington D, Major M, *et al.* Heterogeneity of familial risk in sarcoidosis. *Genet Epidemiol* 1996;**13**:23–33.

9 Rybicki BA, Maliarik MJ, Major M, Popovich J Jr, Iannuzzi MC. Epidemiology, demographics, and genetics of sarcoidosis. *Semin Respir Infect* 1998;**13**:166–73.

10 Ishihara M, Ohno S. Genetic influences on sarcoidosis. *Eye* 1997;**11**:155–61.

11 Peckham DG, Spiteri MA. Sarcoidosis. *Postgrad Med J* 1996;**72**:196–200.

12 American Thoracic Society. Statement on sarcoidosis. *Am J Respir Care Med* 1999;**160**:736–55.

13 Gideon NM, Mannino DM. Sarcoidosis mortality in the United States 1979–1991: an analysis of multiple cause mortality data. *Am J Med* 1996;**100**:423–7.

14 Russo G, Millikan LE. Cutaneous sarcoidosis: diagnosis and treatment. *Comp Therapy* 1994;**20**:418–21.

15 Wilson NJ, King CM. Cutaneous sarcoidosis. *Postgrad Med J* 1998;**74**:649–52.

16 Pietinalho A, Tukiainen P, Haahtela T, Persson T, Selroos O. Oral prednisolone followed by inhaled budesonide in newly diagnosed pulmonary sarcoidosis: a double-blind, placebo-controlled multicenter study. *Chest* 1999;**116**:424–31.

17 Rizzato G, Riboldi A, Imbimbo B, Torresin A, Milani S. The long-term efficacy and safety of two different corticosteroids in chronic sarcoidosis. *Respir Med* 1997;**91**:449–60.

18 Selroos O, Sellergren TL. Corticosteroid therapy of pulmonary sarcoidosis. A prospective evaluation of alternate day and daily dosage in stage II disease. *Scand J Respir Dis* 1979;**60**:215–21.

19 Eule H, Roth I, Ehrke I, Weinecke W. Cortocosteroid therapy of intrathoracic sarcoidosis stages I and II—results of a controlled clinical trial. *Z Erkr Atmungsorgane* 1977;**149**:142–7.

20 Johns CJ, Zachary JB, Ball WC. A ten year study of corticosteroid treatment of pulmonary sarcoidosis. *Johns Hopkins Med J* 1974;**134**:271–83.

21 Israel HL, Fouts DW, Beggs RA. A controlled trial of prednisone treatment of sarcoidosis. *Am Rev Respir Dis* 1973;**107**:609–14.

22 Sharma OP, Colp C, Williams MH. Course of pulmonary sarcoidosis with and without corticosteroid therapy as determined by pulmonary function studies. *Am J Med* 1966;**41**:541–51.

23 Zaki MH, Lyons HA, Leilop L, Huang CT. Corticosteroid therapy in sarcoidosis: a five year controlled follow-up. *NY State J Med* 1987;**87**:496–9.

24 James DG, Carstairs LS, Trowell J, Sharma OP. Treatment of sarcoidosis: report of a controlled therapeutic trial. *Lancet* 1967;**ii**:526–8.

25 Sharma OP. Cutaneous sarcoidosis: clinical features and management. *Chest* 1972;**61**:320–5.

26 Johns CJ, Michele TM. The clinical management of sarcoidosis: a 50-year experience at the Johns Hopkins Hospital. *Medicine* 1999;**78**:65–111.

27 Verdegem TD, Sharma OP. Cutaneous ulcers in sarcoidosis. *Arch Dermatol* 1987;**123**:1531–4.

28 Baughman RP, Sharma OP, Lynch JP 3rd. Sarcoidosis: is therapy effective? *Semin Respir Infect* 1998;**13**:255–73.

29 Zic JA, Horowitz DH, Arzubiaga C, King LE. Treatment of cutaneous sarcoidosis with chloroquine: review of the literature. *Arch Dermatol* 1991;**127**:1034–40.

30 Veien NK. Cutaneous sarcoidosis: prognosis and treatment. *Clin Dermatol* 1986;**4**:75–87.

31 Morse SI, Cohn ZA, Hirsch JG, Sheadler RW. The treatment of sarcoidosis with chloroquine. *Am J Med* 1961;**30**:779–84.

32 Hirsch JG. Experimental treatment with chloroquine. *Am Rev Respir Dis* 1961;**2**:947–8.

33 Siltzbach LE, Teirstein AS. Chloroquine therapy in 43 patients with intrathoracic and cutaneous sarcoidosis. *Acta Med Scand* 1964;**176**:302–8.

34 Brodthagen H. Hydroxychloroquine in the treatment of sarcoidosis. In: Turiaf J, Chabot J, eds. *La Sarcoidose: Rapports de la IV Conference International.* Paris: Masson, 1967: 764–7.

35 Johns CJ, Schonfeld SA, Scott PP, Zachary JB, MacGregor MI. Longitudinal study of chronic sarcoidosis with low-dose maintenance corticosteroid therapy: outcome and complications. *Ann N Y Acad Sci* 1986;**465**:702–12.

36 Jones E, Callen JP. Hydroxychloroquine is effective therapy for control of cutaneous sarcoidal granulomas. *J Am Acad Dermatol* 1990;**23**:487–9.

37 Baughman RP, Lower EE. Alternatives to corticosteroids in the treatment of sarcoidosis. *Sarcoid Vas Diffuse Lung Dis* 1997;**14**:121–30.

38 Baughman RP, Lower EE. Steroid sparing alternative treatments for sarcoidosis. *Clin Chest Med* 1997;**18**:853–64.

39 Millard TP, Smith HR, Black MM, Barker JN. Bullous pemphigoid developing during systemic therapy with chloroquine. *Clin Exp Dermatol* 1999;**24**:263–5.

40 Baughman RP, Winget DB, Lower EE. Methotrexate is steroid sparing in acute sarcoidosis. Results of a double blind, randomized trial. *Sarcoid Vas Diff Lung Dis* 2000;**17**:60–6.

41 Veien NK, Brodthagen H. Treatment of sarcoid with methotrexate. *Br J Dermatol* 1977;**97**:213–6.

42 Lower EE, Baughman RP. Prolonged use of methotrexate for sarcoidosis. *Arch Intern Med* 1995;**155**:846–51.

43 Kaye O, Palazzo E, Grossin M, Bourgeois P, Kahn MF, Malaise MG. Low-dose methotrexate: an effective corticosteroid-sparing agent in the musculoskeletal manifestations of sarcoidosis. *Br J Rheum* 1995;**34**:632–44.

44 Gedalia A, Molina JF, Ellis GS, Galen W, Moore C, Espinoza LR. Low-dose methotrexate therapy for childhood sarcoidosis. *J Pediatr* 1997;**130**:25–9.

45 Lacher MJ. Spontaneous remission or response to methotrexate in sarcoidosis. *Ann Intern Med* 1968;**69**:1247–8.

46 Webster GF, Razsi LK, Sanchez M, Shupack JL. Weekly low-dose methotrexate therapy for cutaneous sarcoidosis. *J Am Acad Dermatol* 1991;**24**:451–4.

47 Henderson CA, Ilchyshyn A, Curry AR. Laryngeal and cutaneous sarcoidosis treated with methotrexate. *J R Soc Med* 1994;**87**:632–3.

48 Gary A, Modeste AB, Richard C, *et al.* Methotrexate for the treatment of patients with chronic cutaneous sarcoidosis: 4 cases. *Ann Dermatol Venereol* 2005;**132**(8–9 Pt 1):659–62.

49 Albertini JG, Tyler W, Miller F. Ulcerative sarcoidosis: case report and review of the literature. *Arch Dermatol* 1997;**133**:215–9.

50 Carlesimo M, Giustini S, Rossi A, Bonaccorsi P, Calvieri S. Treatment of cutaneous and pulmonary sarcoidosis with thalidomide. *J Am Acad Dermatol* 1995;**32**:866–9.

51 Rousseau L, Beylot-Barry M, Doutre MS, Beylot C. Cutaneous sarcoidosis successfully treated with low doses of thalidomide. *Arch Dermatol* 1998;**134**:1045–6.

52 Wu JJ, Huang DB, Pang KR, Hsu S, Tyring SK. Thalidomide: dermatological indications, mechanisms of action and side-effects. *Br J Dermatol* 2005;**153**:254–73.

53 Estines O, Revuz J, Wolkenstein P, Bressieux JM, Roujeau JC, Cosnes A. Sarcoidosis: thalidomide treatment in ten patients. *Ann Dermatol Venereol* 2001;**128**:611–3.

54 Baughman RP, Judson MA, Teirstein AS, Moller DR, Lower EE. Thalidomide for chronic sarcoidosis. *Chest* 2002;**122**:227–32.

55 Nguyen YT, Dupuy A, Cordoliani F, *et al.* Treatment of cutaneous sarcoidosis with thalidomide. *J Am Acad Dermatol* 2004;**50**:235–41.

56 Oliver SJ, Kikuchi T, Krueger JG, Kaplan G. Thalidomide induces granuloma differentiation in sarcoid skin lesions associated with disease improvement. *Clin Immunol* 2002;**102**:225–36.

57 Lee JB, Koblenzer PS. Disfiguring cutaneous manifestation of sarcoidosis treated with thalidomide: a case report. *J Am Acad Dermatol* 1998;**39**:835–8.

58 Hoch O, Muller S, Buttner G, Mensing H. [Thalidomide in the treatment of cutaneous and systemic sarcoidosis; in German.] *Hautarzt* 2001;**52**:962–5.

59 Walter MC, Lochmuller H, Schlotter-Weigel B, Meindl T, Muller-Felber W. Successful treatment of muscle sarcoidosis with thalidomide. *Acta Myol* 2003;**22**:22–5.

60 Baughman RP, Lower EE. Newer therapies for cutaneous sarcoidosis: the role of thalidomide and other agents. *Am J Clin Dermatol* 2004;**5**:385–94.

61 Bachelez H, Senet P, Cadranel J, Kaoukhov A, Dubertret L. The use of tetracyclines for the treatment of sarcoidosis. *Arch Dermatol* 2001;**137**:69–73.

62 Antonovich DD, Callen JP. Development of sarcoidosis in cosmetic tattoos. *Arch Dermatol* 2005;**141**:869–72.

63 Samuel M, Allen GE, McMillan SC, Burrows D, Corbett JR, Beare JM. Sarcoidosis: initial results on six patients treated with allopurinol. *Br J Dermatol* 1984;**111**(Suppl 26):20.

64 Bregnhoej A, Jemec GB. Low-dose allopurinol in the treatment of cutaneous sarcoidosis: response in four of seven patients. *J Dermatolog Treat.* 2005;**16**:125–7.

65 Pfau A, Stolz W, Karrer S, Szeimies RM, Landthaler M. Allopurinol in treatment of cutaneous sarcoidosis. *Hautarzt* 1998;**49**:216–8.

66 Rosof BM. Allopurinol for sarcoid? [letter]. *N Engl J Med* 1976;**294**:447.

67 Pollock JL. Sarcoidosis responding to allopurinol. *Arch Dermatol* 1980;**116**:273–4.

68 Brechtel B, Haas N, Henz BM, Kolde G. Allopurinol: a therapeutic alternative for disseminated cutaneous sarcoidosis. *Br J Dermatol* 1996;**135**:307–9.

69 Antony F, Layton AM. A case of cutaneous acral sarcoidosis with response to allopurinol. *Br J Dermatol* 2000;**142**:1052–3.

70 Voelter-Mahlknecht S, Benez A, Metzger S, Fierlbeck G. Treatment of subcutaneous sarcoidosis with allopurinol. *Arch Dermatol* 1999;**135**:1560–1.

71 Georgiou S, Monastirli A, Pasmatzi E, Tsamboas D. Cutaneous sarcoidosis: complete remission after oral isotretinoin therapy. *Acta Dermatol Venereol* 1998;**78**:457–8.

72 Waldinger TP, Ellis CN, Quint K, Voorhees JJ. Treatment of cutaneous sarcoidosis with isotretinoin. *Arch Dermatol* 1983;**119**:1003–5.

73 Spiteri MA, Taylor SJ. Retinoids in the treatment of cutaneous sarcoidosis [letter]. *Arch Dermatol* 1985;**121**:1486.

74 Vaillant L, Le Marchand D, Bertrand S, Grangeponte MC, Lorette G. Sarcoidose cutanée annulaire du front: traitement par isotrétinoine. *Ann Dermatol Venereol* 1986;**113**:1089–92.

75 Mosam A, Morar N. Recalcitrant cutaneous sarcoidosis: an evidence-based sequential approach. *J Dermatolog Treat* 2004;**15**:353–9.

76 Hoxtermann S, Nuchel C, Altmeyer P. Fumaric acid esters suppress peripheral CD4- and CD8-positive lymphocytes in psoriasis. *Dermatology* 1998;**196**:223–30.

77 Breuer K, Gutzmer R, Volker B, Kapp A, Werfel T. Therapy of noninfectious granulomatous skin diseases with fumaric acid esters. *Br J Dermatol* 2005;**152**:1290–5.

78 Gutzmer R, Kapp A, Werfel T. [Successful treatment of skin and lung sarcoidosis with fumaric acid ester; in German.] *Hautarzt* 2004;**55**:553–7.

79 Nowack U, Gambichler T, Hanefeld C, Kastner U, Altmeyer P. Successful treatment of recalcitrant cutaneous sarcoidosis with fumaric acid esters. *BMC Dermatol* 2002;**2**:15.

80 Dummler U, Rinke M, Sabel R, Gollnick H. Sarkoidose mit kutaner dissemination: Zwei unter fumarsauretherapie. *Allergologie* 1998;**8**:387 [abstract].

81 Hoefnagel JJ, Thio HB, Willemze R, Bouwes Bavinck JN. Long-term safety aspects of systemic therapy with fumaric acid esters in severe psoriasis. *Br J Dermatol* 2003;**149**:363–9.

82 Haley H, Cantrell W, Smith K. Infliximab therapy for sarcoidosis (lupus pernio). *Br J Dermatol* 2004;**150**:146–9.

83 Mallbris L, Ljungberg A, Hedblad MA, Larsson P, Stahle-Backdahl M. Progressive cutaneous sarcoidosis responding to anti-tumor necrosis factor-alpha therapy. *J Am Acad Dermatol* 2003;**48**:290–3.

84 Doty JD, Mazur JE, Judson MA. Treatment of sarcoidosis with infliximab. *Chest* 2005;**127**:1064–71.

85 Heffernan MP, Anadkat MJ. Recalcitrant cutaneous sarcoidosis responding to infliximab. *Arch Dermatol* 2005;**141**:910–1.

86 Baughman RP, Lower EE. Infliximab for refractory sarcoidosis. *Sarcoidosis Vasc Diffuse Lung Dis* 2001;**18**:70–4.

87 Meyerle JH, Shorr A. The use of infliximab in cutaneous sarcoidosis. *J Drugs Dermatol* 2003;**2**:413–4.

88 Pritchard C, Nadarajah K. Tumour necrosis factor alpha inhibitor treatment for sarcoidosis refractory to conventional treatments: a report of five patients. *Ann Rheum Dis* 2004;**63**:318–20.

89 Philips MA, Lynch J, Azmi FH. Ulcerative cutaneous sarcoidosis responding to adalimumab. *J Am Acad Dermatol* 2005;**53**:917.

90 Heffernan MP, Smith DI. Adalimumab for treatment of cutaneous sarcoidosis. *Arch Dermatol* 2006;**142**:17–9.

91 Khanna D, Liebling MR, Louie JS. Etanercept ameliorates sarcoidosis arthritis and skin disease. *J Rheumatol* 2003;**30**:1864–7.

92 Imperato AK, Bingham CO 3rd, Abramson SB. Overview of benefit/risk of biological agents. *Clin Exp Rheumatol.* 2004;**22** (5 Suppl 35):S108–14.

93 Yamada H, Ide AA, Suigiura M. Treatment of cutaneous sarcoidosis with tranilast. *J Dermatol* 1995;**22**:149–52.

94 Cagnoni ML, Lombardi A, Cerinic MM, *et al.* Melatonin for treatment of chronic refractory sarcoidosis. *Lancet* 1995;**346**:1229–30.

95 Schwarzenbach R, Djawari D. Disseminated small-node cutaneous sarcoidosis. *Dtsch Med Wochenschr* 2000;**125**:560–2.

96 Hughes JR, Pembroke AC. Cutaneous sarcoidosis treated with mepacrine. *Clin Exp Dermatol* 1994;**19**:448.

97 Veien NK. Cutaneous sarcoidosis treated with levamisole. *Dermatologica* 1977;**154**:185–9.

98 Khatri KA, Chotzen VA, Burrall BA. Lupus pernio: successful treatment with a potent topical corticosteroid. *Arch Dermatol* 1995;**131**:617–8.

99 Volden G. Successful treatment of chronic skin diseases with clobetasol propionate and a hydrocolloid occlusive dressing. *Acta Derm Venereol* 1992;**72**:69–71.

100 Sullivan RD, Mayock RL, Jones R. Local injection of hydrocortisone and cortisone into skin lesions of sarcoidosis. *J Am Med Assoc* 1953;**152**:308–12.

101 Verbov J. The place of intralesional steroid therapy in dermatology. *Br J Dermatol* 1976;**94**(Suppl 12):51–8.

102 Katoh N, Mihara H, Yasuno H. Cutaneous sarcoidosis successfully treated with topical tacrolimus. *Br J Dermatol* 2002;**147**:154–6.

103 Gutzmer R, Volker B, Kapp A, Werfel T. [Successful topical treatment of cutaneous sarcoidosis with tacrolimus; in German.] *Hautarzt* 2003;**54**:1193–7.

104 Landers MC, Skokan M, Law S, Storrs FJ. Cutaneous and pulmonary sarcoidosis in association with tattoos. *Cutis* 2005;**75**:44–8.

105 Beck LA. The efficacy and safety of tacrolimus ointment: a clinical review. *J Am Acad Dermatol* 2005;**53**(2 Suppl 2):S165–70.

106 Hultsch T, Kapp A, Spergel J. Immunomodulation and safety of topical calcineurin inhibitors for the treatment of atopic dermatitis. *Dermatology* 2005;**211**:174–87.

107 Goodman MM, Alpern K. Treatment of lupus pernio with the flashlamp pulsed dye laser. *Lasers Surg Med* 1992;**12**:549–51.

108 Cliff S, Felix RH, Singh L, Harland CC. The successful treatment of lupus pernio with the flashlamp pulsed dye laser. *J Cutan Laser Ther* 1999;**1**:49–52.

109 Dosik JS, Ashinoff R. Treating lupus pernio with the 585 nm pulsed dye laser. *Skin Aging* 1999;**7**:93–4.

110 Green JJ, Lawrence N, Heymann WR. Generalized ulcerative sarcoidosis induced by therapy with the flashlamp-pumped pulsed dye laser. *Arch Dermatol* 2001;**137**:507–8.

111 Grema H, Greve B, Raulin C. Scar sarcoidosis—treatment with the Q-switched ruby laser. *Lasers Surg Med* 2002;**30**:398–400.

112 O'Donoghue NB, Barlow RJ. Laser remodelling of nodular nasal lupus pernio. *Clin Exp Dermatol* 2006;**31**:27–9.

113 Stack BC Jr, Hall PJ, Goodman AL, Perez IR. CO_2 laser excision of lupus pernio of the face. *Am J Otolaryngol* 1996;**17**:260–3.

114 Young HS, Chalmers RJ, Griffiths CE, August PJ. CO_2 laser vaporization for disfiguring lupus pernio. *J Cosmet Laser Ther* 2002;**4**:87–90.

115 Ekback M, Molin L. Effective laser treatment in a case of lupus pernio. *Acta Derm Venereol* 2005;**85**:521–2.

116 Mahnke N, Medve-Koenigs K, Berneburg M, Ruzicka T, Neumann NJ. Cutaneous sarcoidosis treated with medium-dose UVA1. *J Am Acad Dermatol* 2004;**50**:978–9.

117 Graefe T, Konrad H, Barta U, Wollina U, Elsner P. Successful ultraviolet A1 treatment of cutaneous sarcoidosis. *Br J Dermatol* 2001;**145**:354–5.

118 Patterson JW, Fitzwater JE. Treatment of hypopigmented sarcoidosis with 8-methoxypsoralen and long wave ultraviolet light. *Int J Dermatol* 1982;**21**:476–80.

119 Karrer S, Abels C, Wimmershoff MB, Landthaler M, Szeimies RM. Successful treatment of cutaneous sarcoidosis using topical photodynamic therapy. *Arch Dermatol* 2002;**138**:581–4.

120 O'Brien P. Sarcoidosis of the nose. *Br J Plast Surg* 1970;**23**:242–7.

121 Shaw M, Black MM, Davis PKB. Disfiguring lupus pernio successfully treated with plastic surgery. *Clin Exp Dermatol* 1984;**9**:614–7.

122 Collison DW, Novice F, Banse L, Rodman OG, Kelly AP. Split thickness skin grafting in extensive ulcerative sarcoidosis. *J Dermatol Surg Oncol* 1989;**15**:679–83.

123 Streit M, Bohlen LM, Braathen LR. Ulcerative sarcoidosis successfully treated with Apligraf. *Dermatology* 2001;**202**:367–70.

124 Gogstetter DS, Goldsmith LA. Treatment of cutaneous sarcoidosis using phonophoresis. *J Am Acad Dermatol* 1999;**40**:797–9.

60

Erythema multiforme

Pierre-Dominique Ghislain, Jean-Claude Roujeau

Background

Definition

Erythema multiforme (EM) is an acute, self-limited, feverish eruption characterized by target cutaneous lesions, with a symmetric and mainly acral distribution (Figures 60.1, 60.2). The lesions are rounded, with three zones:
- A central area of dusky erythema or purpura, sometimes bullous
- A middle, paler zone of edema
- An outer ring of erythema with a well-defined edge

The hands and feet are the areas usually most affected and are sometimes selectively involved. Mucous membrane erosions are frequent and are characteristic of erythema multiforme major, in contrast to erythema multiforme minor, in which the mucous membranes are not involved. Histopathological examination shows a predominantly inflammatory pattern characterized by a lichenoid infiltrate and limited epidermal necrosis, which mainly affects the basal layer.

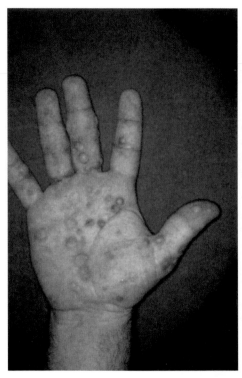

Figure 60.2 Typical targets with central blisters.

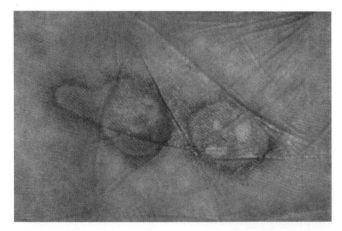

Figure 60.1 Acral lesions (palm).

Incidence/prevalence

Unknown.

Etiology/risk factors

The principal cause is infection with herpes simplex virus (HSV), which probably explains 40–70% of cases. Many other infections can induce occasional cases, especially *Mycoplasma pneumoniae* infection. According to a recent classification, EM-like drug eruption is related to Stevens–Johnson syndrome (see Chapter 61); the clinical signs are quite different.

Prognosis

EM has a low morbidity rate and no mortality. Spontaneous resolution follows in 1–6 weeks. Ocular sequelae may also occur. Recurrences are frequent. Rarely, the recurrences overlap, leading to "continuous" or "persistent" EM. Oral erosions may strongly impair the patients' quality of life.

Aims

To reduce the duration of fever, eruption, and hospitalization; and to prevent or reduce recurrences.

Outcomes

Duration of fever, eruption and hospitalization; frequency of recurrences; number of days with symptoms per year.

Methods

Clinical evidence was searched for and appraised in April 2006 (Cochrane databases with randomized controlled trials and controlled clinical trials, Medline 1966 to April 2006).

Questions

What are the effects of treatment for acute attacks?

Short course of systemic corticosteroids

On the basis of retrospective series and small randomized controlled trials (RCTs), corticosteroids appear to shorten the duration of fever and eruption, but they increase hospitalization periods due to the risk of complications.

Benefits

Sixteen children with erythema multiforme major were included in a randomized controlled prospective study within 3 days of the onset of rash; 10 received bolus infusions of methylprednisolone (4 mg/kg/day), while six only received supportive treatment. Corticosteroids led to a reduction in the period of fever (4.0 vs. 9.5 days), a reduction in the period of acute eruption (7.0 vs. 9.8 days), and milder signs of prostration. Complications were minimal in both groups. The authors suggest that an early and short course of corticosteroids has a favorable influence on the course of erythema multiforme major in children.[1]

Harms

An RCT included nine adult patients with mild, uncomplicated EM major; four received prednisolone and five received placebo. The mean length of the hospital stay was longer in the corticosteroid group (9.5 vs. 8 days). However,

the diagnoses were not clear: histology was consistent with EM; a drug was suspected in five cases; and no information about HSV was given.[2]

In a retrospective study, Rasmussen compared 17 children with EM who were treated with systemic corticosteroids with 15 children who only received supportive care. The two groups were comparable in age, sex, the length of the prodromal period, exposure to drugs, initial fever, extent of oral and cutaneous involvement, and frequency of isolation of pathogens. The group with corticosteroids had a shorter fever period (1.8 vs. 5.5 days) but a longer mean hospitalization period (21 vs. 13 days), as complications were more frequent (53% vs. 0%).[3]

In a series of 51 children, it was claimed that corticosteroids worsened the prognosis: patients treated with corticosteroids had a 74% complication rate, compared with 28% in patients without corticosteroids.[4]

In a series of 25 patients with erythema multiforme minor, corticosteroids did not lead to any clinical improvement except for a shorter duration of fever (2.7 vs. 5.6 days).[5]

Comments

Corticosteroids appear to be of little use, and side effects are frequent. However, the methodology in most of the studies is poor, with small numbers of patients and often with a mixture of idiopathic or viral-associated EM and drug-induced Stevens–Johnson syndrome.

Erythromycin

We found no evidence of the usefulness of erythromycin.

Benefits

No evidence was found.

Harms

No evidence was found.

Comment

Erythromycin is claimed to be useful only when *M. pneumoniae* infection is suspected.

Acyclovir

There are no RCTs, but several series in which it is stated that initiating acyclovir in the treatment of full-blown post herpetic EM was useless.

Benefits

No evidence was found.

Harms

No evidence was found.

Comment

Probably useless.

What are the effects of treatment to prevent recurrences?

Sun protection
No evidence was found regarding the effects of sun protection.

Benefits
Ultraviolet light may induce herpes recurrence. No good evidence was found regarding the effects of sun protection on the recurrence of EM.

Harms
By contrast, it has been suggested that psoralen ultraviolet A (PUVA) can be used in the treatment of persistent EM. We found no good evidence regarding the effectiveness of this.

Comment
The effects of ultraviolet are not clear.

Acyclovir
We found one RCT reporting that continuous oral acyclovir treatment is effective in preventing EM recurrences. Another RCT stated that topical acyclovir is not effective.

Benefits
One RCT was found, in which 19 patients with more than four attacks of EM per year were enrolled in a 6-month double-blind, placebo-controlled trial of acyclovir 400 mg twice daily. The median number of attacks in the acyclovir group was zero (range none to two), compared with three (one to six) in the placebo group (significantly different). At the time of inclusion, five patients had no clinical evidence of disease precipitation by HSV, two of whom were in the acyclovir group; one showed complete disease suppression.[6]

Another RCT reported that topical acyclovir therapy used in a prophylactic manner is not successful in preventing recurrent herpes-associated EM.[7]

Harms
No evidence was found.

Comment
Continuous oral acyclovir is effective in preventing recurrences of herpes-associated EM, but it may also be useful for patients in whom there is no clinical evidence that herpes is the precipitating factor.

Dapsone
We found no evidence on the effects of dapsone.

Benefits
We found no sufficient evidence.

Harms
No evidence was found.

Antimalarials
No evidence was found.

Benefits
No evidence was found.

Harms
No evidence was found.

Azathioprine
We found one small series reporting that azathioprine is beneficial.

Benefits
We did not find any controlled trials. In a series of 65 patients with recurrent EM, 11 were treated with azathioprine when all other treatments had failed. Azathioprine was successfully used in all 11 patients.[8] Another series reported five cases.[9]

Harms
No evidence was found.

Comment
Further trials are needed.

Ciclosporin
We found no good evidence.

Benefits
We found no sufficient evidence.

Harms
No evidence was found.

Thalidomide
We found one series reporting that thalidomide is beneficial in EM.

Benefits
We found one retrospective analysis of thalidomide prescription (1981–1993), which reported good efficacy in the treatment of recurrent or proleptic EM.[10] However, these data were uncontrolled and have not been confirmed.

Harms
No evidence was found.

Comment
No clinical evidence is available.

Potassium iodide

We found insufficient evidence regarding the value of potassium iodide.

Benefits

In a retrospective study, potassium iodide was used for 16 patients with EM (300 mg three times daily). Complete remission was noted in 14 patients, including those with concomitant herpes simplex.[11]

Harms

No evidence was found.

Comment

To date, no conclusions are possible.

Levamisole

In one RCT, levamisole appeared to be useful.

Benefits

We found a double-blind, placebo-controlled cross-over trial, which included 14 patients with chronic or recurrent EM resistant to corticosteroid therapy. The dose of levamisole was 150 mg/day for three consecutive days each week, for at least 4 weeks after the first appearance of a lesion. Levamisole led to a decrease in the severity, duration, and frequency of EM attacks.[12]

An open comparative trial showed that levamisole was similarly effective when used alone (17 patients; 76% with a complete response) in comparison with a combination of prednisone and levamisole (22 patients; 82% with a complete response).[13]

Harms

As agranulocytosis is a severe and not exceptional adverse effect, levamisole is not available in many countries.

Comment

The risk–benefit ratio is probably too low to support the use of levamisole in patients with EM.

Cimetidine

We did not find sufficient evidence.

Benefits

No evidence was found.

Harms

No evidence was found.

Comment

No clinical evidence is available.

Immunoglobulin

No evidence was found.

Benefits

No evidence was found.

Harms

No evidence was found.

Comment

No clinical evidence is available.

Summary

Systemic acyclovir appears to be beneficial in preventing recurrences. With corticosteroids and levamisole, there is a trade-off between benefits and harms.

The effectiveness of the following treatments is unknown: erythromycin, dapsone, antimalarials, azathioprine, ciclosporin, thalidomide, potassium iodide, cimetidine, and immunoglobulins.

Key points

- We found one RCT showing that acyclovir is useful in preventing recurrences of EM.
- We found some, but controversial, evidence of the effectiveness of corticosteroids in treating acute attacks of EM. Early administration reduces the duration of fever, but may have many side effects.
- We found no good evidence regarding any of the other therapeutic choices.

References

1 Kakourou T, Klontza D, Soteropoulou F, Kattamis C. Corticosteroid treatment of erythema multiforme major (Stevens–Johnson syndrome) in children. *Eur J Pediatr* 1997;**156**:90–3.

2 Wright S. The treatment of erythema multiforme major with systemic corticosteroids. *Br J Dermatol* 1991;**124**:612–3.

3 Rasmussen JE. Erythema multiforme in children: response to treatment with systemic corticosteroids. *Br J Dermatol* 1976;**95**:181–6.

4 Ginsburg CM. Stevens–Johnson syndrome in children. *Pediatr Infect Dis* 1982;**1**:155–8.

5 Ting HC, Adam BA. Erythema multiforme: response to corticosteroid. *Dermatologica* 1984;**169**:175–8.

6 Tatnall FM, Schofield JK, Leigh IM. A double-blind, placebo-controlled trial of continuous acyclovir therapy in recurrent erythema multiforme. *Br J Dermatol* 1995;**132**:267–70.

7 Fawcett HA, Wansbrough-Jones MH, Clark AE, Leigh IM. Prophylactic topical acyclovir for frequent recurrent herpes simplex infection with and without erythema multiforme. *Br Med J (Clin Res Ed)* 1983;**287**:798–9.

8 Schofield JK, Tatnall FM, Leigh IM. Recurrent erythema multiforme: clinical features and treatment in a large series of patients. *Br J Dermatol* 1993;**128**:542–5.

9 Farthing PM, Maragou P, Coates M, Tatnall F, Leigh IM, Williams DM. Characteristics of the oral lesions in patients with cutaneous recurrent erythema multiforme. *J Oral Pathol Med* 1995;**24**:9–13.

10 Cherouati K, Claudy A, Souteyrand P, *et al.* Traitement par thalidomide de l'érythème polymorphe chronique (formes récidivantes et subintrantes). Etude rétrospective de 26 malades. *Ann Dermatol Venereol* 1996;**123**:375–7.

11 Horio T, Danno K, Okamoto H, Miyachi Y, Imamura S. Potassium iodide in erythema nodosum and other erythematous dermatoses. *J Am Acad Dermatol* 1983;**9**:77–81.

12 Lozada F. Levamisole in the treatment of erythema multiforme: a double-blind trial in fourteen patients. *Oral Surg Oral Med Oral Pathol* 1982;**53**:28–31.

13 Lozada-Nur F, Cram D, Gorsky M. Clinical response to levamisole in thirty-nine patients with erythema multiforme: an open prospective study. *Oral Surg Oral Med Oral Pathol* 1992;**74**:294–8.

61

Stevens–Johnson syndrome and toxic epidermal necrolysis

Pierre-Dominique Ghislain, Jean-Claude Roujeau

Background

Definition

Stevens–Johnson syndrome (SJS) and toxic epidermal necrolysis (TEN) are variants of the same process, presenting as severe mucosal erosions with widespread purpuric cutaneous macules (atypical targets), often confluent, with a positive Nikolsky sign and epidermal detachment (Figure 61.1). In SJS, epidermal detachment involves less than 10% of the total body skin area; transitional SJS/TEN is defined by epidermal detachment of between 10% and 30% and TEN by detachment greater than 30%. Full-thickness epidermal necrosis is observed on pathological examination.

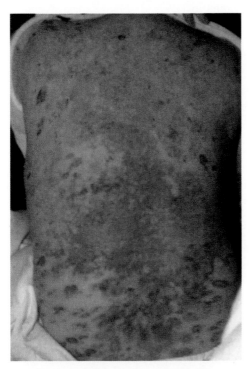

Figure 61.1 A patient with Stevens–Johnson syndrome.

Incidence/prevalence

On the basis of case registries and observational studies, the incidence of TEN is estimated at 1–1.4 cases per million inhabitants per year. The incidence of SJS is probably of the same order (one to three cases per million inhabitants per year).[1–3]

Etiology/risk factors

SJS/TEN is essentially drug-induced (70–90% of cases). Graft-versus-host disease is another well-established etiology, independent of drugs. A few cases are related to infections (*Mycoplasma pneumoniae*); other cases remain unexplained ("idiopathic" forms). The most extensive study of medication use and SJS/TEN mainly implicated anti-infectious sulfonamides, anticonvulsant agents, some nonsteroidal anti-inflammatory drugs, and allopurinol.[4] Human immunodeficiency virus (HIV) infection dramatically increases the risk. A predisposing effect of autoimmune disorders, such as lupus, and HLA-linked genetic susceptibility have been also suggested.

Prognosis

SJS/TEN is an acute disease with high morbidity and mortality rates. The mortality rates are 10% with SJS, 30–40% with TEN, and 10–15% with transitional forms. Epidermal detachment may be extensive. As in severe burns, fluid losses are massive, with electrolyte imbalance. Superinfection, thermoregulation impairment, energy expenditure, alteration of immunologic functions and hematologic abnormalities are usual systemic complications. Mucous membrane involvement (oropharynx, eyes, genitalia, and anus) requires attentive nursing. Gastrointestinal and tracheobronchial epithelium can be involved and can cause severe morbidity.

Age, the percentage of denuded skin, neutropenia, the serum urea nitrogen level, and visceral involvement are prognostic factors. Several scoring systems for predicting the prognosis, such as the Simplified Acute Physiology Score (SAPS and SAPS II) have been proposed, but these have not been validated. The SCORTEN was developed and validated in a single center as a TEN-specific severity-of-illness score.

After healing, scars, pigmentation disorders, ocular lesions, and Sjögren-like syndrome are the principal long-term complications.

Aims

- To reduce the mortality rate
- To block the extent of the disease
- To reduce associated morbidity
- To prevent sequelae

Outcomes

- Mortality rate
- Percentage of epidermal detachment at the peak of the disease
- Infectious complications
- Length of healing
- Length of stay in hospital
- Ocular sequelae

Methods

Clinical evidence was searched for and appraised in April 2006; we used the Cochrane databases for randomized controlled trials (RCTs) and controlled clinical trials (CCTs) and Medline from 1966 to April 2006. No systematic reviews and only one placebo-controlled trial were found. We have therefore also included observational studies and open trials.

Questions

What are the effects of specific treatments?

Prompt withdrawal of all potential culprit drugs
We found limited evidence that early withdrawal of the drug or drugs that cause SJS/TEN alters the clinical course of the disease.

Benefits
We found one observational study reporting that death rates were lower when causative drugs with short elimination half-lives were withdrawn no later than the day on which blisters or erosions first occurred: 2/44 (5%) vs. 11/42 (26%). No differences were observed for drugs with long half-lives.[5]

Harms
We found no controlled data.

Comment
As it would be unethical to carry out an RCT on the effects of prolonging drug administration, observational studies will probably remain the only available clinical evidence for this question.

Corticosteroids
We found no good evidence regarding the use of corticosteroids in patients with SJS/TEN. Beneficial effects are doubtful and may be accompanied by side effects.

Benefits
Only uncontrolled series were identified. A series of 14 patients with skin detachment of 45–100% were treated with high doses of corticosteroids (400 mg prednisone/day in six patients and 200 mg/day in eight, gradually reduced over a 4–6-week period); only one death was observed.[6]

A series of 67 patients with SJS/TEN who were treated with corticosteroids (from prednisolone 40 mg to methylprednisolone 750 mg) reported an excellent survival rate and minor side effects. However, the diagnoses were not clear; only some of the patients had mucous involvement.[7–11]

In a small retrospective study of 14 patients, no differences in the mortality rates or infectious complications were noted in patients who had received steroids before referral.[12] In a retrospective analysis of 39 patients with TEN, steroid treatment was not significantly related to the mortality rate.[13]

Harms
We found poor evidence that the use of corticosteroids is detrimental. It has been suggested that corticosteroids lead to prolonged wound healing, an increased risk of infection, masking of early signs of sepsis, severe gastrointestinal bleeding, and increased mortality.

Thirty patients with SJS or TEN were included in an uncontrolled prospective study. The first 15 patients received corticosteroids and had a mortality rate of 66%. The next 15 patients were therefore treated without corticosteroids; the mortality rate was 33%. The two groups were similar in other respects. However, 11 of the 15 patients without corticosteroids had taken corticosteroids before referral. Thus, no conclusions can be drawn regarding exclusive early administration of corticosteroids.[14]

In a retrospective study, a multivariate analysis of prognostic factors showed that corticosteroid therapy is an independent factor for increased mortality.[15] Other series appear to support the same conclusion.[16] Moreover, many cases of TEN have occurred during treatment with high doses of corticosteroids for preexistent disease. The data for 216 patients with TEN were investigated in a retrospective study; 11 of the patients had been treated with corticosteroids for at least 1 week before the first sign of TEN (from 1 week to several months, at dosages of between 7.5 and 325 mg prednisolone/day).[17] In another series including 179 patients, 13 had been undergoing long-term glucocorticosteroid therapy before developing TEN. In comparison with 166 other patients, these patients had a longer delay between the introduction of the suspect drug and the onset of TEN, and a longer time elapsed between the first symptom of TEN and hospital admission. No other differences were observed.[18]

Comment

The results of many studies are difficult to analyze because drug-induced SJS and erythema multiforme cases are mixed in some series.

These uncontrolled data provide no evidence regarding the potential benefit of corticosteroids early in the disease. Prolonged use of corticosteroids can be harmful.

Intravenous immunoglobulin

We found no good evidence regarding the effects of intravenous immunoglobulin (IVIG) in patients with TEN.

Benefits

We found several uncontrolled clinical trials. The first was based on an *in vitro* demonstration that intravenous immunoglobulins can inhibit Fas-Fas ligand-mediated apoptosis. Ten consecutive patients with TEN of moderate severity were treated with different doses of IVIG (0.2–0.75 g/kg body weight per day for four consecutive days); all survived.[19]

Case reports and multicenter retrospective series have also suggested a positive effect.[20]

In one prospective noncomparative study with 2 g/kg IVIG within 2 days, no beneficial effects on mortality or progression were seen.[21]

In two series from burn units, IVIG was not judged to provide any benefit in comparison with "historical controls."[22,23]

In one retrospective study, no reduction in ocular complications was seen in 10 consecutive TEN patients in comparison with historical controls; the IVIG dosage was 2 g/kg body weight over 2 days.[24]

Harms

We found only case reports and a few series. An expert consensus emphasizes that there is an increased risk of renal failure, particularly in patients with diabetes mellitus and prior impairment of renal function.[25,26]

Comment

Despite theoretically positive aspects and general enthusiasm, no evidence was found in favor of IVIG, with only case reports and short observational series. The potential severity of SJS/TEN does not justify the absence of well-conceived evidence-based trials.

Plasmapheresis

No good evidence was found regarding plasmapheresis/ plasma exchanges in patients with SJS/TEN.

Benefits

A few retrospective or uncontrolled trials on plasmapheresis were identified, but without any good evidence for a positive effect. One trial used plasmapheresis in combination with IVIG.

Harms

We found one open trial with historical controls in which eight consecutive patients with TEN underwent plasma exchange. This series showed no significant differences with regard to mortality, length of hospital stay, or time to reepithelialization.[27]

Comment

The usefulness of plasmapheresis is unknown and doubtful.

Ciclosporin A

We did not find sufficient evidence regarding the effects of ciclosporin.

Benefits

We found a case series of patients with TEN who were treated with ciclosporin A. The treatment was safe and was associated with a more rapid reepithelialization rate and a lower mortality rate (0/11 vs. 3/6) in comparison with a historical series of patients treated with cyclophosphamide and corticosteroid.[28]

Harms

No evidence was found.

Comment

A controlled trial is needed to evaluate the real effectiveness of ciclosporin.

Cyclophosphamide

We found insufficient evidence regarding the therapeutic effectiveness of cyclophosphamide.

Benefits

We found a few trials that used historical controls. Eight patients with TEN were treated with cyclophosphamide alone (initial dose 300 mg/day); all survived.[29] We also found a few series with concomitant therapy with cyclophosphamide and corticosteroids; these are not interpretable.

Harms

A few cases of cyclophosphamide-induced TEN have been reported, one of which occurred with a positive rechallenge test.

Comment

No conclusions are possible.

N-acetylcysteine (NAC)

NAC increases the clearance of several drugs and their metabolites, and *in vitro* it inhibits the production of tumor necrosis factor-α (TNF-α) and interleukin-1β. We found no evidence of clinical effectiveness in TEN.

Benefits

We found no evidence with regard to SJS or TEN.

Harms

High doses of NAC may inactivate not only the culprit drug but also other drugs that are potentially beneficial for the patient.

A randomized trial has shown that NAC is not effective in preventing hypersensitivity reactions to trimethoprim–sulfamethoxazole in patients with HIV infection.[30]

Comment

The usefulness of NAC is unknown and doubtful.

Other medications

We found no evidence regarding granulocyte colony-stimulating factor, heparin, monoclonal antibodies against cytokines, or pentoxifylline.

Benefits

Only case reports were found.

Harms

No evidence was found.

Comment

No conclusions are possible.

Thalidomide

We found one RCT comparing thalidomide with a placebo, which reported excess mortality with thalidomide.

Benefits

Thalidomide has been proposed for the treatment of TEN because it is a potent inhibitor of TNF-α action. We found no clinical evidence regarding the benefits of thalidomide use in patients with SJS/TEN.

Harms

We found a double-blind, randomized, placebo-controlled study of thalidomide in TEN. The regimen was a 5-day course of thalidomide 400 mg daily. Twenty-two patients were included, but the study was stopped because there was an unexplained excess of mortality in the thalidomide group (10 of 12 patients died in comparison with three of 10 in the placebo group). There were no significant differences between the two groups in the causes of death.[31]

Comment

On the basis of a unique but randomized controlled trial, thalidomide appears to be detrimental in TEN.

What are the effects of symptomatic treatments?

Early referral to specialized medical units

We found several retrospective studies reporting a lower risk of infection and a lower mortality if patients are referred to a specialized unit at an early stage.

Benefits

Three retrospective studies pointed out the effects of prompt referral. In the first study, patients who were transferred to a specialized center more than 7 days after the onset of epidermal slough had a period of hospitalization that was more than twice as long as that of patients who were transferred earlier than 7 days, even though other risk factors were comparable.[15] In another study including 44 patients, delayed transfer was associated with high morbidity and mortality rates.[32] Finally, a third retrospective analysis summarized the data for 36 patients with TEN; it showed that patients who survived had been referred earlier than nonsurvivors (4.0 vs. 11.5 days). Patients referred earlier than 7 days had a mortality rate of 4%, compared with 83% for those referred after 7 days. An increased risk of infection in other facilities was claimed to be the critical factor.[33]

However, in a small retrospective study mentioned earlier, no vital or infectious differences were observed in patients who were transferred late.[12]

Harms

No evidence was found.

Comment

Early referral is regarded as a priority for treatment, although good evidence is still lacking.

Supportive care

Most, but not all, symptomatic treatments are the same as those used for severe burns. We did not find any controlled studies of specific care for SJS/TEN.

Benefits

Recommended symptomatic treatments include:
• Careful handling, with intravenous fluid replacement (with the quantity being adjusted daily) via a peripheral

access point distant from the affected areas (a central venous line should not be used).

- Oral rehydration should be started as soon as possible (via nasogastric support), with nutrition.
- Aseptic care should be observed.
- The patient's environment should be kept warm.
- Pain and anxiety should be controlled.
- Sequelae should be prevented.

It has been claimed that the fluid requirements in TEN patients are two-thirds to three-quarters of those of patients with burns covering the same area. We did not find any RCTs or CCTs supporting this claim.

Several trials were found on techniques for helping skin healing, but none of these was comparative: epidermal stripping, biologic skin covers (porcine xenografts or cadaveric allografts), and synthetic dressings have been used. The skin necrosis is more superficial in comparison with burns.

It is suggested that wearing gas-permeable scleral contact lenses reduces photophobia and discomfort; these lenses improved visual acuity and healed corneal epithelial defects in half of the patients in one study.[34]

Harms
The type of fluid used for intravenous fluid replacement varies (e.g., macromolecules and saline solutions); a systematic review of human albumin administration in critically ill patients suggested that albumin and colloids should be replaced with crystalloids, as there was an excess mortality when albumin was used.[35]

Comment
In contrast to TEN, many RCTs have been published on burn care. Several of the most recent trials are potentially relevant for SJS/TEN.

Enteral feeding. Twenty-two patients were randomly assigned to two groups receiving either early enteral feeding or delayed enteral feeding. In the early enteral feeding group, there was a beneficial effect on the reduction of enterogenic infection, as a result of reduced intestinal permeability.[36]

Supplementation. Oxandrolone is an anabolic agent. In comparison with a placebo, it is effective for reducing weight loss and net nitrogenous loss and for increasing donor-site wound healing.[37] In comparison with human growth hormone, oxandrolone was equally effective; however, oxandrolone induced fewer complications (such as hyperglycemia and hypermetabolism).[38] The effectiveness of ornithine alpha-ketoglutarate supplementation of enteral feeding was assessed in comparison with an isonitrogenous control; the wound healing time was reduced by 33% with ornithine.[39] High-dose ascorbic acid (66 mg/kg/h)

during the first 24 hours of burns covering more than 30% of the skin area reduced resuscitation fluid volume requirements.[40]

Topical treatment. A controlled, side-by-side comparative and randomized study showed that frozen cultured human allogeneic epidermal sheets reduced the healing time in partial-thickness burns by 44%.[41] A living skin equivalent, Apligraf, was applied over meshed split-thickness autografts in 38 patients. The Apligraf sites were rated as superior to the control sites in 58% of cases and as worse in 16%. Pigmentation and vascularity were significantly better.[42] In 89 children with burns covering < 25% of the skin area, Biobrane decreased the healing time without an increased risk of infection.[43] Biobrane was found to be superior to topical 1% silver sulfadiazine on pain, pain medication requirements, wound healing time, and length of hospital stay in a trial including 20 children.[44] TransCyte consists of human newborn fibroblasts cultured on the nylon mesh of Biobrane. Sites treated with TransCyte healed more rapidly (11 vs. 18 days) and with less hypertrophic scarring than sites treated with silver sulfadiazine (in 14 patients).[45] A total of 600 patients with second-degree burns were included in one RCT. Topical recombinant bovine basic fibroblast growth factor led to faster granulation-tissue formation and epidermal regeneration than a placebo.[46] The effect of systemic growth hormone is still debated.

Prophylactic antibiotics
We found no evidence on the effects of prophylactic antibiotics.

Benefits
We found no good evidence regarding the type of antibiotic or the appropriate time of administration.

Harms
No evidence was found.

Comment
Most authors do not use prophylactic antibiotics. Preventive isolation, aseptic handling, and the use of sterile fields are suggested. We found no clinical evidence on the benefits or harms of early antibiotic therapy.

Are there any tests for proving drug culpability?
We found no evidence for a reliable test to prove the link between a single case and a specific drug.

Benefits
A study of patch tests and drug reactions found only two patients among 22 with SJS/TEN who had a relevant positive test—one with sulfonamide and one with phenobarbital.

Healthy volunteers were used as controls.[47] In a series of 14 patients, seven patch tests were carried out; three were positive (ethylbutylmalonylureum, phenazone, phenylbutazone). Among four negative tests, three intracutaneous tests were performed; two were positive (phenacetin, chloramphenicol).[6]

We found only case reports, but no clinical trials, on *in vitro* tests (essentially lymphocyte transformation tests).

Harms

Although it is theoretically possible, no cases of reactivation of SJS/TEN have been reported after patch tests. We found only a few case reports of generalized erythema or a sensation of irritation.

Comment

The sensitivity and specificity of patch tests, and thus their clinical usefulness, remain to be determined. *In vitro* tests are not routinely performed.

What happens in case of rechallenge with the causative drug or a related drug?

We found no good evidence regarding the risk of reuse of the culprit drug or on the possibility of desensitization in patients with TEN. Some data are available on prevention and on desensitization in benign cutaneous adverse drug reactions.

Benefits

The first step in prevention is to avoid the culprit drug and compounds that are closely related to it chemically. We found two RCTs on the prevention of drug reactions (not specifically for TEN). In the first trial, the incidence of rash complicating the first few weeks of treatment with nevirapine was significantly diminished by adding corticosteroids (50 mg every other day) for 2 weeks, or by using a slowly escalating dose.[48] The second RCT demonstrated a lower incidence of adverse reactions to sulfamethoxazole in the prevention of pneumocystosis in HIV-infected individuals, when slowly escalating doses were used.[49] These two RCTs only evaluated primary prevention, rather than patients with a previous drug reaction.

In contrast, desensitization with low doses of the culprit drug and progressively increasing the amount was used to prevent drug eruption in patients with a history of previous benign drug eruptions. We found one RCT in which HIV patients with a history of a reaction to trimethoprim–sulfamethoxazole were rechallenged with oral trimethoprim. If no reaction was seen (59 of 73 patients), randomization was carried out and the patient took sulfamethoxazole with a treatment scheme for desensitization, or immediately at the dosage commonly used in prophylaxis. Recurrent adverse effects were seen in 28% of the patients in the desens-

itization group compared with 20.5% of those in the other group. The difference was not statistically significant.[50]

Harms

We found one publication reporting a series of provocation tests in TEN (10 patients) and SJS (eight patients). The dosage was progressively increased to a commonly used daily dose. The test was continued at this level for 2–9 days. Only one test was positive (with a maculopapular eruption) in the TEN patients and four were positive in the SJS patients (with two SJS recurrences). Hypotheses to explain this low rate of recurrence include misdiagnosis, a desensitizing effect of the progressive dosage, or a real lack of systematic recurrence.[51]

Comment

Although the recurrence rate was only 10%, the risk of a life-threatening recurrence is so great that rechallenging the patient with a highly suspect drug is not ethically acceptable.

Summary

Prompt withdrawal of potentially causative drugs is likely to be beneficial. With systemic corticosteroids, there is a trade-off between benefits and harms.

The effectiveness of the following treatments is unknown: intravenous immunoglobulins, plasmapheresis, ciclosporin A, cyclophosphamide, *N*-acetylcysteine, granulocyte-colony stimulating factor, heparin, monoclonal antibodies against cytokines, and pentoxifylline.

Thalidomide is harmful.

Key points

- *Terminology.* the terms erythema multiforme (EM), Stevens–Johnson syndrome (SJS), and toxic epidermal necrolysis (TEN) terms are still used with varying definitions. This diversity of definition does not allow accurate analysis of the literature.
- *Treatments.* We found insufficient evidence for effective treatments. We found only one placebo-controlled RCT, which demonstrated a higher mortality with thalidomide treatment. We found no good evidence on the effects of corticosteroids.
- *Value of tests.* No evidence was found.
- *Drug reintroduction.* We found insufficient evidence.

References

1 Rzany B, Mockenhaupt M, Baur S, *et al.* Epidemiology of erythema exsudativum multiforme majus, Stevens–Johnson syndrome, and toxic epidermal necrolysis in Germany (1990–1992): structure and results of a population-based registry. *J Clin Epidemiol* 1996;**49**:769–73.

2 Roujeau JC, Guillaume JC, Fabre JP, Penso D, Flechet ML, Girre JP. Toxic epidermal necrolysis (Lyell syndrome): incidence and drug etiology in France, 1981–1985. *Arch Dermatol* 1990;126:37–42.

3 Chan HL, Stern RS, Arndt KA, *et al.* The incidence of erythema multiforme, Stevens–Johnson syndrome, and toxic epidermal necrolysis: a population-based study with particular reference to reactions caused by drugs among outpatients. *Arch Dermatol* 1990;**126**:43–7.

4 Roujeau JC, Kelly JP, Naldi L, *et al.* Medication use and the risk of Stevens–Johnson syndrome or toxic epidermal necrolysis. *N Engl J Med* 1995;**333**:1600–7.

5 Garcia-Doval I, LeCleach L, Bocquet H, Otero XL, Roujeau JC. Toxic epidermal necrolysis and Stevens–Johnson syndrome: does early withdrawal of causative drugs decrease the risk of death? *Arch Dermatol* 2000;**136**:323–7.

6 Tegelberg-Stassen MJ, van Vloten WA, Baart de la Faille. Management of nonstaphylococcal toxic epidermal necrolysis: follow-up study of 16 case histories. *Dermatologica* 1990;**180**:124–9.

7 Patterson R, Dykewicz MS, Gonzalzles A, *et al.* Erythema multiforme and Stevens–Johnson syndrome: descriptive and therapeutic controversy. *Chest* 1990;**98**:331–6.

8 Patterson R, Grammer LC, Greenberger PA, *et al.* Stevens–Johnson syndrome (SJS): effectiveness of corticosteroids in management and recurrent SJS. *Allergy Proc* 1992;**13**:89–95.

9 Patterson R, Miller M, Kaplan M, *et al.* Effectiveness of early therapy with corticosteroids in Stevens–Johnson syndrome: experience with 41 cases and a hypothesis regarding pathogenesis. *Ann Allergy* 1994;**73**:27–34.

10 Cheriyan S, Patterson R, Greenberger PA, Grammer LC, Latall J. The outcome of Stevens–Johnson syndrome treated with corticosteroids. *Allergy Proc* 1995;**16**:151–5.

11 Tripathi A, Ditto AM, Grammer LC, *et al.* Corticosteroid therapy in an additional 13 cases of Stevens–Johnson syndrome: a total series of 67 cases. *Allergy Asthma Proc* 2000;**21**:101–5.

12 Engelhardt SL, Schurr MJ, Helgerson RB. Toxic epidermal necrolysis: an analysis of referral patterns and steroid usage. *J Burn Care Rehabil* 1997;**18**:520–4.

13 Schulz JT, Sheridan RL, Ryan CM, MacKool B, Tompkins RG. A 10-year experience with toxic epidermal necrolysis. *J Burn Care Rehabil* 2000;**21**:199–204.

14 Halebian PH, Corder VJ, Madden MR, Finklestein JL, Shires GT. Improved burn center survival of patients with toxic epidermal necrolysis managed without corticosteroids. *Ann Surg* 1986;**204**:503–12.

15 Kelemen JJ, Cioffi WG, McManus WF, Mason ADJ, Pruitt BAJ. Burn center care for patients with toxic epidermal necrolysis. *J Am Coll Surg* 1995;**180**:273–8.

16 Kim PS, Goldfarb IW, Gaisford JC, Slater H. Stevens–Johnson syndrome and toxic epidermal necrolysis: a pathophysiologic review with recommendations for a treatment protocol. *J Burn Care Rehabil* 1983;**4**:91–100.

17 Rzany B, Schmitt H, Schopf E. Toxic epidermal necrolysis in patients receiving glucocorticosteroids. *Acta Derm Venereol* 1991;**71**:171–2.

18 Guibal F, Bastuji-Garin S, Chosidow O, Saiag P, Revuz J, Roujeau JC. Characteristics of toxic epidermal necrolysis in patients undergoing long-term glucocorticoid therapy. *Arch Dermatol* 1995;**131**:669–72.

19 Viard I, Wehrli P, Bullani R, *et al.* Inhibition of toxic epidermal necrolysis by blockade of CD95 with human intravenous immunoglobulin. *Science* 1998;**282**:490–3.

20 Prins C, Kerdel FA, Padilla RS, *et al.* Treatment of toxic epidermal necrolysis with high-dose intravenous immunoglobulins: multicenter retrospective analysis of 48 consecutive cases. *Arch Dermatol* 2003;**139**:26–32.

21 Bachot N, Revuz J, Roujeau JC. Intravenous immunoglobulin treatment for Stevens–Johnson syndrome and toxic epidermal necrolysis: a prospective noncomparative study showing no benefit on mortality or progression. *Arch Dermatol* 2003;**139**:33–6.

22 Brown KM, Silver GM, Halerz M *et al.* Toxic epidermal necrolysis: does immunoglobulin make a difference? *J Burn Care Rehabil* 2004;**25**:81–8.

23 Shortt R, Gomez M, Mittman N, Cartotto R. Intravenous immunoglobulin does not improve outcome in toxic epidermal necrolysis. *J Burn Care Rehabil* 2004;**25**:246–55.

24 Yip LW, Thong BY, Tan AW, Khin LW, Chng HH, Heng WJ. High-dose intravenous immunoglobulin in the treatment of toxic epidermal necrolysis: a study of ocular benefits. *Eye* 2005;**19**:846–53.

25 Levy JB, Pusey CD. Nephrotoxicity of intravenous immunoglobulin. *QJM* 2000;**93**:751–5.

26 Sati HI, Ahya R, Watson HG. Incidence and associations of acute renal failure complicating high-dose intravenous immunoglobulin therapy. *Br J Haematol* 2001;**113**:556–7.

27 Furubacke A, Berlin G, Anderson C, Sjoberg F. Lack of significant treatment effect of plasma exchange in the treatment of drug-induced toxic epidermal necrolysis? *Intensive Care Med* 1999;**25**:1307–10.

28 Arevalo JM, Lorente JA, Gonzalez-Herrada C, Jimenez-Reyes J. Treatment of toxic epidermal necrolysis with cyclosporin A. *J Trauma* 2000;**48**:473–8.

29 Trautmann A, Klein CE, Kampgen E, Brocker EB. Severe bullous drug reactions treated successfully with cyclophosphamide. *Br J Dermatol* 1998;**139**:1127–8.

30 Walmsley SL, Khorasheh S, Singer J, Djurdjev O. A randomized trial of *N*-acetylcysteine for prevention of trimethoprim-sulfamethoxazole hypersensitivity reactions in *Pneumocystis carinii* pneumonia prophylaxis (CTN 057). Canadian HIV Trials Network 057 Study Group. *J Acquir Immune Defic Syndr Hum Retrovirol* 1998;**19**:498–505.

31 Wolkenstein P, Latarjet J, Roujeau JC, *et al.* Randomised comparison of thalidomide versus placebo in toxic epidermal necrolysis. Lancet 1998;**352**:1586–9.

32 Murphy JT, Purdue GF, Hunt JL. Toxic epidermal necrolysis. *J Burn Care Rehabil* 1997;**18**:417–20.

33 McGee T, Munster A. Toxic epidermal necrolysis syndrome: mortality rate reduced with early referral to regional burn center. *Plast Reconstr Surg* 1998;**102**:1018–22.

34 Romero-Rangel T, Stavrou P, Cotter J, Rosenthal P, Baltatzis S, Foster CS. Gas-permeable scleral contact lens therapy in ocular surface disease. *Am J Ophthalmol* 2000;**130**:25–32.

35 Cochrane Injuries Group. Human albumin administration in critically ill patients: systematic review of randomised controlled trials. *BMJ* 1998;**317**:235–40.

36 Peng YZ, Yuan ZQ, Xiao GX. Effects of early enteral feeding on the prevention of enterogenic infection in severely burned patients. *Burns* 2001;**27**:145–9.

37 Demling RH, Orgill DP. The anticatabolic and wound healing effects of the testosterone analog oxandrolone after severe burn injury. *J Crit Care* 2000;**15**:12–7.

38 Demling RH. Comparison of the anabolic effects and complications of human growth hormone and the testosterone analog, oxandrolone, after severe burn injury. *Burns* 1999;**25**:215–21.

39 Coudray-Lucas C, Le Bever H, Cynober L, De Bandt JP, Carsin H. Ornithine alpha-ketoglutarate improves wound healing in severe burn patients: a prospective randomized double-blind trial versus isonitrogenous controls. *Crit Care Med* 2000;**28**:1772–6.

40 Tanaka H, Matsuda T, Miyagantani Y, Yukioka T, Matsuda H, Shimazaki S. Reduction of resuscitation fluid volumes in severely burned patients using ascorbic acid administration: a randomized, prospective study. *Arch Surg* 2000;**135**:326–31.

41 Alvarez-Diaz C, Cuenca-Pardo J, Sosa-Serrano A, Juarez-Aguilar E, Marsch-Moreno M, Kuri-Harcuch W. Controlled clinical study of deep partial-thickness burns treated with frozen cultured human allogeneic epidermal sheets. *J Burn Care Rehabil* 2000;**21**:291–9.

42 Waymack P, Duff RG, Sabolinski M. The effect of a tissue engineered bilayered living skin analog, over meshed split-thickness autografts on the healing of excised burn wounds. The Apligraf Burn Study Group. *Burns* 2000;**26**:609–19.

43 Lal S, Barrow RE, Wolf SE, *et al.* Biobrane improves wound healing in burned children without increased risk of infection. *Shock* 2000;**14**:314–8.

44 Barret JP, Dziewulski P, Ramzy PI, Wolf SE, Desai MH, Herndon DN. Biobrane versus 1% silver sulfadiazine in second-degree pediatric burns. *Plast Reconstr Surg* 2000;**105**:62–5.

45 Noordenbos J, Dore C, Hansbrough JF. Safety and efficacy of TransCyte for the treatment of partial-thickness burns. *J Burn Care Rehabil* 1999;**20**:275–81.

46 Fu X, Shen Z, Chen Y, *et al.* Randomised placebo-controlled trial of use of topical recombinant bovine basic fibroblast growth factor for second-degree burns. *Lancet* 1998;**352**:1661–4.

47 Wolkenstein P, Chosidow O, Flechet ML, *et al.* Patch testing in severe cutaneous adverse drug reactions, including Stevens–Johnson syndrome and toxic epidermal necrolysis. *Contact Dermatitis* 1996;**35**:234–6.

48 Barreiro P, Soriano V, Casas E, *et al.* Prevention of nevirapine-associated exanthema using slow dose escalation and/or corticosteroids. *AIDS* 2000;**14**:2153–7.

49 Para MF, Finkelstein D, Becker S, Dohn M, Walawander A, Black JR. Reduced toxicity with gradual initiation of trimethoprim-sulfamethoxazole as primary prophylaxis for *Pneumocystis carinii* pneumonia: AIDS Clinical Trials Group 268. *J Acquir Immune Defic Syndr* 2000;**24**:337–43.

50 Bonfanti P, Pusterla L, Parazzini F, *et al.* The effectiveness of desensitization versus rechallenge treatment in HIV-positive patients with previous hypersensitivity to TMP-SMX: a randomized multicentric study. C.I.S.A.I. Group. *Biomed Pharmacother* 2000;**54**:45–9.

51 Kauppinen K. Cutaneous reactions to drugs with special reference to severe bullous mucocutaneous eruptions and sulphonamides. *Acta Derm Venereol* 1972;**68**:1–89.

62 Focal hyperhidrosis

Berthold Rzany, Hendrik Zielke, Thomas Sycha, Peter Schnider

Background

Sweating helps control body temperature.[1] However, excessive sweating (hyperhidrosis) can cause physical and social problems. People with excessively sweaty palms may not be able to handle paper without soaking it. They may also experience social stigmatism and discrimination, especially when shaking hands, since their hands may be wet and clammy. People who suffer from excessive underarm sweating have to change clothes frequently. Their clothes may show stains and may not last long (Figure 62.1). Since sweating is commonly associated with insecurity, people with excessive localized sweating may be stereotyped as lacking in confidence. Consequently, patients with excessive localized sweating may exhibit signs of social phobia.[2]

Definition

There are no precise criteria for the definition of hyperhidrosis. Hyperhidrosis is defined on the basis of clinical findings and gravimetry as excessive sweating at rest and during normal temperature. On the basis of the size of the area affected, excessive sweating can be divided into generalized and focal.

In addition, there is no accepted severity grading system for hyperhidrosis. Reinauer *et al.*[3] suggested a four-grade score for palmar hyperhidrosis on the basis of gravimetry and clinical appearance. No such grading system exists for axillary hyperhidrosis.

Incidence/prevalence

A national survey published in 2004 estimated the hyperhidrosis prevalence in the United States at 2.8%. The average age of onset was 25 years, peaking at 40 years and declining after 64 years. The prevalence in males was only

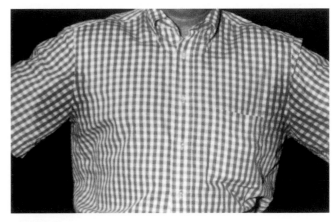

Figure 62.1 A 24-year-old man with excessive axillary hyperhidrosis. Note the significant sweat stains around the axillae.

slightly higher than in females. No ethnic differences have been documented.[4]

Etiology

Generalized excessive sweating can occur over most of the body and may be caused by underlying infections, malignancies, or hormonal imbalances. In contrast, apart from some known trigger factors such as emotional challenges,[5] the reasons for localized (focal) sweating are not readily apparent. It is therefore described as idiopathic. Idiopathic sweating appears to have a genetic background, as patients with focal hyperhidrosis often report a family history of hyperhidrosis. In a study of the effects of sympathectomy, 54% of 91 patients were found to have a positive family history.[6]

Prognosis

No good data are available on the prognosis of focal

hyperhidrosis. The incidence and prevalence are presumed to decrease with age. In an experimental setting, Kenney and Fowler[7] found a decrease in methylcholine-activated eccrine sweating in men aged 58–67 in comparison with men aged 22–24.

Diagnostic tests

Focal hyperhidrosis is a clinical diagnosis, diagnosable by history, a handshake, or stained clothes. In severe localized excessive sweating, pearls of sweat form even when the person is resting. In addition, the amount of sweat and the area affected can be measured. The amount of sweat can be measured using gravimetry (milligrams of sweat produced over a period of time). However, there is no standardization regarding the time period for which sweat should be collected. In the two randomized clinical trials (RCTs) on botulinum toxin A for axillary hyperhidrosis, Heckmann et al.[8] report the sweat rate in milligrams per minute, whereas Naumann and Lowe[9] used units of milligrams per 5 minutes. In other trials, the volume per 10 minutes has been used.[10,11]

The area that is affected by increased sweating can be defined using the ninhydrin test or the iodine starch test. Both tests use a change in color to indicate the hyperhidrotic area. Studies of validity or reproducibility are not available for either test. Particularly in studies evaluating surgical interventions, patient satisfaction is used as a marker of therapeutic success.[5,12]

Aims of treatment

The aim of treatment is to reduce the amount of sweating and to produce patient satisfaction.

Relevant outcomes

Relevant outcomes for the success of treatment are the reduction of sweating as measured by gravimetry, or the iodine starch or ninhydrin tests.

Methods of search

The following key words were used for a systematic search of the literature: "hyperhidrosis," "focal," "localized," "palmar," "hands," "plantar," "feet," "therapy," "treatment," "topical," "surgery," "surgical," "aluminum chloride," "anticholinergic drugs," "methenamine," "bornaprine," "methanthelinum bromide," "botulinum toxin," "triethanolamine," "iontophoresis," "sympathectomy," and "sweat". For the second edition of this chapter, the search was updated (February 2006).

Questions

Which interventions reduce sweating effectively in patients with *axillary* hyperhidrosis?

Case scenario 1
A 24-year-old patient enters the outpatient department complaining about excessive axillary sweating. Significant sweat stains can be found around the axillae (Figure 62.1).

Aluminum chloride
Benefits
There are no systematic reviews or good RCTs on aluminum chloride treatments (25–30% aluminum chloride hexahydrate, 10% aluminum chloride in combination with 5% propantheline bromide) in focal hyperhidrosis. The following treatments have been reported to be beneficial in axillary hyperhidrosis in case series.

Graber[11] reported the successful treatment of axillary hyperhidrosis using a 30% aluminum chloride solution in 10 patients. Sweat production was reduced from 201 mg/10 min to 44 mg/10 min (22% of the baseline value). Brandrup and Larsen[10] reported on 23 women with axillary hyperhidrosis who were treated with 25% aluminum chloride hexahydrate, with (n = 11) and without occlusion (n = 12). The treatment was considered to be effective, with the amount of sweat produced in 10 minutes (measured by gravimetry) decreasing by 60–80% even during exercise for both groups. Ewert and Link[13] reported a good or very good effect in 34 of 49 (70%) soldiers with clinical hyperhidrosis of the axillae, palms, and plantar surfaces by combining 10% aluminum chloride and 5% propantheline bromide in a solution. The effect was less obvious, however, in 27 additional soldiers who lived in the tropics.

Harms
No serious side effects were reported for aluminum chloride. However, reversible skin irritations can occur, and some patients have to discontinue the treatment. Graber[11] reported that one of 10 treated patients had to discontinue treatment. In the study by Brandrup and Larsen,[10] itching was reported in all 23 patients, leading to discontinuation of therapy in two. Irritation and itching were worsened by occlusive dressing. Occlusive dressing had to be discontinued in all 11 patients.

Comments/implications for clinical practice
Although there is not a good RCT, 10–30% aluminum chloride hexahydrate appears likely to be effective. There is a trade-off between efficacy and side effects (i.e., local irritation of the skin). Occlusive dressings appear to increase the irritation.

Botulinum toxin A

Botulinum toxin A (BNT-A) is a bacterial toxin that paralyses muscles and decreases sweating by blocking the release of the acetylcholine from presynaptic vesicles. It is given by injection into the deeper part of the skin where the sweat glands are located. There are two major BNT-A brands available, Botox and Dysport. Botox and Dysport units cannot be directly compared. Each drug will therefore be discussed separately. The data for the BTN-B brand that is also available are so scarce that they will be not discussed for this indication.[14]

Benefits

There are no systematic reviews. In addition to two small RCTs that demonstrated the efficacy of 200 units of botulinum toxin A (Dysport),[15] and of 50 units (Botox),[16] two large RCTs have demonstrated the efficacy of this treatment in axillary hyperhidrosis.[8,9]

Heckmann et al.[8] investigated the efficacy of botulinum toxin A 200 units (two-fifths of a vial of Dysport) in 145 participants with axillary hyperhidrosis. After 2 weeks, the rate of sweating was reduced below 25 mg/min in 64.8% of the axillae treated with botulinum toxin, compared with 1.4% of the axillae treated with placebo. At least a 50% reduction in sweating (in comparison with the baseline) was achieved in 134 of 145 axillae treated with botulinum toxin and 22 of 145 axillae treated with placebo. Based on these data, the numbers needed to treat (NNT) can be calculated as 1.3 to one (i.e., of four patients treated with 200 units of Dysport, three patients will obtain at least a 50% reduction in sweating). In another smaller randomized, unblinded side-by-side within-patient comparison of 100 and 200 units of Dysport in 43 patients, the authors did not see any differences in effectiveness or safety. In this study, it was stated that 100 Dysport units is the optimal dosage for axillary hyperhidrosis.[17]

In another RCT, 320 patients with axillary hyperhidrosis were treated with 50 Botox units. After 3 weeks, 95% (95% CI, 92 to 97) of the active-treatment group and 32% (95% CI, 22 to 44) of the placebo group reported at least a 50% reduction in sweating.[9] On the basis of these data, the NNT for 50 units Botox can be calculated as 1.7 to one (of four patients treated, two would obtain at least a 50% reduction in sweating).

Harms

There is no evidence for systemic side effects. In the study by Naumann and Lowe,[9] 11 patients (4.5%) reported increased nonaxillary (compensatory) sweating after treatment. Heckmann et al.[8] reported one patient (< 1%) with increased sweating.

Comments/implications for clinical practice

Botulinum toxin A is the only drug with proven efficacy for hyperhidrosis of the axilla. On the basis of the available studies, 50 units of Botox or 100 units of Dysport appear to be effective in the treatment of axillary hyperhidrosis.

Oral anticholinergics
Benefits

There are no systematic reviews on the efficacy of oral anticholinergics (bornaprine, methanthelinium bromide) in axillary hyperhidrosis. In addition to a few case series of patients with palmar and plantar hyperhidrosis (see below), one small RCT with 41 patients demonstrated a significant reduction in axillary sweat production about 36 mg/min after treatment with 50 mg methanthelinium bromide (Vagantin) twice per day compared with two in the placebo group.[18]

Harms

In the available RCT, dry mouth was the only adverse event that occurred significantly more often in the active treatment group ($P = 0.01$).[18]

Comments/implications for clinical practice

At present, more evidence is needed to allow a reliable recommendation of systemic anticholinergic treatments with regard to possible side effects. On a case-to-case basis, oral anticholinergics appear to suppress increased sweating for a certain time. Patients might use them to decrease sweating in foreseeable circumstances with high emotional impact.

Iontophoresis
Benefits

In contrast to palmar and plantar hyperhidrosis (see below), there is little evidence on the efficacy of iontophoresis in axillary hyperhidrosis. Akins et al.[19] reported on eight of 27 sites in 22 patients with focal hyperhidrosis that were treated with iontophoresis. Iontophoresis was not effective in two of the eight axillae. Three of the eight axillae (38%) showed a 50% decrease in sweating after 2 weeks, as measured by the starch iodine test. In another case series, Hölzle and Alberti[20] reported an excellent or moderate reduction in one of five patients with axillary sweating.

Harms

In the study by Akins et al.,[19] two of eight treated sites developed vesicles, four developed erythematous papules, and three developed scaling. In three sites, the discomfort was defined as moderate or severe.

Comments/implications for clinical practice

There is little evidence that iontophoresis works in axillary hyperhidrosis. Local side effects such as discomfort and skin inflammation limit the use of iontophoresis in some patients.

Surgical interventions: curettage of the axilla

Several local surgical interventions can be used for hyperhidrosis of the axilla. The idea is to reduce the number of active sweat glands by removing them, or by disturbing the anatomical integrity of the skin. This procedure is only used for axillary hyperhidrosis and cannot be used for palmar or plantar hyperhidrosis.

Benefits

We found no RCTs. The largest case series so far compared subcutaneous curettage (n = 90) with injection of botulinum toxin A (n = 20), and reported equally good results for both interventions.[12] Sixty-seven percent of the patients reported a good or very good outcome after subcutaneous curettage in this study. Hasche et al.[21] reported a reduction of the area of sweating as shown by the starch iodine test. However, no quantitative efficacy data were reported. Subjectively, 18 of 20 patients considered that the intervention had led to good results.

Harms

As with any surgery, curettage of the axillary sweat glands may be accompanied by local infections, hematoma, and scarring. However, the prevalence of these adverse effects appears to be low.[12,21]

Comments/implications for clinical practice

There is no good evidence on the efficacy of axillary surgery on hyperhidrosis. Subjective data from various studies suggest that it is beneficial. Clinical trials using objective outcome measures such as gravimetry are needed.

Surgical interventions: sympathectomy

Sympathectomy is the dissection or coagulation of sympathetic nerve nodes, and it can be carried out to reduce excessive sweating of the axillae. This procedure is now done by endoscopy (introducing instruments through the skin via a narrow tube) rather than by opening the chest surgically, but general anesthesia is still required. The lungs are collapsed by pumping in carbon dioxide, and the sympathetic nerve nodes that transmit the nervous signals to the sweat glands in the upper limb and the face (T1–T4) are destroyed.

Benefits

In a retrospective study of the long-term efficacy and side effects in 270 patients with a total of 480 T1–T4 sympathectomies, Herbst et al.[5] reported results in 39 patients with axillary hyperhidrosis. After surgery, 30 (77%) reported immediate success. However, after a mean follow-up of 15 years, only 13 patients (33%) with axillary hyperhidrosis

remained completely satisfied, in contrast to 167 (73%) with palmar hyperhidrosis (see the following "Harms" comment).

Harms

Acute side effects include bleeding (one of 48 sites) and transient or persistent Horner's syndrome (three of 48 sites).[22] Long-term side effects include compensatory sweating and gustatory sweating, which is reflected in a decrease in long-term satisfaction. The results reported by Herbst et al.[5] (i.e., a decreased proportion of completely satisfied patients) are a reflection of increases in compensatory and gustatory sweating, not loss of efficacy.

Comments/implications for clinical practice

There is insufficient evidence for sympathectomy for axillary hyperhidrosis. The long-term side effects are compensatory or gustatory sweating.

Other interventions: salvia

Salvia (sage) is a herb given in the form of tea or tablets. There are no systematic reviews or RCTs of its use, and no evidence for harm. There is insufficient evidence that salvia works in patients with hyperhidrosis.

Which interventions reduce sweating efficiently in patients with *palmar* hyperhidrosis?

Case scenario 2

A 22-year-old woman complains of severe sweating of the palms. Both palmar areas are covered with sweat drops. Paper is stained as soon as the patient touches it (Figure 62.2).

Topical agents
Benefits

There are no studies on the treatment of patients with palmar hyperhidrosis using exclusively topical agents (10%

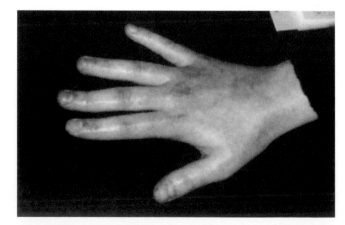

Figure 62.2 Dropping sweat pearls in a 22-year-old woman with grade III hyperhidrosis.

aluminum chloride, 5% methenamine, 5% glutaraldehyde, 5% propantheline bromide). There was one placebo-controlled RCT of 5% methenamine on 109 patients with palmar and plantar hyperhidrosis.[23] In this study, the mean hyperhidrosis score was 1.4 for patients treated for 28 days with 5% methenamine, in comparison with 2.5 in the placebo group ($P \leq 0.001$). Of the treated patients, 71 of 109 (65%) rated the result as good or excellent, compared with 19 of 109 (17%) in the placebo group (response difference 0.48; 95% CI, 0.36 to 0.59; NNT 3, 95% CI, 2 to 3). In another study by Phadke et al.,[24] 60 patients were randomly assigned to treatment with topical 10% methenamine aqueous solution, 5% glutaraldehyde, or tap water iontophoresis with direct current. After 4 weeks, 19 of 20 patients treated with methenamine, 13 of 20 patients treated with glutaraldehyde, and 11 of 20 treated with iontophoresis described good or excellent results. The differences were statistically significant ($P = 0.01$).

The case series by Ewert and Link[13] on the efficacy of 10% aluminum chloride plus 5% propantheline bromide in a solution included patients with axillary hyperhidrosis as well as palmar and plantar hyperhidrosis. In this European study, the efficacy was reported to be good or very good.

Harms

As in the treatment of axillary hyperhidrosis, reversible skin irritations can occur, causing some patients to discontinue the treatment. In the study by Phadke et al.,[24] hyperpigmentation occurred in eight of 20 patients treated with methenamine and in 12 of 20 patients treated with glutaraldehyde. Scaling was provoked in five of 20 patients treated with methenamine.

Comments/implications for clinical practice

There are insufficient data to show that 10–30% aluminum chloride (hexahydrate) is beneficial. Local irritation of the skin may occur.

Botulinum toxin A
Benefits

There are three RCTs demonstrating the efficacy of botulinum toxin A for palmar hyperhidrosis. All RCTs, one of Dysport 120 units and two of Botox, comparing 50 units versus 100 units, had significant flaws in the design or analysis of the study.[25–27] In the most recent small RCT with 19 patients, bilateral injections of 100 units of Botox were compared with placebo. In this study, a significantly greater reduction in sweat production was documented in the Botox-treated hand at day 28 ($P = 0.004$).[27] Other evidence is based on case series. The largest case series included 23 patients treated with Botox 50 units[28] and 21 patients treated with Dysport 240 units (approximately half a vial) per hand.[29] Vadoud-Seyedi et al.[28] reported "significant improvement." Schnider et al.[29] reported a median reduc-

tion of sweat production, as measured by the ninhydrin test, of 42% in comparison with the baseline values. The median overall satisfaction was "very good."

Harms

A decrease in finger pinch strength, resulting from diffusion of the toxin into the palmar muscles, has been documented. Schnider et al.[29] reported a transient measurable reduction in finger power in five of 21 patients after the first treatment. Finger pinch strength appears to decrease with increasing dosage (50 units versus 100 units Botox).[26] In contrast, in a small study by Lowe et al.[27] using a hydraulic hand dynamometer, no difference in grip strength was observed between the verum-treated and placebo-treated hands.

Comments/implications for clinical practice

Although the available data are limited to case series, botulinum toxin A appears to be beneficial in patients with palmar hyperhidrosis. The injections are painful, and regional anesthesia with medial, ulnar, and radial nerve blocks should be administered before the injection of the toxin. Topical local anesthesia—for example, with a eutectic mixture of lidocaine and prilocaine (Emla cream)—may be beneficial in some patients to reduce the pain of the injection.

Oral anticholinergics
Benefits

Evidence on anticholinergics (bornaprine, methanthelinium bromide) is based on case series. In the study by Castells Rodellas et al.,[30] six of 12 patients (50%) with palmar or plantar hyperhidrosis reported that the response to bornaprine was excellent after the first week. In a small pilot study, methanthelinium bromide was found to reduce sweating in four patients by 24–80% in comparison with baseline values.[31] However, in the larger clinical study, in contrast to axillary hyperhidrosis, no significant differences were documented between verum and placebo.[18]

Harms

Oral anticholinergics have well-known systemic side effects (for example, dry mouth and eyes). Only one patient of 10 in the case series by Castells Rodellas et al. had to discontinue bornaprine due to dizziness or dryness of the mucosa.[30]

Comments/implications for clinical practice

So far, there is no good evidence of the efficacy of oral anticholinergics. There is certainly a trade-off between efficacy and anticholinergic side effects.

Iontophoresis
Benefits

In contrast to axillary hyperhidrosis, there are more studies on the efficacy of iontophoresis in palmar and plantar hyperhidrosis. There are two RCTs, one double-blind, including a total of 31 patients. Dahl and Glent-Madsen[32] demonstrated in 11 patients that iontophoresis with direct current reduced sweat production by 38% (median quartiles: 7%, 53%) in comparison with placebo. Phadke et al.[24] reported a good or excellent response in 11 of 20 patients after 4 weeks of iontophoresis with direct current. Iontophoresis was compared with glutaraldehyde and topical methenamine in this study (see above).

Akins et al.,[19] using the Drionic unit, reported a 50% decrease in sweating in comparison with the control site in eight of 10 hands. In a nonrandomized study, Hölzle and Alberti[20] reported that sweating was reduced to normal or to a moderate extent using the Drionic unit in seven of 12 patients. The average reduction of spontaneous palmar sweating was $19 \pm 17\%$ in comparison with the untreated site after 3 weeks' treatment. In another study by Reinauer et al.,[3] different types of current (4.3 kHz and 10 kHz pulsed direct current versus direct current) were investigated in a total of 30 patients. All of the patients were reported to have returned to a normal sweat rate after an average of 10–12 sessions. Treatment failed in two patients in the 4.3-kHz pulse group. However, the generalizability of this study is limited, as only patients with moderate palmar hyperhidrosis were included.

Harms
Dahl et al.[32] reported that one of 11 patients had multiple bullae after direct contact with electrodes. Phadke et al.[24] report scaling in two of 20 patients, but no irritant dermatitis. Akins et al.[19] reported moderate to severe discomfort in six of 10 hands. Reinauer et al.[3] reported that the pulsed current was well tolerated.

Comments/implications for clinical practice
There is some evidence, based mostly on smaller studies, that iontophoresis reduces hyperhidrosis of the palms. Treatment has to be performed on a regular base (from initially three to five times a week to once a week). The treatment is usually safe. However, burns and blisters may occur.

Iontophoresis with combination treatment
Benefits
A small trial including 10 patients reported a greater decrease in the severity of sweating (scored on a five-point scale): −3.1 for the combination of iontophoresis with 2% aluminum chloride and 0.01% glycopyrrolate versus −1.5 for iontophoresis alone.[33] Shimizu et al.[34] compared randomized, but unblinded, alternate-current treatment (AC) alone versus AC in combination with oral anticholinergics (n = 19; oxybutynin hydrochloride 4 mg/day). There were no significant differences in treatment effectiveness between the two groups.

Harms
One patient in the study by Shen et al. 1990 reported transient mouth dryness. Some patients noted peeling or vesiculation after 3–4 days of treatment.[33] AC iontophoresis with or without the combination of oxybutynin hydrochloride was well tolerated, according to Shimizu et al.[34]

Comments
Combination therapy may increase the efficacy of iontophoresis. However, there is a lack of good data to prove this.

Surgical interventions: sympathectomy
Benefits
Sympathectomy is mostly used for palmar hyperhidrosis. When performed correctly, it is effective in almost all patients, resulting in dry hands.[22] In a retrospective study of 270 patients with a total of 480 T1–T4 sympathectomies, sweating was relieved in the majority of patients (98%), and 96% were satisfied initially.[5] Similar efficacy was shown by Yazbek et al., who compared thoracoscopic surgery of the T2 versus the T3 ganglion in 60 patients, with only one failure to achieve complete dryness in the T3 group. The quality of life improved significantly in both groups during the follow-up period.[35]

Harms
In a large study,[5] T1–T4 endoscopic thoracic sympathectomies in 270 patients were found to be associated with rare acute severe side effects such as pneumothorax (n = 11; 2%), Horner syndrome (n = 12; 2%), and ptosis (n = 7; 1%). These data are supported by other smaller studies. Chiou and Chen[6] reported a hemothorax in one of 91 patients with transaxillary T2 sympathectomy.

There is a systematic review looking at the current indications for this intervention and the incidence of late complications, collectively and per indication. A total of 135 articles (no RCT) up to April 1998 reporting 22 458 patients were identified. The main indication found was hyperhidrosis, accounting for 84.3% of procedures. Compensatory hyperhidrosis occurred in 52.3% of patients, gustatory sweating in 32.3%, phantom sweating in 38.6%, and Horner's syndrome in 2.4%. Compensatory sweating occurred three times more often after sympathectomy for hyperhidrosis.[36]

In the study by Herbst et al.,[5] 182 patients (67.4%) reported compensatory sweating, mostly on the feet and face. In the study by Chiou and Chen,[6] 97% of 91 patients reported compensatory sweating in the first year, mostly on the upper back. Some patients regretted undergoing the procedure (13% of 91) because of this side effect.[6] In addition to compensatory sweating, Herbst et al.[5] reported gustatory sweating in 50.7% of patients. In the same study, 10% of the patients reported an increased susceptibility to influenza and rhinitis. Yazbek et al. observed that denervation at the T3 level led to less severe compensatory hyperhidrosis.[35]

Comments/implications for clinical practice

So far, there is no good evidence on the efficacy of sympathectomy. Although it is quite likely that, when performed correctly, sympathectomy is effective in palmar hyperhidrosis, there is increasing evidence regarding harms, especially long-term harms. Sympathectomy should therefore never be considered as a first-line therapy.

Other interventions: salvia

No additional comments can be made regarding salvia in palmar hyperhidrosis. It is unlikely to be an effective drug.

Key points

- Limited data suggest that 10–30% aluminum chloride hexahydrate is effective, but there is a trade-off between efficacy and side effects (local irritation of the skin).

- Evidence from RCTs suggests that botulinum toxin A is effective in focal hyperhidrosis. Botulinum toxin A is a highly effective treatment for axillary hyperhidrosis.

- There is limited evidence on the efficacy of oral anticholinergics, bornaprine, and methanthelinium bromide. These are associated with anticholinergic side effects.

- Iontophoresis of the palm may be moderately effective. The efficacy of iontophoresis of the axillae is questionable. Local irritation is common.

- There is little evidence to support the surgical removal of axillary sweat glands. A formal clinical trial has not yet been conducted, and the real efficacy of the procedure is therefore not clear.

- There is some evidence for the efficacy of sympathectomy, although there is a lack of objective criteria to measure efficacy. Sympathectomy for axillary and palmar sweating is associated with long-term side effects such as compensatory and gustatory sweating. Because of the unknown long-term side effects, sympathectomy should only be considered in very severe cases.

References

1 Lopez M, Sessler DI, Walter K, Emerick T, Ozaki M. Rate and gender dependence of the sweating, vasoconstriction, and shivering thresholds in humans. *Anesthesiology* 1994;**80**:780–8.

2 Weber A, Heger S, Sinkgraven R, Heckmann M, Elsner P, Rzany B. Psychosocial aspects of patients with focal hyperhidrosis: marked reduction of social phobia, anxiety and depression and increased quality of life after treatment with botulinum toxin A. *Br J Dermatol* 2005;**152**:342–5.

3 Reinauer S, Neusser A, Schauf G, Hälzle E. Die gepulste Gleichstrom-Iontophorese als neue Behandlungsmöglichkeit der Hyperhidrosis. *Hautarzt* 1995;**46**:538–75.

4 Strutton DR, Kowalski JW, Glaser DA, Stang PE. US prevalence of hyperhidrosis and impact on individuals with axillary hyper-

hidrosis: results from a national survey. *J Am Acad Dermatol* 2004; **51**:241–8.

5 Herbst F, Plas EG, Fägger R, Fritsch A. Endoscopic thoracic sympathectomy for primary hyperhidrosis of the upper limbs: a critical analysis and long-term results of 480 patients. *Ann Surg* 1994;**220**:86–90.

6 Chiou TSM, Chen SC. Intermediate-term results of endoscopic transaxillary T2 sympathectomy for primary palmar hyperhidrosis. *Br J Surg* 1999;**86**:45–7.

7 Kenney LW, Fowler SR. Methylcholine-activated eccrine sweat gland density and output as a function of age. *J Appl Physiol* 1988;**65**:1082–6.

8 Heckmann M, Ceballos-Baumann AO, Plewig G. Botulinum toxin A for axillary hyperhidrosis (excessive sweating). *N Engl J Med* 2001;**344**:488–93.

9 Naumann M, Lowe NJ. Efficacy and safety of botulinum toxin A in the treatment of bilateral primary axillary hyperhidrosis: a randomised, placebo controlled study. *BMJ* 2001;**323**:596–9.

10 Brandrup F, Larsen PO. Axillary hyperhidrosis: local treatment with aluminium chloride hexahydrate 25% in absolute ethanol. *Acta Derm Venerol* 1978;**58**:461–5.

11 Graber W. Eine einfache, wirksame Behandlung der axillären Hyperhidrose. *Schweiz Rundsch Med (Praxis)* 1977;**66**:1080–4.

12 Rompel R, Scholz S. Subcutaneous curettage *v.* injection of botulinum toxin A for treatment of axillary hyperhidrosis. *Eur J Dermatol* 12001;**15**:207–11.

13 Ewert L, Link A. Neuartiges Antihidrotikum in der Erprobung bei Soldaten der Bundeswehr. *Dermatol Kosmet* 1976;**17**:10–4.

14 Baumann L, Slezinger A, Halem M, *et al.* Pilot study of the safety and efficacy of Myobloc (botulinum toxin type B) for treatment of axillary hyperhidrosis. *Int J Dermatol* 2005;**44**:418–24.

15 Schnider P, Binder M, Kittler H, *et al.* A randomized, double-blind placebo controlled trial of botulinum toxin A for severe axillary hyperhidrosis. *Br J Dermatol* 1999;**140**:677–80.

16 Odderson IR. Long-term quantitative benefits of botulinum toxin type A in the treatment of axillary hyperhidrosis. *Dermatol Surg* 2002;**28**:480–3.

17 Heckmann M, Ceballos-Baumann AO, Plewig G; Hyperhidrosis Study Group. Botulinum toxin A for axillary hyperhidrosis (excessive sweating). *N Engl J Med* 2001;**344**:488–93.

18 Hund M, Sinkgraven R, Rzany B. [Randomized, placebo-controlled, double blind clinical trial on the efficacy and safety of oral methanthelinium bromide (Vagantin) in the treatment of focal hyperhidrosis; in German.] *J Dtsch Dermatol Ges* 2004;**2**:343–9.

19 Akins DL, Meisenheimer JL, Dobson RL. Efficacy of the Drionic unit in the treatment of hyperhidrosis. *J Am Acad Dermatol* 1987;**16**:828–32.

20 Hölzle E, Alberti N. Long-term efficacy and side effects of tap water iontophoresis of palmoplantar hyperhidrosis: the usefulness of home therapy. *Dermatologica* 1987;**175**:126–35.

21 Hasche E, Hagedorn M, Sattler G. Die subkutane Schweissdrüsensaugkürettage in Tumeszenzlokalanästhesie bei Hyperhidrosis axillaris. *Hautarzt* 1997;**48**:817–9.

22 Hashmonai M, Kopelman D, Schein M. Thoracoscopic versus open supraclavicular upper dorsal sympathectomy: a prospective randomised trial. *Eur J Surg Suppl* 1994;**572**:13–6.

23 Bergstresser P, Quero R. Treatment of hyperhidrosis with topical methenamine. *Int J Dermatol* 1976;**15**:452–5.

24 Phadke VA, Joshi RS, Khopar US, Wadhwa SL. Comparison of topical methenamine, glutaraldehyde and tap water iontophoresis for palmoplantar hyperhidrosis. *Ind J Dermatol Venerol Leprol* 1995;**61**:346–8.

25 Schnider P, Binder M, Auff E, Kittler H, Berger T, Wolff K. Double-blind trial of botulinum A toxin for the treatment of focal hyperhidrosis of the palms. *Br J Dermatol* 1997;**136**:548–52.

26 Saadia D, Voustianiouk A, Wang AK, Kaufmann H. Botulinum toxin type A in primary palmar hyperhidrosis: randomized, single blind, two dose study. *Neurology* 2001;**57**:2095–9.

27 Lowe NJ, Yamauchi PS, Lask GP, Patnaik R, Iyer S. Efficacy and safety of botulinum toxin type a in the treatment of palmar hyperhidrosis: a double-blind, randomized, placebo-controlled study. *Dermatol Surg* 2002;**28**:822–7.

28 Vadoud-Seyedi J, Heenen M, Simonart T. Treatment of idiopathic palmar hyperhidrosis with botulinum toxin: report of 23 cases and review of the literature. *Dermatology* 2001;**203**:318–21.

29 Schnider P, Moreau E, Kittler H, *et al.* Treatment of focal hyperhidrosis with botulinum toxin type A: long-term follow-up in 61 patients. *Br J Dermatol* 2001;**145**:289–93.

30 Castells Rodellas A, Moragón Gordon M, Ramírez Bosca A. [Effect of bornaprine in localized hyperhidrosis; in Spanish.] *Med Cutan Ibero Lat Am* 1987;**15**:303–5.

31 Fuchslocher M, Rzany B. Orale anticholinerge Therapie der fokalen Hyperhidrose mit Methanthelinumbromid (Vagantin). Erste Daten zur Wirksamkeit. *Hautarzt* 2002;**53**:151–2.

32 Dahl CJ, Glent-Madsen L. Treatment of hyperhidrosis manuum by tap water iontophoresis. *Acta Derm Venerol* 1989;**69**:343–8.

33 Shen JL, Lin GS, Li WM. A new strategy of iontophoresis for hyperhidrosis. *J Am Acad Dermatol* 1990;**22**:239–41.

34 Shimizu H, Tamada Y, Shimizu J, Ohshima Y, Matsumoto Y, Sugenoya J. Effectiveness of iontophoresis with alternating current (AC) in the treatment of patients with palmoplantar hyperhidrosis. *J Dermatol* 2003;**30**:444–9.

35 Yazbek G, Wolosker N, de Campos JR, Kauffman P, Ishy A, Puech-Leao P. Palmar hyperhidrosis: which is the best level of denervation using video-assisted thoracoscopic sympathectomy: T2 or T3 ganglion? *J Vasc Surg* 2005;**42**:281–5.

36 Furlan AD, Mailis A, Papagapiou M. Critical review: are we paying a high price for surgical sympathectomy? A systematic review of late complications. *J Pain* 2000;**1**:287–9.

63 Polymorphic light eruption (PLE)

Robert S. Dawe, James Ferguson

This condition, also known as polymorphous light eruption, is one of the group of idiopathic photosensitivity disorders that also includes hydroa vacciniforme, chronic actinic dermatitis (photosensitivity dermatitis and actinic reticuloid syndrome), idiopathic solar urticaria, actinic prurigo, and juvenile springtime eruption. Although the cause of each of these conditions remains unknown, there are suggestions that the mechanism for some, especially PLE, may be autoimmune. For the purposes of this book, we discuss some aspects of PLE, the commonest of these conditions, on which there is the largest volume of published literature. Where appropriate—for example, when discussing differential diagnosis—we mention other photodermatoses. Other photodermatoses, such as cutaneous porphyrias, DNA-repair disorders (such as xeroderma pigmentosa) and drug-induced photosensitivity, will be dealt with in future editions of the book and on the accompanying web site (Figure 63.1).

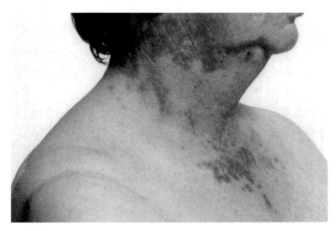

Figure 63.1 A typical papular polymorphic light eruption.

Background

Definition

PLE is a recurrent abnormal reaction to sunlight (or artificial ultraviolet radiation) that occurs after a delay following exposure and heals without scarring.[1-3]

Prevalence

Questionnaire surveys have found that 10–21% of selected northern European and North American populations are affected.[4-6] PLE is less frequent closer to the equator.[7-9]

Etiology

A commonly postulated mechanism is that PLE might be an autoimmune disorder in which there is an abnormal delayed hypersensitivity to an endogenous molecule rendered antigenic by ultraviolet (UV) exposure.[10]

Prognosis

Spontaneous resolution can occur, but is probably infrequent amongst those affected severely enough to be assessed in hospital.[11]

Diagnostic tests

The diagnosis is usually made on the basis of the clinical history. The following investigations are sometimes indicated:

- *Lupus serology*, when cutaneous lupus erythematosus is considered in the differential diagnosis; particularly if treatment with prophylactic phototherapy is being considered, antinuclear antibody and anti-Ro and La antibodies should be requested.[12]
- *Histopathology*, when a superficial and deep, perivascular, dermal inflammatory infiltrate is seen. Histopathology

and direct immunofluorescence can help differentiate PLE and lupus erythematosus.[13,14]

- *Phototesting.* Monochromator phototesting is usually normal in PLE, but can be useful in excluding solar urticaria or chronic actinic dermatitis if these are considered possible alternative, or concomitant, diagnoses. Repeated irradiation provocation testing to 4×4 cm or larger areas is positive in a proportion of patients (< 50% in some series), but can be helpful in cases of diagnostic uncertainty.
- *Patch testing and photopatch testing to sunscreens.* These are useful when sunscreen photoallergy or contact allergy is suspected as a coexistent diagnosis.[15–18]
- *Porphyrin plasma spectrofluorometry.* Cutaneous porphyrias occasionally feature as differential diagnoses, and can be excluded if this simple test is negative.
- *HLA class II typing* can help distinguish actinic prurigo (see below).[19,20]

Aims of treatment

Treatments can be divided into prophylactic and suppressive. Prophylactic measures include sunlight avoidance and "desensitization" prophylactic phototherapy. Sunlight avoidance measures include advice on behavior (for example, avoiding outdoor exposure between 10 a.m. and 3 p.m.), clothing (long sleeves and hat), topical broad-spectrum sunscreens, and environmental measures (such as applying UV-absorbing "museum film" to house and car windows for those severely sensitive to UV wavelengths). The aim of these measures is to reduce the frequency of and severity of the eruption.

The aim of prophylactic phototherapy is to increase the duration of sunlight exposure required to elicit PLE, and so improve the quality of life for those severely affected patients who cannot carry out normal activities (for example, putting out washing during daytime) because very limited sunlight exposure triggers the eruption. Suppressive treatment should alleviate symptoms (particularly itch), and speed the resolution of PLE when it occurs.

Relevant outcomes

For prophylactic treatments, important outcomes are number of episodes of PLE (and their severity) and quality of life. For symptomatic suppressive therapies, the main outcomes are symptom severity (primarily itch) and the speed of resolution of the eruption.

Methods of search

Studies were identified using the Medline (1966 to January 2006) and Embase (1988 to January 2006) databases, with search terms including "polymorphic/polymorphous light eruption AND treatment OR prognosis." Abstracts were read to determine which were likely to be relevant.

Questions

What is the prognosis for resolution of PLE for a severely affected patient living in a temperate country?

Follow-up of 94 Finnish patients (by questionnaire, supplemented by repeat clinical assessments of a subgroup) up to a mean of 32 years after onset found that 24% (95% confidence interval, 16–34%) experienced resolution of their PLE and that 51% (95% CI, 41–62%) had milder PLE.[11] A recent report suggested that those with negative provocation tests may be more likely to proceed to remission than those with positive provocation tests.[21]

Comments
We have very limited information on the prognosis of PLE, and this one well-conducted follow-up study[11] involved a selected group of patients—those assessed in a hospital department and willing to attend for review. Our experience in Dundee (based on another severely affected patient group) is that a substantial proportion of those with PLE severe enough to require repeated yearly prophylactic phototherapy do, after several years, experience resolution, or marked improvement, so that they can then stop attending for treatment.[22] We do not know whether this is spontaneous resolution or whether it is a result of repeated phototherapy courses.

Implications for practice
We can advise patients that spontaneous resolution is possible, but cannot reliably indicate how likely it is to occur. We still do not know whether repeated yearly courses of prophylactic phototherapy influence the long-term prognosis.

Which form of prophylactic phototherapy—psoralen UVA photochemotherapy or UVB monotherapy—should be prescribed for severely affected patients?

Efficacy
A randomized, patient-masked, controlled trial[23] including 25 adults found that narrowband (TL-01) UVB was as effective as psoralen ultraviolet A (PUVA) in preventing episodes of PLE following a treatment course, and that it was possibly be more effective in reducing post-treatment subjective PLE severity scores. PUVA is more effective than broadband UVB.[24]

Drawbacks

Both TL-01 UVB and PUVA produced PLE during the treatment course in about half of those treated.[23] High cumulative PUVA exposures administered to psoriasis patients increase the risk of later development of skin cancers, particularly squamous cell carcinomas.[25] Although the risks with UVB have not been well defined, it is probable that high cumulative UVB exposure will also result in some increased skin cancer risk (but less than with PUVA).

Comments

The analysis of each of these studies comparing PUVA with UVB (narrowband and broadband) as prophylactic therapies for PLE took into account natural UV exposure measured with polysulfone badges after the treatment courses. Even with randomization (methods for which were not defined in either paper), differences in subsequent sunlight seeking or avoidance behavior in the groups compared could have influenced the findings. Insufficient raw data were presented to allow retrospective calculations of the power of either study. Nevertheless, it can be safely concluded that PUVA is not much more effective than TL-01 UVB, and may even be less effective.

Implications for practice

TL-01 UVB is the prophylactic phototherapy of choice for patients severely affected by PLE. When this fails to provide useful benefit, or when repeated episodes of PLE are provoked during therapy, PUVA can be considered.

Should corticosteroids be prescribed for a mildly affected patient to use if PLE develops while he or she is on holiday?

Efficacy

A randomized controlled trial of prednisolone 25 mg/day in a presumably mildly affected group (only 10 of 21 patients needed to take the study drug while on vacation) showed that it had an effect. PLE resolved more quickly (by a mean of 3.6 days; 95% CI, 0.6 to 6.1 days) with prednisolone than with placebo, despite the fact that for this study patients were encouraged to continue sun exposure after they developed PLE.[26]

It is unclear whether moderately potent or potent topical steroids help to suppress established PLE, but potent topical steroids may be of value prophylactically if applied immediately after exposure.[27]

Drawbacks

One of 10 patients who took a short course of oral prednisolone for PLE experienced "mild gastrointestinal disturbance and slight depression of mood."[26]

Comments

For most patients with mild PLE, it is doubtful whether the small improvement produced by systemic prednisolone is sufficient to outweigh concerns about side effects. We do not know whether a potent topical steroid is of benefit for established PLE, but as systemic steroids have an effect it is possible that, at least for some patients, this may be beneficial.

Implications for practice

Corticosteroids can have a small to modest effect on established PLE. While there is a lack of evidence that topical steroids have a similar effect, it may be appropriate to prescribe a potent topical steroid to use if PLE develops for patients whose problem is mild and confined to episodes induced by holiday sunlight.

Can HLA class II typing distinguish PLE from actinic prurigo?

Actinic prurigo is strongly associated with HLA-DR4, and particularly HLA-DRB1*0407 in the UK[19,20] and Mexico.[28]

Comments

Polymorphic light eruption is distinguished from actinic prurigo on the basis of history and clinical features. The finding of a strong HLA association with actinic prurigo, but not PLE, strengthened the evidence that these are distinct diseases. A study to determine the value of HLA class II typing as a diagnostic test in cases of clinical uncertainty about the diagnosis has not been performed, but such testing could be helpful.

Implications for practice

In cases in which the diagnosis is in doubt, a negative HLA-DR4 test makes actinic prurigo less likely than PLE, while a positive HLA-DR4 is of limited value, as this antigen is common (about 25%) in most populations. A positive HLA-DRB1*0407 test (rare in most populations) may help to rule in a diagnosis of actinic prurigo (and exclude PLE), whereas a negative test result (found in almost 40% of UK cases of actinic prurigo) is of limited value.

Key points

- PLE can improve over the years. This improvement may be spontaneous or partly due to repeated prophylactic phototherapy.
- Narrowband UVB and PUVA are similarly effective in preventing episodes of PLE.
- Oral prednisolone has a small or modest beneficial effect in PLE.
- Is not clear whether topical corticosteroids are of help in suppression of established PLE.
- HLA typing may occasionally be helpful in classifying a photodermatosis with features of both PLE and actinic prurigo.

References

1 Elpern DJ, Morison WL, Hood AF. Papulovesicular light eruption: a defined subset of polymorphous light eruption. *Arch Dermatol* 1985;**121**:1286–8.

2 Holzle E, Plewig G, von Kries R, Lehmann P. Polymorphous light eruption. *J Invest Dermatol* 1987;**88**(Suppl 3):32–8.

3 Dover JS, Hawk JLM. Polymorphic light eruption sine eruptione. *Br J Dermatol* 1988;**118**:73–6.

4 Morison WL, Stern RS. Polymorphous light eruption: a common reaction uncommonly recognized. *Acta Derm Venereol* 1982;**62**:237–40.

5 Millard TP, Bataille V, Snieder H, Spector TD, McGregor JM. The heritability of polymorphic light eruption. *J Invest Dermatol* 2000;**115**:467–70.

6 Ros AM, Wennersten G. Current aspects of polymorphous light eruptions in Sweden. *Photodermatology* 1986;**3**:298–302.

7 Pao C, Norris PG, Corbett M, Hawk JLM. Polymorphic light eruption: prevalence in Australia and England. *Br J Dermatol* 1994;**130**:62–4.

8 Olumide YM. Photodermatoses in Lagos. *Int J Dermatol* 1987;**26**:295–9.

9 Khoo SW, Tay YK, Tham SN. Photodermatoses in a Singapore skin referral centre. *Clin Exp Dermatol* 1996;**21**:263–8.

10 Norris PG, Morris J, McGibbon DM, Chu AC, Hawk JL. Polymorphic light eruption: an immunopathological study of evolving lesions. *Br J Dermatol* 1989;**120**:173–83.

11 Hasan T, Ranki A, Jansen CT, Karvonen J. Disease associations in polymorphous light eruption: a long-term follow-up study of 94 patients. *Arch Dermatol* 1998;**134**:1081–5.

12 Murphy GM, Hawk JL. The prevalence of antinuclear antibodies in patients with apparent polymorphic light eruption. *Br J Dermatol* 1991;**125**:448–51.

13 Panet-Raymond G, Johnson WC. Lupus erythematosus and polymorphous light eruption: differentiation by histochemical procedures. *Arch Dermatol* 1973;**108**:785–7.

14 Weedon D. Polymorphous light eruption. In: Weedon D. *Skin Pathology*. Edinburgh: Churchill Livingstone, 1997: 509–10.

15 Green C, Norris PG, Hawk JL. Photoallergic contact dermatitis from oxybenzone aggravating polymorphic light eruption. *Contact Dermatitis* 1991;**24**:62–3.

16 Bilsland D, Ferguson J. Contact allergy to sunscreen chemicals in photosensitivity dermatitis/actinic reticuloid syndrome (PD/AR) and polymorphic light eruption (PLE). *Contact Dermatitis* 1993;**29**:70–3.

17 Thune P. Contact and photocontact allergy to sunscreens. *Photodermatology* 1984;**1**:5–9.

18 Allan SJR, Ray RE, Savin JA. The optimal management of polymorphic light eruption in a non-photobiological unit. *J Dermatol Treat* 1999;**10**:3–6.

19 Grabczynska SA, McGregor JM, Kondeatis E, Vaughan RW, Hawk JLM. Actinic prurigo and polymorphic light eruption: common pathogenesis and the importance of HLA-DR4/DRB1*0407. *Br J Dermatol* 1999;**140**: 232–6.

20 Dawe RS, Collins P, O'Sullivan A, Ferguson J. Actinic prurigo and HLA-DR4 1. *J Invest Dermatol* 1997;**108**: 233–4.

21 Leroy D, Dompmartin A, Faguer K, Michel M, Verneuil L. Polychromatic phototest as a prognostic tool for polymorphic light eruption. *Photodermatol Photoimmunol Photomed* 2000;**16**:161–6.

22 Man I, Dawe RS, Ferguson J. Artificial hardening for polymorphic light eruption: practical points from ten years' experience. *Photodermatol Photoimmunol Photomed* 1999;**15**:96–9.

23 Bilsland D, George SA, Gibbs NK, Aitchison T, Johnson BE, Ferguson J. A comparison of narrow band phototherapy (TL-01) and photochemotherapy (PUVA) in the management of polymorphic light eruption. *Br J Dermatol* 1993;**129**:708–12.

24 Murphy GM, Logan RA, Lovell CR, Morris RW, Hawk JL, Magnus IA. Prophylactic PUVA and UVB therapy in polymorphic light eruption: a controlled trial. *Br J Dermatol* 1987;**116**:531–8.

25 Stern RS, Lunder EJ. Risk of squamous cell carcinoma and methoxsalen (psoralen) and UV-A radiation (PUVA): a meta-analysis. *Arch Dermatol* 1998;**134**: 1582–5.

26 Patel DC, Bellaney GJ, Seed PT, McGregor JM, Hawk JLM. Efficacy of short-course oral prednisolone in polymorphic light eruption: a randomized controlled trial. *Br J Dermatol* 2000;**143**: 828–31.

27 Man I, Dawe RS, Ibbotson SH, Ferguson J. Is topical steroid effective in polymorphic light eruption? *Br J Dermatol* 2000;**143**(Suppl 57): 113.

28 Hojyo-Tomoka T, Granados J, Vargas-Alarcon G, *et al.* Further evidence of the role of HLA-DR4 in the genetic susceptibility to actinic prurigo. *J Am Acad Dermatol* 1997;**36**:935–7.

64

Infantile hemangiomas and port-wine stains

Kapila Batta, Sean W. Lanigan

Infantile hemangiomas

Background (Figure 64.1)

Definition

Infantile hemangiomas (IHs) are benign endothelial tumors that characteristically have an initial rapid proliferative and later slower involutional phase. Superficial IHs are the most common type and have the characteristic bright strawberry red color. Deep IHs lie deeper in the dermis and subcutis and appear as bluish soft swellings with little involvement of the overlying skin. IHs frequently have both superficial and deep components. Extracutaneous IHs will not be discussed in this chapter.

Incidence/prevalence

The estimated incidence in white children is 1.1–2.6% at birth,[1,2] rising to 10% at 1 year of age.[3,4] The true incidence is not known, as they are often not present at birth, and the few prospective studies that have been conducted have methodological flaws and were undertaken prior to the accurate classification of vascular birthmarks. IHs are three times more common in females and less common in black[5] and Japanese[6] infants. They are more common in premature infants and those with low birth weight; the incidence has been reported to be as high as 20% in premature infants with a birth weight of less than 1000 g.[7,8]

Etiology

The etiology of IHs is not well understood, but one current theory is that IHs have a placental origin. Immunohistochemical studies have shown that IHs share several unique markers with placental blood vessels, including glucose transporter protein-1 (GLUT-1). These findings have led to speculation that IHs may arise from embolization of placental cells, or that vascular precursor cells may aberrantly differentiate towards the placental vascular phenotype.[9] Other theories on their origin include a mutation in

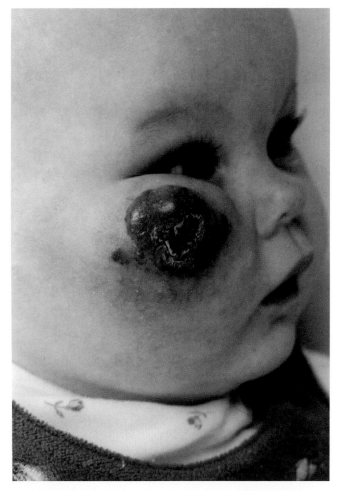

Figure 64.1 In this 4-month-old child, a red mark was first noted on the right cheek at the age of 3 days. The mark grew rapidly during the first few months, despite early laser treatment. The mixed superficial and deep hemangioma involved the infraorbital area and ulcerated at the age of 3 months. As it was growing rapidly close to the eye and was likely to leave residual deformity, it was treated with a course of oral prednisolone, with stabilization of growth. Ophthalmic assessments were normal. The ulceration healed with wound care. At the age of 4 years, there was a residual fibroadipose structure, which was surgically corrected.

a cytokine regulatory pathway, developmental field defects, and a derangement of angiogenesis.[10]

Prognosis

IHs are clinically heterogeneous with regard to growth characteristics and involution. Some barely grow at all, while others reach very large sizes. Their exact behavior is very difficult to predict, particularly in early infancy. Superficial IHs usually reach their maximum size by 6–8 months, but deep IHs may proliferate for longer. The majority of IHs will resolve with minimal or no residual changes and without complications. Hospital-based studies have shown that approximately 50% have resolved by the age of 5 years, 75% by the age of 7 years, and 90% by the age of 10 years,[11] although involution may be complete by 2–3 years. It is estimated that at least 20% of IHs will leave residual changes in the skin. These include skin pallor, telangiectasia, atrophic wrinkling, or altered skin texture.[12] More significant changes are redundant skin with underlying residual fibrofatty tissue, which may need surgical correction, or scarring due to ulceration. IHs in hair-bearing areas may leave scarring alopecia. These residual changes may cause psychosocial problems at school age. IHs at certain sites, such as the lips, nose, and parotid, and large facial lesions with deep components are particularly slow to involute and more likely to leave permanent scarring.[13]

A minority of IHs, particularly at certain locations, may develop complications. These include painful ulceration, infection, and bleeding. Periorbital IHs are at risk of ophthalmological complications, the most serious of which is amblyopia. Lesions obstructing other vital structures, such as the nose, mouth, and auditory canal, may also cause complications.

Diagnostic tests

In most cases, the diagnosis of IHs can be made clinically, but imaging studies such as magnetic resonance imaging (MRI), ultrasonography, and even biopsy may be required for atypical cases. MRI scanning is also useful to define the extent of IH. Although not discussed in this chapter, certain presentations of IH are indicators of systemic associations and require further investigations. These associations include large segmental plaque-like facial IHs with PHACE(S) syndrome (posterior fossa malformations, hemangioma, arterial anomalies, coarctation of the aorta and cardiac defects, eye abnormalities, sternal defects), midline lumbosacral IHs with spinal dysraphism and genitourinary abnormalities, beard IHs with airway hemangiomas, and multiple cutaneous IHs with visceral involvement, particularly of the liver.[12]

Aims of treatment

The aims of treatment are clearance of IHs with no or minimal scarring before school age, when psychosocial morbidity from residual lesions is most likely to be a problem; to reduce complications such as ulceration and obstruction of vital structures; and to select the most appropriate therapy for complicated IHs.

Relevant outcomes

- Clearance before school age
- Parental assessment of clearance
- Residual skin changes such as skin hypopigmentation, atrophy, fibrofatty tissue, telangiectasia
- Objective measures of resolution, such as redness, surface area, height
- Incidence of complications such as ulceration
- Improvement in complications

Methods of research

The Cochrane Library to issue 1, 2006, and Medline and Pubmed until May 2006 were searched for terms including hemangiomas and treatment. Abstracts were read and all potentially relevant studies were obtained in hard copy.

Questions

Does early pulsed dye laser treatment of uncomplicated IHs result in fewer complications and a better long-term cosmetic outcome in comparison with leaving the lesions untreated and waiting for natural resolution?

The pulsed dye laser (PDL) is the gold standard treatment for port-wine stains. However, its use in IHs has been more controversial. A single prospective randomized controlled trial (RCT) compared early PDL treatment with a wait-and-see policy in 121 children with a median age of 5 weeks.[14] Sixty infants were assigned to PDL and 61 to observation, and they were followed up to 1 year of age. The number of lesions completely clear or almost clear at 1 year did not differ significantly between the PDL-treated and observation groups (42% vs. 44%; $P = 0.92$). The frequency of complications was similar in the two groups. The most common complication, ulceration, occurred in 7% of both groups. The only objective measure of resolution that improved with PDL treatment was hemangioma redness. The number of children whose parents considered the hemangioma to be a problem at 1 year was similar in both groups, and an independent parent panel validated this result.

Several uncontrolled studies had previously claimed advantages for early PDL treatment. A prospective study of 165 children with 225 separate IHs at varying stages reported their results with PDL.[15] The mean follow-up period was 5 months. Of the 153 flat IHs, 34% completely cleared and 52% had good results (defined as slower involution or incomplete lightening). Treatment was less successful in treating deeper lesions. In a retrospective series of 617 early or proliferating IHs treated with PDL, assessments were made from documentation in case notes or questionnaires sent to parents with infants at ages varying from 0 to 55 months. Complete or marked regression was achieved in 28.7% of all lesions and approximately 60% of small superficial lesions.[16]

Drawbacks

The results of the RCT showed that there was an increased risk of skin atrophy (28% vs. 8%; $P = 0.008$) and hypopigmentation (45% vs. 9%; $P = 0.001$) in the PDL-treated group.[14] These residual skin changes can be seen in naturally resolved IHs and may have been noted earlier in the treated group. In the 7% of IHs that ulcerated in the treated group, this complication developed immediately after the first treatment, suggesting that laser skin injury may have caused this. Other studies have also noted ulceration and atrophic scarring in previously intact hemangiomas treated with PDL.[17,18]

Comments

This RCT[14] used a variety of outcome measures that are likely to be important to children and parents, including clear definitions of clearance, parental assessments, objective quantitative measures of resolution, complications, and blinded assessment of photographs by a panel of parents. The results were assessed at 1 year of age and showed no useful benefit of PDL in early uncomplicated lesions. This suggests that IHs that have responded well to PDL in uncontrolled studies[15,16] are likely to be superficial lesions that would have shown excellent natural resolution. Extensive facial and eyelid IHs were excluded due to ethical difficulties, but the poor results seen in this RCT suggest that they are also unlikely to benefit from early PDL. Treatment did significantly reduce redness at 1 year. However, PDL is already widely accepted as a treatment for erythema or telangiectasias that remain after natural resolution of IHs,[15,19,20] and treatment is best undertaken at this later stage if necessary.

The children in this RCT were treated with traditional 585-nm PDL with a pulse width of 0.45 ms.[14] PDLs with wavelengths of up to 600 nm, pulse widths of up to 1.5 ms, and attached cooling devices are available, but no further RCTs with these newer lasers have been undertaken.

Implications for clinical practice

There is no useful benefit of early PDL treatment in uncomplicated hemangiomas. In addition, treated lesions are at increased risk of skin atrophy, hypopigmentation, and possible ulceration. PDL is likely to be effective for removing any residual erythema after spontaneous involution.

What are the most effective treatments for ulcerated IHs?

Ulceration is the most common complication of IHs, occur-

ring in 5–13% of lesions.[17] The nappy and perioral areas are the most frequent sites, probably because of recurrent friction, maceration, and—in the case of the perineum—repeated exposure to urine and feces. Ulceration can lead to other significant complications, including pain, scarring, infection, and bleeding. Several treatments have been reported to be effective, but none have been tested in a prospective RCT.

Although no trials have been undertaken, most physicians would agree that the first-line treatment is local wound care and pain management, which may be the only treatment required. Wound care includes gentle cleaning and application of topical antibiotics, barrier creams, and occlusive dressings. In a retrospective study of 60 ulcerated IHs, metronidazole gel or mupirocin were the preferred topical antibiotics.[17] A variety of occlusive dressings were advocated, including DuoDerm, Tegaderm, and Allevyn. In areas where dressing adherence was difficult, such as the anus, Vaseline-impregnated gauze was found to be helpful. In one case series of eight ulcerated IHs, prompt pain relief and healing was reported within 1–2 months with the use of a polyurethane film dressing.[21]

Treatment of ulcerated IHs with PDL has been found to speed healing and reduce pain in several case series. A prospective case series of 78 children with ulcerated IHs treated with PDL alone at 3–4-week intervals showed a 91% response rate and a mean of only two treatments needed for healing.[22] Morelli et al. treated 37 infants with ulcerated hemangiomas with the PDL at 2-week intervals.[23] All healed within three treatments and 68% healed within 2 weeks following a single treatment. Pain also subjectively decreased within days of a single treatment. However, one retrospective analysis reported only a 50% response rate in 22 ulcerated IHs.[17]

A topical platelet-derived growth factor, becaplermin gel, which is licensed for diabetic neuropathic ulcers, has been reported to be effective in a retrospective case series of eight ulcerated IHs.[24] In three cases, this was the only medication used; two patients had had previous wound care and three had had previous wound care and corticosteroid treatment. All eight patients healed within 3–21 days, with an average of 10 days.

Corticosteroids and surgery are also considered treatment options in resistant cases,[19] but have not be assessed specifically in ulcerated IHs.

Drawbacks

In the retrospective review of 22 ulcerated IHs treated with PDL, one definitely worsened.[17]

Comments

Although PDL has been reported to be effective in ulcerated IHs, many of the lesions in these large case series had not previously been managed with local wound care treatment and might have healed with this conservative treatment alone. RCTs comparing first-line local wound care treatment with other therapies such as PDL or becaplermin gel are required in order to assess their efficacy.

Interpretation

The first-line treatment of ulcerated IHs is local wound care. PDL has been shown to be of benefit in uncontrolled studies and should be considered in refractory cases. Becaplermin gel may be beneficial and could also be considered in resistant cases.

Are corticosteroids effective in the treatment of problematic IHs, and what are the optimum doses, treatment regimens, and methods of delivery?

IHs that are interfering with normal function, usually because of their location (e.g., vision, feeding) or are cosmetically disfiguring and unlikely to spontaneously involute, or otherwise problematic (e.g., ulceration refractory to other therapies) require treatment, usually with corticosteroids, during the proliferative growth phase.

Oral corticosteroids. There are no RCTs, but several case series have been published. A meta-analysis of 10 case series with 184 patients analyzed the efficacy of systemic steroids in the treatment of cutaneous IHs.[25] A mean prednisolone dose equivalent to 2.9 mg/kg given over 1.8 months before tapering had a response rate (defined as "shrinkage or cessation of growth of an actively growing IH coincident with initiation of systemic corticosteroid therapy") of 84%. The mean rate of rebound growth after treatment cessation was 36%. A significant difference was found between the mean dose administered to responders and nonresponders. Doses of 2–3 mg/kg resulted in a 75% response; this increased to 94% at more than 3 mg/kg/day, but with greater adverse effects.

Intralesional and topical corticosteroids. There are no RCTs, but most specialists agree that intralesional corticosteroids are best used for smaller localized problematic lesions. Many authors use 40 mg/mL triamcinolone acetonide combined with either 6 mg/mL betamethasone or 4 mg dexamethasone, which can be repeated a few times at 4–8-weekly intervals.[26] Others recommend triamcinolone alone at a 10–20 mg/mL concentration to a maximum dosage of 3–5 mg/kg per treatment session.[12] There are several case series, mainly from the ophthalmology literature, that report benefit based on reduced size and visual complications. A study by Kushner reviewed 25 periorbital IHs treated with intralesional corticosteroids; 84% showed a marked or moderate response based on estimated lesion size at least 6 months after the first injection.[27] The incidence of amblyopia or strabismus was 16%. A study by Morrell and Wilshaw showed that 81.5% of 27 patients with

periorbital IHs treated with intralesional steroids experienced marked improvement, with the lesion reducing to 25% or less of its original size, while 53.8% showed a marked reduction in astigmatism.[28] A nonrandomized study compared four conservatively treated and five steroid-injected patients with periorbital IHs who were at risk of amblyopia due to astigmatism and concluded that the visual outcomes were similar.[29] A literature review of corticosteroid treatment of periorbital hemangiomas found that few studies measured relevant ophthalmological outcomes.[30] Only 28 patients from four case series met the inclusion criteria; 23 received intralesional steroids and five received topical corticosteroids. Patients receiving intralesional steroids tended to have reduced astigmatism at the follow-up examinations. The efficacy of intralesional steroids at other sites, based on a reduction in volume, has been reported in a retrospective case series of 155 hemangiomas of the head and neck. After a mean follow-up of 40 months, 84.5% showed greater than 50% reduction in volume; the best response was seen in superficial IHs.[31]

There are three case series on the use of topical steroids in the management of IHs. In two small series including three and five patients with vision-threatening periorbital IHs, topical clobetasol propionate was used, with a reduction in the size of the IHs and clearing of the visual axis.[32,33] However, the authors noted that topical treatment was not as successful as intralesional steroids, with only one of five patients in one series having a reduced refractive error after treatment.[33] A larger case series of 34 infants with IHs at various sites used potent and very potent topical corticosteroids and showed that 35% had a good response (defined as two of the following: cessation of growth, shrinkage or flattening, and lightening of the surface color) during a follow-up period of up to 18 months.[34]

Drawbacks

The average incidence of side effects in the meta-analysis of systemic corticosteroid treatment was 35%—most commonly behavior changes, irritability, a cushingoid appearance, and transient growth delay.[25] One patient was reported to have osteoporosis, but no other serious long-term side effects were seen. Boon *et al.* retrospectively evaluated the side effects of systemic corticosteroid therapy in 62 children with problematic IHs, from case notes and questionnaires sent to parents.[35] The initial prednisolone dosage was 2–3 mg/kg/day and the treatment period ranged from 2 to 21 months. Short-term side effects were common, including cushingoid facies in 71%, personality changes in 29%, gastric irritation in 21%, fungal infection in 6%, hypertension in 2%, diminished height gain in 35%, and diminished weight gain in 42%. One child developed corticosteroid myopathy, which resolved by 6 years of age. Another retrospective study of 22 infants found hypertension in 45% and evidence of hypothalamic–pituitary–adrenal axis suppression in 87%.[36]

Serious local complications with injections into periocular lesions have been described in case reports, including retinal artery occlusion[37] and eyelid necrosis.[38] Minor reversible complications include hematomas,[27] eyelid depigmentation,[39] dystrophic periocular calcification,[40] and linear subcutaneous atrophy.[41] Adrenal suppression has also been documented with intralesional corticosteroids.[42]

Comments
No RCTs are available comparing corticosteroid treatment with observation, and it is therefore not possible to exclude spontaneous stabilization of treated lesions. However, it would be difficult compare treatment with observation in complicated IHs. RCTs are required in order to confirm the response and determine the optimum dosage, tapering regimens, and adverse effects of oral corticosteroids. There have been no comparative RCTs of oral, topical, and intralesional corticosteroids to establish which route of administration is safer and more effective.

Interpretation
Analysis of case series suggests that oral corticosteroids are effective for problematic IHs and that the optimum dosage is 2–3 mg/kg prednisolone. Careful monitoring for side effects, including growth charts and hypertension assessment, is required. Intralesional corticosteroids are probably effective for localized problematic lesions. Special care should be taken in the periorbital area, as serious complications have been reported. The efficacy of topical corticosteroids is unclear.

Key points: infantile hemangiomas

- IHs are completely heterogeneous with regard to growth characteristics and involution and many are self-limiting. However, only one study has compared an active treatment with observation in an RCT.
- There are no RCTs comparing treatments for complicated IHs, and all the evidence comes from case series.
- Many investigators have used short-term outcome measures, although it is the long-term results that are clinically meaningful for children and parents.
- There is no useful benefit of early PDL treatment in uncomplicated IHs. PDL is likely to improve residual erythema after spontaneous involution.
- Evidence from case series suggests that PDL may be effective for ulcerated IHs that have failed to respond to local wound care.
- Evidence from case series suggests that oral corticosteroids are effective for problematic IHs and that the optimum dose is 2–3 mg/kg/day prednisolone. Intralesional corticosteroids are likely to be of benefit for localized problematic lesions, but special care is needed in the periorbital area.

Treatment for port-wine stains

Background

Definition
Port-wine stains (PWSs) are benign vascular birthmarks that consist of abnormal, ectatic capillaries in the superficial dermis.

Incidence/prevalence
PWSs affect 0.3% of the population. Unlike strawberry hemangiomas, PWSs do not involute and persist throughout life.

Etiology
Although defined as vascular birthmarks, PWSs are thought to be due to a deficiency of perivascular nerve endings, leading to passive dilation of the dermal capillaries.

Prognosis
PWSs are usually flat and pink during infancy, becoming darker, more purple, and nodular with advancing age. They can lead to significant morbidity, especially when they are located over the face.

Aims of treatment
Treatment is aimed at improving the appearance of the affected skin by eradicating the nevus or significantly lightening the color. Secondary aims are the prevention of hypertrophic changes seen in adults with untreated PWSs.

Relevant outcomes
Measurable outcomes after treatment have mainly involved subjective visual assessment of improvement by an observer in comparison with baseline color photography.

Quantifiable measurement of improvement involves methods of recording changes in redness or hemoglobin content, such as reflectance spectrophotometry and spectrophotometric intracutaneous analysis (SIAscopy), or through visualization of blood vessels by video microscopy.

Search methods
A search of the Cochrane Library database was made for randomized controlled trials and systematic reviews for port-wine stains and treatment, or laser treatment, or pulsed dye laser treatment, as pulsed dye laser treatment is considered the current treatment of choice.

Questions

How does laser treatment improve the appearance of PWS?
Lasers deliver powerful and short bursts of light of a single wavelength. Most lasers produce light in the ultraviolet,

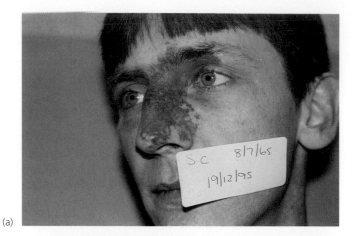

(a)

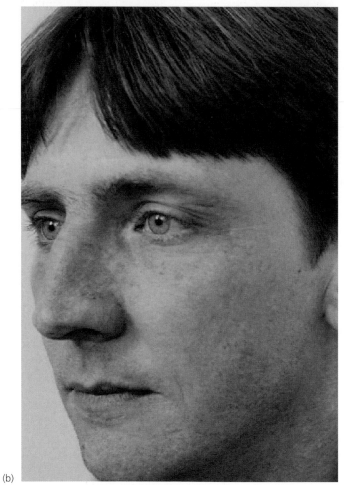

(b)

Figure 64.2 Port wine stain (a) on face before and (b) after pulsed dye laser treatment.

visible, or infrared spectrum. The light energy is absorbed by target structures in the skin and converted to heat energy, which produces the desired effect. Different targets absorb different colors of light. When the appropriate color is chosen, thermal damage is restricted to target structures, sparing surrounding tissue. The main targets in the skin are oxyhemoglobin, melanin, and water.

Another important laser parameter is pulse duration, which is the duration of each burst of energy. Small structures, such as tattoo particles, heat up and cool down quickly and need energy in small bursts lasting nanoseconds. Large structures such as hair shafts heat up more slowly and need energy in milliseconds. For PWS treatment, laser light is absorbed by hemoglobin within ectatic vessels. The pulse duration of around 1 ms allows damage to be confined to the capillary wall.

Which lasers improve the appearance of PWS?

Currently, the main lasers used for the treatment of vascular lesions, including port-wine stains, are the pulsed dye laser (PDL) and the potassium titanyl phosphate (KTP) laser. Recent work has also demonstrated that long-pulsed alexandrite and neodymium–yttrium aluminum garnet (Nd:YAG) lasers at 1064 nm may be valuable in the treatment of hypertrophic PWS.

The flashlamp pulsed dye laser (PDL) was the first laser specifically designed for selective photothermolysis of cutaneous blood vessels and is considered to be the best laser for the treatment overall of a population of patients with PWS, although individuals may benefit from other lasers. The PDL produces yellow light at 577 or 585 nm. Most lasers emit the longer wavelength, which has greater depth of penetration and retains vascular selectivity. The pulse duration was fixed at 450 ms.

A number of studies have reported on the efficacy of the PDL in the treatment of PWS. Results are generally reported in terms of lightening the PWS rather than clearance, as complete clearance only occurs in the minority. The vast majority of studies use subjective criteria for improvement in comparison with baseline photography. There are no placebo-controlled studies, nor any randomized prospective clinical trials using other nonlaser treatments. Approximately 40% of patients with PWS achieved 75% lightening or more after laser treatment, and more than 80% of PWSs lightened by at least 50%. Several prognostic criteria have been put forward to assist in predicting the outcome of treatment. Some authors have reported the best results in pink lesions,[43] while others have reported better results in red lesions.[44] In a study of 261 patients treated over a 5-year period, the color of PWSs was not found to be a prognostic value.[45]

Two features that may affect outcome are the site of the PWS and the size of the nevus. PWSs on the face and neck respond better than those on the leg and hand.[46] On the face, PWSs on the forehead and lateral face respond better than those centrally.[47] The chest, upper arm, and shoulder generally respond well. PWSs less than 20 cm^2 at initial examination cleared more than those greater than 20 cm^2, irrespective of age.[48]

The tunable pulsed dye laser has become the treatment of choice for PWS. However, complete clearance cannot be achieved in the majority of cases, and a significant proportion of lesions are resistant to treatment. In recent years, increased understanding of the interaction between lasers and PWSs has led to modification of the original PDL. The most important modifications include longer pulse widths, longer wavelengths, higher fluences, and use of cooling. Many of these lasers have proved to be useful in the treatment of PWS. Again, most studies use subjective clinical end points, and there are no placebo-controlled trials.

Geronemus et al.[49] used the ScleroLaser, which has a 595-nm wavelength, 1.5-ms pulse width, and fluences up to 11–12 J/cm^2 with a dynamic cooling spray, and obtained greater than 75% clearing of PWS in 10 of 16 patients (63%) after four treatments. All of the patients were children under 12 months of age.

Longer-wavelength lasers, such as alexandrite (755 nm) and Nd:YAG (1064 nm) may have a role in PWS treatment. In the millisecond modes, these lasers have been widely used for hair removal and leg vein telangiectasia. These lasers may have a particular role in the treatment of bulky malformations and mature PWSs, lesions that are typically more resistant to PDL due to the predominance of larger and deeper vessels and higher content of deoxygenated hemoglobin. No et al.[50] used a 3-ms alexandrite laser with dynamic cooling to treat three patients with hypertrophic PWS, using fluences ranging from 30 to 85 J/cm^2. All lesions significantly lightened without side effects.

Intense pulsed light (IPL) has also been used to treat PWS. Unlike laser systems, these flashlamps produce non-coherent broadband light with wavelengths in the range of 515–1200 nm and permit various pulse widths. Filters are used to remove unwanted wavelengths. A study of 37 patients treated with IPL showed subjective clearance of pink and red PWSs and lightening in purple PWS.[51]

Are there comparative studies of laser treatment of PWS?

In a study comparing PDL at 585 nm, 7 mm spot, and 0.45 ms pulse width with a second-generation long-pulsed tunable dye laser (LPTDL) with a 1.5-ms pulse width, 5-mm spot, and wavelength settings ranging from 585 to 600 nm, optimal subjective fading in 30 of 62 patients was seen with the LPTDL in comparison with only 12 patients with the shorter pulse width laser.[52] The authors compensated for the reduced light absorption at longer wavelengths by increasing the fluence.

In another study using a PDL with a wavelength of 600 nm, superior lightening of PWS was seen in 11 of 22 patients in comparison with treatment with 585 nm when compensatory fluences 1.5–2 times higher were used.[53] Blinded investigators assessed the sites of each laser treat-

ment. At equal fluences, 585 nm produces significantly greater lightening than the longer wavelength.

Longer pulse widths, as opposed to the 0.45-ms duration delivered by first-generation PDLs, may be more appropriate for larger-caliber PWS vessels. Longer wavelengths penetrate deeper, allowing targeting of deeper vessels. Higher fluences are needed in part because the wavelength is further from the β absorption peak of oxyhemoglobin.

However, higher fluences increase the potential for epidermal heating due to absorption by epidermal melanin, necessitating the use of cooling devices to minimize epidermal damage (and consequent side effects).

Yang et al.[54] treated 17 patients with PWS, comparing a 595-nm PDL to a long-pulsed Nd:YAG laser with contact cooling. Similar clearance rates were achieved by blinded assessment, and scarring was only noted in one patient in whom fluences exceeded the minimum purpura dose. Patients preferred the Nd:YAG laser because of the shorter recovery period between treatments.

Overall, the findings of various studies with second-generation PDLs and longer-wavelength lasers indicate a modest improvement over the results with first-generation PDLs. Individual patients appear to benefit from the options of varying wavelengths, pulse widths and higher fluences, but there is no evidence from large population studies to suggest significant improvements in the majority of PWSs treated compared with earlier PDLs. In addition, with so many variables uncontrolled in the plethora of small studies, it is often difficult to clarify which modification contributed to improved outcomes.

Can new lasers improve treatment-resistant PWSs?

Further evidence of improved efficacy of second-generation PDLs comes from responses in PWSs that have proven to be resistant to first-generation PDLs. In a case report, PDL treatment with a longer pulse width of 1.5 ms was effective in further lightening a PWS previously resistant to a 0.5-ms PDL.[55] Work using high-fluence long-pulsed dye laser with cryogen cooling (V beam) in the treatment of resistant PWSs has demonstrated that further lightening can be obtained, although this may be at the expense of increased side effects.

Laube et al.[56] treated 12 patients with PWS who had received multiple treatments with a first-generation PDL. Treatments were performed with a long-pulsed dye laser at 600 nm. The test area with the best response in the majority of patients was the setting of highest fluence and shortest pulse–i.e., 14 J/cm^2 and 1.5 ms. Of nine patients who completed the study, three had 50% improvement of their PWSs, and a further three achieved 25–50% lightening. The authors used two objective measures of response: reflectance spectrophotometry and spectrophotometric intracutaneous analysis (SIAscope, Astron Clinica, Cambridge, UK). Both devices provide derived measurements of redness and hemoglobin content in the superficial dermis. Objective measures correlated with the clinical assessments. One patient developed an atrophic scar.

The same group investigated the use of shorter treatment intervals in PDL treatment of resistant PWSs. Blinded observation and reflectance spectrophotometry suggested that short (2-week) treatment intervals might be beneficial.[57]

The Nd:YAG laser is a solid-state laser with a primary wavelength in the infrared range at 1064 nm. A frequency-doubling crystal can be placed in the beam path to emit green light at 532 nm. This is the KTP laser. High fluences are available with this laser, and the pulse durations may be more appropriate for some PWSs. The KTP laser has been shown to produce further lightening in PDL-resistant lesions.[58] In this study, 30 patients with PWSs that had failed to lighten after at least five treatments with PDL were treated with the KTP laser. Subjective assessments were supported by reflectance spectrophotometry and video microscopy. Five patients (17%) had a greater than 50% response. In general, patients preferred the KTP laser, as it led to less discomfort and purpura. However, two patients (7%) developed scarring.

A study comparing the PDL with a frequency-doubled Nd:YAG (KTP) laser showed similar response rates among the 43 patients with regard to observer-rated lightening, but a substantially higher scarring rate with the 532-nm Nd:YAG laser was noted.[59] It would appear that the KTP laser has a role to play in the treatment of PWS, but the long pulses employed with this laser may increase the incidence of adverse effects in comparison with modern PDLs.

The potential role of IPL for treating PDL-resistant PWS has been confirmed by a recent study showing responses in seven of 15 patients previously resistant to PDL, with six patients showing between 75% and 100% improvement, as assessed by nonblinded observers.[60] Twelve patients with PDL-resistant PWSs were treated with an IPL. Some fading was noted by the authors in eight of the 12. The authors point out the limitations of their study, including only 12 patients.[61]

There is a multiplicity of choices of treatment parameters with noncoherent light sources, and further research is necessary to determine the optimum settings.

Evidence summary

The available evidence from published research suggests that pulsed dye lasers using various treatment parameters are of value in improving the appearance of PWS by fading the birthmark. Reasonable expectations are noticeable fading of the birthmark to a "satisfactory" degree as assessed by the treating clinician in the majority, but less than 10% of patients can expect complete clearance. An individual patient may benefit from alteration of the pulsed dye laser parameters or treatment intervals, or from changing to another laser or intense pulsed light source.

As the natural history of PWS is persistence unchanged or with gradual darkening, studies have not included a placebo arm. It has been argued that there is no need for randomized trials of laser treatment for PWSs, as this is a treatment whose effects have been widely accepted on the basis of evidence from case series or nonrandomized trials.[62] However, there are very few published studies in which investigators have attempted to record objective as well as subjective improvement. This is a major weakness in the body of literature relating to the treatment of PWS. Although indirect measurements of PWS response to treatment have been made using laser Doppler flowmetry, video microscopy, thermography, and ultrasound, only color measurements such as reflectance spectrophotometry record what can actually be seen when looking at the patient—i.e., color and brightness.[63]

A study by Currie and Monk[64] comparing intraobserver concordance in three commonly used subjective scoring systems demonstrated that judges could only consistently score results at the extremes of outcome—i.e., poor clearance and excellent (near-clear) clearance. It seems clear from this research that determining the differences in "fair" and "good," or between > 25% to < 75% lightening, is relatively meaningless. For comparative studies, greater emphasis should be placed on clearance and failure rates supported by objective measurements.

It may be more important in assessing the outcomes of laser treatment for PWS to assess patient-reported measures, which are infrequently recorded. Gupta and Bisland[65] have attempted this with standardized questionnaires, and future work should assess the correlation between observer-rated and subjectively rated outcomes against the reduction in patient morbidity levels.

References

1 Jacobs AH, Walton RG. The incidence of birthmarks in the neonate. *Pediatrics* 1976;**58**:218–22.

2 Pratt AG. Birthmarks in infants. *Arch Dermatol* 1953;**67**:302–5.

3 Jacobs AH. Strawberry nevi: natural history of the untreated lesion. *Calif Med* 1957;**86**:8–10.

4 Holmdahl K. Cutaneous hemangiomas in premature and mature infants. *Acta Paediatr* 1955;**44**:370–9.

5 Alper JC, Holmes LB. The incidence and significance of birthmarks in a cohort of 4641 newborns. *Pediatr Dermatol* 1983;**1**:58–68.

6 Hidano A, Nakajma S. Earliest features of the strawberry mark in the newborn. *Br J Dermatol* 1972;**87**:138–44.

7 Powell TG, West CR, Pharoah PO, Cooke RW. Epidemiology of strawberry haemangioma in low birthweight infants. *Br J Dermatol* 1987;**116**:635–41.

8 Amir J, Metzker A, Krikler R, Reisner SH. Strawberry hemangioma in preterm infants. *Pediatr Dermatol* 1986;**3**:331–2.

9 North PE, Waner M, Mizeracki A, *et al.* A unique microvascular phenotype shared by juvenile hemangiomas and human placenta. *Arch Dermatol* 2001;**137**:559–70.

10 Bauland CG, van Steensel MA, Steijlen PM, Rieu PN, Spauwen PH. The pathogenesis of hemangiomas: a review. *Plast Reconstr Surg* 2006;**117**:29e–35e.

11 Bowers RE, Graham EA, Tomlinson KM. The natural history of the strawberry nevus. *Arch Dermatol* 1960;**82**:667–80.

12 Bruckner AL, Frieden IJ. Hemangiomas of infancy. *J Am Acad Dermatol* 2003;**48**:477–93.

13 Frieden IJ. Management of hemangiomas. Special symposium. *Pediatr Dermatol* 1997;**14**:57–83.

14 Batta K, Goodyear HM, Moss C, Williams HC, Hiller L, Waters R. Randomised controlled study of early pulsed dye laser treatment of uncomplicated childhood haemangiomas: results of a 1-year analysis. *Lancet* 2002;**360**:521–7.

15 Poetke M, Philipp C, Berlien HP. Flashlamp-pumped pulsed dye laser for hemangiomas in infancy: treatment of superficial vs mixed hemangiomas. *Arch Dermatol* 2000;**136**:628–32.

16 Hohenleutner S, Bandur-Ganter E, Landthaler M, Hohenleutner U. Long-term results in the treatment of childhood hemangioma with the flashlamp-pumped pulsed dye laser: an evaluation of 617 cases. *Lasers Surg Med* 2001;**28**:273–7.

17 Kim HJ, Colombo M, Frieden IJ. Ulcerated hemangiomas: clinical characteristics and response to therapy. *J Am Acad Dermatol* 2001;**44**:962–72.

18 Witman PM, Wagner AM, Scherer K, Waner M, Frieden IJ. Complications following pulsed dye laser treatment of superficial hemangiomas. *Lasers Surg Med* 2006;**38**:116–23.

19 Frieden IJ, Haggstrom AN, Drolet BA, *et al.* Infantile hemangiomas: current knowledge, future directions. Proceedings of a research workshop on infantile hemangiomas, April 7–9, 2005, Bethesda, Maryland, USA. *Pediatr Dermatol* 2005;**22**:383–406.

20 Scheepers JH, Quaba AA. Does the pulsed tunable dye laser have a role in the management of infantile hemangiomas? Observations based on 3 years' experience. *Plast Reconstr Surg* 1995;**95**:305–12.

21 Oranje AP, de Waard-van der Spek FB, Devillers AC, de Laat PC, Madern GC. Treatment and pain relief of ulcerative hemangiomas with a polyurethane film. *Dermatology* 2000;**200**:31–4.

22 David LR, Malek MM, Argenta LC. Efficacy of pulse dye laser therapy for the treatment of ulcerated haemangiomas: a review of 78 patients. *Br J Plast Surg* 2003;**56**:317–27.

23 Morelli JG, Tan OT, Yohn JJ, Weston WL. Treatment of ulcerated hemangiomas in infancy. *Arch Pediatr Adolesc Med* 1994;**148**:1104–5.

24 Metz BJ, Rubenstein MC, Levy ML, Metry DW. Response of ulcerated perineal hemangiomas of infancy to becaplermin gel, a recombinant human platelet-derived growth factor. *Arch Dermatol* 2004;**140**:867–70.

25 Bennet ML, Fleisher AB, Chamlin SL, Frieden IJ. Oral corticosteroid use is effective for cutaneous hemangiomas. *Arch Dermatol* 2001;**137**:1208–13.

26 Reyes BA, Vazquez-Botet M, Capo H. Intralesional steroids in cutaneous hemangioma. *J Dermatol Surg Oncol* 1989;**15**:828–32.

27 Kushner BJ. The treatment of periorbital infantile hemangioma with intralesional corticosteroid. *Plast Reconstr Surg* 1985;**76**:517–26.

28 Morrell AJ, Wilshaw HE. Normalisation of refractive error after steroid injections for adnexal haemangiomas. *Br J Ophthamol* 1991;**75**:301–5.

29 Motwani MV, Simon JW, Pickering JD, Catalano RA, Jenkins PL. Steroid injection versus conservative treatment of anisometropia amblyopia in juvenile adnexal hemangioma. *J Pediatr Ophthalmol Strabismus* 1995;**32**:26–8.

30 Ranchod TM, Frieden IJ, Fredrick DR. Corticosteroid treatment of periorbital haemangioma. *Br J Opthalmol* 2005;**89**:1134–8.

31 Chen MT, Yeong EK, Horng SY. Intralesional corticosteroid therapy in proliferating head and neck hemangiomas: a review of 155 cases. *J Pediatr Surg* 2000;**35**:420–3.

32 Cruz OA, Zarnegar SR, Myers SE. Treatment of periocular capillary hemangioma with topical clobetasol propionate. *Ophthalmology* 1995;**102**: 2012–5.

33 Elsas FJ, Lewis AR. Topical treatment of periocular capillary hemangioma. *J Paediatr Ophthalmol Strabismus* 1994;**31**:153–6.

34 Garzon M, Lucky AW, Hawrot A, Friedon IJ. Ultrapotent topical corticosteroid treatment of hemangiomas of infancy. *J Am Acad Dermatol* 2005;**52**:281–6.

35 Boon LM, MacDonald DM, Mulliken JB. Complications of systemic corticosteroid therapy for problematic hemangioma. *Plast Reconstr Surg* 1999;**104**:1616–23.

36 George ME, Sharma V, Jacobson J, Simpson S, Nopper AJ. Adverse effects of systemic of systemic glucocorticosteroid therapy in infants with hemangiomas. *Arch Dermatol* 2004;**140**:963–9.

37 Shorr N, Seiff SR. Central retinal artery occlusion associated with periocular corticosteroid injection for juvenile hemangioma. *Ophthalmic Surg* 1986;**17**:229–31.

38 Sutula FC, Glover AT. Eyelid necrosis following intralesional corticosteroid injection for capillary hemangioma. *Ophthalmic Surg* 1987;**18**:103–5.

39 Cogen MS, Elsas FJ. Eyelid depigmentation following corticosteroid injection for infantile adnexal hemangioma. *J Pediatr Ophthalmol* 1988;**105**:65–9.

40 Carruthers J, Jevon G, Prendiville J. Localized dystrophic periocular calcification: a complication of intralesional corticosteroid therapy for infantile periocular hemangioma. *Pediatr Dermatol* 1998;**15**:23–6.

41 Vasquez-Botet R, Reyes BA, Vasquez-Botet M. Sclerodermiform linear atrophy after the use of intralesional steroids for periorbital hemangiomas: a review of complications. *J Pediatr Ophthalmol Strabismus* 1989;**26**:124–7.

42 Goyal R, Watts P, Lane CM, Beck L, Gregory JW. Adrenal suppression and failure to thrive after steroid injections for periocular hemangioma. *Ophthalmology* 2004;**111**:389–95.

43 Fitzpatrick RE, Lowe NJ, Goldman MP, Borden H, Behr KL, Ruiz-Esparza J. Flashlamp-pumped pulsed dye laser treatment of port-wine stains. *J Dermatol Surg Oncol* 1994;**20**:743–8.

44 Taieb A, Touati L, Cony M, *et al.* Treatment of port-wine stains with the 585-nm flashlamp-pulsed tunable dye laser: a study of 74 patients. *Dermatology* 1994;**188**:276–81.

45 Katugampola GA, Lanigan SW. Five years' experience of treating port wine stains with the flashlamp-pumped pulsed dye laser. *Br J Dermatol* 1997;**137**:750–4.

46 Lanigan SW. Port wine stains on the lower limb: response to pulsed dye laser therapy. *Clin Exp Dermatol* 1996;**21**:88–92.

47 Renfro L, Geronemus RG. Anatomical differences of port-wine stains in response to treatment with the pulsed dye laser. *Arch Dermatol* 1993;**129**:182–8.

48 Morelli JG, Weston WL, Huff JC, Yohn JJ. Initial lesion size as a predictive factor in determining the response of port-wine stains

in children treated with the pulsed dye laser. *Arch Pediatr Adolesc Med* 1995;**149**:1142–4.

49 Geronemus RG, Quintana AT, Lou WW, Kauvar AN. High-fluence modified pulsed dye laser photocoagulation with dynamic cooling of port wine stains in infancy. *Arch Dermatol* 2000;**136**:942–3.

50 No D, Dierickx C, McClaren M, Chotzen V, Kilmer S. Pulsed alexandrite treatment of bulky vascular malformations. *Lasers Surg Med* 2003;**15**(Suppl):26.

51 Raulin C, Schroeter CA, Weiss RA, Keiner M, Werner S. Treatment of port-wine stains with a noncoherent pulsed light source: a retrospective study. *Arch Dermatol* 1999;**135**:679–83.

52 Scherer K, Lorenz S, Wimmershoff M, Landthaler M, Hohenleutner U. Both the flashlamp-pumped dye laser and the long-pulsed tunable dye laser can improve results in port-wine stain therapy. *Br J Dermatol* 2001;**145**:79–84.

53 Edstrom DW, Ros AM. The treatment of port wine stains with the pulsed dye laser at 600 nm. *Br J Dermatol* 1997;**136**:360–3.

54 Yang MU, Yaroslavsky AN, Farinelli WA, *et al.* Long-pulsed neodymium:yttrium-aluminum-garnet laser treatment for port-wine stains. *J Am Acad Dermatol* 2005;**52**:480–90.

55 Bernstein EF. Treatment of a resistant port-wine stain with the 1.5-msec pulse duration, tunable, pulsed dye laser. *Dermatol Surg* 2000;**26**:1007–9.

56 Laube S, Taibjee SM, Lanigan SW. Treatment of resistant port wine stains with the V Beam pulsed dye laser. *Lasers Surg Med* 2003;**33**:282–7.

57 Tomson N, Lim SP, Abdullah A, Lanigan SW. The treatment of port-wine stains with the pulsed-dye laser at 2-week and 6-week intervals: a comparative study. *Br J Dermatol* 2006;**154**:676–9.

58 Chowdhury MM, Harris S, Lanigan SW. Potassium titanyl phosphate laser treatment of resistant port-wine stains. *Br J Dermatol* 2001;**144**:814–7.

59 Lorenz S, Scherer K, Wimmershoff MB, Landthaler M, Hohenleutner U. Variable pulse frequency-doubled Nd:YAG laser versus flashlamp-pumped pulsed dye laser in the treatment of port wine stains. *Acta Derm Venereol* 2003;**83**:210–3.

60 Bjerring P, Christiansen K, Troilius A. Intense pulsed light source for the treatment of dye laser resistant port-wine stains. *J Cosmet Laser Ther* 2003;**5**:7–13.

61 Reynolds N, Exley J, Hills S, Falder S, Duff C, Kenealy J. The role of the Lumina intense pulsed light system in the treatment of port wine stains—a case controlled study. *Br J Plast Surg* 2005;**58**:968–80.

62 Glasziou P, Chalmers I, Rawlins M, McCulloch P. When are randomised trials unnecessary? Picking signal from noise. *BMJ* 2007;**334**:349–51.

63 Lanigan SW. Measuring the improvement in pulsed dye laser treated port wine stains. *Br J Dermatol* 2000;**143**:237–43.

64 Currie CLA, Monk BE. Can the response of port wine stains to laser treatment be reliably assessed using subjective methods? *Br J Dermatol* 2000;**143**:360–4.

65 Gupta G, Bilsland D. A prospective study of the impact of laser treatment on vascular lesions. *Br J Dermatol* 2000;**143**:356–9.

65 Psychocutaneous disease

Dennis Linder

What is psychocutaneous medicine?

Psychocutaneous diseases are conditions often described as lying in between the fields of psychiatry and dermatology. A broader definition encompasses all those skin diseases in which social and/or psychological factors play an important etiopathogenetic role, and/or have important psychological and social implications for the patient.

Taken to an extreme, in a modern, psychosomatic vision of medicine in which psychosocial factors (affecting vulnerability, course, and outcome) are taken into account, in which there is a holistic view of patient care and in which psychological and social interventions in prevention and treatment are considered an option whenever possible,[1] this broader definition might imply considering any skin disease as "psychocutaneous."

This broader understanding of the word "psychocutaneous" is legitimate both because of the tight biological links between the nervous system, the immune system, the endocrine system, and the skin (covering the field of what has been termed "psychoneuroendocrinoimmunodermatology") and because of the relevant psychosocial impact of practically any skin disease. Hence, the practice of psychocutaneous medicine should also be seen as an ethical attitude,[2] rather than just dealing with a particular distinct field of dermatology comprising certain diseases (e.g., trichotillomania for its purely psychogenic origin, or psoriasis for its psychophysiological nature—exacerbation by stress—and heavy psychosocial implications) and excluding others (such as genodermatoses or infectious skin diseases).

From a practical point of view, a working classification of psychocutaneous disease can be based on the one given by Koo and Lee:[3]

• Psychophysiological disorders (such as psoriasis and atopic eczema, etc.) for which sound data at both the epidemiological and biological level are available, showing or making it plausible that exogenous factors (such as "stress") act on the psyche, triggering the disease onset or influencing its course. However, one should be aware that in many skin diseases—such as vitiligo, acne, pemphigus, and others—the influence of exogenous psychological factors such as stress may have been overestimated for some time, as has been shown by Picardi *et al.*[4]

• Primary psychiatric disorders, in which patients may present with self-inflicted skin lesions that are actually due to a primary psychiatric condition (trichotillomania, neurotic excoriations, delusions of parasitosis).

• Secondary psychiatric disorders, which are the consequence of stigmatizing (e.g., psoriasis) or incapacitating conditions (e.g., epidermolysis bullosa). These can include depression or anxiety—e.g., as a consequence of diseases such as psoriasis or vitiligo.

• Cutaneous sensory disorders, such as burning, itching, pain without an apparent organic substrate.

Some primary psychiatric diseases may not necessarily lead to self-inflicted cutaneous lesions; still, it is important to remember that a high percentage of patients with body dysmorphic disorder (BDD), for instance, may consult dermatologists or plastic surgeons. A study in 2000 by Phillips *et al.* estimated the rate of BDD in patients seeking dermatological treatment at about 12%.[5] Similarly, self-smell delusions or delusions of seborrhea can lead psychiatric patients to seek dermatological advice.

Moreover, psychodermatology encompasses skin conditions arising or worsening due to the intake of psychotropic drugs, hence the need for the awareness of possible psychiatric conditions resulting from the intake of dermatological medications (such as confusion deriving from antihistamine intake or the alleged depression and suicidal thoughts caused by isotretinoin—for which no final conclusions have yet been drawn).[6]

Some aspects of dermatology commonly encountered in laboratory research, clinical or epidemiological research, and public health research, or even in daily practice, and not necessarily related to particular diseases are also to be considered domain of psychocutaneous medicine—for instance:

- Advances in "psychoneuroimmunoendocrinodermatology"—exciting and important as these results are, this field has unfortunately not yet engendered practical consequences in clinical dermatology. A better understanding of the deep interconnections between the various functional entities and their pathologies has yet to be translated into a different, less reductionist approach to the diagnosis and therapy of skin diseases.
- Planning and carrying out psycho(socio)logical and educational interventions in chronic skin diseases such as atopic dermatitis and psoriasis, and assessing the efficacy of such interventions.[7]
- Coping with life-threatening skin diseases such as melanoma, with a possible effect on enhanced survival in patients with advanced melanoma receiving adjuvant psychotherapy.
- Lifestyle drugs in dermatology—dermatological drugs applied to "dermatological nondisease."[8]
- Use of psychotropic drugs (such as antidepressants) for treating skin disease.
- Psychological diagnosis (e.g., psychometric tests) in dermatological patients.
- Psychotherapy in dermatology, including psychoanalytic approaches.
- Quality-of-life (QoL) research in dermatology.
- Liaison consultation in dermatology.

The above list shows that psychodermatology, as already mentioned, also involves an ethical attitude to the discipline. From the perspective of psychodermatologists, any part of dermatology can (and should) therefore be approached with an effort to take psychosocial aspects into account.

Clinical psychodermatology

In the absence of a satisfactory, widely applicable epistemological model for psychodermatological issues, most research in the fields concerned has so far been dedicated to psychometric issues such as the development of skin-related questionnaires, measurements of QoL, assessment of particular personality traits associated with selected skin diseases, assessment of relationships between psychological parameters, and the course of skin diseases. A considerable amount of research has also been done in the field of psychoneuroimmunoendocrinodermatology. Nevertheless, very little of such research has been of value for immediate clinical application. The evidence about an association between psoriasis and depression has led to a couple of promising clinical studies to assess the possible benefit of antidepressants for this skin disease. Trials of psychological or educational interventions in skin diseases have shown interesting and promising results, but such studies are expensive, and finding financial support for the collection

of further evidence is difficult—let alone turning such interventions into part of everyday clinical practice.

Collecting the "best evidence" on any theoretical result, with no immediate implications for therapy in psychocutaneous medicine, is obviously beyond the scope of this chapter. Hence, for instance, results on associations of psychocutaneous diseases with certain personality types—for example, the alleged association between psoriasis and alexithymic personality—have so far not produced any practical consequences for clinical management of the disease and will not be discussed. The remaining part of this chapter will therefore be devoted to the available evidence on the treatment of selected "classical" psychocutaneous diseases, classified as above. For some psychophysiological disorders, such as psoriasis, some relevant data on psychological or educational interventions or pharmaceutical interventions with psychotropic drugs will also be reviewed.

Epidemiological data on psychocutaneous diseases are generally scarce, despite the strong evidence overall for an interconnection between psychiatric and dermatological conditions—the estimated 30% level of psychiatric comorbidity in dermatological patients is evidence of the close interrelationship between the two fields.

Clinical studies in psychocutaneous medicine, ranging from case reports to randomized double blind trials, were searched. The available data regarding the efficacy of treatment for psychocutaneous disease were obtained from Medline, Ovid, and Cochrane database searches using the terms "name of the disease", "psychological" or "psychosomatic" or "psyche." The literature references in the identified articles were also accessed whenever reasonable and possible. Five major comprehensive works in book form published between 1987 and 2006 were also consulted and searched for relevant data, as well as one recently published exhaustive review, an issue of a dermatological journal dedicated wholly to psychocutaneous disease, and all issues of the journal *Dermatology and Psychosomatics*, which ceased publication in December 2004.[2,3,9–12]

Psychophysiological diseases

The main cutaneous diseases in which psychological factors are thought to trigger the onset or substantially influence the course are:

- *Psoriasis*
- *Alopecia areata*
- *Atopic dermatitis*
- *Urticaria*
- Lichen planus
- Vitiligo
- Acne
- Rosacea

- Seborrheic dermatitis
- Pemphigus

The review by Picardi *et al.*[4] found only limited evidence for a causal influence of stressful life events on these diseases. For the first group of diseases (in italics above), the role seems clearer, although more research is generally needed.

Psychological and educational interventions

"A Cochrane Review of RCT of psychological or educational interventions, or both, used to manage children with atopic exema[53] showed, with one exception,[7] only limited evidence of the effectiveness of educational and psychological interventions in the management of the condition of children affected by atopic eczema. (Of originally 338 identified studies, only 5 RCT could be included in the review). The authors of the review stress that there is significant scope in undertaking robustly designed trials to evaluate effectiveness of theoretically based psychological interventions." The positive outcome of the trial by Staab *et al.*[7] on educational interventions in atopic eczema may partly be due to increased compliance,[13] but the results are nevertheless promising. We found no similar trial on other chronic inflammatory skin diseases.

Several case series or case reports are available suggesting beneficial effects of relaxation techniques, meditation, hypnosis, and various forms of psychotherapy on psychophysiological diseases.[14–16] We found no controlled studies comparing such interventions with pharmacological therapy alone.

A controlled study in which the intervention was "writing about stressful events" showed positive results in asthma and rheumatoid arthritis. This type of trial would definitely also be worth attempting in the field of inflammatory chronic dermatoses.[17]

Psychopharmacological interventions

One open-label study showed a beneficial effect of bupropion-SR (an aminoketone antidepressant) on a small group of psoriasis and atopic eczema patients (10 patients in each arm).[18] However, a case report suggests that the same drug may trigger pustular psoriasis.[19]

Analogous paradoxical effects may occur during treatment with anti-tumor necrosis factor drugs for psoriasis; the underlying mechanism may be the same.[20,21]

A randomized, placebo-controlled, double-blind study showed a beneficial effect of an antidepressant agent, moclobemide, if used together with topical steroid therapy in patients with psoriasis.[22] There are theoretical considerations suggesting a link between inflammation and depression, and several mediators, such as substance P or tumor necrosis factor-α, are involved in both diseases.[23] This link may possibly explain the beneficial effects of antidepressants.

The antidepressant doxepin has been shown to be effective in chronic urticaria, but we did not find a randomized controlled trial. The efficacy is likely to be due to the drug's antihistamine properties.[24]

Primary psychiatric disorders with dermatological manifestations

These include trichotillomania, trichophagia, and other rarer "psychotrichologic" disorders, including trichoteiromania and trichotemnomania.

Trichotillomania (TTM) is a condition characterized by chronic hair-pulling. It is considered to be self-limiting, without no need for intervention in young children (under the age of 5). It is comparatively harmless in children and young adolescents, but when it is present in adults, referral to a psychiatrist may be indicated. The compulsion can present along with major depression, anxiety disorders, and phobias. Lifetime estimates are in the range of 0.6–3.4%. There have been a few controlled studies suggesting the efficacy of pharmacotherapy (clomipramine, selective serotonin reuptake inhibitor) and/or cognitive–behavioral therapy in TTM.[25] Serotonin reuptake inhibitors (SRIs) have shown less convincing results in the treatment of TTM than they do in the treatment of obsessive compulsive disorder (OCD), in which they are the treatment of choice, supporting the view that TTM cannot be clearly regarded as a form of OCD.

Dermatologists should be trained to recognize lesions caused by hair-pulling and to be aware of the danger of gastrointestinal obstruction due to trichobezoars (hair balls) when the disorder presents along with the habit of hair-eating (trichophagia). However, the pharmacological and psychological treatment is better left in the hands of the psychiatrist and clinical psychologist, since patients do not usually object to being referred to the proper specialist (in contrast to those with the delusion of parasitosis). A systematic review of the efficacy of the various treatments is therefore beyond the scope of this text.

Delusion of parasitosis

Delusion of parasitosis is defined as an unshakable and objectively wrong belief that one is infested with parasites or other microorganisms. We found no recent controlled studies or sound data on the incidence and duration of the illness, and evidence of the efficacy of treatments is lacking. A survey carried out in two regions of Poland indicates that about 15% of the dermatologists involved in the survey had never diagnosed a case of the syndrome, while one-third of them had treated three to five patients with the condition during the course of their careers.[26] In 1995, the syndrome was the subject of a meta-analysis including more than 1200 case reports.[27] The best data on the topic are probably found in this meta-analysis, which suggests that, contrary to common belief, the delusion may eventually resolve with full remission (half of the patients in the pharmacological era, compared to about one-third in the prepharmacological period (before 1960). A small double-blind crossover study[28] and many case series suggest that pimozide, which is widely used for the disease, is an effective treatment. Other commonly employed drugs are olanzapine and risperidone. Because of the rarity of the disorder, no large-scale controlled studies are available. The main difficulty lies in the fact that patients refuse referral to the psychiatrist, and dermatologists need to be familiar enough with the use of antipsychotic drugs to be able to manage the patient in their own practice. It has been recently suggested that the disease should be renamed pseudoparasitic dysesthesia, in an attempt to make the diagnosis more acceptable and less offensive to the patient.[29]

Self-inflicted skin lesions: neurotic excoriations/dermatitis artefacta

Self-inflicted skin lesions can be divided into *neurotic excoriations* (caused "involuntarily" but consciously—e.g., nail-biting, hair-pulling, *acné excoriée*, etc.) or *dermatitis artefacta*, in which the lesions result from more or less conscious but "voluntary" manipulation of the skin and patients almost always deny responsibility for the lesions.[30] The classification and definition of self-inflicted lesions in the literature is not always unequivocal, leading to difficulties in conducting meta-analyses of case reports.

The strategy for treating neurotic excoriations essentially follows the same lines as treatment for trichotillomania, and prescription of SRIs directly by the dermatologist may seem advisable in certain cases (especially in the context of an underlying dermatological disease—e.g., *acné excoriée*, pruritus), but sound evidence is lacking.[31]

By contrast, dermatitis artefacta may be associated with severe psychological discomfort and can have an exacerbating course, eventually developing into a chronic condition, with considerable psychiatric morbidity.[3] Although cases of dermatitis artefacta belong unequivocally to the domain of psychiatry, dermatologists may be confronted with patients who cannot, at least for a certain time, tolerate being confronted with the psychiatric etiology of their illness. Awareness of the psychogenic origin of the disturbance, skill in establishing an appropriate therapeutic relationship, having an instinct for the "right" way of dealing with the patient and gaining his or her confidence to allow eventual referral to a mental health professional, all belong to the capabilities of the "well-informed dermatologist" as defined by Poot *et al.*[32]

The reviews on dermatitis artefacta available are case series in which the authors attempt to assess the prevailing clinical context and the patients' psychological profile.[33–35] We did not find any controlled studies assessing the efficacy of interventions.

Body dysmorphic disorder

Body dysmorphic disorder is defined as a mental disorder manifesting itself in excessive concern about one's own physical appearance. An underlying physical defect may sometimes be present, but in a BDD patient the concern has to be definitely excessive in relation to the underlying defect. The preoccupation causes significant psychological distress, and impairment in many areas of social function (e.g., occupation, relationships, or sex).

The disease may have a component of delusion, when no physical defect is present.

Epidemiological data in the general population show a prevalence of between 0.7% and 13%.[36]

The high prevalence of BDD symptoms among dermatology patients[5] mentioned above, and the high prevalence of suicidal ideation associated with it—with a mean of 57.8% of the patients per year reporting suicidal ideation, according to Phillips and Menard[37]—makes it imperative for dermatologists to familiarize themselves with this condition. Dermatological treatment is the most frequent form of nonpsychiatric therapy sought and received, followed by surgery (most frequently, rhinoplasty).

We found two controlled pharmacotherapy studies, one of which showed that the SRI clomipramine was more effective than the non-SRI antidepressant desimipramine.[38] In a placebo-controlled study including 67 randomized patients, the SRI fluoxetine was found to be more effective than placebo.[39] Cognitive–behavioral therapy appears to be effective, but available studies are limited. There is an ongoing Cochrane protocol[40] to assess the efficacy of psychotherapy, pharmacotherapy, or both combined in the treatment of body dysmorphic disorders.[36,38,39]

SRIs appear to be effective both for delusional and non-delusional forms of BDD, but even delusional BDD does not seem to respond to antipsychotics alone. There is a lack of dose-finding studies.[36]

Patients may not accept the fact that they need psychopharmaceutical treatment, and they may refuse to be referred to a psychiatrist. Dermatologists need to be able to recognize BDD and initiate suitable psychopharmacological therapy if appropriate.

Secondary psychiatric disorders after dermatological diseases

Skin diseases such as psoriasis or alopecia areata can be disfiguring and may lead to severe social and psychological discomfort. Other diseases, such as atopic eczema, may also be associated with heavy itching and sleep disturbances and can lead to severe psychosocial impairment both for patients and their relatives.

Favorable outcomes have been reported after psychosocial interventions such as educational interventions, encouragement of self-help, support groups, cognitive–behavioral therapy, hypnosis, and biofeedback.

We found no specific controlled studies on pharmacological treatments for secondary psychiatric disorders after dermatological diseases, such as anxiety in psoriasis.

Acné excoriée des jeunes filles

This disease, defined as the urge to pick real or imagined acne lesions, is generally regarded as an overlapping of acne partly with neurotic excoriations and partly with body dysmorphic disorder. In this view, it is regarded basically as a primary psychiatric condition causing skin lesions. On the other hand, however, it could also be the result of anxiety deriving from real past or present acne lesions, and could therefore be seen as a secondary psychiatric disorder after a dermatological illness.

There is no definite evidence-based treatment, and the definition of the disease itself is rather blurred. There have been single case reports of benefit from behavioral therapy, olanzapine, or hypnosis. Due to the similarity of the condition with neurotic excoriations, which can improve with SRI treatment, this class of drugs may be of some help.[31,41]

Cutaneous sensory disorders

Unexplained itch is discussed in Chapter 66.

Vulvodynia

There are no recent epidemiological data, but it has been claimed that the prevalence of chronic vulvar pain is as high as 18%. Although the importance of psychological factors in the etiology of vulvar pain is widely recognized, it is not matched by an even remotely appropriate number of randomized clinical studies. We found only one randomized comparison of group cognitive–behavioral therapy, electromyographic biofeedback, and vestibulectomy in the treatment of dyspareunia resulting from vulvar vestibulitis. A recent literature review states that "all patients with vulvodynia should undergo psychologic and sexual evaluation, since in some instances psychotherapy may offer the only successful approach to the alleviation of vulvar pain."[42–44] Recent data suggest that there is altered central pain processing in patients with vulvodynia, so that the effectiveness of psychological interventions appears to be worthy of further investigation.[45]

Glossodynia

Essential glossodynia—a burning sensation in the mouth in which no underlying medical causes are identifiable and no oral signs are found—is also known as burning mouth syndrome. Reported prevalence rates are as high as 15%. Nine trials were identified in a recent Cochrane review. Two of these examined the use of antidepressants, and one investigated cognitive–behavioral therapy (CBT). The trial of CBT, but not the two trials on antidepressants, demonstrated a significant reduction in burning mouth symptoms, although the differences might have been due to methodological flaws. The studies also suggested that alpha-lipoic acid (three trials) and the anticonvulsant clonazepam (one trial) were effective.[46]

Other cutaneous sensory disorders

Reports on localized pain or other unpleasant sensations —different from itching, without medical explanation, and located in other surface areas than the vulva and oral mucosa—are only anecdotal in character and evidence of the efficacy of any sort of intervention is lacking.

Effect of psychiatric interventions on melanoma patients

A brief structured psychiatric intervention in melanoma patients in the USA was initially found to be associated with a survival benefit. However, there was weakening, but not complete disappearance, of the benefit at the 10-year follow-up. The results of a replication study conducted in Denmark and published in 2005 have so far failed to confirm any efficacy for this intervention in terms of improved survival, although the study suggested that such interventions may reduce psychological distress and enhance coping.[47–49]

Conclusions

The growing field of psychodermatology is fostering a more holistic approach to patients on the part of clinical dermatologists. Laboratory and clinical studies are providing increasing data on the biological kinship of mind and skin, and we are steadily gaining a better understanding of the way in which exogenous and endogenous processes that take place mainly in one system may influence the other. There is increasing public awareness of the importance of taking quality-of-life issues into account in the prevention and treatment of skin diseases.

If the problem of financing this type of research can be solved,[13] there are likely to be increasing numbers of studies on the beneficial effects of educational interventions in chronic skin diseases,[50] which will hopefully lead to reduced drug consumption and fewer side effects of pharmaceutical therapy.

However, a word of caution on the "psychodermatological approach" is warranted. Symptoms may have a protective effect for patients who may not be able to tolerate the disclosure of underlying conflicts. For instance, Sneddon and Sneddon reported in 1983 on patients presenting with *acné excoriée* over several years, who had been treated successfully with phenothiazines and psychotherapy. Psychiatric investigations showed that in a large proportion of the patients, the excoriations had been used as a protective device to conceal an emotional failure, and treatment ended by revealing a phobic state in many of them that had previously been hidden even from the patients.[51]

As Ring puts it,[52] the medical principle of *primum non nocere* also—and in particular—applies to psychosomatic investigations and therapy. It is certainly much easier to identify emotional difficulties and conflicts than to solve them.

References

1 Fava GA. A different medicine is possible. *Psychother Psychosom* 2006;**75**:1–3.
2 Walker C, Papadoupolos L. *Psychodermatology*. Cambridge: Cambridge University Press, 2005.
3 Koo JYM, Lee CS. *Psychocutaneous Medicine*. New York: Dekker, 2003.
4 Picardi A, Abeni D, Phillips KA, Dufresne RG Jr, Wilkel CS, Vittorio CC. Stressful life events and skin diseases: disentangling evidence from myth. *Psychother Psychosom* 2001;**70**:118–36.
5 Phillips KA, Dufresne RG Jr, Wilkel CS, Vittorio CC. Rate of body dysmorphic disorder in dermatology patients. *J Am Acad Dermatol* 2000;**42**:436–41.
6 Strahan JE, Raimer S. Isotretinoin and the controversy of psychiatric adverse effects. *Int J Dermatol* 2006;**45**:789–99.
7 Staab D, Diepgen TL, Fartasch M, Kupfer J, *et al.* Age related, structured educational programmes for the management of atopic dermatitis in children and adolescents: multicentre, randomised controlled trial. *BMJ* 2006;**332**:933–8.
8 Cotterill JA. Dermatological non-disease: a common and potentially fatal disturbance of cutaneous body image. *Br J Dermatol* 1981;**104**:611–9.
9 Koblenzer C. *Psychocutaneous Disease*. New York: Grune & Stratton, 1987.
10 Grimalt F, Cotterill JA. *Dermatología y Psiquiatría: Historias Clínicas Comentadas*. Madrid: Aula Medica, 2002.
11 Gupta MA, ed. [Special issue of journal.] *Dermatol Clin* 2005; **23**(4):591–755.
12 Harth W, Gieler U. *Psychosomatische Dermatologie*. Heidelberg: Springer, 2006.
13 Williams HC. Educational programmes for young people with eczema. *BMJ* 2006;**332**:923–4.
14 Lange S, Zschocke I, Langhardt S, Amon U, Augustin M. [Effects of combined dermatological and behavioral medicine therapy in hospitalized patients with psoriasis and atopic dermatitis; in German.] *Hautarzt* 1999;**50**:791–7.
15 Price ML, Mottahedin I, Mayo PR. Can psychotherapy help patients with psoriasis? *Clin Exp Dermatol* 1991;**16**:114–7.
16 Kabat-Zinn J, Wheeler E, Light T, *et al.* Influence of a mindfulness meditation–based stress reduction intervention on rates of skin clearing in patients with moderate to severe psoriasis undergoing phototherapy (UVB) and photochemotherapy (PUVA). *Psychosom Med* 1998;**60**:625–32.
17 Smyth JM, Stone AA, Hurewitz A, Kaell A. Effects of writing about stressful experiences on symptom reduction in patients with asthma or rheumatoid arthritis: a randomized trial. *JAMA* 1999;**281**:1304–9.
18 Modell JG, Boyce S, Taylor E, Katholi C. Treatment of atopic dermatitis and psoriasis vulgaris with bupropion-SR: a pilot study. *Psychosom Med* 2002;**64**:835–40.
19 Cox NH, Gordon PM, Dodd H. Generalized pustular and erythrodermic psoriasis associated with bupropion treatment. *Br J Dermatol* 2002;**146**:1061–3.
20 Sfikakis PP, Iliopoulos A, Elezoglou A, Kittas C, Stratigos A. Psoriasis induced by anti-tumor necrosis factor therapy: a paradoxical adverse reaction. *Arthritis Rheum* 2005;**52**:2513–8.
21 Brustolim D, Ribeiro-dos-Santos R, Kast RE, Altschuler EL, Soares MB. A new chapter opens in anti-inflammatory treatments: the antidepressant bupropion lowers production of tumor necrosis factor-alpha and interferon-gamma in mice. *Int Immunopharmacol* 2006;**6**:903–7.
22 Alpsoy E, Ozcan E, Cetin L, *et al.* Is the efficacy of topical corticosteroid therapy for psoriasis vulgaris enhanced by concurrent moclobemide therapy? A double-blind, placebo-controlled study. *J Am Acad Dermatol* 1998;**38**:197–200.
23 O'Brien SM, Scully P, Scott LV, Dinan TG. Cytokine profiles in bipolar affective disorder: focus on acutely ill patients. *J Affect Disord* 2006;**90**:263–7.
24 Tilles SA. Approach to therapy in chronic urticaria: when Benadryl is not enough. *Allergy Asthma Proc* 2005;**26**:9–12.
25 Chamberlain SR, Menzies L, Sahakian BJ, Fineberg NA. Lifting the veil on trichotillomania. *Am J Psychiatry* 2007;**164**:568–74.
26 Szepietowski JC, Salomon J, Hrehorow E, Pacan P, Zalewska A, Sysa-Jedrzejowska A. Delusional parasitosis in dermatological practice. *J Eur Acad Dermatol Venereol* 2007;**21**:462–5.
27 Trabert W. 100 years of delusional parasitosis. Meta-analysis of 1223 case reports. *Psychopathology* 1995;**28**:238–46.
28 Hamann K, Avnstorp C. Delusions of infestation treated by pimozide: a double-blind crossover clinical study. *Acta Derm Venereol* 1982;**62**:55–8.
29 Walling HW, Swick BL. Psychocutaneous syndromes: a call for revised nomenclature. *Clin Exp Dermatol* 2007;**32**:317–9.
30 Grant JE, Potenza MN. Compulsive aspects of impulse-control disorders. *Psychiatr Clin North Am* 2006;**29**:539–51.
31 Linder MD. Existe-t-il un traitement evidence-based pour l'acné excoriée? *Nouv Dermatol* 2004;**23**(Suppl 6):1–32.
32 Poot F, Sampogna F, Onnis L. Basic knowledge in psychodermatology. *J Eur Acad Dermatol Venereol* 2007;**21**:227–34.
33 Haenel T, Rauchfleisch U, Schuppli R, Battegay R. The psychiatric significance of dermatitis artefacta. *Eur Arch Psychiatry Neurol Sci* 1984;**234**:38–41.
34 Nielsen K, Jeppesen M, Simmelsgaard L, Rasmussen M, Thestrup-Pedersen K. Self-inflicted skin diseases. A retrospective

analysis of 57 patients with dermatitis artefacta seen in a dermatology department. *Acta Derm Venereol* 2005;**85**:512–5.

35 Verraes-Derancourt S, Derancourt C, Poot F, Heenen M, Bernard P. [Dermatitis artefacta: retrospective study in 31 patients; in French.] *Ann Dermatol Venereol* 2006;**133**:235–8.

36 Phillips KA. Body dysmorphic disorder: recognizing and treating imagined ugliness. *World Psychiatry* 2004;**3**:12–7.

37 Phillips KA, Menard W. Suicidality in body dysmorphic disorder: a prospective study. *Am J Psychiatry* 2006;**163**:1280–2.

38 Hollander E, Allen A, Kwon J, *et al.* Clomipramine vs desipramine crossover trial in body dysmorphic disorder: selective efficacy of a serotonin reuptake inhibitor in imagined ugliness. *Arch Gen Psychiatry* 1999;**56**:1033–9.

39 Phillips KA, Albertini RS, Rasmussen SA. A randomized placebo-controlled trial of fluoxetine in body dysmorphic disorder. *Arch Gen Psychiatry* 2002;**59**:381–8.

40 Ipser JC, Stein DJ. Pharmacotherapy and psychotherapy for body dysmorphic disorder [protocol stage]. Cochrane Depression, Anxiety and Neurosis Group. *Cochrane Database Syst Rev* 2007;(**3**):CD005332.

41 Nicolay D, Jadoulle V. Pour une approche multidimensionnelle de l'acné juvénile compliquée de troubles psychopathologiques. *Louvain Méd* 2005;**124**:329–37.

42 Bergeron S, Binik YM, Khalife S, *et al.* A randomized comparison of group cognitive–behavioral therapy, surface electromyographic biofeedback, and vestibulectomy in the treatment of dyspareunia resulting from vulvar vestibulitis. *Pain* 2001;**91**:297–306.

43 Mascherpa F, Bogliatto F, Lynch PJ, Micheletti L, Benedetto C. Vulvodynia as a possible somatization disorder. More than just an opinion. *J Reprod Med* 2007;**52**:107–10.

44 Bachmann GA, Rosen R, Pinn VW, *et al.* Vulvodynia: a state-of-the-art consensus on definitions, diagnosis and management. *J Reprod Med* 2006;**51**:447–56.

45 Zakrzewska JM, Forssell H, Glenny AM. Interventions for the treatment of burning mouth syndrome. *Cochrane Database Syst Rev* 2005;(**1**):CD002779.

46 Giesecke J, Reed BD, Haefner HK, Giesecke T, Clauw DJ, Gracely RH. Quantitative sensory testing in vulvodynia patients and increased peripheral pressure pain sensitivity. *Obstet Gynecol* 2004;**104**:126–33.

47 Fawzy FI, Fawzy NW, Huyn CS, *et al.* Effects of an early structured psychiatric intervention, coping and affective state on recurrence and survival 6 years later. *Arch Gen Psychiatry* 1993;**50**:681–9.

48 Fawzy FI, Canada AL, Fawzy NW. Malignant melanoma: effects of a brief, structured psychiatric intervention on survival and recurrence at 10-year follow-up. *Arch Gen Psychiatry* 2003;**60**:100–3.

49 Boesen EH, Ross L, Frederiksen K, *et al.* Psychoeducational intervention for patients with cutaneous malignant melanoma: a replication study. *J Clin Oncol* 2005;**23**:1270–7.

50 Staab D, Diepgen TL, Fartasch M, *et al.* Age related, structured educational programmes for the management of atopic dermatitis in children and adolescents: multicentre, randomised controlled trial. *BMJ* 2006;**332**:933–8.

51 Sneddon J, Sneddon I. *Acné excoriée*: a protective device. *Clin Exp Dermatol* 1983;**8**:65–8.

52 Ring J. *Angewandte Allergologie*. 3rd ed. Munich: Urban & Vogel, 2004.

53 Ersser SJ, Latter S, Sibley A, *et al.* Psychological and educational interventions for atopic eczema in children. *Cochrane Database Syst Rev.* 2007 Jul 18;(3).

66 Pruritus

Elke Weisshaar, Malcolm W. Greaves

Background

At first sight, pruritus (itch) and the scratching or rubbing it induces might seem valueless and even detrimental to the survival or continued health of the sufferer, but teleologically it has an important purpose in removing unwanted cutaneous parasite infestation.

Recent important advances in understanding the pathophysiology of itch include the identification by microneurography of sensory neurons dedicated to the transmission of itch but not pain, and definition by functional positron-emission tomography of a matrix of cerebral cortical loci that become activated in response to itch.

The consequences of pruritus range from trivial discomfort to excruciating distress, and when persistent it causes substantial impairment of the quality of life.[1] Occasionally, heavy excoriation caused by intense pruritus can lead to serious secondary skin infection.

Most skin diseases itch, especially if they have an inflammatory or epidermal component, and these are discussed in the relevant chapters elsewhere in the present volume.

Definition

Pruritus is defined conventionally as a poorly localized, nonadapting, usually unpleasant sensation that provokes a desire to rub or scratch.

With a view to facilitating investigation and treatment, pruritus has recently been classified[2,3] into four categories, which are not mutually exclusive:
- Pruritoceptive: itch generated in the skin due to skin disease
- Neuropathic: due to lesion(s) in the central or peripheral nervous system
- Neurogenic: caused by presumed circulating pruritogens, without evident disease of the nervous system
- Psychogenic, including delusional and affective disorder.

Measurement of pruritus remains a challenge. Pruritus is subjective and therefore difficult to quantify, resort usually being made to a digital visual analogue scale. Pruritus has also been measured indirectly by quantification of scratching or rubbing—for example, by using limb movement meters. However, the specificity of this method in distinguishing between restlessness and pruritus is unclear. Animal models of itch depend on the unsafe and unverifiable assumption that the sensation perceived by the scratching animal resembles human itch.

Incidence and prevalence

Epidemiological data on pruritus are rare. A community survey in 1976 of a UK (London) urban population revealed a prevalence of pruritus of up to 20% in a population of 2120 adults studied.[4] Due to the increasingly aged population in the developed countries, the prevalence of pruritus is likely to have increased. Idiopathic pruritus of old age occurs in 30–60% of people over the age of 60 within any 1-week period.[5] There are no recognized sex or ethnic differences.

Causation

Apart from being the most common symptom of skin disease, pruritus is also an important manifestation of systemic disease, including chronic renal failure, cholestasis, and human immunodeficiency virus (HIV) infection, or less commonly underlying malignancy, especially of the lymphoreticular system. A few patients present with intractable widespread pruritus with no discernible skin or systemic disease. These patients usually represent a major management problem, and the condition is designated as "idiopathic generalized pruritus."

Prognosis

If a cause can be identified and dealt with (e.g., relief of biliary tract obstruction in pruritus of cholestasis), the itch should remit. However, even when a cause has been identified (e.g., pruritus of chronic renal failure), the itch may persist unabated despite best efforts. Itch of senescence is also notoriously intractable, and in these cases treatment is essentially palliative.

Diagnosis

A careful history and examination are crucial. The quality, diurnal or nocturnal periodicity, and duration are very important. Itch that the patient likens to "ants crawling over the skin" (formication) should raise a suspicion of delusional parasitosis. Itching often occurs in brief bouts—e.g., at bedtime—and this information allows appropriate fine-tuning of treatment. The Eppendorf itch questionnaire[6] has proved useful in evaluating the intensity of itch and the resulting handicap.

Examination for scabies burrows and for symptomatic dermographism (firm stroking of skin causes wheal, flare, and itch) should be done routinely. Care should be taken not to confuse induced secondary eczematous changes—as a consequence of rubbing or scratching due to a systemic cause of itch—with a pruritoceptive itch consequent upon primary skin disease.

Aims of treatment

The aim of treatment is to alleviate the itching, the distress it causes to the patient, and the secondary changes wrought in the skin by scratching.

Relevant outcomes

In practice, total abolition of itching in the chronically pruritic patient is rarely achieved, and its partial amelioration is a more or less acceptable compromise outcome. For example, it is often possible to relieve itching to the extent that it does not interfere significantly with the patient's daily activities or cause excessive sleep disturbance at night.

Methods of search

The following key words were used in a literature search: itch, pruritus, prurigo, scratch, excoriation.

Pruritus of chronic renal failure

Definition

Pruritus of chronic renal failure is multifactorial in causation and variable in its clinical presentation and therefore eludes precise definition. It is often unremitting, sometimes episodic, generalized in distribution in 25–50% of patients, and localized in the remainder—often to the shunt arm in dialysis patients. It is frequently associated with secondary skin complications, often with infection, due to scratching.

Incidence

The incidence of pruritus in chronic renal failure patients on dialysis has fallen in recent years (about 70% 20–25 years ago; now 15–20%).[7] It is unrelated to sex, the duration of dialysis, or the cause of the renal failure. It is very rare in children. It is more common in patients receiving hemodialysis than in those receiving continuous ambulatory peritoneal dialysis (CAPD).[8] In patients on dialysis, it is an independent risk factor for mortality. Acute renal failure does not cause itching.

Etiology

The cause of pruritus in chronic renal failure is unknown. Causative factors proposed include proliferation of dermal mast cells, elevated histamine levels, secondary hyperparathyroidism, and peripheral neuropathy. Xerosis is very common in chronic renal failure patients and probably contributes to itching in many.

Prognosis

There are no systematic studies of the natural history of pruritus of chronic renal failure, but it is widely perceived to be unremitting and poorly responsive to treatment.

Treatment aims

The primary object of treatment is to remove or mitigate any identifiable cause and abolish or at least ameliorate the itching. Patients with pruritus of chronic renal failure are frequently depressed and despairing of any effective remedy, so any treatment strategy needs to take this into account, including counseling and the use of antidepressants. The only reliably effective treatment for pruritus of chronic renal failure is a kidney transplant.

Outcomes

Reduction or abolition of pruritus should lead to resolution of the secondary manifestations of itching, including excoriation, eczematization, and secondary infection and relief of xerosis. Successful treatment should be reflected in an improvement in the patient's sense of well-being and quality of life.

What are the guiding principles in choosing treatments for pruritus of chronic renal failure?

General measures

Treatment of xerosis by emollients brings about some symptomatic relief in most patients. Secondary infection and eczematization can usually be controlled by topical treatment with a combination of antibiotics and corticosteroids. The intensity of pruritus correlates with skin temperature, so a cool environment, tepid showering, and wearing of light, loose-fitting clothes is beneficial.

Efficacy

Recent usage of dialysis membranes with improved biocompatibility has reduced the frequency and severity of pruritus in patients receiving hemodialysis treatment. However, dialysis itself has an inconsistent effect, since itching is unrelated to blood urea or creatinine levels.

Although no results are available from controlled studies, oral antihistamines are of little or no value in the management of pruritus of renal failure. However, because of its sedative and antidepressant properties, the tricyclic antihistamine doxepin is useful, especially in the elderly. It should be prescribed initially at a low dosage (e.g.,10 mg at night) and gradually increased. Abrupt withdrawal should be avoided, and care should be exercised in patients with a history of heart disease.

Opioid μ-receptor antagonists, which have been found to be effective in pruritus of cholestasis (see below), have also been advocated in the treatment of pruritus of renal failure. However, the published results have been conflicting. A randomized, placebo-controlled crossover study by Peer et al.[9] showed that the oral μ-receptor antagonist naltrexone (50 mg per day) was effective, with all of 15 patients responding with reduced itching. However, a subsequent placebo-controlled double-blind crossover study including 23 patients taking oral naltrexone 50 mg daily, with a visual analogue scale and a detailed score to measure pruritus intensity, showed no difference in comparison with placebo.[10] On the basis of these apparently conflicting data, it is reasonable to try administration of naltrexone when other measures have failed.

The efficacy of broadband ultraviolet B (UVB) phototherapy in pruritus of renal failure was first suggested by Gilchrest et al. in a large open study.[11] Since generalized pruritus abated even though only half of the body was treated, a systemic effect was inferred. A subsequent meta-analysis of the results of randomized controlled trials came to the conclusion that broadband UVB is the treatment of choice for moderate or severe uremic pruritus.[12]

Odansetron is a serotonin type 3 receptor antagonist that is administered orally. The results with its use in pruritus of chronic renal failure have been conflicting. Balaskas et al. treated 11 patients with 4 mg odansetron daily for 3 months in an open study, and all of the patients responded.[13] However, a further small placebo-controlled study failed to substantiate this finding.[14]

Other treatments for which only sparse anecdotal evidence exists include parenteral lidocaine,[15] oral activated charcoal,[16] and topical tacrolimus, a calcineurin inhibitor with immunosuppressive properties.[17]

Drawbacks

Doxepin, a tricyclic antidepressant and potent H_1 antihistamine, also possesses anticholinergic properties. In the elderly, there is therefore a risk of glaucoma and, in males, of urinary retention. Patients with a history of ischemic heart disease who are given doxepin run a risk of developing arrhythmia. Doxepin interacts with other drugs metabolized via the cytochrome P-450A liver enzyme system.

Opioid μ-receptor antagonists carry a risk of hepatotoxicity, and they inactivate opioid pain killers that are being given concurrently.

Comments

Although sometimes inconvenient, broadband UVB phototherapy three times weekly, supplemented by generous use of emollients and a low night-time oral dose of doxepin, is probably the most effective treatment strategy for moderate to severe pruritus of chronic renal failure. Doxepin has the additional advantage of alleviating the depression frequently associated with pruritus due to this cause.

Implications for clinical practice

The causes of pruritus in chronic renal failure are obscure, so it is unsurprising that there are no highly effective treatments. Despite best efforts, treatment is often at best only moderately successful.

Key points: pruritus of chronic renal failure

- The cause of the itch is probably multifactorial, and generally poorly responsive to treatment.
- Broadband UVB combined with a small night-time dose of doxepin and copious emollients is helpful in most cases.
- Care must be exercised in administering doxepin in the elderly, especially in those with preexisting heart disease.
- Naltrexone is probably worth trying in recalcitrant cases.

Pruritus of cholestasis and hepatic disease

Definition

This itch—often intense and unbearable in cholestasis—is frequently widespread, but unlike generalized pruritus due to other causes, symmetrical involvement of the palms of the hands and soles of the feet is common and typical. When due to cholestasis it is often, but not invariably, accompanied by jaundice. Patients usually rub rather than scratch, and secondary excoriation, eczematization, and skin infection are therefore less common than in pruritus of chronic renal failure.

Incidence

Itching occurs in 20–25% of patients with cholestasis[18] and is severe and invariable in cholestasis due to primary biliary cirrhosis.[19] It is less common and more variable in liver disease, such as hepatitis C. If liver failure supervenes, pruritus remits.

Etiology

Recognized causes of pruritus include primary biliary cirrhosis, primary sclerosing cholangitis, obstructive choledocholithiasis, carcinoma of the bile duct or head of the pancreas, and viral hepatitis. Less common causes include cirrhosis. Cholestasis and associated itch can also be drug-induced.[20] The cause of the itching, originally thought to be due to bile acids, is now also believed to be due to opioid peptides synthesized in the liver and acting on μ-opioid receptors located mainly in the central nervous system.[21]

Prognosis

Relief of biliary obstruction by surgery or a stent causes rapid abatement of pruritus. In patients with itch due to parenchymal liver disease such as hepatitis C infection, itching is variable and persistent, with a capricious response to treatment.

Diagnosis

The combination of jaundice and generalized pruritus, the skin being otherwise essentially normal, is highly suggestive of a cholestatic cause for the itch. However, cholestatic itching can occur without jaundice, as in pregnancy cholestasis. In such cases, the presence of elevated plasma bilirubin and alkaline phosphatase and bile acids in plasma and urine strengthens the diagnosis.

Treatment aims

When an obstructive cause can be identified and relieved, treatment of the itch is symptomatic and short-term. In patients in whom the pruritus is secondary to hepatitis or cirrhosis, the aim is to alleviate or if possible abolish the itching.

Outcomes

Amelioration or abolition of itching.

What are the guiding principles in choosing treatment for pruritus of cholestasis or liver disease?

General measures

These include a cool environment, tepid showers, and wearing light, loose-fitting clothes.

Frequent application of a lotion of calamine with 1% menthol is also well appreciated by most patients.

Efficacy

Any obstruction of the biliary tract should be relieved, and this will be followed by rapid remission of the pruritus. Interferon therapy may relieve pruritus in hepatitis C virus infection. Oral antihistamines are generally ineffective. In selected cases in which pruritus is intractable and severe, liver transplantation should be considered.

Oral cholestyramine (4 g administered before and after breakfast) is hallowed by tradition but not by controlled clinical trials.[22] Since it works by binding intestinal bile acids and other anions, thereby decreasing enterohepatic circulation, it is ineffective in the presence of total biliary obstruction.

Oral ursodeoxycholic acid, a naturally occurring hydrophilic bile salt, was found to be effective in pruritus of primary biliary cirrhosis in only two of 11 trials reported in a recent meta-analysis of randomized controlled trials.[23]

Rifampicin, which induces cytochrome P-450 enzymes in the liver, thereby reducing putative liver-derived pruritogens, was found to be effective in the treatment of cholestatic pruritus at a dosage of 350–450 mg per day in two randomized and controlled trials.[24,25]

The oral opioid antagonists nalmefene (5–20 mg twice daily) and naltrexone (50 mg/day) were shown to be effective in reducing pruritus in two controlled studies, which both used a visual analogue scale and a scratching activity monitoring system to quantify itch.[26,27] A reduction in itch by 50–90% was seen in these studies. Naloxone, a parenterally administered opioid antagonist (infused at 0.2 μg/kg/min) was also found to be effective in a double-blind, randomized, placebo-controlled trial.[28]

Other treatment modalities advocated include odansetron (8 mg daily orally in one randomized controlled trial)[29] and an open study of bright light therapy directed into the eyes up to 60 min twice daily.[30]

Drawbacks

Cholestyramine, although probably mildly effective, is unsatisfactory due to poor patient compliance (due to the taste and constipation). Rifampicin and the opioid μ-receptor antagonists, although of proven effectiveness, are associated with a high frequency of liver toxicity. The latter also cause opioid withdrawal symptoms, which can be largely prevented by starting with a low dose and increasing gradually.[31]

Comments

Rifampicin, opioid antagonists, and possibly cholestyramine are effective in the treatment of cholestatic itch, but the incidence of adverse effects is high with rifampicin and opioid antagonists, and they should be used cautiously.

Implications for clinical practice

Patients receiving active treatment for cholestatic pruritus with rifampicin or opioid antagonists should be regularly and frequently monitored for adverse effects, especially in the liver. With this caveat, the results are usually reasonably good.

Key points: pruritus of cholestasis and hepatic disease

- General nonspecific antipruritic measures are valuable and in some cases may be all that is required.
- Where there is an identifiable obstruction, its removal will result in rapid relief of pruritus.
- Rifampicin and opioid antagonists are of proven value as second-line measures, but they should be used cautiously, owing to the frequency of adverse side effects.

Pruritus in hematological diseases

Definition

Itching is frequently a presenting symptom of polycythemia vera and occasionally also occurs in other hematological disorders, including myelodysplasia and lymphoblastic leukemia, and is characteristically triggered by contact with water. Pruritus, often localized, also occurs in association with iron deficiency.

Incidence

In polycythemia vera, itching occurs in about 40% of the patients.[32] Figures from an epidemiological study in Finland involving a survey of over 40 000 adults showed that 13.6% of iron-deficient men complained of frequent pruritus, contrasting with 5.3% in men who were not iron-deficient ($P < 0.001$).[33] The corresponding figures for adult women were 7.4% and 5.1% ($P < 0.01$).

Etiology

Pruritus in polycythemia vera is significantly associated with a low mean corpuscular volume and raised leukocyte count.[32] Other proposed pathogenetic factors include elev-

ated plasma histamine levels and elevated tissue fibrinolytic activity.[34] The pathogenesis of itching in iron deficiency is unknown.

Prognosis

Treatment of polycythemia vera often improves the pruritus, but in 20% of patients the itch is persistent.[35] Symptomatic treatment also greatly improves the quality of life for affected patients. The benefits conferred by iron supplements in patients with pruritus associated with iron deficiency are unclear, since no controlled trials have been done.

Diagnosis

Any patient complaining of pruritus triggered by contact with water at any temperature, and without a rash, should be suspected of having polycythemia vera. The diagnosis is confirmed by demonstrating raised hemoglobin, hematocrit, red cell mass, platelet count, and leukocytosis. Iron deficiency is established by demonstrating a lowered serum iron and total iron-binding capacity.

Treatment aims

Water-induced itching is a distressing symptom, and the aim should be to achieve its abolition or at least reduction to tolerable levels. Iron deficiency should be corrected in order to ameliorate itching.

Outcomes

Reduction or abolition of itching.

What treatments are available for pruritus of polycythemia vera? Is there any evidence that correction of iron deficiency reduces pruritus?

General measures

Pruritus in polycythemia vera, sometimes water-induced ("bath-time itch"), is distressing and disabling. Because there is often no visible accompanying eruption, the sufferer receives scant sympathy. Explaining this to family members and carers forms an important part of the management of these patients.

Efficacy

Although blood histamine levels are often elevated, H_1 antihistamines are rarely effective. Aspirin has anecdotally been found effective in some patients with polycythemia vera.[36] Narrowband UVB administered three times weekly (10 patients) and photochemotherapy with 8-methoxypsoralen ultraviolet A (PUVA) two or three times weekly, with 15 treatments (in 11 patients) have been claimed to be effective in open studies of polycythemia vera.[37,38]

The efficacy of oral iron supplements in patients with pruritus and iron deficiency has not been established in clinical trials.

Drawbacks
PUVA and narrowband UVB are usually well tolerated, but relapse occurs within weeks of the end of treatment.

Comments
Although the published evidence is weak, it is likely that phototherapy or photochemotherapy is effective in ameliorating pruritus in some patients with polycythemia vera. The value of iron supplements in the treatment of pruritus associated with iron deficiency is questionable.

Implications for clinical practice
Phototherapy and photochemotherapy offer safe and often effective, although temporary, relief of pruritus in polycythemia vera.

Key points: pruritus in polycythemia vera and patients with iron deficiency

- Pruritus in polycythemia vera, often triggered by contact with water, can be effectively relieved in some patients using either narrowband UVB or PUVA.
- There is no evidence from clinical trials to support the value or otherwise of iron supplements in the management of itching in iron-deficient patients.

Aquagenic pruritus

Definition
Episodic intense itching provoked by contact with water at any temperature and without physical signs in the skin and with a normal full blood count.

Incidence
There are no extant figures for the incidence or prevalence of aquagenic pruritus but, since it was first described in the early 1970s, its worldwide prevalence has become evident. Due to the absence of visible disease, under-recognition is common. The condition is familial in one-quarter to one-third of patients. It characteristically affects middle-aged adults and is very rare in children.

Etiology
The cause is unknown. Associations with myelodysplasia,

hypereosinophilic syndrome, juvenile xanthogranuloma, squamous carcinoma of the cervix, and acute lymphoblastic leukemia have been reported in isolated cases. Aquagenic pruritus has also occasionally been attributed to an adverse reaction to drugs. Increased cutaneous acetylcholinesterase and fibrinolytic activity in symptomatic skin has also been reported.[39]

Prognosis
The condition is chronic and unremitting. About 5% of patients with initially normal blood pictures subsequently develop polycythemia vera.[40]

Treatment aims
This condition is surprisingly distressing to sufferers and their families. Treatment is palliative, and aims to enable patients to bathe without experiencing unbearable itching.

Outcomes
Patients can wash and shower without undue discomfort.

What treatments are available to mitigate this excruciating itch?

General measures
A full blood count should be performed initially and subsequently at regular intervals to identify the occasional patient who subsequently develops polycythemia vera in the course of the disease. Some patients achieve an acceptable compromise by sponging small areas of skin at a time during bathing.

Efficacy
Bathing in water alkalinized by sodium bicarbonate (500 g per bath, achieving pH 8) was found to prevent itching in several small uncontrolled studies,[41] but is of inconsistent value.[42] Although no controlled studies have been done, phototherapy represents the best treatment option. Suberythemal UVB (290–320 nm) was used in 29 patients, half of whom responded satisfactorily.[43] PUVA is also effective.[44] In all of five patients, remission occurred after an average of 15 treatments, but relapse supervened during the follow-up. Narrowband UVB was also recently reported to be effective in two patients, who required 12–21 treatments for remission. Both required maintenance treatment.[45] Other treatments proposed anecdotally include propranolol and topical capsaicin.

Drawbacks
Aquagenic pruritus tends to be a chronic condition, so there is concern over the potential risk of phototherapy-induced

skin cancer, especially as long-term maintenance is normally required.

Comments

The risk of skin cancer favors use of narrowband UVB rather than broadband UVB or PUVA. In any case, the policy should be to minimize ultraviolet dosage, especially during maintenance.

Key points: aquagenic pruritus

- The condition is chronic and unremitting, and treatment is palliative.
- Phototherapy is effective, but requires long-term maintenance.
- Maintenance dosage should be kept as low as possible, due to the risk of skin cancer.
- Patients should be monitored regularly for the onset of polycythemia vera.

Pruritus of endocrine diseases

Definition

When pruritus occurs in diabetes mellitus, it is usually a localized, persistent symptom, most commonly anogenital. It may be more widespread if diabetes is complicated by chronic renal failure. In contrast, pruritus in both hypothyroidism and hyperthyroidism is usually widespread, and in hyperthyroidism it may be a severe presenting symptom.

Incidence

Most textbooks cite diabetes as an important cause of chronic generalized pruritus. This belief dates from 1927, when a study of the skin in 500 patients with diabetes reported an incidence of pruritus of 6.5%, with about half of the cases being generalized; however, there was no control group.[46] A more recent study of 300 diabetic and 100 matched nondiabetic patients reported that pruritus vulvae was more common in the diabetic group (18.4% vs. 5.6% in controls), but the frequency of generalized pruritus did not differ between the two groups.[47]

Although itching is a widely recognized symptom of overactive and underactive thyroid disease, figures for the incidence and prevalence are scarce. A recent study in 120 hyperthyroid patients reported pruritus, often generalized, in 60%.[47] In hypothyroidism, the incidence of pruritus is unknown, but it is likely to be significant due to the frequency of skin dryness.

Etiology

Pruritus in diabetes is commonly localized to the anogenital area, especially the vulva, is frequently due to candidosis,

and is directly related to poor diabetes control.[47] Occasionally, it can be due to diabetic neuropathy, xerosis, or chronic renal failure. The cause of itching in thyrotoxicosis is unclear. In myxedema, the skin is usually dry, and anogenital candidosis is an additional factor in some patients.

Prognosis

The prognosis in anogenital pruritus of diabetes depends on the effectiveness of control of underlying hyperglycemia. Correction of thyroid dysfunction leads to remission of the itch in thyrotoxicosis, but the itch of hypothyroidism tends to be more recalcitrant.

Treatment aims

The achievable aim should be complete abolition of localized pruritus in diabetics, and of generalized pruritus in thyrotoxicosis. The itching in hypothyroidism can be reduced, but complete relief is often difficult to attain.

Outcomes

Freedom from itching in diabetics and patients with thyrotoxicosis, and significant improvement in patients with myxedema.

How can anogenital itch of diabetics be effectively treated? How should the patient with generalized itching due to hypothyroidism or hyperthyroidism be managed?

General measures

Anogenital pruritus in diabetics is helped by careful drying after bathing, use of loose-fitting underwear, and most importantly, adequate control of diabetes. Mitigation of generalized pruritus of thyrotoxicosis can be achieved by measures to cool the warm moist itchy skin. These include wearing light clothing, tepid showering, a cool ambient temperature, and calamine lotion.

Efficacy

There are no clinical trials of treatment of anogenital pruritus in diabetics, but since the majority are due to candidosis, anti-*Candida* treatment using topical imidazole antifungals is usually effective if combined with adequate management of the diabetes. Oral antifungals are rarely required. Pruritus in hypothyroidism and hyperthyroidism should be treated by correction of thyroid function. Liberal use of emollients is valuable in patients with dry skin due to hypothyroidism.

Drawbacks

Since diabetics are strongly predisposed to mucocutaneous candidosis, the relapse rate of anogenital candidosis and its associated pruritus is high even if the diabetes is controlled.

Comments

Oral antihistamines are ineffective in relieving of pruritus due to endocrine disease. Topical antihistamines and local anesthetics should be avoided in anogenital pruritus in diabetics, due to risk of sensitization. Topical corticosteroids should also not be used for this indication.

Implications for clinical practice

Sustained remission of anogenital pruritus of diabetes mellitus can be difficult to achieve, especially in women with vulvovaginal candidosis. Reservoirs of reinfection, such as *Candida* paronychia, also need to be vigorously treated.

Key points: pruritus in thyroid disease and diabetes mellitus

- In diabetes, pruritus is usually localized, anogenital, and due to candidosis.
- In hyperthyroidism or hypothyroidism, pruritus is generalized and multifactorial.
- Treatment of diabetic anogenital pruritus includes adequate control of diabetes, combined with local or occasionally systemic anti-*Candida* therapy.
- Apart from general measures, the treatment of pruritus of thyrotoxicosis or myxedema consists of correcting the thyroid dysfunction.

Anogenital pruritus

Definition

This is defined as chronic localized intense pruritus affecting the perianal area (pruritus ani) and the vulva (pruritus vulvae). Although frequently idiopathic, anogenital pruritus may be a manifestation of either skin or systemic disease. If persistent, it leads to lichenification locally, and it also causes severe distress and sleep disturbance.

Incidence

Pruritus ani occurs in 1–5% of the adult population, and males are more commonly affected than females.[48] Precise figures for the incidence and prevalence of pruritus vulvae are unavailable, but most women will suffer from it at one time or another during their lives. It can occur at any age, but in its chronic presentation it is common postmenopausally.

Etiology

Common dermatoses that involve the anogenital area and cause pruritus include psoriasis, atopic dermatitis, lichen sclerosus, lichen planus, scabies, pediculosis, allergic contact dermatitis (especially with perfumed soaps; 18 of 40 patients with pruritus ani had positive patch tests),[49] and seborrheic dermatitis. Dermatitis medicamentosa due to contact allergic sensitization to long-continued topical application of antipruritics, especially local anesthetics and antihistamines, is common.[50] Local problems causing pruritus include threadworms, virus warts, hemorrhoids, lichen simplex chronicus, carcinoma, and urinary or fecal incontinence. In women, vaginitis—especially vaginal candidosis—is an important local cause, and estrogen deficiency is an important systemic cause. In one study of 1104 patients with pruritus vulvae, 946 (85%) had candidal or trichomonal vaginitis.[51] Diabetes mellitus is a common systemic cause in both sexes.

Psychogenic factors ("stress") are often cited in cases in which none of the above causes are found, but this is probably a rare cause.[51]

Prognosis

Anogenital pruritus is characteristically chronic and poorly responsive to treatment, even when a cause has been identified and treated. The itch–scratch–itch cycle is especially hard to break at this site. Although anogenital pruritus is intensely distressing for many patients, for others, scratching in this area causes significant (albeit temporary) gratification.

Treatment aims

Treatment should be targeted at breaking the itch–scratch cycle. This allows restoration of effective stratum corneum barrier function.

Outcomes

Effective treatment should lead to gradual lessening of the compulsive desire to rub or scratch, with accompanying resolution of lichenification, pigmentation, and excoriation. Sleep disturbance should diminish. Restoration of an effective barrier function enables the anogenital skin to resist normal "wear and tear" as well as minor irritancy.

What are the roles of local and systemic treatments in the management of anogenital pruritus?

General measures

Overenthusiastic cleansing and use of irritant toiletries,

perfumed soaps, foam baths, or sensitizing topical medicaments should be discontinued. The anogenital area should be washed regularly with plain water and air-dried or gently dabbed with cotton wool. For pruritus vulvae, wiping should always be from front to back. In severe cases of anogenital pruritus, sitz baths (warm plain water hip baths) bring about rapid relief. Ointments are preferable to creams, owing to the presence of potentially irritant preservatives in the latter. Silicone barrier and zinc oxide ointments help retain moisture in affected skin, thereby enhancing healing.

Efficacy

When anogenital pruritus is a manifestation of a primary skin disease or local lesion such as hemorrhoids, threadworms, or vaginitis, apart from general measures the management is that of the causative dermatosis or local pathology. Adequate control of underlying diabetes mellitus is essential, together with treatment of the invariable underlying candidosis. In postmenopausal pruritus vulvae, systemic hormone replacement therapy should be considered.

Vaginal candidosis is also an important cause of pruritus vulvae in nondiabetic women. In one study, 17 of 38 women (45%) with pruritus vulvae were found to have *Candida albicans* infection.[52] Although underlying local or systemic disease can be identified in many patients, the cause in some patients with pruritus vulvae is elusive (idiopathic vulval pruritus). Most of these patients receive topical steroid treatment. There are no controlled trials, but one open study of 65 patients showed that 56 of these reported complete relief in 2 days following topical fluocinolone acetonide.[53] Intralesional injection of triamcinolone has been proposed for recalcitrant pruritus vulvae. Of 45 patients, 35 experienced relief for at least 1 month (mean 5.8 months) following a single injection.[54] For exceptionally resistant and handicapped patients, multiple local intradermal injections of ethanol have been reported to be effective by several authors. In one double-blind study,[55] 14 of 17 patients reported complete relief by undermining the skin of the vulva, the vaginal mucosa, and perianal skin.[56,57] Of 16 women, 15 experienced immediate relief of itching and no relapse occurred after follow-up periods ranging from 3 months to 3 years.

Topical corticosteroids are the orthodox treatment for perianal pruritus if it persists despite the removal or treatment of the underlying causes, or when no cause can be found. Controlled trials are lacking, but in a recent study in idiopathic perianal pruritus, one group of 28 patients applied topical methylprednisolone cream twice daily for 2 weeks, with a second group of 32 patients using a liquid cleanser only.[58] The results were similar in the two groups, with over 90% of patients responding ($P > 0.05$). Intralesional triamcinolone has also been used for recalcitrant pruritus ani. Nineteen patients with idiopathic pruritus ani were treated with triamcinolone hexacetonide intralesionally for 4 weeks (dosage 5–20 mg weekly).[59] Very good improvement occurred in 14 patients and fair improvement in two. No skin atrophy was noted. Topical capsaicin is a recognized treatment for various types of localized pruritus. It appears to work via vanilloid receptors on unmyelinated sensory nerve endings, causing depletion of the neuropeptide substance P. A recent double-blind placebo-controlled crossover study compared capsaicin 0.006% cream with 1% menthol cream in idiopathic intractable pruritus ani.[60] Use of the capsaicin cream three times daily for a month led to partial relief of pruritus in 31 of 44 patients, and the menthol cream was invariably ineffective. Intralesional 5% phenol has also been used with success in patients with idiopathic pruritus ani resistant to conventional modalities. In an open study of 67 patients, 62 (92.5%) experienced complete relief.[61] Five of them subsequently relapsed, but sustained remission followed after a repeat injection.

Drawbacks

Potent topical corticosteroids are widely prescribed for most types of anogenital pruritus, often for long periods of time. Although usually effective, they may mask underlying primary pathology, including neoplasia, infection, and allergic contact sensitization. Local steroid atrophy may also occur. Similar caveats apply to intralesional triamcinolone injections. Although safe, patient compliance with topical capsaicin is poor due to its burning action. Experience with intralesional injection of ethanol or phenol is too limited to warrant consideration except in the most intractable cases.

Comments

Careful history-taking, clinical examination, and investigation of patients with pruritus vulvae or ani will frequently be rewarded by discovery of an underlying primary cause. Embarking on prolonged topical potent steroid application should be delayed until these avenues have been thoroughly explored.

Implications for clinical practice

Anogenital pruritus is usually a symptom rather than a specific disorder, and diabetes mellitus should always be considered. Failure to respond to general measures and topical steroids should prompt a skin biopsy in order to exclude underlying malignancy. A patient presenting with pruritus ani or vulvae should also always undergo rectal and/or vaginal examination, for the same reason. Patients with a long history of poor response to topical medications should be considered to have dermatitis medicamentosa until proved otherwise by patch testing.

Key points: anogenital pruritus

- Anogenital pruritus is usually a symptom of underlying skin disease, systemic disease, or local disease.
- Diabetes mellitus, candidosis, and rectal or vaginal malignancy should be sought and treated.
- Dermatitis medicamentosa is very common, and patch testing should be carried out in treatment-resistant patients.
- General measures, especially avoidance of irritants, and skin-friendly anogenital hygiene encourages restoration of the stratum corneum barrier.
- In idiopathic cases, topical corticosteroids may be helpful, but they may mask malignancy and other underlying disease.

Drug-induced itch

Definition

Drug-induced itch is defined as generalized itching without skin lesions, caused by a drug.

Incidence/prevalence

In the Boston Collaborative Drug Surveillance Program (BCDSP) studies which were published in the *Journal of the American Medical Association*, drug-induced itch without a rash accounted for approximately 5% of adverse cutaneous reaction in prospectively followed hospitalized patients. Adverse cutaneous reactions occurred in 3% of the patients,[62,63] except for itch induced by hydroxyethyl starch (HES). The latter is described as occurring in 12.6–42% of patients treated with HES.[64,65] Opioid-induced itch is a common problem after epidural and intrathecal administration of opioids, usually localized on the face, neck, and upper thorax. No reliable data are available on the incidence and prevalence rates. The variation in the incidence has been reported to range from 50% to 90%.[66,67]

Etiology

Many drugs must be used with caution in HIV patients, who may be susceptible to hypersensitivity reactions, drug interactions, and idiosyncratic reactions. Some of them may present with pruritus without skin lesions.

Severe generalized or localized itching can be induced via the following mechanisms:
- Cholestasis—e.g., oral contraceptives or other estrogens, captopril, chlorpromazine, valproic acid, erythromycin, sulfonamide, minocycline
- Hepatotoxicity: oral contraceptives or other estrogens, testosterone and other anabolic steroids, phenothiazine,

phenytoin, acetaminophen, isoniazid, halothane, sulfonamide, minocycline, cyclooxygenase-2 (COX-2) inhibitors (e.g. celecoxib)
- Deposition: hydroxyethyl starch (HES)
- Sebostasis, xerosis cutis: retinoids, beta-blockers, tamoxifen, busulfan, clofibrate
- Phototoxicity: 8-methoxypsoralen, doxycycline
- Neurologic: tramadol, codeine, cocaine, morphine, butorphanol, fentanyl, topiramate
- Idiopathic: chloroquine, quinidine, clonidine, gold salts, lithium, angiotensin-converting enzyme inhibitors

Prognosis

If the offending drug is discontinued, the itching resolves. There are no studies on the prognosis, except for HES-induced itch. The mean duration of HES-induced itching is 15 months, mainly depending on the amount of HES deposited. Tissue deposition of HES is dose-dependent and time-dependent.[68] Neural deposition of HES was confined to a total dose of HES exceeding 210 g. After administration of 414 g, 32% of the patients suffered from pruritus, in comparison with 1% after a dosage of 150 g.[65,69]

Diagnostic tests

In HES-induced itch, a skin biopsy with immunoelectron microscopy may demonstrate HES deposits in the skin.

Aims of treatment

The aim of treatment is to abolish or reduce itching.

Relevant outcomes

- Abolition of drug-induced itch
- Prevention of drug-induced itch

Methods of search

We reviewed Pubmed, Medline, Embase, and the Cochrane Library. In addition, a hand-search of the major German dermatology journals was carried out.

Are there any drugs more likely to induce pruritus? Are there any treatment options other than discontinuing the offending drug?

Evidence summary: efficacy

There are no controlled trials investigating the mechanisms and treatment options for drug-induced itch, except for opioid-induced itch. The literature shows that cholestasis and hepatotoxicity appear to be the most frequently reported triggers of this type of pruritus.

In HES-induced itch, topical capsaicin therapy at concentrations ranging from 0.025% to 0.5% four to six times daily showed antipruritic potency in a case report[70] and case series.[71] Single patients were reported to respond to oral naltrexone 50 mg daily in HES-induced itch.[72,73] Two cases of intractable pruritus in drug-induced cholestasis were successfully treated by extracorporeal albumin dialysis using the Molecular Adsorbent Recirculating System (MARS).[74]

According to a quantitative systematic review of randomized trials on the pharmacological control of opioid-induced pruritus, there is a lack of valid data on the efficacy of interventions for the treatment of established pruritus.[75] Naloxone 0.25 μg/kg/h was found to be efficacious in relieving postoperative pruritus in children and adolescents in a double-blind, prospective, randomized controlled study.[76] Celecoxib 200 mg failed to relieve pruritus in a prospective randomized placebo-controlled trial involving 60 women undergoing cesarean section.[77]

Naloxone 2 μg/kg/h i.v., naltrexone 6 mg orally, nalbuphine i.v. (the optimal dose remains to be determined) and droperidol 2.5 mg or 5 mg i.v. or epidurally are effective in preventing opioid-induced pruritus.[75,76] The optimal dose is one that provides adequate relief of pruritus without increasing pain scores. There was a lack of evidence for any antipruritic efficacy with prophylactic propofol, epidural and intrathecal epinephrine, epidural clonidine, epidural prednisone, intravenous ondansetron, and intramuscular hydroxyzine.[75] A case report suggests rifampicin 300 mg i.v. twice daily in pruritus after morphine treatment in a cancer patient.[78]

Key points: drug-induced itch

- Drug-induced pruritus has multiple mechanisms. The treatment of drug-induced pruritus centers on discontinuation of the triggering drug.
- To prevent opioid-induced itch, naloxone, naltrexone, nalbuphine, and droperidol are efficacious.
- According to case reports, topical capsaicin therapy and oral naltrexone may be used to treat HES-induced pruritus.

HIV and itch

Definition

HIV-related itch is defined as generalized or localized itching in patients with HIV infection or acquired immune deficiency syndrome (AIDS).

Incidence/prevalence

Itching is a very common symptom in this population, but epidemiological data about the incidence and prevalence of itch in HIV and AIDS populations are scarce. A recent study in 897 American HIV-infected patients revealed a pruritus prevalence rate of 6%.[79] HIV viral loads higher than 55 000 copies/mL had a higher prevalence of pruritus.[79] When the prevalence of pruritus in 310 patients with chronic HIV and hepatitis B and C virus infection was prospectively determined, the prevalence rate was 28% in patients with hepatitis C and HIV and 25% in those with hepatitis B and HIV.[80] When 84 Ugandan pruritus patients were investigated, 19% were found to be HIV-positive.[81]

Etiology

HIV/AIDS patients are prone to develop a number of pruritic dermatoses.[82,83] Systemic causes of pruritus in HIV are relatively uncommon, but may occur in HIV nephropathy, hepatic failure due to hepatitis B or C, and systemic lymphoma.[82,83] Severe pruritus may lead to lichenification. Localized areas of lichenified dermatitis are relatively common in HIV patients. Lichenification is often triggered by other pruritic dermatoses. Prurigo nodularis can be caused by HIV-related dermatoses or HIV-related systemic diseases, but may also occur without any known cause. Generalized asteatosis clinically presents as xerosis or dry skin, accompanied by pruritus. It increases with disease progression, and CD4 counts decline.[82]

As many as half of AIDS patients may never have specific causative or categoric diagnoses identified. Some authors term this "idiopathic pruritus."[82] In these cases, it is most likely that itching is directly related to the HIV infection—e.g., HIV viral load, immune dysregulation, reduced Th1, increased Th2, increasing levels of immunoglobulin A (IgA) and immunoglobulin E (IgE), increased eosinophils.[84]

Prognosis

The prognosis depends on the prognosis of the HIV infection and on the stage of the AIDS disease, as well as on optimum antiviral therapy.

Diagnostic tests

The tests performed depend on the relevant differential diagnoses concerning the etiology. They may include HIV viral load, CD4 count, IgE, eosinophils, bile acids, transaminases, alkaline phosphatase, creatinine, blood urea nitrogen, and radiographic and sonographic examinations.

Aims of treatment

Abolition of itching, reducing ichthyosis, reducing discomfort, improving the quality of life.

Relevant outcomes

Abolition of itch, improvement of the quality of life.

Methods of search

We reviewed Pubmed, Medline, Embase, and the Cochrane Library. In addition, a hand-search of the major German dermatology journals was carried out.

Are there any treatment options for HIV-induced itch? Is one therapy superior to the others in improving quality of life in HIV-induced itch?

Evidence summary: efficacy

In a controlled but nonrandomized study, treatment of pruritus in HIV-1 disease did not reveal any difference between indomethacin 25 mg t.i.d., pentoxifylline 400 mg t.i.d., hydroxyzine hydrochloride 25 mg t.i.d., and 0.025% triamcinolone lotion (120 mL/week).[85]

In a noncontrolled, nonrandomized study, UVB phototherapy produced significant relief of pruritus and improved the quality of life in HIV-positive patients suffering from primary pruritus (n = 7) and pruritic eosinophilic folliculitis.[86] The safety of phototherapy in HIV-positive patients has been debated, but it is considered to be safe.[87,88]

Thalidomide has been used to relieve HIV-related pruritus in the setting of prurigo nodularis. A randomized study in 10 HIV patients suffering from prurigo nodularis showed a greater than 50% response in reduction of itch over 3.4 months when thalidomide was taken for longer than 1 month (eight of the 10 patients). The dosage ranged from 33 to 200 mg daily.[89] Three patients developed thalidomide peripheral neuropathy.[89]

A case report describes the use of hypnosis in the treatment of generalized itching in three HIV-positive men.[90]

Key points: HIV and itch

- Pruritus is an important cause of discomfort and morbidity in HIV and AIDS patients.
- Treatment of pruritus in HIV and AIDS depends on the underlying etiology. Patients need careful evaluation in order to determine the underlying cause. In these cases, causative treatment is possible (e.g., treatment of an underlying systemic cause, treatment of underlying specific dermatoses, discontinuation of a drug).
- In pruritus that is not related to a specific dermatological or systemic disease, optimal antiviral treatment is best.
- Very limited data suggesting that symptomatic relief can be achieved with UVB phototherapy and that thalidomide may be helpful for pruritus associated with HIV-related prurigo nodularis need confirmation.

Psychogenic itch

Definition

Psychogenic itch refers to pruritus associated with psychiatric diseases and psychological factors (e.g., the delusional state of parasitophobia or neurotic excoriations). It may be generalized or localized.

Incidence/prevalence

There are no data on the incidence and prevalence of psychogenic itch. It is estimated that psychogenic excoriation occurs in 2% of dermatology clinic patients.[91]

Etiology

Depression, anxiety, and schizophrenia have been described as causes of psychogenic itch. Neurotic excoriations and the delusional state of parasitophobia can be accompanied by psychogenic itch. Neurotic excoriations are characterized by excessive scratching and picking of normal skin, but this is not necessarily associated with pruritus. One study revealed that 58% of patients with psychogenic excoriations had a current major depressive syndrome and that 45% of patients with psychogenic excoriations had obsessive-compulsive disorder.[92]

Prognosis

There are no data on the prognosis of psychogenic itch. It is most likely that the prognosis depends on the underlying psychiatric disease and its treatment.

Diagnostic tests

Psychiatric consultation and counseling for diagnosis or verification of the underlying psychiatric disease.

Aims of treatment

Abolition of itching, reducing discomfort, improving the quality of life.

Relevant outcomes

Abolition of itch and improving the quality of life.

Methods of search

We reviewed Pubmed, Medline, Embase, and the Cochrane Library. In addition, a hand-search of the major German dermatology journals was carried out.

Which treatment options are efficacious for psychogenic itch?

Evidence summary: efficacy

There are no controlled trials investigating the treatment of psychogenic itch. Serotonin reuptake inhibitors (SSRIs) such as paroxetine 20 mg or 30 mg daily or fluoxetine 20 mg daily showed efficacy in case reports.[93,94] In elderly patients, cardiac side effects may occur and these drugs should therefore be applied with caution.

Mirtazapine, a nonadrenergic and specific serotonergic antidepressant, was associated with significant relief in a case of chronic neurotic excoriations at a dosage of 15 mg/day.[95] Dry mouth, sedation, and weight gain are the most commonly reported side effects, but its advantages are once-daily dosing and its lack of addictive potential.

There are no controlled trials of behavioral or psychotherapeutic treatments for neurotic excoriations. In case reports, behavioral techniques such as "habit reversal" have been found to be effective.[91]

Key points: psychogenic itch

- Treatment of psychogenic pruritus depends on the underlying etiology.
- Paroxetine and mirtazapine were found to be useful in case reports of psychogenic pruritus and neurotic excoriations.

Itch and senescence

Definition

Generalized or localized itching in patients over the age of 65 may be called senescent pruritus or elderly itching.

Incidence/prevalence

A Turkish study investigating 4099 elderly patients found that pruritus ranked first in the distribution of skin diseases, with 11.5% complaining about pruritus. Women were more frequently affected (12.0%) than men (11.2%).[96] With regard to the age group, patients aged over 85 had the highest prevalence rate (19.5%). With regard to seasonal variations, senescent pruritus was among the five most frequent diagnoses in all seasons and was most frequent in winter (12.8%) and fall (12.7%).[96] Pruritic diseases were the most common in a study from Thailand (41%) that identified xerosis (which for the authors was identical with senescent pruritus) as being the most frequent condition (38.9%) in a total of 149 elderly patients.[97]

Etiology

Aging skin is characterized by a decline in the regular functions of the skin (e.g., cell replacement capacity, barrier function, immune responsiveness, sebum production, sweat production, sensory perception, and wound healing). Current theories of senescent pruritus range from xerosis cutis to degenerative changes in the peripheral nerve endings. One study detected increased histamine release and skin hypersensitivity to histamine in pruritus of the elderly.[98]

Prognosis

No data are available on the prognosis.

Diagnostic tests

The elderly are more likely to take multiple medications that may cause itching (see also the section on drug-induced itch above). As the elderly are also more likely to have systemic diseases that can potentially cause itching, a precise dermatological and general examination should exclude an underlying systemic disorder. Laboratory studies may include erythrocyte sedimentation rate (ESR), a complete blood cell count with differential leukocyte count, blood urea nitrogen, creatinine, liver transaminases, alkaline phosphatase, bilirubin, thyroid function test, serum iron, ferritin, and radiographic and sonographic examinations. The diagnosis of senescent pruritus is made on the basis of chronic pruritus after other causes of itching have been excluded.

Aims of treatment

Abolition of itching, reducing discomfort, improving the quality of life.

Relevant outcomes

Abolition of itch.

Methods of search

We reviewed Pubmed, Medline, Embase, and the Cochrane Library. In addition, a hand-search of the major German dermatology journals was carried out.

What are the major causes of senescent pruritus? Are there any effective therapies for itch in the elderly?

Evidence summary

Therapy depends on an underlying systemic disease, if present.

A double-blind placebo-controlled trial including 19 patients with senile pruritus who were treated with oxatomide 30 mg b.i.d. for 2 months showed complete suppression or marked improvement of pruritus in 79% of the patients.[99]

A controlled nonrandomized study in 60 patients suffering from senescent pruritus and 20 control individuals (20 patients unaffected by pruritus in the elderly, aged 63–83, median age 77) was carried out and showed complete or marked improvement in 41% of patients treated with loratadine 10 mg and in 38% of patients treated with terfenadine 120 mg orally. There were no significant differences between the groups.[98] Exact results for the control group were not given in the study.

Ten patients with essential senescent pruritus were treated with ciclosporin A 5 mg/kg body weight per day for 8 weeks in an open uncontrolled study. Ciclosporin A treatment significantly reduced the itch intensity in all patients. In eight patients, pruritus ceased in the fourth week of treatment. No relapses occurred until 3 months after discontinuation, except for one patient suffering from mild localized pruritus.[100]

The antipruritic effect of thalidomide 200 mg given on two nights was investigated in 11 patients, one of whom was suffering from senescent pruritus. Thalidomide decreased the itch, assessed subjectively and measured objectively as nocturnal scratch movements.[101]

From the clinical point of view, it is well known that the elderly frequently suffer from itching caused by xerosis cutis, asteatotic dermatitis, or stasis dermatitis. Topical emollients (also with urea and/or anesthetic agents) are usually very helpful, but there is a paucity of published quantitative evidence of its role. Ultraviolet light phototherapy is known to relieve pruritus, but there are no clinical trials for these therapies.

Key points: itch and senescence

- Pruritus in the elderly is quite frequent, with a gradually increasing prevalence in increasing age.
- Therapy may include treatment of an underlying systemic disease, if present.
- Everyday experience suggests that xerosis cutis plays an important role.

Neuropathic itch

Definition

Neuropathic itch is defined as pruritus that is caused by a disease at any point along the afferent pathway of the nervous system.

Incidence/prevalence

Itching is reported by up to 58% of patients suffering from herpes zoster and up to 30% of patients suffering of postherpetic neuralgia, mainly affecting the head, face and neck.[102] There are no epidemiological data on notalgia paresthetica, brachioradial pruritus, or pruritus in multiple sclerosis.

Etiology

Notalgia paresthetica, brachioradial pruritus, postherpetic neuralgia/itch, and pruritus in multiple sclerosis are clinical forms of neuropathic itch.

Notalgia paresthetica is characterized as localized pruritus medial to the scapular area, frequently accompanied by a hyperpigmented patch. It is described as being caused by degenerative changes in the vertebrae corresponding to the dermatome of itching.[103] When 43 patients with notalgia paresthetica were evaluated, 61% had spinal changes judged to be relevant.[104] The striking correlation between the localization of notalgia paresthetica and spinal pathology suggests that spinal nerve entrapment may contribute to notalgia paresthetica.[103,104]

Brachioradial pruritus is characterized by intense pruritus of the dorsal and lateral parts of the underarms and elbows. The symptoms are frequently temporal—appearing in August, for example, and disappearing during winter in European countries. Brachioradial pruritus may be attributed to neuropathic conditions such as chronic cervical radiculopathy, cervical spondylosis, transverse myelitis.[105–107] A spinal cord tumor has been reported in a patient with brachioradial pruritus.[108] The occurrence of brachioradial pruritus in several members of one family affecting two generations has been described.[109] The temporal course of itching in brachioradial pruritus and the histological changes in the skin, similar to those caused by ultraviolet light, indicate that sunlight is most likely to be an eliciting factor and cervical spine disease to be a predisposing factor.[110] It is believed that both cervical spine disease and sun-induced cutaneous nerve injury are important contributors, acting to variable degrees in individual patients.[106,110]

In 20 patients suffering from anogenital pruritus without any skin disease or anorectal pathology, lumbosacral radiculopathy and degenerative changes of the lower spine were confirmed in 80% of cases.[111]

Prognosis

The prognosis depends on identifying an underlying cause, such as cervical radiculopathy (brachioradial pruritus) and degenerative changes in the vertebrae (notalgia paresthetica).

Diagnostic tests

These depend on the underlying etiology and may include radiological examinations of the spine (notalgia paresthetica, brachioradial pruritus) and brain (multiple sclerosis).[106,112]

Aims of treatment

Abolition of itching, reducing discomfort, improving the quality of life.

Relevant outcomes

Abolition of itch.

Methods of search

We reviewed Pubmed, Medline, Embase, and the Cochrane Library. In addition, a hand-search of the major German dermatology journals was carried out.

What are the major causes of neuropathic itch? Are there any effective treatments for it?

Evidence summary: efficacy

Topical capsaicin 0.025% three times daily showed significant antipruritic efficacy in a randomized, double-blind, crossover, placebo-controlled 10-week study in 20 patients with notalgia paresthetica. Seventy percent of the patients treated with capsaicin and 30% of those treated with placebo improved.[113]

In 24 patients with notalgia paresthetica, relief of up to 90% was achieved in 70% in a noncontrolled, nonrandomized study with topical capsaicin 0.025% four times daily.[114]

When 15 patients were treated with capsaicin 0.025% four times daily for 3 weeks, 10 of 13 patients who completed the study experienced significant or complete relief after 3 weeks in comparison with an untreated arm that served as a control.[115]

Case reports have described antipruritic effects of topical capsaicin 0.025% four to five times daily in brachioradial pruritus. In both patients, pruritus had resolved within 2 weeks, and in one pruritus was continuing to be controlled with once-weekly application of capsaicin 4 months after the start of therapy.[116]

When 16 patients with notalgia paresthetica or brachioradial pruritus were treated with cutaneous field stimulation once daily, 20–30 min a time for 5 weeks in an open trial, pruritus was reduced by 49% at the end of the fifth week in comparison with baseline values.[117]

Gabapentin is an anticonvulsant structurally related to the neurotransmitter gamma-aminobutyric acid (GABA). The mechanism of action is unclear. Several case reports

demonstrated efficacy of gabapentin for brachioradial pruritus. The dosage needed ranged from 6×100 mg daily or 3×300 mg daily up to $3–6 \times 600$ mg daily.[118–121]

Oxcarbazepine, a keto-analogue of the anti-convulsant carbamazepine, decreased pruritus when administered to a group of five patients at a dosage of 300 mg twice daily.[122]

Fifteen patients with neuropathic scrotal pruritus were treated with paravertebral injections consisting of 2.5 mL triamcinolone and 2.5 mL lidocaine 1% divided into five or six separate injections, with a significant decrease in the mean pruritus scores assessed by the patients before and after therapy.[111]

In a retrospective case series, 16 patients with segmental pruritus were treated with deep intramuscular stimulation acupuncture to the paravertebral muscles in the dermatomal segments of the body affected. Twelve patients had complete resolution and four had partial resolution of the pruritus. Relapses occurred in 37% of patients within 1–12 months, requiring further acupuncture. The author described this form of pruritus as "neurogenic pruritus."[123]

Key points: neuropathic itch

- In the real world, almost no patients with notalgia paresthetica undergo radiography.
- Topical capsaicin 0.025% four times daily appears to be effective for pruritus in notalgia paresthetica and brachioradial pruritus. However, the data may be too weak for conclusions to be drawn.

Pruritus in pregnancy unrelated to skin diseases (Table 66.1)

Definition

Pruritus during pregnancy unrelated to skin diseases, especially unrelated to pregnancy-specific dermatoses and without skin lesions, can occur as pruritus gravidarum with or without intrahepatic cholestasis. The latter may be associated with clinical jaundice. There is no clear terminology. Particularly in the older literature, some authors used the terms "pruritus gravidarum" and "intrahepatic cholestasis of pregnancy." Both forms may lead to scratching, resulting in papules, nodules, excoriations, and crusts. Some authors have suggested that pruritus gravidarum in women with an atopic predisposition can result in prurigo of pregnancy.[124]

Incidence/prevalence

Epidemiological studies focusing on the prevalence of pruritus during pregnancy unrelated to skin diseases are limited. Interestingly, pruritus is described as the main

Table 66.1 Pruritus in pregnancy not related to dermatoses

	Occurrence	Etiology and laboratory findings	Fetal risk	Location of pruritus	Therapy
Pruritus gravidarum (without cholestasis)	1st trimester	Not clear Increased bile acids and decreased itch threshold due to prostaglandins Normal liver function	No	Generalized	Topical—e.g., emollients, menthol, polidocanol
Pruritus gravidarum (with cholestasis)	2nd and 3rd trimesters	Not clear, genetic predisposition and altered bile duct and hepatocytes Increased bile acids, transaminases, alkaline phosphatase, cholesterol, lipids	Yes	Generalized, especially hands and feet; deterioration at night	Topical Cholestyramine Phenobarbital Activated carbon UVB therapy Ursodeoxycholic acid 450–1200 mg/day
Prurigo gestationis	Early and late forms possible	Not clear (atopy?)	No	Extensor sides of extremities	Topical

UVB, ultraviolet B.

dermatological symptom during pregnancy and is observed in approximately 18% of pregnancies.[125]

A French prospective study of 3192 pregnant women showed that 1.6% had pruritus.[126] Seventeen patients (0.5%) had pruritus gravidarum, while all of the other cases were pregnancy-specific dermatoses.[126] The prevalence of pruritus in pregnancy was reported to be 4.6% in an Indian study of 500 pregnant women, but with the exception of four cases of pruritus gravidarum all of them were suffering from specific dermatosis of pregnancy.[127] The prevalence of pruritus gravidarum was 0.8%.[127] The rate of intrahepatic cholestasis is higher in Chile, related to ethnic and dietary factors. A prevalence rate of 13.2% was found for pruritus gravidarum and 2.4% for cholestatic jaundice of pregnancy.[128]

Etiology

Pruritus gravidarum can occur with or without intrahepatic cholestasis. Intrahepatic cholestasis is associated with dyslipidemia, which may contribute to the pathogenesis of intrahepatic cholestasis.[129] The elevation of low-density lipoprotein cholesterol and the reduction of high-density lipoprotein cholesterol may prove to be a useful marker for the early identification of intrahepatic cholestasis of pregnancy and differentiation from pruritus gravidarum without intrahepatic cholestasis.[129]

It is estimated that pregnant women take three to eight different medications—some over-the-counter ones, some prescribed by physicians.[130] Drug-induced pruritus during pregnancy is not one of the more probable differential diagnoses, but in tropical regions, chloroquine-induced

pruritus in malaria therapy during pregnancy is a frequent cause, with a prevalence rate of 65%. According to one study, it occurred in 75% of those affected within 24 hours after consumption and was described as severe by over 60% of the patients.[131]

Prognosis

In pruritus gravidarum with cholestasis and prurigo gestationis, there is a possibility of recurrence during a subsequent pregnancy. Pruritus gravidarum can imply an increased risk to the fetus, such as impaired development, intrauterine death, or premature birth.[127] One population-based study compared pregnancies in women with and without pruritus gravidarum. Among 159 197 deliveries, 376 (0.2%) occurred in patients with pruritus gravidarum. Using a multivariate analysis, the following conditions were found to be significantly associated with pruritus gravidarum: twin pregnancies, fertility treatments, diabetes mellitus, and nulliparity. No significant differences were noted between the groups with regard to perinatal outcomes, such as birth weight, low Apgar scores, or perinatal mortality. Pruritus gravidarum, associated with multiple gestations, fertility treatments, diabetes mellitus, and nulliparity, is not associated with adverse perinatal outcomes. However, there are higher rates of labor induction and cesarean delivery.[132]

Diagnostic tests

These include bile acids, transaminases, alkaline phosphatase, cholesterol, and lipids. Measurement of glutathione

S-transferase α (GSTA), a marker of hepatocellular integrity, provides a test of liver dysfunction that distinguishes between pruritus gravidarum with and without intrahepatic cholestasis.[133]

Aims of treatment

Abolition of itching, reducing discomfort, improving the quality of life.

Relevant outcomes

Abolition of itch.

Methods of search

We reviewed Pubmed, Medline, Embase, and the Cochrane Library. In addition, a hand-search of the major German dermatology journals was carried out.

What are the major causes of pruritus during pregnancy unrelated to skin diseases? Are there any effective treatments?

Evidence summary: efficacy

Aspirin showed significant antipruritic efficacy in a systematic review when it was administered at a dosage of 600 mg four times daily in comparison with chlorpheniramine 4 mg three times daily applied during late pregnancy. Aspirin was more effective in relieving itch, but chlorpheniramine was more effective than aspirin when a rash was present.[134] Aspirin may not be given during the last trimester, as it can lead to early occlusion of the ductus arteriosus.

There are no studies on the efficacy of antihistamines for the treatment of pruritus during pregnancy, but there are studies concerning their safety. The older sedating antihistamines, such as chlorpheniramine, dimetindene, diphenhydramine, and hydroxyzine are considered relatively safe during pregnancy, on the basis of long-term experience and several independent animal studies, and these agents have not shown any teratogenic effects.[130] In animal studies during pregnancy, astemizole, terfenadine, and cetirizine did not show any notable effects in influencing the fetus, but terfenadine and fexofenadine led to decreased fetal weight gain. In younger-generation antihistamines (e.g., levocetirizine), animal studies so far have not demonstrated any impairment of pregnancy or of embryonic and fetal development. Second- and third-generation antihistamines should not be administered during the first trimester of pregnancy. If antihistamines are necessary during this period of pregnancy, the older sedating ones are preferable. Fexofenadine, terfenadine, and astemizole are not suitable for treatment during pregnancy.[130]

If needed, nonmethylated glucocorticosteroids are preferable, as they pose a very small risk to the fetus. Prednisolone (or alternatively prednisone) is the glucocorticosteroid of choice if systemic therapy is required in pregnant women, mostly for short-term therapy (< 4 weeks).[130] There have been no studies investigating the efficacy of glucocorticosteroids in patients with pruritus gravidarum.

Cholestyramine binds bile acids. According to uncontrolled studies, it may be effective in up to 70% of patients suffering from pruritus gravidarum and intrahepatic cholestasis.[124] Ursodeoxycholic acid enhances the excretion of bile acids. It is very effective when administered at daily doses of between 450 and 1200 mg, as shown in four small controlled trials.[124] A case report showed complete disappearance of pruritus in intrahepatic cholestasis of pregnancy using ursodeoxycholic acid 900 mg daily.[135]

The administration of ultraviolet therapy during pregnancy is not generally contraindicated, but it should be carried out with caution. It should be limited to late pregnancy and should be performed only after the patient has been provided with thorough information. PUVA therapy with oral psoralen administration is contraindicated.

Key points: pruritus in pregnancy

- Pruritus during pregnancy without any skin lesions presents as pruritus gravidarum, which may occur with or without intrahepatic cholestasis.
- The prevalence of pruritus during pregnancy shows substantial geographical variation.
- There are too few controlled studies investigating treatment for pruritus during pregnancy for conclusions to be drawn.

Pruritus of unknown origin

Definition

Itching without any underlying etiology after precise history-taking and examination of the skin and general examination is termed pruritus of unknown etiology. Some authors also use the terms "idiopathic pruritus" and "idiopathic itch." Pruritus of unknown origin is rare in children but common in adults, especially the elderly. This type of pruritus is characterized by prolonged persistence, lasting months to years.

Incidence/prevalence

There are limited epidemiological data on the incidence and prevalence of pruritus of unknown origin. In 132 patients suffering from pruritus as a leading symptom, it was impossible to identify an underlying etiology in 8%.[81] A study investigating outpatients presenting with pruritus of unknown origin identified an underlying systemic disease in 11 of 50 patients.[136] In 20 patients suffering from anogenital pruritus without any skin disease or anorectal pathology, lumbosacral radiculopathy and degenerative changes in the lower spine were confirmed in 80% of cases.[111]

Prognosis

According to one clinical study, the prognosis is poorer and the quality of life is significantly more impaired in comparison with pruritus in dermatological and systemic diseases.[81]

Aims of treatment

Abolition of itching, reducing discomfort, improving the quality of life.

Relevant outcomes

Abolition of itch.

Methods of search

We reviewed Pubmed, Medline, Embase, and the Cochrane Library. In addition, a hand-search of the major German dermatology journals was carried out.

Have any effective therapies been reported for pruritus of unknown origin?

Evidence summary

Gabapentin is an anticonvulsant structurally related to the neurotransmitter GABA. The mechanism of action is unclear. When two patients with pruritus of unknown origin were treated with gabapentin 300 mg daily on day 1, increased to 600 mg daily and up to 1800 mg daily, itching was completely controlled within the first month.[137] Both patients continued with a maintenance dosage of gabapentin based on symptom control, without any side effects.[137]

In an open-label study, one patient had a 50% reduction in pruritus when treated with oral naltrexone 50 mg daily, but three patients did not respond to this form of treatment.[72]

Sixty patients with "idiopathic perianal pruritus" were treated either with topical steroids twice daily (methylprednisolone) for 2 weeks (n = 28) or with a liquid cleanser twice daily for 2 weeks (n = 32). Treatment was effective in 93% of the patients receiving topical steroid treatment and in 91% of those treated with the liquid cleanser. There were no significant differences between the two treatments, suggesting that perianal cleansing is as effective as topical corticosteroids.[58] Fifteen patients with idiopathic anogenital

pruritus were treated with paravertebral injections consisting of 2.5 mL triamcinolone and 2.5 mL lidocaine 1% divided into five or six separate injections, with a significant decrease in the mean pruritus scores assessed by the patients before and after treatment.[111]

There have been no studies on ultraviolet phototherapy in patients with pruritus of unknown origin.

Key points: pruritus of unknown origin

- Pruritus of unknown origin has a major impact on patients' quality of life and mood. Therapy is a challenge in this group of patients, as no effective treatments are available. The available data are insufficient for conclusions to be drawn.

References

1 Yosipovitch G, Zucker I, Boner, G, *et al.* A questionnaire for the assessment of pruritus: validation in uraemic patients. *Acta Derm Venereol* 2001;**81**:108–11.

2 Yosipovitch G, Greaves MW, Schmelz M. Itch. *Lancet* 2003; **361**:690–4.

3 Bernhard JD. Itch and pruritus: what are they and how should itches be classified? *Dermatol Ther* 2005;**18**:288–91.

4 Rea JN, Newhouse ML, Halil T. Skin disease in Lambeth. A community study of prevalence and use of medical care. *Br J Prev Soc Med* 1976;**30**:107–14.

5 Beauregard S, Gilchrest BA. A survey of skin problems and skin care regimens in the elderly. *Arch Dermatol* 1987;**123**:1638–43.

6 Darsow U, Scharein E, Simon D, *et al.* Component analysis of atopic itch using the "Eppendorf itch questionnaire." *Int Arch Allergy Immunol* 2001;**124**:326–31.

7 Mettang T, Pauli-Magnus C, Alscher DM. Uraemic pruritus—new perspectives from recent trials. *Nephrol Dial Transplant* 2002;**17**:1558–63.

8 Mettang T, Fritz P, Weber J, Machleidt C, Hubel E, Kuhlmann U. Uremic pruritus in patients on hemodialysis or continuous ambulatory peritoneal dialysis (CAPD). The role of plasma histamine and skin mast cells. *Clin Nephrol* 1990;**34**:136–41.

9 Peer G, Kivity S, Agami O, *et al.* Randomised crossover trial of natrexone in uraemic pruritus. *Lancet* 1996;**348**:1552–4.

10 Pauli-Magnus C, Mikus G, Alscher DM, *et al.* Naltrexone does not relieve uremic pruritus: results of a randomized placebo-controlled crossover study. *J Am Soc Nephrol* 2000;**11**:514–9.

11 Gilchrest BA, Rowe J, Brown RS, *et al.* Relief of uremic pruritus with ultraviolet phototherapy. *N Engl J Med* 1977;**297**:136–8.

12 Tan KL, Haberman HF, Coldman AJ Identifying effective treatments for uremic pruritus *J Am Acad Dermatol* 1991;**24**:811–8.

13 Balaskas EV, Bamihas GI, Karamouzis M, Voyiatzis G, Tourkantonis A. Histamine and serotonin in uremic pruritus: effect of odansetron in CAPD-pruritic patients. *Nephron* 1998; **78**:395–401.

14 Murphy M, Reaich D, Pai P, *et al.* Randomised placebo-controlled double blind trial of odansetron in renal itch. *Br J Dermatol* 2003;**148**:314–7.

15 Tapia L, Cheigh JS, David DS, *et al.* Pruritus in dialysis patients treated with parenteral lidocaine *N Engl J Med* 1997;**296**:261–2.

16 Pederson JA, Matter BJ, Czerwinski AW, *et al.* Relief of idiopathic generalized pruritus in dialysis patients treated with oral charcoal. *Ann Intern Med* 1980;**93**:446–8.

17 Pauli-Magnus C, Klumpp S, Alscher DM, *et al.* Short-term efficacy of tacrolimus ointment in severe uremic pruritus. *Perit Dial Int* 2000;**20**:802–3.

18 Botero F. Pruritus as a manifestation of systemic disorders. *Cutis* 1978;**21**:873–80.

19 Prince MI, Jones DE. Primary biliary cirrhosis: new perspectives in diagnosis and treatment. *Postgrad Med J* 2000;**76**:199–206.

20 Nunes ACR, Amaro P, Macoas F, *et al.* Fosinopril-induced prolonged cholestatic jaundice and pruritus: a first case report. *Eur J Gastroentrerol Hepatol* 2001;**13**:279–82.

21 Bergasa NV, Thomas DA, Vergalla J, *et al.* Plasma from patients with pruritus of cholestasis induces opioid receptor-mediated scratching in monkeys. *Life Sci* 1993;**53**:1253–7.

22 Thompson W. Cholestyramine. *Can Med Assoc J* 1971;**104**:305–9.

23 Goulis J, Leandro G, Burroughs AK. Randomised controlled trials of ursodeoxycholic acid therapy for primary biliary cirrhosis: a meta-analysis. *Lancet* 1999;**355**:657–8.

24 Ghent CN, Carruthers SG. Treatment of pruritus in primary biliary cirrhosis with rifampin: results of a double-blind, crossover, randomized trial. *Gastroenterology* 1988;**94**:488–93.

25 Bachs L, Parés A, Elena M, Piera C, Rodés J. Comparison of rifampicin with phenobarbitone for treatment of pruritus in biliary cirrhosis. *Lancet* 1989;**i**:574–6.

26 Bergasa N, Alling DW, Talbot TL, *et al.* Oral nalmefene therapy reduces scratching activity due to the pruritus of cholestasis: a controlled study. *J Am Acad Dermatol* 1999;**41**:431–4.

27 Wolfhagen, FHJ, Sternieri E, Hop WCJ, *et al.* Oral naltrexone treatment for cholestatic pruritus: a double-blind placebo-controlled study. *Gastroenterology* 1997;**113**:1264–9.

28 Bergasa, N, Alling DW, Talbot TL, *et al.* Effects of naloxone infusions in patients with the pruritus of cholestasis. A double-blind, randomized, controlled trial. *Ann Intern Med* 1995;**123**:161–7.

29 O'Donohue JW, Haigh C, Williams R. Odansetron in the treatment of pruritus of cholestasis: a randomized controlled trial. *Gastroenterology* 1997;**112A**:1349.

30 Bergasa N, Link MJ, Keogh M, *et al.* Pilot study of bright light therapy reflected towards the eyes for pruritus of chronic liver disease. *Am J Gastroenterol* 2001;**96**:1563–70.

31 Jones EA, Neuberger J, Bergasa N. Opiate antagonist therapy for the pruritus of cholestasis: the avoidance of opioid withdrawal-like reactions. *QJM* 2002;**95**:547–52.

32 Diehn F, Tefferli A. Pruritus in polycythemia vera: prevalence, laboratory correlates and management. *Br J Haematol* 2001;**115**:619–21.

33 Takkunen H. Iron deficiency in the Finnish adult population: an epidemiological survey from 1967 to 1972 inclusive. *Scand J Haematol Suppl* 1976;**25**:1–91.

34 Steinman HK, Black AK, Lotti TM, *et al.* Polycythaemia rubra vera and water-induced pruritus: blood histamine levels and cutaneous fibrinolytic activity before and after water challenge. *Br J Dermatol* 1987;**116**:329–33.

35 Wasserman L. The treatment of polycythaemia vera. *Semin Haematol* 1976;**13**:57–78.

36 Fjellner B, Hagermark O. Pruritus in polycythaemia rubra vera: treatment with aspirin and possibility of platelet involvement. *Acta Derm Venereol* 1979;**59**:505–12.

37 Baldo A, Sammarco E, Plaitano R, *et al.* Narrow band (TL-01) ultraviolet B phototherapy for pruritus in polycythaemia rubra vera. *Br J Dermatol* 2002;**147**:979–81.

38 Jeanmougin M, Rain JD, Najean Y. Efficacy of photochemotherapy on severe pruritus in polycythaemia vera. *Ann Haematol* 1996;**73**:91–3.

39 Menage H du P, Greaves MW. Aquagenic pruritus. *Semin Dermatol* 1995;**14**:313–6.

40 Archer CB, Camp RDR, Greaves MW. Polycythaemia vera can present with aquagenic pruritus. *Lancet* 1988;**ii**:1451.

41 Bayoumi A, Highet AS. Baking soda baths for aquagenic pruritus *Lancet* 1986;**ii**:464.

42 Danamaker CJ, Greenway H. Failure of sodium bicarbonate baths in the treatment of aquagenic pruritus. *J Am Acad Dermatol* 1989;**20**:1136.

43 Greaves MW, Handfield Jones SE. Aquagenic pruritus: pharmacological findings and treatment. *Eur J Dermatol* 1992;**2**:482–4.

44 Menage H du P, Norris PG, Hawk JLM, *et al.* The efficacy of psoralen photochemotherapy in aquagenic pruritus. *Br J Dermatol* 1993;**129**:163–5.

45 Xifra A, Carrascosa JM, Ferrándiz C. Narrow-band ultraviolet B in aquagenic pruritus. *Br J Dermatol* 2005;**153**:1233–4.

46 Greenwood AM. A study of the skin in five hundred cases of diabetes. *J Am Med Assoc* 1927;**89**:774–7.

47 Neilly JB, Martin A, Simpson N, MacCuish AC. Pruritus in diabetes mellitus: investigation of prevalence and correlation with diabetes control. *Diabetes Care* 1986;**9**:273–5.

48 Daniel GL, Longo WE, Vernava AM. Pruritus ani: causes and concerns. *Dis Colon Rectum* 1994;**37**:670–4.

49 Dasan S, Neill SM, Donaldson DR, *et al.* Treatment of persistent pruritus ani in a combined colorectal and dermatological clinic. *Br J Surg* 1999;**86**:1337–40.

50 Bauer A, Geier J, Elsner P. Allergic contact dermatitis in patients with anogenital complaints. *J Reprod Med* 2000;**45**:649–54.

51 Rumpianske R, Shiskin J. Pruritus vulvae: a five year survey. *Dermatologica* 1965;**131**:446–51.

52 Wright HJ, Palmer AJR. The prevalence and clinical diagnosis of vaginal candidosis in non-pregnant patients with vaginal discharge and pruritus vulvae. *J R Coll Gen Pract* 1978;**28**:719–23.

53 Fleckner AN, Anderson C, Yersansian J, *et al.* Pruritus vulvae and its treatment with fluocinolone acetonide *J Am Med Women's Assoc* 1967;**22**:460–1.

54 Kelly RA, Foster DC, Woodruff JD. Subcutaneous injection of triamcinolone acetonide in the treatment of chronic vulvar pruritus. *Am J Obstet Gynecol* 1993;**169**:568–70.

55 Sutherst JR. Treatment of pruritus vulvae by multiple intradermal injections of alcohol. A double-blind study. *Br J Obstet Gynecol* 1979;**86**:371–3.

56 Woodruff JD, Thompson B. Local alcohol injection in the treatment of vulvar pruritus. *Obstet Gynecol* 1972;**40**:18–20.

57 Mering JH. A surgical approach to intractable pruritus vulvae. *Am J Obstet Gynecol* 1952;**64**:619–27.

58 Oztas MO, Oztas P, Onder M. Idiopathic perianal pruritus: washing compared with topical corticosteroids. *Postgrad Med J* 2004;**80**:295–7.

59 Minvielle L, Hernandez VL. The use of intralesional triamcinolone hexacetonide in the treatment of idiopathic pruritus ani. *Dis Colon Rectum* 1969;**12**:340–3.

60 Lysy J, Sistiery-Ittah M, Israelit Y, *et al.* Topical capsaicin: a novel and effective treatment for idiopathic intractable pruritus ani: a randomized placebo controlled crossover study. *Gut* 2003;**52**: 1323–6.

61 Shafik A. A new concept of the anatomy of the anal sphincter mechanism and physiology of defaecation. XXIII. An injection technique for the treatment of idiopathic pruritus ani. *Int Surg* 1990;**75**:43–6.

62 Bigby M, Jick S, Jick H, Arndt K. Drug-induced cutaneous reactions. A report from the Boston Collaborative Drug Surveillance Program on 15,438 consecutive inpatients, 1975 to 1982. *JAMA* 1986;**256**:3358–63.

63 Arndt KA, Jick H. Rates of cutaneous reactions to drugs: a report from the Boston Collaborative Drug Surveillance Program. *JAMA* 1976;**235**:918–22.

64 Murphy M, Carmichael AJ, Lawler PG, White M, Cox NH. The incidence of hydroxyethyl starch-associated pruritus. *Br J Dermatol* 2001;**144**:973–6.

65 Metze D, Reimann S, Szepfalusi Z, Bohle B, Kraft D, Luger TA. Persistent pruritus after hydroxyethyl starch infusion therapy. Results of a long-term starch in cutaneous nerves. *Br J Dermatol* 1997;**136**:553–9.

66 Ballantyne JC, Losch AB, Carr DB. Itching after epidural and spinal opioids. *Pain* 1988;**33**:149–60.

67 Ballantyne JC, Loach AB, Carr DB. The incidence of pruritus after epidural morphine. *Anaesthesia* 1989;**44**:863.

68 Sirtl C, Laubenthal H, Zumtobel V, Kraft D, Jurecka W. Tissue deposits of hydroxyethyl starch (HES): dose-dependent and time related. *Br J Anaesth* 1999;**82**:510–5.

69 Ständer S, Szepfalusi Z, Bohle B, *et al.* Differential storage of hydroxyethyl starch (HES) in the skin: an immunoelectron-microscopical long-term study. *Cell Tissue Res* 2001;**304**:261–9.

70 Szeimies RM, Stolz W, Wlotzke U, Korting HC, Landthaler M. Successful treatment of hydroxyethyl starch-induced pruritus with topical capsaicin. *Br J Dermatol* 1994;**131**:380–2.

71 Reimann S, Luger T, Metze D. [Topical administration of capsaicin in dermatology for treatment of itching and pain; in German.] *Hautarzt* 2000;**51**:164–72.

72 Metze D, Reimann S, Beissert S, Luger T. Efficacy and safety of natrexone, an oral opiate receptor antagonist, in the treatment of pruritus in internal and dermatological diseases. *J Am Acad Dermatol* 1999;**41**:533–9.

73 Brune A, Metze D, Luger TA, Stander S. [Antipruritic therapy with the oral opioid receptor antagonist naltrexone. Open, non-placebo controlled administration in 133 patients; in German.] *Hautarzt* 2004;**55**:1130–6.

74 Bellmann R, Feistrizer C, Zoller H, *et al.* Treatment of intractable pruritus in drug induced cholestasis with albumin dialysis: a report of two cases. *ASAIO J* 2004;**50**:387–91.

75 Kjellberg F, Tramèr MR. Pharmacological control of opioid-induced pruritus: a quantitative systematic review of randomized trials. *Eur J Anaesthesiol* 2001;**18**:346–57.

76 Maxwell LG, Kaufmann SC, Bitzer S, *et al.* The effects of small-dose naloxone infusion on opioid-induced side effects and analgesia in children and adolescents treated with intravenous patient-controlled analgesia: a double-blind, prospective, randomized, controlled study. *Anesth Analg* 2005;**100**:953–8.

77 Lee LHY, Irwin MG, Lim J, Wong CK. The effect of celecoxib on intrathecal morphine-induced pruritus in patients undergoing Caesarean section. *Anaesthesia* 2004;**59**:876–80.

78 Mercadente S, Villari P, Fulfaro F. Rifampicin in opioid-induced itching. *Support Care Cancer* 2001;**9**:467–8.

79 Zancanaro PSQ, McGirt LY, Mamelak AJ, Nguyen RHN, Martins CR. Cutaneous manifestation of HIV in the era of highly active antiretroviral therapy: an institutional urban clinic experience. *J Am Acad Dermatol* 2006;**54**:581–8.

80 Bonacini M. Pruritus in patients with chronic human immunodeficiency virus, hepatitis B and C virus infections. *Drug Liver Dis* 2000;**32**:621–5.

81 Weisshaar E, Apfelbacher C, Jäger G, *et al.* Pruritus as a leading symptom: clinical characteristics and quality of life in German and Ugandan patients. *Br J Dermatol* 2006;**155**:957–64.

82 Gelfand JM, Rudikoff D. Evaluation and treatment of itching in HIV-infected patients. *Mount Sinai J Med* 2001;**68**:298–308.

83 Weisshaar E, Kucenic MJ, Fleischer AB Jr. Pruritus: a review. *Acta Derm Venereol Suppl (Stockh)* 2003;**213**:5–32.

84 Milazzo F, Piconi S, Trabattoni D, *et al.* Intractable pruritus in HIV interaction: immunologic characterization. *Allergy* 1999;**54**: 226–72.

85 Smith KJ, Skelton HG, Yeager J, Lee RB, Wagner KF. Pruritus in HIV-1 disease: therapy with drugs which may modulate the pattern of immune dysregulation. *Dermatology* 1997;**195**:353–8.

86 Lim HW, Vallurupalli S, Meola T, Soter NA. UVB phototherapy is an effective treatment for pruritus in patients infected with HIV. *J Am Acad Dermatol* 1997;**37**:414–7.

87 Gelfand JM, Rudikoff D, Lebwohl M, Klotman ME. Effect of UV-B phototherapy on plasma HIV type 1 RNA viral level: a self-controlled prospective study. *Arch Dermatol* 1998;**134**:940–5.

88 Akaraphanth R, Lim HW. HIV, UV, and immunosuppression. *Photodermatol Photoimmunol Photomed* 1999;**15**:28–31.

89 Maurer T, Poncelet A, Berger T. Thalidomide treatment for prurigo nodularis in human immunodeficiency virus-infected subjects: efficacy and risk of neuropathy. *Arch Dermatol* 2004;**140**:845–9.

90 Rucklidge JJ, Saunders D. The efficacy of hypnosis in the treatment of pruritus in people with HIV/AIDS. a time-series analysis. *Int J Clin Exp Hypn* 2002;**50**:149–69.

91 Arnold LM, Auchenbach MB, McElroy SL. Psychogenic excoriation. Clinical features, proposed diagnostic criteria, epidemiology and approaches to treatment. *CNS Drugs* 2001;**15**:351–9.

92 Calikusu C, Yucel B, Polat A, Baykal C. The relation of psychogenic excoriations with psychiatric disorders: a comparative study. *Compr Psychiatry* 2003;**44**:256–61.

93 Biondi M, Arcangeli T, Petrucci RM. Paroxetine in a case of psychogenic pruritus and neurotic excoriations. *Psychother Psychosom* 2000;**69**:165–6.

94 Gupta MA, Gupta AK. Fluoxetine is an effective treatment for neurotic excoriations: case report. *Cutis* 1993;**51**:386–7.

95 Hundley JL, Yosipovitch G. Mirtazapine for reducing nocturnal itch in patients with chronic pruritus. *J Am Acad Dermatol* 2004; **50**:889–91.

96 Yalcm B, Tamer E, Toy GG, Öztas P, Hayran M, Alli N. The prevalence of skin diseases in the elderly: analysis of 4099 geriatric patients. *Int J Dermatol* 2006;**45**:672–6.

97 Thaipisuttikul Y. Pruritic skin diseases in the elderly. *J Dermatol* 1998;**25**:153–7.

98 Guillet G, Zampetti A, Czarlewski W, Guillet MH. Increased histamine release and skin hypersensitivity to histamine in senile pruritus: study of 60 patients. *J Eur Acad Dermatol Venereol* 2000;**14**:65.

99 Dupont C, de Maubeuge J, Kotlar W, Lays Y, Masson M. Oxatomide in the treatment of pruritus senilis. A double-blind placebo-controlled trial. *Dermatologica* 1984;**169**:348–53.

100 Teofoli P, De Pita O, Frezzolini A, Lotti T. Antipruritic effect of oral cyclosporin A in essential senile pruritus. *Acta Derm Venereol* 1998;**78**:232.

101 Daly BM, Shuster S. Antipruritic action of thalidomide. *Acta Derm Venereol* 2000;**80**:24–5.

102 Oaklander AL, Bowsher D, Galer B, Haanpaa M, Jensen MP. Herpes zoster itch: preliminary epidemiological data. *J Pain* 2003;**4**:338–43.

103 Savk E, Savk SÖ, Bolukbasi O, *et al.* Notalgia paresthetica: a study on pathogenesis. *Int J Dermatol* 2000;**39**:754–9.

104 Savk O, Savk E. Investigation of spinal pathology in notalgia paresthetica. *J Am Acad Dermatol* 2005;**52**:1085–7.

105 Cohen AD, Masalha R, Medvedovsky E, Vardy DA. Brachioradial pruritus: a symptom of neuropathy. *J Am Acad Dermatol* 2003; **48**:825–8.

106 Goodkin R, Wingard E, Bernhard JD. Brachioradial pruritus: cervical spine disease and neurogenic/neurogenic pruritus. *J Am Acad Dermatol* 2003;**48**:521–4.

107 Bond LD, Keough GC. Neurogenic pruritus: a case of pruritus induced by transverse myelitis. *Br J Dermatol* 2003;**149**:193–4.

108 Kavak A, Dosoglu M. Can a spinal cord tumor cause brachioradial pruritus? *J Am Acad Dermatol* 2002;**46**:437–40.

109 Wallengren J, Dahlbäck K. Familial brachioradial pruritus. *Br J Dermatol* 2005;**153**:1016–8.

110 Wallengren J, Sundler F. Brachioradial pruritus is associated with reduction in cutaneous innervation that normalizes during the symptom-free remission. *J Am Acad Dermatol* 2005;**52**:142–5.

111 Cohen AD, Vander T, Medvendovsky E, *et al.* Neuropathic scrotal pruritus. Anogenital pruritus is a symptom of lumbosacral radiculopathy. *J Am Acad Dermatol* 2005;**52**:61–6.

112 Raison-Peyron N, Meunier L, Acevedo M, Meynadier J. Notalgia paresthetica: clinical, physiopathological and therapeutic aspects. A study of 12 cases. *J Eur Acad Dermatol Venereol* 1999;**12**:215–21.

113 Wallengren J, Klinker M. Successful treatment of notalgia paresthetica with topical capsaicin: vehicle-controlled, double-blind, crossover study. *J Am Acad Dermatol* 1995;**32**:287–9.

114 Leibsohn E. Treatment of nostalgia paresthetica with capsaicin. *Cutis* 1992;**49**:335–6.

115 Knight TE, Hayashi T. Solar (brachioradial) pruritus: response to capsaicin cream. *Int J Dermatol* 1994;**33**:206–9.

116 Goodless DR, Eaglstein WH. Brachioradial pruritus: treatment with topical capsaicin. *J Am Acad Dermatol* 1993;**29**:783–4.

117 Wallengren J, Sundler F. Cutaneous field stimulation in the treatment of itch. *Arch Dermatol* 2001;**137**:1323–5.

118 Bueller HA, Bernhard JD, Dubroff LM. Gabapentin treatment for brachioradial pruritus. *J Eur Acad Dermatol Venereol* 1999; **13**:227–30.

119 Winhoven SM, Coulson IH, Bottomley WW. Brachioradial pruritus: response to treatment with gabapentin. *Br J Dermatol* 2004;**150**:786–7.

120 Schürmeyer-Horst F, Fischbach R, Nabavi D, Metze D, Ständer S. [Brachioradial pruritus: a rare, localized, neuropathic form of itching; in German.] *Hautarzt* 2006;**57**:523–7.

121 Kanitakis J. Brachioradial pruritus: report of a new case responding to gabapentin. *Eur J Dermatol* 2006;**16**:311–2.

122 Savk E, Bolukbasi O, Akyol A, Karaman G. Open pilot study on oxcarbazepine for the treatment of notalgia paresthetica. *J Am Acad Dermatol* 2001;**45**:630–2.

123 Stellon A. Neurogenic pruritus: an unrecognized problem? A retrospective case series of treatment by acupuncture. *Acupuncture Med* 2002;**20**:186–90.

124 Kroumpouzos G, Cohen LM. Specific dermatoses of pregnancy: an evidence-based systematic review. *Am J Obstet Gynecol* 2003; **188**:1083–92.

125 Black MM, McKay M, Braude PR. *Color Atlas and Text of Obstetric and Gynecologic Dermatology*. 2nd ed. London: Times Mirror International, 2001.

126 Roger D, Vaillant L, Fignon A, *et al.* Specific pruritic dermatoses of pregnancy. A prospective study of 3192 pregnant women. *Arch Dermatol* 1994;**130**:734–9.

127 Shanmugam S, Thappa DM, Habeebullah S. Pruritus gravidarum: a clinical and laboratory study. *J Dermatol* 1998;**25**:582–6.

128 Reyes H, Gonzales MC, Ribalta J, *et al.* Prevalence or intrahepatic cholestasis of pregnancy in Chile. *Ann Intern Med* 1978;**88**:487–93.

129 Dann AT, Kenyon AP, Wierzbicki AS, Seed PT, Shennan AH, Tribe RM. Plasma lipid profiles of women with intrahepatic cholestasis of pregnancy. *Obstet Gynecol* 2006;**107**:106–14.

130 Schaefer C, Spielmann H. *Arzneiverordnung in Schwangerschaft und Stillzeit*. Munich: Urban & Fischer, 2001.

131 Olayemi O, Fehintola FA, Osungbade A, Aimakhu CO, Udoh ES, Adeniji AR. Pattern of chloroquine-induced pruritus in antenatal patients at the University College Hospital, Ibadan. *J Obstet Gynaecol* 2003;**23**:490–5.

132 Sheiner E, Ohel I, Levy A, Katz M. Pregnancy outcome in women with pruritus gravidarum. *J Reprod Med* 2006;**51**:394–8.

133 Dann AT, Kenyon AP, Seed PT, Poston L, Shennan AH, Tribe RM. Glutathione *S*-transferase and liver function in intrahepatic cholestasis of pregnancy and pruritus gravidarum. *Hepatology* 2004;**40**:1406–14.

134 Young GL, Jewell D. Antihistamines versus aspirin for itching in late pregnancy. *Cochrane Database Syst Rev* 2000;(**2**):CD000027.

135 den Dulk M, Valentijn RM, Welten CA, Beyer GP. Intrahepatic cholestasis of pregnancy. *Neth J Med* 2002;**60**:366–9.

136 Zirwas MJ, Seraly MP. Pruritus of unknown origin: a retrospective study. *J Am Acad Dermatol* 2001;**45**:892–96.

137 Yesudian PD, Wilson NJE. Efficacy of gabapentin in the management of pruritus of unknown origin. *Arch Dermatol* 2005;**141**: 1507–9.

67

Other skin diseases for which trials exist

Sinéad Langan, Hywel Williams

Why a chapter on "everything else"?

Any textbook purporting to guide clinical dermatological practice that fails to cover the majority of skin diseases is open to major criticism. Yet, as Naldi points out in Chapter 1, around 1000–2000 skin conditions have been described to date, and trying to cover them all in just one textbook and in sufficient detail is challenging. In the first edition of this textbook, we aspired to cover as many of the common or important conditions as possible—the words "common" or "important" being defined empirically by the editors on the basis of epidemiological studies and clinical practice around the world. Although we included 54 chapters in that book, there were still prominent omissions with respect to some fairly common conditions, such as "moles" or "pityriasis versicolor," which we have now endeavored to cover in this edition or in the accompanying web chapters that will follow between this second edition and the next. But what happens to the remaining 1900 or so less common or ignored skin diseases?

Many of these other skin conditions may be rare in relative terms, yet collectively they make up a significant component of the dermatologist's workload, and diagnosing and managing them may take up a disproportionate amount of time relative to the everyday conditions seen in clinical practice. Previous research on the use of Internet resources in dermatology suggests that many hits/requests are concerned with less common skin diseases.[1] From a patient's perspective, being told that you have a rare skin disease is of little consolation, especially if your doctor knows little about it and you need to find out about effective treatments. So there is a clear case for including as many less common skin disorders as possible in a book such as this—but if possible without resulting in an unwieldy four-volume edition.

The importance of mapping all randomized controlled trials

As well as the requirement to ensure at least some degree of coverage for less common skin diseases, there is a need to point health-care providers and patients to the most reliable sources of evidence—i.e., randomized controlled trials or systematic reviews of such trials. This book is, after all, a textbook on evidence-based dermatology. Predictably, there is a lack of such randomized controlled trials (RCTs) for less common skin diseases, possibly due to the difficulties in recruiting sufficient people with the same condition in order to obtain enough statistical power to answer the questions posed on the therapeutic interventions. Such trials are not impossible, however, as has been proved by a trial on toxic epidermal necrolysis (TEN) conducted by a European group.[2] That study found that a treatment for TEN that was fashionable at the time (thalidomide) was associated with increased rather than decreased mortality in comparison with placebo. As such, it was a very important trial in preventing doctors from inadvertently killing patients with a drug they thought would benefit them. The trial also underscores the importance of conducting randomized controlled trials to identify harms in addition to benefits, and why it is important not to base clinical practice on empirical logic alone based on the known mechanisms of thalidomide and its potential to reduce tumor necrosis factor. Other trials highlighted in this chapter have also shown that it is possible to recruit modest numbers of participants with less common skin disorders such as Jessner's lymphocytic infiltrate, recessive dystrophic epidermolysis bullosa, and notalgia paresthetica into clinical trials. Like other clinical trial research networks that have pioneered trials of rare childhood tumors, national networks such as the United Kingdom Dermatology Clinical Trials Network (www.ukdctn.org) are now working together to try and answer important primary questions about diseases such as pyoderma gangrenosum and cutaneous vasculitis.

Drawbacks of mapping randomized controlled trials

In this chapter, we have started by trying to map out where all the RCTs have been done for conditions that have not been covered elsewhere in this book, and we have included 72 so far. This does not mean to say that in the absence of RCTs, treatments currently used in practice do not work, but simply that their use has yet to be backed up by the most reliable form of evidence. Our choice of drawing a line in the evidence hierarchy (Chapter 7) at the level of RCTs does not mean to say that data from case series and other observational studies should be discarded if no RCT evidence is forthcoming. But as Albrecht and Bigby point out in Chapter 11, assessing the quality of such observational studies can be tricky. It also should be stressed that just because a study is an RCT, it does not necessarily mean that it provides reliable evidence. Authors can fail to report essential study features, report only the data that they want to show, and use the wrong statistical tests, which is why some comment about the study's quality is also important in the table presented in this chapter.[3] As the RCTs included in the table show (Table 67.1), most of the studies are inconclusive and are far too small to exclude even very large treatment differences, although even small studies can be used in future systematic reviews and pooled together in meta-analyses if they are sufficiently similar.

A further problem in trying to find and report all dermatology RCTs in one resource in a book such as this is that such a strategy may inadvertently collude with external forces that dictate the current research agenda in dermatology, which tends to reflect new drug developments generated by the pharmaceutical industry (or alternative uses for "new" drugs), instead of drawing attention to the large gaps in information and collective ignorance on the many interventions already in use for skin disease. It is like a man who has lost his wallet in a dark street crossing the road to look under a street lamp, simply because "the light is better over there." Thus, teams conducting systematic reviews in the Cochrane Skin Group (Chapter 4) are encouraged not to "peep" at the external data beforehand and end up with a data-driven review, but instead to ask important questions about interventions for skin disease and then to seek the evidence to address those questions.

Seek and ye shall find

Despite the above caveats, we have not been deterred in our attempts at starting to describe the RCTs for "everything else" not covered in the rest of this text book, and we have summarized a reasonable collection of RCTs to hopefully inform clinical practice and future research. And there are some surprises there. It is easy to assume that there are no RCTs present for most skin diseases, but you will not know unless you look. For example, we were surprised to find quite a good RCT on aphthous stomatitis and another on chronic paronychia.[4,5] The study on aphthous ulceration demonstrated a clear benefit for thalidomide over placebo, offering a useful intervention for severe cases, while the paronychia study showed that topical methylprednisone acetonide was more effective than terbinafine or itraconazole. The point is that unless you search following the principles of evidence-based dermatology outlined in Chapter 6, you will not find answers—the human mind is fallible and cannot hope to passively assimilate important information from the 200 or so specialist dermatology journals that are currently in existence.[6]

Informing future trials

In addition to informing clinical practice, another important use of this chapter is in looking to see how existing studies can inform future, better RCTs. Even small inconclusive studies can provide valuable data on recruitment rates, acceptability of interventions, the logistics of procedures, and the choice and variability of outcome measures, as well as common adverse effects. Too many times, well-intentioned clinicians have gone ahead with a new clinical trial without recourse to reviewing what has previously been done in that area, only to repeat the same mistakes pointed out in previous work. Thankfully, many commissioning bodies, such as the Medical Research Council in the United Kingdom, now insist that new trial applications must be accompanied by a previous systematic review that summarizes previous trials and relevant evidence, and groups such as the Cochrane Skin Group are filling important gaps with systematic reviews on rare disorders such as mucous membrane pemphigoid and epidermolysis bullosa acquisita.[7] Unnecessary overlap in future trials is also likely to decline as more and more journals insist on prospective trial registration in a publicly accessible database.[8]

How to use the table

Although some readers might find some interesting snippets after scanning through some of the trials in this chapter, it is not our intention for the reader to work through this chapter from start to finish like a novel. Apart from being a bit boring, the type of quantitative data included is difficult to recall and its immediate utility is unclear. Instead, it is hoped that in the true spirit of evidence-based dermatology, driven by questions following a patient consultation, readers will turn to this section as a first stop when they encounter a less common condition, in case there is a good

Table 67.1 Other skin diseases for which trials exist

First author, year, ref.	Interventions (co-treatments)	Study population and sample size	Trial design description and follow-up	Outcome measures	Main reported results	Quality of reporting	Comments
Aphthous stomatitis							
Revuz 1990[4]	Thalidomide 100 mg daily or placebo, each for period of 2 months in crossover fashion. No wash-out period	73 adults (45 men, 28 women aged 28 to 58 years. Typical painful aphthous ulcers (multiple shallow or giant) present for 6 months. Sample size of 80 calculated to detect significance at 5% level	Multicenter randomized double-blinded crossover study, 4 months	Primary outcome measure: complete clearing of all aphthae within 1 month and maintenance for second month. Secondary measures: mean number of aphthae per day and degree of functional impairment by daily self-evaluation	Complete remission (CR) in 17 (45%) of 38 patients (thalidomide) and 1 (3%) placebo during first period; $P < 0.0001$. 15 (44%) of 34 patients (thalidomide) and 5 (15%) of 33 patients (placebo) had CRs during the second period. 95% confidence interval for difference in treatments 25 to 53%. NNT period 1 = 2, period 2 = 3. Mean number of aphthae thalidomide 3.3 to 0.3 (first period) and 2.4 to 0.2 (second period). Mean number of aphthae placebo group 3.3 to 2.4 (first period) and 0.3 to 1.7 (second period)	Unclear how randomization done at each center. Allocation concealment and blinding adequate. Analysis by ITT. Adverse events clearly reported. Six drop-outs (two paresthesia with electrical abnormalities, one constipation), 10 treatment interruptions secondary to adverse events	The sample size was adequate. A significant improvement in aphthae was seen with thalidomide in comparison with placebo. Adverse events necessitating interruption in 10 (15%) of thalidomide group; two patients (3%) had persisting abnormal peripheral nerve electrical activity. Duration to relapse 19 days (range 1–35 days)
Collier 1992[12]	5% 5-aminosalicylic acid (5-ASA) cream vs. placebo three times daily for up to 14 days (or clearance of ulcers)	22 patients (11 males and 11 females, aged 20–73 years) with recurrent active aphthous ulcers	Randomized double-blind placebo-controlled study, 28 days	Pain and difficulty eating assessed on 0–100 mm VAS. Number and site of ulcers recorded. Daily diary recording of ulcer numbers	84% reduction in pain in treatment group vs. placebo group at day 7; day 15: 0 of 5 in treatment group vs. 6 of 8 in placebo group experienced pain ($P = 0.032$). Days to clearing 7 in treatment group vs. 11 in placebo group ($P < 0.01$). Difficulty eating: at day 14 none of treatment group, half of placebo group had difficulty eating ($P < 0.01$)	Randomization and treatment allocation poorly described. Blinding appeared adequate. Analysis by ITT. Three drop-outs	Small study group and short duration of study limit conclusions. Treatment did not appear to provide benefit

Table 67.1 Cont'd

First author, year, ref.	Interventions (co-treatments)	Study population and sample size	Trial design description and follow-up	Outcome measures	Main reported results	Quality of reporting	Comments
Femiano 2003[13]	*Group A:* Systemic sulodexide (500 lipidic units) 250 mg twice daily 1 month, once daily 1 month *Group B:* Oral prednisolone 25 mg (1 week) on reducing schedule *Group C:* Cellulose starch 100 mg twice daily 1 month, once daily for 1 month	30 adults (24 women, six men, aged 21–48 years) with frequent minor recurrent aphthous stomatitis (RAS) for > 4 months unresponsive to topical corticosteroids	Randomized double-blind placebo-controlled study, 5 months	Primary outcome measures: days to recovery from pain and ulceration during first month and numbers of aphthae during rest of study period	Both treatment groups were compared to controls only. Days to resolution of pain 4 (Group A), 2–3 (Group B), 4–5 (Group C); $P < 0.03$. Days to reepithelialization 7–8 (Group A), 4–5 (Group B), 10–11 (Group C); $P < 0.05$. No comparison between active treatments (A and B). Authors state that results suggest lower efficacy in the latter in comparison with the former, but did not compare the two groups, so this conclusion cannot be drawn	Randomization and treatment allocation concealment are inadequately described. Blinding appeared adequate. No drop-outs. Authors state that adverse events described in prednisolone group, but list an equal number of events in sulodexide group	Number of aphthae given in tabular format, but no analysis of significance of difference between groups. Small sample size and no validation of outcome measures
Alidaee 2005[14]	Chemical cautery with the tip of a silver nitrate stick or sugar stick (placebo) once off	85 adults (43 men, 42 women, aged 16–40 years) with a single minor aphthous ulceration	Randomized double-blind placebo-controlled study, 7 days	Change in severity of pain from baseline (3-point scale from no pain to severe pain that interferes with eating) Change in size of ulcers and time to reepithelialization	No difference in size of ulcers or time to reepithelialization. Difference in change in severity of pain day 1 (treatment group: before 47 severe pain; days 1–14 severe pain; no severe pain by day 3; placebo group: before 38 severe pain, days 1–34 severe pain, days 3–20 severe pain) to day 6. Pain resolved in both groups by day 7	Randomization, allocation concealment, and blinding well described (treating physician not blinded, assessing physician blinded). 12 patients excluded from analysis. No ITT analysis. No adverse events. Sample size calculated	Adequate sample size and well-conducted study showing reduced pain, but no effect on healing of ulcers

Chilblains—prophylaxis

Reference	Intervention	Patients	Study design	Outcome measures	Results	Methodological comments	Conclusion
Langtry 1989[15]	One limb treated with UVB, one with visible light three times per week for 2 weeks in October	Nine female patients (aged 11–75 years) with chilblains of the hands and/or feet	Randomized double-blind placebo-controlled study, 3 months	Severity assessed on ordinal scale 0–4 (nil to ulcerated). Patients assessed severity on VAS (0–100)	No difference between treatment and placebo sides	Details of randomization not given. Allocation concealment adequate. Blinding described, may not have been effective due to erythema and subsequent pigmentation of treatment side. No drop-outs.	No benefit in UV prophylaxis shown for chilblains

Chilblains—treatment*

Reference	Intervention	Patients	Study design	Outcome measures	Results	Methodological comments	Conclusion
Rustin 1989[16]	Nifedipine retard 20 mg three times daily or placebo tablets for 6 weeks followed by crossover, no wash-out	10 patients (eight females, two males, aged 21–64 years) with severe recurrent acral perniosis for 5 months per annum in the last 5 years with established lesions	Randomized double-blind, placebo-controlled crossover study, 12 weeks	Symptoms of pain and irritation (better, same or worse) Duration of established lesions and appearance of new lesions	7/10 patients clear of lesions on nifedipine in a mean of 8 days. All patients on placebo developed new lesions, which resolved over a mean of 24 days. Severe relapse in three patients on switch to placebo led to breaking the code and restarting nifedipine. Pain and irritation resolved in a mean of 5 and 4 days, respectively, in comparison with 25 and 23 days on placebo.	Randomization and allocation concealment not described. Blinding appeared adequate. No statistical analysis done. Adverse events seen in two of nifedipine group	Study was followed by open study which confirmed findings with histology and laser Doppler velocimetry. Study suggests benefit, but sample size small, follow-up short, and no statistical analysis done

Diabetic foot ulcers*

Reference	Intervention	Patients	Study design	Outcome measures	Results	Methodological comments	Conclusion
Tom 2005[17]	Topical 0.05% tretinoin solution or placebo saline solution applied for 10 min once daily, then rinsed off. Cadexomer iodine gel then applied to wound bed until the next day	24 male volunteers (aged 57–65 years) with diabetic foot ulcers	Randomized double-blind placebo-controlled study, 16 weeks	The proportion of ulcers that healed in each group and the degree of change in ulcer size	2/11 (18%) of control and 6/13 (46%) of tretinoin group completely healed ($P = 0.03$). Percentage change in surface area: +2 in control, −54.7% in active group. Change in depth: −29.6 in control, −60.1 in active group, $P < 0.01$	Randomization, allocation concealment, and blinding well described and appeared effective. Two drop-outs. No ITT analysis. Pain described in one control and two in active treatment group	Small, well-conducted study using volunteers suggesting that short contact tretinoin 0.05% may be useful for diabetic ulcers. Needs large RCT to confirm

Table 67.1 Cont'd

First author, year, ref.	Interventions (co-treatments)	Study population and sample size	Trial design description and follow-up	Outcome measures	Main reported results	Quality of reporting	Comments
Disorders of keratinization							
Christophersen 1992[18]	Acitretin or etretinate 30 mg for 4 weeks, followed by dose adjustment for individual patients	26 patients (10 males, 16 females, aged 17–69 years) with Darier's disease	Randomized multicenter double-blind study, 16 weeks	Scores (0–3) for hyperkeratosis, papulosis, and erythema. Estimate of body surface area involved. Overall efficacy by investigator and patients	Reduction in body surface area to 5% (from 30% in acitretin and 10% in etretinate group. A satisfactory response was seen in 77% of patients on acitretin and 73% on etretinate. (95% CI for a +4% difference, –30 to 38%). No difference in tolerability between groups	Randomization and allocation concealment poorly described. Blinding appeared adequate. Results of primary outcome reported, but no statistical analysis given. No definition given for "satisfactory response." Two drop-outs in etretinate group (one adverse events, one improved)	Small sample size. No statistical analysis given of primary outcome. Treatments appear equally effective
Kragballe 1995[19]	Randomized double-blind, right–left comparative study of calcipotriol (50 μg/g) and placebo ointment twice daily, to either right or left arm.	67 patients (aged 11–69 years) with ichthyosis vulgaris (9), X-linked ichthyosis (8), congenital ichthyosis (10), hereditary palmoplantar keratoderma (20), keratosis pilaris (9), Darier's disease (11)	Randomized, double-blind, placebo-controlled right–left comparative study, 12 weeks	Extent of dyskeratotic involvement (percentage body surface area). Mean total sign score (scales, roughness, hyperpigmentation, papules, crust, excoriation, thickness erythema and fissuring. Signs assessed varied for each disease). Investigator and patient global assessment (6-point scale from worse to cleared)	Investigator assessment: marked improvement or clearance in 5/9 with ichthyosis vulgaris (1/9 in placebo), 4/8 with X-linked ichthyosis (0/8 with placebo) and 8/10 with congenital ichthyosis (1/10 in placebo). Difference in total sign score between treatment sides for congenital ichthyosis (–2 with placebo, –4 with active treatment), ichthyosis vulgaris (–3 vs. –4 placebo vs. active), X-linked ichthyosis (0 vs. –3 placebo vs. active)	No details given of randomization and allocation concealment. Unable to assess the efficacy of blinding. 15 withdrawals. No ITT analysis. Adverse events described. Reduction in sign scores interpreted from figure (not given in text).	Small subgroups, short study duration. No benefit seen in keratosis pilaris or palmoplantar keratoderma. Darier's disease worsened in 8/11 patients. Possibly useful in congenital ichthyosis and X-linked ichthyosis, although clinical correlation of change in severity scores unclear
Ganemo 1999[20]	Four 500-g jars of cream labeled "left" or "right arm" or "leg" containing 5% urea in Locobase fatty cream	20 adults (13 women, seven men aged 16–64 years) with widespread lamellar ichthyosis	Randomized double-blind within-patient study	Weekly patient evaluation of skin symptoms on VAS. Scoring 0–4 for scaling, dryness and	Results given were comparison with UL. PL no significant difference seen. LPL scores scaling 1.7 (2.1 UL), dryness 1.3	Randomization, allocation concealment, and blinding adequate. Two drop-outs (one deterioration in skin after stopping acitretin,	Small sample size and short study duration limit study conclusions. Reductions in scaling and dryness

Epidermolysis bullosa simplex

Reference	Intervention	Patients	Study design	Outcome measures	Results	Methodological quality	Comments
	(UL), 20% propylene glycol in Locobase fatty cream (PL), 5% lactic acid and 20% propylene glycol in Locobase fatty cream (LPL), and 5% lactic acid and 20% propylene glycol in Essex cream (LPE)			erythema on days 1 and 28. Photographs, skin molding, skin capacitance, and transepidermal water loss (TEWL) were measured	(1.8 UL) and erythema 1.3 (0.9UL); all $P < 0.01$. LPE scaling 1.4, dryness 1.1, and erythema 1.3; $P < 0.001$ first two variables and < 0.01 latter variable. Significant increases in capacitance and TEWL with LPL and LPE	one irritation all extremities). Unclear if ITT analysis	accompanied by increases in erythema and decreased barrier function. Long-term tolerability would be of interest
Fine 1988[21]	Bufexamac 5% cream vs. placebo four times daily for 4 weeks each; no wash-out	10 patients (four male, six female, aged 15–74 years) with EBS	Randomized double-blind placebo-controlled crossover study	Weekly lesion counts by investigators. Patient weekly grading of pain and improvement. Daily diaries of symptoms and blister counts	Mean difference in lesion counts 3.44 (lesions); $P = 0.62$. No difference in pain, healing time, or activity time between groups	Randomization and allocation concealment poorly described. Blinding appeared adequate. Two patients not included in analysis (reduced activity), no drop-outs	Small sample size lacking power to detect effect; results suggest a lack of efficacy
Younger 1990[22]	Topical aluminum chloride hexahydrate (Drichlor) vs. placebo once daily to soles of feet for 4 weeks each treatment period, 1 week wash-out	23 patients (4–63 years) with Weber–Cockayne EBS	Randomized double-blind placebo-controlled crossover study, 9 weeks	New bullae counts by patients and weekly by investigators	First month: mean blister count 6.5 both groups, second month: mean blister count 5.4 (placebo) and 5.1 (active); not significant	Randomization and allocation concealment poorly described. Blinding appeared adequate. Eight drop-outs, reasons not given. Authors state no adverse events	Small sample size; results suggest a lack of efficacy
Hansen 1996[23]	Oral oxytetracycline 1 g daily vs. placebo in 3-week blocks with 2-week wash-out period	21 patients (12 men and nine women, mean age 36.6 years) with EBS	Randomized double-blind placebo-controlled cross-over study.	New bullae counts at 3, 5 and 8 weeks	Six of 18 improved with tetracycline, seven of 18 with placebo; $P > 0.05$.	Randomization, allocation concealment, and blinding poorly described. Three drop-outs inadequately described. Authors state no adverse events	Small sample size and results suggest a lack of efficacy
Weiner 2004[24]	Oral tetracycline 1500 mg daily vs. placebo in four month blocks with 2-month wash-out	12 patients (eight males, four females, aged 13–47) with Weber–Cockayne EBS	Randomized double-blind placebo-controlled crossover study, 10 months	Total counts of discrete EB lesions (blisters, erosions and crusts) every 2 months	Authors state that four of six patients had a reduction in lesions on tetracycline, while two experienced an increased number. Authors state that no patients had decreased lesion counts on placebo, but results and significance test results not given	Block randomization described. Allocation concealment poorly described. Blinding appeared adequate. Unclear how many were in each treatment group in each arm of the study. Drop-outs (two completed full trial) and adverse events poorly described	Sample size small, with inconclusive results and increased adverse events with tetracycline

Table 67.1 Cont'd

First author, year, ref.	Interventions (co-treatments)	Study population and sample size	Trial design description and follow-up	Outcome measures	Main reported results	Quality of reporting	Comments
Recessive dystrophic epidermolysis bullosa							
Caldwell-Brown 1992[25]	Phenytoin (initial dose 5 mg/kg body weight per day) given once daily as 50 mg tablets or placebo for 5–7 months (phenytoin for 4 months once blood concentration 8–20 µg/mL)	36 patients (12 male, 24 female aged up to 26 years) with recessive dystrophic EB	Randomized double-blind placebo-controlled crossover study, 16 months	Total number of blisters and erosions; size, number of erosions and blisters of three chronic plaques; global score (−3 = markedly worse to +3 = markedly improved)	*Change in number of blisters and erosions:* phenytoin −2 (−7%), placebo +2 (6%), 95% CI, −11 to +4 *Area of plaques (cm²):* phenytoin −1 (−0.4%), placebo +1 (+0.2%) *Number of blisters and erosions in plaques:* phenytoin −1 ± 20 (−12%), placebo +2 ± 12 (+31%) No difference for patients with blood phenytoin > 6 µg/mL for at least 4 months	Randomization and treatment allocation poorly described. Blinding seemed effective. 14 drop-outs. No ITT analysis. Adverse events described (three patients developed phenytoin toxicity)	Power of study to detect differences 65%. No benefit seen with phenytoin over placebo
Erythromelalgia							
Kalgaard 2003[26]	Patients were hospitalized and given either iloprost 0.2 µg/mL (dose 10–40 mL/h) in saline or placebo (normal saline). Treatment was for 6 hours on 3 consecutive days	12 patients (eight female, four male) aged 17–74 years with a diagnosis of primary erythromelalgia (EM) localized to the feet	Double-blind placebo-controlled parallel-group study; Doppler repeated at 1 month	Disease severity was rated on an 8-point Likert scale (subjective cooling score) Secondary measures included tests of sympathetic function (contralateral cooling and Valsalva) and Doppler flowmetry	Authors compared pre- and post-treatment results, but did not compare treatment vs. placebo results	Details of randomization and allocation concealment not clear. Blinding well described, although compromised by side effects in iloprost group. ITT not specified. but no drop-outs. Adverse events clearly reported	Small study population with inconclusive results. Long-term follow-up not described
Erythropoietic protoporphyria							
Mathews-Roth 1994[27]	500 mg cysteine or placebo twice daily for 8 weeks, followed by wash-out and crossover	16 adults (aged 18–68 years) with erythropoietic protoporphyria	Randomized double-blind crossover study, 17 weeks	Time to erythema using xenon arc lamp (380–560 nm). Subjective assessment of time to symptoms following self-reported sun exposure	Seven of eight took longer to develop erythema with cysteine in first period (one took longer with placebo), all of seven did so in the second period (P < 0.001). By subjective assessment, four patients	Randomization, allocation concealment and blinding appear adequate. One drop-out, no ITT analysis. Five patients did not complete diaries. Adverse events clearly described	Small sample size. Study does appear to demonstrate some benefit from use of cysteine, although the clinical significance of some of these changes—e.g., from 5 to

Reference	Intervention	Patients	Study design	Outcome measures	Results	Methodological comments	Comments
Norris 1995[28]	Subjects were given either N-acetylcysteine (NAC) 600 mg t.i.d. or placebo in a crossover fashion, with 4 weeks in each treatment period and 1 week wash-out	15 patients aged 12–68 years with erythropoietic protoporphyria	Double-blind, placebo-controlled crossover study, 9 weeks	VAS scores for itch, pain, redness, swelling and sensitivity to sunlight completed before treatment and weekly throughout. Patient overall assessment of treatment completed at the end of each period	reported prolonged time to symptoms with all daylight exposure with placebo and seven with cysteine; the same findings were obtained when exposure from 11.00 to 15.00 h was assessed No significant difference in symptom scores comparing treatment to placebo. No order effect reported. The same percentage of patients felt that both NAC (9/15) and placebo (9/15) provided moderate, very good or total photoprotection	Randomization, concealment allocation, and blinding poorly described. Measurement of VAS not clearly described. ITT not specified, but no drop-outs. Adverse events clearly reported. Summary measure of overall difference between NAC and placebo and 95% CI not given	7 minutes—is unclear. The patients' subjective records are less convincing The short duration, small sample size, and lack of objective measures limit the conclusions. The authors describe no significant difference with active treatment. Mean scores look very similar in both groups, but confidence intervals are needed to exclude a plausible range of potentially useful clinical differences
Boffa 1996[29]	Oral vitamin C 1 g or placebo daily 4 weeks with 3-day wash-out period	14 patients (eight male, six female, aged 10–76 years) with erythropoietic protoporphyria	Randomized double-blind placebo-controlled crossover trial, 8 weeks	Overall sunlight tolerance change on VAS (–5 = max. deterioration to +5 = max. improvement)	Eight improved in vitamin C period, two in placebo period and two no difference, $P = 0.055$. Median change in VAS with vitamin C 1.2 cm, $P = 0.067$; 95% CI, 0 to 2.3.	Unclear how randomization done. Allocation concealment appeared adequate. Blinding of patients and observer, unclear if blinding effective. Two drop-outs, no ITT analysis. No adverse events	Small sample size. Results do not suggest benefit. Primary outcome measure is not validated
Granuloma annulare							
Smith 1994[30]	Oral potassium iodide (KI) or placebo three drops, increasing to 10 drops (1500 mg daily) three times day	10 adults (five women and five men, aged 17–75 years) with biopsy proven disseminated granuloma annulare (GA)	Randomized double-blind placebo-controlled crossover study, 12 months	Scoring 0–4 for diameter and induration of three representative lesions on different body sites. Five-point global score (much improved to much worse)	3/5 improved on placebo; 4/5 on KI. Results of scores not given by authors and statistical significance not assessed	Randomization and allocation concealment poorly described. Blinding attempted but due to KI adverse events, probably not effective. Adverse events described. Four drop-outs, no ITT analysis	Small study, unlikely to have power to detect effects. Results suggested no benefit from KI

Table 67.1 Cont'd

First author, year, ref.	Interventions (co-treatments)	Study population and sample size	Trial design description and follow-up	Outcome measures	Main reported results	Quality of reporting	Comments
Hidradenitis suppurativa							
Jemec 1998[31]	Minimum of 3 months' active systemic treatment (tetracycline 1 g daily) with placebo topical treatment or 3 months' placebo systemic treatment with active topical treatment (1% clindamycin phosphate)	46 patients (39 women and 7 men) with stage 1 or 2 hidradenitis suppurativa	Double-blind, double-dummy, placebo-controlled trial. Three-month follow-up	Patient global assessment, soreness and physician global assessment on 100-mm VAS and counts of abscesses and nodules	No significant differences between treatments. No quantitative results given except in five graphs	Randomization, concealment allocation and blinding well described. 12 drop-outs; these patients were replaced. No ITT analysis. Adverse events not described	Visual inspection of responses in figures suggests no consistent difference between topical and systemic antibiotics, but actual results and uncertainty limits not reported. Sample size rationale unclear. No long-term follow-up or ITT analysis
Hypertrophic and keloid scars—prophylaxis*							
Gold 2001[32]	Routine postoperative care (polymyxin ointment and tape dressing) or topical silicone gel sheeting (48 h after surgery, worn for up to 24 h/day for 6 months)	96 patients: 50 in low-risk group (30 males, 20 females, mean age 38.5 years), 46 in high-risk group (nine men, 37 women, mean age 34.8 years) having dermatologic surgery. High-risk group had previous hypertrophic or keloid scar (27 revisions, 19 other lesion)	Randomized controlled trial, 6 months	Physician observation, patient opinions, and scaled photographic analysis	*Low-risk group:* one hypertrophic scar (routine group). *High-risk group:* 12/35 normal scars (71%; 17 silicone, 18 routine 5/35 (29%) developed hypertrophic scars. *Routine high-risk group:* 7/18 normal, 3/18 keloid, 8/18 hypertrophic scars. *Silicone high-risk group:* 12/17 normal scars, 5/17 hypertrophic scars (P = 0.072). *High-risk revision group:* 4/11 abnormal scar in silicone group, 10/12 in routine group (P = 0.035)	Randomization not described. Not blinded. 30 drop-outs (19 low-risk, 11 high-risk). No ITT analysis. No sample size calculations	Small study size. Results suggest benefit from silicone dressings following revision surgery in high-risk patients, but results based on very small numbers as subgroup analysis
Hypertrophic and keloid scars—treatment*							
Layton 1994[33]	Cryosurgery as two 15-second freeze–thaw cycles vs. 1 mL	11 patients (seven male and four female, mean age 20 years for men	Randomized controlled study, 16 weeks	Palpability of keloids (0 = nil, 1 = minimal, 2 = moderate and	No change in diameter with either treatment. No response to treatment in	Randomization not described. Method of allocation not clear. No	Actual palpability scores not produced, only P values. Small study with

	Intervention	Participants	Study design	Outcome measures	Results	Comments
	triamcinolone (5 mg/mL). Single treatment to each keloid. Two groups of keloids were identified in each site and treatment was randomly allocated	and 28 years for women) with acne keloids		3 = severe). Diameter was measured using calipers and depth using ultrasound	grossly palpable keloids (> 6 mm depth). Only two patients had facial keloids (50% of which completely unresponsive, others minimal response). Lesions on back flattened more than chest lesions ($P < 0.03$). Correlation between palpability scores ($P < 0.04$). Better response in moderately palpable than flatter lesions ($P < 0.05$). Better response in more vascular lesions ($P < 0.04$), particularly to cryosurgery ($P < 0.03$)	blinding possible. No adverse events described ... short follow-up. Single treatment only
Palmieri 1995[34]	*Group A*: Silicone plates with added vitamin E (3% per plate) *Group B*: Silicone gel sheets. Each sheet (110 × 150 × 3 mm) worn for 10 h at night, attached with adhesive tape	80 patients (18–63 years) with hypertrophic scars and keloids	Randomized parallel group blinded study, 2 months	Scott–Husskinson (VAS) scale for pain and itching	Percentage of patients reporting > 50% improvement at 8 weeks: group A 95%, group B 75% ($P < 0.01$)	Randomization and allocation concealment not described. Unclear who was blinded (single or double?) or how blinding was achieved. Objective assessment of response with photography scoring, but results not given. No placebo-control group ... Subjective scoring only given, although objective measures taken, not reported in paper. No placebo control group, so we cannot compare to the natural history of the disease. Some of the scars 3 months old; pain and itching may resolve spontaneously
Phillips 1996[35]	Hydrocolloid dressing (replaced every 7 days) or emollient once daily	20 patients (11 females, nine males, mean age 33.3 years) with hypertrophic or keloid scars	Randomized controlled study, 3 months	Scar pigmentation, vascularity, pliability and elevation	Results at 8 weeks: no change in pigmentation or elevation with treatments. *Itch* (VAS): dressing = 1.3 (baseline 3.1), cream = 0.8 (baseline 1.7). *Pain*: dressing = 0 (baseline 0.3), cream = 0.8, *Erythema*: dressing 1.2 (baseline 1.8), cream 1.0 (baseline 1.8)	Randomization and allocation concealment procedures not described. Single-blind (physician assessing results was unaware of allocation). No drop-outs. Adverse events described. Mean scar elevation in groups not given (minimum and maximum are reported) ... No control group. Small study with short follow-up. Benefit only shown for symptoms but study probably not powered to detect any effect

Table 67.1 *Cont'd*

First author, year, ref.	Interventions (co-treatments)	Study population and sample size	Trial design description and follow-up	Outcome measures	Main reported results	Quality of reporting	Comments
Berman 1999[36]	Silicone gel-filled cushion vs. silicone gel sheeting applied to scars for at least 10 hours per day to one lesion per patient	32 patients (28 women, four men aged 25–70 years; 14 black, 18 white) with hypertrophic or keloid scars present for at least 7 months	Randomized parallel-group study, 4 months	Mean scar volume reduction, symptoms, color (pink, red, and black) and induration (slight, moderate and severe)	Mean scar volumes decreased by 53% and 36.3% with gel cushion and gel sheet, respectively. One patient had increased scar volume with gel cushion. No statistically significant difference between groups. Similar improvement in symptoms between groups. One patient in each group had improved color; five and three patients had scar softening, respectively	Unclear how randomization performed. No blinding. Nine drop-outs, no ITT analysis. Adverse events described.	Small study group. The lack of a control group makes it impossible to determine the efficacy of the intervention
De Oliveira 2001[37]	Silicone gel sheeting (applied 24 h/day, replacing every 30 days), non-silicone gel sheeting (applied 24 h/day, replacing every week), or nothing	26 patients with 41 hypertrophic or keloid scars (23 females and 3 males, aged 15–53 years) present for at least 3 months	Randomized parallel-group study, 4.5 months	Scar size, induration and symptoms. Scar color (assessed using a color palate) and pressure (intracicatricial pressure measured in a subset)	*Proportional decrease in length:* silicone 0.07, non-silicone 0.09, control 0 *Proportional decrease in width:* silicone 0.18, non-silicone 0.21, control 0 (*P* = 0.01 for length and *P* = 0.001 for width for the difference between groups) *Proportional decrease in intracicatricial pressure:* silicone 1.38, non-silicone 1.29, control 2.59 (*P* = 0.015 for difference between groups)	Randomization not described. No blinding. No drop-outs. Adverse events described. Intracicatricial data based on 20 scars only.	Small study. Difference between any dressings compared to no dressing, but no difference between silicone vs. non-silicone dressings
Manuskiatti 2001[38]	Scars divided into four segments. Three of four segments treated with 585-nm PDL at fluences of 3, 5 and 7 J/cm², respectively, every 4 weeks for a	10 patients with untreated hypertrophic medial sternotomy scars (six women and four men, aged 34–72 years) present for at least 6 months	Randomized paired-comparison controlled trial, 32 weeks	Mean scar height, erythema and pliability	Reduction in mean scar height at week 16 on 3 and 5 J/cm² segments (*P* = 0.01) and at week 24 for 7 J/cm² segments (*P* = 0.028). No difference in mean height between	Randomization poorly described. No blinding. No drop-outs. Investigators reported results in comparison with baseline and control groups only. Thus it is not possible to	Small study. Spontaneous improvement in erythema seen in control group suggests that this relates to natural history, not intervention.

Study	Intervention	Participants	Design	Outcomes	Results	Comments
	total of six sessions. One segment used as control				different fluence groups at 32 months. No flattening in control segments. No difference in erythema between laser-treated areas and non-treated areas. Better softening with 3 J/cm² , but also seen in control group	draw any conclusions regarding the comparable efficacy of the different interventions. Data shown graphically only. Adverse events described, but unclear in what proportion of patients	PDL at any fluence appears to result in scar flattening
Manuskiatti 2002[39]	Scars divided into five segments separated by 1-cm sections. Four regimens used on 4/5 segment of each scar: laser radiation with 585-nm pulsed-dye laser (PDL) 5 J/cm² six treatment sessions at 4-weekly intervals; intralesional triamcinolone acetonide (TAC) 20 mg/mL every 4 weeks for six sessions; intralesional 5-FU 50 mg/mL for 10 treatments, and intralesional TAC 1 mg/mL mixed with 5-FU 45 mg/mL for 10 treatments. One segment of each scar received no treatment (control area)	10 patients (six women, four men, aged 25–74 years) with untreated hypertrophic midline sternotomy scars present for at least 6 months	Randomized paired-comparison controlled trial, 32 weeks	Mean scar height, erythema and pliability	Flattening: laser, significant flattening compared with baseline at week 16 and control at week 32 ($P = 0.01$), TAC segment, significant compared to baseline at week 8 ($P = 0.003$) and control at week 16 ($P = 0.02$) 5-FU segment, significant compared to baseline at week 8 ($P = 0.02$) and control at week 16 ($P = 0.003$). 5-FU+TAC segment, flattening compared to baseline at week 8 ($P = 0.004$) and control at week 8 ($P = 0.02$). Erythema: Degree of erythema compared to baseline: laser at week 32 ($P = 0.02$), 5-FU at week 16 ($P = 0.01$), control ($P = 0.03$) and TAC+5-FU at week 24 (reported as significant, P not given). Pliability improved in all groups (including control) except laser segments	Randomization poorly described. No blinding. No drop-outs. Investigators reported results compared to baseline and control groups only. Thus it is not possible to conclude regarding the comparable efficacy of the different interventions. Data shown graphically only. Adverse events: discomfort 90% PDL, 100% of intralesional segments and purpura in all of laser group. TAC alone: 20% hypopigmentation, 10% atrophy and 20% telangiectasia; adverse events persisted to 32 weeks	Small study. Spontaneous improvement in erythema seen in control group suggests that this relates to natural history, not intervention. Need longer-term follow-up, blinding, and allocation concealment to assess impact of interventions. TAC adverse events do not support its use

Table 67.1 Cont'd

First author, year, ref.	Interventions (co-treatments)	Study population and sample size	Trial design description and follow-up	Outcome measures	Main reported results	Quality of reporting	Comments
Hypopigmented scars and striae alba							
Alexiades-Armenakas 2004[40]	Xenon chloride excimer laser 308 nm. Minimum erythema dose (MED) minus 50 mJ/cm² was starting dose (increased by 50 mJ/cm² if no erythema). Treated twice weekly until 50–75% repigmentation and 2-weekly after until 10 treatments. Each patient had a site-matched control area.	Volunteer sample of 31 adults with hypopigmented scars (22) and striae alba (9) on the face, torso or extremities	Randomized controlled single-blinded study, 4 months	Visual assessment of pigment correction (0–100% scale). Spectrophotometer used to compare color with site matched normal skin	Visual assessment: mean percentage repigmentation relative to matched control area 61% (95% CI, 55–67%) for scars and 68% (95% CI, 62–74%) for striae, declining to baseline at 6 months. Spectrophotometer: mean percentage repigmentation relative to control site: 101% (95% CI, 99–103%) for scars and 102% (95% CI, 99–104%) for striae after nine treatments, declining to baseline during follow-up	Randomized by alternate allocation with site-matched control areas. Observer blinded only. No drop-outs. Adverse events included transient erythema only	Small study group with heterogeneous presentations. Excimer laser was effective for hypopigmented scars and striae alba, but the benefits were short-lived, with values returning to baseline at 6 months. Possibility of long-term risk of skin cancer if maintenance treatment given
Idiopathic erythema nodosum							
Liu 1999[41]	Sulfasalazine + usual treatment Usual treatment (herbs, antibacterial and local therapy)	131 patients with idiopathic erythema nodosum N1 = 70 N2 = 61	Open randomized study, 4–8 weeks	Primary: reduction of skin damage > 60% Secondary: relapse in 1 year	66/70 vs. 50/61 14/65 vs. 19/48	Method of randomization not described. No blinding	No benefit with use of active treatment vs. placebo
Jessner's lymphocytic infiltrate							
Guillaume 1995[42]	Thalidomide 100 mg or placebo daily for 2 months in each period	28 patients (20 men, eight women aged 30–53 years with Jessner's lymphocytic infiltrate	Randomized double-blind placebo-controlled crossover study, 4 months	Complete remission (CR) of lesions	*First period:* 11/13 CR in active group, 0/15 in placebo group (P < 0.0001). NNT = 1 (but small study) *Second period:* 9/14 CR in active group. In placebo group, 10/11 in CR to start: 4/10 remained in CR. 95% CI for difference between treatments, 37–82%	Randomization and allocation concealment not described. Blinding described, but adverse effects from active agent may have compromised this. Five drop-outs. ITT analysis. Adverse events described	Small study, results suggest good efficacy, but use may be limited by neuropathy (seen in 2/27)

Lichen sclerosus

Buxton 1990[43]	25 adults (22 females and three males, mean age 53–59 years with LSA (11 genital and extragenital, six genital only and eight extragenital only)	Para-aminobenzoic acid 3 g capsules or placebo four times daily	Randomized double-blind placebo-controlled study, 8 weeks	Response assessed by dermatologist before and after on five-point scale (worse to marked improvement)	6/10 had some improvement on treatment, 7/11 on placebo	Randomization appeared adequate, but poorly described. Concealment allocation adequate. Blinding may not have been effective (taste of para-aminobenzoic acid). Four drop-outs. Adverse events well described	Small study, results suggest no benefit, but low study power
Bousema 1994[44]	78 adult females (18–83 years) with severe histologically confirmed lichen sclerosis et atrophicus (LSA) of the vulva present for > 3 months and refractory to treatment	Acitretin 30 mg (reduced to 20 mg if adverse events) or placebo once daily for 16 weeks	Multicenter randomized placebo-controlled double-blind study, 20 weeks	"Responder" rate: based on symptoms (0–4), signs (0–3) and extent (grade 0–3). "Responder" decrease ≥ 2 grades in a symptom and ≥ 1 grade in two signs with no increase in extent	Pruritus reduced in 22/22 (acitretin) and 19/24 (placebo), $P < 0.05$. No change in secondary features. Atrophy reduced in 19/22 (acitretin) and 13/24 (placebo), $P < 0.05$; hyperkeratosis reduced in 12/21 (acitretin) and 9/23 (placebo), $P < 0.05$ and extent reduced in 8/22 vs. 2/24, $P < 0.05$. Probability of response in acitretin group = 0.64 vs. 0.25 in placebo group, NNT = 3	25 patients excluded following randomization (did not fulfil inclusion criteria). Randomization and concealment allocation not described. Blinding described, but due to acitretin, adverse events unlikely to have been effective. Twelve drop-outs reported (seven adverse events, two no response, two refused and one lost to follow-up); however in figure 1, only 10 drop-outs described and eight drop-outs excluded from analysis. No ITT analysis	Good duration of follow-up. Acitretin appeared effective, but use limited by side effects

Lichen simplex chronicus

Geraldez 1989[45]	60 patients (age and sex not given) with lichen simplex chronicus (LSC)	Diflucortolone valerate (DFV) 0.3% ointment with and without occlusion applied twice daily	Randomized parallel group study, 2 weeks	Percentage improvement from baseline in pruritus (0–4) and lichenification (0–3).	Pruritus: without occlusion, improvement of 72 and 90% at 1 and 2 weeks, compared with 20% to 68 and 81% with occlusion, $P < 0.001$ for former vs. latter. Lichenification: without occlusion, improvement of 52 and 81%, respectively, compared to 44 and 62% with occlusion, $P < 0.001$	Randomization not described. Unclear how assessments were undertaken and if assessor was blind to allocation. Adverse events in occlusion group, none in the other group. Baseline characteristics not given	Short follow-up. Results suggest no benefit from the addition of occlusion

Table 67.1 Cont'd

First author, year, ref.	Interventions (co-treatments)	Study population and sample size	Trial design description and follow-up	Outcome measures	Main reported results	Quality of reporting	Comments
Molluscum contagiosum*							
Syed 1994[46]	0.3%, 0.5% podophyllotoxin creams or placebo cream twice a day for 3 days, repeated weekly up to a maximum of 4 weeks	150 males aged 10 to 26 years (45 aged 10–12 years) with molluscum contagiosum	Randomized double-blind placebo-controlled study, 9 months	Complete elimination (clinical, histological and dot blot hybridization) vs. partial cure or treatment failure	At 4 weeks, 46/50 (92%) of 0.5% group, 26/50 (52%) of 0.3% group and 8/50 (16%) of the placebo group were cured, $P < 0.00$. 9-month results not given. NNT with 0.5% = 1	Randomization and treatment allocation poorly described. Blinding measures taken, but adverse events may have compromised this. No drop-outs. Erythema and/or pruritus seen in 58/150 (38.6%)	Results given for 0.5% podophyllotoxin vs. 0.3% and placebo. Unclear if significant benefit with 0.3% cream. 9-month results would have been useful to assess rates of spontaneous remission
Syed 1998[47]	Analogue of imiquimod 1% cream or placebo three times daily for 5 days for maximum 4 weeks	100 male patients (aged 9–27 years)	Randomized double-blind placebo-controlled study, 1 year	Cure rates (100% = complete, 50% = partial)	82% of patients and 86.3% of the lesions (309/358) were cured with imiquimod; 16% of patients and 63 of the lesions with placebo, $P < 0.001$. NNT = 2	Randomization poorly described. Allocation concealment and blinding appeared adequate. No drop-outs. Side effects referred to but not described	Imiquimod 1% appeared effective in treating mollusca
Ormerod 1999[48]	5% sodium nitrite with 5% salicylic acid under occlusion or placebo with 5% salicylic acid topically applied every night	30 children (22 girls, eight boys, median age 6 months, interquartile range 4 years)	Randomized double-blind group-sequential design, 3 months	Cure rate	12 (75%) cures in active treatment group, three (21%) in control group, $P < 0.01$. NNT = 2	Randomization and treatment allocation poorly described. Blinding described, but may been less effective due to brown staining with active treatment in six of 16. Only nine of 30 completed 3 months. Nine drop-outs after 1 month. ITT analysis. Adverse events described	Small sample size and large numbers of drop-outs
He 2001[49]	Group 1: curettage Group 2: cryotherapy Group 3: electrocautery Group 4: coagulation	1656 patients with molluscum contagiosum n1 = 423 n2 = 415 n3 = 397 n4 = 421	Open randomized study, 7–10 days	Primary: clinically cured (i.e., > 95% MC reduction)	Group 1: 402/423 Group 2: 365/415 Group 3: 381/397 Group 4: 396/421	Method of randomization not described. No blinding. Adverse events described	Large study, but very short follow-up period. Unclear if remission maintained or if any long-term adverse outcomes (e.g., pigmentation)

Study	Intervention	Study design	Participants	Outcome measures	Results	Methods	Comment
Barton 2002[50]	Cryotherapy (10 s every 2 weeks) vs. cryotherapy plus podophyllotoxin (three times weekly for 4 weeks)	Randomized open study, 1 month	40 patients with facial molluscum contagiosum and HIV infection	Percentage lesion-free at 1 month. Reduction in the number of individual lesions	16.7% of combined group and 0% of cryotherapy group were lesion free at 1 month, $P = 0.136$. Authors state that difference in log reduction in number of individual lesions at 1 month, $P = 0.007$	Methods of randomization not described. No blinding. Adverse events described. Six drop-outs (reasons not given). No ITT analysis. Results for reduction in number of lesions not given	Small study, underpowered to detect a difference between treatments. No blinding and very short follow-up limit conclusions
Theos 2004[51]	Imiquimod 5% cream or placebo three times a week for 12 weeks	Randomized double-blind placebo controlled pilot study, 12 weeks	23 children (11 female, 12 male, aged 1–9 years)	Complete or partial (≥ 30% decrease from baseline lesion count) clearance rates	Partial clearance 8/12 (66.7%) of imiquimod vs. 2/11 (18.2%) of placebo group. Complete clearance 4/12 (33.3%) and 1/11 (9.1%) in imiquimod and placebo groups ($P = 0.32$). At week 12, average 45.9% decrease from baseline and mean increase of 26.9% in active and placebo groups ($P = 0.03$)	Randomization, allocation concealment and blinding not described. Two drop-outs ITT analysis used. Adverse events described	Very small sample size; no difference in primary outcome measure, but study may have lacked power to detect a difference
Burke 2004[52]	10% essential oil of Australian lemon myrtle leaf (MLE) or vehicle, one drop at bedtime	Randomized double-blind placebo-controlled study, 21 days	31 children (mean age 1.5–7.7 years)	Complete clearance or reduction in number of lesions 90% reduction in number of lesions defined as "successful"	9/16 with > 90% reduction in MLE group, vs. 0/15 in placebo group, $P < 0.05$	Randomization and allocation concealment clearly described. Blinding appeared adequate. Four drop-outs. No ITT analysis. Adverse events erythema only	Small numbers and short study duration. Results do suggest benefit, but authors allude to need for further safety testing due to in vitro fibroblast toxicity

Morphea and systemic scleroderma*

Study	Intervention	Study design	Participants	Outcome measures	Results	Methods	Comment
Hulshof 2000[53]	Calcitriol (0.75 µg/day for 6 months plus 1.25 µg/day for 3 months) or placebo	Randomized double-blind placebo-controlled study, 9 months	27 patients (seven with systemic sclerosis (SSc) and 20 with morphea, 25 women, two men, aged 22.7–70.1 years)	Skin score (0–66). Serum markers of collagen synthesis and degradation. In SSc, oral aperture measurements, lung function studies, and esophageal motility	No difference in skin score between calcitriol and placebo (−19.4 vs. −29.3) in morphea. In SSc, 2/7 had improved skin scores, no improvement in lung function, oral aperture or esophageal manometry. No change in markers of collagen synthesis or degradation	Block randomization, allocation concealment and blinding well described. Four drop-outs. ITT analysis. Adverse events described (reversible hypercalciuria)	No benefit of calcitriol over placebo in morphea. Numbers of SSc too small to detect a difference

Table 67.1 Cont'd

First author, year, ref.	Interventions (co-treatments)	Study population and sample size	Trial design description and follow-up	Outcome measures	Main reported results	Quality of reporting	Comments
El-Mofty 2004[54]	Different low doses of broadband UVA *Group 1:* 5 J/cm²/session *Group 2:* 10 J/cm²/session *Group 3:* 20 J/cm²/session All were for 20 sessions	67 patients with morphea (43 females, 20 males aged 3–66 years; four drop-outs, data not given) and 17 patients with systemic sclerosis (15 completed study, of which there were 12 females and three males, aged 18–63 years)	Randomized parallel group study, 7 weeks	Clinical response graded as very good, good, fair, or poor based on softening and texture assessed by palpation. Skin biopsies from subsample of morphea group	No difference in onset or degree of improvement between 3 morphea groups. *Group 1:* Very good (18.8%), good (18.8%), fair (50%), and poor (12.5%) *Group 2:* Very good (19%), good (28.6%), fair (38.1%), and poor (12.5%) *Group 3:* Very good (30.8%), good (26.9%), fair (34.6%), and poor (7.7%), P = 0.881. No difference between collagen appearances in subgroup. No difference in responses in SSc group, P = 0.678	Methods of randomization not described. No blinding. Four drop-outs in morphea group, two in SSc group. Adverse events pruritus in morphea group	Small study. Lack of allocation concealment and blinding. No placebo group
Napkin dermatitis*							
Bowring 1984[55]	*Group 1:* miconazole (2%) and hydrocortisone (1%) compared to *Group 2:* nystatin (100 000 IU/g) mixed with benzalkonium chloride (0.2%), dimethicone (10%), and hydrocortisone (0.5%); each cream applied three times daily for 7 days	62 infant patients (29 male and 33 female, aged 1–34 months)	Randomized double-blind parallel group study, 7 days	Erythema, weeping, bleeding, maceration, and irritability assessed (4-point scale from absent to severe). Time to improvement	24/30 of group 1 and 27/32 of group 2 had complete resolution of signs and symptoms at 7 days. 19/30 and 17/32 had significant improvement in symptoms by 48 h	Randomization and allocation concealment poorly described. Blinding appears adequate	Short study duration and lack of placebo control limit conclusions of study

Study	Intervention	Participants	Study design	Outcome measure	Results	Methodology	Comments
Seymour 1987[56]	Six groups: atopic dermatitis patients wearing cloth, cellulose, or absorbent cellulose (A, B, and C); and controls wearing cloth, cellulose, and absorbent cellulose (D, E, and F)	85 babies with atopic dermatitis and 87 controls	Randomized double-blind (with cellulose napkin groups) parallel group study, 26 weeks	Atopic dermatitis scale modified from Queille (0–100) Diaper rash grading scale (0–4)	Atopic dermatitis group: diaper rash in absorbent cellulose group 0.4, compared to 0.5 in cellulose group and 1.1 in cloth group Controls: diaper rash in cellulose group 0.4 as compared to 0.7 in cloth and absorbent cellulose groups	Stratified randomization described. Allocation concealment and blinding poorly reported. Six drop-outs, no ITT analysis. Adverse events not described	Small allocation groups. More diaper rash in atopic dermatitis babies using cloth nappies as opposed to cellulose nappies
Bosch-Banyeras 1988[57]	Control group: cream with Lassar's paste, lanolin and petrolatum. Active group: cream with same ingredients and vitamin A ester palmitate 1000 IU/g. Both creams were applied at diaper change	114 newborn infants (48 boys, 66 girls)	Randomized double-blind placebo-control study, 12 weeks	Diaper rash severity 0–4 (none to severe) and duration	No significant difference in severity or duration of symptoms between groups. Mean severity in control = 0.2; in active group = 0.3	Randomization unclear. Adequate allocation concealment and blinding. No drop-outs. No adverse events described	Reviewed by Davies et al. in Cochrane review of topical vitamin A for treating or preventing napkin dermatitis; conclusion was that no evidence to suggest that it alters the development of napkin dermatitis
Davis 1989[58]	Two groups: diapers containing fluff absorbent (high or low weight) or an absorbent polymer	150 infants between 4 and 12 months of age with no dermatological history	Randomized parallel-group study, 15 weeks	Rating scale of diaper dermatitis (0–5). Investigators also measured transepidermal water loss (TEWL)	Investigators report higher rash scores with low weight fluff diaper than high weight or absorbent diapers	Stratified randomization described. No blinding. 22 drop-outs, no ITT analysis. Differences are 0.1 of a score between low-weight fluff diapers and other groups; unclear if this is clinically relevant	Unclear if difference of 0.1 in scores between groups is clinically relevant
Arad 1999[59]	Zinc oxide paste 6/day, clobetasone butyrate 0.05% 3/day, and aqueous solution of eosin 2% 6/day	54 infants (29 males, 25 females) with diaper dermatitis ≥ grade 3	Randomized controlled study, 10 days	Severity assessed using 0–5 scale (healthy to extreme irritation or rash) and diameter of individual lesions	After 5 days of treatment, partial and complete healing in 14/18 (eosin), 6/18 (corticosteroid), 5/18 (zinc paste), $P = 0.02$. Results of lesion size not given. No definition given of what constituted partial response	Randomization not described. No blinding or allocation concealment. No adverse events. No drop-outs	Open study of short duration. Long-term effects not known. Subjective assessment was primary outcome measure
Baldwin 2001[60]	Group 1: control diaper with absorbent cellulose core Group 2: identical diaper except for the inclusion of top sheet incorporating	304 children, average age 9.9 months (excluded children with severe diaper dermatitis)	Randomized double-blind parallel group study, 4 weeks	Diaper rash and erythema scoring scale (0–3.0, 6-point scale, 0.5 intervals)	Severity of diaper rash: Genital region score 0.3 at baseline to 0.4 (group 2) and 0.3 (control group) Perianal region score: Group 2: 0.9 to 0.9 Group 1: 0.85 to 0.875	Randomization and allocation concealment poorly described. Blinding appeared adequate. Results only given graphically. Results only given for 268 children	Authors compared scores in the two groups at the end of the study period and commented that group 2 (active group) had reduced diaper dermatitis.

Table 67.1 *Cont'd*

First author, year, ref.	Interventions (co-treatments)	Study population and sample size	Trial design description and follow-up	Outcome measures	Main reported results	Quality of reporting	Comments
	petrolatum, stearyl alcohol and zinc oxide (ZnO/Pet)				Buttocks: *Group 2*: 0.2 to 0.4 *Group 1*: 0.2 to 0.2 Leg folds: *Group 2*: 0.8 to 0.8 *Group 1*: 0.8 to 0.8	(number of drop-outs not stated). No ITT analysis. Conclusions different to results shown graphically	However, the difference appears to be either unchanged scores in each group or worse in the active group
Concannon 2001[61]	Miconazole nitrate 0.25% in zinc oxide/petrolatum base or ointment base only at each diaper change	202 infants (107 boys, 95 girls, aged 2–13 months) with diaper dermatitis	Randomized double-blind placebo-controlled parallel group trial, 7 days	Severity of rash at different sites recorded using 5-point scale (none to extreme erythema with erosions or ulcers)	Mean rash scores at baseline, day 3, 5 and 7 in active group were 6.5, 5.03, 3.27 and 2.28 compared to 6.7, 6.95, 6.58 and 6.69, $P < 0.001$. In *Candida albicans*–positive participants, mean score reduced from 7.77 at baseline to 1.36 at day 7, compared to a reduction from 8.42 to 8.22 ($P < 0.001$)	Unclear how randomization and allocation concealment achieved. Blinding appeared adequate. 14 drop-outs (five active, nine ointment group). No ITT analysis	Large sample size, short duration. Results suggest benefit, especially with *Candida albicans*–positive cultures. No follow-up, unclear if implications for azole resistance, although authors state rare

Necrobiosis lipoidica

First author, year, ref.	Interventions (co-treatments)	Study population and sample size	Trial design description and follow-up	Outcome measures	Main reported results	Quality of reporting	Comments
Statham 1981[62]	Aspirin 300 mg and 75 mg dipyridamole combination or placebo three times daily	14 patients with necrobiosis lipoidica aged 17–63 years (two male, 12 female)	Randomized double-blind matched-pair study, 8 weeks	Tracing of lesions, skin biopsy before and after. Patient global assessment (better, unchanged, or worse)	Only one patient improved, in the placebo group. Two patients developed new lesions during the study (one in placebo and one in active group). No biopsy changes seen	Unclear how randomization and allocation concealment achieved. Blinding appeared adequate. Two drop-outs. No ITT analysis. No adverse events described	Small sample size. No benefit with use of aspirin–dipyridamole combination
Beck 1985[63]	40 mg acetylsalicylic acid or placebo daily for 24 weeks	18 patients with clinical and histologically confirmed necrobiosis lipoidica (NL) aged 17–75 (three males and 15 females)	Randomized double-blind placebo-controlled study, 24 weeks	Tracings of the lesions were taken before and after treatment. Patient global assessment (better, unchanged, or worse)	Tracings grew larger in both groups ($P < 0.02$ ASA and $P < 0.05$ in placebo group). 44% reported improvement in ASA group vs. 11% in placebo group	Unclear how randomization and allocation concealment achieved. Blinding appeared adequate. Two patients excluded because of wrong tablet administration. No ITT analysis. No description of adverse events	Small sample size. No benefit with use of ASA in NL

Neurodermatitis

Yosipovitch 2001[64]	Twice daily 3% aspirin vs. placebo for 2 weeks	29 patients aged 23 to 69 with lichen simplex chronicus (3 cm diameter) unresponsive to topical corticosteroids	Double-blind crossover study with 2 week wash-out period	Itch questionnaire and VAS. Photographic assessment (5-point scale)	Aspirin patients experienced average decrease in VAS of 2.2 compared to 0.7 ($P = 0.03$). No order effect seen. Positive correlation to photographic evaluation ($r = 0.5$, $P = 0.006$)	Details of randomization unclear. Allocation concealment and blinding appears adequate. Sample size calculated. Results of photographic evaluation described, but not given	Small sample size. Results suggest reduced symptoms with active treatment. Short study duration

Notalgia paresthetica

Wallengren 1995[65]	Capsaicin 0.025% or vehicle applied five times daily 1 week and three times daily for 3 weeks. Crossover with two 4-week treatment periods and 2 weeks' wash-out	20 adults (16 women, four men aged 35–70 years) with intermittent intense itch or pain localized to patch at scapular border (0.1 to 10 years)	Double-blind placebo controlled study 10 weeks	Itch score (0–100mm) on VAS	*Capsaicin first group*: VAS 60.9 to 34.7 (first period; capsaicin); 8 of 10 improved. VAS 35 to 30.7 (second period; vehicle); 2 of 9 improved. *Vehicle first group*: VAS 68.3 to 55.2 (first period; vehicle); 3 of 10 improved. VAS 52.5 to 26.6 (second period; capsaicin). Difference between vehicle and capsaicin significant at end of first week only ($P < 0.05$)	Randomization by computer-generated schedule. Allocation concealment inadequately described. Blinding attempted with identical unmarked tubes; however, five patients identified constituents). ITT not specified. Two drop-outs (one contact urticaria, the other improved). Adverse events described. No overall summary measure given	Small sample size limits conclusions. Results suggest reduced symptoms with active treatment, although lack of overall summary measure makes conclusions difficult

Paronychia

Wong 1984[66]	Oral ketoconazole 200 mg once daily or topical econazole (2 mL QDS) to the nail fold	24 adults (19 women, five men, aged 28–68 years) with chronic paronychia and positive cultures for *Candida* species	Randomized parallel group study, 6 months	Categorized as "clinical cure" or "partial responders"	Cure is 8/12 in ketoconazole group and 7/12 in econazole group. No difference in cure rate between groups, $P > 0.5$. No difference in cure rate with *Candida albicans* eradication	Details of randomization not given. No blinding. No drop-outs. Adverse events described	Results claim equivalence between oral ketoconazole and topical econazole in treatment of paronychia, but confidence intervals are likely to be large from such a small study
Roberts 1992[67]	Terbinafine 250 mg daily vs. placebo	27 patients (age and sex not given) with chronic paronychia stratified into mycologically positive and negative	Randomized double-blind stratified parallel group study, 24 weeks	Four categories: clinically and mycologically cured; mycological cure and clinical improvement; clinically improved, mycologically positive; and clinical failure.	No statistically significant difference between terbinafine and placebo at 12 weeks. Authors suggest improvement in *Candida parapsilosis* group	Details of randomization and allocation concealment not given. Four drop-outs. ITT analysis. No summary table of clinical results. Results of significance testing described but not given. No adverse events	Results suggest no benefit of terbinafine over placebo in chronic paronychia, but power was low

Table 67.1 Cont'd

First author, year, ref.	Interventions (co-treatments)	Study population and sample size	Trial design description and follow-up	Outcome measures	Main reported results	Quality of reporting	Comments
Tosti 2002[5]	Three treatments: itraconazole 200 mg daily, terbinafine 250 mg daily, or topical methylprednisolone aceponate (MPA) cream 0.1% 5 mg daily. Each patient took a capsule of A or B or placebo and applied C or placebo for 3 weeks	45 patients (six men, 39 women, aged 22–69 years) with chronic paronychia	Randomized double-blind placebo-controlled study, 9 weeks	Nail cured, improved, stable or worse. Mycological examination	Nails improved/cured at 3 weeks: itraconazole 22 (34.4%), terbinafine 19 (33.3%), and MPA 42 (87.5%), $P < 0.01$. At 9 weeks, itraconazole 29 (45.3%), terbinafine 30 (52.7%), and 41 (85.3%). No correlation between clinical cure and eradication of *Candida*	Randomization and treatment allocation poorly described. Blinding seemed effective. Three drop-outs. ITT analysis. Adverse events described in one patient on itraconazole	Short study, but appears to demonstrate superiority of topical MPA over itraconazole and terbinafine in chronic paronychia
Perniosis							
Rustin 1986[68]	Nifedipine retard 20 mg or placebo three times daily	10 patients with severe idiopathic perniosis for 5 months per year for 3 years	Randomized, double-blind placebo-controlled crossover study, 6 months	Daily irritation, pain, soreness (all 3-point scales—better, same, or worse). Duration of lesions, development of new lesions	7/10 lesions resolved within 7–10 days with active (vs. 20–28 days with placebo). No new lesions with active treatment, new lesions in placebo group (numbers not given). Improvement in self-ratings with active, none with placebo	Randomization and allocation concealment not described. Blinding may have been compromised by nifedipine adverse events. Unclear if drop-outs. No statistical analysis done	Small study, results not adequately described although some benefit appears to have been seen with nifedipine
Pityriasis rosea*							
Lazaro-Medina 1996[69]	*Intervention 1:* dexchlorpheniramine 4 mg twice daily for 2 weeks, once daily for 2 weeks (n = 27) *Intervention 2:* Betamethasone 500 µg twice daily for 2 weeks, once daily for 2 weeks (n = 31). *Intervention 3:* Betamethasone 250 µg and	85 patients with pityriasis rosea, 38 men and 47 women, mean age 22.1 years	Randomized double-blind placebo-controlled trial, 12 weeks	Subjective resolution of itch. Proportion with good or excellent improvement of rash as rated by doctor	No difference in itch between treatment groups. No difference between interventions 1 and 2 at 2 weeks (RR 0.66; 95% CI, 0.42 to 1.06). Intervention 2 better than intervention 3 at 2 weeks (RR 12.31; 95% CI, 1.81 to 83.52). Intervention 1 better than intervention 3 at 2 weeks (RR 8.16; 95% CI, 1.17 to 57.05)	Randomization well described. Allocation concealment and blinding not clearly outlined. Drop-outs described although reasons not clear. No ITT analysis	Many drop-outs, reason unclear. There does not appear to be an advantage to using oral corticosteroids in comparison with antihistamines. No placebo control group

Study	Intervention	Study design	Outcome measures	Results	Allocation/methods	Comments
	dexchlorpheniramine 2 mg twice daily for 2 weeks, once daily for 2 weeks (n = 27)					
Sharma 2000[70]	Oral erythromycin stearate 1 g daily in four doses (adults) or 25–40 mg/kg in four doses (children) compared to placebo tablets/syrup	Patients age 1.5–45 years with a clinical diagnosis of pityriasis rosea. Double-blind placebo-controlled trial, 6 weeks	Global response assessed by investigator, three categories (complete, partial, or no response)	Complete response in 33 patients (73.3%) of treatment group compared to none in placebo group at 2 weeks. In placebo group, 11% (5) complete response, 22% (10) partial response by week 6	Allocation was by alternate assignment, treatment allocation and blinding appear adequate. Adverse events clearly reported. No sample size calculation given	Alternate assignment could result in prediction of treatment group. It is not clear if severity was equivalent in groups at baseline. Unclear how assessments were done and by whom. Conclusion unclear

Porphyria cutanea tarda

Study	Intervention	Study design	Outcome measures	Results	Allocation/methods	Comments
Cainelli 1983[71]	Hydroxychloroquine (HCQ) 200 mg twice weekly or twice-monthly phlebotomy of 400 mL of whole blood	62 male alcoholic patients. Randomized open study comparing two treatments, 12 months	Serum iron, ferritin and transferrin levels. Urinary porphyrin levels and before and after liver biopsy examination	Serum iron and ferritin reduced in both groups, more marked in phlebotomy group (P < 0.001). Reduction in total urinary porphyrins and/or coproporphyrin ratios in both groups, significantly greater in HCQ group, P < 0.01. 22 patients receiving HCQ (73%) and eight patients receiving phlebotomy (25%) achieved normal pattern and normal total urinary porphyrin levels, P < 0.001. Activity of liver disease worsened in 12 HCQ patients and 7 phlebotomy patients	Unclear how randomization done. No blinding or allocation concealment. One drop-out. Only adverse event reported was anemia in phlebotomy group	Open design makes conclusions difficult. Alcohol reduction may have contributed. HCQ is more effective in reducing porphyrins; its effect on liver histology requires further study
Marchesi 1984[72]	Desferrioxamine 30 mg/kg body weight/day for 1 week every 3 months either by intramuscular injection or subcutaneous infusion or hydroxychloroquine	40 male alcoholic patients (aged 38–60 years) with porphyria cutanea tarda. Randomized open study comparing two treatments, 12 months	Serum iron, transferring and ferritin levels, and liver function tests. Urine porphyrin levels and patterns	Fall in iron (greater in desferrioxamine group, P < 0.01), transferrin and ferritin levels in both groups. Decrease in urinary total porphyrin in both groups, more marked in HCQ group:	Unclear how randomization done. No blinding or allocation concealment. No drop-outs. No adverse events reported.	Open design makes conclusions difficult. Alcohol reduction may have contributed. It is surprising that there were no adverse events related to the routes of administration of

Table 67.1 Cont'd

First author, year, ref.	Interventions (co-treatments)	Study population and sample size	Trial design description and follow-up	Outcome measures	Main reported results	Quality of reporting	Comments
	(HCQ) 200 mg twice weekly for 12 months				1571 ± 356 to 262 ± 98 and 155 ± 62 µg/24 h at 6 and 12 months, respectively, compared to a drop from 1559 to 634 and 451 µg/24 h at the same time periods. Porphyrin pattern normalized in 16 patients in HCQ group and four in desferrioxamine group (P < 0.01)		desferrioxamine. HCQ 200 mg twice weekly appears to be a safe and effective treatment for PCT in alcoholics
Prurigo nodularis							
Wong 2000[73]	Calcipotriol or 0.1% betamethasone valerate ointment (< 50 g per week of each) twice daily to nodules on legs in right–left comparison	10 patients (five male and five female) aged 8–55 years with symmetrical nodules (> 0.5 cm diameter) on lower legs. None had atopic dermatitis	Double-blind right–left randomized controlled trial, 8 weeks. Followed for further 2 months. 4-week wash-out period	Number of palpable nodules and size of nodules (mean diameter of three largest nodules) recorded at 0, 2, 4, and 8 weeks. Global response recorded for each leg (−1 to +4)	Percentage change in number of nodules from baseline greater in calcipotriol side at week 4 and 8 (49.1% calcipotriol vs. 18.1% betamethasone side, P < 0.05). Significant reduction in size both treatments but greater percentage change in calcipotriol side (56.1% reduction calcipotriol vs. 25.0% betamethasone side, P < 0.05)	Randomization, concealment allocation and blinding well described. One drop-out due to noncompliance	Investigators comment that global scores better in calcipotriol side, but sample size too small to assess significance
Maurer 2004[74]	Thalidomide 100 mg daily for first month, then randomized to receive either 100 mg or 200 mg daily	10 HIV-positive patients (aged 37–65 years) with refractory prurigo nodularis	Open study followed by randomized study at different dosages, 13 weeks	Modified Psoriasis Area and Severity Index (PASI) VAS for pruritus (10-point scale)	No correlation between dose and response in RCT phase of study. All patients able to discontinue other therapies	Randomization, allocation concealment and blinding not described. Two drop-outs, no ITT analysis. Results from RCT part of study not clearly described. Adverse events described. Peripheral neuropathy in one-third of cases	Small study. High adverse event rate

Pseudofolliculitis barbae

Study	Intervention	Participants	Design	Outcomes	Results	Methods/Quality	Comments
Perricone 1993[75]	Twice-daily 8% buffered glycolic acid compared to base lotion (study 1 oil-in-water lotion, study 2 acid in nonlipid liquid soap)	35 men aged 19–37 years with pseudofolliculitis barbae for at least 1 year	Double-blind placebo controlled trial, 8 weeks	Photography, papule and pustule count. Subjective patient evaluation	Significant reduction in number of papules and pustules in active side vs. placebo (27 to four on glycolic oil and water side vs. 29 to 22 placebo side at 8 weeks ($P < 0.0001$). In study 2, pustules and papules reduced by 25 in nonlipid soap group vs. 16 in placebo side ($P < 0.0001$)	Randomization and concealment allocation alluded to but not described. Blinding well described. Four drop-outs: two lost to follow-up, two irritation on placebo side. No ITT analysis. Quantitative results only given graphically	Results suggest beneficial effect from use of glycolic acid; unclear if assessor aware of treatment allocation
Cook-Bolden 2004[76]	Twice-daily benzoyl peroxide 5%/clindamycin 1% gel or vehicle	88 men (aged 18–65 years, 77.3% black) with pseudofolliculitis barbae (PFB) with at least 16 but no more than 100 lesions on the face and neck	Randomized double-blind pilot study, 12 weeks (preceded by run-in study to identify patients with lesion counts varying by ≤ 20%)	Percentage change from baseline in lesion counts. Physician global improvement score (0–6) PFB severity score (0–4) Patient global assessment (+2 to –2)	No difference in mean percentage reduction from baseline of number of papules and pustules at 10 weeks ($P = 0.4$). In black patients, no difference at 10 weeks ($P = 0.08$), difference at weeks 2–8. PGI score, improvements in 74.5% active and 68.1% vehicle groups. Only patient global assessment showed better satisfaction: 76.7 vs. 47.2% in active and vehicle groups, $P = 0.002$	Randomization and allocation concealment not described. Blinding appeared adequate. Eight drop-outs, ITT analysis. Adverse events described	Power of study 47% at 5% level of significance. No difference in primary outcome measures, except in subgroup analysis of black patients. Further study is required to confirm the findings of subgroup analyses. Some of the improvements may have been due to the introduction of a new shaving regimen

Seborrheic warts

Study	Intervention	Participants	Design	Outcomes	Results	Methods/Quality	Comments
Long 1994[77]	*Treatment 1*: curettage with the sharp end of a disposable curette, followed by aluminum chloride 25% in 70% isopropyl alcohol (no anesthetic), vs. *Treatment 2*: Curettage with a spoon curette preceded and followed by light cautery (0.5% preservative-free lignocaine as local anesthetic)	31 patients (10 male, 21 female, mean age 65 years) with multiple basal cell papillomas	Randomized controlled study (patient acting as their own control), 2 months	Treatment duration Preferred treatment by patient and physician Convenience for physician Cosmetic result at 2 months Patient preferred treatment at 2 months	Mean duration of treatments: 16 s (treatment 1), 53 s (treatment 2), $P < 0.001$. Patient preference at time of treatment: 7/31 (technique 1), 15/31 (technique 2), n.s. Physician preference and convenience: technique 1 was preferred by 25/31 and most convenient for 29/31	Method of randomization not described. No blinding. No drop-outs. No adverse events described	Small study. The use of disposable curettage was quicker and preferred by physicians. The investigator assessing the site at 2 months was not blinded to treatment allocation and this might lead to observer bias regarding the outcomes

Table 67.1 Cont'd

First author, year, ref.	Interventions (co-treatments)	Study population and sample size	Trial design description and follow-up	Outcome measures	Main reported results	Quality of reporting	Comments
					(P < 0.001). At 2 months: Appearance better in 21/31 (technique 1) and 1/31 (technique 2), patient preference 13/21 (technique 1), 1/31 (technique 2) and residual lesion present in 2/31 (technique 1), 4/31 (technique 2)		
Striae distensae							
Pribanich 1994[78]	Treatment with tretinoin 0.025% vs. placebo applied once daily	32 women aged 18–31 years with grade 4 striae distensae	Randomized double-blind placebo-controlled study, 7 months	Striae were graded in an area of 8.5 × 8.5 cm. Severity grading 0–4 (0 = absent, 4 = severe, > 4 striae of any width)	No change in grade of striae following treatment. No difference between active treatment and placebo	Randomization, treatment allocation and blinding appeared adequate. 21 women were not seen at follow-up (65% drop-out rate). No ITT analysis. Adverse events poorly described	No benefit seen with the use of tretinoin 0.025% vs. placebo
Morganti 2001[79]	Group A: twice-weekly dermal injections with Active A (containing hyaluronic acid 2 mg and ascorbic acid 0.5 mg 1–4 mL per area with 3% Carbocaine) with twice-daily application of Active B (ascorbyl phosphate and	66 women aged 18–24 years with striae distensae over the abdomen and buttocks	Randomized single-blind placebo-controlled study, 16 weeks	Striae assessed on scale of 0–3 (0 = normal color and dermatoglyphic pattern to 3 = violaceous color, flat skin). Profilometry of skin done and skin biopsies taken	Results shown graphically only. Mean clinical score 2.9 prior to treatment, reduced to 0.5 (group B) and < 0.5 (group A) vs. 2.1 (placebo) at 16 weeks, P < 0.05	Randomization and treatment allocation poorly described. Blinding mentioned, but in view of injections, may not have been effective. Authors do not comment on drop-outs. Results only given graphically, no confidence intervals given. Authors report increased	Authors report benefit with injection of combined hyaluronic and ascorbic acid product. Insufficient information given and results not clear

Study	Treatment	Patients	Design	Outcome measures	Results	Comments
(continued)	hyaluronic acid) Group B: twice-daily Active B Group C: twice-daily placebo solution					elastin and change in architecture, but actual data not given. Only reported adverse event light burning at the moment of injection (? number)
Urticaria pigmentosa Czarnetzki 1983[80]	3 months of either ketotifen (2 mg) or placebo twice daily. Data were compared to a previous study: Disodium cromoglycate vs. placebo, duration unclear	12 adults (six men, six women) with biopsy-proven urticaria pigmentosa, all of whom had itching and urtication	Double-blind placebo control crossover study with multiple crossovers (number not clear). Patients reviewed at 3 months	Patients recorded daily intensity of whealing and pruritus on a 0–3 + score. A mean daily score was used as a summary measure	Two drop-outs (reasons given). Mean daily whealing and pruritus scores shown diagrammatically; whealing was 0.25 and for ketotifen and 0.75 for placebo; pruritus was 0.5 and 1.3 for ketotifen and placebo, respectively. Significant improvements for whealing and pruritus reported (P < 0.03 and < 0.01, respectively)	Details of randomization, allocation concealment, and blinding not clear. Investigators state that randomization was done by an independent party. Unclear how effective blinding was. Difficult to determine time course of study from paper. ITT not used for analysis. The small size of this study and poor reporting of methods and results makes interpretation difficult. At face value, effects of ketotifen seem quite large but short-lived; 40% on active treatment experienced tiredness
Venous eczema Haeger 1975[81]	5% oxyphenbutazone in an indifferent base or placebo cream applied twice daily with compression therapy	60 patients (32–64 years) with venous eczema and venous incompetence	Randomized, double-blind placebo-controlled study, duration of study not stated	Index scale (Bjornberg and Hellgren) from 0 (normal skin) to 5 (erythema, papules, vesicles and infiltration)	Difference in mean scores (before and after) between active and placebo group = 1.30 (95% CI, 0.56 to 2.04), 0.01 < P < 0.05	Randomization, allocation concealment and blinding not described. 14 drop-outs, no ITT analysis. Small study, duration unclear. 23% drop-out rate, results might have changed if ITT analysis used

* Cochrane systematic review published or in progress.

CI, confidence intervals; DFV, diflucortolone valerate; EBS, epidermolysis bullosa simplex; HIV, human immunodeficiency virus; ITT, intention to treat; LSA, lichen sclerosus et atrophicus; LSC, lichen simplex chronicus; n.s., not significant; NL, necrobiosis lipoidica; NNT, number needed to treat; PDL, pulsed dye laser; PFB, pseudofolliculitis barbae; PGI, physician global improvement; RAS, recurrent aphthous stomatitis; RCT, randomized controlled trial; SSc, systemic sclerosis; UV, ultraviolet; UVA, ultraviolet A; UVB, ultraviolet B; VAS, visual analogue scale.

RCT there that can help inform and improve patient outcomes. We searched the Cochrane Central Register of Controlled Trials (Central) database of the Cochrane Library and the Cochrane special skin database using the abridged British Association of Dermatologists index from the National Electronic Library for Health/Skin Disorders Specialist Library from its inception until April 2006.

The inclusion criteria were as follows: randomized controlled trials only, rare diseases, diseases primarily treated by dermatologists and not covered in the other chapters of this textbook.

The exclusion criteria were: other study designs, including controlled clinical trials, studies in abstract format only, disorders with significant overlap with other specialties, and disorders covered in other chapters of this book.

The summary table follows a common format that has been used in other systematic reviews describing the essential study details—author, date, country, what was studied, who was studied, what outcomes were used, and what the main results were (Table 67.1).[9] We also assess the quality of reporting of those studies using the same methods as those recommended by the Cochrane Collaboration and described more fully in Chapter 9, which evaluate how randomization was generated and subsequently concealed from investigators, blinding (i.e., masking of participants and those assessing outcomes), and ensuring that the analysis included all those initially randomized (intention-to-treat analysis).[10] Finally, at the end of each trial, having described the data as accurately and as impartially as we could from the published papers (which was sometimes very difficult, given that crucial data were sometimes completely missing), we have then made our own comments on how the trial might inform clinical practice or otherwise. Your conclusions might well be very different from our own, but at least our opinions are separated from the data to enable you to make up your own mind up. We have also indicated where a Cochrane systematic review has been done or is being done, so that readers can refer to such reviews rather than read individual RCTs.

Your opportunity to contribute

Inevitably, we have missed many important RCTs in this first attempt to mop up all previously published RCTs that are not covered elsewhere in this book. We have done this either deliberately—e.g., we have not described the 19 or so RCTs that we identified on the topic of "flushing," as these referred almost exclusively to postmenopausal hot flushes. Perhaps that was unfair, as dermatologists in some countries may well deal with such patients. Other trials referred to multisystem disorders such as systemic sclerosis, Still's disease, Marfan's syndrome, histiocytosis, Lyme disease, chancroid, and lymphedema, and these are not included

mainly because such conditions are normally dealt with primarily by nondermatologists, or because the trials we found did not contain dermatological outcomes. But if you, the reader, have identified an important RCT that we have missed in the topics that we covered, or if you feel that we should include a topic that we have excluded, then please write to us at the book's web site so that we can look at it and include it in future versions if it is appropriate.

As with other chapters in this book, we plan to use the accompanying web site to build on the table included in this hard-copy version, so that they can grow in real time and then be decanted into the third edition of the book when the time comes. Now is your opportunity to help in our collective effort to summarize all randomized controlled trials relevant to dermatology. That would make the late Professor Archie Cochrane very happy.[11]

References

1 Grindlay D, Kamel Boulos MN, Williams HC. Introducing the National Library for Health Skin Conditions Specialist Library. *BMC Dermatol* 2005;**5**:4.

2 Wolkenstein P, Latarjet J, Roujeau JC, *et al.* Randomised comparison of thalidomide versus placebo in toxic epidermal necrolysis. *Lancet* 1998;**352**:1586–9.

3 Williams HC. Hywel Williams' top 10 deadly sins of clinical trial reporting. *Ned Tijdschr Dermatol Venereol* 1999;**9**:372–3.

4 Revuz J, Guillaume JC, Janier M, *et al.* Crossover study of thalidomide vs placebo in severe recurrent aphthous stomatitis. *Arch Dermatol* 1990;**126**:923–7.

5 Tosti A, Piraccini BM, Ghetti E, Colombo MD. Topical steroids versus systemic antifungals in the treatment of chronic paronychia: an open, randomized double-blind and double-dummy study. *J Am Acad Dermatol* 2002;**47**:73–6.

6 Collier A, Johnson KR, Delamere F, Leonard T, Dellavalle RP, Williams H. The Cochrane Skin Group: promoting the best evidence. *J Cutan Med Surg* 2005;**9**:324–31.

7 Kirtschig G, Murrell D, Wojnarowska F, Khumalo N. Interventions for mucous membrane pemphigoid and epidermolysis bullosa acquisita. *Cochrane Database Syst Rev* 2003;(**1**):CD004056.

8 Ormerod AD, Williams HC. Compulsory registration of trials. *Br J Dermatol* 2005;**152**:859–60.

9 Hoare C, Li Wan Po A, Williams H. Systematic review of treatments for atopic eczema. *Health Technol Assess* 2000;**4**(37):1–191.

10 Jüni P, Altman DG, Egger M. Systematic reviews in health care: assessing the quality of controlled clinical trials. *BMJ* 2001;**323**:42–6.

11 Cochrane AL. *Effectiveness and Efficiency: Random Reflections on Health Services.* London: Nuffield Provincial Hospitals Trust, 1972.

12 Collier PM, Neill SM, Copeman PW. Topical 5-aminosalicylic acid: a treatment for aphthous ulcers. *Br J Dermatol* 1992;**126**:185–8.

13 Femiano F, Gombos F, Scully C. Recurrent aphthous stomatitis unresponsive to topical corticosteroids: a study of the comparative therapeutic effects of systemic prednisone and systemic sulodexide. *Int J Dermatol* 2003;**42**:394–7.

14 Alidaee MR, Taheri A, Mansoori P, Ghodsi SZ. Silver nitrate cautery in aphthous stomatitis: a randomized controlled trial. *Br J Dermatol* 2005;**153**:521–5.

15 Langtry JA, Diffey BL. A double-blind study of ultraviolet phototherapy in the prophylaxis of chilblains. *Acta Derm Venereol* 1989;**69**:320–2.

16 Rustin MH, Newton JA, Smith NP, Dowd PM. The treatment of chilblains with nifedipine: the results of a pilot study, a double-blind placebo-controlled randomized study and a long-term open trial. *Br J Dermatol* 1989;**120**:267–75.

17 Tom WL, Peng DH, Allaei A, Hsu D, Hata TR. The effect of short-contact topical tretinoin therapy for foot ulcers in patients with diabetes. *Arch Dermatol* 2005;**141**:1373–7.

18 Christophersen J, Geiger JM, Danneskiold-Samsoe P, *et al.* A double-blind comparison of acitretin and etretinate in the treatment of Darier's disease. *Acta Derm Venereol* 1992;**72**:150–2.

19 Kragballe K, Steijlen PM, Ibsen HH, *et al.* Efficacy, tolerability, and safety of calcipotriol ointment in disorders of keratinization. Results of a randomized, double-blind, vehicle-controlled, right/left comparative study. *Arch Dermatol* 1995;**131**:556–60.

20 Ganemo A, Virtanen M, Vahlquist A. Improved topical treatment of lamellar ichthyosis: a double-blind study of four different cream formulations. *Br J Dermatol* 1999;**141**:1027–32.

21 Fine JD, Johnson L. Evaluation of the efficacy of topical bufexamac in epidermolysis bullosa simplex. A double-blind placebo-controlled crossover trial. *Arch Dermatol* 1988;**124**:1669–72.

22 Younger IR, Priestley GC, Tidman MJ. Aluminum chloride hexahydrate and blistering in epidermolysis bullosa simplex. *J Am Acad Dermatol* 1990;**23**(5 Pt 1):930–1.

23 Hansen S. Oxytetracycline in epidermolysis bullosa simplex. A double-blind, placebo-controlled trial. *J Eur Acad Dermatol Venereol* 1996;**6**:277.

24 Weiner M, Stein A, Cash S, de Leoz J, Fine JD. Tetracycline and epidermolysis bullosa simplex: a double-blind, placebo-controlled, crossover randomized clinical trial. *Br J Dermatol* 2004;**150**:613–4.

25 Caldwell-Brown D, Stern RS, Lin AN, Carter DM. Lack of efficacy of phenytoin in recessive dystrophic epidermolysis bullosa. Epidermolysis Bullosa Study Group. *N Engl J Med* 1992;**327**:196–7.

26 Kalgaard OM, Mork C, Kvernebo K. Prostacyclin reduces symptoms and sympathetic dysfunction in erythromelalgia in a double-blind randomized pilot study. *Acta Derm Venereol* 2003;**83**:442–4.

27 Mathews-Roth MM, Rosner B. Long-term treatment of erythropoietic protoporphyria with cysteine. *Photodermatol Photoimmunol Photomed* 2002;**18**:307–9.

28 Norris PG, Baker CS, Roberts JE, Hawk JL. Treatment of erythropoietic protoporphyria with N-acetylcysteine. *Arch Dermatol* 1995;**131**:354–5.

29 Boffa MJ, Ead RD, Reed P, Weinkove C. A double-blind, placebo-controlled, crossover trial of oral vitamin C in erythropoietic protoporphyria. *Photodermatol Photoimmunol Photomed* 1996;**12**:27–30.

30 Smith JB, Hansen CD, Zone JJ. Potassium iodide in the treatment of disseminated granuloma annulare. *J Am Acad Dermatol* 1994;**30**(5 Pt 1):791–2.

31 Jemec GB, Wendelboe P. Topical clindamycin versus systemic tetracycline in the treatment of hidradenitis suppurativa. *J Am Acad Dermatol* 1998;**39**:971–4.

32 Gold MH, Foster TD, Adair MA, Burlison K, Lewis T. Prevention of hypertrophic scars and keloids by the prophylactic use of topical silicone gel sheets following a surgical procedure in an office setting. *Dermatol Surg* 2001;**27**:641–4.

33 Layton AM, Yip J, Cunliffe W. A comparison of intralesional triamcinolone and cryosurgery in the treatment of acne keloids. *Br J Dermatol* 1994;**130**:498–501.

34 Palmieri B, Gozzi G, Palmieri G. Vitamin E added silicone gel sheets for treatment of hypertrophic scars and keloids. *Int J Dermatol* 1995;**34**:506–9.

35 Phillips TJ, Gerstein AD, Lordan V. A randomized controlled trial of hydrocolloid dressing in the treatment of hypertrophic scars and keloids. *Dermatol Surg* 1996;**22**:775–8.

36 Berman B, Flores F, Gold MH. Comparison of a silicone gel-filled cushion and silicon gel sheeting for the treatment of hypertrophic or keloid scars. *Dermatol Surg* 1999;**25**:484–6.

37 De Oliveira GV, Nunes TA, Magna LA, *et al.* Silicone versus non-silicone gel dressings: a controlled trial. *Dermatol Surg* 2001;**27**:721–6.

38 Manuskiatti W, Fitzpatrick RE, Goldman MP. Energy density and numbers of treatment affect response of keloidal and hypertrophic sternotomy scars to the 585-nm flashlamp-pumped pulsed-dye laser. *J Am Acad Dermatol* 2001;**45**:557–65.

39 Manuskiatti W, Fitzpatrick RE. Treatment response of keloidal and hypertrophic sternotomy scars: comparison among intralesional corticosteroid, 5-fluorouracil, and 585-nm flashlamp-pumped pulsed-dye laser treatments. *Arch Dermatol* 2002;**138**:1149–55.

40 Alexiades-Armenakas MR, Bernstein LJ, Friedman PM, Geronemus RG. The safety and efficacy of the 308-nm excimer laser for pigment correction of hypopigmented scars and striae alba [SR-SKIN]. *Arch Dermatol* 2004;**140**:955–60.

41 Liu DX, Zhou LY. Clinical randomized and controlled study on the effect of sulfasalazine on the erythema nodosum. *Chin J Pharmacoepidemiol* 1999;**8**:1–2.

42 Guillaume JC, Moulin G, Dieng MT, *et al.* Crossover study of thalidomide vs placebo in Jessner's lymphocytic infiltration of the skin. *Arch Dermatol* 1995;**131**:1032–5.

43 Buxton PK, Priestley GC. Para-aminobenzoate in lichen sclerosus et atrophicus. *J Dermatol Treat* 1990;**1**:255–6.

44 Bousema MT, Romppanen U, Geiger JM, *et al.* Acitretin in the treatment of severe lichen sclerosus et atrophicus of the vulva: a double-blind, placebo-controlled study. *J Am Acad Dermatol* 1994;**30**(2 Pt 1):225–31.

45 Geraldez MC, Carreon Gavino M, Hoppe G, Costales A. Diflucortolone valerate ointment with and without occlusion in lichen simplex chronicus. *Int J Dermatol* 1989;**28**:603–4.

46 Syed TA, Lundin S, Ahmad M. Topical 0.3% and 0.5% podophyllotoxin cream for self-treatment of molluscum contagiosum in males. A placebo-controlled, double-blind study. *Dermatology* 1994;**189**:65–8.

47 Syed TA, Goswami J, Ahmadpour OA, Ahmad SA. Treatment of molluscum contagiosum in males with an analog of imiquimod 1% in cream: a placebo-controlled, double-blind study. *J Dermatol* 1998;**25**:309–13.

48 Ormerod AD, White MI, Shah SA, Benjamin N. Molluscum contagiosum effectively treated with a topical acidified nitrite, nitric oxide liberating cream. *Br J Dermatol* 1999;**141**:1051–3.

49 He H, Lv JY, Fang J, *et al.* Observation on effect of four kinds of therapy for molluscum contagiosum [in Chinese]. *Chin J Dermatovenereol* 2001;**15**:308–9.

50 Barton SE, Chard S. Facial molluscum: treatment with cryotherapy and podophyllotoxin. *Int J STD AIDS* 2002;**13**:277–8.

51 Theos AU, Cummins R, Silverberg NB, Paller AS. Effectiveness of imiquimod cream 5% for treating childhood molluscum contagiosum in a double-blind, randomized pilot trial. *Cutis* 2004;**74**:134–8, 141–2.

52 Burke BE, Baillie JE, Olson RD. Essential oil of Australian lemon myrtle (*Backhousia citriodora*) in the treatment of molluscum contagiosum in children. *Biomed Pharmacother* 2004;**58**:245–7.

53 Hulshof MM, Bouwes Bavinck JN, Bergman W, *et al.* Double-blind, placebo-controlled study of oral calcitriol for the treatment of localized and systemic scleroderma. *J Am Acad Dermatol* 2000;**43**:1017–23.

54 El-Mofty M, Mostafa W, El-Darouty M, *et al.* Different low doses of broad-band UVA in the treatment of morphea and systemic sclerosis. A clinico-pathologic study. *Photodermatol Photoimmunol Photomed* 2004;**20**:148–56.

55 Bowring AR, Mackay D, Taylor FR. The treatment of napkin dermatitis: a double-blind comparison of two steroid-antibiotic combinations. *Pharmatherapeutica* 1984;**3**:613–7.

56 Seymour JL, Keswick BH, Hanifin JM, Jordan WP, Milligan MC. Clinical effects of diaper types on the skin of normal infants and infants with atopic dermatitis. *J Am Acad Dermatol* 1987;**17**:988–97.

57 Bosch-Banyeras JM, Catala M, Mas P, Simon JL, Puig A. Diaper dermatitis. Value of vitamin A topically applied. *Clin Pediatr* 1988;**27**:448–50.

58 Davis JA, Leyden JJ, Grove GL, Raynor WJ. Comparison of disposable diapers with fluff absorbent and fluff plus absorbent polymers: effects on skin hydration, skin pH, and diaper dermatitis. *Pediatr Dermatol* 1989;**6**:102–8.

59 Arad A, Mimouni D, Ben Amitai D, Zeharia A, Mimouni M. Efficacy of topical application of eosin compared with zinc oxide paste and corticosteroid cream for diaper dermatitis. *Dermatology* 1999;**199**:319–22.

60 Baldwin S, Odio MR, Haines SL, O'Connor RJ, Englehart JS, Lane AT. Skin benefits from continuous topical administration of a zinc oxide/petrolatum formulation by a novel disposable diaper. *J Eur Acad Dermatol Venereol* 2001;**15**(Suppl 1):5–11.

61 Concannon P, Gisoldi E, Phillips S, Grossman R. Diaper dermatitis: a therapeutic dilemma. Results of a double-blind placebo controlled trial of miconazole nitrate 0.25%. *Pediatr Dermatol* 2001;**18**:149–55.

62 Statham B, Finlay AY, Marks R. A randomised double blind comparison of an aspirin dipyridamole combination versus a placebo in the treatment of necrobiosis lipoidica. *Acta Derm Venereol (Stockh)* 1981;**61**:270–1.

63 Beck HI, Bjerring P, Rasmussen I, Zachariae N, Sternbjerg S. Treatment of necrobiosis lipoidica with low-dose acetylsalicylic acid. *Acta Derm Venereol (Stockh)* 1985;**65**:230–4.

64 Yosipovitch G, Sugeng MW, Chan YH, Goon A, Ngim S, Goh CL. The effect of topically applied aspirin on localized circumscribed neurodermatitis. *J Am Acad Dermatol* 2001;**45**:910–3.

65 Wallengren J, Klinker M. Successful treatment of notalgia paresthetica with topical capsaicin: vehicle-controlled, double-blind, crossover study. *J Am Acad Dermatol* 1995;**32**(2 Pt 1):287–9.

66 Wong ES, Hay RJ, Clayton YM, Noble WC. Comparison of the therapeutic effect of ketoconazole tablets and econazole lotion in the treatment of chronic paronychia. *Clin Exp Dermatol* 1984;**9**:489–96.

67 Roberts DT, Richardson MD, Dwyer PK, Donegan R. Terbinafine in chronic paronychia and candida onychomycosis. *J Dermatol Treat* 1992;**3**(Suppl 1):39–42.

68 Rustin MHA, Newton JA, Smith NP, Dowd PM. The treatment of chilblains with nifedipine: the results of a pilot study, a double-blind placebo-controlled randomized study and a long-term open trial. *Br J Dermatol* 1989;**120**:267–75.

69 Lazaro-Medina A, Villena-Amurao C, Dy-Chua NS, Sit-Toledo MSW, Villanueva B. A clinicohistopathologic study of a randomized double-blind clinical trial using oral dexchlorpheniramine 4 mg, betamethasone 500 mcg and betamethasone 250 mcg with dexchlorpheniramine 2 mg in the treatment of pityriasis rosea: a preliminary report. *J Philipp Dermatol Soc* 1996;**5**:3–7.

70 Sharma PK, Yadav TP, Gautam RK, Taneja N, Satyanarayana L. Erythromycin in pityriasis rosea: a double-blind, placebo-controlled clinical trial. *J Am Acad Dermatol* 2000;**42**:241–4.

71 Cainelli T, Di Padova C, Marchesi L, *et al.* Hydroxychloroquine versus phlebotomy in the treatment of porphyria cutanea tarda. *Br J Dermatol* 1983;**108**:593–600.

72 Marchesi L, Di Padova C, Cainelli T, *et al.* A comparative trial of desferrioxamine and hydroxychloroquine for treatment of porphyria cutanea tarda in alcoholic patients. *Photodermatology* 1984;**1**(6):286–92.

73 Wong SS, Goh CL. Double-blind, right/left comparison of calcipotriol ointment and betamethasone ointment in the treatment of prurigo nodularis. *Arch Dermatol* 2000;**136**:807–8.

74 Maurer T, Poncelet A, Berger T. Thalidomide treatment for prurigo nodularis in human immunodeficiency virus-infected subjects: efficacy and risk of neuropathy. *Arch Dermatol* 2004;**140**:845–9.

75 Perricone NV. Treatment of pseudofolliculitis barbae with topical glycolic acid: a report of two studies. *Cutis* 1993;**52**:232–5.

76 Cook-Bolden FE, Barba A, Halder R, Taylor S. Twice-daily applications of benzoyl peroxide 5%/clindamycin 1% gel versus vehicle in the treatment of pseudofolliculitis barbae. *Cutis* 2004;**73**:18–24.

77 Long CC, Motley RJ, Holt PJ. Curettage of small basal cell papillomas with the disposable ring curette is superior to conventional treatment [letter]. *Br J Dermatol* 1994;**131**:732–3.

78 Pribanich S, Simpson FG, Held B, Yarbrough CL, White SN. Low-dose tretinoin does not improve striae distensae: a double-blind, placebo-controlled study. *Cutis* 1994;**54**:121–4.

79 Morganti P, Palombo P, Fabrizi G, Palombo M, Persechino S. Biweekly in-office injectable treatment of striae distensae vs a long-term daily use of topical vitamin C. *J Appl Cosmetol* 2001;**19**:107–12.

80 Czarnetzki BM, Behrendt H. Urticaria pigmentosa: clinical picture and response to oral disodium cromoglycate. *Br J Dermatol* 1981;**105**:563–7.

81 Haeger K. The efficacy of five per cent oxyphenbutazone cream in the treatment of venous eczema of the leg. *Angiology* 1975;**26**:524–7.

IV The future of evidence-based dermatology

Luigi Naldi, Editor

68 Where do we go from here?

Hywel Williams

What is the point of discussing evidence-based dermatology?

The idea that doctors should base their treatment decisions on good evidence seems such an obvious notion that it might be taken for granted. Who can really be opposed to the central tenet of evidence-based medicine—that of using the best evidence wisely?[1] It is not as if there is one group of dermatologists "over there" practicing evidence-based dermatology and another group "over here" who choose not to (Figure 68.1). Yet, if the practice of evidence-based dermatology (EBD) goes without saying, what is point of discussing and promoting EBD?

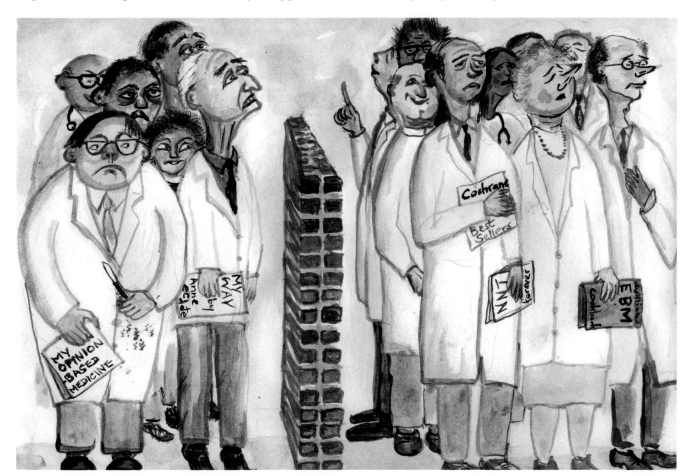

Figure 68.1 It's not as if there are two distinct groups of dermatologists separated by a brick wall: one evidence-based and the other not. All dermatologists practice evidence-based dermatology to some degree. But like learning how to perform skin surgery, learning the basics of formulating questions, searching, critical appraisal and interpretations are skills that have to be acquired and practised.

Medicine is advancing very rapidly, creating major changes in the way we treat our patients. Although there is a clinical need to keep up to date with the exponential growth of such new external evidence, we frequently fail to do this when we rely on passive sources such as a visit from a pharmaceutical representative or an occasional flick through the main journals that arrive in our post. This leads to a deterioration of our knowledge with time. Attempts to overcome this deficiency by attending clinical education programs fail to improve our performance, whereas the practice of evidence-based medicine (EBM) has been shown to keep its practitioners up to date.[2] New skills need to be learnt on how to search electronic bibliographic databases efficiently and how to critically appraise the different types of study, as outlined in the "toolbox" section of this book (Part 2). Yet time for such activities is limited in a busy clinical schedule. Dermatologists cannot be expected to read and appraise every new randomized controlled trial published in dermatology, especially as reliance on just one early randomized controlled trial can be hazardous, even when published in a prestigious journal.[3,4] Instead, high-quality systematic reviews that have searched for all relevant data are needed to update dermatologists on current best treatments.

It is important to point out that the acquisition of new information technology skills does not mean that they replace the attributes of being a good doctor, such as history and examination skills, often described as the "art" of medicine.[5] As the original definition of evidence-based dermatology developed in Chapter 2 implies, the practice of EBM is an integration of knowledge management skills with clinical skills. The aim is to create an emergent, knowledgeable, up-to-date, skillful, caring, and efficient doctor.

What exactly are the advantages of evidence-based dermatology?

Being systematic, explicit and up-to-date

At the top of the evidence hierarchy tree discussed in Chapter 7 stands the systematic review. Systematic reviews of randomized clinical trials (RCTs) developed after it was realized that traditional reviews were done in quite arbitrary ways.[6] Traditional expert reviews are fine for raising issues for discussion and debate, but they are less suitable for summarizing treatment effects. The unsystematic approach used in such traditional reviews often means that they are more prone to bias and influence from hidden agendas.[6] Many have written "traditional" review articles in the past containing a biased selection of citations to support pre-determined views, and I confess to having used the "file drawer" method to search for articles for my review of atopic eczema in 1995 (Figure 68.2).[7]

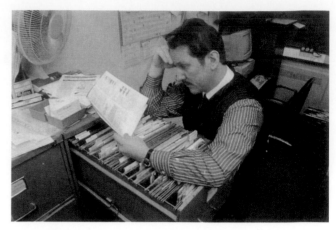

Figure 68.2 The good old "file drawer" method for locating studies is still the method used and preferred by some authors of traditional "expert" reviews.

Systematic reviews, such as those produced by the Cochrane Collaboration, summarize accurate, up-to-date, high-quality external evidence of the effectiveness and drawbacks of interventions for treating and preventing human disease.[2] Systematic reviewers use a protocol to describe precisely how they will search, appraise, and synthesize data concerning a specific clinical question, as described in Chapter 8. Such an explicit structure and methodology means that another researcher could replicate the review if necessary. Good systematic reviews will publish their protocol beforehand in order to prevent being driven by data when putting the studies together. For example, it is easy to collude with seven RCTs that have measured a clinically dubious outcome measure by providing a meta-analysis of such data, instead of pointing out that none of the studies has measured what is really important to patients according to a pre-specified primary outcome published in a protocol. A recent clinical trial of levamisole measured serum tumor necrosis factor levels as the sole outcome in patients with oral lichen planus rather than symptom control—when did you last see a serum tumor necrosis factor walk into your clinic?[9]

Keeping up to date and increasing precision

Evidence from cardiovascular medicine has shown that doctors have failed to use effective treatments, such as intravenous streptokinase, for acute myocardial infarction even when there was overwhelming evidence for their effectiveness.[10] Conversely, they continued to recommend medicines such as intravenous lidocaine for post-infarction arrhythmias long after the evidence suggested that they were ineffective or even harmful.[11] With over 260 specialist dermatology journals (F. Delamere, personal written communication, May 15th, 2007), it has become increasingly difficult for the dermatologist to keep up with the literat-

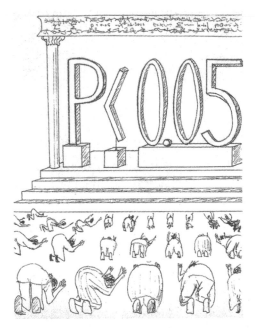

Figure 68.3 As dermatologists, we must overcome our slavish obsession for dividing the results of all clinical trials into those that are statistically significant at the 5% level and those that are not, and instead use confidence intervals to estimate a range of likely effects.

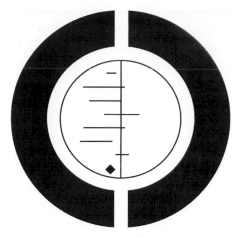

Figure 68.4 The Cochrane Collaboration logo depicts a systematic review of seven placebo-controlled trials evaluating the efficacy of a short course of oral corticosteroids for women in premature labour to prevent fetal death. Each horizontal line represents a single RCT; the shorter the line, the more certain are the results. If an RCT touches the vertical line, it means that particular trial found no clear evidence of treatment benefit. The diamond at the bottom represents the combined results, and its position to the left of the vertical line of no treatment difference indicates that the treatment was clearly beneficial in reducing premature infant mortality by 30–50%.

The first of these RCTs was done in 1972. The figure depicts what would have been revealed had a systematic review of the available evidence been done a decade later. By 1991, another seven RCTs had been done. Because no systematic review of these studies had been produced until 1989, most obstetricians had not realized that the treatment was so effective, but instead interpreted each individual study as "conflicting." As a result, tens of thousands of premature babies around the world have probably died or suffered unnecessarily. This is an example of the human costs of failing to perform an up-to-date systematic review of apparently "conflicting" studies. (*Source:* the Cochrane Collaboration.)

ure.[12] Systematic reviews such as those supported by the Cochrane Skin Group that track down all possible published and unpublished studies are needed to keep us up to date.[13] Cochrane Skin Group reviews have been shown to be of higher quality than non-Cochrane reviews dealing with dermatology,[14] and they are also updated as new evidence and criticisms become available.

Systematic reviews can also reduce uncertainty and confusion created by the apparently conflicting results of several small inconclusive studies by combining their results—provided they are sufficiently similar. This may overcome our current obsession with dividing all clinical trials into those that are significant at the arbitrary 5% level and those that are not (Figure 68.3), instead of pooling studies that are sufficiently alike in terms of patients, interventions, and outcomes into summary estimates that indicate a range of plausible treatment effects by means of confidence intervals. Studies that reach the "magic" $P < 0.05$ significance level are commonly claimed as being "positive" and those that fail to reach that level are often considered "negative," whereas in reality many of the latter trials are far too small to detect even quite large changes.[15] Instead of concluding that such studies are "conflicting," a meta-analysis performed within the context of a carefully conducted systematic review may show that they are all compatible with a clear overall treatment benefit. The Cochrane Collaboration logo shows a good example of this (Figure 68.4).

Minimizing bias and identifying research gaps

Systematic reviews are powerful tools for minimizing bias, because they use explicit methods. When assessing an intervention for skin disease, a pre-published protocol provides an opportunity to state which participants should ideally be studied, which comparators are appropriate, and which outcomes would make a difference clinically and at what time point. This "bottom-up" and nonreductionist approach also provides the opportunity of consulting users (people with a condition, or their carers) to ensure that the perspective of the review and outcome measures are appropriate. The beneficial role of such service-user involvement is extolled in Chapter 3. Specifying analysis plans in protocols also helps minimize the problem of data-driven reviews that amplify features of studies that may interest the pharmaceutical industry more than patients or healthcare professionals. Even for rare skin diseases, producing a systematic review that finds no reliable evidence to inform practice may still be useful, in that we can be reassured that as practitioners we are not missing some important new development. Systematic reviews also have an important role to play in highlighting possible research gaps for future study,[16–18] and most funding bodies now will not commit to funding an RCT without a systematic review being done first. It should be noted that, like any other study design, there are good and bad systematic reviews, and even the better ones have room for improvement.[19]

The basic unit of analysis in most systematic reviews is the RCT. As pointed out in Chapter 9, like any study design, RCTs can also be done badly and used in the wrong situations.[20,21] Nevertheless, the RCT remains one of the strongest designs in modern medicine for assessing treatment efficacy, because of its potential to minimize bias.[20] As Bigby points out in his essay on "Snake oil for the 21st century," studies of inferior design, such as case series, have many times led to overly optimistic claims of treatment efficacy in dermatology that were not borne out by subsequent RCTs.[22]

Influencing the agenda of future dermatology trials

Perhaps the most important and subtle advantage of EBD is its propensity to help change the RCT agenda. It is quite clear from a systematic review of 272 RCTs in atopic eczema that most trials have reflected the agenda of the drug industry in order to license a particular "me-too" product, and that many questions that are important to clinicians and patients remain unanswered.[17] Similar conclusions have been voiced in a review of all RCTs conducted in the field of psoriasis by the European Dermato-Epidemiology Network (EDEN).[23] Many of the outcome measures used in these trials are clinical scoring systems that may show up minor differences in disease scores in the short term, yet their clinical significance in practice is often obscure, especially in chronic diseases where disease remission and quality of life may be more important.

What are the potential limitations of evidence-based dermatology?

Poor coverage

Given that groups such as the Cochrane Skin Group are less than 10 years old, it is not surprising that many of the questions that interest dermatologists have not yet been the subject of fully published systematic reviews. Such lack of comprehensiveness is a phenomenon of time rather than intent. The range of Cochrane reviews has already increased substantially since the first edition of this book, with nearly all priority dermatology topics in development as registered protocols. Even in 2004, Parker and colleagues found 54 Cochrane reviews of relevance to dermatology,

and 65 in the Database of Abstracts of Review of Effectiveness.[24] Moreover, most of these reviews dealt with the 10 most common dermatologic diagnoses. In 2007, at least 100 Cochrane reviews are available that are relevant to the practicing dermatologist. Given that dermatology involves around 2000 skin diseases, large gaps in evidence are bound to exist. This book is itself an attempt at filling in some of the evidence gaps not covered by existing systematic reviews, especially in the new Chapter 67, which lists other skin diseases for which some RCT evidence exists.

The threat of reductionism

Meta-analysis, which refers to the statistical pooling of results drawn from several studies, is prone to dangerous reductionism if used to add studies together which it is not sensible to combine in the first place.[25,26] Thus, before contemplating playing with any statistical techniques, it may be wise not to consider combining studies of childhood atopic dermatitis with those dealing exclusively with adult atopic dermatitis, as they may belong to a different disease group in terms of the etiology of treatment responsiveness. It may also be sensible not to combine studies of atopic eczema that evaluate one sort of dietary exclusion with another. It may not make any sense to pool a clinically obscure outcome measure such as a "doctor-assessed itch," simply because it was the only outcome that was common to all trials.[17] Meta-analyses are only as good as the data from the individual studies that make up such analyses, and great care needs to be taken to avoid adding together things that should not be combined, especially when the statistical output may give rise to a spurious air of precision to those less experienced in assessing the quality of such analyses. It is for this reason that we recommend that meta-analyses should always be performed within the context of a systematic review.[27] The involvement of users is another important aspect that may protect against reductionism—for example, in the choice of outcomes. Another criticism of meta-analyses is that, as more and more data are pooled and aggregated, it becomes more difficult to apply such "average" summary measures to individual patients—in other words, evidence-based medicine applies to populations and not to individuals.[28] This is a somewhat specious argument, given that extrapolation from groups to individuals is a paradox that is fundamental to all scientific studies on groups of people. The paradox of groups and individuals is also applicable to "clinical experience," which by definition relies on recall of aggregated experiences with groups of patients. It can also be argued that combining several studies containing a broad range of people with different ethnic backgrounds, sex, and co-morbidities actually *increases* external validity to a wider and more typical group of patients, rather than relying on a single trial that describes a narrow range of trial participants.

Cheating

As with any research methodology, it is possible for those with a vested interest to twist the methods and conclusions of a systematic review to their own advantage.[29] Thus, one could conveniently fail to include one crucial study that contradicted the results one wanted to show, or if the study is declared within the review, find a weak excuse to exclude it *post hoc*. Because many trials never see the light of day in terms of publication, or are held as "data on file" by many pharmaceutical companies, it is possible for a review to include or exclude such additional unpublished data in a way that favors the product.[30] As with any written document assessing drug treatments, there is plenty of scope for undue emphasis on positive effects and lack of discussion of relevant adverse events. Readers need to develop a "good nose" for what constitutes a good systematic review and clinical trial; some pointers are given in Chapters 8 and 9. This includes starting with a peep at the acknowledgments to see who sponsored the review or study and assess possible conflicts of interest[31]—if, in fact, sponsorship has been declared.[32,33]

Overemphasis on RCTs

Whilst RCTs may be the most robust study design for minimizing bias in conventional evaluation of the effectiveness of interventions for skin diseases, they have their limitations.[34] In some circumstances, it may be impossible or unethical to perform an RCT. For example, it is unlikely that mothers will agree to be randomized to breastfeeding or bottle-feeding to see whether either prevents atopic eczema. Similarly, it would be impractical to randomize medical students to one form of education and others to another within the same class, because they would not be blinded to the interventions, and there might be considerable "contamination" of the intervention from one group as students talk together. Just because it is an RCT does not mean that it is a good RCT, and attention to quality and relevance is important, rather than just blindly following the concept of the hierarchy of evidence.[20] Rare but serious events, which are extremely important when evaluating the pros and cons of a new treatment, are not well characterized in RCTs, but instead require other approaches such as case reports, case–control studies, and wide-scale pharmaceutical surveillance methods, as Naldi points out in Chapter 10. Frequently, there is asymmetry in the way that systematic reviews devote a lot of space to treatment efficacy and less or none to issues such as potentially serious side effects.[35]

The concept of only using RCTs as the basic building blocks of evidence for systematic reviews has been criticized because it implies that all other evidence that contributes to our understanding of treatment efficacy, such as case series, case reports, and "clinical experience," are not

valid.[36] This is clearly inappropriate. Ideally, the totality of evidence should be considered when conducting a systematic review, so that evidence from observational studies can contribute to the conclusions from RCTs. Approaches such as hierarchical modeling, likelihood estimations, and Bayesian statistics have been used in attempts to address these gaps. It is likely that the concept of a good informative study design is more of a continuum representing the risk of bias, rather than a dichotomy of "good" (i.e., RCTs) and "bad" (for example, a large case series). This continuum needs to be tempered by the added but crucial dimension of study quality.

There are challenges, therefore, for future systematic reviewers to find ways of incorporating informative data from nonrandomized studies, and a methodology group has been set up within the Cochrane Collaboration specifically to address such challenges. In the meantime, it is best that we learn to walk before we run, by adhering to the RCT as the basic study design for assessing treatment efficacy in dermatology, at least until better methodological approaches have evolved that enable us to integrate evidence from a wider range of designs.

Reviews always end with the phrase "insufficient evidence"

A common criticism of Cochrane skin reviews by dermatology trainees is that they always end up with the same conclusion—that there is "insufficient evidence" to inform current practice. Whilst this may be true for some reviews, a glance at the reviews in the Cochrane Database of Systematic Reviews shows that at least 40% of those relevant to a practicing dermatologist make specific and clear recommendations for therapy.[24] Even "null reviews" that do not find any good evidence to make specific treatment recommendations have their uses. Thus, a systematic review evaluating the evidence for antistreptococcal treatments for guttate psoriasis found no reliable evidence, despite confident textbook recommendations in favor of such a treatment approach.[18] Not only does this identify a major gap needing research, it also reassures doctors and their patients that they are not missing some important study. It empowers doctors to feel more confident in relying on other levels of evidence, such as case series and empirical reasoning based on mechanism, until better studies are done. It also empowers patients with guttate psoriasis, by allowing them to challenge doctors who insist that they must take prolonged courses of antibiotics or who threaten to take out their tonsils (Figure 68.5).

Evidence-based paralysis

Absence of RCT evidence does not mean we become paralyzed into doing nothing—so-called therapeutic nihilism.[37]

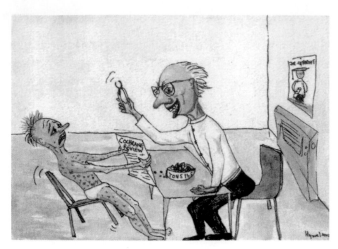

Figure 68.5 A recent Cochrane systematic review found no good evidence to support the use of antistreptococcal interventions (prolonged antibiotics or tonsillectomy) for treating guttate psoriasis. Sometimes such a "negative" systematic review can be useful, by empowering patients to question doctors on the evidential basis for their treatment decisions

Failure to find any RCTs for the treatment of acne agminata, for instance, does not mean that we tell our patients to go away because there is no treatment. We may come across a well-conducted case series, a convincing case report, or trust the anecdotal evidence of a senior colleague—all of forms of evidence that are entirely appropriate to use in the absence of better sources. It is just that for many years, the evidence hierarchy has been inverted in everyday dermatology practice—starting with muddling along and experimenting on individual patients on empirical grounds, or asking a colleague, or referring to an out-of-date textbook.

Progress and future prospects for evidence-based dermatology

The potential limitations of evidence-based dermatology are diverse and only partly justified.[36,38] Some—such as inadequate coverage—are a function of time, while some —such as reductionism, a refusal to consider non-RCT evidence, and cheating—belong predominantly to those conducting and publishing systematic reviews. Other aspects, such as evidence-based paralysis, are a misunderstanding that belongs to those using the evidence. Many of the commonly cited criticisms, such as "all skin reviews are negative," fall down when challenged by objective data and when the original tenets of evidence-based practice are revisited.

So is it all just another fashion that will come and go?

For some, the whole concept of EBD might seem like just another new management-driven fad that will come and go like others.[25] Perhaps it is the human factor of shame in admitting that some of our previous treatment beliefs might be wrong that prevents progress—the "elephant in the front room" that doctors keep bumping into without seeing.[39] Yet what is the alternative to EBD? Is it anecdote-based medicine ("I once treated a patient with such and such with remarkable effect . . ."), entropy-based medicine ("let's try this cream today . . ."), arrogance-based medicine ("I know best"), or propaganda-based dermatology driven by powerful cartels with vested interests? I cannot believe that any caring dermatologist would not wish to base his or her treatments on the best external evidence. Two studies have already shown that dermatologists use as much high-quality external evidence to inform their treatment decisions as other specialists.[40,41] Since the first edition of this book, considerable progress has been made to incorporate evidence-based medicine into continual professional development and clinical practice. Major dermatology journals such as *Archives of Dermatology* have sections dedicated to evidence-based dermatology, whilst others, including the *British Journal of Dermatology,* have been forthright in adopting the Consolidated Standards of Reporting Trials (CONSORT) statement for improving the reporting of trials.[42,43] The *Journal of Investigative Dermatology* has opened its door to high-quality clinical trials, but only if they have been registered prospectively, and the *Journal of the American Academy of Dermatology* has started a section on summaries of Cochrane reviews.[44,45] Taboo issues such as conflict of interest are now being openly discussed at dermatology journals and meetings, with appropriate declarations during presentations.[31] Evidence-based medicine principles form part of many teaching curricula in dermatology, and specific courses that use dermatological examples are appearing at most major dermatology meetings and centers (http://www.bees.org.uk/about/). Dermatology is no longer a backwater for evidence-based medicine, although it still has a long way to go. One of the most difficult challenges common to all evidence-based medicine is how to ensure that the findings of well-conducted studies are incorporated into practice.[46]

It is reasonable at this point to ask, "What is the evidence for EBD?" An entire theme issue of the *British Medical Journal* was dedicated to this topic in 2004, although it came up with more questions than answers, given the methodological difficulties in linking EBM teaching to clinical outcomes.[47] In some senses, it is a tautological question, as it implies that there is a group of doctors who are evidence-based and another group who are not, as pointed out at the start of this chapter (Figure 68.1)—whereas the reality is that we belong to a dynamic and complex continuum. Such a continuum makes the evaluation of "EBM" as an intervention in its own right almost impossible to assess by means of an RCT. In-depth discussions on the epistemology and ethical issues posed by the name and concept of evidence-based medicine can be found elsewhere.[28,48,49]

Trying to divide physicians into those who are evidence-based and those who are not is a form of binary thought disorder and not an accurate reflection of real life. Like Molière's bourgeois gentilhomme, who, after 40 years, discovered that he had been speaking prose without realizing it, many dermatologists have been practicing, and will continue to practice, high-quality EBD. Yet we all need to learn new skills in searching, appraising, and translating the evidence. Now it's up to you.

References

1 Sehon SR, Stanley DE. A philosophical analysis of the evidence-based medicine debate. *BMC Health Serv Res* 2003;**3**:14–24.

2 Sackett DL, Richardson WS, Rosenberg Q, Haynes RB. *Evidence-based Medicine. How to Practise and Teach EBM.* London: Churchill Livingstone, 1997.

3 Ioannides JPA. Contradicted and initially stronger effects in highly cited clinical research. *JAMA* 1995;**294**: 218–28.

4 Williams HC. Two "positive" studies of probiotics for atopic dermatitis—or are they? *Arch Dermatol* 2006;**142**:1201–3.

5 Cook HJ. What stays constant at the heart of medicine. *Br Med J* 2006;**333**:1281–2.

6 Ladhani S, Williams HC. Management of postherpetic neuralgia: a comparison of the quality and content of traditional versus systematic reviews. *Br J Dermatol* 1998;**139**:66–72.

7 Williams HC. Atopic eczema—we should look to the environment. *BMJ* 1995;**311**:1241–2.

8 Greenhalgh T. *How to Read a Paper.* London: BMJ Publishing Group, 1997.

9 Sun A, Chia JS, Wang JT, Chiang CP. Levamisole can reduce the high serum tumour necrosis factor-alpha level to a normal level in patients with erosive oral lichen planus. *Clin Exp Dermatol* 2007;**32**:308–10.

10 Lau J, Antman EM, Jimenez-Silva J, Kupelnick B, Mosteller F, Chalmers TC. Cumulative meta-analysis of therapeutic trials for myocardial infarction. *N Engl J Med* 1992;**327**:248–54.

11 Echt DS, Liebson PR, Mitchell LB, *et al.* Mortality and morbidity in patients receiving encainide, flecainide, or placebo. The Cardiac Arrhythmia Suppression Trial. *N Engl J Med* 1991;**324**:781–8.

12 Delamere FM, Williams HC. How can hand searching the dermatological literature benefit people with skin problems? *Arch Dermatol* 2001;**137**:332–5.

13 Freeman SR, Williams HC, Dellavalle RP. The increasing importance of systematic reviews in dermatology clinical trial research and publication. *J Invest Dermatol* 2006;**126**:2357–60.

14 Collier A, Heilig L, Schilling L, Williams H, Dellavalle RP. Cochrane Skin Group systematic reviews are more methodologically rigorous than other systematic reviews in dermatology. *Br J Dermatol* 2006;**155**:1230–5.

15 Williams HC, Seed P. Inadequate size of "negative" clinical trials in dermatology. *Br J Dermatol* 1993;**128**:317–26.

16 Griffiths CEM, Clark CM, Chalmers RJG, Li Wan Po A, Williams HC. A systematic review of treatments for severe psoriasis. *Health Technol Assess* 2000;**4**(40):1–125.

17 Hoare C, Li Wan Po A, Williams H. Systematic review of treatments for atopic eczema. *Health Technol Assess* 2000;**4**(37):1–191.

18 Owen CM, Chalmers RJ, O'Sullivan T, Griffiths CE. Antistreptococcal interventions for guttate and chronic plaque psoriasis. *Cochrane Database Syst Rev* 2000;(2):CD001976.

19 Jadad AR, Cook DJ, Jones A, *et al.* Methodology and reports of systematic reviews and meta-analyses: a comparison of Cochrane reviews with articles published in paper-based journals. *JAMA* 1998;**280**:278–80.

20 Barton S. Which clinical studies provide the best evidence? The best RCT still trumps the best observational study. *BMJ* 2000;**321**: 255–6.

21 Rees J. The nature of clinical evidence: floating currencies rather than gold standards. *J Invest Dermatol* 2007;**127**:499–500.

22 Bigby M. Snake oil for the 21st century. *Arch Dermatol* 1998;**134**: 1512–4.

23 Naldi N, Svensson A, Diepgen T, *et al.* Randomized clinical trials for psoriasis 1987–2000: the EDEN Survey. *J Invest Dermatol* 2003;**120**:738–741.

24 Parker ER, Schilling LM, Diba V, Williams HC, Dellavalle RP. What's the point of databases of reviews in dermatology if all they compile is "insufficient evidence"? *J Am Acad Dermatol* 2004;**50**:635–9.

25 Rees J. Evidence-based medicine: the epistemology that isn't. *J Am Acad Dermatol* 2000;**43**:727–9.

26 Goodman NW. Who will challenge evidence-based medicine? *J R Coll Phys Lond* 1999;**33**:249–51.

27 Egger M, Smith GD, Sterne JA. Uses and abuses of meta-analysis. *Clin Med* 2001;**1**:478–84.

28 Tonelli MR. The philosophical limits of evidence-based medicine. *Acad Med* 1998;**73**:1234–40.

29 Jorgensen AW, Hilden J, Gotzsche PC. Cochrane reviews compared with industry supported meta-analyses and other meta-analyses of the same drugs: systematic review. *BMJ* 2006;**333**:782–5.

30 Melander H, Ahlqvist-Rastad J, Meijer G, Beermann B. Evidence b(i)ased medicine—selective reporting from studies sponsored by pharmaceutical industry: review of studies in new drug applications. *BMJ* 2003;**326**:1171–3.

31 Williams HC, Naldi L, Paul C, Vahlquist A, Schroter S, Jobling R. Conflicts of interest in dermatology. *Acta Derm Venereol* 2006;**86**: 485–97.

32 Bero LA. Accepting commercial sponsorship. Disclosure helps—but is not a panacea. *BMJ* 1999;**319**:653–4.

33 Perlis CS, Harwood M, Perlis RH. Extent and impact of industry sponsorship conflicts of interest in dermatology research. *J Am Acad Dermatol* 2005;**52**:967–71.

34 Hampton JR. Evidence-based medicine, practice variations and clinical freedom. *J Eval Clin Pract* 1997;**3**:123–31.

35 Ernst E, Pittler MH. Assessment of therapeutic safety in systematic reviews: literature review. *BMJ* 2001;**323**:546.

36 Straus SE, McAlister FA. Evidence-based medicine: a commentary on common criticisms. *Can Med Assoc J* 2000;**163**:837–41.

37 Hill D. Efficacy of sunscreens in protection against skin cancer. *Lancet* 1999;**354**:699–700.

38 Dickersin K, Straus SE, Bero LA. Evidence based medicine: increasing, not dictating, choice. *BMJ* 2007;**334**(Suppl 1):s10.

39 Davidoff F. Shame: the elephant in the room. *BMJ* 2002;**324**:623–4.

40 Jemec GB, Thorsteinsdottir H, Wulf HC. Evidence-based dermatologic out-patient treatment. *Int J Dermatol* 1998;**37**:850–4.

41 Abeni D, Girardelli CR, Masini C, *et al*. What proportion of dermatological patients receive evidence-based treatment? *Arch Dermatol* 2001;**137**:771–6.

42 Abeni D, Bigby M, Pasquini P, Szklo M, Williams H. "Evidence-Based Dermatology" section in the *Archives of Dermatology*. *Arch Dermatol* 2000;**136**:1148–9.

43 Cox N, Williams HC. Can you COPE with CONSORT? *Br J Dermatol* 2000;**142**:1–7.

44 Williams HC, Goldsmith L. The JID opens its doors to high quality randomised controlled clinical trials. *J Invest Dermatol* 2006;**126**: 1683–4.

45 Weinstock MA, Williams HC. JAAD commentary on "From the Cochrane Library". *J Am Acad Dermatol* 2007;**56**:105–6.

46 Guyatt G, Cook D, Haynes B. Evidence based medicine has come a long way. *BMJ* 2004;**329**:990–1.

47 Coomarasamy A, Khan KS. What is the evidence that postgraduate teaching in evidence based medicine changes anything? A systematic review. *BMJ* 2004;**329**:1017–22.

48 Gupta M. A critical appraisal of evidence-based medicine: some ethical considerations. *J Eval Clin Pract* 2003;**9**:111–21.

49 Straus SE, Jones G. What has evidence based medicine done for us? *BMJ* 2004;**329**:987–8.

Index

Page numbers in *italics* represent figures, those in **bold** represent tables.

urticaria
  acute 197–201
    definition 197
    diagnostic tests 198
    etiology 197
    incidence/prevalence 197
    management 198–200, **199**
    outcomes 198
    prognosis 197
    treatment aims 198
  chronic 202–10
    definition 202, *202*
    diagnosis *205*
    diagnostic tests 204
    etiology 202–4, *203*
    incidence/prevalence 202
    management 205–8, **206, 207**
    outcomes 204
    prognosis 204
    treatment aims 204
urticaria pigmentosa **697**
UVA1
  lupus erythematosus 554
  sarcoidosis 603–4
UVB
  hand eczema 121–2
  polymorphic light eruption 630–1
  psoriasis 176

validity 44–5
venom immunotherapy 483–4
  antihistamine pretreatment 484
venous ulcers 539–45
  definition 539, *539*
  etiology 539
  incidence/prevalence 539
  management
    compression 540
    intermittent pneumatic compression 543
    pentoxifylline 540–1
    skin grafting 541–2
    ultrasound, laser and electromagnetic therapy 542–3
    vitamins and minerals 542
  outcomes 539
  prognosis 539
  reducing recurrence risk 543–4
  treatment aims 539
visibility of skin disease 14–15
vitamins
  melasma 507–8
  photoaging 328
vitamin D derivatives, psoriasis 174–5
vitiligo 489–96
  definition 489
  etiology 489
  incidence/prevalence 489
  management
    antioxidants 492
    cognitive-behavioral therapy 492
    corticosteroids 491–2
    depigmentation therapy 493
    immunomodulators 491–2
    levamisole 492
    melagenine 492
    phototherapy/photochemotherapy 490–1, *490*
    pseudocatalase 492
    surgery 492–3
  outcomes 489
  prognosis 489
  treatment aims 489
vulvodynia 647

warts 347–53
  definition 347, *347*
  diagnostic tests 347
  etiology and risk factors 347
  incidence/prevalence 347
  management
    bleomycin 351–2
    cryotherapy 348–9
    dinitrochlorobenzene 350
    occlusive management with duct tape 349–50
    photodynamic therapy 350–1
    salicylic acid 348
  outcomes 348
  prognosis 347
  treatment aims 348
washing powders, and atopic eczema 150–1
well-built clinical questions
  advantages of 29–30, **30**
  structuring of 29
whiteheads 83
within-patient control studies 5–6
wrong parameters 48
wrong tests 48

zinc sulfate, leishmaniasis 453